DISEASE MANAGEMENT

for NURSE

PRACTITIONERS

• • • • • • •

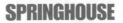

SPRINGHOUSE

Springhouse, Pennsylvania

STAFF

Publisher
Judith A. Schilling McCann, RN, MSN

Creative Director
Jake Smith

Editorial Director
David Moreau

Clinical Director
Joan M. Robinson, RN, MSN, CCRN

Clinical Editors
Kate McGovern, RN, BSN, CCRN (project manager); Melissa M. Devlin, PharmD (drug information editor); Elaine G. Lange, RN, MSN, CCRN, ANP-C; Norma Mann, RN, NP,C

Editors
Julie Munden (senior editor),
Cynthia C. Breuninger, Pat Wittig

Copy Editors
Jaime L. Stockslager (supervisor),
Virginia Baskerville, Kimberly Bilotta,
Scotti Cohn, Priscilla DeWitt, Heather
Ditch, Amy Furman, Shana Harrington,
Dona Hightower, Fruma Klass, Malinda
LaPrade, Judith Orioli, Marcia Ryan,
Dorothy P. Terry, Pamela Wingrod,
Helen Winton

Designers
Arlene Putterman (associate design
director), Lesley Weissman-Cook
(book designer and project manager),
Joseph John Clark, Donna S. Morris

Projects Coordinator
Liz Schaeffer

Electronic Production Services
Diane Paluba (manager), Joyce Rossi Biletz

Manufacturing
Patricia K. Dorshaw (manager), Otto Mezei
(book production manager)

Editorial Assistants
Beverly Lane, Beth Janae Orr,
Elfriede Young

Indexer
Manjit Sahai

Library of Congress Cataloging-in-Publication Data
Disease management for nurse practitioners.
  p. ; cm.
  Includes bibliographical references and index.
  ISBN 1-58255-069-7 (alk. paper)
  1. Nurse practitioners — Handbooks, manuals, etc. 2. Disease management — Handbooks, manuals, etc. 3. Nursing — Handbooks, manuals, etc. I. Lippincott Williams & Wilkins. Springhouse Division.
  [DNLM: 1. Nursing Care — Handbooks. 2. Nurse practitioners — Handbooks. 3. Nursing Diagnosis — Handbooks. WY 49 D611 2002]
  RT82.8 .D57 2002
  610.73′06′92 — dc21   2001040098

CONTENTS

· · · · · · · · ·

CONTRIBUTORS

• • • • • • • •

Ivy M. Alexander, RN, MS, PhD, ANP, APRN
Assistant Professor
Yale University
New Haven, Conn.

Mary Milano Carter, RN, MS, ANP, CS
Nurse Practitioner and Pain
  Management Coordinator
North Shore Pain Services at North
  Shore University Hospital
Syosset, N.Y.

JoAnn Coleman, RN, MS, ACNP, ANP, AOCN
Acute Care Nurse Practitioner—
  Gastrointestinal Surgery
Johns Hopkins Hospital
Baltimore

Jennifer E. DiMedio, MSN, CRNP
Family Nurse Practitioner
West Chester (Pa.) Family Practice

Joseph L. DuFour, RN,CS, MS, FNP
Lecturer
State University of New York at New
  Paltz

Susan F. Galiczynski, RN, MSN, CRNP
Temple University Hospital
Philadelphia

Shelton M. Hisley, PhD, RNC, ACCE, WHNP
Assistant Professor
School of Nursing
University of North Carolina at
  Wilmington

Nona Holmes, RN, MS, CARN, CS, NPP
Assistant Professor, Psychiatric NPP
Molloy College at South Oaks Hospital
Amityville, N.Y.

April L. Lewis, MS, NP
Adult Nurse Practitioner
Johns Hopkins Urgent Care Center
Baltimore

Norma Mann, RN, MSN, NPC
Nurse Practitioner
Private office, Neil Levin, D.O.
Sewell, N.J.

Maureen Mathews, RN, MS, CS
Family Nurse Practitioner
OSF Medical Group
Chillicothe, Ill.

Lourdes "Cindy" Santoni-Reddy,
  MSN, MEd, CPP, FAAPM, NPC
Faculty, Nurse Practitioner, Legal Nurse
  Consultant
EMCARE Inc.
Horsham, Pa.

Alexander John Siomko, RN,C, MSN, CRNP
Staff Nurse
Methodist Division, Thomas Jefferson
    University Hospital
Philadelphia

Leonora P. Thomas, RN, MS, CS
Acute Care Nurse Practitioner
Department of Cardiology, Hartford
    (Conn.) Hospital

Denise A. Vanacore-Netz, MSN, ANP, CRNP, CS
Coordinator Nurse Practitioner Program
Gwynedd Mercy College
Lower Gwynedd, Pa.

Dianne Weyer, RN, MS, CFNP
Assistant Professor
Georgia State University School of
    Nursing
Atlanta

FOREWORD

• • • • • • • • •

Disease management is a complex and challenging undertaking. Not only are new pathologies and treatments constantly being discovered but effective disease management requires the recognition and understanding of complex clinical presentations, knowledge of multiple differential diagnoses, familiarity with laboratory and diagnostic evaluations, and the ability to critically analyze findings to determine an appropriate course of action. These challenges must be accomplished in a health care setting that's increasingly fraught with time demands, cost concerns, and disease complexity — all without losing sight of your patients and their unique concerns.

Nurse practitioners (NPs) are particularly well poised to accomplish this undertaking. Recognized as exceptional clinicians, NPs are also known for providing patient-focused care. This care includes focusing on your patients within the context of their lifestyles and circumstances, educating them to maximize their wellness, and assisting them in regaining control of their health.

Disease Management for Nurse Practitioners provides an excellent clinical resource to aid you in providing state-of-the-art, patient-focused care. It includes nearly 300 diseases frequently encountered in ambulatory, subacute, and acute clinical settings — far more than found in other disease references for primary care

clinicians. Chapters are organized according to a specific body system or disease category. Each chapter begins with a description of the appropriate physical examination for the body system or disease category involved, including information for interpreting abnormal findings.

For your convenience, a consistent format for each entry includes essential facts about the disease process and management strategies. First, the text presents a succinct definition of the problem and a description of the causes and pathophysiology of the disease. Next, each entry provides the clinical presentation of the disease, including signs and symptoms and possible clinical examination findings, and a list of potential differential diagnoses to consider. Specific guidelines are then discussed for establishing the diagnosis, including appropriate diagnostic testing and interpretation of results. The management section includes pharmacologic and nonpharmacologic treatments as well as surgical intervention, follow-up, and referral guidelines.

The final sections of each entry provide useful and clinically relevant information to assist you with individualizing management strategies for your patients. Patient teaching includes recommendations for advising patients about self-care techniques, dietary and activity alterations, treatment information and options, and when to seek reevaluation. A comprehensive list of complications alerts you to problems patients may encounter. Finally, special considerations offer solutions to monitoring and managing treatment-related problems and special patient situations. These sections cover useful approaches for counseling your patients and their families.

Disease Management for Nurse Practitioners also includes hundreds of quick-reference charts and illustrations offering vital information that further clarifies pathophysiology and treatment options. Helpful logos are also featured, such as *Healthy Living* (covers lifestyle and health behaviors, including stress management, social support, nutrition, exercise, safety, and environment), *Age Alert* (addresses physiologic and psychosocial considerations specific to certain age-groups with certain disorders, and treatments), and *Clinical Caution* (alerts the NP to crucial considerations to prevent severe complications).

Today's health care market requires rapid, accurate, and cost-effective provision of services. *Disease Management for Nurse Practitioners* provides an essential tool to assist you in meeting this demand. This valuable resource can aid you in making rapid and accurate diagnoses and determining appropriate clinical management plans for your patients.

Ivy M. Alexander, RN, MS, PhD,
   ANP, APRN
Assistant Professor
Yale University
New Haven, Conn.

Psychosocial disorders

Providing care for psychiatric patients requires that you develop a practical, orderly method for dealing with problems as diverse and complex as humanity itself. Your responsibilities include not only planning, implementing, and evaluating care but also establishing a meaningful therapeutic relationship with the patient. When you encounter intractable psychiatric problems, you also need to be keenly aware of your own attitudes and feelings to prevent frustration from hobbling your efforts.

Make sure you're familiar with the revised fourth edition of the American Psychiatric Association's *Diagnostic and Statistical Manual of Mental Disorders (DSM-IV)*. (See *Understanding the DSM-IV,* page 2.)

• • • • • • • • • • •

ASSESSMENT

Psychiatric assessment refers to the scientific process of identifying a patient's psychosocial problems, strengths, concerns, and treatment goals and evaluating therapeutic interventions. Recognizing psychosocial problems and how they affect health is important in any clinical setting.

Mental status examination

The mental status examination (MSE) is a tool for assessing psychological dysfunction and for identifying the causes of psychopathology. Your responsibilities may include conducting all or a portion of the MSE. The MSE examines the patient's level of consciousness (LOC), general appearance, behavior, speech, mood and affect, intellectual performance, judgment, insight, perception, and thought content.

Level of consciousness

Begin by assessing the patient's LOC, a basic brain function. Identify the intensity of stimulation needed to arouse the patient.

Describe the patient's response to stimulation, including the degree and quality of movement, the content and coherence of speech, and the level of eye opening and eye contact. Finally, describe the patient's actions after the stimulus is removed.

1

Understanding the DSM-IV

The revised fourth edition of the American Psychiatric Association's *Diagnostic and Statistical Manual of Mental Disorders (DSM-IV)* defines a mental disorder as a clinically significant behavioral or psychological syndrome or pattern that's associated with current distress (a painful symptom) or disability (impairment in one or more important areas of functioning) or with a significantly greater risk of suffering, death, pain, disability, or an important loss of freedom. This syndrome or pattern isn't merely an expected, culturally sanctioned response such as grief over the death of a loved one. Whatever its original cause, it must currently be considered a sign of behavioral, psychological, or biological dysfunction.

To add diagnostic detail, the *DSM-IV* uses a multiaxial approach. This flexible approach specifies that every patient must be evaluated on each of five axes.

AXIS I
Clinical disorders — the diagnosis (or diagnoses) that best describes the presenting complaint

AXIS II
Personality disorders; mental retardation

AXIS III
General medical conditions — a description of any concurrent medical conditions or disorders

AXIS IV
Psychosocial and environmental problems that may affect the diagnosis, treatment, and prognosis of the mental disorder

AXIS V
Global assessment of functioning, which is based on a scale of 1 to 100 that allows evaluation of the patient's overall psychological, social, and occupational function

A patient's diagnosis after being evaluated on these five axes may look like this:
Axis I: adjustment disorder with anxiety
Axis II: obsessive-compulsive personality disorder
Axis III: Crohn's disease, acute bleeding episode
Axis IV: death of a father and homelessness
Axis V: GAF — 53 (current).

Impaired LOC may indicate the presence of a medical disorder. If you discover an alteration in consciousness, refer the patient for a more complete medical examination.

General appearance
Appearance helps to indicate the patient's overall mental status. Answer these questions:

- Is the patient's appearance appropriate to his age, sex, and situation?
- Are his skin, hair, nails, and teeth clean?
- Is his manner of dress appropriate?
- If the patient wears cosmetics, are they applied appropriately?
- Does the patient maintain direct eye contact?

Behavior

Describe the patient's demeanor and way of relating to others. Does the patient appear sad, joyful, or expressionless? Does he use appropriate gestures? Does he keep an appropriate distance between himself and others? Does he have distinctive mannerisms, such as tics or tremors?

Indicate the patient's interactions with others. Is he cooperative, mistrustful, embarrassed, hostile, or overly revealing about his personal life? Describe the patient's level of activity. Is he tense, rigid, restless, or calm?

Note extraordinary behavior. Disconnected gestures may indicate that the patient is hallucinating. Pressured, rapid speech or a heightened level of activity may indicate that the patient is in the manic phase of a bipolar disorder.

Speech

Observe the content and quality of the patient's speech. Note an illogical choice of topics, irrelevant or illogical replies to questions, speech defects such as stuttering, excessively fast or slow speech, sudden interruptions, excessive volume, and barely audible speech. Also watch for slurred speech, use of an excessive number of words, or minimal, monosyllabic responses.

Mood and affect

Mood refers to a person's pervading feeling or state of mind. Usually, a patient projects a prevailing mood, though this mood may change throughout the course of a day. Affect refers to a person's expression of his mood. Variations in affect are referred to as range of emotion.

To assess mood and affect, begin by asking the patient about his current feelings. Also look for indications of mood in facial expressions and posture.

Does the patient seem able to keep mood changes under control? Mood swings may indicate a physiologic disorder. Medications, recreational drug or alcohol use, stress, dehydration, electrolyte imbalance, or disease may induce mood changes. After childbirth and during menopause, many women experience profound depression.

Other signs of mood disorders include:
■ lability of affect — rapid, dramatic changes in the range of emotion
■ flat affect — unresponsive range of emotion
■ inappropriate affect — inconsistency between expression (affect) and mood.

Intellectual performance

To develop a picture of the patient's intellectual abilities, test the patient's orientation, immediate and delayed recall, recent and remote memory, attention level, comprehension, concept formation, and general knowledge.

Judgment

Assess the patient's ability to evaluate choices and draw appropriate conclusions. Defects in judgment may also become apparent while the patient tells his history. Pay attention to how the patient handles interpersonal relationships and occupational and economic responsibilities.

Insight

To assess insight, ask "What do you think has caused your anxiety?" or "Have you noticed a recent change in yourself?" Expect patients to show varying degrees of insight. Severe lack of insight may indicate a psychotic state.

Perception

Perception refers to interpretation of reality as well as use of the senses. Proponents of the cognitive theory of depression have suggested that depression arises from distorted perception.

If the patient has a sensory perception disorder, he may experience hallucinations, in which he perceives nonexistent external stimuli, or illusions, in which he misinterprets external stimuli. Tactile, olfactory, and gustatory hallucinations usually indicate organic disorders.

Not all visual and auditory hallucinations are associated with psychological disorders. Patients may also experience mild and transitory hallucinations. Constant visual and auditory hallucinations may, however, give rise to strange or bizarre behavior. Disorders associated with hallucinations include schizophrenia and acute organic brain syndrome after withdrawal from alcohol or barbiturate addiction.

Thought content

Assess the patient's thought patterns. Are the patient's thoughts well connected to reality? Are the patient's ideas clear, and do they progress in a logical sequence? Observe for indications of morbid thoughts and preoccupations or abnormal beliefs.

Delusions, which are usually associated with schizophrenia, are grandiose or persecutory false beliefs. Delusions may be obvious or may have a slight basis in reality.

Obsessions are intense preoccupations from which some patients suffer; they may interfere with daily living. For example, patients may constantly think about hygiene. Compulsions are also preoccupations that patients act out, such as constantly washing their hands.

Observe patients for suicidal, self-destructive, violent, or superstitious thoughts; recurring dreams; distorted perceptions of reality; and feelings of worthlessness.

Additional psychological assessment
Sexual drive

Changes in sexual drive provide valuable information in psychological assessment. Prepare yourself for patients who are uncomfortable discussing their sexuality. Avoid language that implies a heterosexual orientation. Introduce the subject tactfully but directly.

Follow-up questions might include:
■ Are you currently sexually active?
■ Have you noticed recent changes in your interest in sex?
■ Do you have the same pleasure from sex now as before?

Competence

Can the patient understand reality and the consequences of his actions? Does the patient understand the implications of his illness, its treatment, and the consequences of avoiding treatment? Use extreme caution when assessing changes in competence. Unless behavior strongly indicates otherwise, assume that the patient is competent. Remember that legally, only a judge has the power or right to declare a person incompetent.

Assessing self-destructive behavior

Suicide — intentional, self-inflicted death — may be carried out with guns, drugs, poisons, rope, automobiles, or razor blades or by drowning, jumping, or refusing food, fluid, or medications. In a subintentional suicide, a person has no conscious intention of dying but nevertheless engages in self-destructive acts.

Not all self-destructive behavior is suicidal in intent. A patient who has lost touch with reality may cut or mutilate body parts to focus on physical pain. Such behavior may indicate a borderline personality disorder.

Assess depressed patients for suicidal tendencies. A higher percentage of depressed patients commit suicide than pa-

Recognizing and responding to suicidal patients

Be alert for these warning signs of impending suicide:
- withdrawal
- social isolation
- signs of depression (constipation, crying, fatigue, helplessness, hopelessness, poor concentration, reduced interest in sex and other activities, sadness, and weight loss)
- farewells to friends and family
- putting affairs in order
- giving away prized possessions
- expression of covert suicide messages and death wishes
- obvious suicide messages, (such as "I'd be better off dead").

ANSWERING A THREAT

If a patient shows signs of impending suicide, assess the seriousness of the intent and the immediacy of the risk. A patient with a chosen method who plans to commit suicide in the next 48 to 72 hours is considered a high risk.

Tell the patient that you're concerned. Then urge the patient to avoid self-destructive behavior until the staff has an opportunity to help him. You may specify a time for the patient to seek help.

Next, consult with the treatment team about arranging for psychiatric hospitalization or a safe equivalent such as having someone watch the patient at home. Initiate safety precautions for those at high suicide risk:
- Provide a safe environment. Check and correct conditions that could be dangerous for the patient. Look for exposed pipes, windows without safety glass, and access to the roof or open balconies.
- Remove dangerous objects, such as belts, razors, suspenders, light cords, glass, knives, nail files, and clippers.
- Make the patient's specific restrictions clear to staff members, plan for observation of the patient, and clarify day- and night-staff responsibilities.

A patient may ask you to keep his suicidal thoughts confidential. Remember that such a request is ambivalent; a suicidal patient wants to escape the pain of life, but he also wants to live. A part of him wants you to tell other staff members so he can be kept alive. Tell the patient that you can't keep a secret that endangers his life or conflicts with his treatment. You have a duty to keep him safe and to ensure the best care.

In addition to observing the patient, maintain personal contact with him. Encourage continuity of care and consistency of primary nurses. Helping the patient build emotional ties to others is the best technique for preventing suicide.

tients with other diagnoses. Chemical dependence and a history of schizophrenia are also risk factors for suicide.

Suicidal schizophrenics may be agitated instead of depressed. Voices may tell them to kill themselves. Alarmingly, some schizophrenics provide only vague behavioral clues before taking their lives.

If you perceive signals of hopelessness, perform a direct suicide assessment. (See *Recognizing and responding to suicidal patients*.) Protect patients from self-harm during a suicidal crisis. After treatment, the patient should think more clearly and find reasons for living.

Physical examination

Because psychiatric problems may stem from organic causes or medical treatment, a physical examination should be completed for psychiatric patients. Observe for key signs and symptoms and examine the patient by using inspection, palpation, percussion, and auscultation.

•••••••••••

ALCOHOL DEPENDENCE AND ABUSE

Alcohol dependence is a progressive, chronic disorder characterized by tolerance and withdrawal symptoms. Impairment in one or more of the following areas of life with continued use indicates alcohol abuse: social and family relationships, occupational responsibilities, physical or mental health, educational pursuits, or legal issues. Alcoholism cuts across all social and economic groups, involves both sexes, and occurs at all stages of the life cycle, beginning as early as elementary school. About two-thirds of the adult population in the United States consumes alcohol regularly. Of these, more than 10% have a problem with alcohol use. Males are two to five times more likely to abuse alcohol than females. According to some statistics, alcohol abuse is a factor in 60% of all automobile accidents.

AGE ALERT Drinking is most prevalent between the ages of 21 and 34, but current statistics show that up to 19% of 12- to 17-year-olds have serious drinking problems.

Causes

Numerous biological, psychological, and sociocultural factors appear to be involved in alcohol dependence. An offspring of one parent with alcohol dependence is seven to eight times more likely to become alcohol-dependent than a peer without such a parent. Biological factors may include genetic or biochemical abnormalities, nutritional deficiencies, endocrine imbalances, and allergic responses.

Psychological factors may include the urge to drink alcohol to reduce anxiety or symptoms of mental illness; the desire to avoid responsibility in familial, social, and work relationships; the need to bolster self-esteem; and the inability to cope with stress in everyday life.

Sociocultural factors include the availability of alcoholic beverages, group or peer pressure, an excessively stressful lifestyle, and social attitudes that approve of frequent drinking.

Clinical presentation

Because people with alcohol dependence may hide or deny their addiction and may temporarily manage to maintain a functional life, assessing for alcoholism can be difficult. Note physical and psychosocial symptoms that suggest alcoholism such as:
- need for daily or episodic alcohol use to maintain adequate functioning
- inability to discontinue or reduce alcohol intake
- episodes of anesthesia or amnesia (blackouts) during intoxication
- episodes of violence during intoxication
- interference with social and familial relationships and occupational responsibilities.

Complaints may be alcohol-related, such as:
- malaise
- dyspepsia
- mood swings
- depression
- increased incidence of infection.

Observe the patient for poor personal hygiene and untreated injuries, such as:
- cigarette burns
- fractures
- bruises.

Additional signs include:
- unusually high tolerance for sedatives and narcotics
- secretive or manipulative behavior
- use of inordinate amounts of aftershave or mouthwash.

When confronted, the patient may deny or rationalize the problem. Alternatively, he may be guarded or hostile in his response and may even sign himself out of the health care facility against medical advice. He also may project his anger or feelings of guilt or inadequacy onto others to avoid confronting his illness.

Chronic alcohol abuse brings with it an array of physical complications, including:
- malnutrition
- cirrhosis of the liver
- peripheral neuropathy
- brain damage
- cardiomyopathy.

Assess for these complications in a patient with an alcohol-related disorder. (See *Complications of alcohol use*, page 8.) Also assess for alcohol dependence and abuse when these medical conditions are present.

After abstinence or reduction of alcohol intake, signs and symptoms of withdrawal may begin as early as 12 hours after drinking has stopped and last up to 7 days. The patient may experience:
- anorexia
- nausea
- anxiety
- fever
- insomnia
- diaphoresis
- tremor

- severe tremulousness
- agitation
- hallucinations
- violent behavior
- major motor seizures (known as "rum fits"). (See *Signs and symptoms of alcohol withdrawal*, page 9.)

Remember to consider the possibility of alcohol abuse when evaluating older patients. Research suggests that alcoholism affects 2% to 10% of adults over age 60. More than half of all geriatric hospital admissions are due to alcohol-related problems.

Differential diagnoses
- Depression
- Anxiety disorders
- Bipolar disorder
- Peptic ulcer disease
- Gastroenteritis
- Viral hepatitis
- Pancreatitis
- Cholelithiasis
- Primary seizure disorder

Diagnosis
For characteristic findings in patients with alcoholism, see *Diagnosing substance dependence and related disorders*, page 10.

Clinical findings may help support the diagnosis of alcohol dependence. These laboratory tests may confirm alcohol use or recent alcohol ingestion:
- Blood alcohol level (BAL) ranges from 0.08% to 0.10% weight/volume (200 mg/dl).
- Blood urea nitrogen level is increased in severe hepatic disease.
- Serum glucose level may be increased or decreased.
- Serum ammonia is increased.
- Urine toxicology studies may help to determine other types of drug abuse in patients.
- Liver function studies may reveal increased levels of serum cholesterol, lac-

Complications of alcohol use

Alcohol can damage body tissues by direct irritating effects, changes that take place in the body during its metabolism, aggravation of existing disease, accidents occurring during intoxication, and interactions between the substance and drugs. Such tissue damage can cause numerous complications.

CARDIOPULMONARY COMPLICATIONS
- Cardiac arrhythmias
- Cardiomyopathy
- Chronic obstructive pulmonary disease
- Essential hypertension
- Impaired respiratory diffusion
- Increased incidence of pulmonary infections
- Increased risk of tuberculosis
- Pneumonia

GI COMPLICATIONS
- Chronic diarrhea
- Esophageal cancer
- Esophageal varices
- Esophagitis
- Gastric ulcers
- Gastritis
- GI bleeding
- Malabsorption
- Pancreatitis

HEMATOLOGIC COMPLICATIONS
- Anemia
- Coagulopathy
- Leukopenia
- Reduced number of phagocytes

HEPATIC COMPLICATIONS
- Alcoholic hepatitis
- Cirrhosis
- Fatty liver

MYOPATHIES
- Prostatitis
- Sexual performance difficulty

NEUROLOGIC COMPLICATIONS
- Alcoholic dementia
- Alcoholic hallucinosis
- Alcohol withdrawal delirium
- Korsakoff's syndrome
- Peripheral neuropathy
- Seizure disorders
- Subdural hematoma
- Wernicke's encephalopathy

OTHER COMPLICATIONS
- Beriberi
- Hypoglycemia
- Infertility
- Leg and foot ulcers

PSYCHIATRIC COMPLICATIONS
- Amotivational syndrome
- Depression
- Fetal alcohol syndrome
- Impaired social and occupational functioning
- Multiple substance abuse
- Suicide

tate dehydrogenase, alanine aminotransferase, aspartate aminotransferase, and creatine kinase, which may indicate liver damage

- Serum amylase and lipase levels may be elevated with acute pancreatitis.
- A hematologic workup can identify anemia, thrombocytopenia, increased

Signs and symptoms of alcohol withdrawal

Withdrawal signs and symptoms may vary in degree from mild (morning hangover) to severe (alcohol withdrawal delirium). Formerly known as delirium tremens (or DTs), alcohol withdrawal delirium is marked by acute distress following abrupt withdrawal after prolonged or massive use.

SIGNS AND SYMPTOMS	MILD	MODERATE	SEVERE
Motor impairment	Hand tremor	Visible tremors	Gross, uncontrollable bodily shaking
Anxiety	Mild restlessness	Obvious motor restlessness and anxiety	Extreme restlessness and agitation with intense fearfulness
Sleep disturbance	Restless sleep or insomnia	Marked insomnia and nightmares	Total wakefulness
Appetite	Impaired appetite	Marked anorexia	Rejection of all food and fluid except alcohol
GI symptoms	Nausea	Nausea and vomiting	Dry heaves and vomiting
Confusion	None	Variable	Marked confusion and disorientation
Hallucinations	None	Vague, transient visual and auditory hallucinations and illusions (commonly nocturnal)	Visual and occasionally auditory hallucinations, usually of fearful or threatening content; misidentification of people and frightening delusions related to hallucinatory experiences
Pulse rate	Tachycardia	Pulse rate of 100 to 120 beats/minute	Pulse rate of 120 to 140 beats/minute
Blood pressure	Normal or slightly elevated systolic	Usually elevated systolic	Elevated systolic and diastolic
Sweating	Slight	Obvious	Marked hyperhidrosis
Seizures	None	Possible	Common

prothrombin time, and increased partial thromboplastin time. Coagulopathy is indicative of advanced disease.

Other diagnostic findings:

■ A computed tomography scan or magnetic resonance imaging of the brain may reveal cortical atrophy or structural lesions.

Diagnosing substance dependence and related disorders

The *Diagnostic and Statistical Manual of Mental Disorders,* Fourth Edition, identifies the following diagnostic criteria for substance dependence, abuse, intoxication, and withdrawal.

SUBSTANCE DEPENDENCE

▪ A maladaptive pattern of substance use leading to clinically significant impairment or distress, as manifested by three or more of the following criteria, occurring within a 12 month period:

– tolerance — defined as need for increased amounts of the substance to achieve intoxication or desired effect or a markedly diminished effect with continued use of the same amount of the substance

– withdrawal — manifested by characteristic withdrawal syndrome for the substance or the same or a similar substance is taken to relieve or avoid withdrawal symptoms

– taking the substance in larger amounts or over a longer period than was intended

– experiencing a persistent desire or unsuccessful efforts to cut down or control substance use

– spending a great deal of time in activities needed to obtain, use, or recover from the effects of the substance

– abandoning or reducing important social, occupational, or recreational activities because of substance use

– continuing to use the substance despite knowledge of having a persistent or recurrent physical or psychological problem that's likely to have been caused or exacerbated by the substance

SUBSTANCE ABUSE

▪ A maladaptive pattern of substance use leading to clinically significant impairment or distress, as manifested by one or more of the following criteria, occurring within a 12-month period:

– recurrent substance use resulting in a failure to fulfill major role obligations at work, school, or home

– recurrent substance use in situations in which using the substance is physically hazardous

– recurrent substance-related legal problems

– continued substance use despite persistent or recurrent social or interpersonal problems caused or exacerbated by the effects of the substance

(Symptoms have never met the criteria for substance dependence for this class of substance.)

SUBSTANCE INTOXICATION

▪ Development of a reversible substance-specific syndrome resulting from recent ingestion of, or exposure to, a substance

▪ Clinically significant maladaptive behavioral or psychological changes resulting from the effect of the substance on the central nervous system and developing during or shortly after its use

▪ Symptoms not caused by a mental disorder or another general medical condition

SUBSTANCE WITHDRAWAL

▪ Development of a substance-specific syndrome resulting from the cessation or reduction of substance use that has been heavy and prolonged

▪ Substance-specific syndrome that causes clinically significant distress or impairment in social, occupational, or other important areas of functioning

▪ Symptoms not caused by a mental disorder or another general medical condition

- A liver biopsy may disclose alcohol-related hepatitis and cirrhosis.

Management
General
Total abstinence from alcohol is the only known effective treatment. Supportive programs that offer detoxification, rehabilitation, and aftercare, including continued involvement in Alcoholics Anonymous (AA), may produce good long-term results.

Acute intoxication is treated symptomatically by supporting respiration, preventing aspiration of vomitus, replacing fluids, administering I.V. glucose to prevent hypoglycemia (if the patient can't eat), correcting hypothermia or acidosis, and initiating emergency treatment for trauma, infection, or GI bleeding.

Treatment of alcohol dependence relies on medications to deter alcohol use and treat effects of withdrawal; psychotherapy, consisting of behavior modification techniques, group therapy, and family therapy; and appropriate measures to relieve associated physical problems.

Detoxification may be undertaken in either an inpatient or outpatient setting. Site selection depends on the severity of alcohol withdrawal, associated medical conditions, and the presence of significant psychiatric symptoms. Presence or absence of an adequate social support network, patient commitment to abstain from alcohol, and complications such as alcohol withdrawal delirium during prior detoxification attempts may also be criteria for site selection. Pregnancy indicates a need for inpatient detoxification.

Medication
Tranquilizers, particularly benzodiazepines, are used to alleviate acute physical withdrawal symptoms, such as seizures and alcohol withdrawal delirium, during detoxification. However, these drugs have addictive potential (may result in substituting one substance abuse problem for another). Decreasing doses are administered during a 3- to 5-day detoxification period. Combining alcohol and benzodiazepines has been fatal.

To alleviate extreme physical withdrawal symptoms, give 25 to 100 mg of chlordiazepoxide every 3 to 6 hours P.O., I.M., or I.V. initially; taper to 25 mg every 6 hours on the 2nd and 3rd day and continue tapering until withdrawal is complete.

Alternate regimens over 3 to 6 days include:
- oxazepam — 15 to 30 mg P.O. every 6 hours
- lorazepam — 2 to 6 mg/day P.O. in divided doses

If tachycardia or high blood pressure occurs, these are indicated:
- atenolol — 50 mg/day P.O. for 3 to 7 days
- clonidine — 0.1 mg/day P.O. for 3 to 7 days.

For nutritional deficiencies, these medications are used:
- thiamine — 100 mg/day P.O.
- folic acid — 1 mg/day P.O.
- multivitamins with minerals daily.

Aversion or deterrent therapy is rarely used. In rare instances, however, disulfiram is administered daily. Alcohol in any form will then cause illness.

Referral
- Supportive counseling or individual, group, or family psychotherapy may help. Ongoing support groups such as AA are fairly successful. About 40% of AA's members stay sober as long as 5 years, and 30% stay sober longer than 5 years.
- Refer spouses of alcoholics to Al-Anon and children of alcoholics to Alateen.
- Refer adult children of alcoholics to the National Association for Children of Alcoholics.

■ Refer the patient to a partial hospitalization program, an intensive outpatient program, or professional therapy as needed after detoxification.

Follow-up

Patients undergoing outpatient detoxification should be followed daily during the beginning stages of recovery. Follow-up referrals can then proceed according to the patient's clinical status. Patients who are unsuccessful with an outpatient detoxification program should be referred to an inpatient facility that specializes in substance abuse treatment.

Patient teaching

■ Make the patient and his family members aware of possible withdrawal symptoms and the need to report them.
■ Teach the patient the disease process of alcohol abuse as well as the psychosocial consequences of alcohol dependence.

Complications

■ Seizures
■ Hypertension
■ Depression
■ Trauma
■ Poisoning
■ Nutritional deficiencies
■ Pancreatitis
■ Gastritis
■ Dilated cardiomyopathy
■ Cirrhosis
■ Fetal alcohol syndrome

Special considerations

■ For individuals who have lost all contact with family and friends and who have a long history of unemployment, trouble with the law, or other problems associated with alcohol abuse, rehabilitation may involve job training, sheltered workshops, halfway houses, and other supervised facilities.

• • • • • • • • • • •

ANOREXIA NERVOSA

The key feature of anorexia nervosa is self-imposed starvation, resulting from a distorted body image and an intense, irrational fear of gaining weight, even when the patient is obviously emaciated. An anorexic patient is preoccupied with her body size, describes herself as "fat," and commonly expresses dissatisfaction with a particular aspect of her physical appearance. Although the term anorexia suggests that the patient's weight loss is associated with a loss of appetite, this is rare. Anorexia nervosa and bulimia nervosa can occur simultaneously. In anorexia nervosa, the refusal to eat may be accompanied by compulsive exercising, self-induced vomiting, or abuse of laxatives or diuretics. Bulimia indicates bingeing and purging with self-induced vomiting.

Anorexia occurs in 5% to 10% of the population; about 95% of those affected are women. This disorder occurs primarily in adolescents and young adults, but it may also affect older women. The occurrence among males is rising. The prognosis varies but improves if the patient is diagnosed early or if she wants to overcome the disorder and seeks help voluntarily. Mortality ranges from 5% to 15% — the highest mortality is associated with a psychiatric disturbance. One-third of these deaths can be attributed to suicide.

Causes

No one knows what causes anorexia nervosa. Researchers in neuroendocrinology are seeking a physiologic cause but have found nothing definite. Clearly, social attitudes that equate slimness with beauty play some role in provoking this disorder; family factors also are implicated. Most theorists believe that refusing to eat is a subconscious effort to exert personal control over one's life. Major depression or dysthymia occurs in 50% to 75% of these patients; obsessive-compulsive disorder is present in approximately 10% to 13% of cases. Both are probably factors in the development of the disorder.

Clinical presentation

The patient's history usually reveals a 25% or greater weight loss for no organic reason, coupled with a morbid dread of being fat and a compulsion to be thin. Such a patient tends to be angry and ritualistic. Females report amenorrhea or infertility. Other complaints include loss of libido, fatigue, sleep alterations, intolerance to cold, and constipation. Hypotension and bradycardia may be present.

Inspection may reveal:
- emaciated appearance
- skeletal muscle atrophy
- loss of fatty tissue
- atrophy of breast tissue
- blotchy or sallow skin
- lanugo on the face and body
- dryness or loss of scalp hair.

If the patient is also bulimic, additional signs include:
- calluses on the knuckles
- abrasions and scars on the dorsum of the hand.

Signs of associated vomiting include:
- dental caries
- oral or pharyngeal abrasions. (See *Complications of anorexia nervosa*, page 14.)

Further assessment may disclose:
- painless salivary gland enlargement
- bowel distention
- slowed reflexes
- hyperactivity and vigor (despite malnourishment).

During psychosocial assessment, the anorexic patient may express:
- morbid fear of gaining weight
- obsession with her physical appearance
- obsession with food

- social regression (including poor sexual adjustment)
- fear of failure
- feelings of despair, hopelessness, and worthlessness
- suicidal thoughts.

Differential diagnoses
- Depressive disorders
- Body dysmorphic disorder
- Conversion disorder
- Food phobia
- Schizophrenic disorder
- Brain tumor

Diagnosis

For characteristic findings in patients with this condition, see *Diagnosing anorexia nervosa*, page 15.

Laboratory tests help to identify various disorders and deficiencies and help to rule out endocrine, metabolic, and central nervous system abnormalities; cancer; malabsorption syndrome; and other disorders that cause physical wasting.

Abnormal findings that may accompany a weight loss that exceeds 30% of normal body weight include:
- low hemoglobin level, platelet count, and white blood cell count
- prolonged bleeding time due to thrombocytopenia
- decreased erythrocyte sedimentation rate
- decreased levels of serum creatinine, blood urea nitrogen, uric acid, cholesterol, total protein, albumin, sodium, potassium, chloride, calcium, and fasting blood glucose (resulting from malnutrition)
- elevated levels of alanine aminotransferase and aspartate aminotransferase in severe starvation states
- elevated serum amylase levels when pancreatitis isn't present

Complications of anorexia nervosa

Serious medical complications can result from the malnutrition, dehydration, and electrolyte imbalances caused by prolonged starvation, frequent vomiting, or laxative abuse that's typical with anorexia nervosa.

MALNUTRITION AND RELATED PROBLEMS

Malnutrition may cause hypoalbuminemia and subsequent edema or hypokalemia, leading to ventricular arrhythmias and renal failure.

Poor nutrition and dehydration, coupled with laxative abuse, produce changes in the bowel similar to those in chronic inflammatory bowel disease. If the patient is frequently vomiting, it can cause esophageal erosion, ulcers, tears, and bleeding as well as tooth and gum erosion and dental caries.

CARDIOVASCULAR CONSEQUENCES

Cardiovascular complications, which can be life-threatening, include decreased left ventricular muscle mass, chamber size, and myocardial oxygen uptake; reduced cardiac output;

hypotension; bradycardia; electrocardiographic changes, such as a nonspecific ST interval, T-wave changes, and a prolonged PR interval; heart failure; and sudden death, possibly caused by ventricular arrhythmias.

INFECTION AND AMENORRHEA

Anorexia nervosa may increase the patient's susceptibility to infection.

In addition, amenorrhea, which may occur when the patient loses about 25% of her normal body weight, is usually associated with anemia. Possible complications of prolonged amenorrhea include estrogen deficiency (increasing the risk of calcium deficiency and osteoporosis) and infertility. Menses usually return to normal when the patient weighs at least 95% of her normal weight.

- decreased levels of serum luteinizing hormone and follicle-stimulating hormone (in females)
- decreased triiodothyronine levels resulting from a lower basal metabolic rate
- dilute urine caused by the kidneys' impaired ability to concentrate urine
- prolonged PR interval, nonspecific ST interval, T-wave changes and, possibly, ventricular arrhythmias on the electrocardiogram
- elevated levels of growth hormone, vasopressin, and cortisol
- decreased $CD4^+$ to $CD8^+$ ratio
- decreased plasma tryptophan.

Management
General

Appropriate treatment aims to promote weight gain or control the patient's compulsive binge eating and purging. Malnutrition and the underlying psychological dysfunction must be corrected. Admission to either a medical or psychiatric health care facility may be required to improve the patient's precarious physical condition. The admission stay may be as brief as 2 weeks or may stretch from a few months to 2 years or longer. Admission is absolutely indicated when the patient has the following conditions:

- weight that's 75% of normal for height and age

- hypotension
- bradycardia
- tachycardia
- inability to maintain normal body temperature
- expression of suicidal ideation
- failure to progress with outpatient treatment.

A team approach to care — combining aggressive medical management, nutritional counseling, and individual, group, or family psychotherapy or behavior modification therapy — is most effective in treating anorexia. Treatment results may be discouraging. Many clinical centers are now developing inpatient and outpatient programs aimed specifically at managing eating disorders.

Treatment may include behavior modification (privileges depend on weight gain); curtailed activity for physical reasons (such as arrhythmias); vitamin and mineral supplements; a reasonable diet with or without liquid supplements; subclavian, peripheral, or enteral hyperalimentation (enteral and peripheral routes carry less risk of infection); and group, family, or individual psychotherapy.

Medication
No drug has proven efficacy in the treatment of this disorder.

Medications that may be used to treat anorexia nervosa include:
- oxazepam — 15 mg P.O. a.c.
- alprazolam — 0.25 to 0.5 mg P.O. a.c.
- fluoxetine — 10 to 60 mg/day P.O.
- metoclopramide — 10 mg P.O. a.c. and h.s.

Referral
- Overeaters Anonymous may address some issues regarding bingeing and purging.
- Anorexia Nervosa and Related Eating Disorders organization may help the pa-

Diagnosing anorexia nervosa

A diagnosis of anorexia nervosa is made when the patient meets the following criteria put forth in the *Diagnostic and Statistical Manual of Mental Disorders,* Fourth Edition.
- The patient refuses to maintain body weight over a minimal normal weight for age and height (for instance, weight loss leading to maintenance of body weight 15% below that expected) or failure to achieve expected weight gain during a growth period, leading to body weight 15% below that which is expected.
- The patient experiences intense fear of gaining weight or becoming fat, despite her underweight status.
- The patient has a distorted perception of body weight, size, or shape (that is, the person claims to feel fat even when emaciated or believes that one body area is too fat even when it's obviously underweight).
- In women, absence of at least three consecutive menstrual cycles when they're otherwise expected to occur.

tient and her family to uncover and correct dysfunctional patterns as well as offer guidance and support information.
- Psychological counseling should continue after the treatment regimen is instituted.

Follow-up
Patient monitoring depends on the severity of physical symptoms and the progress of psychological interventions. All laboratory tests with abnormal values should be repeated at weekly or monthly intervals until stable. Weekly weight should be obtained until an appropriate gain of 1 to 2 lb per week is evident; weight may then be obtained on a monthly basis. Ac-

tivity levels should be closely monitored and increased or decreased according to weight gain or loss.

Patient teaching
■ Negotiate an adequate food intake with the patient. Make sure she understands that she'll need to comply with this contract or lose certain established privileges.
■ Teach the patient how to keep a food journal that includes the types of food eaten, eating frequency, and feelings associated with eating and exercise.

Complications
■ Arrhythmias
■ Cardiac arrest
■ Cardiomyopathy
■ Heart failure
■ Peripheral neuropathy
■ Seizures
■ Premature osteoporosis
■ Compromised growth and bone marrow hypoplasia
■ Delayed gastric emptying
■ Necrotizing colitis
■ Infertility
■ Esophageal strictures and erosive esophagitis

Special considerations
■ Advise family members to avoid discussing food with the patient because control issues are commonly expressed with food.

• • • • • • • • • • • •

ANXIETY DISORDER, GENERALIZED

Anxiety is a feeling of apprehension that some describe as an exaggerated feeling of impending doom, dread, or uneasiness. Unlike fear — a reaction to danger from a specific external source — anxiety is a re-action to an internal threat, such as an unacceptable impulse or a repressed thought that's straining to reach a conscious level.

A rational response to a real threat, occasional anxiety is a normal part of life. Overwhelming anxiety, however, can result in generalized anxiety disorder (GAD) — uncontrollable, unreasonable worry that persists for at least 6 months and narrows perceptions or interferes with normal functioning. It can begin at any age but typically has an onset in persons in their twenties and thirties and is equally common in men and women. Recent evidence indicates that the prevalence of GAD is greater than previously thought and may be even greater than that of depression.

Causes
Theorists share a common premise that conflict, whether intrapsychic, sociopersonal, or interpersonal, promotes an anxiety state. It's now accepted that genetic factors as well as neurotransmitter abnormalities also play a role in the development of anxiety states.

Clinical presentation
Psychological or physiologic symptoms of anxiety states vary with the degree of anxiety. Mild anxiety mainly causes psychological symptoms, with unusual self-awareness and alertness to the environment. Moderate anxiety leads to selective inattention but with the ability to concentrate on a single task. Severe anxiety causes an inability to concentrate on more than scattered details of a task. A panic state with acute anxiety causes a complete loss of concentration, often with unintelligible speech.

Physical examination of the patient with GAD may reveal:
■ signs or symptoms of motor tension, such as trembling, muscle aches and

spasms, headaches, or an inability to relax
■ autonomic signs and symptoms, such as shortness of breath, tachycardia, sweating, or abdominal complaints.

Additionally, the patient may display:
■ easy startling
■ complaints of feeling apprehensive, fearful, or angry
■ difficulty concentrating, eating, and sleeping.

Differential diagnoses
■ Ischemic heart disease, arrhythmias, cardiomyopathies, valvular heart disease, and myocarditis
■ Asthma, emphysema, pulmonary embolism, Hamman-Rich syndrome, and scleroderma
■ Cerebral insufficiency, psychomotor epilepsy, and essential tremor
■ Hyperthyroidism, hypoglycemia, hypokalemia, hyperparathyroidism, adrenal insufficiency, Cushing's syndrome, pheochromocytoma, and myasthenia gravis
■ Thiamine, pyridoxine, or folate deficiency; iron deficiency anemia
■ Caffeine, alcohol, cocaine, sympathomimetic, and amphetamine intoxication
■ Alcohol and sedative-hypnotic withdrawal
■ Other psychiatric disorders, such as depression and panic disorder

Diagnosis
For characteristic findings in patients with this condition, see *Diagnosing generalized anxiety disorder,* page 18.

Laboratory tests must exclude organic causes of the patient's signs and symptoms.

An electrocardiogram can rule out a cardiac source.

Because anxiety is the central feature of other mental disorders, psychi-

atric evaluation must rule out phobias, obsessive-compulsive disorders, depression, and acute schizophrenia.

Behaviors commonly associated with a diagnosis of anxiety may have cultural origins or acceptance. For example, Hispanics may experience *susto* — a state of anxiety, insomnia, anorexia, and social withdrawal following a frightening stimulus. Koreans may experience *Hwabyung* — a state of anxiety and irritability with various physiologic symptoms, such as headache and palpitations. African Americans may experience *blockout,* involving collapse, dizziness, and reduced physical movement in time of stress.

Management
General
A combination of drug therapy and psychotherapy may help a patient with GAD. Psychotherapy for GAD has two goals: helping the patient identify and deal with the cause of the anxiety and eliminating environmental factors that precipitate an anxious reaction. In addition, the patient can learn relaxation techniques, such as deep breathing, progressive muscle relaxation, focused relaxation, and visualization.

Medication
Benzodiazepines may relieve mild anxiety and improve the patient's ability to cope. Commonly prescribed benzodiazepines include:
■ alprazolam — 0.25 mg P.O. b.i.d. to t.i.d.
■ clonazepam — 0.25 mg P.O. b.i.d. to a maximum of 4.5 mg/day
■ diazepam — 2 to 10 mg b.i.d. to q.i.d.
■ lorazepam — 0.5 to 1 mg P.O. b.i.d to t.i.d.
■ buspirone — 5 mg P.O. t.i.d. increasing to a maximum of 60 mg/day.

Tricyclic antidepressants (TCAs) or higher doses of short-acting benzodi-

Diagnosing generalized anxiety disorder

When the patient's symptoms match criteria documented in *Diagnostic and Statistical Manual of Mental Disorders,* Fourth Edition, the diagnosis of generalized anxiety disorder is confirmed. The criteria include:

- excessive anxiety and worry about a number of events or activities that occur more often than not for at least 6 months
- difficulty controlling worry
- anxiety and worry associated with at least three of the following six symptoms:
 – restlessness or feeling keyed up or on edge
 – easily fatigued
 – difficulty concentrating or mind going blank
 – irritability
 – muscle tension
 – sleep disturbances (difficulty falling or staying asleep or restless, unsatisfying sleep).
- focus of the anxiety not confined to features of an axis I disorder
- anxiety, worry, or physical symptoms, causing clinically significant distress or impairment in social, occupational, or other important areas of functioning
- disturbance not due to the direct physiologic effects of a substance or general medical condition and not occurring exclusively during a mood disorder, psychotic disorder, or pervasive developmental disorder.

azepines may relieve the patient of severe anxiety and panic attacks. Commonly prescribed TCAs include:
- imipramine—10 to 25 mg P.O. t.i.d. with increasing dosage by 25 to 50 mg/day every 2 weeks for a maximum of 200 mg/day

- clomipramine—25 mg/day P.O. with gradual increase to a maximum of 250 mg/day.

Selective serotonin reuptake inhibitors (SSRIs) have become the drugs of choice for long-term antianxiety therapy. Commonly prescribed SSRIs include:
- citalopram—20 mg/day P.O. with weekly increases of 10 mg to a maximum of 40 mg/day
- fluoxetine—20 mg/day P.O. with weekly increases of 10 mg to a maximum of 80 mg/day
- paroxetine—10 mg/day P.O. with gradual increases to maximum dose of 60 mg/day
- sertraline—25 mg/day P.O. with weekly increases of 25 mg to a maximum of 200 mg/day.

Referral
- The patient may need a referral to a recovery program such as Recovery Anonymous or Emotions Anonymous for information and support.

Follow-up
Regular office visits, monitoring and adjustment of medication dosages (if prescribed), and assessment for depression and substance abuse should occur.

If TCAs are administered, serum levels should be obtained periodically and blood pressure and heart rate should be monitored. Additionally, the patient should be monitored for anticholinergic adverse effects of TCAs.

Patient teaching
- Teach the patient about prescribed medications, including the need for compliance with the medication regimen. Review adverse reactions.
- Teach the patient effective coping strategies and relaxation techniques. Help him identify stressful situations that trigger his anxiety, and provide positive

reinforcement when he uses alternative coping strategies.

- Stress management should be taught to the patient. This includes limiting caffeine and alcohol, getting proper rest, and balancing work with family and social life.

Complications
- Drug dependence
- Impaired social functioning
- Suicide risk
- Sexual dysfunction

Special considerations
- Benzodiazepines are contraindicated during pregnancy and breast-feeding and in patients with a history of drug and alcohol abuse.
- Patients taking SSRIs should never take St. John's wort, because concomitant use can precipitate a fatal serotonin syndrome.
- SSRIs are contraindicated with monoamine oxidase inhibitors; a wash-out period is required. SSRIs may also raise serum levels of other medications.

• • • • • • • • • • • •

ATTENTION DEFICIT HYPERACTIVITY DISORDER

The patient with attention deficit hyperactivity disorder (ADHD) has difficulty focusing his attention; engaging in quiet, passive activities; or both. Although the disorder is present at birth, diagnosis before age 5 is difficult unless the child shows severe symptoms. Some patients aren't diagnosed until adulthood. Males are three times more likely to be affected than females.

Causes
ADHD is thought to be a physiologic brain disorder with a familial tendency.

Some studies indicate that it may result from disturbances in neurotransmitter levels in the brain due to reduced blood flow in the striated area of the brain.

Clinical presentation
Typically, the patient is characterized as a fidgeter and a daydreamer. Other descriptive terms include:
- inattentive
- lazy
- inconsistent school or work performance patterns
- jumping from one partly completed project, thought, or task to another.

Some patients have attention deficit without hyperactivity; they're less likely to be diagnosed and treated.

In a younger child, signs and symptoms include:
- inability to wait in line
- difficulty remaining seated
- inability to wait his turn
- lack of concentration on one activity until its completion.

An older child or an adult may be described as:
- impulsive
- easily distracted by irrelevant thoughts, sounds, or sights
- emotionally labile
- inattentive
- prone to daydreaming
- having difficulty meeting deadlines
- unable to keep track of school or work tools and materials.

Differential diagnoses
- Bipolar disorder
- Dysfunctional family situation
- Learning disability
- Hearing disorder
- Vision disorder
- Oppositional-defiant disorder
- Conduct disorder
- Lead poisoning
- Medication adverse effects

- Tourette syndrome
- Autism
- Hyperthyroidism
- Absence seizures in attention deficit without hyperactivity

Diagnosis

For characteristic findings in patients with ADHD, see *Diagnosing attention deficit hyperactivity disorder*.

Most children are referred for evaluation by the school. Diagnosis of this disorder usually begins by obtaining data from several sources, including parents, teachers, and the child himself. Complete psychological, medical, and neurologic evaluations rule out other problems; then the child undergoes tests that measure impulsiveness, attention, and the ability to sustain a task.

In areas where older homes are present, serum lead levels are evaluated to rule out lead poisoning as the source of the child's behavioral problems.

The combined findings portray a clear picture of the disorder and the areas of support the child will need.

Management

General

Education is the first step in effective treatment. The entire treatment team (which ideally includes parents, teachers, and therapists as well as the patient and the health care provider) must understand the disorder and its effect on the individual's functioning.

Treatment varies, depending on the severity of symptoms and their effects on the ability to function. Behavior modification, coaching, external structure, use of planning and organizing systems, and supportive psychotherapy help the patient cope with the disorder.

Medication

Some patients benefit from medication to relieve symptoms.

Medications commonly prescribed include these stimulants:

- methylphenidate — children age 6 and older, 5 to 10 mg P.O. at breakfast and lunch, up to 60 mg/day
- pemoline — children age 6 and older, 18.75 mg P.O. in morning with weekly increases of 18.75 mg to maximum of 112.5 mg/day
- dextroamphetamine — adults and children age 6 and older, 5 mg P.O. with weekly increases of 5 mg to maximum of 40 mg/day in divided doses; children ages 3 to 6, 2.5 mg/day P.O.

Antipsychotics sometimes may be combined with stimulants. Other drugs, however, including tricyclic antidepressants (such as desipramine and nortriptyline), beta-adrenergic blockers, and mood stabilizers, may sometimes help control symptoms. Selective serotonin reuptake inhibitors, such as fluoxetine and paroxetine, are sometimes used.

Referral

- Refer the patient to a neurologist to rule out absence seizures and other neurologic disorders.
- Refer the patient and family to Children and Adults with Attention Deficit Disorder for information and support.

Follow-up

Medical follow-up consists mainly of monitoring adverse effects and titration of medications. When medication has been instituted, the patient should be evaluated in 2 weeks. Regular parent-child follow-up visits should be established to provide emotional support and track progress. Yearly contact with the child's school is also advisable, because this disorder requires a team approach for optimal results.

Diagnosing attention deficit hyperactivity disorder

The *Diagnostic and Statistical Manual of Mental Disorders*, Fourth Edition, groups a selection of symptoms into inattention and hyperactivity-impulsivity categories. The diagnosis of attention deficit hyperactivity disorder is based on the person's demonstration of at least six symptoms from the inattention group or at least six symptoms from the hyperactivity-impulsivity group. The symptoms must have persisted for at least 6 months to a degree that is maladaptive and inconsistent with the person's developmental level.

SYMPTOMS OF INATTENTION

The person manifesting inattention often:

- fails to give close attention to details or makes careless mistakes in schoolwork, work, or other activities
- has difficulty sustaining attention in tasks or play activities
- doesn't seem to listen when spoken to directly
- doesn't follow through on instructions and fails to finish schoolwork, chores, or duties in the workplace (not because of oppositional behavior or failure to understand instructions)
- has difficulty organizing tasks and activities
- avoids, dislikes, or is reluctant to engage in tasks that require sustained mental effort (such as schoolwork or homework)
- loses things necessary for tasks or activities (for example, toys, school assignments, pencils, books, or tools)
- becomes distracted by extraneous stimuli
- demonstrates forgetfulness in daily activities.

SYMPTOMS OF HYPERACTIVITY-IMPULSIVITY

The person manifesting hyperactivity often:

- fidgets with hands or feet or squirms in seat

- leaves his seat in the classroom or in other situations in which remaining seated is expected
- runs about or climbs excessively in situations in which remaining seated is expected
- has difficulty playing or engaging in leisure activities quietly
- is characterized as "on the go" or acts as if "driven by a motor"
- talks excessively.

The person manifesting impulsivity often:

- blurts out answers before questions have been completed
- has difficulty awaiting his turn
- interrupts or intrudes on others.

ADDITIONAL FEATURES

- Some symptoms that caused impairment were evident before age 7.
- Some impairment from the symptoms is present in two or more settings.
- Clinically significant impairment in social, academic, or occupational functioning must be clearly evident.
- The symptoms don't occur exclusively during the course of a pervasive developmental disorder, schizophrenia, or another psychotic disorder and aren't better accounted for by another mental disorder.

Patient teaching

- Set realistic expectations and limits because the patient with ADHD is easily frustrated, which leads to decreased self-control.
- Keep instructions short and simple.

Complications

- Abdominal pain
- Headaches
- Decreased appetite
- Delayed growth
- Work or school failure
- Low self-esteem
- Social isolation

Special considerations

- The child with ADHD is at risk for abuse, depression, and social difficulties. Work with the individual to develop external structure and controls.

• • • • • • • • • • • •

BIPOLAR DISORDER

Marked by severe pathologic mood swings from hyperactivity and euphoria to sadness and depression, bipolar disorders involve various symptom combinations. Type I bipolar disorder is characterized by alternating episodes of mania and depression, whereas type II is characterized by recurrent depressive episodes and occasional manic episodes. In some patients, bipolar disorder assumes a seasonal pattern, marked by a cyclic relation between the onset of the mood episode and a particular 60-day period of the year.

The American Psychiatric Association estimates that 0.4% to 1.2% of adults experience bipolar disorder. It affects women and men equally, is more common in higher socioeconomic groups, and is associated with high levels of creativity. Before the onset of overt symptoms, many patients with bipolar disorder

have an energetic and outgoing personality with a history of wide mood swings.

AGE ALERT Bipolar disorder can begin any time after adolescence, but onset usually occurs between ages 20 and 35; about 35% of patients experience onset between ages 35 and 60.

Bipolar disorder recurs in 80% of patients; as they grow older, the episodes recur more frequently and last longer. This illness is associated with a significant mortality; 20% of patients commit suicide, many just as the depression lifts. Older adults at highest risk for suicide are at least 85 years old, are depressed, have high self-esteem, and have a need to control their own lives. Even a frail nursing home resident with these characteristics may have the strength to kill himself.

Causes

The cause of bipolar disorder is unclear, but hereditary and biological and psychological factors may play a part. For example, the incidence of bipolar disorder among relatives of affected patients is higher than in the general population and highest among maternal relatives — the closer the relationship, the greater the susceptibility.

CLINICAL CAUTION A child with one affected parent has a 25% chance of developing bipolar disorder; a child with two affected parents, a 50% chance. The incidence of this illness in siblings is 20% to 25%; in identical twins, the incidence is 66% to 96%.

Although certain biochemical changes accompany mood swings, it isn't clear whether these changes cause the mood swings or result from them. In both mania and depression, intracellular sodium concentration increases during illness and returns to normal with recovery.

Patients with mood disorders have a defect in the way the brain handles certain neurotransmitters — chemical mes-

sengers that shuttle nerve impulses between neurons. Low levels of the chemicals dopamine and norepinephrine, for
example, have been linked to depression,
whereas excessively high levels of these
chemicals are associated with mania.

Changes in the concentration of
acetylcholine and serotonin also may
play a role. Although neurobiologists
have yet to prove that these chemical
shifts cause bipolar disorder, it's widely
assumed that most antidepressant medications work by modifying these neurotransmitter systems.

New data suggest that changes in the
circadian rhythms that control hormone
secretion, body temperature, and appetite
may contribute to the development of
bipolar disorder.

Emotional or physical trauma, such
as bereavement, disruption of an important relationship, or a serious accidental
injury, may precede the onset of bipolar
disorder; however, bipolar disorder commonly appears without identifiable predisposing factors.

Manic episodes may follow a stressful
event, but they're also associated with
antidepressant therapy and childbirth.
Major depressive episodes may be precipitated by chronic physical illness, psychoactive drug dependence, psychosocial
stressors, and childbirth. Other familial
influences, especially the early loss of a
parent, parental depression, incest, or
abuse, may predispose a person to depressive illness. (See *Cyclothymic disorder*,
page 24.)

Clinical presentation

Signs and symptoms vary widely, depending on whether the patient is experiencing a manic or depressive episode.

During the assessment interview, the
manic patient typically appears:
- grandiose
- euphoric
- expansive
- irritable
- impulsive.

He may describe:
- hyperactive or excessive behavior
- efforts to renew old acquaintances by
telephoning friends at all hours of the
night
- spending sprees
- promiscuous sexual activity
- starting projects for which he has little
aptitude.

The patient's activities may have a
bizarre quality, such as:
- dressing in colorful or strange garments
- wearing excessive makeup
- giving advice to passing strangers.

He often expresses an inflated sense
of self-esteem, ranging from uncritical
self-confidence to marked grandiosity,
which may be delusional.

Note if the patient's speech patterns
and concentration level resemble the following:
- accelerated and pressured speech
- frequent changes of topic and flight of
ideas (common features of the manic
phase)
- easy distraction
- rapid response to external stimuli, such
as background noise or a ringing tele-
phone.

Physical examination of the patient
in the manic phase may reveal:
- signs of malnutrition
- poor personal hygiene.

He may report:
- sleeping and eating less
- being more physically active than usual.

Hypomania, more common than
acute mania, can be recognized during
the assessment interview by three classic
symptoms:
- euphoric but unstable mood
- pressured speech
- increased motor activity.

Cyclothymic disorder

A chronic mood disturbance of at least 2 years' duration, cyclothymic disorder involves numerous episodes of hypomania or depression that aren't of sufficient severity or duration to qualify as a major depressive episode or a bipolar disorder.

Cyclothymia commonly starts in adolescence or early adulthood. Beginning insidiously, this disorder leads to persistent social and occupational dysfunction.

SIGNS AND SYMPTOMS

In the hypomanic phase, the patient may experience insomnia; hyperactivity; inflated self-esteem; increased productivity and creativity; overinvolvement in pleasurable activities, including an increased sexual drive; physical restlessness; and rapid speech. Depressive symptoms may include insomnia, feelings of inadequacy, decreased productivity, social withdrawal, loss of libido, loss of interest in pleasurable activities, lethargy, slow speech, and crying.

DIAGNOSIS

A number of medical disorders (for example, endocrinopathies, such as Cushing's syndrome, cerebrovascular accident, brain tumors, and head trauma) and drug overdose can produce a similar pattern of mood alteration. These organic causes must be ruled out before a cyclothymic disorder is diagnosed.

The patient with hypomania may appear:
- elated
- hyperactive
- easily distracted
- talkative
- irritable
- impatient
- impulsive
- full of energy.

Delusions and other symptoms of psychotic intensity are never present. They seldom exhibit flight of ideas.

The patient who experiences a depressive episode may report:
- loss of self-esteem
- overwhelming inertia
- social withdrawal
- feelings of hopelessness, apathy, or self-reproach
- believing that he's wicked and deserves to be punished.

His growing sadness, guilt, negativity, and fatigue place extraordinary burdens on his family.

During the assessment interview, the depressed patient:
- may speak and respond slowly
- may complain of difficulty concentrating or thinking clearly
- usually isn't obviously disoriented
- isn't intellectually impaired.

Physical examination may reveal:
- reduced psychomotor activity
- lethargy
- low muscle tonus
- weight loss
- slowed gait
- constipation.

The patient also may report:
- sleep disturbances
- sexual dysfunction
- headaches
- chest pains
- heaviness in the limbs.

Typically, symptoms are worse in the morning and gradually subside as the day goes on.

The patient's concerns about his health may become hypochondriacal: He may worry excessively about having cancer or some other serious illness. In an elderly patient, physical symptoms may be the only clues to depression.

Suicide is an ever-present risk, especially as the depression begins to lift. At that point, a rising energy level may strengthen the patient's resolve to carry out suicidal plans. The suicidal patient may also harbor homicidal ideas, for example, thinking of killing his family either in anger or to spare them pain and disgrace.

Differential diagnoses
- Mood disorders, such as dysthymia, major depression, personality disorders, cyclothymic disorder, or psychosis
- Substance abuse, particularly alcohol or cocaine
- Endocrine disorders
- Medication overdose
- Organic brain syndrome
- Renal disease
- Cardiac disease

Diagnosis
For characteristic findings in patients with this condition, see *Diagnosing bipolar disorders*, pages 26 to 28.

Physical examination and laboratory tests, such as endocrine function studies, rule out medical causes of the mood disturbances, including intra-abdominal neoplasm, hypothyroidism, heart failure, cerebral arteriosclerosis, parkinsonism, psychoactive drug abuse, brain tumor, and uremia. Moreover, a review of the medications prescribed for other disorders may point to drug-induced depression or mania.

Management
General
Acutely manic patients require immediate hospitalization for stabilization and to prevent harm to themselves and others.

Medication
Lithium is widely used to treat bipolar disorder. The typical dosage is 300 to 600 mg P.O. q.i.d. or 900 mg (controlled-release tablets) P.O. every 12 hours.

Anticonvulsants may be used with lithium to treat bipolar disorder and include:
- carbamazepine — adults, 200 mg P.O. b.i.d. may be increased by 200 mg at weekly intervals to a maximum of 1,600 mg/day; children ages 6 to 12, 100 mg P.O. b.i.d. may be increased by 100 mg at weekly intervals to a maximum of 1 g/day
- valproic acid — 750 mg P.O. in divided doses
- clonazepam — 0.75 to 16 mg/day P.O.

Antidepressants used to treat bipolar disorder include:
- imipramine — 10 to 25 mg P.O. h.s. with increasing dosage of 10 to 25 mg/day every 2 weeks for a maximum of 300 mg/day
- fluoxetine — 10 mg/day P.O. with weekly increases of 10 mg/day to a maximum of 80 mg/day.

Referral
- Patient needs to be managed by a psychiatrist for lifelong monitoring.
- Refer the patient and family to the National Alliance for the Mentally Ill for information and support.

Follow-up
Medication and patient compliance need to be monitored. Blood levels for lithium and valproic acid should be obtained weekly or biweekly. Thyroid and renal

(*Text continues on page 28.*)

Diagnosing bipolar disorders

The diagnosis of a bipolar disorder is confirmed when the patient meets the criteria documented in the *Diagnostic and Statistical Manual of Mental Disorders,* Fourth Edition.

FOR A MANIC EPISODE
- A distinct period of abnormally and persistently elevated, expansive, or irritable mood lasts at least 1 week (or any duration if hospitalization is needed).
- During the mood disturbance period, at least three of the following symptoms must have persisted (four, if the mood is only irritable) and must have been present to a significant degree:
  – inflated self-esteem or grandiosity
  – decreased need for sleep
  – more talkativeness than usual or pressure to keep talking
  – flight of ideas or subjective experience that thoughts are racing
  – distractibility
  – increased goal-directed activity or psychomotor agitation
  – excessive involvement in pleasurable activities that have a high potential for painful consequences.
- The symptoms don't meet the criteria for a mixed episode.
- The mood disturbance is sufficiently severe to cause one of the following to occur:
  – marked impairment in occupational functioning or in usual social activities or relationships with others
  – hospitalization to prevent harm to self or others
  – evidence of psychotic features.
- The symptoms aren't due to the direct physiologic effects of a substance or a general medical condition.

FOR A HYPOMANIC EPISODE
- A distinct period of abnormally and persistently elevated, expansive, or irritable mood lasts at least 4 days and is clearly different from the usual nondepressed mood.

- During the mood disturbance period, at least three of the following symptoms must have persisted (four, if the mood is only irritable) and have been present to a significant degree:
  – inflated self-esteem or grandiosity
  – decreased need for sleep
  – more talkativeness than usual or pressure to keep talking
  – flight of ideas or subjective experience that thoughts are racing
  – distractibility
  – increased goal-directed activity or psychomotor agitation
  – excessive involvement in pleasurable activities that have a high potential for painful consequences.
- The episode is associated with an unequivocal change in functioning that is uncharacteristic of the person when not symptomatic.
- Others can recognize the disturbance in mood and the change in functioning.
- The episode isn't severe enough to markedly impair social or occupational functioning or to necessitate hospitalization to prevent harm to self or others. No psychotic features are evident.
- The symptoms aren't due to the direct physiologic effects of a substance or a general medical condition.

FOR A BIPOLAR I SINGLE MANIC EPISODE
- Presence of only one manic episode and no past major depressive episodes.
- The manic episode isn't better accounted for by schizoaffective disorder and isn't superimposed on schizophrenia, schizophreniform disorder, delusional disorder, or psychotic disorder not otherwise specified.

Diagnosing bipolar disorders (continued)

FOR A BIPOLAR I DISORDER, MOST RECENT EPISODE HYPOMANIC

- The person is currently (or most recently) in a hypomanic episode.
- The person previously had at least one manic episode or mixed episode.
- The mood symptoms cause clinically significant distress or impairment in social, occupational, or other important areas of functioning.
- The first two exacerbations of the mood episode (above) aren't better accounted for by schizoaffective disorder and aren't superimposed on schizophrenia, schizophreniform disorder, delusional disorder, or psychotic disorder not otherwise specified.

FOR A BIPOLAR I DISORDER, MOST RECENT EPISODE MANIC

- The person is currently (or most recently) in a manic episode.
- The person previously had at least one major depressive episode, manic episode, or mixed episode.
- The first two exacerbations of mood episode (above) aren't better accounted for by schizoaffective disorder and aren't superimposed on schizophrenia, schizophreniform disorder, delusional disorder, or psychotic disorder not otherwise specified.

FOR A BIPOLAR I DISORDER, MOST RECENT EPISODE MIXED

- The person is currently (or most recently) in a mixed episode.
- The person previously had at least one major depressive episode, manic episode, or mixed episode.
- The first two exacerbations of mood episode (above) aren't better accounted for by schizoaffective disorder and aren't superimposed on schizophrenia, schizophreniform disorder, delusional

disorder, or psychotic disorder not otherwise specified.

FOR A BIPOLAR I DISORDER, MOST RECENT EPISODE DEPRESSED

- The person is currently (or most recently) in a major depressive episode.
- The person previously had at least one manic episode or mixed episode.
- The first two exacerbations of mood episode (above) aren't better accounted for by schizoaffective disorder and aren't superimposed on schizophrenia, schizophreniform disorder, delusional disorder, or psychotic disorder not otherwise specified.

FOR A BIPOLAR I DISORDER, MOST RECENT EPISODE UNSPECIFIED

- Criteria, except for duration, are currently (or most recently) met for a manic, hypomanic, mixed, or major depressive episode.
- The person previously had at least one manic episode or mixed episode.
- The mood symptoms cause clinically significant distress or impairment in social, occupational, or other important areas of functioning.
- The first two exacerbations of mood episode (above) aren't better accounted for by schizoaffective disorder and aren't superimposed on schizophrenia, schizophreniform disorder, delusional disorder, or psychotic disorder not otherwise specified.
- The first two exacerbations of mood episode (above) aren't due to the direct physiologic effects of a substance or a general medical condition.

FOR A BIPOLAR II DISORDER

- The person has the presence (or history) of one or more major depressive episodes.

(continued)

Diagnosing bipolar disorders *(continued)*

- The person has the presence (or history) of at least one hypomanic episode.
- The person has never had a manic episode or a mixed episode.
- The first two exacerbations of mood episode (above) aren't better accounted for by schizoaffective disorder and aren't superimposed on schizophrenia, schizophreniform disorder, delusional disorder, or psychotic disorder not otherwise specified.
- The symptoms cause clinically significant distress or impairment in social, occupational, or other important areas of functioning.

function studies need to be done periodically and electrocardiograms should be done frequently.

Patient teaching

- Teach the patient the importance of compliance with the medication schedule established. Any adverse effects should be reported immediately.
- Tell the patient to avoid caffeine.
- The patient needs to drink approximately 2 to 3 L of fluid per day, with consistent sodium intake.
- The patient should know to consult health care professional prior to taking any over-the-counter medications.
- If the patient is taking lithium, tell him and his family to temporarily discontinue the drug if signs or symptoms of toxicity, such as diarrhea, abdominal cramps, vomiting, unsteadiness, drowsiness, muscle weakness, polyuria, and tremors, occur.

Complications

- Harm to self
- Harm to others
- Recurrence of symptoms
- Disruption of lifestyle

Special considerations

- Because lithium has a narrow therapeutic range, treatment must be initiated cautiously and the dosage adjusted slowly. Therapeutic blood levels during the active manic period are 0.4 to 1.4 mEq/L. For safety, the level should never exceed 1.5 mEq/L. Therapeutic blood levels must be maintained for 7 to 10 days before the drug's beneficial effects appear.
- If the patient is taking an antidepressant, watch for signs of mania.
- Nonsteroidal anti-inflammatory drugs may increase lithium toxicity.

• • • • • • • • • • • •

BULIMIA NERVOSA

The essential features of bulimia nervosa include eating binges followed by feelings of guilt, self-deprecation, and humiliation. These feelings cause the patient to engage in self-induced vomiting, use laxatives or diuretics, follow a strict diet, or fast to overcome the effects of the binges. Unless the patient spends an excessive amount of time bingeing and purging, bulimia nervosa seldom is incapacitating. However, electrolyte imbalances (such as metabolic alkalosis, hypochloremia, and hypokalemia) and dehydration can occur, increasing the risk of physical complications.

Bulimia nervosa usually begins in adolescence or early adulthood and can occur simultaneously with anorexia nervosa. It affects nine women for every man. Nearly 2% of adult women meet the diagnostic criteria for bulimia nervosa; 5% to 15% have some symptoms of the disorder.

Causes
The cause of bulimia is unknown, but psychosocial factors may contribute to its development. These factors include family disturbance or conflict, sexual abuse, maladaptive learned behavior, struggle for control or self-identity, cultural overemphasis on physical appearance, and parental obesity. Bulimia nervosa is associated with depression, anxiety, phobias, and obsessive-compulsive disorder.

Eating disorders are most prevalent in affluent cultural groups and are essentially unknown in cultural groups where poverty and malnutrition are prevalent. In developing countries, almost no cases of eating disorders have been recognized.

Clinical presentation
The history of a patient with bulimia nervosa is characterized by episodes of binge eating that may occur up to several times a day. The patient commonly reports a binge-eating episode during which she continues eating until abdominal pain, sleep, or the presence of another person interrupts it. The preferred food usually is sweet, soft, and high in calories and carbohydrate content.

The patient with bulimia may appear thin and emaciated. Typically, however, although her weight frequently fluctuates, it usually stays within normal limits — through the use of diuretics, laxatives, vomiting, and exercise. So, unlike the anorexic patient, the bulimic patient can usually hide her eating disorder.

Overt clues to this disorder include:
- hyperactivity
- peculiar eating habits or rituals
- frequent weighing
- a distorted body image. (See *Characteristics of bulimia nervosa*.)

> ## Characteristics of bulimia nervosa
>
> Recognizing a patient with bulimia nervosa isn't always easy. Unlike those with anorexia, patients with bulimia nervosa don't deny that their eating habits are abnormal, but they commonly conceal their behavior out of shame. If you suspect bulimia nervosa, be on the lookout for the following features:
> - difficulty with impulse control
> - chronic depression
> - exaggerated sense of guilt
> - low tolerance for frustration
> - recurrent anxiety
> - feelings of alienation
> - self-consciousness
> - difficulty expressing feelings such as anger
> - impaired social or occupational adjustment.

The patient may complain of the following:
- abdominal and epigastric pain
- painless swelling of the salivary glands
- hoarseness
- throat irritation or lacerations
- dental erosion.

The patient may also exhibit calluses on the knuckles or abrasions and scars on the dorsum of the hand that result from tooth injury during self-induced vomiting, although many bulimic persons induce vomiting chemically, such as with ipecac.

A bulimic patient is commonly perceived by others as a "perfect" student, mother, or career woman; an adolescent may be distinguished for participation in competitive activities such as sports. However, the patient's psychosocial history may reveal:
- an exaggerated sense of guilt
- symptoms of depression

Diagnosing bulimia nervosa

The diagnosis of bulimia is made when the patient meets criteria put forth in the *Diagnostic and Statistical Manual of Mental Disorders,* Fourth Edition. Both of the behaviors listed below must occur at least twice per week for 3 months:
- recurrent episodes of binge eating (rapid consumption of a large amount of food in a discrete period of time and a feeling of lack of control over eating behavior during the eating binges)
- recurrent inappropriate compensatory behavior to prevent weight gain (self-induced vomiting; misuse of laxatives, diuretics, enemas, or other medications; fasting; excessive exercise).

- childhood trauma (especially sexual abuse)
- parental obesity
- history of unsatisfactory sexual relationships.

Differential diagnoses
- Kleine-Levin syndrome
- Major depressive disorder
- Borderline personality disorder
- Acquired immunodeficiency syndrome
- Hyperthyroidism
- Cancer

Diagnosis
For characteristic findings in this condition, see *Diagnosing bulimia nervosa.*

Additional diagnostic tools include the Beck Depression Inventory, which may identify coexisting depression. Laboratory tests may help determine the presence and severity of complications:

- Serum electrolyte studies may show elevated bicarbonate, decreased potassium, and decreased sodium levels.
- Complete blood count may show anemia, leukopenia, and thrombocytopenia.
- Calcium level may be low.
- Magnesium level may be low.

A baseline electrocardiogram may be done in the presence of malnutrition or abuse of syrup of ipecac, which may also induce cardiomyopathy due to emetine toxicity.

Management
General
Treatment of bulimia nervosa may continue for several years. Interrelated physical and psychological symptoms must be treated simultaneously. Merely promoting weight gain isn't sufficient to guarantee long-term recovery. A patient whose physical status is severely compromised by inadequate or chaotic eating patterns is difficult to engage in the psychotherapeutic process.

Medication
Antidepressant drugs may be used as an adjunct to psychotherapy and include:
- imipramine — 10 to 25 mg P.O. h.s. with increasing dosage of 10 to 25 mg/day every 2 weeks to a maximum of 300 mg/day
- fluoxetine — 10 mg/day P.O. with weekly increases of 10 mg/day to a maximum of 60 mg/day.

Referral
- The patient should be referred for psychological counseling.
- The patient may benefit from participation in self-help groups, such as Overeaters Anonymous, or in a drug rehabilitation program if she has a concurrent substance-abuse problem.
- Refer the patient and family to the Anorexia Nervosa and Related Eating

Disorders organization for information and support.

Follow-up
Patient monitoring depends on the severity of physical symptoms and the progress of psychological interventions. All laboratory tests with abnormal values should be repeated at weekly or monthly intervals until stable.

Patient teaching
- Teach the patient how to keep a food journal to monitor treatment progress.
- Outline the risks of laxative, emetic, and diuretic abuse for the patient.

Complications
- Cardiac arrest
- Cardiac arrhythmia
- Harm to self
- Drug and alcohol abuse
- Esophageal strictures and erosive esophagitis

Special considerations
- Provide assertiveness training to help the patient gain control over her behavior and achieve a realistic and positive self-image.

• • • • • • • • • • • •

DEPRESSION, MAJOR

Also known as unipolar disorder, major depression is a syndrome of persistently sad, dysphoric mood, accompanied by disturbances in sleep and appetite, lethargy, and an inability to experience pleasure (anhedonia). Major depression occurs in up to 17% of adults, affecting all racial, ethnic, and socioeconomic groups. It affects both sexes but is more common in women.

About half of all depressed patients experience a single episode and recover completely; the rest have at least one recurrence. Major depression can profoundly alter social, family, and occupational functioning. However, suicide is the most serious consequence of major depression—the patient's feelings of worthlessness, guilt, and hopelessness are so overwhelming that she no longer considers life worth living. Nearly twice as many women as men attempt suicide, but men are far more likely to succeed.

Causes and pathophysiology
The multiple causes of depression aren't completely understood. Current research suggests possible genetic, familial, biochemical, physical, psychological, and social causes. Psychological causes (the focus of many nursing interventions) may include feelings of helplessness and vulnerability, anger, hopelessness and pessimism, and low self-esteem. They may be related to abnormal character and behavior patterns and troubled personal relationships. In many patients, the history identifies a specific personal loss or severe stressor that probably interacts with the person's predisposition to provoke major depression.

Depression may be secondary to a specific medical condition—for example, metabolic disturbances, such as hypoxia and hypercalcemia; endocrine disorders, such as diabetes and Cushing's syndrome; neurologic diseases, such as Parkinson's and Alzheimer's diseases; cancer (especially of the pancreas); viral and bacterial infections, such as influenza and pneumonia; cardiovascular disorders, such as heart failure; pulmonary disorders, such as chronic obstructive pulmonary disease; musculoskeletal disorders, such as degenerative arthritis; GI disorders, such as irritable bowel syndrome; genitourinary problems, such as incontinence; collagen vascular diseases, such as lupus; and anemias.

Dysthymic disorder

Dysthymic disorder is characterized by a chronic dysphoric mood (irritable mood in children), persisting at least 2 years in adults and 1 year in children and adolescents.

SIGNS AND SYMPTOMS
During periods of depression, the patient also may experience poor appetite or overeating, insomnia or hypersomnia, low energy or fatigue, low self-esteem, poor concentration or difficulty making decisions, and feelings of hopelessness.

DIAGNOSIS
Dysthymic disorder is confirmed when the patient exhibits at least two of the signs or symptoms listed above nearly every day, with intervening normal moods lasting no more than 2 months during a 2-year period.

The disorder typically begins in childhood, adolescence, or early adulthood and causes only mild social or occupational impairment. In adults, it's more common in women; in children and adolescents, it's equally common in both sexes.

Drugs prescribed for medical and psychiatric conditions as well as many commonly abused substances can also cause depression. Examples include antihypertensives, psychotropics, narcotic and nonnarcotic analgesics, antiparkinsonian drugs, numerous cardiovascular medications, oral antidiabetics, antimicrobials, steroids, chemotherapeutic agents, cimetidine, and alcohol.

Clinical presentation
The primary features of major depression are a predominantly sad mood and a loss of interest or pleasure in daily activities. The patient may report:
- feeling "down in the dumps"
- doubts about her self-worth or ability to cope
- feeling angry or anxious.

Symptoms tend to be more severe than those caused by dysthymic disorder, which is a milder, chronic form of depression. (See *Dysthymic disorder.*)

Other common signs include:
- difficulty concentrating or thinking clearly
- distractibility
- indecisiveness
- slow physiologic and psychological processes
- anergia and fatigue
- anhedonia (inability to experience pleasure)
- insomnia.

Take special note if the patient reveals suicidal thoughts, a preoccupation with death, or previous suicide attempts.

The psychosocial history may reveal life problems or losses that can account for the depression. Alternatively, the patient's medical history may implicate a physical disorder or the use of prescription, nonprescription, or illegal drugs that can cause depression.

The patient may report:
- an increase or a decrease in appetite
- sleep disturbances (for example, insomnia or early awakening)
- a lack of interest in sexual activity
- constipation or diarrhea.

Other signs that you may note during a physical examination include:
- agitation (such as hand wringing or restlessness)
- reduced psychomotor activity (for example, slowed speech).

Differential diagnoses
- Manic, mixed, or hypomanic episode
- Mood disorder

Diagnosing major depression

A patient is diagnosed with major depression when he fulfills the criteria for a single major depressive episode put forth in *Diagnostic and Statistical Manual of Mental Disorders,* Fourth Edition.

■ At least five of the following symptoms must have been present during the same 2-week period and must represent a change from previous functioning; one of these must be either depressed mood or loss of interest in previously pleasurable activities:
– depressed mood (irritable mood in children and adolescents) most of the day, nearly every day, as indicated by either subjective account or observation by others
– markedly diminished interest or pleasure in all, or almost all, activities most of the day, nearly every day
– significant weight loss or weight gain when not dieting or decrease or increase in appetite nearly every day (in children, consider failure to make expected weight gains)
– insomnia or hypersomnia nearly every day
– psychomotor agitation or retardation nearly every day
– fatigue or loss of energy nearly every day

– feelings of worthlessness or excessive or inappropriate guilt nearly every day
– diminished ability to think or concentrate, or indecisiveness, nearly every day
– recurrent thoughts of death, recurrent suicidal ideation without a specific plan, a suicide attempt, or a specific plan for committing suicide.
■ The symptoms don't meet criteria for a mixed episode.
■ The symptoms cause clinically significant distress or impairment in social, occupational, or other important areas of functioning.
■ The symptoms aren't due to the direct physiologic effects of a substance or a general medical condition.
■ The symptoms aren't better accounted for by bereavement, they persist for longer than 2 months, or they're characterized by marked functional impairment, morbid preoccupation with worthlessness, suicidal ideation, psychotic symptoms, or psychomotor retardation.

■ Dysthymic disorder
■ Schizophrenic disorder

Diagnosis

For characteristic findings in patients with this condition, see *Diagnosing major depression.*

The diagnosis is supported by psychological tests, such as the Beck Depression Inventory, which may help determine the onset, severity, duration, and progression of depressive symptoms. A

toxicology screening may suggest drug-induced depression.

Management
General

Depression is difficult to treat, especially in children, adolescents, elderly patients, and those with a history of chronic disease. The primary treatment methods are drug therapy, electroconvulsive therapy (ECT), and psychotherapy. When a depressed patient is incapacitated, suicidal, or psychotically depressed or when antidepressants are contraindicated or ineffective, ECT is commonly the treatment of choice. Short-term psychotherapy is also effective in treating major depression. Many psychiatrists believe that the best results are achieved with a combination of individual, family, or group psychotherapy and medication. After resolution of the acute episode, patients with a history of recurrent depression may be maintained on low doses of antidepressants as a preventive measure.

Depression may be experienced differently by members of different cultures. For instance, in some Asian cultures, there are more somatic manifestations of depression than overt psychological signs or symptoms.

Medication
Drug therapy includes tricyclic antidepressants (TCAs), the most widely used class of antidepressant drugs. These TCAs may be used to treat depression:
- amitriptyline — 50 to 100 mg/day P.O. for a maximum of 300 mg/day
- imipramine — 10 to 25 mg P.O. h.s. with increasing dosage of 10 to 25 mg/day every 2 weeks for a maximum of 300 mg/day P.O.
- clomipramine — 25 mg/day with a gradual dose increase to a maximum of 250 mg/day.

Selective serotonin reuptake inhibitors (SSRIs) are increasingly becoming the drugs of choice for depression. These SSRIs may be used to treat depression:
- fluoxetine — 20 to 80 mg/day P.O.
- paroxetine — 20 to 50 mg/day P.O.

Other medications that may be utilized include:
- trazodone — 150 to 400 mg/day P.O.
- bupropion — 200 to 400 mg/day P.O.

Pharmacologic interventions should be continued from 9 months to 1 year.

Referral
- Refer the patient for psychiatric counseling or consultation with a collaborating physician when ECT therapy is a consideration, the patient fails to adequately respond, psychosis is suspected, the diagnosis is unclear, or suicidal tendencies surface.

Follow-up
Follow-up visits should occur every 2 weeks after the initiation of pharmacotherapy to evaluate its effectiveness, titrate the dosage, and monitor for adverse effects. Once significant improvement occurs, follow-up appointments can be decreased to every 3 months.

Patient teaching
- Inform the patient that antidepressants may take several weeks to produce an effect.
- Teach the patient about depression. Emphasize that effective methods are available to relieve his symptoms. Help him to recognize distorted perceptions that may contribute to the depression.
- Instruct the patient about prescribed medications. Stress the need for compliance, and review adverse effects.

Complications
- Harm to self
- Failure to improve

Special considerations
- Caution the patient taking a TCA to avoid drinking alcoholic beverages or taking other CNS depressants during therapy.

• • • • • • • • • • • •
PAIN DISORDER

The most striking feature of pain disorder is a persistent complaint of pain in the absence of appropriate physical findings. The symptoms are either inconsistent with the normal anatomic distribution of the nervous system or they mimic a disease (such as angina) in the absence of diagnostic validation. Although the pain has no physical cause, it's real to the patient. The disorder is more common in women than men. The pain usually is chronic, in many cases interfering with interpersonal relationships or employment.

AGE ALERT Pain disorder usually has an onset in patients ages 30 to 40.

Causes
Pain disorder has no specific cause, but it may be related to severe psychological stress or conflict. The pain provides the patient with a means to cope with upsetting psychological issues. For example, a person with dependency needs may develop this disorder as an acceptable way to receive care and attention. The pain may have special significance, such as leg pain in the same leg a parent lost through amputation.

Clinical presentation
The cardinal feature of pain disorder is a history of chronic, consistent complaints of pain without confirming physical disease. The patient may relate a long history of evaluations and procedures at multiple settings without much pain relief. Because of frequent hospitalizations, the patient may:
■ be familiar with pain medications and tranquilizers
■ ask for a specific drug

■ know correct dosages and administration routes.
■ openly behave like an invalid.

Physical examination of the painful site reveals that the pain doesn't follow anatomic pathways. The patient may not display typical nonverbal signs of pain, such as grimacing or guarding. (Sometimes such reactions are absent in patients with chronic organic pain.) Palpation, percussion, and auscultation may not reveal expected associated signs. Psychosocial assessment may reveal a patient who's angry with health care professionals because they've failed to relieve his pain.

Differential diagnoses
■ Fibromyalgia
■ Chronic fatigue syndrome
■ Lyme disease
■ Conversion disorder
■ Hypochondriasis
■ Somatization disorder
■ Malingering
■ Body dysmorphic disorder

Diagnosis
For characteristic findings in patients with this condition, see *Diagnosing pain disorder*, page 36.

Management
General
In pain disorder, the goal of treatment is to ease the pain and help the patient live with it. Thus, long, invasive evaluations and surgical interventions are avoided. Treatment at a comprehensive pain center may be helpful. Supportive measures for pain relief may include hot or cold packs, physical therapy, distraction techniques, and cutaneous stimulation with massage or transcutaneous electrical nerve stimulation. Measures to reduce the patient's anxiety may help, as may an

Diagnosing pain disorder

The diagnosis of pain disorder is difficult because the perception of pain is subjective. Diagnosis is based on fulfillment of the criteria put forth in the *Diagnostic and Statistical Manual of Mental Disorders,* Fourth Edition.

■ Pain in one or more body sites is the predominant focus of the patient and is sufficiently severe to warrant clinical attention.

■ The pain causes clinically significant distress or impairment in social, occupational, or other important areas of functioning.

■ Psychological factors are judged to have an important role in the onset, severity, exacerbation, and maintenance of the pain.

■ The symptom or deficit isn't intentionally produced or feigned.

■ The pain isn't better accounted for by a mood, anxiety, or psychotic disorder and doesn't meet criteria for dyspareunia.

antidepressant medication such as a tricyclic antidepressant.

A continuing, supportive relationship with an understanding health care professional is essential for effective management; regularly scheduled follow-up appointments are helpful.

Medication

Analgesics become an issue because the patient believes that he has to "fight to be taken seriously." The patient should be clearly told what medication he'll receive in addition to supportive pain-relief measures. Regularly scheduled analgesic doses can be more effective than scheduling medication as needed. Regular doses combat pain by reducing anxiety about asking for medication, and they elimi-

nate unnecessary confrontations. The use of placebos will destroy trust when the patient discovers deceit.

Narcotic analgesics generally aren't employed in this patient population because of dependency issues and questionable appropriateness. Nonnarcotic drug choices may include:

■ acetaminophen — 325 to 650 mg P.O. every 4 to 6 hours p.r.n.

■ aspirin — 325 to 650 mg P.O. every 4 to 6 hours, p.r.n.

■ ibuprofen — 400 mg P.O. every 4 to 6 hours p.r.n.

■ naproxen sodium — 250 to 500 mg P.O. every 6 to 8 hours

■ diclofenac potassium — 50 mg t.i.d. P.O.

■ etodolac — 200 to 400 mg P.O. every 6 to 8 hours p.r.n.

■ ketoprofen — 25 to 50 mg P.O. every 6 to 8 hours p.r.n.

Referral

■ Consider psychiatric referrals; however, realize that the patient may resist psychiatric intervention, and don't expect it to replace analgesic measures.

■ Consider referral for noninvasive, drug-free methods of pain control, such as guided imagery, relaxation techniques, hypnosis, and biofeedback.

Patient teaching

■ Teach the patient about the medications prescribed and their potential adverse effects.

Complications

■ Psychoactive substance dependence

■ Multiple surgical interventions

Special considerations

■ Observe and record characteristics of the pain: severity, duration, and any precipitating factors. Continue to reassess for possible physical disorders.

•••••••••••••
PANIC DISORDER

Characterized by recurrent episodes of intense apprehension, terror, and impending doom, panic disorder represents anxiety in its most severe form. Initially unpredictable, panic attacks may become associated with specific situations or tasks. The disorder often exists concurrently with agoraphobia. Equal numbers of men and women are affected by panic disorder alone, whereas panic disorder with agoraphobia occurs in about twice as many women than men.

Panic disorder typically has an onset in late adolescence or early adulthood, often in response to a sudden loss. It also may be triggered by severe separation anxiety experienced during early childhood. Without treatment, panic disorder can persist for years, with alternating exacerbations and remissions. The patient with panic disorder is at high risk for a psychoactive substance abuse disorder: He may resort to alcohol or anxiolytics in an attempt to relieve his extreme anxiety.

Causes

Like other anxiety disorders, panic disorder may stem from a combination of physical and psychological factors. For example, some theorists emphasize the role of stressful events or unconscious conflicts that occur early in childhood.

Recent evidence indicates that alterations in brain biochemistry, especially in norepinephrine, serotonin, and gamma-aminobutyric acid activity, may also contribute to panic disorder.

Clinical presentation

The patient with panic disorder typically complains of:
- repeated episodes of unexpected apprehension
- fear
- rarely, intense discomfort.

These panic attacks may last for minutes or hours and leave the patient shaken, fearful, and exhausted. They occur several times a week, sometimes even daily. Because the attacks occur spontaneously, without exposure to a known anxiety-producing situation, the patient generally worries between attacks about when the next episode will occur.

Physical examination of the patient during a panic attack may reveal signs of intense anxiety, such as:
- hyperventilation
- tachycardia
- trembling
- profuse sweating
- difficulty breathing
- digestive disturbances
- chest pain.

Differential diagnoses
- Anxiety disorder
- Substance-induced anxiety disorder
- Separation anxiety disorder

Diagnosis

For characteristic findings in patients with this condition, see *Diagnosing panic disorder*, page 38.

Because many medical conditions can mimic panic disorder, additional tests may be ordered to rule out an organic basis for the symptoms. For example, tests of serum glucose levels rule out hypoglycemia, studies of urine catecholamines and vanillylmandelic acid rule out pheochromocytoma, and thyroid function tests rule out hyperthyroidism.

Urine and serum toxicology tests may reveal the presence of psychoactive substances that can precipitate panic attacks, including barbiturates, caffeine, and amphetamines.

Diagnosing panic disorder

The diagnosis of panic disorder is confirmed when the patient meets the criteria put forth in the *Diagnostic and Statistical Manual of Mental Disorders,* Fourth Edition.

PANIC ATTACK

The person experiences a discrete period of intense fear or discomfort in which at least four of the following symptoms develop abruptly and reach a peak within 10 minutes:

- palpitations, pounding heart, or tachycardia
- sweating
- trembling or shaking
- shortness of breath or smothering sensations
- feeling of choking
- chest pain or discomfort
- nausea or abdominal distress
- dizziness or faintness
- depersonalization or derealization
- fear of losing control or going crazy
- fear of dying
- numbness or tingling sensations (paresthesia)
- hot flashes or chills.

PANIC DISORDER WITHOUT AGORAPHOBIA

- The person experiences recurrent unexpected panic attacks and at least one of the attacks has been followed by 1 month (or more) of one (or more) of the following:
  - persistent concern about having additional attacks
  - worry about the implications of the attack or its consequences

  - significant change in behavior related to the attacks.
- The panic attacks aren't due to the direct physiologic effects of a substance or a general medical condition.
- The panic attacks aren't better accounted for by another mental disorder, such as social phobia, specific phobia, obsessive-compulsive disorder, posttraumatic stress disorder, or separation anxiety disorder.

PANIC DISORDER WITH AGORAPHOBIA

- The person experiences recurrent unexpected panic attacks and at least one of the attacks has been followed by 1 month (or more) of one (or more) of the following:
  - persistent concern about having additional attacks
  - worry about the implications of the attack or its consequences
  - significant change in behavior related to the attacks.
- The person exhibits agoraphobia.
- The panic attacks aren't due to the direct physiologic effects of a substance or a general medical condition.
- The panic attacks aren't better accounted for by another mental disorder, such as social phobia, specific phobia, obsessive-compulsive disorder, posttraumatic stress disorder, or separation anxiety disorder.

Management

General

Panic disorder may respond to behavioral therapy, supportive psychotherapy, or drug therapy, alone or in combination.

Behavioral therapy works best when agoraphobia accompanies panic disorder because the identification of anxiety-inducing situations is easier.

Medications for treating panic disorder

DRUG	DOSAGE
alprazolam	Initially 0.5 mg P.O. t.i.d., mean range 5 to 6 mg/day in divided doses
buspirone	Severe symptoms: 5 mg P.O. t.i.d. increase every 3 days to a maximum of 60 mg/day
chlordiazepoxide	Moderate anxiety: 5 to 10 mg P.O. t.i.d. to q.i.d. Severe anxiety: 20 to 25 mg P.O. t.i.d. to q.i.d.
clonazepam	Initially 0.25 mg P.O. b.i.d.; after 3 days increase to 1 mg/day P.O. ; maximum dose 4 mg/day P.O.
diazepam	2 to 10 mg/day P.O. b.i.d. to q.i.d.
lorazepam	2 to 10 mg P.O. q.d. in divided doses
oxazepam	10 to 15 mg P.O. t.i.d. to q.i.d.
paroxetine	Initially 10 mg/day P.O.; usual dose 40 mg/day P.O.; maximum dose 60 mg/day P.O.
sertraline	Initially 25 mg/day P.O.; may increase weekly by 25 mg P.O. to maximum dose of 200 mg/day P.O.
venlafaxine	Initially 37.5 mg/day for 4 to 7 days, then increase to 75 mg/day P.O.; maximum dose 225 mg/day P.O.

Psychotherapy commonly uses cognitive techniques to enable the patient to view anxiety-provoking situations more realistically and to recognize panic symptoms as a misinterpretation of essentially harmless physical sensations.

Medication

Drug therapy includes antianxiety drugs, such as diazepam, alprazolam, and clonazepam, and beta blockers, such as propranolol, to provide symptomatic relief. Antidepressants, including tricyclic antidepressants, selective serotonin reuptake inhibitors (SSRIs), and monoamine oxidase inhibitors, are also effective. (See *Medications for treating panic disorder*.)

Referral

■ For extremely anxious patients, particularly agoraphobics, referral to a psychiatrist is recommended.
■ Encourage the patient and his family to use community resources such as the Anxiety Disorders Association of America.

Follow-up

Follow-up of patients with panic disorder is similar to that for those with generalized anxiety. Follow-up should consist of regular office visits to evaluate effects of prescribed medications and to monitor for adverse effects. Regular office visits also build a trusting relationship that offers hope for improvement and emotional support.

Patient teaching
- Teach the patient relaxation techniques, and explain how he can use them to relieve stress or avoid a panic attack.
- Review with the patient any adverse effects of the drugs he'll be taking. Caution him not to discontinue the medication unless directed because abrupt withdrawal could cause severe symptoms.
- Stress the importance of avoiding over-the-counter medicines and herbal preparations because they frequently interact with antianxiolytics. Patients taking SSRIs should never take St. John's wort as this may potentiate a fatal serotonin syndrome.

Complications
- Impaired occupational functioning
- Impaired social functioning

Special considerations
- The patient may be so overwhelmed that he can't follow lengthy or complicated instructions. Speak in short, simple sentences, and slowly give one direction at a time. Avoid giving lengthy explanations and asking too many questions.
- Avoid touching the patient until you have established rapport. Unless he trusts you, he may be too stimulated or frightened to find touch reassuring.

• • • • • • • • • • • •

PERSONALITY DISORDERS

Defined as individual traits that reflect chronic, inflexible, and maladaptive patterns of behavior, personality disorders cause social discomfort and impair social and occupational functioning. Although no statistics document the number of cases of personality disorders, these disorders are known to be widespread. Most patients with a personality disorder don't receive treatment; when they do, they're typically managed as outpatients.

Personality disorders fall on axis II of the *DSM-IV* classification. Personality notations help provide a fuller picture of the patient and a more accurate diagnosis. For example, many features characteristic of personality disorders are apparent during an episode of another mental disorder (such as a major depressive episode in a patient with compulsive personality features).

Personality disorders typically have an onset before or during adolescence and early adulthood, and they persist throughout adult life affecting both men and women. Approximately 5% to 15% of the general population is affected. The prognosis is variable.

Causes
Only recently have personality disorders been categorized in detail, and research continues to identify their causes.

Various theories attempt to explain the origin of personality disorders. Biological theories hold that these disorders may stem from chromosomal and neuronal abnormalities or head trauma. Social theories hold that the disorders reflect learned responses, having much to do with reinforcement, modeling, and aversive stimuli as contributing factors. According to psychodynamic theories, personality disorders reflect deficiencies in ego and superego development and are related to poor mother-child relationships characterized by unresponsiveness, overprotectiveness, or early separation.

Clinical presentation
Each specific personality disorder produces characteristic signs and symptoms, which may vary among patients and within the same patient at different

times. In general, the history of the patient with a personality disorder reveals :
■ long-standing difficulties in interpersonal relationships, ranging from dependency to withdrawal
■ trouble with occupational functioning, with effects ranging from compulsive perfectionism to intentional sabotage.
■ any degree of self-confidence, ranging from no self-esteem to arrogance.
■ a conviction that his behavior is normal, thus he avoids responsibility for its consequences, commonly resorting to projections and blame.

Differential diagnoses
■ Major depression
■ Bipolar disorder
■ Schizophrenia
■ General anxiety disorder
■ Obsessive-compulsive disorder
■ Posttraumatic stress disorder
■ Phobic disorders
■ Substance abuse

Diagnosis
For characteristic findings in patients with this condition, see *Diagnosing personality disorders*, pages 42 to 45.

Management
General
Personality disorders are difficult to treat. Successful therapy requires a trusting relationship in which the therapist can use a direct approach. The type of therapy chosen depends on the patient's symptoms. Family and group therapies usually are effective. Hospital inpatient milieu therapy can be effective in crisis situations and possibly for long-term treatment of borderline personality disorders. Inpatient treatment is controversial, however, because most patients with personality disorders don't comply with extended therapeutic regimens; for such patients, outpatient therapy may be more useful.

Medication
Drug therapy is ineffective but may be used to relieve acute anxiety and depression.

Referral
■ Referral to a psychiatrist for therapy may be helpful.

Follow-up
Follow-up for patients with personality disorders includes monitoring for complications and adverse effects of medication (if utilized). Encourage active participation in ongoing psychotherapy.

Patient teaching
■ Teach the patient social skills, and reinforce appropriate behavior.
■ Teach the patient about administered medications and their potential adverse effects.

Complications
■ Harm to self
■ Social impairment
■ Occupational impairment
■ Anxiety
■ Depression
■ Substance use disorder

Special considerations
■ Provide consistent care. Take a direct, involved approach to ensure the patient's trust. Keep in mind that many of these patients don't respond well to interviews, whereas others are charming and convincing.
■ Encourage expression of feelings, self-analysis of behavior, and accountability for actions.
■ Specific care measures vary with the particular personality disorder.

(*Text continues on page 46.*)

Diagnosing personality disorders

The diagnosis of a recognized personality disorder is made when a patient's symptoms match the diagnostic criteria put forth in the *Diagnostic and Statistical Manual of Mental Disorders,* Fourth Edition.

PARANOID PERSONALITY DISORDER

■ The person must exhibit a pervasive and unwarranted tendency, beginning by early adulthood and present in various contexts, to interpret the actions of people as deliberately demeaning or threatening, as indicated by at least four of the following criteria:
– The person suspects, without sufficient basis, that he's being exploited, deceived, or harmed by others.
– The person questions, without justification, the loyalty or trustworthiness of friends or associates.
– The person is reluctant to confide in others because of unwarranted fear that the information will be used against him.
– The person finds hostile or evil meanings in benign remarks.
– The person bears grudges or is unforgiving of insults or slights.
– The person is easily slighted and quick to react with anger or to counterattack.
– The person questions without justification the fidelity of a spouse or sexual partner.
■ The symptoms don't occur exclusively during the course of schizophrenia or other psychotic disorders and aren't the direct physiologic effect of a general medical condition.

SCHIZOID PERSONALITY DISORDER

■ The person must exhibit a pervasive pattern of indifference to social relationships and a restricted range of emotional experience and expression, beginning by early adulthood and present in various contexts, as indicated by at least four of the following criteria:

– The person neither desires nor enjoys close relationships, including being part of a family.
– The person almost always chooses solitary activities.
– The person seldom, if ever, claims or appears to experience strong emotions, such as anger and joy.
– The person indicates little, if any, desire to have sexual experiences with another person.
– The person is indifferent to the praise and criticism of others.
– The person has no close friends or confidants other than immediate relatives.
– The person displays flat affect.
■ The symptoms don't occur exclusively during the course of schizophrenia, another psychotic disorder, or a pervasive developmental disorder and aren't the direct physiologic effect of a general medical condition.

SCHIZOTYPAL PERSONALITY DISORDER

■ This pervasive pattern of social and interpersonal deficits is marked by acute discomfort with, and reduced capacity for, close relationships as well as by cognitive or perceptual distortions and eccentricities of behavior, beginning by early adulthood and present in various contexts. The person with schizotypal personality disorder has at least five of the following symptoms:
– ideas of reference (excluding delusions of reference)
– odd beliefs or magical thinking influencing behavior and inconsistent with subcultural norms

Diagnosing personality disorders (continued)

– unusual perceptual experiences, including bodily illusions
– odd thinking and speech
– suspiciousness or paranoid thinking
– inappropriate or flat affect
– odd behavior or appearance
– no close friends or confidants other than first-degree relatives
– excessive social anxiety that doesn't diminish with familiarity and tends to be associated with paranoid fears rather than negative self-judgment.
■ The symptoms don't occur exclusively during the course of schizophrenia, a mood disorder with psychotic features, another psychotic disorder, or a pervasive developmental disorder.

ANTISOCIAL PERSONALITY DISORDER
■ This disorder manifests as a pervasive disregard for and violation of the rights of others occurring since age 15, as indicated by at least three of the following criteria:
– The person fails to conform to social norms with respect to lawful behavior, as demonstrated by repeatedly performing acts that are grounds for arrest.
– The person exhibits deceitfulness, as indicated by repeated lying, using aliases, or conning others for personal profit or pleasure.
– The person demonstrates impulsivity or failure to plan ahead.
– The person is irritable and aggressive, as indicated by repeated physical fights or assaults.
– The person has reckless disregard for the safety of self or others.
– The person shows consistent irresponsibility, as indicated by repeated failure to sustain consistent work behavior or honor financial obligations.
– The person lacks remorse, as indicated by being indifferent to or rationalizing

having hurt, mistreated, or stolen from others.
■ The person is at least age 18.
■ The person's history includes evidence of a conduct disorder with onset before age 15.
■ The antisocial behavior doesn't occur exclusively during the course of schizophrenia or a manic episode.

BORDERLINE PERSONALITY DISORDER
This pervasive pattern of instability of interpersonal relationships, self-image and affect, and marked impulsivity, beginning by early adulthood and present in various contexts, is indicated by at least five of the following features:
■ The person makes frantic efforts to avoid real or imagined abandonment (excluding suicidal or self-mutilating behavior).
■ The person has a pattern of unstable and intense interpersonal relationships characterized by alternating extremes of overidealization and devaluation.
■ The person has an identity disturbance characterized by a markedly and persistently unstable self-image or sense of self.
■ The person shows impulsiveness in at least two areas that are potentially self-damaging, such as spending, sexual activity, substance abuse, shoplifting, reckless driving, and binge eating (excluding suicidal or self-mutilating behavior).
■ The person engages in recurrent suicidal threats, gestures, or behavior or in self-mutilating behavior.
■ The person has affective instability resulting from marked mood reactivity (for example, depression, irritability, or anxiety, lasting usually a few hours and seldom more than a few days).

(continued)

Diagnosing personality disorders (continued)

- The person has chronic feelings of emptiness or boredom.
- The person has inappropriate intense anger or difficulty controlling anger.
- The person has transient, stress-related paranoid ideation or severe dissociative symptoms.

HISTRIONIC PERSONALITY DISORDER

This pervasive pattern of excessive emotionality and attention-seeking behavior, beginning by early adulthood and present in various contexts, is indicated by at least four of the following features:
- The person is uncomfortable in situations in which he isn't the center of attention.
- The person's interaction with others is often characterized by inappropriately sexually seductive or provocative behavior.
- The person displays rapidly shifting and shallow expression of emotions.
- The person consistently uses physical appearance to draw attention to self.
- The person has a style of speech that is excessively impressionistic and lacking in detail.
- The person shows self-dramatization, theatricality, and exaggerated emotional expression.
- The person is suggestible (easily influenced by others or circumstances).
- The person considers relationships to be more intimate than they actually are.

NARCISSISTIC PERSONALITY DISORDER

This pervasive pattern of grandiosity, need for admiration, and lack of empathy, beginning by early adulthood and present in various contexts, is indicated by at least five of the following criteria:
- The person has a grandiose sense of self-importance.

- The person is preoccupied with fantasies of unlimited success, power, brilliance, beauty, or ideal love.
- The person believes that he's special and unique and can only be understood by, or should associate with, other special or high-status people (or institutions).
- The person requires excessive admiration.
- The person has a sense of entitlement (an unreasonable expectation of especially favorable treatment or automatic compliance with his expectations).
- The person is interpersonally exploitive, taking advantage of others to achieve his own ends.
- The person lacks empathy.
- The person is often envious of others or believes that others are envious of him.
- The person shows arrogant, haughty behaviors or attitudes.

AVOIDANT PERSONALITY DISORDER

This pervasive pattern of social inhibition, feelings of inadequacy, and hypersensitivity to negative evaluation, beginning by early adulthood and present in a variety of contexts, is indicated by at least four of the following criteria:
- The person avoids social or occupational activities that involve significant interpersonal contact because of fears of criticism, disapproval, or rejection.
- The person is unwilling to get involved with people unless he's certain that they'll like him.
- The person shows restraint within intimate relationships because of the fear of being shamed or ridiculed.
- The person is preoccupied with being criticized or rejected in social situations.

Diagnosing personality disorders (continued)

- The person's feelings of inadequacy inhibit him in new interpersonal situations.
- The person views himself as socially inept, personally unappealing, or inferior to others.
- The person is unusually reluctant to take personal risks or to engage in any new activities because they may prove embarrassing.

DEPENDENT PERSONALITY DISORDER

This pervasive and excessive need to be taken care of that leads to submissive and clinging behavior and fears of separation, beginning by early adulthood and present in a variety of contexts, is indicated by at least five of the following criteria:

- The person has difficulty making everyday decisions without an excessive amount of advice or reassurance from others.
- The person needs others to assume responsibility for most major areas of his life.
- The person has difficulty expressing disagreement with others because of fear of loss of support or approval (excluding realistic fears of retribution).
- The person has difficulty initiating projects or doing things on his own (because of a lack of self-confidence in his judgment or abilities rather than a lack of motivation or energy).
- The person goes to excessive lengths to obtain nurture and support from others, to the point of volunteering to do things that are unpleasant.
- The person feels uncomfortable or helpless when alone because of exaggerated fears of inability to care for himself.
- The person urgently seeks another relationship as a source of care and support when a close relationship ends.

- The person is unrealistically preoccupied with fears of being left to take care of himself.

OBSESSIVE-COMPULSIVE PERSONALITY DISORDER

This pervasive pattern of preoccupation with orderliness, perfectionism, and mental and interpersonal control at the expense of flexibility, openness, and efficiency, beginning by early adulthood and present in a variety of contexts, is indicated by at least four of the following criteria:

- The person is preoccupied with details, rules, lists, order, organization, or schedules to the extent that the core point of the activity is lost.
- The person shows perfectionism that interferes with task completion.
- The person is excessively devoted to work and productivity to the exclusion of leisure activities and friendships (not accounted for by obvious economic need).
- The person exhibits overconscientiousness, scrupulousness, and inflexibility about matters of morality, ethics, or values (not accounted for by cultural or religious identification).
- The person can't discard worn-out or worthless objects even when they have no sentimental value.
- The person is reluctant to delegate tasks or to work with others unless they submit exactly to his way of doing things.
- The person adopts a miserly spending style toward self and others; money is viewed as something to be hoarded in preparation for future catastrophes.
- The person shows rigidity and stubbornness.

• • • • • • • • • • • • •
POSTTRAUMATIC STRESS DISORDER

Characteristic psychological consequences that persist for at least 1 month after a traumatic event outside the range of usual human experience are classified as posttraumatic stress disorder (PTSD). This disorder can follow almost any distressing event, including a natural or man-made disaster, physical or sexual abuse, or an assault or a rape. Psychological trauma, which accompanies the physical trauma, is characterized by intense fear and feelings of helplessness and loss of control. PTSD can be acute, chronic, or delayed. When the precipitating event is of human design, the disorder is more severe and more persistent. Onset can occur at any age, even during childhood.

Causes
PTSD occurs in response to an extremely distressing event, including a serious threat of harm to the patient or his family, such as war, abuse, or violent crime. It may be triggered by sudden destruction of his home or community by a bombing, fire, flood, tornado, earthquake, or similar disaster. It may also follow witnessing the death or serious injury of another person by torture, in a death camp, by natural disaster, or by a motor vehicle or airplane crash.

Preexisting psychopathology can predispose some patients to this disorder, but anyone can develop it, especially if the stressor is extreme.

Any person who has experienced traumatic relocation due to such events as rioting or other civil strife, extreme natural disasters, or war should be assessed for signs of PTSD.

Clinical presentation
The psychosocial history of a patient with PTSD may reveal early life experiences, interpersonal factors, military experiences, or other incidents that suggest the precipitating event. Typically, the patient may report that his symptoms began immediately or soon after the trauma, although they may not develop until months or years later. In such a case, avoidance symptoms have usually been present during the latency period.

Symptoms include:
- pangs of painful emotion and unwelcome thoughts
- intrusive memories
- dissociative episodes (flashbacks)
- a traumatic reexperience of the event
- difficulty falling or staying asleep
- frequent nightmares of the traumatic event
- aggressive outbursts on awakening
- emotional numbing (diminished or constricted response)
- chronic anxiety or panic attacks (with physical signs and symptoms).

The patient may display:
- rage and survivor guilt
- use of violence to solve problems
- depression and suicidal thoughts
- phobic avoidance of situations that arouse memories of the traumatic event (such as hot weather and tall grasses for the Vietnam veteran)
- memory impairment or difficulty concentrating
- feelings of detachment or estrangement that destroy interpersonal relationships.

Some have physical symptoms, fantasies of retaliation, and substance abuse. Children may:
- engage in repetitive play in which aspects of trauma are expressed
- regress to an earlier stage of development.

Differential diagnoses
- Organic brain disorders
- Generalized anxiety disorder
- Phobic disorder
- Depressive disorder
- Panic disorder
- Conversion disorder
- Somatization disorder
- Personality disorders
- Substance abuse

Diagnosis
For characteristic findings in patients with this condition, see *Diagnosing posttraumatic stress disorder,* page 48.

The Minnesota Multiple Personality Inventory can reveal pathologic signs and symptoms affecting the personality. More extensive neuropsychological testing as well as computed tomography scanning, magnetic resonance imaging, EEG, or sleep studies may be required to exclude organic brain syndromes. A psychiatric examination should then be obtained if the diagnosis isn't clear.

Management
General
Treatment of PTSD aims to reduce the target symptoms, prevent chronic disability, and promote occupational and social rehabilitation. Specific treatments may emphasize behavioral techniques (such as relaxation therapy to decrease anxiety and induce sleep or progressive desensitization). Treatment is conducted on an outpatient basis unless the patient is suicidal or unable to perform activities of daily living.

Medication
Selective serotonin reuptake inhibitors may be used and include:
- fluoxetine — 10 to 80 mg/day P.O.
- sertraline — 50 to 200 mg/day P.O.
- paroxetine — 20 to 50 mg/day P.O.

- venlafaxine — 75 to 225 mg/day P.O.
Tricyclic antidepressants and monoamine oxidase inhibitors may also be employed in the treatment of PTSD.

Referral
- The patient should be referred for psychiatric counseling.
- Support groups are highly effective and are provided through many Veterans Administration centers and crisis clinics.
- Rehabilitation programs in physical, social, and occupational settings are available for victims of chronic PTSD.
- Many patients need treatment for depression, alcohol or drug abuse, or medical conditions before psychological healing can take place and should be referred to the appropriate facility.
- Refer the patient to a spiritual counselor as appropriate.

Follow-up
In general, medical follow-up is provided according to the severity of the symptoms. If medications are utilized, you should monitor the patient for tolerance, effectiveness, and adverse effects. During volatile periods and in the early phases of treatment, the patient should attend weekly psychotherapy sessions. Close collaboration with the patient's mental health care provider is necessary. Suicidal ideation merits immediate admission to an inpatient psychiatric facility.

Patient teaching
- Teach the patient about administered medications and their potential adverse effects.
- Teach the patient relaxation techniques that may help during volatile periods.

Complications
- Ongoing social problems
- Substance abuse

Diagnosing posttraumatic stress disorder

The diagnosis of posttraumatic stress disorder is made when the patient's signs and symptoms meet the following criteria documented in the *Diagnostic and Statistical Manual of Mental Disorders,* Fourth Edition.

- The person was exposed to a traumatic event in which both of the following situations occurred:
– The person experienced, witnessed, or was confronted with an event or events that involved actual or threatened death or serious injury or a threat to the physical integrity of self or others.
– The person's response involved intense fear, helplessness, or horror (in children, the response may be expressed by disorganized or agitated behavior).
- The person persistently reexperiences the traumatic event in at least one of the following ways:
– recurrent and intrusive distressing recollections of the event, including images, thoughts, or perceptions
– recurrent distressing dreams of the event
– acting or feeling as if the traumatic event were recurring (includes a sense of reliving the experience, illusions, hallucinations, and dissociative episodes that occur even when awakening or intoxicated)
– intense psychological distress with exposure to internal or external cues that symbolize or resemble an aspect of the traumatic event.
- The person persistently avoids stimuli associated with the traumatic event and experiences numbing of general responsiveness (not present before the traumatic event), as indicated by at least three of the following actions:
– efforts to avoid thoughts or feelings associated with the trauma
– efforts to avoid activities, places, or people that arouse recollections of the trauma
– inability to recall an important aspect of the traumatic event
– markedly diminished interest in significant activities
– feeling of detachment or estrangement from other individuals
– restricted range of affect, such as inability to love others
– sense of foreshortened future.
- The person has persistent symptoms of increased arousal (not present before the trauma), as indicated by at least two of the following actions:
– difficulty falling or staying asleep
– irritability or outbursts of anger
– difficulty concentrating
– hypervigilance
– exaggerated startle response.
- The disturbance must be of at least 1 month's duration.
- The disturbance causes clinically significant distress or impairment in the patient's social, occupational, or other important areas of functioning.

- Flashbacks
- Depression
- Harm to self

Special considerations
- Know and practice crisis intervention techniques as appropriate in PTSD.

- Establish trust by accepting the patient's current level of functioning and assuming a positive, consistent, honest, and nonjudgmental attitude toward the patient.

• • • • • • • • • • • •

PSYCHOACTIVE DRUG ABUSE AND DEPENDENCE

The National Institute on Drug Abuse defines psychoactive drug abuse and dependence as the use of a legal or an illegal drug that causes physical, mental, emotional, or social harm. Examples of abused drugs include narcotics, stimulants, depressants, antianxiety agents, and hallucinogens. Chronic drug abuse, especially I.V. use, can lead to life-threatening complications, such as cardiac and respiratory arrest, intracranial hemorrhage, acquired immunodeficiency syndrome, tetanus, subacute infective endocarditis, hepatitis, vasculitis, septicemia, thrombophlebitis, pulmonary emboli, gangrene, malnutrition and GI disturbances, respiratory infections, musculoskeletal dysfunction, trauma, depression, increased risk of suicide, and psychosis. Materials used to "cut" street drugs also can cause toxic or allergic reactions.

Psychoactive drug abuse can occur at any age. Experimentation with drugs commonly begins in adolescence or even earlier. In many cases, drug abuse leads to addiction, which may involve physical or psychological dependence, or both. The most dangerous form of abuse occurs when users mix several drugs simultaneously — including alcohol.

Causes

Psychoactive drug abuse commonly results from a combination of low self-esteem, peer pressure, inadequate coping skills, and curiosity. Most people who are predisposed to drug abuse have few mental or emotional resources against stress, an overdependence on others, and a low tolerance for frustration. Taking the drug gives them pleasure by relieving tension,

abolishing loneliness, allowing them to achieve a temporarily peaceful or euphoric state, or simply relieving boredom.

Drug dependence may follow experimentation with drugs in response to peer pressure. It may also follow the use of drugs to relieve physical pain, but this is uncommon.

Clinical presentation

The signs and symptoms of acute intoxication vary, depending on the drug. The drug user seldom seeks treatment specifically for his drug problem. Instead, he may seek emergency treatment for drug-related injuries or complications, such as:
- a motor vehicle accident
- burns from freebasing
- an overdose
- physical deterioration from illness or malnutrition
- symptoms of withdrawal.

Friends, family members, or law enforcement officials may bring the patient to a health care facility because of respiratory depression, unconsciousness, acute injury, or a psychiatric crisis. Signs and symptoms of substance may differ (See *Understanding commonly abused substances*, pages 50 to 54.)

The hospitalized drug abuser may be uncooperative, disruptive, or even violent. He may experience:
- mood swings
- anxiety
- impaired memory
- sleep disturbances
- flashbacks
- slurred speech
- depression
- thought disorders.

Some patients resort to plays on sympathy, bribery, or threats to obtain drugs. They may try to manipulate caregivers.

(*Text continues on page 54.*)

Understanding commonly abused substances

SUBSTANCE	SIGNS AND SYMPTOMS	IMMEDIATE INTERVENTIONS
Stimulants		

Cocaine
- *Street names:* coke, flake, snow, nose candy, hits, gold dust, toot, crack (hardened form), rock, crank
- *Routes:* ingestion, injection, sniffing, smoking
- *Dependence:* psychological
- *Duration of effect:* 15 minutes to 2 hours; with crack, rapid high of short duration followed by down feeling
- *Medical uses:* local anesthetic

- *Of use:* abdominal pain; alternating euphoria and fear; anorexia; cardiotoxicity, such as ventricular fibrillation or cardiac arrest; coma; confusion; diaphoresis; dilated pupils; excitability; fever; grandiosity; hyperpnea; hypotension or hypertension; insomnia; irritability; nausea and vomiting; pallor or cyanosis; perforated nasal septum with prolonged use; pressured speech; psychotic behavior with large doses; respiratory arrest; seizures; spasms; tachycardia; tachypnea; visual, auditory, and olfactory hallucinations; weight loss
- *Of withdrawal:* anxiety, depression, fatigue

For acute intoxification:
- If drug was ingested, induce vomiting or perform gastric lavage; follow with activated charcoal and saline cathartic.
- If drug was inhaled, remove residual drug from mucus membranes, if present.
- Give propranolol for tachycardia.
- Give anticonvulsants for seizures.
- Give lidocaine for ventricular arrhythmias.

Amphetamines
- *Street names:* for amphetamine sulfate — bennies, cartwheels, greenies; for methamphetamine — speed, meth, crystal; for dextroamphetamine sulfate — dexies, hearts, oranges
- *Routes:* ingestion, injection
- *Dependence:* psychological
- *Duration of effect:* 1 to 4 hours
- *Medical uses:* hyperkinesis, narcolepsy, weight control

- *Of use:* altered mental status (from confusion to paranoia), coma, diaphoresis, dilated reactive pupils, dry mouth, exhaustion, hallucinations, hyperactive deep tendon reflexes, hypertension, hyperthermia, paradoxical reaction in children, psychotic behavior with prolonged use, seizures, shallow respirations, tachycardia, tremors
- *Of withdrawal:* abdominal tenderness, apathy, depression, disorientation, irritability, long periods of sleep, muscle aches, suicide (with sudden withdrawal)

For acute intoxification:
- If drug was ingested, induce vomiting or perform gastric lavage; give activated charcoal and saline or magnesium sulfate cathartic.
- Add ammonium chloride or ascorbic acid to I.V. solution to acidify urine to pH of 5. Also, administer mannitol to induce diuresis.
- Give short-acting barbiturate such as pentobarbital for seizures; haloperidol for assaultive behavior; phentolamine for hypertension; propranolol for tachyarrhythmias; lidocaine for ventricular arrhythmias.
- Institute suicide precautions.

Understanding commonly abused substances *(continued)*

SUBSTANCE	SIGNS AND SYMPTOMS	IMMEDIATE INTERVENTIONS

Hallucinogens

Lysergic acid diethylamide (LSD)
- *Street names:* acid, blue dots, cube, D, owsleys, gel tabs, microdot
- *Routes:* ingestion, smoking
- *Dependence:* possibly psychological
- *Duration of effect:* 8 to 12 hours
- *Medical uses:* none

- *Of use:* abdominal cramps, arrhythmias, chills, depersonalization, diaphoresis, diarrhea, distorted visual perception and perception of time and space, dizziness, dry mouth, fever, grandiosity, hallucinations, heightened sense of awareness, hyperpnea, hypertension, illusions, increased salivation, muscle aches, mystical experiences, nausea, palpitations, seizures, tachycardia, vomiting
- *Of withdrawal:* none

For acute intoxification:
- If drug was ingested, induce vomiting or perform gastric lavage. Follow with activated charcoal and cathartic.
- Give diazepam for seizures.

Phencyclidine
- *Street names:* PCP, hog, angel dust, peace pill, dummy mist, aurora, bust bee, guerrilla, rocket fuel
- *Routes:* ingestion, injection, smoking
- *Dependence:* possibly psychological
- *Duration of effect:* 30 minutes to several days
- *Medical uses:* veterinary anesthetic

- *Of use:* amnesia; blank stare; cardiac arrest; decreased awareness of surroundings; delusions; distorted body image; distorted sense of sight, hearing, and touch; drooling; euphoria; excitation and psychoses; fever; gait ataxia; hallucinations; hyperactivity; hypertensive crisis; individualized unpredictable effects; muscle rigidity; nystagmus; panic; poor perception of time and distance; possible chromosomal damage; psychotic behavior; recurrent coma; renal failure; seizures; sudden behavioral changes; tachycardia; violent behavior
- *Of withdrawal:* none

For acute intoxification:
- If drug was ingested, induce vomiting or perform gastric lavage. Follow with activated charcoal.
- Add ascorbic acid to I.V. solution to acidify urine.
- Give diuretic; propranolol for hypertension or tachycardia; nitroprusside for severe hypertensive crisis; diazepam for seizures; diazepam or haloperidol for agitation or psychotic behavior; physostigmine salicylate, diazepam, chlordiazepoxide, or chlorpromazine for "bad trip."

(continued)

Understanding commonly abused substances *(continued)*

SUBSTANCE	SIGNS AND SYMPTOMS	IMMEDIATE INTERVENTIONS

Depressants

Alcohol

- *Found in:* beer, wine, distilled spirits; also in cough syrup, aftershave, mouthwash
- *Route:* ingestion
- *Dependence:* physical, psychological
- *Duration of effect:* varies with individual and amount ingested; metabolized at rate of 10 ml/hour
- *Medical uses:* neurolysis (absolute alcohol); emergency tocolytic; treatment of ethylene glycol and methanol poisoning

- *Of acute use:* coma, decreased inhibitions, euphoria followed by depression or hostility, impaired judgment, incoordination, respiratory depression, slurred speech, unconsciousness, vomiting
- *Of withdrawal:* delirium, hallucinations, seizures, tremors

For acute intoxification:
- If alcohol was ingested within 4 hours, induce vomiting or perform gastric lavage; give activated charcoal and a saline cathartic.
- Give diazepam for seizures; chlordiazepoxide, chloral hydrate, or paraldehyde for hallucinations and delirium.
- Give I.V. fluid replacement and dextrose, thiamine, B-complex vitamins, and vitamin C to treat dehydration, hypoglycemia, nutritional deficiencies.
- Assess for aspiration pneumonia.
- Consider dialysis if vital functions are severely depressed.

Benzodiazepines

(alprazolam, chlordiazepoxide, clonazepam, clorazepate, diazepam, flurazepam, halazepam, lorazepam, midazolam, oxazepam, prazepam, quazepam, temazepam, triazolam)
- *Street names:* dolls, yellow jackets
- *Routes:* ingestion, injection
- *Dependence:* physical, psychological
- *Duration of effect:* 4 to 8 hours
- *Medical uses:* antianxiety agent, anticonvulsant, sedative, hypnotic

- *Of use:* ataxia, drowsiness, hypotension, increased self-confidence, relaxation, slurred speech
- *Of overdose:* confusion, coma, drowsiness, respiratory depression
- *Of withdrawal:* abdominal cramps, agitation, anxiety, diaphoresis, hypertension, tachycardia, tonic-clonic seizures, tremors, vomiting

For acute intoxification:
- If drug was ingested, induce vomiting or perform gastric lavage. Follow with activated charcoal and cathartic.
- Give supplemental oxygen for hypoxia-induced seizures.
- Give I.V. fluids for hypertension and physostigmine salicylate for respiratory or central nervous system (CNS) depression.

Understanding commonly abused substances *(continued)*

SUBSTANCE	SIGNS AND SYMPTOMS	IMMEDIATE INTERVENTIONS

Depressants *(continued)*

Barbiturates

(amobarbital, phenobarbital, secobarbital)
- *Street names:* for barbiturates — barbs, downers; for amobarbital — blue angels, blue devils; for phenobarbital — goofballs, purple hearts; for secobarbital — reds, red devils
- *Routes:* ingestion, injection
- *Dependence:* physical, psychological
- *Duration:* 1 to 16 hours
- *Medical uses:* anesthetic, anticonvulsant, sedative, hypnotic

- *Of use:* absent reflexes, blisters or bullous lesions, cyanosis, depressed level of consciousness (from confusion to coma), fever, flaccid muscles, hypotension, hypothermia, nystagmus, paradoxical reaction in children and elderly people, poor pupil reaction to light, respiratory depression
- *Of withdrawal:* agitation, anxiety, fever, insomnia, orthostatic hypotension, tachycardia, tremors
- *Of rapid withdrawal:* anorexia, apprehension, hallucinations, orthostatic hypotension, tonic-clonic seizures, tremors, weakness

For acute intoxification:
- If ingestion was recent, induce vomiting or perform gastric lavage. Follow with activated charcoal.
- Give I.V. fluid bolus for hypotension and alkalinize urine.
- Relieve withdrawal symptoms as appropriate.
- Use hypothermia or hyperthermia blanket for temperature alterations.

Opiates

(codeine, heroin, morphine, meperidine, and opium)
- *Street names:* for heroin — junk, horse, H, smack, Chinese white, Mexican mud; for morphine — morph, M, microdots
- *Routes:* for codeine, meperidine, and morphine — ingestion, injection, smoking; for heroin — ingestion, injection, inhalation, smoking; for opium — ingestion, smoking
- *Dependence:* physical, psychological
- *Duration of effect:* 3 to 6 hours
- *Medical uses:* for codeine — analgesia, antitussive; for heroin — none; for morphine and meperidine — analgesia; for opium — analgesia, antidiarrheal

- *Of use:* anorexia, arrhythmias, clammy skin, constipation, constricted pupils, decreased level of consciousness, detachment from reality, drowsiness, euphoria, hypotension, impaired judgment, increased pigmentation over veins, lack of concern, lethargy, nausea, needle marks, respiratory depression, seizures, skin lesions or abscesses, slurred speech, swollen or perforated nasal mucosa, thrombotic veins, urine retention, vomiting
- *Of withdrawal:* abdominal cramps, anorexia, chills, diaphoresis, dilated pupils, hyperactive bowel sounds, irritability, nausea, panic, piloerection, runny nose, sweating, tremors, watery eyes, yawning

For acute intoxification:
- If drug was ingested, induce vomiting or perform gastric lavage.
- Give naloxone until CNS effects are reversed.
- Give I.V. fluids to increase circulatory volume.
- Use extra blankets for hypothermia; if ineffective, use hyperthermia blanket.
- Assess pulmonary edema.
- Assess signs and symptoms of withdrawal.

(continued)

Understanding commonly abused substances *(continued)*

SUBSTANCE	SIGNS AND SYMPTOMS	IMMEDIATE INTERVENTIONS
Cannabinoids		

Marijuana
- *Street names:* pot, grass, weed, Mary Jane, roach, reefer, joint, muggles, Acapulco gold, Texas tea, Yesca, hemp
- *Routes:* ingestion, smoking
- *Dependence:* psychological
- *Duration of effect:* 2 to 3 hours
- *Medical uses:* antiemetic for chemotherapy

- *Of use:* acute psychosis; agitation; amotivational syndrome; anxiety; asthma; bronchitis; conjunctival reddening; decreased muscle strength; delusions; distorted sense of time and self-perception; dry mouth; euphoria; hallucinations; impaired cognition, short-term memory, and mood; incoordination; increased hunger; increased systolic pressure when in supine position; orthostatic hypotension; paranoia; spontaneous laughter; tachycardia; vivid visual imagery
- *Of withdrawal:* chills, decreased appetite, increased rapid-eye-movement sleep, insomnia, irritability, nervousness, restlessness, tremors, weight loss

For acute intoxification:
- Give supplemental oxygen for respiratory depression and I.V. fluids for hypotension.
- Give diazepam for extreme agitation and acute psychosis.

Psychoactive substances may be used in cultural practices. For instance, some Native Americans use hallucinatory drugs to help achieve spiritual experiences. Therefore, use and abuse must be carefully distinguished.

Differential diagnoses
- Hypoxia
- Hypothyroidism, hyperthyroidism
- Hypoglycemia
- Delirium
- Syphilis
- Thiamine deficiency
- Other altered mental states

Diagnosis
For characteristic findings in patients with this condition, see *Diagnosing substance dependence and related disorders*, page 10. Various tests can confirm drug use, determine the amount and type of drug taken, and reveal complications. For example, a serum or urine drug screen can detect recently ingested substances.

Characteristic findings in other tests include:
- elevated serum globulin levels
- decreased blood glucose levels
- leukocytosis
- abnormal liver function studies
- positive rapid plasma reagin test due to elevated protein fractions

- elevated mean corpuscular hemoglobin levels
- elevated uric acid levels
- decreased blood urea nitrogen levels.

Management
General
The patient with acute drug intoxication should receive symptomatic treatment based on the drug ingested. Measures include supporting respirations, fluid replacement therapy, and nutritional and vitamin supplements. Additional treatments may include gastric lavage, induced emesis, administration of medication and, possibly, hemoperfusion or hemodialysis. If physical signs of withdrawal occur or are known by history, detoxification with the same drug or a pharmacologically similar drug must be initiated and tapered over an appropriate amount of time. Exceptions include cocaine and hallucinogens, which aren't used for detoxification. Marijuana has no dangerous physical withdrawal.

Treatment of drug dependence commonly involves a triad of care: detoxification, short- and long-term rehabilitation, and aftercare. The latter means a lifetime of abstinence, usually aided by participation in Narcotics Anonymous or a similar self-help group.

Medication
Sedatives (except those that are addicting) may be administered to induce sleep. For example, diphenhydramine 25 to 100 mg P.O. h.s.

Common drugs that are used to treat overdoses of drugs include:
- naloxone hydrochloride — 0.4 to 2 mg I.V. repeated every 2 minutes up to 10 mg until desired response is achieved for an opiate overdose
- flumazenil — 0.2 mg I.V. over 30 seconds, followed by 0.3 mg over 30 seconds; if response is inadequate, 0.5 mg

I.V. over 30 seconds, then repeat over 1-minute intervals to maximum of 3 mg for benzodiazepine overdose
- activated charcoal — 1 to 2 g/kg P.O. or 10 times the amount of medication ingested as a suspension in 120 to 240 ml of water.

Detoxification, the controlled and gradual withdrawal of an abused drug, is achieved through substitution of a drug with similar action. Such gradual replacement of the abused drug controls the effects of withdrawal, thereby reducing the patient's discomfort and associated risks.

Opioid withdrawal causes severe physical discomfort but isn't usually life-threatening. To minimize these effects, chronic opioid abusers commonly are detoxified with small doses of methadone (20 to 120 mg/day P.O., [highly individualized] decreased by 5 mg/day over a 5- to 7-day period).

Referral
- The patient should be referred to an appropriate rehabilitation facility for drug withdrawal.
- Support groups, such as Narcotics Anonymous, may be beneficial in maintaining drug-free status.
- In a suspected overdose, immediately refer the patient to the hospital.

Patient teaching
- Educate the patient and his family about drug abuse and dependence.
- Teach the patient about withdrawal medications and the importance of following the prescribed regimen.

Complications
- Hepatitis
- HIV
- Tuberculosis
- Abscesses
- Pneumonia

- Malnutrition
- Social dysfunction
- Harm to self
- Overdose

Special considerations

- Emphasize the importance of using a condom during sexual intercourse to prevent disease transmission and pregnancy. If necessary, teach the female drug abuser about other methods of birth control. Explain the devastating effects of drugs on the developing fetus.

• • • • • • • • • • • •
VIOLENCE, DOMESTIC

Domestic violence refers to the intentional infliction of physical, verbal, emotional, or sexual abuse by one party in a relationship upon another. This relationship is usually a family unit, but abuse can also occur between dating couples, same-sex partners, and paid or informal caregivers and their charges. In the case of elder abuse, domestic violence can also take the form of financial exploitation, neglect, unreasonable confinement, or deprivation of needed services. In addition to nonaccidental physical or mental injuries, child abuse involves parental failure to provide for basic necessities or lack of supervision or care. People who abuse others come from all socioeconomic levels, racial and ethnic groups, and religions.

Spouses, disabled persons, and elderly parents or relatives are the most common victims of adult abuse. It's estimated that 2 million adults over age 60 are abused annually; for every reported incident, about five go unreported. Elderly females and those having mental impairments are more likely to be victims of domestic violence. Among younger women,

30% of those seen in the emergency department have injuries inflicted as a result of domestic violence and 50% of all female deaths occur at the hands of their male partners. No reliable data exists detailing domestic violence against heterosexual men or homosexual couples, but it's known to occur. Among children, approximately 1.5 million cases of neglect and 600,000 cases of physical abuse are reported annually; of these, 1,000 end in death. Approximately 30% of females and 20% of males report that they had been sexually assaulted by age 18.

Causes and pathophysiology
The abuser
No specific psychiatric diagnosis encompasses the abuser's personality or behavior. However, many abusers have a history of being abused when young or having witnessed abuse of parents and siblings. In many cases, abusive persons lack self-esteem and the security of being loved, qualities that help nonabusive persons cope with stress. In times of crisis, abusers resort to the behavior they learned in childhood. They abuse as they were abused, in an attempt to restore their own feelings of self-control and self-esteem. Abusers are usually unable to tolerate personal failure or disapproval from spouses, children, or friends, and they commonly have unrealistic expectations of the people they abuse. When an individual fails to live up to those expectations, the abuser feels a compulsion to control, mortify, reject, and physically injure that individual. Parental child abusers may view children as extensions of persons they hate and abuse them accordingly.

CLINICAL CAUTION While alcohol and drug dependency haven't been shown to cause abusers to abuse, they're frequently implicated in instances of abusive activity.

Low self-esteem may prompt an abuser to choose a partner much like himself. Each will then feed into the other's form of abuse. If the couple has children, in many cases they become targets of their parents' abusive behavior. What the children witness and suffer often begins another cycle of abused child to child abuser or abused child to abused adult.

The abused

In cases of partner abuse, the abused spouse suffers from low self-esteem. The abused spouse's parents may have abused each other, or one parent may have abused the other. Having witnessed these attacks as a child, the present-day abused spouse accepts that she too will be abused. By behaving passively, spouses make it easy for their partners to abuse them repeatedly without fear of retaliation.

Children with behavior problems are particularly vulnerable to abuse, as are malformed or developmentally disabled children and children born prematurely or to unmarried parents. Like children, adults can become abuse victims if they're viewed as too dependent, too sickly, or too much like a hated person. Ill or elderly persons who make financial, emotional, or personal demands in many cases end up injured when the stress they create becomes intolerable for their abusers.

Abused men in most cases show the same low self-esteem and passivity as abused women. Sometimes an abused man is the less aggressive and more subservient member of the relationship and accepts a certain level of abuse in the hope that it won't get worse. At other times, he may be so ashamed by his inability to provide adequately that he invites abuse to give himself a feeling of atonement.

Clinical presentation
Child abuse

Physical indicators include:
- skin markings, such as lacerations, burns, contusions, bites, finger compression points, ecchymosis in various stages of healing, welts, or bald spots
- unexplained or inadequately explained fractures, especially if in various stages of healing
- injuries present under areas normally covered by clothing
- retinal hemorrhages, especially in infants
- oral trauma, particularly loose teeth
- abdominal blunt trauma
- vague physical complaints such as abdominal pain
- bruises, bleeding, or unexplained injury of external genitalia
- hymenal lacerations or asymmetry
- presence of sexually transmitted diseases
- pregnancy
- perianal lacerations or circumferential edema.

There may also be no apparent physical signs, especially in cases of sexual abuse, because abuse involving fondling or other contact leaves no detectable injury.

Behavioral indicators include:
- withdrawn demeanor
- extreme concern for siblings' health or safety
- school problems, especially if sudden
- self-destructive behaviors such as substance abuse
- isolation
- behavior regression such as thumb-sucking
- anxiety or depression

- sleep disturbances or nightmares
- sexual acting out or promiscuity
- running away from home
- wearing clothing to cover injuries.

Indicators of other abuse such as neglect include:
- abnormal growth and developmental patterns
- poor hygiene, inappropriate dress
- failure to thrive, poor nutritional status
- unmet medical needs
- fear or clinging
- avoidance of parents
- too much trusting.

Partner abuse
Physical indicators include:
- injuries of various types, such as bites, burns, lacerations, contusions, or fractures
- vague complaints, such as of chronic pain, headaches, or sleep disturbances
- blunt trauma to abdomen
- Battle's sign or "raccoon eyes"
- patchy hair loss
- discrepancy between injury and explanation
- blood behind tympanic membranes.

Behavioral indicators include:
- stress-related conditions, such as anxiety, depression, or suicidal ideation
- substance abuse
- fearfulness
- long interval between injury and seeking medical intervention.

Elder abuse
Physical indicators are the same as for partner abuse with the addition of:
- oddly, distinctly shaped injuries
- injuries to external genitalia
- sexually transmitted diseases
- failure to thrive, poor nutritional status, or dehydration
- pressure sores

- injuries that aren't congruent with explanations.

Behavioral indicators include:
- lethargy or listlessness (may be due to overmedication)
- withdrawal or fearful affect
- anxiety or depression
- sleep disorders
- decreased appetite.

Indicators of other abuse such as neglect include:
- unmet medical needs, such as for eyeglasses or dentures
- poor hygiene
- inappropriate dress.

Differential diagnoses
Differential diagnoses for abuse must rule out pathologic etiologies, although suspected cases of abuse should never go unreported.

Child abuse
Physical
- Accidental trauma such as falls
- Bleeding disorders, such as hemophilia, vitamin K deficiency, platelet aggregation disorders, or disseminated intravascular coagulation
- Congenital disorders
- Other origins of cutaneous manifestations, such as Mongolian spots, erythema multiforme, Schönlein-Henoch purpura, phytophotodermatitis, staphylococcal scalded skin syndrome, congenital syphilis, hypersensitivity vasculitis, purpura fulminans of meningococcemia, osteogenesis imperfecta
- Obstetric trauma

Neglect
- Endocrine disorders such as diabetes, thyroid disorders, or adrenal or pituitary disorders
- Cystic fibrosis
- Liver disorders

- Renal disorders
- Central nervous system (CNS) disorders such as fetal alcohol syndrome or accidental poisoning
- Nutritional or metabolic disorders, such as scurvy or rickets
- GI disorders, such as inflammatory bowel disease, reflux, or celiac disease
- Prematurity
- Leukemia
- Metastatic neuroblastoma
- Histiocytosis X
- Infantile cortical hyperostosis

Elder and partner abuse
- Accidental injury
- Self-inflicted injury
- Self-neglect secondary to mental or physical impairments
- Poor hygiene or inappropriate clothing because of poverty

Diagnosis
In all cases of suspected abuse, diagnostic testing is based upon clinical indicators as well as the patient history. In general, such standard laboratory tests as urinalysis, complete blood count, and electrolyte, blood urea nitrogen, creatinine, and glucose levels are routinely obtained. Suspected bleeding disorders warrant evaluation of prothrombin time, partial thromboplastin time, platelet count factor XIII, and bleeding time. Toxicology screens are appropriate in patients with CNS manifestations.

Imaging studies—particularly X-rays—should be obtained as the patient's symptoms dictate. Some health care facilities employ a standard series of X-rays in cases of suspected nonaccidental trauma. Fractures in various stages of healing, spiral fractures in nonambulatory patients, chip or "bucket-handle" fractures, and rib fractures, especially in infants, highly suggest abuse. In some cases,

a bone scan may provide additional information. Photographs of injuries should be obtained in all suspected cases of abuse to meet legal requirements.

Patients with suspected sexual abuse should be examined only by a health care provider who is highly trained and experienced in obtaining forensic specimens in order to maintain the chain of evidence necessary for legal proceedings. A wet mount for motile sperm and an acid phosphatase test of secretions for sperm should be obtained during the pelvic examination. The presence of sperm in a child is diagnostic for sexual abuse. Serum pregnancy, syphilis, gonorrhea, chlamydia, and human immunodeficiency virus tests should also be obtained.

In cases of suspected neglect, a calorie count and stool examination are appropriate. Other tests and special studies, depending on what type of injury was found, may be helpful in ruling out the physical causes of presenting symptoms.

While the physical examination is important, the patient's history is equally important, particularly in suspected cases of abuse. A thorough social history frequently gives clues that narrow the differential diagnosis list. The approach in identifying abuse varies based on age.

Child abuse
In cases of child abuse, parents should be questioned regarding child-rearing difficulties, discipline practices, family stressors, and safety in and out of the home (including previous trauma or ingestions). Additionally, parents should be asked about difficulties with toilet training (in the older child, enuresis or encopresis), feeding, and behavior (especially if the onset is recent). Questions regarding the perinatal period may also provide relevant clues. If possible, children should be interviewed without the par-

ents present. The interviewer should inquire whether the child is afraid of anyone, if anyone has attempted to hurt her, and if anyone has ever told her to keep activities secret. Affirmative responses require more detailed information. When, where, how, and who did what questions should then be asked by the interviewer. An anatomically correct doll may help the child to express herself. Red flags of abuse include a long interval between the injury and seeking help; inconsistent or contradictory stories; or explanations that don't adequately correlate with the presenting signs and symptoms.

Elder abuse

In cases of elder abuse or neglect, the social history should elicit information regarding the patient's caregivers, living arrangements, and family functioning. Questions should focus attention on stressors within the family unit; feelings of safety with caregivers and family members; and perceived threats to safety. If any questions are answered affirmatively, further attempts should be made to elicit information regarding the patient's support network (other family members, friends), whether the patient has attempted to notify others in the support network of the situation and if help could be expected, and if the patient has a safe place to go in an emergency. If the patient is willing to discuss mistreatment, the interviewer should inquire as to the perpetrator, when and how the abuse occurs, and the patient's means of coping. Inappropriate behavior should prompt inquiry as to whether caregivers make the patient do things he doesn't want to do willingly, if he's denied assistance when it's needed, or if he's left alone inappropriately or for prolonged periods of time. Again, affirmative responses require further investigation. It's important for

the interviewer to determine if the patient is able to provide reliable information because cognitive impairment may require the assistance of other sources for an accurate history.

Partner abuse

Suspected partner abuse tends to be more difficult to diagnose because the victims are predominately female, usually have children, and perceive themselves as being dependent on their partners. The social history should elicit information regarding current living arrangements and significant relationships. Stressors within the relationship and methods of handling disagreements should be discussed. Additionally, the patient should be questioned regarding her feelings of safety, whether or not there have been threats or incidents of abuse in the past, and if unwanted sexual acts have been forced on her. Any positive responses require further inquiry as to how and when the abuse occurs, who inflicts it, how the patient deals with it, and how she plans to protect herself (and her children) from future episodes. Additionally, the patient should be asked if friends or family members are aware of the abuse and whether or not she can expect help from them. Female victims of abuse are frequently reluctant to disclose their abuse. Red flags include a long interval between the incident and seeking help; a contradictory, inconsistent, or changing story; or injuries that are inconsistent with the explanation. Females tend to blame injuries on household accidents such as falls.

Management
General

Treatment for an abuse victim focuses on treating the physical injuries, psychological dysfunction, and safety of the abused individual. In the case of elder and child abuse, the goals of treatment are to provide protection from continuing harm, to identify risk factors for abuse or neglect and determine the best method of dealing with them, and to comply with statutory requirements. All cases of suspected elder and child abuse must be reported to state adult and child protection agencies. Incidents of abuse or neglect don't need to be confirmed; health care providers are protected from liability in reporting their suspicions in good faith. Thorough documentation is key because the patient's chart will be used during legal proceedings. If protective service agencies determine that the child or elder isn't in immediate harm, the victim most likely will remain in his home environment and supportive services will be implemented.

In the case of partner abuse, competent adults may refuse to take legal action or to leave their living situation. In some cases, this may not be practical.

Referral
There is no legal requirement for health care providers to report suspected cases of partner abuse to protective agencies as long as the adult is competent and no injuries were inflicted by weapons. In such cases, referral to appropriate community resources is appropriate.

Follow-up
In the case of child or elder abuse, frequent follow-up appointments should be scheduled to screen for abuse. For partner abuse, follow-up consists of monitoring physical injuries accordingly, maintaining confidentiality, and encouraging involvement in support groups.

Patient teaching
- Stress to the patient the need to seek outside assistance to cope with the domestic situation.

- Teach the patient about alternative resources if needed.

Complications
- Death
- Traumatic injury
- Depression
- Social impairment

Special considerations
- Most child victims of sexual abuse have no detectable genital injury.
- Female victims of partner abuse may experience new or escalating incidents of battering during pregnancy.
- Abdominal injuries caused by blunt trauma may leave no visible signs.
- Serious intracranial injuries may not be immediately evident.
- Accidental injuries usually manifest on extensor surfaces.
- Domestic violence victims may need treatment for depression or substance abuse.
- Victims of partner abuse who leave their abusers are more likely to suffer fatal injuries.

•••••••••••
SELECTED REFERENCES

Copel, L.C. *Nurse's Clinical Guide: Psychiatric and Mental Health Care.* 2nd ed. Springhouse, Pa.: Springhouse Corp., 2000.

Diagnostic and Statistical Manual of Mental Disorders, 4th ed. Washington, D.C.: American Psychiatric Association, 1994.

Greinenko, A. "Rapid Screening for Disordered Eating in College-Aged Females in the Primary Care Setting," *Journal of Adolescent Health* 26(5):338-42, 2000.

Isaacs, A. *Lippincott's Review Series: Mental Health and Psychiatric Nursing.* Philadelphia: Lippincott Williams & Wilkins, 2000.

Ketner, K. "Identifying the Adolescent at Risk." In: *Summary of 23rd Annual California Coalition of Nurse Practitioners Educational Conference.* Santa Rosa, Calif.: California Coalition of Nurse Practitioners, 2000.

Pomerantz, J. "Managed Care and Suicide Prevention," *Drug Benefit Trends* 12(6):5-6, 2000.

Stuart, G. and Laraia, M. *Principles and Practice of Psychiatric Nursing,* 7th ed., St. Louis: Mosby–Year Book, Inc., 2001.

Townsend, M.C. *Psychiatric Mental Health Nursing: Concepts of Care,* 3rd ed., Philadelphia: F.A. Davis Co., 1999.

Cardiovascular disorders

In North America, more than 70 million people suffer from some form of cardiovascular disorder, and many of them suffer from a combination of disorders. Year after year, the number of affected patients continues to rise.

This chapter will help you to provide effective care for these patients, promote recovery, improve patient compliance, and ensure adequate home care.

• • • • • • • • • • • •
ASSESSMENT

Performed correctly, assessment helps to identify and evaluate changes in the patient's cardiac function — changes that may disrupt or threaten his life. Baseline information obtained during assessment can be used to guide your intervention and follow-up care. (See *Key questions for assessing cardiac function*, page 64.)

Note, however, that if your patient is in a cardiac crisis, you must quickly rethink your assessment priorities. The patient's condition and the clinical situation dictate the steps you need to take.

See the section on cardiac emergencies at the end of this chapter.

Inspection
Inspect the patient's chest and thorax. Expose the anterior chest and observe its general appearance. Normally, the lateral diameter is twice the anteroposterior diameter. Note deviations from typical chest shape.

Checking for jugular vein distention
When the patient is in a supine position, the neck veins normally protrude; when the patient stands, they normally lie flat. To check for jugular vein distention, place the patient in semi-Fowler's position with the head turned slightly away from the side being examined. Use tangential lighting (side lighting) to cast small shadows along the neck. This allows you to see pulse wave movement better. If jugular veins appear distended, it indicates high right atrial pressure and an increase in fluid volume caused by right heart dysfunction.

Characterize distention as mild, moderate, or severe. Determine the level of distention in fingerbreadths above the

Key questions for assessing cardiac function

Ask these questions to help the patient more accurately describe the symptoms of cardiovascular illness:
- Can you point to the site of your pain?
- Do you get a burning or squeezing sensation in your chest?
- What relieves the pain?
- Do you ever feel short of breath? Does a particular body position seem to bring this on? Which one? How long does any shortness of breath last? What relieves it?
- Has sudden breathing trouble ever woken you up?
- Do you ever wake up coughing? How often?
- Have you ever coughed up blood?
- Does your heart ever pound or skip a beat? If so, when does this happen?
- Do you ever get dizzy or faint? What brings this on?
- Do your feet or ankles swell? At what time of day? Does anything relieve the swelling?
- Do you urinate more frequently at night?
- Do any activities tire you? Which ones? Have you had to limit your activities or rest more often while doing them?

Inspecting the precordium

Place the patient in a supine position with the head flat or elevated as needed for respiratory comfort. Stand to the right of the patient. Then identify the necessary anatomic landmarks. (See *Inspecting and palpating the precordium*, page 66.)

Using tangential lighting to cast shadows across the chest, watch for chest wall movement, visible pulsations, and exaggerated lifts or heaves (strong outward thrusts palpated over the chest during systole) in all areas of the precordium.

Normally, pulsations are seen at the point of maximal impulse (PMI) of the apical impulse. The apical impulse (pulsations at the apex of the heart) normally appears in the fifth intercostal space at or just medial to the midclavicular line. This impulse reflects the location and size of the heart, especially of the left ventricle.

Palpation

Palpate the peripheral pulses and precordium. Remember to warm your hands and to use gentle to moderate pressure.

Palpating pulses

Palpate the carotid, brachial, radial, femoral, popliteal, dorsalis pedis, and posterior tibial pulses. These arteries are close to the body surface, making palpation easier. Press gently over the pulse sites; excess pressure can obliterate the pulsation, making the pulse appear absent. Also, palpate only one carotid artery at a time; simultaneous palpation can slow the pulse or decrease blood pressure, causing the patient to faint.

Look for these signs:
- pulse rate — this varies with age and other factors; in adults, it usually ranges from 60 to 100 beats/minute
- pulse rhythm — should be regular

clavicle or in relation to the jaw or clavicle. Also, note the amount of distention in relation to head elevation.

You can use jugular vein distention to obtain a rough estimate of central venous pressure. In addition, observing pulsations of the right internal jugular vein helps you to assess right heart dynamics. (See *Assessing jugular venous pulse*.)

Assessing jugular venous pulse

Inspecting the right jugular venous pulse can provide information about the dynamics of the right side of the heart. The jugular venous pulse consists of five waves: three positive, or ascending, waves (*a*, *c*, and *v*) and two negative, or descending, waves (*x* and *y*).

The following pulsations of the positive waves occur ⅜″ to ¾″ (1 to 2 cm) above the clavicle, just medial to the sternocleidomastoid muscle. Use the carotid pulse or heart sounds to time venous pulsations with the cardiac cycle:

■ The *a* wave marks the initial pulsation of the jugular vein. Occurring just before the first heart sound, it results from right atrial contraction and transmission of pressure to the jugular veins.

■ The c wave occurs shortly after the first heart sound. It results from the tricuspid valve's closing at the beginning of ventricular systole.

■ The *v* wave peaks during ventricular contraction as the tricuspid valve bulges into the right atrium.

Although the negative waves aren't visible as pulsations, they help define the ascending pulses and are shown when the jugular venous pulse is recorded as a waveform. The negative waves occur as follows:

■ The *x* descent follows the *a* and *c* waves. It results from right atrial relaxation, ventricular filling, and falling right atrial pressure.

■ The *y* descent reflects the drop in right atrial pressure from the *v* wave peak that occurs with ventricular systole and the opening of the tricuspid valve.

IMPLICATIONS

Abnormal jugular vein pulsations may signal an arrhythmia. For example, an exaggerated *a* wave may indicate pulmonic or tricuspid stenosis — conditions that elevate right atrial pressure. A giant *a* wave, or cannon wave, may signal serious conduction defects. A giant *v* wave may indicate tricuspid valve insufficiency with regurgitant blood flow.

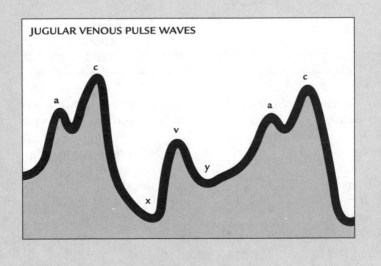

JUGULAR VENOUS PULSE WAVES

Inspecting and palpating the precordium

Use these guidelines when inspecting and palpating the precordium:

■ Locate the six precordial areas by using the anatomic landmarks named for the underlying structures.

■ Palpate (or inspect) the sternoclavicular area, which lies at the top of the sternum at the junction of the clavicles.

■ Move to the aortic area, located in the second intercostal space on the right sternal border.

■ Assess the pulmonic area, found in the second intercostal space on the left sternal border.

■ Palpate the right ventricular area, the point where the fifth rib joins the left sternal border.

■ Then assess the left ventricular area (apical area), which falls at the fifth intercostal space at the midclavicular line.

■ Finally, palpate the epigastric area at the base of the sternum between the cartilage of the left and right seventh ribs.

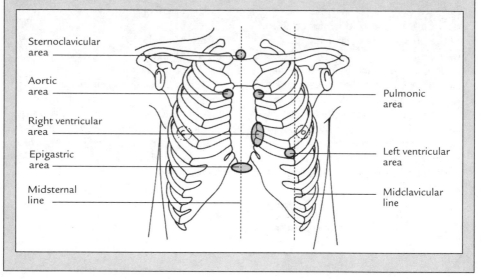

■ symmetry — pulses should be equally strong bilaterally

■ contour — the wavelike flow of the pulse, the upstroke and downstroke, should be smooth

■ strength — pulses should be easily palpable; obliterating the pulse should require strong finger pressure.

Grade the pulse amplitude bilaterally at each site. Use a pulse rating scale, such as a 3+ scale in which 0 is absent, 1 is weak, 2 is normal, and 3 is bounding.

Document any variations in rate, rhythm, contour, symmetry, and strength.

Palpating the precordium
Follow a systematic palpation sequence covering the sternoclavicular, aortic, pulmonic, right ventricular, left ventricular (apical), and epigastric areas. Use the pads of the fingers to effectively assess large pulse sites. Finger pads prove especially sensitive to vibrations.

Start at the sternoclavicular area and move methodically through the palpation sequence down to the epigastric area. At the sternoclavicular area, you may feel pulsation of the aortic arch, especially in a thin or average-build patient.

To locate the apical impulse, place your fingers in the fifth intercostal space at or just medial to the midclavicular line. Usually, the apical pulse is palpated best at the PMI; light palpation should reveal a tap with each heartbeat over a space roughly ¾″ (2 cm) in diameter.

Moderately strong, the apical impulse demonstrates a swift upstroke and downstroke early in systole, caused by left ventricular movement. It normally lasts for about one-third of the cardiac cycle if the heart rate is under 100 beats/minute. It should correlate with the first heart sound and carotid pulsation.

You shouldn't be able to palpate pulsations over the aortic, pulmonic, or right ventricular area.

Auscultation
The cardiovascular system requires more auscultation than any other body system.

Auscultating the precordium
Practice auscultating for and identifying heart sounds in the precordium. First practice identifying normal heart sounds, rates, and rhythms. Then auscultate patients with known abnormal sounds, seeking help from experts to identify findings.

Expect some difficulty. Fat, muscle, and air tend to reduce sound transmission.

Make sure the room is quiet. Use the diaphragm of the stethoscope to detect the normal higher-pitched heart sounds (first and second heart sounds [S_1 and S_2]). Use the bell to identify low-pitched

sounds, such as mitral murmurs and gallops.

Help the patient into a supine position. Use alternative positions, as needed, to improve heart sound auscultation.

Instruct the patient to breathe normally, inhaling through the nose and exhaling through the mouth. Warm the stethoscope chestpiece by rubbing it between your hands.

Identify cardiac auscultation sites. Most normal heart sounds result from vibrations created by the opening and closing of the heart valves. Auscultation sites don't lie directly over the valves, but over the pathways the blood takes as it flows through chambers and valves. (See *Auscultation sites,* page 68.)

Now auscultate, listening selectively for each cardiac cycle component. Move the stethoscope slowly and methodically over the four main auscultation sites.

You must concentrate to hear these relatively quiet sounds. Keep your hand steady, and ask the patient to remain as still as possible.

Begin by listening for a few cycles to become accustomed to the rate and rhythm of the sounds. Two sounds normally occur: S_1 and S_2. They sound relatively high pitched and are separated by a silent period.

Characterize the patient's heart sounds by their pitch (frequency), intensity (loudness), duration, quality (such as musical or harsh), location, and radiation. The timing of heart sounds in relation to the cardiac cycle is especially important. Normal heart sounds last only a fraction of a second, followed by slightly longer periods of silence.

S_1
S_1—the lub of the lub-dub sound—marks the beginning of systole. It occurs as the mitral and tricuspid valves close.

Auscultation sites

When auscultating for heart sounds, place the stethoscope over four different sites. Follow the same auscultation sequence during every cardiovascular assessment:

■ Place the stethoscope in the second intercostal space along the right sternal border. In the aortic area, blood moves from the left ventricle during systole, crossing the aortic valve and flowing through the aortic arch.

■ Move to the pulmonic area, located in the second intercostal space at the left sternal border. In the pulmonic area, blood ejected from the right ventricle during systole crosses the pulmonic valve and flows through the main pulmonary artery.

■ Assess the third auscultation site, the tricuspid area, which lies in the fifth intercostal space along the left sternal border. In the tricuspid area, sounds reflect blood movement from the right atrium across the tricuspid valve, filling the right ventricle during diastole.

■ Finally, listen in the mitral area, located in the fifth intercostal space near the midclavicular line. (If the patient's heart is enlarged, the mitral area may be closer to the anterior axillary line.) In the mitral, or apical, area, sounds represent blood flow across the mitral valve and left ventricular filling during diastole.

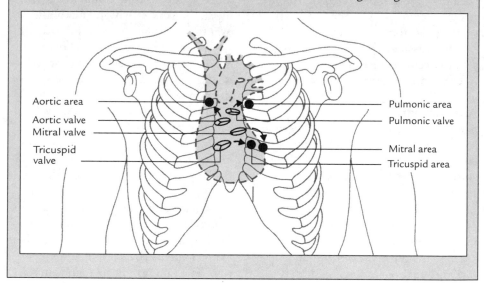

The closing of these valves immediately precedes elevation of ventricular pressure, aortic and pulmonic valve opening, and ejection of blood into the circulation. All this occurs within one-third of a second.

The mitral valve actually closes slightly before the tricuspid valve. An experienced examiner may be able to discriminate the corresponding sound (split S_1), which sounds somewhat like li-lub. However, an inexperienced examiner may confuse a split S_1 with an abnormal extra sound occurring just before S_1.

S_1 is louder in the mitral and tricuspid listening areas (LUB-dub) and softer in the aortic and pulmonic areas (lub-DUB). Compare the loudness of the normal heart sounds at each site to help you differentiate systole from diastole. Learning to identify phases of the cardiac cycle enables you to time abnormal sounds.

S_2

S_2 — the dub of the lub-dub sound — occurs at the beginning of diastole. S_2 coincides with the closing of the aortic and pulmonic valves; it's louder in the aortic and pulmonic areas of the chest. At these sites, the sequence sounds like lub-DUB. S_2 coincides with the pulse downstroke. At normal rates, the diastolic pause between S_2 and the next S_1 exceeds the systolic pause between S_1 and S_2.

During auscultation, S_2 may have a split sound, like that of a broken syllable. This may occur normally when aortic and pulmonic valves don't close at exactly the same time. Split S_2 commonly occurs in healthy children and young adults.

At each auscultatory site, use the diaphragm to listen closely to S_1 and S_2 and compare them. Next, listen to the systolic period and the diastolic period. Then auscultate again, using the bell of the stethoscope. If you hear any sounds during the systolic or diastolic period, or any variations in S_1 and S_2, document the characteristics of the sound. Note the auscultatory site and the part of the cardiac cycle in which it occurred.

S_3

S_3 is also known as the third heart sound or ventricular gallop. Its rhythm resembles the sound of a galloping horse and its cadence resembles the word Ken-tuc-ky (lub-dub-by). Listen for S_3 with the patient in a supine position or in the left-lateral decubitus position.

S_3 usually occurs during early to mid-diastole, at the end of the passive filling phase of either ventricle. It may signify that the ventricle isn't compliant enough to accept the filling volume without additional force. If the right ventricle is noncompliant, the sound occurs in the tricuspid area; if the left ventricle is noncompliant, it occurs in the mitral area. A heave may be palpable when the sound occurs.

S_3 may occur normally in a child or young adult. In a patient over age 30, it usually indicates a disorder such as right-sided heart failure, left-sided heart failure, pulmonary congestion, intracardiac shunting of blood, myocardial infarction (MI), anemia, or thyrotoxicosis.

S_4

The fourth heart sound (S_4), occurs late in diastole, just before the pulse upstroke. It immediately precedes the S_1 of the next cycle and is associated with acceleration and deceleration of blood entering a chamber that resists additional filling. Known as the atrial or presystolic gallop, it occurs during atrial contraction.

S_4 shares the same cadence as the word Ten-nes-see (le-lub-dub). Heard best with the bell of the stethoscope and with the patient in a supine position, S_4 may occur in the tricuspid or mitral area, depending on which ventricle is dysfunctional.

In many cases, S_4 indicates cardiovascular disease, such as acute MI, hypertension, coronary artery disease, cardiomyopathy, angina, anemia, elevated left ventricular pressure, or aortic stenosis. If the sound persists, it may indicate impaired ventricular compliance or volume overload. It commonly appears in elderly patients with age-related systolic hypertension and aortic stenosis.

Occasionally, a patient has both S_3 and S_4, which is known as a summation gallop. Auscultation may reveal two separate abnormal heart sounds and two normal sounds. Usually, the patient has tachycardia and diastole is shortened. S_3 and S_4 occur so close together that they appear to be one sound.

Murmurs

Murmurs are longer than a heart sound and occur as a vibrating, blowing, or rumbling noise. Turbulent blood flow produces a murmur.

If you detect a murmur, identify where it's loudest, pinpoint the time it occurs during the cardiac cycle, and describe its pitch, pattern, quality, and intensity.

Abnormal heart sounds

During auscultation, three other abnormal sounds may occur: clicks, snaps, and rubs. These sounds may indicate a need for diagnostic examination.

Clicks

A click usually precedes a late systolic murmur caused by regurgitation of a little blood from the left ventricle into the left atrium.

To detect the high-pitched click of mitral valve prolapse, place the stethoscope diaphragm at the apex and listen during midsystole to late systole. To enhance the sound, change the patient's position to sitting or standing, and listen along the lower left sternal border.

Snaps

With the stethoscope diaphragm medial to the apex along the lower left sternal border, you may detect an opening snap immediately after S_2. The snap resembles the normal S_1 and S_2 in quality; its high pitch helps differentiate it from an S_3.

The opening snap usually precedes a midsystolic to late diastolic murmur, which is a classic sign of stenosis.

Rubs

To detect a pericardial friction rub, use the diaphragm of the stethoscope to auscultate in the third left intercostal space along the lower left sternal border. Listen for a harsh, scratchy, scraping, or squeaking sound that occurs throughout systole, diastole, or both. Have the patient sit upright and lean forward or exhale to enhance the sound. A rub usually indicates pericarditis.

Auscultating the arteries

Auscultate the carotid, femoral, and popliteal arteries as well as the abdominal aorta. Over the carotid, femoral, and popliteal arteries, auscultation should reveal no sounds; over the abdominal aorta, you may detect bowel sounds, but no vascular sounds.

During auscultation of the central and peripheral arteries, you may notice a bruit, which is a continuous sound caused by turbulent blood flow. A bruit over the carotid artery usually indicates atherosclerosis; over the femoral or popliteal arteries, narrowed vessels; over the abdominal aorta, an aneurysm or a dissection

• • • • • • • • • • • •

AORTIC ANEURYSM, ABDOMINAL

An abdominal aortic aneurysm (AAA) is an abnormal dilation in the arterial wall that generally occurs in the aorta between the renal arteries and iliac branches. Such aneurysms are four times more common in men than in women. More than 50% of all people with untreated abdominal aneurysms die, primarily from aneurysmal rupture, within 2 years of diagnosis; more than 85% die within 5 years.

 AGE ALERT AAAs are most prevalent in whites ages 50 to 80.

Causes and pathophysiology

About 95% of AAAs result from arteriosclerosis; the rest, from cystic medial necrosis, trauma, syphilis, and other infections. These aneurysms develop slowly. First, a focal weakness in the muscular layer of the aorta (tunica media), due to degenerative changes, allows the inner layer (tunica intima) and outer layer (tunica adventitia) to stretch outward. Blood pressure within the aorta progressively weakens the vessel walls and enlarges the aneurysm. Aneurysms may be fusiform or saccular formations and are generally comprised of clots.

CLINICAL CAUTION Hypertension is strongly associated with progressive weakness and expansion of AAAs.

Clinical presentation

Although AAAs usually don't produce symptoms, most are evident (unless the patient is obese) as a pulsating mass in the periumbilical area, accompanied by a systolic bruit over the aorta. Some tenderness may be present on deep palpation. A large aneurysm may produce symptoms that mimic renal calculi, lumbar disk disease, and duodenal compression. AAAs rarely cause diminished peripheral pulses or claudication, unless embolization occurs.

Significant signs of AAA include:
■ lumbar pain that radiates to the flank and groin from pressure on lumbar nerves (signifies enlargement and imminent rupture)

■ severe, persistent abdominal and back pain, mimicking renal or ureteral colic (signifies rupture).

Signs of hemorrhage include:
■ weakness
■ sweating
■ tachycardia
■ hypotension

Patients with a rupture into the retroperitoneal space may remain stable for hours before shock and death occur (although 20% die immediately) because of a tamponade effect that's created.

Differential diagnoses

■ Renal colic or renal artery dissection
■ Appendicitis
■ Bowel obstruction
■ Gallbladder disease
■ Peptic ulcer disease and gastritis
■ Intra-abdominal or retroperitoneal masses
■ Myocardial infarction or angina
■ Diverticular disease
■ Pancreatitis
■ Urinary tract infection or pyelonephritis

Diagnosis

Because AAAs seldom produce symptoms, they're commonly detected accidentally as the result of an X-ray or a routine physical examination. Several tests can confirm a suspected abdominal aneurysm:
■ Ultrasonography allows accurate determination of aneurysm size, shape, and location and the presence of free peritoneal blood. It serves as the most useful test for diagnosing and monitoring AAAs.
■ Anteroposterior and lateral X-rays of the abdomen can detect aortic calcification, which outlines the aneurysm, at least 50% to 75% of the time.
■ Aortography (angiogram) shows the condition of vessels proximal and distal

to the aneurysm and the extent of the aneurysm but may underestimate the aneurysm's diameter because it visualizes only the flow channel and not the surrounding clot.

- Computed tomography scanning detects almost 100% of AAAs and is superior in defining size of the aorta and extent of aneurysm involvement in the surrounding blood vessels.
- Magnetic resonance imaging allows better imaging of the aorta without the need for dye but doesn't assess the suprarenal vessels well and is unsuitable for very unstable patients.

Management
General
Medical treatment is geared toward controlling contributing factors: optimal control of hypertension, smoking cessation, and administration of lipid-lowering agents.

Medication
Beta-adrenergic blockers have been found to decrease the rate of growth of aneurysms and are the preferred antihypertensive agent; they include:
- atenolol — 25 to 50 mg P.O. q.d.
- labetalol — 100 mg P.O. b.i.d., which may be increased from 1.2 to 2.4 g/day.

Controlled trials are under way to determine the benefits of beta-adrenergic blockers for this population.

Surgical intervention
AAAs usually require surgical intervention. The current surgical procedure involves resecting the affected vessel and replacing the damaged aortic section with a Dacron graft. Some surgeons are using endovascular stent grafts to bridge the aneurysm. This procedure is still investigational and the long-term outcome for these patients is unknown. In sympto-

matic patients, immediate surgical repair is indicated regardless of the diameter of the aneurysm. In asymptomatic patients, elective surgery is advised when the aneurysm is greater than 5 cm or the rate of aneurysm expansion is greater than 0.5 cm in 6 months. In patients who are poor surgical risks, surgery can be delayed until the aneurysm reaches 6 cm, but the risk of rupture is greatly increased. Serial ultrasounds are recommended for every 6 months to 1 year (if the aneurysm is stable and little expansion is noted) to monitor the aneurysm's diameter and shape and blood flow.

Referral
Refer the patient to a vascular surgeon when or if the AAA exceeds 3 cm.

Follow-up
The patient should be monitored for adequate blood pressure control, with medications adjusted as needed. Lipid levels should be monitored periodically. Postoperatively, the patient should be monitored for graft infection or occlusion. For stable aneurysms, evaluate by ultrasound yearly. Mean expansion is 0.4 cm per year.

HEALTHY LIVING To decrease the risk of AAA, the patient should follow treatment regimens established for control of hypertension and atherosclerotic disease. If the patient smokes, measures should be taken to stop smoking.

Patient teaching
- Advise the patient and family of signs and symptoms of rupture such as shock, pulsating abdominal mass, and abdominal or flank pain. Inform them that this is a surgical emergency.

Complications
- Death
- Rupture
- Associated dissection
- Thrombosis
- Distal embolization

Special considerations
Baseline studies should be done when a diagnosis of AAA is made, in case of an emergency situation, such as: renal function tests, complete blood count with differential, an electrocardiogram and cardiac evaluation, pulmonary function tests, arterial blood gas analysis, blood typing, and crossmatching.

• • • • • • • • • • • •

AORTIC ANEURYSM, THORACIC

Thoracic aortic aneurysm is an abnormal widening of the ascending, transverse, or descending part of the aorta. Aneurysm of the ascending aorta is the most common type and has the highest mortality. Aneurysms may be dissecting, a hemorrhagic separation in the aortic wall, usually within the medial layer; saccular, an outpouching of the arterial wall, with a narrow neck; or fusiform, a spindle-shaped enlargement encompassing the entire aortic circumference. (See *Types of aortic aneurysms,* page 74.) Some aneurysms progress to serious and, eventually, lethal complications, such as rupture of an untreated thoracic dissecting aneurysm into the pericardium, with resulting tamponade.

Causes
Thoracic aortic aneurysms commonly result from atherosclerosis, which weakens the aortic wall and gradually distends the lumen. An intimal tear in the ascending aorta initiates dissecting aneurysm in about 60% of the patients.

Ascending aortic aneurysms, the most common type, are usually seen in men under age 60 who are hypertensive. Descending aortic aneurysms, usually found just below the origin of the subclavian artery, are most common in elderly hypertensive men.

Descending aortic aneurysms are also seen in younger patients with a history of traumatic chest injury; less often in those with infection. Transverse aortic aneurysms are the least common type.

Other causes include:
- fungal infection (mycotic aneurysms) of the aortic arch and descending segments
- congenital disorders, such as coarctation of the aorta and Marfan syndrome
- trauma, usually of the descending thoracic aorta, from an accident that shears the aorta transversely (acceleration-deceleration injuries)
- syphilis, usually of the ascending aorta (uncommon because of antibiotics)
- hypertension (in dissecting aneurysm).

Clinical presentation
The most common symptom of thoracic aortic aneurysm is pain. With an ascending aneurysm, the pain is described as severe, boring, and ripping. It extends to the neck, shoulders, lower back, or abdomen but seldom radiates to the jaw and arms. Pain is more severe on the right side.

Other signs of an ascending aneurysm may include:
- bradycardia
- aortic insufficiency
- pericardial friction rub caused by a hemopericardium
- unequal intensities of the right carotid and left radial pulses

Types of aortic aneurysms

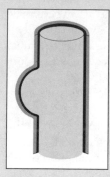

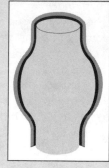

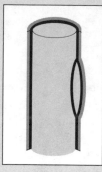

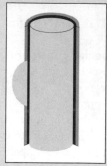

SACCULAR
Unilateral pouch-like bulge with a narrow neck

FUSIFORM
Spindle-shaped bulge encompassing the entire diameter of the vessel

DISSECTING
Hemorrhagic separation of the medial layer of the vessel wall, which creates a false lumen

FALSE ANEURYSM
Pulsating hematoma resulting from trauma and often mistaken for an abdominal aneurysm

- differing blood pressures between the right and left arms.

These signs are absent in a descending aneurysm. If dissection involves the carotids, an abrupt onset of neurologic deficits may occur.

With a descending aneurysm, pain usually starts suddenly between the shoulder blades and may radiate to the chest; it's described as sharp and tearing. A transverse aneurysm may cause:

- a sudden, sharp, tearing pain radiating to the shoulders
- hoarseness
- dyspnea
- dysphagia
- dry cough. (See *Clinical characteristics of thoracic dissection.*)

Differential diagnoses
- Myocardial infarction (MI)
- Brain attack

- Pericarditis
- Peptic ulcer disease and gastritis

Diagnosis
Diagnosis relies on patient history, clinical features, and appropriate tests. In an asymptomatic patient, diagnosis often occurs accidentally when chest X-rays show widening of the aorta. Other tests help confirm an aneurysm:

- Aortography, the most definitive test, shows the lumen of the aneurysm, its size and location, and the false lumen in a dissecting aneurysm.
- Electrocardiography helps distinguish a thoracic aneurysm from an MI.
- Echocardiography may help identify a dissecting aneurysm of the aortic root.
- Hemoglobin levels may be normal or because of blood loss from a leaking aneurysm.

Clinical characteristics of thoracic dissection

ASCENDING AORTA	DESCENDING AORTA	TRANSVERSE AORTA
Character of pain		
Severe, boring, ripping; extending to neck, shoulders, lower back, or abdomen (rarely to jaw and arms); more severe on right side	Sudden onset, sharp, tearing, usually between the shoulder blades; may radiate to the chest; most diagnostic feature	Sudden onset, sharp, boring, tearing, radiates to shoulders
Other symptoms and effects		
If dissection involves carotids, abrupt onset of neurologic deficit (usually intermittent); bradycardia, aortic insufficiency, and hemopericardium detected by pericardial friction rub; unequal intensity of right and left carotid pulses and radial pulses; difference in blood pressure, especially systolic, between right and left arms	Aortic insufficiency without murmur, hemopericardium, or pleural friction rub; carotid and radial pulses and blood pressure in both arms tend to stay equal	Hoarseness, dyspnea, pain, dysphagia, and dry cough resulting from compression of surrounding structures
Diagnostic features		
Chest X-ray Best diagnostic tool; shows widening of mediastinum, enlargement of ascending aorta	Shows widening of mediastinum; descending aorta larger than ascending	Shows widening of mediastinum; descending aorta larger than ascending, widened transverse arch
Aortography Shows false lumen; narrowing of lumen of aorta in ascending section	Shows false lumen; narrowing of lumen of aorta in descending section	Shows false lumen; narrowing of lumen of aorta in transverse arch
Treatment		
This is a medical emergency requiring immediate, aggressive treatment to reduce blood pressure (usually with nitroprusside or trimethaphan). Surgical repair is also required.	Surgical repair is required but is less urgent than for an ascending dissection. Nitroprusside and propranolol may be used to control hypertension if bradycardia and heart failure are absent.	Immediate surgical repair (mortality as high as 50%) and control of hypertension are required.

■ Computed tomography scanning can confirm and locate the aneurysm and may be used to monitor its progression.
■ Magnetic resonance imaging may aid diagnosis.
■ Transesophageal echocardiography is used to diagnose and determine the size of an aneurysm in either the ascending or the descending aorta.

Management
General
Once a thoracic aneurysm is detected, careful monitoring for enlargement needs to be done. Decisions must be made regarding management of the aneurysm and the potential for surgery. If the aneurysm results from MI, it must be determined whether the patient would be able to tolerate surgery.

Medication
The following medications may be given for a thoracic aortic aneurysm:
■ beta-adrenergic blockers such as:
–atenolol, 25 to 50 mg/day P.O.
–labetalol, 100 mg P.O. b.i.d., or 20 mg I.V. with repeated doses of 40 to 80 mg I.V. every 10 minutes until the maximum dose of 300 mg
■ negative inotropic agents such as propranolol 80 mg P.O. q.d. in two to four divided doses
■ analgesics such as morphine sulfate 2 to 4 mg I.V. every 1 to 3 hours, p.r.n.

Surgical intervention
A dissecting aortic aneurysm is an emergency that requires prompt surgery and stabilization. Surgery consists of resecting the aneurysm, restoring normal blood flow through a Dacron or Teflon graft replacement and, with aortic valve insufficiency, replacing the aortic valve.

Referral
■ Refer the patient to a cardiothoracic surgeon for monitoring of the aneurysm and potential surgery.
■ Refer the patient to community agencies for continued support and assistance as needed.

Follow-up
The patient should be monitored for adequate blood pressure control, with medication adjustment as needed. Serial ultrasounds should be done yearly to monitor the size of the aneurysm.

Patient teaching
■ Prepare the family for potential measures that would need to be instituted in the event of dissection or rupture of the aneurysm.
■ If the patient is unable to undergo elective surgery, teach the patient and family about symptoms that would indicate an emergent situation.
■ Explain the importance of following any antihypertensive therapy that has been instituted. Instruct the patient and family on how to monitor blood pressure.

Complications
■ Dissection
■ Rupture
■ Death

Special considerations
■ Make sure laboratory tests include complete blood count with differential, electrolyte levels, type and crossmatching for whole blood, arterial blood gas studies, and urinalysis.

•••••••••••

ARTERIAL OCCLUSIVE DISEASE

Arterial occlusive disease is the obstruction or narrowing of the lumen of the aorta and its major branches, causing an interruption of blood flow, usually to the legs and feet. This disorder may affect the carotid, vertebral, innominate, subclavian, mesenteric, and celiac arteries. (See *Possible sites of major artery occlusion*, page 78.) Occlusions may be acute or chronic and commonly cause severe ischemia, skin ulceration, and gangrene.

Arterial occlusive disease is more common in males than females. The prognosis depends on the location of the occlusion, the development of collateral circulation to counteract reduced blood flow and, in acute disease, the time elapsed between occlusion and its removal.

Causes

Arterial occlusive disease is a common complication of atherosclerosis. The occlusive mechanism may be endogenous, due to emboli formation or thrombosis, or exogenous, due to trauma or fracture. Predisposing factors include smoking; aging; such conditions as hypertension, hyperlipidemia, and diabetes; and a family history of vascular disorders, myocardial infarction, or cerebrovascular accident.

Clinical presentation

Evidence of this disease varies widely, according to the occlusion site. (See *Clinical features of arterial occlusive disease*, page 79.)

Differential diagnoses

- Thrombophlebitis obliterans
- Raynaud's disease
- Scleroderma
- Hypokalemia

Diagnosis

Diagnosis of arterial occlusive disease is usually indicated by patient history and physical examination.

Pertinent supportive diagnostic tests include:

- Arteriography demonstrates the type (thrombus or embolus), location, and degree of obstruction and the collateral circulation; it's particularly useful in chronic disease or for evaluating candidates for reconstructive surgery.
- Doppler ultrasonography and plethysmography are noninvasive tests that show decreased blood flow distal to the occlusion in acute disease.
- Ophthalmodynamometry helps determine degree of obstruction in the internal carotid artery by comparing ophthalmic artery pressure with brachial artery pressure on the affected side. More than a 20% difference between pressures suggests insufficiency.
- Electroencephalography and computed tomography scanning may be necessary to rule out brain lesions.
- Ankle-Brachial Index (ABI) — a comparison of ankle and brachial systolic blood pressure — is used as a screening test to determine the presence of intermittent claudication. Normal is 1.0; having an ABI under 0.9 suggests peripheral vascular disease

Management
General

Treatment depends on the cause, location, and size of the obstruction. For mild chronic disease, nonpharmacologic treatment includes smoking cessation, hypertension control, cholesterol management, graduated exercise program, weight control, and infection control.

Possible sites of major artery occlusion

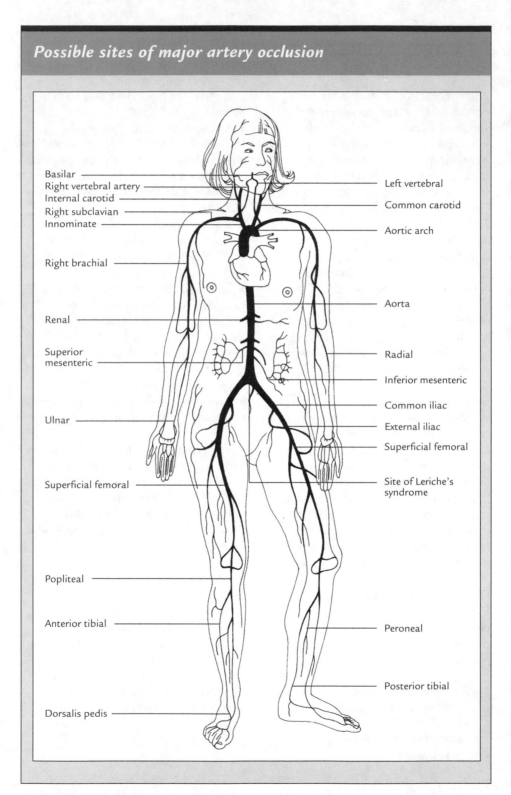

Basilar
Right vertebral artery
Internal carotid
Right subclavian
Innominate

Left vertebral
Common carotid
Aortic arch

Right brachial

Aorta

Renal

Superior mesenteric

Radial

Inferior mesenteric

Common iliac

Ulnar

External iliac

Superficial femoral

Superficial femoral

Site of Leriche's syndrome

Popliteal

Anterior tibial

Peroneal

Posterior tibial

Dorsalis pedis

Clinical features of arterial occlusive disease

SITE OF OCCLUSION	SIGNS AND SYMPTOMS
Carotid arterial system • Internal carotid arteries • External carotid arteries	Neurologic dysfunction (transient ischemic attacks [TIAs] due to reduced cerebral circulation produce unilateral sensory or motor dysfunction [transient monocular blindness, hemiparesis], possible aphasia or dysarthria, confusion, decreased mentation, and headache; usually last 5 to 10 minutes but may persist up to 24 hours and may herald a stroke); absent or decreased pulsation with an auscultatory bruit over the affected vessels
Vertebrobasilar system • Vertebral arteries • Basilar arteries	Neurologic dysfunction (TIAs of brain stem and cerebellum produce binocular visual disturbances, vertigo, dysarthria, and "drop attacks" [falling down without loss of consciousness]); less common than carotid TIA
Innominate Brachiocephalic artery	Neurologic dysfunction (signs and symptoms of vertebrobasilar occlusion); indications of ischemia (claudication) of right arm; possible bruit over right side of neck
Subclavian artery	Subclavian steal syndrome (characterized by the backflow of blood from the brain through the vertebral artery on the same side as the occlusion, into the subclavian artery distal to the occlusion); clinical effects of vertebrobasilar occlusion and exercise-induced arm claudication; possible gangrene, usually limited to the digits
Mesenteric artery • Superior (most commonly affected) • Celiac axis • Inferior	Bowel ischemia, infarct necrosis, and gangrene; sudden, acute abdominal pain; nausea and vomiting; diarrhea; leukocytosis; shock due to massive intraluminal fluid and plasma loss
Aortic bifurcation (saddle block occlusion, an emergency associated with cardiac embolization)	Sensory and motor deficits (muscle weakness, numbness, paresthesia, paralysis), and signs of ischemia (sudden pain; cold, pale legs with decreased or absent peripheral pulses) in both legs
Iliac artery (Leriche's syndrome)	Intermittent claudication of lower back, buttocks, and thighs relieved by rest; absent or reduced femoral or distal pulses; possible bruit over femoral arteries; impotence in males
Femoral and popliteal artery (associated with aneurysm formation)	Intermittent claudication of the calves on exertion, ischemic pain in feet, pretrophic pain (heralds necrosis and ulceration), leg pallor and coolness, blanching of feet on elevation, gangrene, no palpable pulses in ankles and feet

Medication

For carotid artery occlusion, initiate antiplatelet therapy, which may begin with one aspirin daily.

For intermittent claudication of chronic occlusive disease, the following medications may be ordered:

• pentoxifylline — 400 mg P.O. t.i.d. with meals

- cilostazol — 100 mg P.O. b.i.d. 30 minutes a.c. or 2 hours p.c.

Surgical intervention

Acute arterial occlusive disease with ischemic pain usually requires surgery to restore circulation to the affected area. Possible procedures include:

- embolectomy — a balloon-tipped Fogarty catheter used to remove thrombotic material from the artery; used mainly for mesenteric, femoral, or popliteal artery occlusion
- thromboendarterectomy — opening the occluded artery and directly removing the obstructing thrombus and medial layer of the arterial wall; usually performed after angiography and often used with autogenous vein or Dacron bypass surgery (femoral-popliteal or aortofemoral).
- patch grafting — removal of the thrombosed arterial segment and replacement with an autogenous vein or Dacron graft
- bypass graft — diverting blood flow through an anastomosed autogenous or Dacron graft past the thrombosed segment
- thrombolytic therapy — lysis of any clot around or in the plaque by urokinase, streptokinase, or alteplase
- atherectomy — excision of plaque using a drill or slicing mechanism
- balloon angioplasty — compression of the obstruction using balloon inflation
- laser angioplasty — use of excision and hot tip lasers to vaporize the obstruction
- stents — insertion of a mesh of wires that stretch and mold to the arterial wall to prevent reocclusion; this new adjunct follows laser angioplasty or atherectomy
- combined therapy — concomitant use of any of the above treatments
- lumbar sympathectomy — removal of the sympathetic nerve in the lumbar region; an adjunct to surgery, depending on the condition of the sympathetic nervous system.

Amputation becomes necessary with the failure of arterial reconstructive surgery or with the development of gangrene, persistent infection, or intractable pain.

Other therapy includes heparin to prevent emboli (for embolic occlusion) and bowel resection after restoration of blood flow (for mesenteric artery occlusion).

Referral

- Refer patients with peripheral vascular disease to a vascular surgeon if the patient develops any of the following conditions: severe, disabling, and lifestyle-altering claudication; pain at rest; gangrene or nonhealing leg ulcers; and an ABI of less than 0.5.

Follow-up

If the occlusion is acute and surgery has occurred, the patient should be monitored for the development of infection or reocclusion. If the occlusion is chronic, follow the patient at regular 3- to 6-month intervals depending on the severity of the symptoms. Prophylactic foot and limb care is important to avoid ulcers and sources of infection. If the patient is diabetic, careful monitoring of blood glucose levels should be done in order to maintain control of the disease.

HEALTHY LIVING The patient with arterial occlusive disease should be encouraged to stop smoking, follow recommendations for cholesterol management, and maintain control of diabetes and hypertension. Proper diet and exercise should be recommended.

Patient teaching

- Tell the patient to return to the provider if symptoms worsen or if breaks in the skin surface, inflammation, or infection occur.

■ Stress the importance of proper foot care, proper apparel for cold weather, and nonrestrictive clothing on limbs.

■ Patients should be instructed not to drink grapefruit juice when taking Pletal, and patients taking diltiazem, omeprazole, erythromycin, or antifungal agents (CYP3A4 or 2C19 inhibitors) should have the dose of Pletal reduced to 50 mg twice per day.

Complications
■ Gangrene
■ Necrosis
■ Limb amputation
■ Impaired nail and hair growth
■ Stroke or transient ischemic attacks
■ Peripheral or systemic embolism

Special considerations
■ If the patient has carotid, innominate, vertebral, or subclavian artery occlusion, monitor him for signs of stroke.

• • • • • • • • • • •

CARDIAC ARRHYTHMIAS

In cardiac arrhythmias (sometimes called cardiac dysrhythmias), abnormal electrical conduction or automaticity changes heart rate and rhythm. (See *Normal cardiac conduction.*) Arrhythmias vary in severity, from those that are mild, or asymptomatic, and require no treatment such as sinus arrhythmia to catastrophic ventricular fibrillation, which necessitates immediate resuscitation. Arrhythmias are generally classified according to their origin (ventricular or supraventricular). Their effect on cardiac output and blood pressure, partially influenced by the site of origin, determines their clinical significance.

Normal cardiac conduction

Each electrical impulse travels from the sinoatrial node (1) through the intra-atrial tracts (2), producing atrial contraction. The impulse slows momentarily as it passes through the atrioventricular junction (3) to the bundle of His (4). Then, it descends the left and right bundle branches (5) and reaches the Purkinje fibers (6), stimulating ventricular contraction.

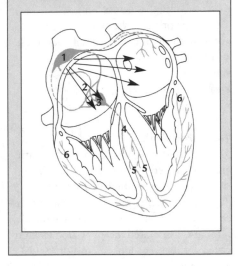

Causes
Arrhythmias may be congenital or they may result from one of several factors, including myocardial ischemia, myocardial infarction, or organic heart disease. Drug toxicity or degeneration of the conductive tissue necessary to maintain normal heart rhythm (sick sinus syndrome) sometimes can also precipitate arrhythmias.

Clinical presentation
Bradyrhythmias
Symptoms are reflective of the ventricular rate in relation to any preexisting cardiac disease as well as metabolic demands

of the individual. Bradyrhythmias are classified as either absolute or relative:

- Absolute — heart rate is below 60 beats per minute.
- Relative — heart rate is too slow to maintain normal blood pressure or adequate cardiac output, even if the rate is over 60 beats per minute.

Bradycardia may be an incidental finding on examination and may be asymptomatic and nonpathologic. Athletes frequently have bradycardia. Bradycardia that causes the following conditions is defined as symptomatic:

- syncope or near-syncope
- transient dizziness or light-headedness
- confusion
- fatigue
- exercise intolerance
- heart failure.

Tachyarrhythmias

Tachyarrhythmias may be asymptomatic and an incidental finding on examination. Symptomatic tachyarrhythmia is dependent on any preexisting cardiac disease, ventricular function, ventricular rate, and associated factors (such as anxiety and tobacco, alcohol, and drug use). These symptoms are common:

- palpitations
- confusion
- hypotension
- light-headedness
- chest pain
- syncope
- heart failure
- shortness of breath.

Differential diagnoses
Bradyrhythmias

- Sinus bradycardia
- First-degree atrioventricular (AV) block
- Second-degree AV block
- Third-degree AV block
- Bundle-branch block

Tachyarrhythmias

- Sinus tachycardia
- Multifocal atrial tachycardia
- Paroxysmal atrial tachycardia
- Atrial flutter
- Atrial fibrillation
- Supraventricular tachycardia
- Ventricular tachycardia
- Ventricular fibrillation

Diagnosis

- Electrocardiography (ECG) identifies arrhythmias and cardiac damage.
- Holter monitoring (also known as ambulatory ECG monitoring) may identify sporadic arrhythmias or arrhythmias triggered by specific events.
- Exercise ECG reveals ischemia, arrhythmias, or conduction abnormalities induced by increased workload of the heart.
- Electrophysiology studies allow precise location of bundle-branch blocks, detection of arrhythmias, and evaluation of antiarrhythmic drugs.

Management
General

Treatment of cardiac arrhythmias depends on many variables. Asymptomatic arrhythmias may remain untreated. Hemodynamically unstable patients need emergency measures to restore homeostasis. These measures may include administration of medications as well as cardioversion or defibrillation. If arrhythmia results from an underlying cause, such as hypoxia, correction of this disorder may restore normal cardiac function.

Medication

The medication prescribed depends on the type of arrhythmia. If an electrolyte disorder is present, it needs to be corrected appropriately. (See *Types of cardiac arrhythmias.*)

(Text continues on page 90.)

Types of cardiac arrhythmias

Use a normal electrocardiogram strip, if available, to compare normal cardiac rhythm configurations with the rhythm strips depicted here. (Note the various features, causes, and treatments of these common cardiac arrhythmias.) Characteristics of normal rhythm include:

- ventricular and atrial rates of 60 to 100 beats/minute
- regular and uniform QRS complexes and P waves
- PR interval of 0.12 to 0.20 second
- QRS duration less than 0.12 second
- identical atrial and ventricular rates, with constant PR interval.

ARRHYTHMIA AND FEATURES	CAUSES	TREATMENT
Sinus arrhythmia 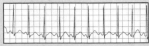 ■ Irregular atrial and ventricular rhythms ■ Normal P wave preceding each QRS complex	■ A normal variation of normal sinus rhythm in athletes, children, and elderly people ■ Also seen in digoxin toxicity and inferior wall myocardial infarction (MI)	■ Atropine (0.5 to 1 mg I.V. push, repeated every 3 to 5 minutes to maximum of 2 mg) if rate decreases below 40 beats/minute and patient is symptomatic (for example, has hypotension)
Sinus tachycardia ■ Atrial and ventricular rhythms regular ■ Rate > 100 beats/minute; rarely, > 160 beats/minute ■ Normal P wave preceding each QRS complex	■ Normal physiologic response to fever, exercise, anxiety, pain, dehydration; may also accompany shock, left-sided heart failure, cardiac tamponade, hyperthyroidism, anemia, hypovolemia, pulmonary embolism, anterior wall MI ■ May also occur with atropine, epinephrine, isoproterenol, quinidine, caffeine, alcohol, and nicotine use	■ Correction of underlying cause
Sinus bradycardia ■ Regular atrial and ventricular rhythms ■ Rate < 60 beats/minute ■ Normal P wave preceding each QRS complex	■ Normal in well-conditioned heart, as in an athlete ■ Increased intracranial pressure; increased vagal tone due to straining during defecation, vomiting, intubation, mechanical ventilation; sick sinus syndrome; hypothyroidism; inferior wall MI ■ May also occur with anticholinesterase, beta-adrenergic blocker, digoxin, and morphine use	■ For low cardiac output, dizziness, weakness, altered level of consciousness, or low blood pressure: atropine (0.5 to 1 mg I.V. push, repeated every 3 to 5 minutes to maximum of 2 mg) ■ Temporary or permanent pacemaker ■ Dopamine 5 to 20 mg/kg per minute ■ Epinephrine 2 to 10 mg per minute

(continued)

Types of cardiac arrhythmias *(continued)*

ARRHYTHMIA AND FEATURES	CAUSES	TREATMENT

Sinoatrial (SA) arrest or block *(sinus arrest)*

- Atrial and ventricular rhythms normal except for missing complex
- Normal P wave preceding each QRS complex
- Pause not equal to a multiple of the previous sinus rhythm

Causes:
- Acute infection
- Coronary artery disease (CAD), degenerative heart disease, acute inferior wall MI
- Vagal stimulation, Valsalva's maneuver, carotid sinus massage
- Digoxin, quinidine, or salicylate toxicity
- Pesticide poisoning
- Pharyngeal irritation caused by endotracheal intubation
- Sick sinus syndrome

Treatment:
- Treatment of symptoms with atropine I.V. (0.5 to 1 mg I.V. push, repeated every 3 to 5 minutes to maximum of 2 mg)
- Temporary or permanent pacemaker for repeated episodes

Wandering atrial pacemaker

- Atrial and ventricular rhythms vary slightly
- Irregular PR interval
- P waves irregular with changing configuration, indicating that they aren't all from SA node or single atrial focus; may appear after the QRS complex
- QRS complexes uniform in shape but irregular in rhythm

Causes:
- Rheumatic carditis due to inflammation involving the SA node
- Digoxin toxicity
- Sick sinus syndrome

Treatment:
- No treatment if patient is asymptomatic
- Treatment of underlying cause if patient is symptomatic

Premature atrial contraction (PAC)

- Premature, abnormal-looking P waves that differ in configuration from normal P waves
- QRS complexes after P waves, except in very early or blocked PACs
- P wave often buried in the preceding T wave or identified in the preceding T wave

Causes:
- Coronary or valvular heart disease, atrial ischemia, coronary atherosclerosis, heart failure, acute respiratory failure, chronic obstructive pulmonary disease (COPD), electrolyte imbalance, and hypoxia
- Digoxin toxicity; use of aminophylline, adrenergics, or caffeine
- Anxiety

Treatment:
- Usually no treatment needed
- Treatment of underlying cause

Types of cardiac arrhythmias (continued)

ARRHYTHMIA AND FEATURES	CAUSES	TREATMENT

Paroxysmal atrial tachycardia (paroxysmal supraventicular tachycardia)

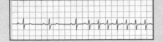

- Atrial and ventricular rhythms regular
- Heart rate > 160 beats/ minute; rarely exceeds 250 beats/minute
- P waves regular but aberrant; difficult to differentiate from preceding T wave
- P wave preceding each QRS complex
- Sudden onset and termination of arrhythmia

- Intrinsic abnormality of AV conduction system
- Physical or psychological stress, hypoxia, hypokalemia, cardiomyopathy, congenital heart disease, MI, valvular disease, Wolff-Parkinson-White syndrome, cor pulmonale, hyperthyroidism, systemic hypertension
- Digoxin toxicity; use of caffeine, marijuana, or central nervous system stimulants

- If patient is unstable: immediate cardioversion.
- If patient is stable: vagal stimulation, Valsalva's maneuver, carotid sinus massage
- Adenosine (6 mg) by rapid I.V. bolus injection to convert arrhythmia
- If cardiac function is preserved: advanced cardiac life support (ACLS) treatment priority — calcium channel blocker, digoxin, and cardioversion; then possibly procainamide, amiodarone, or sotolol
- If ejection fraction is less than 40% or the patient is in heart failure: ACLS treatment order — digoxin, amiodarone, and then diltiazem.

Atrial flutter

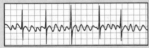

- Atrial rhythm regular rate; 250 to 400 beats/minute
- Ventricular rate variable, depending on degree of atrioventricular (AV) block (usually 60 to 100 beats/minute)
- Sawtooth P-wave configuration possible (F waves)
- QRS complexes uniform in shape, but often irregular in rate

- Heart failure, tricuspid or mitral valve disease, pulmonary embolism, cor pulmonale, inferior wall MI, carditis
- Digoxin toxicity

- If patient is unstable with a ventricular rate > 150 beats/minute: immediate cardioversion
- If atrial flutter is greater than 48 hours and heart function is normal: calcium channel blocker or beta-adrenergic blockers to control rate
- If atrial flutter is less than 48 hours and heart function is normal: amiodarone, ibutilide, flecainide, propafenone, or procainamide to convert rhythm
- If atrial flutter is greater than 48 hours and heart function is impaired: digoxin, diltiazem, or amiodarone, if appropriate
- Possibly synchronized cardioversion and anticoagulation therapy

(continued)

Types of cardiac arrhythmias *(continued)*

ARRHYTHMIA AND FEATURES	CAUSES	TREATMENT
Atrial fibrillation ■ Atrial rhythm grossly irregular; rate > 400 beats/minute ■ Ventricular rhythm irregular ■ QRS complexes of uniform configuration and duration ■ PR interval indiscernible ■ No P waves, or P waves that appear as erratic, irregular, baseline fibrillary waves	■ Heart failure, COPD, thyrotoxicosis, constrictive pericarditis, ischemic heart disease, sepsis, pulmonary embolus, rheumatic heart disease, hypertension, mitral stenosis, atrial irritation, complication of coronary bypass or valve replacement surgery	■ If patient is unstable with ventricular rate > 150 beats/minute: immediate cardioversion ■ If atrial fibrillation (AF) is greater than 48 hours and heart function is normal: calcium channel blocker or beta-adrenergic blockers to control rate ■ If AF is less than 48 hours and heart function is normal: amiodarone, ibutilide, flecainide, propafenone, or procainamide to convert rhythm ■ If AF is greater than 48 hours and heart function is impaired: digoxin, diltiazem, or amiodarone ■ Possibly elective cardioversion for rapid ventricular rate and anticoagulation therapy ■ Treatment of underlying cause
Junctional rhythm ■ Atrial and ventricular rhythms regular ■ Atrial rate 40 to 60 beats/minute ■ Ventricular rate usually 40 to 60 beats/minute (60 to 100 beats/minute is accelerated junctional rhythm) ■ P waves preceding, hidden within (absent), or after QRS complex; usually inverted if visible ■ PR interval (when present), < 0.12 second ■ QRS complex configuration and duration normal, except in aberrant conduction	■ Inferior wall MI or ischemia, hypoxia, vagal stimulation, sick sinus syndrome ■ Acute rheumatic fever ■ Valve surgery ■ Digoxin toxicity	■ Atropine (0.5 to 1 mg I.V. push, repeated every 3 to 5 minutes to maximum of 2 mg) for symptomatic slow rate ■ Pacemaker insertion if patient is refractory to drugs ■ Discontinuation of digoxin, if appropriate

Types of cardiac arrhythmias (continued)

ARRHYTHMIA AND FEATURES	CAUSES	TREATMENT
Junctional contractions (junctional premature beats) ■ Atrial and ventricular rhythms irregular ■ P waves inverted; may precede, be hidden within, or follow QRS complex ■ PR interval < 0.12 second if P wave precedes QRS complex ■ QRS complex configuration and duration normal	■ MI or ischemia ■ Digoxin toxicity and excessive caffeine or amphetamine use	■ Correction of underlying cause ■ Usually no interventions needed
First-degree AV block ■ Atrial and ventricular rhythms regular ■ PR interval > 0.20 second ■ P wave preceding each QRS complex ■ QRS complex normal	■ May be seen in a healthy person ■ Inferior wall myocardial ischemia or infarction, hypothyroidism, hypokalemia, hyperkalemia ■ Digoxin toxicity; use of quinidine, procainamide, or propranolol	■ Cautious use of digoxin ■ Correction of underlying cause ■ Possibly atropine (0.5 to 1 mg I.V. push, repeated every 3 to 5 minutes to maximum of 2 mg) if PR interval exceeds 0.26 second or symptoms of bradycardia develops
Second-degree AV block Mobitz I (Wenckebach) ■ Atrial rhythm regular ■ Ventricular rhythm irregular ■ Atrial rate exceeds ventricular rate ■ PR interval progressively, but only slightly, longer with each cycle until QRS complex disappears (dropped beat); PR interval shorter after dropped beat	■ Inferior wall MI, cardiac surgery, acute rheumatic fever, and vagal stimulation ■ Digoxin toxicity; use of propranolol, quinidine, or procainamide	■ Treatment of underlying cause ■ Atropine (0.5 to 1 mg I.V. push, repeated every 3 to 5 minutes to maximum of 2 mg) or temporary pacemaker for symptomatic bradycardia ■ Discontinuation of digoxin, if appropriate

(continued)

Types of cardiac arrhythmias *(continued)*

ARRHYTHMIA AND FEATURES	CAUSES	TREATMENT

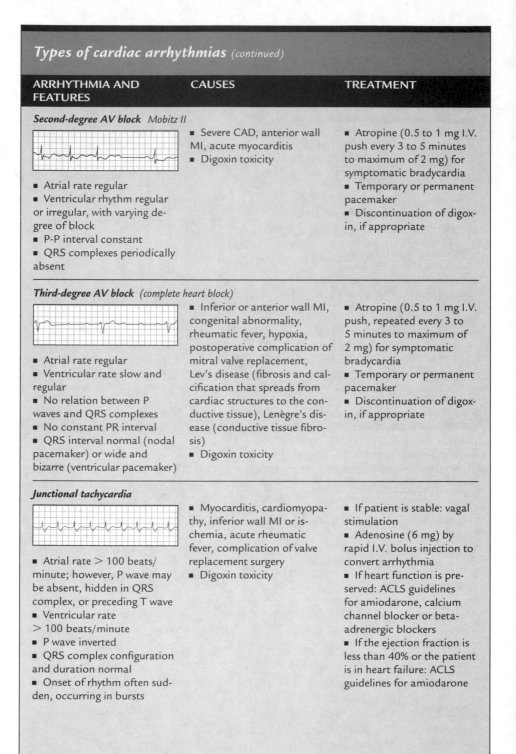

Second-degree AV block *Mobitz II*

- Atrial rate regular
- Ventricular rhythm regular or irregular, with varying degree of block
- P-P interval constant
- QRS complexes periodically absent

• Severe CAD, anterior wall MI, acute myocarditis
• Digoxin toxicity

• Atropine (0.5 to 1 mg I.V. push every 3 to 5 minutes to maximum of 2 mg) for symptomatic bradycardia
• Temporary or permanent pacemaker
• Discontinuation of digoxin, if appropriate

Third-degree AV block *(complete heart block)*

- Atrial rate regular
- Ventricular rate slow and regular
- No relation between P waves and QRS complexes
- No constant PR interval
- QRS interval normal (nodal pacemaker) or wide and bizarre (ventricular pacemaker)

• Inferior or anterior wall MI, congenital abnormality, rheumatic fever, hypoxia, postoperative complication of mitral valve replacement, Lev's disease (fibrosis and calcification that spreads from cardiac structures to the conductive tissue), Lenègre's disease (conductive tissue fibrosis)
• Digoxin toxicity

• Atropine (0.5 to 1 mg I.V. push, repeated every 3 to 5 minutes to maximum of 2 mg) for symptomatic bradycardia
• Temporary or permanent pacemaker
• Discontinuation of digoxin, if appropriate

Junctional tachycardia

- Atrial rate > 100 beats/minute; however, P wave may be absent, hidden in QRS complex, or preceding T wave
- Ventricular rate > 100 beats/minute
- P wave inverted
- QRS complex configuration and duration normal
- Onset of rhythm often sudden, occurring in bursts

• Myocarditis, cardiomyopathy, inferior wall MI or ischemia, acute rheumatic fever, complication of valve replacement surgery
• Digoxin toxicity

• If patient is stable: vagal stimulation
• Adenosine (6 mg) by rapid I.V. bolus injection to convert arrhythmia
• If heart function is preserved: ACLS guidelines for amiodarone, calcium channel blocker or beta-adrenergic blockers
• If the ejection fraction is less than 40% or the patient is in heart failure: ACLS guidelines for amiodarone

Types of cardiac arrhythmias *(continued)*

ARRHYTHMIA AND FEATURES	CAUSES	TREATMENT

Premature ventricular contraction (PVC)

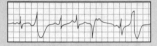

- Atrial rhythm regular
- Ventricular rhythm irregular
- QRS complex premature, followed by a complete compensatory pause
- QRS complex wide and distorted, > 0.14 second
- Premature QRS complexes occurring with normal beats
- Ominous when clustered, multifocal, with R wave on T pattern

- Heart failure; old or acute myocardial ischemia, infarction, or contusion; myocardial irritation by ventricular catheter, such as a pacemaker; hypercapnia; hypokalemia, hypocalcemia
- Drug toxicity (digoxin, aminophylline, tricyclic antidepressants, beta-adrenergics [isoproterenol or dopamine])
- Caffeine, tobacco, or alcohol use
- Psychological stress, anxiety, pain, exercise

- If symptomatic, lidocaine (1 to 1.5 mg/kg I.V. bolus followed by continuous infusion 1 to 4 mg/minute), or procainamide (50 to 100 mg slow I.V. push up to 500 mg followed by continuous infusion of 1 to 6 mg/minute).
- Treatment of underlying cause
- Discontinuation of drug causing toxicity
- Potassium chloride (40 mg rider) I.V. if PVC induced by hypokalemia

Ventricular tachycardia

- Ventricular rate 140 to 220 beats/minute, rhythm may be regular or irregular
- QRS complexes wide, bizarre, and independent of P waves
- P waves not discernible
- May start and stop suddenly

- Myocardial ischemia, infarction, or aneurysm; CAD; rheumatic heart disease; mitral valve prolapse; heart failure; cardiomyopathy; ventricular catheters; hypokalemia; hypercalcemia; pulmonary embolism
- Digoxin, procainamide, epinephrine, or quinidine toxicity
- Anxiety

- Cardioversion at any time to convert the rhythm
- If rhythm is monomorphic VT with normal heart function: procainamide or sotalol; amiodarone and lidocaine
- If rhythm is monomorphic VT with impaired heart function: amiodarone or lidocaine; then synchronized cardioversion to convert rhythm
- If rhythm is polymorphic VT with normal baseline QT interval: treatment of ischemia, correction of electrolytes and, if appropriate, beta-adrenergic blockers, lidocaine, amiodarone, procainamide, or sotalol
- If rhythm is polymorphic VT with prolonged baseline QT interval (suggests torsades de pointes): correction of electrolytes and magnesium, overdrive pacing, isoproterenol, phenytoin, or lidocaine
- Cardiopulmonary resuscitation (CPR) if pulses are absent, after ACLS protocol

(continued)

Types of cardiac arrhythmias *(continued)*

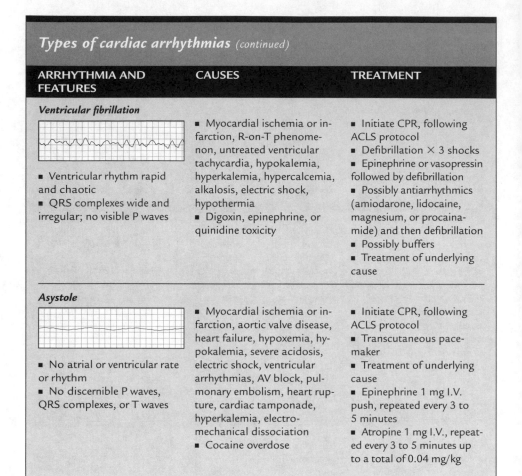

ARRHYTHMIA AND FEATURES	CAUSES	TREATMENT
Ventricular fibrillation • Ventricular rhythm rapid and chaotic • QRS complexes wide and irregular; no visible P waves	• Myocardial ischemia or infarction, R-on-T phenomenon, untreated ventricular tachycardia, hypokalemia, hyperkalemia, hypercalcemia, alkalosis, electric shock, hypothermia • Digoxin, epinephrine, or quinidine toxicity	• Initiate CPR, following ACLS protocol • Defibrillation × 3 shocks • Epinephrine or vasopressin followed by defibrillation • Possibly antiarrhythmics (amiodarone, lidocaine, magnesium, or procainamide) and then defibrillation • Possibly buffers • Treatment of underlying cause
Asystole • No atrial or ventricular rate or rhythm • No discernible P waves, QRS complexes, or T waves	• Myocardial ischemia or infarction, aortic valve disease, heart failure, hypoxemia, hypokalemia, severe acidosis, electric shock, ventricular arrhythmias, AV block, pulmonary embolism, heart rupture, cardiac tamponade, hyperkalemia, electromechanical dissociation • Cocaine overdose	• Initiate CPR, following ACLS protocol • Transcutaneous pacemaker • Treatment of underlying cause • Epinephrine 1 mg I.V. push, repeated every 3 to 5 minutes • Atropine 1 mg I.V., repeated every 3 to 5 minutes up to a total of 0.04 mg/kg

Referral
• The patient should be referred to a cardiologist.
• If the patient is hemodynamically unstable, emergency measures should be instituted.

Follow-up
Monitor heart rate and rhythm and medication effects. Follow-up and evaluation of benign arrhythmias should be every 6 months to 1 year unless symptoms develop.

   If the patient is receiving anticoagulation therapy, monitor International Normalized Ratio (goal, 2.0 to 3.0) and signs and symptoms of bleeding.

Patient teaching
• Stress the importance of taking medications as ordered and reporting any adverse effects for appropriate adjustment of regimen.
• If the patient has a permanent pacemaker, warn him about environmental hazards that can cause inappropriate sensing and firing of impulses, as indicated by the pacemaker manufacturer.
• Tell the patient to report palpitations, light-headedness, syncope, shortness of breath, or chest pain, and stress the importance of regular checkups.
• Teach the patient how to take his own pulse.

Complications
- Sudden cardiac death
- Thromboembolism
- Decreased organ perfusion
- Syncope
- Myocardial infarction or ischemia
- Heart failure or pulmonary edema

Special considerations
- Suggest to the patient's family that certification in cardiopulmonary resuscitation may be beneficial.
- If the patient has a pacemaker, a medical identification bracelet should be worn at all times.

• • • • • • • • • • • •

CARDIOMYOPATHY, DILATED

Dilated cardiomyopathy results from extensively damaged myocardial muscle fibers. This disorder interferes with myocardial metabolism and grossly dilates all four chambers of the heart, giving the heart a globular appearance and shape. In this disorder, hypertrophy may be present. Dilated cardiomyopathy leads to intractable heart failure, arrhythmias, and emboli. Because this disease usually isn't diagnosed until it's in the advanced stages, the patient's prognosis is generally poor.

Causes and pathophysiology
The origin of most cardiomyopathies is unknown. Occasionally, dilated cardiomyopathy results from myocardial destruction by toxic, infectious, or metabolic agents, such as certain viruses, endocrine and electrolyte disorders, and nutritional deficiencies. Other causes include muscle disorders (myasthenia gravis, progressive muscular dystrophy, and myotonic dystrophy), infiltrative disorders (hemochromatosis and amyloidosis), and sarcoidosis.

Cardiomyopathy may also be a complication of alcoholism. The condition may improve with abstinence from alcohol but recurs if the patient resumes drinking.

Thiamine deficiencies can be a cause of heart failure and should be evaluated in alcoholic patients. Chemotherapeutic agents (such as doxorubicin [Adriamycin], cyclophosphamide, amacrine, and interferon) have been associated with the development of left ventricular dysfunction and dilated cardiomyopathy.

How viruses induce cardiomyopathy is unclear, but investigators suspect a link between viral myocarditis and subsequent dilated cardiomyopathy, especially after infection with poliovirus, coxsackievirus B, influenza virus, or human immunodeficiency virus.

Metabolic cardiomyopathies are related to endocrine and electrolyte disorders and nutritional deficiencies. Thus, dilated cardiomyopathy may develop in patients with hyperthyroidism, pheochromocytoma, beriberi (thiamine deficiency), or kwashiorkor (protein deficiency). Cardiomyopathy may also result from rheumatic fever, especially among children with myocarditis.

Antepartum or postpartum cardiomyopathy may develop during the last trimester or within months after delivery. Its cause is unknown, but it occurs most frequently in multiparous women over age 30, particularly those with malnutrition or preeclampsia. In these patients, cardiomegaly and heart failure may reverse with treatment, allowing a subsequent normal pregnancy. If cardiomegaly persists despite treatment, the prognosis is poor. If dilated cardiomyopathy persists, there is a 50% mortality rate after 5 years. 50% of patients improve to normal within the first few months of delivery.

Clinical presentation

In dilated cardiomyopathy, the heart ejects blood less efficiently than normal; therefore the metabolic and oxygen demands of the body aren't being met adequately. Consequently, a large volume of blood remains in the left ventricle after systole. If this occurs, signs of either left-sided or right-sided heart failure may occur.

Signs of left-sided heart failure include:

- shortness of breath
- orthopnea
- dyspnea on exertion
- paroxysmal nocturnal dyspnea
- fatigue
- irritating dry cough at night.

Signs of right-sided heart failure include:

- edema
- liver engorgement
- jugular vein distention.

Additional signs include:

- peripheral cyanosis
- sinus tachycardia or atrial fibrillation at rest
- diffuse apical impulses
- pansystolic murmur
- S_3
- S_4.

Differential diagnoses

- Severe pulmonary disease (chronic obstructive pulmonary disease, emphysema, or cor pulmonale)
- Primary pulmonary hypertension
- Hypothyroidism
- Peripartum heart disease
- Collagen vascular disease
- Neuromuscular disease

Diagnosis

- Echocardiography confirms the presence of dilated cardiomyopathy and assesses left ventricular ejection fraction and right ventricular function, chamber enlargement, heart valve dysfunction, wall motion abnormalities, pulmonary hypertension, and estimated filling pressures.
- Exercise thallium-201 scintigraphy may identify underlying coronary artery disease.
- Electrocardiography (ECG) and angiography rule out ischemic heart disease; the ECG may also show biventricular hypertrophy, sinus tachycardia, atrial enlargement and, in 20% of patients, atrial fibrillation and bundle-branch block.
- Chest X-ray demonstrates cardiomegaly — usually affecting all heart chambers — and may demonstrate pulmonary congestion, pleural or pericardial effusion, or pulmonary venous hypertension.
- Echocardiography identifies left ventricular thrombi, global hypokinesia, and degree of left ventricular dilation.
- Multiple-gated acquisition (MUGA) scanning reveals left ventricular and right ventricular muscle performance and calculates left ventricular ejection fraction. A MUGA scan isn't optimal in patients with rapid and irregular rhythms because the scan is triggered by the R-R interval.
- Coronary angiogram reveals left ventricular dysfunction, decreased cardiac output and ejection fraction, valvular (mitral and tricuspid) regurgitation if present, and elevated filling pressures.

Management

General

If a reversible etiology for dilated cardiomyopathy is identified, treatment is first directed toward the cause.

Nonpharmacologic therapy consists of checking daily weight, restricting sodium (less than 2 g/day), and restricting fluid (especially in the setting of hyponatremia). Immunizations against influenza and pneumococcal pneumonia are strongly encouraged.

Medication
Standard therapy for dilated cardiomyopathy consists of a combination of medications: All patients with left ventricular dysfunction should be on an angiotensin-converting enzyme (ACE) inhibitor unless there is a clear contraindication. Beta-adrenergic blockers are also indicated with this population and should be initiated as tolerated. The following ACE inhibitors may be used to treat dilated cardiomyopathy:
- captopril — 25 to 100 mg t.i.d. P.O.
- ramipril — 2.5 to 20 mg/day P.O.
- enalapril —2.5 to 20 mg b.i.d. P.O.
- lisinopril — 5 to 20 mg/day P.O.

The following angiotensin-receptor blockers may be used in patients who have severe and intractable cough from ACE inhibitors:
- candesartan — 16 to 32 mg/day P.O.
- losartan — 25 to 100 mg/day P.O.
- irbesartan — 150 to 300 mg/day P.O.
- valsartan — 80 to 320 mg/day P.O.

For patients who have a documented contraindication to ACE inhibitors, both of the following should be prescribed:
- hydralazine — 25 to 100 mg t.i.d. P.O.
- isosorbide dinitrate — 20 to 40 mg P.O. every 4 hours.

The following beta-adrenergic blockers may be used:
- carvedilol — 3.125 to 25 mg b.i.d. (50 mg b.i.d. P.O. if the patient weighs more than 180 lb [82 kg])
- metoprolol — 50 to 100 mg/day (extended release).

Additional appropriate medications include:
- digoxin — 0.125 to 0.25 mg/day P.O.
- furosemide — 20 to 80 mg/day P.O. and up to 600 mg/day in divided doses
- spironolactone — 25 to 200 mg/day P.O. in divided doses
- hydrochlorothiazide — 25 to 100 mg/day P.O.
- warfarin — 2 to 5 mg for 2 to 4 days, then dosage based on the target INR of 2.0 to 3.5
- amiodarone — loading dose of 800 to 1,600 mg/day P.O. for 1 to 3 weeks. Reduce to 600 to 800 mg/day for 1 month. Maintenance dose is 200 to 600 mg/day P.O.

Surgical intervention
Severe cardiomyopathy may warrant a heart transplant. As a bridge to a transplant, a left ventricular assist device may be inserted. Two other surgical procedures are also being evaluated — cardiomyoplasty and transmyocardial laser revascularization.

Referral
- Ventricular arrhythmias should be evaluated by a cardiologist or an electrophysiologist for risk stratification and arrhythmia inducibility and appropriate medical therapy or implantation of an internal cardiac defibrillator.
- Refer patients to heart failure outpatient clinics, the Heart Failure Society of America, the American College of Cardiology, and the American Heart Association, if available.

Follow-up
Monthly follow-up is advised or follow-up with the cardiologist.

Patient teaching
- Advise the patient to follow the medication regimen set up for him. Tell him to report any abnormal symptoms.
- Medications should be held only if the patient experiences symptomatic hypotension. Systolic blood pressure be-

tween 80 and 90 mm Hg is usually well tolerated in this population.
• Have the patient follow dietary restrictions, monitor his blood pressure at home, and weigh himself daily to determine fluid retention.

Complications
• Progressive heart failure
• Syncope
• Arrhythmias
• Sudden death
• Systemic embolization

Special considerations
• Encourage the patient's family members to learn cardiopulmonary resuscitation.
• Initiate discussions regarding advanced directives and patient wishes about end-of-life care.

• • • • • • • • • • • •

CARDIOMYOPATHY, HYPERTROPHIC

This primary disease of cardiac muscle, also called idiopathic hypertrophic subaortic stenosis, is characterized by disproportionate, asymmetrical thickening of the interventricular septum, particularly in the free wall of the left ventricle. In hypertrophic cardiomyopathy, cardiac output may be low, normal, or high, depending on whether stenosis is obstructive or nonobstructive. If cardiac output is normal or high, the disorder may go undetected for years; low cardiac output may lead to potentially fatal heart failure. The disease course varies; some patients progressively deteriorate; others remain stable for years. Sudden death, especially during exercise, may be the initial event in up to 30% of cases, as has occurred in athletes.

CLINICAL CAUTION Approximately half of the cases of hypertrophic cardiomyopathy are familially linked and are associated with specific chromosomal abnormality patterns. Because of this link, first-degree family members of persons with hypertrophic cardiomyopathy should be evaluated by echocardiography and genetic analysis.

Causes
Despite being designated as idiopathic, in almost all cases, hypertrophic cardiomyopathy may be inherited as a non–sex-linked autosomal-dominant trait. Most patients have obstructive disease, resulting from effects of ventricular septal hypertrophy and the movement of the anterior mitral valve leaflet into the outflow tract during systole. Eventually, left ventricular dysfunction, from rigidity and decreased compliance, causes pump failure.

Clinical presentation
Clinical features of the disorder may not appear until it's well advanced, when atrial dilation and, possibly, atrial fibrillation abruptly reduce blood flow to the left ventricle. Reduced inflow and subsequent low output produces the following:
• chest pain
• arrhythmias
• dyspnea
• orthopnea
• syncope
• heart failure
• death.

The most frequent symptoms of hypertrophic cardiomyopathy are exertional dyspnea and chest pain. Syncope or near-syncope is present in up to 50% of cases, usually occurring after exertion.

Other signs include:
• a medium-pitched systolic ejection murmur along the left sternal border (increases with Valsalva's maneuver and decreases with squatting)

- a holosystolic murmur heard at the apex (in patients with mitral insufficiency)
- peripheral pulse with a rapid upstroke and a characteristic double impulse (pulsus biferiens)
- irregular pulse (with atrial fibrillation).

Differential diagnoses
- Aortic stenosis
- Pulmonary disease
- Angina pectoris

Diagnosis
Diagnosis depends on typical clinical findings and the following test results:
- Echocardiography (most useful) shows increased thickness of the intraventricular septum and abnormal motion of the anterior mitral leaflet during systole, occluding left ventricular outflow in obstructive disease.
- Cardiac catheterization reveals elevated left ventricular end-diastolic pressure and, possibly, mitral insufficiency.
- Electrocardiography usually demonstrates left ventricular hypertrophy, T-wave inversion, left anterior hemiblock, Q waves in precordial and inferior leads, ventricular arrhythmias and, possibly, atrial fibrillation.
- Auscultation confirms an early systolic murmur.

Management
General
The goals of treatment are to relax the ventricle and relieve outflow tract obstruction.

Medication
Medications that may be used include:
- propranolol — 30 to 120 mg P.O. b.i.d. to t.i.d. for adults and 1 mg/kg/day P.O. for children, not to exceed 16 mg/day
- verapamil — 80 to 120 mg P.O. t.i.d. to q.i.d.

- warfarin — 2 to 5 mg for 2 to 4 days, then dosage based on the target INR of 2.0 to 3.5
- amiodarone — loading dose of 800 to 1,600 mg/day P.O. for 1 to 3 weeks. Reduce to 600 to 800 mg/day for 1 month. Maintenance dose is 200 to 600 mg/day P.O.
- furosemide — 20 to 80 mg/day P.O.

For patients with atrial fibrillation, vasodilators should be avoided because they reduce venous return by permitting pooling of blood in the periphery, decreasing ventricular volume and chamber size, and may cause further obstruction of the outflow tract. Also contraindicated are digoxin and sympathetic stimulators, which enhance cardiac contractility and myocardial demands for oxygen, intensifying the obstruction.

Surgical intervention
If drug therapy fails, surgery may be indicated. Ventricular myotomy (resection of the hypertrophied septum) alone or combined with mitral valve replacement may ease outflow tract obstruction and relieve symptoms. However, ventricular myotomy may cause complications, such as complete heart block and ventricular septal defects. This procedure has mixed results and the long-term effects are unknown.

Dual chamber pacing may prevent progression of hypertrophy and obstruction. Placing the pacing lead in the right ventricular apex, which alters the way the ventricle contracts, theoretically decreasing the outflow obstruction, is being done in many centers and is still being studied for long-term efficacy. Implantable defibrillators may be indicated in patients with malignant ventricular arrhythmias.

Referral
■ Patients who are suspected of having hypertrophic cardiomyopathy should be referred to a cardiologist for evaluation and initiation of treatment.
■ Refer the patient for psychosocial counseling to help him and his family accept his restricted lifestyle and the poor prognosis.

Follow-up
Monthly follow-up is advised or follow-up with the cardiologist.

Patient teaching
■ Advise the patient to follow the medication regimen.
■ Encourage the patient's family to become certified in cardiopulmonary resuscitation.
■ Because syncope or sudden death may follow normal exercise, warn such patients against any strenuous physical activity, such as running or weight lifting.

Complications
■ Atrial fibrillation
■ Sudden death
■ Endocarditis
■ Heart failure or pulmonary edema

Special considerations
■ Before dental work or surgery, administer prophylactic antibiotics for the prevention of subacute bacterial endocarditis.

• • • • • • • • • • • • •

CORONARY ARTERY DISEASE

The primary effect of coronary artery disease (CAD) is the loss of oxygen and nutrients to myocardial tissue because of diminished coronary blood flow. Angina pectoris, a clinical sign of CAD, is defined as pain in the substernal region of the chest and is the result of insufficient oxygen supply to the heart muscle. This disease is near epidemic in the Western world. CAD occurs more often in men than in women, in whites, and in middle-aged and elderly persons. In the past, this disorder seldom affected women who were premenopausal, but this is no longer the case, perhaps because many women now take oral contraceptives, smoke cigarettes, and are employed in stressful jobs that used to be held exclusively by men.

Causes and pathophysiology
Atherosclerosis is the usual cause of CAD. In this form of arteriosclerosis, fatty, fibrous plaques, possibly including calcium deposits, narrow the lumen of the coronary arteries, reduce the volume of blood that can flow through them, and lead to myocardial ischemia. Plaque formation also predisposes to thrombosis, which can provoke myocardial infarction (MI).

Atherosclerosis usually develops in high-flow, high-pressure arteries, such as those in the heart, brain, kidneys, and in the aorta, especially at bifurcation points. It has been linked to many risk factors: family history, hypertension, obesity, smoking, diabetes mellitus, stress, sedentary lifestyle, high serum cholesterol (particularly low-density lipoprotein cholesterol) or triglyceride levels, and low high-density lipoprotein cholesterol levels. In patients with known stable angina, an increase in pain can be precipitated by such problems as anemia, uncontrolled hypertension, atrial fibrillation, and infection. These problems affect the oxygen supply to the heart.

Less common causes of reduced coronary artery blood flow include dis-

Coronary artery spasm

In coronary artery spasm, a spontaneous, sustained contraction of one or more coronary arteries causes ischemia and dysfunction of the heart muscle. This disorder also causes Prinzmetal's angina and even myocardial infarction in patients with unoccluded coronary arteries. Its cause is unknown, but possible contributing factors include:

■ intimal hemorrhage into the medial layer of the blood vessel
■ hyperventilation
■ elevated catecholamine levels
■ fatty buildup in lumen
■ cocaine use.

SIGNS AND SYMPTOMS

The major symptom of coronary artery spasm is angina. Unlike classic angina, however, this pain often occurs spontaneously and may not be related to physical exertion or emotional stress; it's also more severe, usually lasts longer, and may be cyclic, frequently recurring every day at the same time. Such ischemic episodes may cause arrhythmias, altered heart rate, lower blood pressure and, occasionally, fainting due to diminished cardiac output. Spasm in the left coronary artery may result in mitral insufficiency, producing a loud systolic murmur and, possibly, pulmonary edema, with dyspnea, crackles, hemoptysis, or sudden death.

TREATMENT

After diagnosis by coronary angiography and electrocardiography (ECG), the patient may receive calcium channel blockers (verapamil, nifedipine, or diltiazem) to reduce coronary artery spasm and vascular resistance; and nitrates (nitroglycerin or isosorbide dinitrate) to relieve chest pain.

When caring for a patient with coronary artery spasm, explain all necessary procedures and teach him how to take his medications safely. For calcium antagonist therapy, monitor blood pressure, pulse rate, and ECG patterns to detect arrhythmias. For nifedipine and verapamil therapy, monitor digoxin levels and check for signs of digoxin toxicity. Because nifedipine may cause peripheral and periorbital edema, watch for fluid retention.

Because coronary artery spasm is sometimes associated with atherosclerotic disease, advise the patient to stop smoking, avoid overeating, use alcohol sparingly, and maintain a balance between exercise and rest.

---

secting aneurysms, infectious vasculitis, syphilis, and congenital defects in the coronary vascular system. Coronary artery spasms may also impede blood flow. (See *Coronary artery spasm.*)

Clinical presentation

The classic symptom of CAD is angina, which may be accompanied by:

■ nausea
■ vomiting
■ fainting
■ sweating
■ cool extremities.

Anginal episodes most often follow physical exertion but may also follow emotional excitement, exposure to cold, or a large meal.

Angina has three major forms:
■ stable — pain that is predictable in frequency and duration and can be relieved with nitrates and rest

- unstable — pain that increases in frequency and duration and is more easily induced
- Prinzmetal's or variant — causes unpredictable coronary artery spasm.

Severe and prolonged anginal pain generally suggests MI, with potentially fatal arrhythmias and mechanical failure.

Differential diagnoses
- Acute MI
- Esophagitis, esophageal spasm, or peptic or duodenal ulcer disease
- Musculoskeletal pain
- Cholecystitis
- Pulmonary embolus
- Pericarditis
- Costochondritis
- Aortic dissection
- Pleuritis and pneumothorax

Diagnosis
The patient's history — including the frequency and duration of angina and the presence of associated risk factors — is crucial in evaluating CAD. Additional diagnostic measures include:
- Electrocardiography (ECG) during angina may show ischemia and, possibly, arrhythmias such as premature ventricular contractions. The ECG is apt to be normal when the patient is pain-free. Arrhythmias may occur without infarction, secondary to ischemia.
- Treadmill or bicycle exercise test may provoke chest pain and ECG signs of myocardial ischemia.
- Coronary angiography reveals coronary artery stenosis or obstruction, possible collateral circulation, and the arteries' condition beyond the narrowing.
- Myocardial perfusion imaging with thallium-201, Cardiolite, or Myoview during treadmill exercise detects ischemic areas of the myocardium, visualized as "cold spots."

- Stress echocardiography may show wall motion abnormalities.

Management
General
The goal of treatment in patients with angina is to either reduce myocardial oxygen demand or increase oxygen supply.

HEALTHY LIVING Smoking cessation, weight loss, stress avoidance, and a low-fat, low-cholesterol diet are the cornerstones of prevention and treatment. Good control of hypertension and diabetes is important to reduce symptoms and prevent further disease.

Medication
The following nitrates are used in the treatment of CAD:
- nitroglycerin — 0.15 to 0.6 mg given sublingually, or 2.5 to 9 mg P.O. sustained release every 8 to 12 hours; transdermal patches, 0.1 to 0.6 mg/hour with 10 to 14 hours medication-free (This route isn't used routinely.)
- isosorbide dinitrate — 10 to 20 mg P.O. t.i.d. to q.i.d. or 40 mg long-acting P.O. b.i.d.

The following beta-adrenergic blockers are used:
- atenolol — 50 to 100 mg/day P.O.
- propranolol — 10 to 20 mg P.O. t.i.d to q.i.d.; dosage adjusted according to the severity of angina and titrated to a resting heart rate of 50 to 60 beats/minute.

Calcium channel blockers used include:
- amlodipine — 5 to 10 mg/day P.O.
- verapamil — 80 to 120 mg P.O. t.i.d.
- diltiazem CD — 120 to 480 mg/day P.O.

Calcium channel blockers aren't indicated in patients with left ventricular dysfunction. Also, short-acting calcium channel blockers shouldn't be used because they increase cardiac mortality.

Aspirin (325 mg/day P.O.) is indicated for all patients with CAD; 81-mg or coated tablets may be used in patients with a history of peptic ulcer disease or gastritis.

Surgical intervention
Obstructive CAD may necessitate coronary artery bypass grafting and percutaneous transluminal coronary angioplasty (PTCA) to restore blood flow to the myocardium. Surgery is favored for patients with severe CAD (triple vessel disease and decreased left ventricular ejection fraction or left main occlusion) and diabetics with more than one occluded vessel because of improved survival. Internal mammary arteries should be used for the bypasses whenever feasible secondary to superior patency over vein grafts at 10 years. PTCA is preferred for patients with single vessel disease or occlusions amenable to angioplasty.

Referral
- If angina becomes unstable, refer the patient to a cardiologist.

A patient with unstable angina generally needs to be admitted to a hospital for monitoring and diagnostic evaluation.

Follow-up
Frequency of follow-up varies depending on the severity of the disease and the presence or absence of compounding problems, such as hypertension or heart failure. For uncomplicated angina, follow-up every 2 to 4 months should be adequate.

Patient teaching
- Advise the patient to have nitroglycerin available for immediate use.

- Instruct the patient to call immediately whenever he feels chest, arm, or neck pain.
- Advise the patient that nitroglycerin remains maximally effective for 6 months after the bottle is opened.
- Teach the patient how to change any controllable risk factors.

Complications
- MI
- Arrhythmias
- Cardiac arrest
- Heart failure
- Cardiogenic shock
- Death

Special considerations
- Sildenafil shouldn't be prescribed for this population.
- Patients with diabetes and women tend not to experience typical angina and need to be assessed closely for silent ischemia.

• • • • • • • • • • • •

ENDOCARDITIS

Endocarditis (also known as infective or bacterial endocarditis) is an infection of the endocardium, heart valves, or cardiac prosthesis resulting from bacterial or fungal invasion. This invasion produces vegetative growths on the heart valves, endocardial lining of a heart chamber, or endothelium of a blood vessel that may embolize to the spleen, kidneys, central nervous system, and lungs. In endocarditis, fibrin and platelets aggregate on the valve tissue and engulf circulating bacteria or fungi that flourish and produce friable verrucous vegetations. (See *Degenerative changes in endocarditis*, page 100.) Such vegetations may cover the valve surfaces, causing ulceration and necrosis;

Degenerative changes in endocarditis

This illustration depicts typical vegetations on the endocardium produced by fibrin and platelet deposits on infection sites.

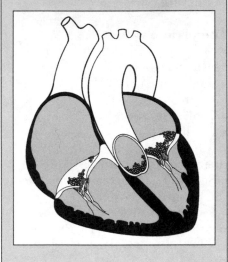

they may also extend to the chordae tendineae, leading to their rupture and subsequent valvular insufficiency. Untreated endocarditis is usually fatal but, with proper treatment, 70% of patients recover. The prognosis is worst when endocarditis causes severe valvular damage, leading to insufficiency and heart failure, or when it involves a prosthetic valve.

Causes

Most commonly, endocarditis occurs in I.V. drug abusers, patients with prosthetic heart valves, those with previous infective endocarditis, and those with degenerative heart disease, mitral valve prolapse with regurgitation, or rheumatic heart disease.

Other predisposing conditions include coarctation of the aorta; tetralogy of Fallot; subaortic and valvular aortic stenosis; ventricular septal defects; pulmonary stenosis; Marfan syndrome; degenerative heart disease, especially calcific aortic stenosis; and, rarely, syphilitic aortic valve. However, some patients with endocarditis have no underlying heart disease.

Infecting organisms differ among these groups. In patients with native valve endocarditis who aren't I.V. drug abusers, causative organisms usually include — in order of frequency — streptococci (especially *Streptococcus viridans*), staphylococci, or enterococci. Although many other bacteria occasionally cause the disorder, fungal causes are rare in this group. The mitral valve is involved most commonly, followed by the aortic valve.

In patients who are I.V. drug abusers, *Staphylococcus aureus* is the most common infecting organism. Less commonly, streptococci, enterococci, gram-negative bacilli, or fungi cause the disorder. The tricuspid valve is involved most commonly, followed by the aortic and then the mitral valve.

In patients with prosthetic valve endocarditis, early cases (those that develop within 60 days of valve insertion) are usually due to staphylococcal infection. However, gram-negative aerobic organisms, fungi, streptococci, enterococci, or diphtheroids may also cause the disorder. The course is usually fulminant and is associated with a high mortality rate. Late cases (occurring after 60 days) present similarly to native valve endocarditis.

Clinical presentation

Endocarditis commonly causes a loud, regurgitant murmur typical of the underlying heart lesion. A suddenly changing murmur or the discovery of a new murmur in the presence of fever is a classic physical sign. Early clinical features of endocarditis are usually nonspecific and include:

- malaise
- weakness
- fatigue
- weight loss
- anorexia
- arthralgia
- night sweats
- chills
- valvular insufficiency
- intermittent fever that may recur for weeks.

A more acute onset is associated with organisms of high pathogenicity, such as *S. aureus*.

In about 30% of patients, embolization from vegetating lesions or diseased valvular tissue may produce the following typical features of splenic, renal, cerebral, or pulmonary infarction or of peripheral vascular occlusion:

- splenic infarction — pain in the left upper quadrant, radiating to the left shoulder, and abdominal rigidity
- renal infarction — hematuria, pyuria, flank pain, and decreased urine output
- cerebral infarction — hemiparesis, aphasia, or other neurologic deficits
- pulmonary infarction (most common in right-sided endocarditis, which commonly occurs among I.V. drug abusers and after cardiac surgery) — cough, pleuritic pain, pleural friction rub, dyspnea, and hemoptysis
- peripheral vascular occlusion — numbness and tingling in an arm, leg, finger, or toe or signs of impending peripheral gangrene.

Other signs may include:

- splenomegaly
- petechiae of the skin (especially common on the upper anterior trunk) and the buccal, pharyngeal, or conjunctival mucosa
- splinter hemorrhages under the nails.

Rare symptoms include:

- Osler's nodes (tender, raised, subcutaneous lesions on the fingers or toes)
- Roth's spots (hemorrhagic areas with white centers on the retina)
- Janeway lesions (purplish macules on the palms or soles).

Acute bacterial endocarditis has a rapid onset, high fevers, and systemic signs of infection. Peripheral signs of endocarditis, with the possible exception of Janeway lesions, aren't often present in acute bacterial endocarditis.

Differential diagnoses
- Pneumonia
- Heart failure
- Fever of unknown origin
- Rheumatic fever
- Lupus erythematosus

Diagnosis
- Echocardiography reveals valvular heart damage and the presence of vegetations and abscesses. It's often necessary to perform a transesophageal echocardiography to better visual the presence of disease. An echocardiogram is also used serially to determine the success or failure of antibiotic treatment.
- Chest X-ray may be normal or show pulmonary edema. It also reveals the presence of prosthetic heart valves.
- Electrocardiography shows hypertrophy, atrioventricular block, or ischemia or infarction in the presence of emboli.
- Three or more blood cultures in a 24- to 48-hour period identify the causative organism in up to 90% of patients. The remaining 10% may have negative blood cultures, possibly suggesting fungal infection or infections that are difficult to diagnose, such as *Haemophilus parainfluenzae*.

Nonspecific laboratory results include:

- normal or elevated white blood cell count
- abnormal histiocytes (macrophages)
- elevated erythrocyte sedimentation rate
- normocytic, normochromic anemia (in 70% to 90% of endocarditis cases)
- positive serum rheumatoid factor (in about one-half of all patients with endocarditis after the disease is present for 3 to 6 weeks)
- serology for *Chlamydia, Coxiella,* and *Bartonella,* which may be useful in negative blood cultures
- urinalysis, which discloses hematuria and proteinuria.

Management
General
Patients with endocarditis may require hospitalization for stabilization of symptoms and initiation of antibiotic therapy. If hemodynamically stable, most patients may be appropriate for outpatient treatment. Close monitoring and follow-up are required. Upon discharge from the health care facility, the patient has a peripherally inserted central catheter or intravascular access device (such as a Hickman catheter) inserted for the duration of I.V. antibiotic therapy. Supportive treatment includes bed rest, aspirin for fever and aches, and sufficient fluid intake.

The goal of treatment is to eradicate the infecting organism. If the patient is hemodynamically stable and not acutely ill, you can wait until cultures are back before starting empiric therapy. If cultures remain negative, repeat blood cultures and start empiric therapy.

Medication
Empiric therapy for native valve includes either of the following regimens:

- penicillin G — 12 to 24 million U I.V. or I.M. q.d. in divided doses every 4 hours, *or* ampicillin, 12 g/day I.V. in divided doses every 4 hours, in addition to nafcillin or oxacillin, 2 to 12 g I.V. every 4 hours, *or* gentamicin, 1 mg/kg I.V. every 8 hours
- vancomycin — 15 mg/kg I.V. every 12 hours (not to exceed 2 g/day), in addition to gentamicin, 1 mg/kg I.V. every 8 hours.

Empiric therapy for prosthetic valve includes vancomycin, 15 mg/kg I.V. every 12 hours, in addition to gentamicin, 1 mg/kg I.V. every 8 hours, and rifampin, 300 mg every 8 hours.

When blood cultures reveal an infecting organism, modify the regimen based on results. Duration of treatment is 2 to 8 weeks, depending on the type of valve and the organism involved.

Antimicrobial prophylaxis, which is required prior to certain procedures, consists of amoxicillin, 3 g P.O. 1 hour prior to the procedure and 1.5 g 6 hours later, or 2 g P.O. 1 hour prior to procedure.

For patients with penicillin allergies, use one of the following drugs 1 hour before the procedure for antimicrobial prophylaxis:

- clindamycin — 600 mg P.O. or I.V.
- azithromycin — 500 mg P.O.
- clarithromycin — 500 mg P.O.

Surgical intervention
Severe valvular damage, especially aortic or mitral insufficiency, may necessitate corrective surgery if refractory heart failure develops or in cases in which an infected prosthetic valve must be replaced.

Referral
- Any patient with suspected endocarditis should be referred to a cardiologist or infectious disease specialist.

Follow-up
Close follow-up is imperative to allow for monitoring the effectiveness of antibiotic therapy and to observe for complications, especially the development of heart failure. Additionally, relapse or reinfection is fairly common and requires monitoring for up to 8 weeks posttreatment. Patients should have serial echocardiograms to determine resolution of vegetations or abscesses and to assess valvular function.

Monitor blood urea nitrogen and creatinine levels twice per week while the patient is taking gentamicin.

Patient teaching
- Inform the patient that he needs to relate any history of heart disease that would make him susceptible to endocarditis when receiving any invasive procedures. Prophylactic antibiotics should be administered in these situations.
- Inform the patient that he needs to complete all antibiotic therapy as prescribed.
- Instruct the patient on how to recognize symptoms of endocarditis and to report them immediately.

Complications
- Death
- Heart failure
- Aortic root abscesses
- Myocardial abscesses
- Pericarditis
- Cardiac arrhythmia
- Meningitis
- Cerebral emboli
- Brain abscesses
- Septic pulmonary infarcts
- Arthritis
- Glomerulonephritis
- Acute renal failure

Special considerations
- In staphylococcal endocarditis, fever and positive blood cultures may persist for up to 10 days.
- In streptococcal endocarditis, there should be a clinical response within approximately 48 hours.
- The following procedures require prophylaxis: Dental work that is likely to cause bleeding (root canal, periodontal work, oral surgery, extractions, major cleaning and scaling), tonsillectomy and adenoidectomy, rigid bronchoscopy, endoscopy with biopsy, sclerotherapy of esophageal varices, esophageal dilatation, gallbladder surgery, surgeries involving infected tissue or abscesses, prostate surgery, urethral dilatation or catheterization, and cystoscopy. The following are optional for high-risk patients: vaginal delivery or hysterectomy and transesophageal echocardiography.

• • • • • • • • • • • •

HEART FAILURE

Heart failure is a syndrome characterized by myocardial dysfunction that leads to impaired pump performance (diminished cardiac output) or to frank heart failure and abnormal circulatory congestion. Congestion of systemic venous circulation may result in peripheral edema or hepatomegaly; congestion of pulmonary circulation may cause pulmonary edema, an acute life-threatening emergency. Pump failure usually occurs in a damaged left ventricle (left-sided heart failure) but can occur in the right ventricle (right-sided heart failure) either as a primary disorder or secondary to left-sided heart failure. Sometimes, left- and right-sided heart failure develop simultaneously (see *What happens in heart failure.*)

Although heart failure may be acute (as a direct result of myocardial infarction [MI]), it's generally a chronic disorder associated with retention of sodium and water by the kidneys. Advances in diagnostic and therapeutic techniques have greatly improved the outlook for patients with heart failure, but the prognosis still depends on the underlying cause and the response to treatment.

Heart failure affects approximately 2 million people in the United States with a mortality rate of 10% after 1 year and 50% after 5 years. The greatest incidence of heart failure occurs after age 65.

Causes and pathophysiology

Heart failure may result from a primary abnormality of the heart muscle (such as an infarction), inadequate myocardial perfusion due to coronary artery disease, or cardiomyopathy. Other causes include:
■ diastolic dysfunction, preserved ejection fraction, or impairment of ventricular filling by diminished relaxation or reduced compliance seen with hypertrophic cardiomyopathy, myocardial hypertrophy, and pericardial restriction
■ mechanical disturbances in ventricular filling during diastole when there is too little blood for the ventricle to pump, as in mitral stenosis secondary to rheumatic heart disease or constrictive pericarditis and atrial fibrillation
■ systolic hemodynamic disturbances, such as excessive cardiac workload due to volume overload or pressure overload, that limit the heart's pumping ability; these disturbances can result from mitral or aortic insufficiency, which causes volume overload, and aortic stenosis or systemic hypertension, which results in increased resistance to ventricular emptying.

Reduced cardiac output triggers compensatory mechanisms, such as ventricular dilation, hypertrophy, increased sympathetic activity, and activation of the renin-angiotensin-aldosterone system. These mechanisms improve cardiac output at the expense of increased ventricular work. In cardiac dilation, an increase in end-diastolic ventricular volume (preload) causes increased stroke work and stroke volume during contraction, stretching cardiac muscle fibers beyond optimum limits and producing pulmonary congestion and pulmonary hypertension, which in turn lead to right-sided heart failure.

In ventricular hypertrophy, an increase in muscle mass or the diameter of the left ventricle allows the heart to pump against increased resistance (impedance) to the outflow of blood. An increase in ventricular diastolic pressure necessary to fill the enlarged ventricle may compromise diastolic coronary blood flow, limiting the oxygen supply to the ventricle and causing ischemia and impaired muscle contractility.

Increased sympathetic activity occurs as a response to decreased cardiac output and blood pressure by enhancing peripheral vascular resistance, contractility, heart rate, and venous return. Signs of increased sympathetic activity, such as cool extremities and clamminess, may indicate impending heart failure. Increased sympathetic activity also restricts blood flow to the kidneys, which respond by reducing the glomerular filtration rate and increasing tubular reabsorption of salt and water, in turn expanding the circulating blood volume. This renal mechanism, if unchecked, can aggravate congestion and produce overt edema.

Chronic heart failure may worsen as a result of respiratory tract infections, pulmonary embolism, stress, increased

What happens in heart failure

Heart failure occurs when cardiac output is inadequate to meet the body's needs. The pathophysiology of heart failure is illustrated in the flow chart below.

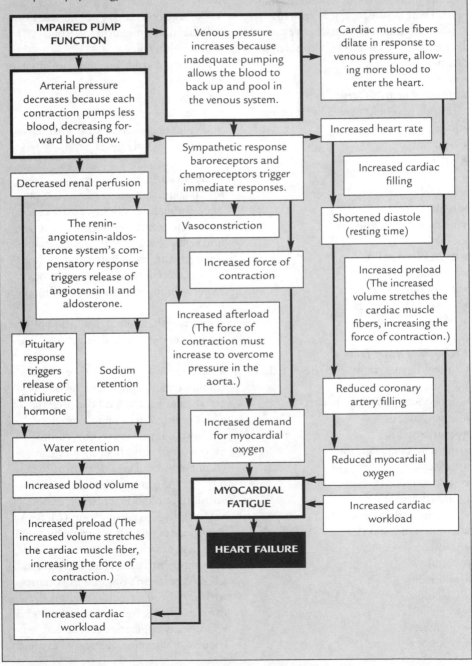

sodium or water intake, or failure to adhere to the prescribed treatment regimen.

Clinical presentation

Left-sided heart failure produces primarily pulmonary signs and symptoms; right-sided heart failure produces primarily systemic signs and symptoms. However, heart failure often affects both sides of the heart.

Left-sided heart failure

Clinical signs of left-sided heart failure include:

- dyspnea
- orthopnea
- crackles
- possibly wheezing
- hypoxia
- respiratory acidosis
- cough
- cyanosis or pallor
- palpitations
- arrhythmias
- elevated blood pressure
- pulsus alternans.

Right-sided heart failure

Clinical signs of right-sided heart failure include:

- dependent peripheral edema
- hepatomegaly
- splenomegaly
- jugular vein distention
- ascites
- slow weight gain
- arrhythmias
- hepatojugular reflex
- abdominal distention
- nausea
- vomiting
- anorexia
- weakness
- fatigue
- dizziness
- syncope.

Differential diagnoses

- MI
- Valvular disease
- Hypertrophic cardiomyopathy
- Complete heart block or bradyrhythmias
- Chronic obstructive pulmonary disease
- Pulmonary embolism
- Cor pulmonale
- Nephrotic syndrome or acute glomerulonephritis
- Cirrhosis
- Asthma
- Venous occlusive disease with subsequent peripheral edema

Diagnosis

- Echocardiography confirms the presence of dilated cardiomyopathy and assesses left ventricular ejection fraction and right ventricular function, chamber enlargement, heart valve dysfunction, wall motion abnormalities, pulmonary hypertension, and estimated filling pressures.
- Exercise thallium-201 scintigraphy may identify underlying coronary artery disease.
- Electrocardiography may reveal biventricular hypertrophy, sinus tachycardia, atrial enlargement, and the presence of atrial fibrillation or bundle-branch block.
- Chest X-ray demonstrates cardiomegaly—usually affecting all heart chambers—and may demonstrate pulmonary congestion, pleural or pericardial effusion, or pulmonary hypertension.
- Multiple-gated acquisition (MUGA) scanning reveals left ventricle and right ventricle muscle performance and calculates left ventricular ejection fraction. A MUGA scan isn't optimal in patients with rapid and irregular rhythms because the scan is triggered by the R-R interval.
- Coronary angiogram reveals left ventricular dysfunction, decreased cardiac

output and ejection fraction, valvular (mitral and tricuspid) regurgitation if present, and elevated filling pressures.

Management
General
The aim of therapy is to improve pump function by reversing the compensatory mechanisms producing the clinical effects.

Nonpharmacologic therapy consists of checking daily weights, restricting sodium (less than 2 g/day), and restricting fluid (especially in the setting of hyponatremia). Immunizations against influenza and pneumococcal pneumonia are strongly encouraged.

Medication
Standard therapy for heart failure consists of a combination of the following medications:
- spironolactone—25 to 200 mg/day P.O.
- furosemide—20 to 80 mg/day P.O. up to 600 mg/day in divided doses
- hydrochlorothiazide—25 to 100 mg/day P.O.
- warfarin—2 to 5 mg/day P.O. for 2 to 4 days; then dosage based on a target INR of 2.0 to 3.5
- amiodarone— loading dose of 800 to 1,600 mg/day P.O. for 1 to 3 weeks. Reduce to 600 to 800 mg/day for 1 month. Maintenance dose is 200 to 600 mg/day P.O.

Surgical intervention
Left ventricular remodeling surgery may be performed. This surgical technique involves cutting a wedge about the size of a small slice of pie out of the left ventricle of an enlarged heart. The remainder of the heart is sewn together. The result is a smaller organ that is able to pump blood more efficiently. This procedure offers promising results, especially for those whose only alternative may be a heart transplant.

Referral
- Ventricular arrhythmias should be evaluated by a cardiologist or an electrophysiologist for risk stratification and arrhythmia inducibility and appropriate medical therapy or implantation of an internal cardiac defibrillator.
- If the patient is having trouble with dietary restrictions, refer him to a nutritionist.

Follow-up
All patients with a new diagnosis of heart failure should have a cardiology referral. Once the patient is stable, you may follow the patient and alter the regimen as needed. Initial follow-up should be within 24 hours of any hospital discharge and then every 1 to 3 weeks until the patient is stable. Once stable, the patient should be monitored every 3 months.

Patient teaching
- Teach the patient about the need for fluid and sodium dietary restrictions.
- Advise the patient to monitor his weight daily as a way to detect fluid retention.
- Emphasize the importance of taking digoxin exactly as prescribed. Tell the patient to watch for and immediately report signs of toxicity, such as anorexia, vomiting, and yellow vision.
- Tell the patient to promptly report any pulse irregularities. He should also report dizziness, blurred vision, shortness of breath, persistent dry cough, palpitations, increased fatigue, paroxysmal nocturnal dyspnea, swollen ankles, decreased urine output, and rapid weight gain (5 to 21 lb [2.25 to 9.5 kg] in 1 week).

Complications
- Electrolyte imbalance
- Atrial and ventricular arrhythmias
- Mesenteric insufficiency
- Digoxin toxicity
- Pulmonary embolism
- Renal failure
- Death
- Cor pulmonale

Special considerations
- Closely follow chest X-rays and electrolyte, blood urea nitrogen, and creatinine levels for changes that may indicate worsening heart failure.
- Consider initiating discussions regarding advanced directives and patient wishes about end-of-life care.

• • • • • • • • • • • •

HYPERTENSION

Hypertension, an intermittent or sustained elevation in diastolic or systolic blood pressure, occurs as two major types: essential (idiopathic) hypertension, the most common, and secondary hypertension, which results from renal disease or another identifiable cause. Malignant hypertension is a severe, fulminant form of hypertension common to both types. Hypertension is a major cause of cerebrovascular accident, cardiac disease, and renal failure. The prognosis is good if this disorder is detected early and treatment begins before complications develop. Severely elevated blood pressure (hypertensive crisis) may be fatal. (See *What happens in hypertensive crisis.*)

Causes and pathophysiology
Hypertension affects 15% to 20% of adults in the United States. If untreated, it carries a high mortality. Risk factors for hypertension include family history, race (most common in blacks), stress, obesity, a high intake of saturated fats or sodium, use of tobacco and alcohol, sedentary lifestyle, and aging. Over 90% of hypertension has no identified causes.

Secondary hypertension may result from renal vascular disease; pheochromocytoma; primary hyperaldosteronism; Cushing's syndrome; thyroid, pituitary, or parathyroid dysfunction; coarctation of the aorta; pregnancy; neurologic disorders; and use of oral contraceptives or other drugs, such as cocaine, epoetin alfa (erythropoietin), and cyclosporine.

Cardiac output and peripheral vascular resistance determine blood pressure. Increased blood volume, cardiac rate, and stroke volume as well as arteriolar vasoconstriction can raise blood pressure. The link to sustained hypertension, however, is unclear. Hypertension may also result from failure of intrinsic regulatory mechanisms:
- Renal hypoperfusion causes release of renin, which is converted by angiotensinogen, a liver enzyme, to angiotensin I. Angiotensin I is converted to angiotensin II, a powerful vasoconstrictor. The resulting vasoconstriction increases afterload. Angiotensin II stimulates adrenal secretion of aldosterone, which increases sodium reabsorption. Hypertonic-stimulated release of antidiuretic hormone from the pituitary gland follows, increasing water reabsorption, plasma volume, cardiac output, and blood pressure.
- Autoregulation changes the diameter of an artery to maintain perfusion despite fluctuations in systemic blood pressure. The intrinsic mechanisms responsible include stress relaxation (vessels gradually dilate when blood pressure rises to reduce peripheral resistance) and capillary fluid shift (plasma moves between vessels and extravascular spaces to maintain intravascular volume).

What happens in hypertensive crisis

Hypertensive crisis is a severe rise in arterial blood pressure caused by a disturbance in one or more of the regulating mechanisms. If left untreated, hypertensive crisis may result in renal, cardiac, or cerebral complications and, possibly, death.

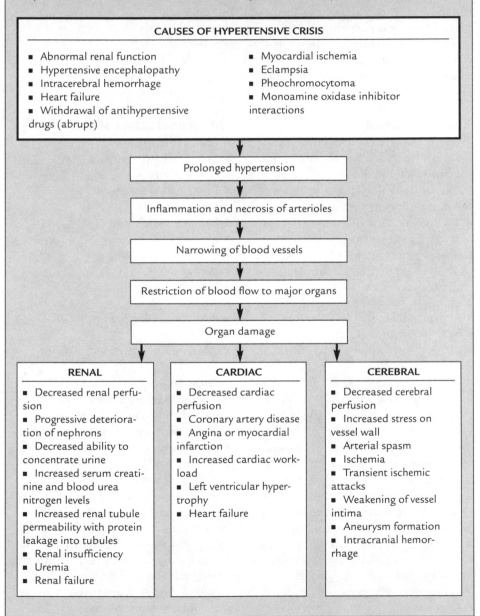

CAUSES OF HYPERTENSIVE CRISIS

- Abnormal renal function
- Hypertensive encephalopathy
- Intracerebral hemorrhage
- Heart failure
- Withdrawal of antihypertensive drugs (abrupt)

- Myocardial ischemia
- Eclampsia
- Pheochromocytoma
- Monoamine oxidase inhibitor interactions

Prolonged hypertension

Inflammation and necrosis of arterioles

Narrowing of blood vessels

Restriction of blood flow to major organs

Organ damage

RENAL

- Decreased renal perfusion
- Progressive deterioration of nephrons
- Decreased ability to concentrate urine
- Increased serum creatinine and blood urea nitrogen levels
- Increased renal tubule permeability with protein leakage into tubules
- Renal insufficiency
- Uremia
- Renal failure

CARDIAC

- Decreased cardiac perfusion
- Coronary artery disease
- Angina or myocardial infarction
- Increased cardiac workload
- Left ventricular hypertrophy
- Heart failure

CEREBRAL

- Decreased cerebral perfusion
- Increased stress on vessel wall
- Arterial spasm
- Ischemia
- Transient ischemic attacks
- Weakening of vessel intima
- Aneurysm formation
- Intracranial hemorrhage

- When the blood pressure drops, baroreceptors in the aortic arch and carotid sinuses decrease their inhibition of the medulla's vasomotor center, which increases sympathetic stimulation of the heart by norepinephrine. This, in turn, increases cardiac output by strengthening the contractile force, increasing the heart rate, and augmenting peripheral resistance by vasoconstriction. Stress can also stimulate the sympathetic nervous system to increase cardiac output and peripheral vascular resistance.

Clinical presentation

Hypertension usually doesn't produce clinical effects until vascular changes in the heart, brain, or kidneys occur. Severely elevated blood pressure damages the intima of small vessels, resulting in fibrin accumulation in the vessels, development of local edema and, possibly, intravascular clotting. Symptoms produced by this process depend on the location of the damaged vessels:

- brain — cerebrovascular accident
- retina — blindness
- heart — myocardial infarction (MI)
- kidneys — proteinuria, edema and, eventually, renal failure.

Hypertension increases the heart's workload, causing left ventricular hypertrophy and, later, left- and right-sided heart failure and pulmonary edema.

Hypertensive crisis is a disorder in which diastolic blood pressure is greater than 120 to 130 mm Hg. Hypertensive urgency exists when the blood pressure is greatly elevated without acute or progressing target organ damage. Hypertensive emergency is when there's not only elevated blood pressure but also acute or progressing target organ damage.

Examples of hypertensive emergencies include:

- hypertensive encephalopathy

- intracranial hemorrhage
- acute left-sided heart failure with pulmonary edema
- dissecting aortic aneurysm.

Hypertensive emergencies are also associated with:

- eclampsia and severe pregnancy-related hypertension
- unstable angina
- acute MI.

Any hypertensive emergency should be evaluated and treated by the collaborating physician.

Differential diagnoses

- Primary hypertension
- Secondary hypertension
- Renal failure
- Primary aldosteronism
- Drug reaction
- Cushing's syndrome
- Pheochromocytoma
- Headaches and dizziness from other causes
- Hyperthyroidism
- Anxiety
- Arteriovascular disease
- Alcohol abuse
- Coarctation of the aorta

Diagnosis

Serial blood pressure measurements are obtained and compared with previous readings and trends to reveal an increase in diastolic and systolic pressures. (See *Classifying blood pressure readings.*)

Auscultation may reveal bruits over the abdominal aorta and the carotid, renal, and femoral arteries; ophthalmoscopy reveals arteriovenous nicking and, in hypertensive encephalopathy, papilledema. Patient history and the following additional tests may show predisposing factors and help identify an underlying cause such as renal disease.

Classifying blood pressure readings

In 1997, the National Institutes of Health issued a revised method of classifying blood pressure according to stages. The former categories — mild, moderate, severe, and very severe — were replaced by stages 1 through 4, respectively, in part because the old terms "mild" and "moderate" failed to convey the true impact of high blood pressure on the risk of developing cardiovascular disease.

The revised categories are based on the average of two or more readings taken on separate visits after an initial screening. They apply to adults age 18 and older who aren't taking antihypertensives and aren't acutely ill. (If the systolic and diastolic pressures fall into different categories, use the higher of the two pressures to classify the reading. For example, a reading of 160/92 mm Hg should be classified as stage 2.)

Optimal blood pressure with respect to cardiovascular risk is a systolic reading below 120 mm Hg and a diastolic reading below 80 mm Hg. Isolated systolic hypertension is defined as a systolic blood pressure of 140 mm Hg or higher and a diastolic pressure lower than 90 mm Hg.

In addition to classifying stages of hypertension based on average blood pressure readings, clinicians should also take note of target organ disease and any additional risk factors. For example, a patient with diabetes, left ventricular hypertrophy, and a blood pressure reading of 144/98 mm Hg would be classified as "stage I hypertension with target-organ disease (left ventricular hypertrophy) and another major risk factor (diabetes)." This additional information is important to obtain a true picture of the patient's cardiovascular health.

CATEGORY	SYSTOLIC	DIASTOLIC
Normal	< 130 mm Hg	< 85 mm Hg
High normal	130 to 139 mm Hg	85 to 89 mm Hg
Hypertension Stage 1 (mild) hypertension	140 to 159 mm Hg	90 to 99 mm Hg
Stage 2 (moderate) hypertension	160 to 179 mm Hg	100 to 109 mm Hg
Stage 3 (severe) hypertension	180 to 209 mm Hg	110 to 119 mm Hg
Stage 4 (very severe) hypertension	≥ 210 mm Hg	≥ 120 mm Hg

■ Urinalysis: Protein levels and red and white blood cell counts may indicate glomerulonephritis.
■ Excretory urography: Renal atrophy indicates chronic renal disease; one kidney more than ⅝" (1.5 cm) shorter than the other suggests unilateral renal disease.
■ Serum potassium: Levels under 3.5 mEq/L may indicate adrenal dysfunction (primary hyperaldosteronism).

- Blood urea nitrogen (BUN) and serum creatinine: A BUN level that is normal or elevated to more than 20 mg/dl and a serum creatinine level that is normal or elevated to more than 1.5 mg/dl suggest renal disease.

Other tests help detect cardiovascular damage and other complications:
- Electrocardiography may show left ventricular hypertrophy or ischemia.
- Chest X-ray may show cardiomegaly.
- Echocardiography may show left ventricular hypertrophy.
- Oral captopril challenge test or captopril renogram for renovascular hypertension is a functional diagnostic test that depends on the abrupt inhibition of circulating angiotensin II by angiotensin-converting enzyme (ACE) inhibitors, removing the major support for perfusion through a stenotic renal artery. The acutely ischemic kidney immediately releases more renin and undergoes a marked decrease in glomerular filtration rate and renal blood flow.
- Renal arteriography may show renal artery stenosis.

Management
General
The National Institutes of Health recommends a stepped-care approach. (See *Stepped-care approach to antihypertensive therapy.*)
- Treatment of secondary hypertension focuses on correcting the underlying cause and controlling hypertensive effects.

Medication
A patient with hypertension without accompanying symptoms or target organ disease seldom requires emergency drug therapy. Multidrug therapy is often needed to obtain adequate control of blood pressure. The following medications are used to treat patients with hypertension:

Diuretics include:
- hydrochlorothiazide — 12.5 to 50 mg/day P.O.
- chlorthalidone — adults, 25 to 100 mg/day P.O.; children, 2 mg/kg/day P.O. three times weekly.

Beta-adrenergic blockers include:
- propranolol — 40 to 240 mg/day P.O. in divided doses
- atenolol — 50 to 100 mg/day P.O.

Calcium channel blockers include:
- nifedipine — 30 to 120 mg/day P.O. (extended-release tablets)
- diltiazem — 60 to 120 mg P.O. b.i.d.; sustained release.

ACE inhibitors include:
- quinapril — 5 to 20 mg P.O. b.i.d., if also taking a diuretic; 10 to 80 mg/day P.O., if not
- captopril — 25 to 50 mg P.O. b.i.d. or t.i.d.

Vasodilators include:
- hydralazine — 10 to 50 mg P.O. q.i.d.
- clonidine — 0.1 to 0.6 mg/day P.O. in divided doses.

Alpha-adrenergic blockers include:
- labetalol — 100 to 400 mg P.O. b.i.d.
- terazosin — 1 to 20 mg/day P.O.

Hypertensive emergencies require parenteral administration of a vasodilator or an adrenergic inhibitor or oral administration of a selected drug, such as nifedipine, captopril, clonidine, or labetalol, to rapidly reduce blood pressure. The initial goal is to reduce mean arterial blood pressure by no more than 25% (within minutes to hours), then to 160/110 within 2 hours, while avoiding excessive falls in blood pressure that can precipitate renal, cerebral, or myocardial ischemia. Dosage would be guided by presenting blood pressure and response to administered medications.

Stepped-care approach to antihypertensive therapy

The diagram below illustrates the four-step approach to antihypertensive therapy that is recommended by the National Institutes of Health for treating pulmonary hypertension. The progression of therapy is based on the patient's response, which is defined in two ways: the patient has achieved the target blood pressure set by the health care provider, or the patient is making considerable progress toward the goal.

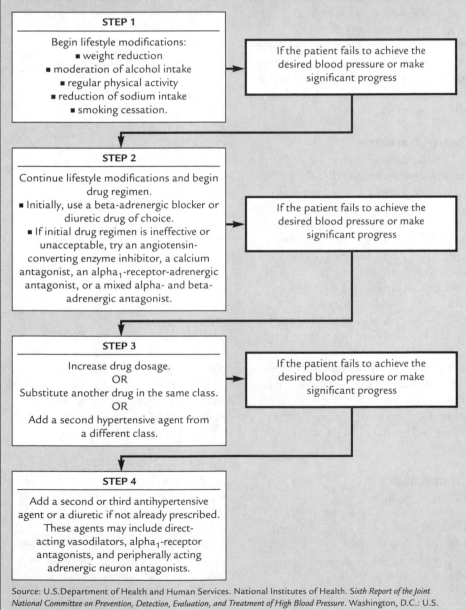

STEP 1

Begin lifestyle modifications:
- weight reduction
- moderation of alcohol intake
- regular physical activity
- reduction of sodium intake
- smoking cessation.

If the patient fails to achieve the desired blood pressure or make significant progress

STEP 2

Continue lifestyle modifications and begin drug regimen.
- Initially, use a beta-adrenergic blocker or diuretic drug of choice.
- If initial drug regimen is ineffective or unacceptable, try an angiotensin-converting enzyme inhibitor, a calcium antagonist, an $alpha_1$-receptor-adrenergic antagonist, or a mixed alpha- and beta-adrenergic antagonist.

If the patient fails to achieve the desired blood pressure or make significant progress

STEP 3

Increase drug dosage.
OR
Substitute another drug in the same class.
OR
Add a second hypertensive agent from a different class.

If the patient fails to achieve the desired blood pressure or make significant progress

STEP 4

Add a second or third antihypertensive agent or a diuretic if not already prescribed. These agents may include direct-acting vasodilators, $alpha_1$-receptor antagonists, and peripherally acting adrenergic neuron antagonists.

Source: U.S. Department of Health and Human Services. National Institutes of Health. *Sixth Report of the Joint National Committee on Prevention, Detection, Evaluation, and Treatment of High Blood Pressure.* Washington, D.C.: U.S. Government Printing Office, 1997.

Referral
- Refer the patient to local support programs for individuals with hypertension.
- In episodes of hypertensive crisis, refer the patient to the emergency department for immediate I.V. treatment.

Follow-up
The patient should be monitored every 1 to 2 weeks until the target blood pressure is achieved, then every month for 3 months, then every 6 months indefinitely, unless the blood pressure becomes unstable. Creatinine and potassium levels and urinalysis should be evaluated annually as part of a screening panel.

Patient teaching
- To encourage adherence to antihypertensive therapy, suggest that the patient establish a daily routine for taking his medication. Warn that uncontrolled hypertension may cause stroke and heart attack. Tell him to report adverse drug effects. Also, advise him to avoid high-sodium antacids and over-the-counter cold and sinus medications, which contain harmful vasoconstrictors.
- Help the patient examine and modify his lifestyle to reduce risk factors as appropriate.
- Emphasize the asymptomatic nature of hypertension and the importance of lifetime treatment.
- Review the patient's present dietary habits and suggest changes as appropriate.

Complications
- Angina pectoris
- Heart failure or cardiomyopathy
- Transient ischemic attack or stroke
- Renal failure
- Hypertensive heart disease
- Poor response to therapy
- Blindness

Special considerations
- Diuretics may worsen gout and diabetes.
- Beta-adrenergic blockers are contraindicated in severe reactive airway disease and type II heart block or sick sinus syndrome.
- ACE-I can be used in renovascular disease but follow renal function closely.

• • • • • • • • • • • •
MYOCARDIAL INFARCTION

Myocardial infarction (MI), commonly known as a heart attack, results from prolonged myocardial ischemia due to reduced blood flow through one of the coronary arteries. In cardiovascular disease, the leading cause of death in the United States and Western Europe, death usually results from the cardiac damage or complications of MI. Mortality is high when treatment is delayed, and almost half of sudden deaths due to MI occur before hospitalization, within 1 hour of the onset of symptoms. An MI is an acute situation that requires hospitalization in an intensive or coronary care unit. Prognosis improves if vigorous treatment begins immediately. Men and postmenopausal women are more susceptible to MI than premenopausal women, although incidence is rising among females, especially those who smoke and take oral contraceptives.

Causes and pathophysiology
Predisposing risk factors include:
- positive family history
- hypertension
- smoking
- elevated serum triglyceride, total cholesterol, and low-density lipoprotein levels
- diabetes mellitus

- obesity or excessive intake of saturated fats, carbohydrates, or salt
- sedentary lifestyle
- stress or a type A personality (aggressive, ambitious, competitive, addicted to work, and chronically impatient)
- drug use, especially cocaine.

HEALTHY LIVING If possible, reduce risk factors for MI. Additionally, one baby aspirin per day (81 mg) is recommended to impede clotting in blood vessels.

The site of the MI depends on the vessels involved. Occlusion of the circumflex branch of the left coronary artery causes a lateral wall infarction; occlusion of the anterior descending branch of the left coronary artery causes an anterior wall infarction. True posterior or inferior wall infarctions generally result from occlusion of the right coronary artery or one of its branches. Right ventricular infarctions can also result from right coronary artery occlusion, can accompany inferior infarctions, and may cause right-sided heart failure. In Q-wave (transmural) MI, tissue damage extends through all myocardial layers; in non–Q-wave (subendocardial) MI, tissue damage occurs only in the innermost and possibly the middle layers.

Clinical presentation

The cardinal symptom of MI is persistent, crushing substernal pain that may radiate to the left arm, jaw, neck, or shoulder blades. Such pain is often described as heavy, squeezing, or crushing and may persist for 12 hours or more. However, in some MI patients — particularly elderly or diabetic — pain may not occur at all; in others, it may be mild and confused with indigestion. In patients with coronary artery disease, angina of increasing frequency, severity, or duration (especially if not provoked by exertion, a

heavy meal, or cold and wind) that is unrelieved by nitroglycerin may signal impending infarction.

Other clinical effects include:
- a feeling of impending doom
- fatigue
- nausea
- vomiting
- shortness of breath.

Some patients may have no symptoms.

The patient may experience catecholamine responses, such as:
- coolness in the extremities
- perspiration
- anxiety
- restlessness.

Fever is unusual at the onset of an MI, but a low-grade temperature elevation may develop during the next few days. Blood pressure varies; hypotension or hypertension may be present.

Differential diagnoses

- Unstable angina pectoris
- Pericarditis
- Myocarditis
- Acute aortic dissection
- Pneumothorax
- Pulmonary embolism
- Acute cholecystitis
- Esophageal spasm or reflux disease

Diagnosis

Persistent chest pain, elevated ST segment on the electrocardiogram (ECG), and elevated total creatine kinase (CK) and CK-MB levels over a 72-hour period usually confirm MI. Tropin T or troponin are also used in the diagnosis because both are specific to cardiac necrosis and levels rise 6 to 8 hours after onset of ischemia.

When clinical features are equivocal, assume that the patient had an MI until tests rule it out. Diagnostic laboratory results include:

■ serial 12-lead ECG—ECG abnormalities may be absent or inconclusive during the first few hours after an MI; when present, characteristic abnormalities include serial ST-segment depression in non–Q-wave (subendocardial) MI and ST-segment elevation in Q-wave (transmural) MI

■ serial serum enzyme levels—elevated CK and CK-MB levels or troponin levels

■ echocardiography—may show ventricular wall motion abnormalities in patients with a Q-wave (transmural) MI

■ angiogram—determine presence of thrombus or occlusive coronary disease

■ nuclear cardiology perfusion studies—identify damaged muscle by picking up radioactive nucleotide, which appears as a "hot spot" on the film. They're useful in localizing heart muscle defects, but aren't specific for acute MI.

Management
General
The goals of treatment are to relieve chest pain, stabilize heart rhythm, reduce cardiac workload, revascularize the coronary artery, and preserve myocardial tissue. Arrhythmias, the predominant problem during the first 48 hours after the infarction, may require antiarrhythmics, possibly a pacemaker and, rarely, cardioversion. Oxygen is administered at a modest flow rate for 3 to 6 hours (a lower concentration is necessary if the patient has chronic obstructive pulmonary disease).

Cardiac rehabilitation is a key component. Its aims are to improve the functional capacity in patients with known heart disease and to intervene to prevent the progression of the coronary atherosclerotic process.

Medication
Treatment depends on the clinical symptoms and extent of complications of MI. The management plan for a patient with MI may be complex and include the following medications.

Analgesics include:

■ nitroglycerin—0.15 to 0.6 mg S.L.; may repeat every 5 minutes for three doses *or* 20 to 100 mcg/minute I.V., for pain control

■ morphine sulfate—2 to 4 mg I.V. every 1 to 2 hours, p.r.n.

Antiplatelet-active drugs include aspirin (160 to 325 mg P.O.), which should be given immediately at onset of symptoms.

Thrombolytics (if appropriate) include:

■ alteplase—adults weighing more than 143 lb (65 kg), 60 mg in 1st hour, with 6 to 10 mg I.V. bolus over 1st 1 to 2 minutes; then 20 mg/hr for an additional 2 hours. Total dose is 100 mg. Adults weighing less than 143 lbs, 1.25 mg/kg given over 3 hours as described above.

■ streptokinase—loading dose of 20,000 IU I.V. bolus, then infusion of 2,000 IU/minute over 60 minutes; (via coronary catheter).

Anticoagulants include:

■ heparin I.V. infusion therapy—initially 5,000 U I.V. bolus, then 750 to 1,500 U/hour by I.V. infusion; hourly rate then titrated every 8 hours based on patient's results

■ enoxaparin—1 mg/kg S.C. b.i.d. 5 to 7 days.

Antiarrhythmics include:

■ lidocaine—1 to 1.5 mg/kg I.V. bolus, then I.V. infusion of 1 to 4 mg/minute

■ amiodarone—loading dose 150 I.V. infusion over 10 minutes, then 360 mg over the next 6 hours followed by 540 mg over next 18 hours; after 24 hours, maintenance I.V. infusion of 720 mg/24 hours.

Beta-adrenergic blockers include:
- atenolol — 5 mg I.V. over 5 minutes, then another 5 mg after 10 minutes. After an additional 10 minutes, 50 mg P.O., then 50 mg P.O. in 12 hours, then 100 mg/day P.O. for at least 7 days
- propranolol — 180 to 240 mg/day P.O. in divided doses beginning 5 to 21 days after MI.

Angiotensin-converting enzyme inhibitors include:
- captopril — initially 6.25 to 12.5 mg P.O. t.i.d.; gradually increase to 50 mg P.O. t.i.d.
- quinapril — 5 to 20 mg P.O. b.i.d.

Calcium channel blockers include:
- nifedipine — 10 to 20 mg P.O. t.i.d.
- diltiazem — 30 mg to a maximum of 360 mg/day P.O. in divided doses t.i.d. to q.i.d.

Inotropic agents include:
- digoxin — loading dose is 0.5 to 1 mg I.V. or P.O. in divided doses over 24 hours. Maintenance dose is 0.125 to 0.5 mg/day I.V. infusion or P.O.
- inamrinone — 0.75 mg/kg I.V. bolus, then maintenance I.V. infusion of 5 to 10 mcg/kg/minute.

Surgical intervention
If PTCA is performed soon after the onset of symptoms, the thrombolytic agent may be administered directly into the coronary artery.

Referral
- Refer the patient to a cardiologist when an MI is suspected.
- Provide counseling referrals as needed. Depression is common in post-MI patients.
- Refer the patient to a cardiac rehabilitation program.
- For information and support, refer the patient and family to the American Heart Association.

Follow-up
Follow-up is determined by the needs of the patient. He should be seen 1 week posthospitalization, then 3 to 6 weeks later for an exercise stress test. A follow-up ECG should be done after 3 months.

Additionally, the patient should be monitored for depression.

Patient teaching
- Promote adherence measures by thoroughly explaining the prescribed medication regimen and other treatment measures.
- Instruct the patient in dietary restrictions. If he must follow a low-sodium or low-fat and low-cholesterol diet, provide a list of foods that he should avoid. Refer the patient to a dietitian.
- Advise the patient to resume sexual activity progressively.
- Advise the patient to report typical or atypical chest pain. Postinfarction syndrome may develop, producing chest pain that must be differentiated from recurrent MI, pulmonary infarct, or heart failure.
- Stress the need to stop smoking and control lipids and hypertension.

Complications
- Recurrent or persistent chest pain (most common)
- Arrhythmias
- Left-sided heart failure (resulting in heart failure or acute pulmonary edema)
- Cardiogenic shock
- Thromboembolism
- Papillary muscle dysfunction or rupture, causing mitral insufficiency
- Rupture of the ventricular septum, causing ventricular septal defect
- Rupture of the myocardium and ventricular aneurysm
- Dressler's syndrome (pericarditis, pericardial friction rub, chest pain, fever,

Complications of myocardial infarction

COMPLICATION	DIAGNOSIS	TREATMENT
Arrhythmias	▪ Electrocardiogram (ECG) shows premature ventricular contractions, ventricular tachycardia, or ventricular fibrillation; in inferior wall myocardial infarction (MI), bradycardia and junctional rhythms or atrioventricular block; in anterior wall MI, tachycardia or heart block.	▪ Antiarrhythmics, atropine, cardioversion, and pacemaker
Heart failure	▪ In left-sided heart failure, chest X-rays show venous congestion, cardiomegaly, and Kerley's B lines. ▪ Catheterization shows increased pulmonary artery pressure (PAP) and central venous pressure.	▪ Angiotensin-converting enzyme inhibitors, beta-adrenergic blockers, diuretics, vasodilators, inotropic agents, and cardiac glycosides
Cardiogenic shock	▪ Catheterization shows decreased cardiac output and increased PAP and pulmonary artery wedge pressure (PAWP) ▪ Signs include hypertension, tachycardia, S_3, S_4, decreased levels of consciousness, decreased urine output, neck vein distension, and cool, pale skin.	▪ I.V. fluids, vasodilators, diuretics, cardiac glycosides, intra-aortic balloon pump (IABP), and beta-adrenergic stimulants
Rupture of left ventricular papillary muscle	▪ Auscultation reveals apical holosystolic murmur. Inspection of jugular vein pulse or hemodynamic monitoring shows increased V waves. ▪ Dyspnea is prominent. ▪ Color-flow and Doppler echocardiogram show mitral insufficiency. Pulmonary artery catheterization shows increased PAP and PAWP.	▪ Nitroprusside ▪ IABP ▪ Surgical replacement of the mitral valve with possible concomitant myocardial revascularization (in patients with significant coronary artery disease)
Ventricular septal rupture	▪ In left-to-right shunt, auscultation reveals holosystolic murmur and thrill. ▪ Catheterization shows increased PAP and PAWP. ▪ Confirmation by increased oxygen saturation of right ventricle and pulmonary artery.	▪ Surgical correction, IABP, nitroglycerin, nitroprusside, low-dose inotropic agents, or pacemaker
Pericarditis or Dressler's syndrome	▪ Auscultation reveals a friction rub. ▪ Chest pain is relieved by sitting up.	▪ Nonsteroidal anti-inflammatory drugs or corticosteroids

Complications of myocardial infarction *(continued)*

COMPLICATION	DIAGNOSIS	TREATMENT
Ventricular aneurysm	■ Chest X-ray may show cardiomegaly. ■ ECG may show arrhythmias and persistent ST-segment elevation. ■ Left ventriculography shows altered or paradoxical left ventricular motion.	■ Cardioversion, defibrillation, antiarrhythmics, vasodilators, anticoagulants, cardiac glycosides, and diuretics. If conservative treatment fails, surgical resection is necessary.
Thromboembolism	■ Severe dyspnea and chest pain or neurologic changes. ■ Nuclear scan shows ventilation-perfusion mismatch. ■ Angiography shows arterial blockage.	■ Oxygen and heparin

leukocytosis and, possibly, pleurisy or pneumonitis) (See *Complications of myocardial infarction.*)

Special considerations

■ Encourage the patient's family to become certified in cardiopulmonary resuscitation.

• • • • • • • • • • • •

MYOCARDITIS

Myocarditis is focal or diffuse inflammation of the cardiac muscle (myocardium). It may be acute or chronic and affects men 1.5 times more than women. In many cases, myocarditis fails to produce specific cardiovascular symptoms or electrocardiogram abnormalities, and recovery is usually spontaneous, without residual defects. Occasionally, myocarditis is complicated by heart failure; in rare cases, it leads to cardiomyopathy.

 AGE ALERT Myocarditis occurs more often after age 42.

Causes

Myocarditis may result from:
■ viral infections (most common cause in the United States and Western Europe) — coxsackievirus A and B strains and, possibly, poliomyelitis, influenza, rubeola, rubella, and adenoviruses and echoviruses
■ bacterial infections — diphtheria, tuberculosis, typhoid fever, tetanus, and staphylococcal, pneumococcal, and gonococcal infections
■ hypersensitive immune reactions — acute rheumatic fever and postcardiotomy syndrome
■ radiation therapy — large doses of radiation to the chest in treating lung or breast cancer
■ chemical poisons — such as chronic alcoholism
■ parasitic infections — especially South American trypanosomiasis (Chagas' disease) in infants and immunosuppressed adults; also, toxoplasmosis
■ helminthic infections — such as trichinosis.

Clinical presentation

Myocarditis usually causes nonspecific symptoms that reflect accompanying systemic infection such as:

- fatigue
- dyspnea
- palpitations
- fever.

Occasionally, it may produce mild, continuous pressure or soreness in the chest (unlike the recurring, stress-related pain of angina pectoris). Although myocarditis is usually self-limiting, it may induce myofibril degeneration that results in:

- right- and left-sided heart failure with cardiomegaly
- neck vein distention
- dyspnea
- persistent fever with resting or exertional tachycardia disproportionate to the degree of fever
- supraventricular and ventricular arrhythmias
- S_3 and S_4 gallops
- a faint S_1
- possibly a murmur of mitral insufficiency
- pericardial friction rub (if pericarditis is present).

Differential diagnoses

- Coronary artery disease
- Cardiomyopathy
- Arrhythmia etiologies
- Valvular heart disease

Diagnosis

Patient history commonly reveals recent febrile upper respiratory tract infection, viral pharyngitis, or tonsillitis. Laboratory tests can't unequivocally confirm myocarditis, but the following findings support this diagnosis:

- cardiac enzymes: elevated creatine kinase (CK), CK-MB, aspartate aminotransferase, and lactate dehydrogenase levels

- increased white blood cell count and erythrocyte sedimentation rate
- elevated antibody titers (such as anti-streptolysin O titer in rheumatic fever).

Endomyocardial biopsy remains the gold standard for diagnosing myocarditis; however, the procedure is invasive, costly, and controversial. A negative biopsy doesn't exclude the diagnosis; a repeat biopsy may be needed.

Electrocardiography typically shows diffuse ST-segment and T-wave abnormalities as in pericarditis, conduction defects (prolonged PR interval), and other supraventricular arrhythmias. Echocardiography demonstrates some degree of left ventricular dysfunction, and radionuclide scanning may identify inflammatory and necrotic changes characteristic of myocarditis.

Stool and throat cultures may identify bacteria.

Management

General

Treatment includes modified bed rest to decrease heart workload and careful management of complications. Heart failure requires restriction of activity to minimize myocardial oxygen consumption. Oxygen therapy should be initiated as needed to maintain pulse oximetry less than 92%.

Medication

Medication is administered based on the patient's symptoms and may include:

- penicillin — 1.6 to 3.2 million U/day P.O. every 6 hours, or 1.2 to 2.4 million U I.M. or I.V. per day every 4 to 6 hours
- furosemide — 20 to 80 mg/day I.V.
- quinidine — 200 to 400 mg P.O. every 6 hours
- procainamide — 50 mg/kg/day P.O. in divided doses every 3 hours

- heparin—5,000 U S.C. every 12 hours
- warfarin—2 to 10 mg/day P.O. based on a target INR of 2.0 to 3.0.

Nonsteroidal anti-inflammatory drugs are contraindicated during the acute phase (first 2 weeks) because they increase myocardial damage.

Surgical intervention
Cardiac transplant may be indicated in severe cases of myocarditis.

Referral
- The patient may require a cardiology consult.

Follow-up
The patient should be seen 1 week post-hospitalization and if tachycardia or palpitations recur. He should be assessed periodically to rule out development of cardiomyopathies.

Patient teaching
- During recovery, recommend that the patient resume normal activities slowly and avoid competitive sports.
- Stress the need for rest to allow adequate recovery.
- Teach the patient how to detect signs of recurrence.

Complications
- Sudden death
- Heart block
- Heart failure
- Cardiac arrhythmia
- Thromboembolism
- Cardiomyopathy
- Recurrence of disorder
- Chronic valvulitis

• • • • • • • • • • • •
PERICARDITIS

Pericarditis is an inflammation of the pericardium, the fibroserous sac that envelops, supports, and protects the heart. It occurs in both acute and chronic forms. Acute pericarditis can be fibrinous or effusive, with purulent serous or hemorrhagic exudate; chronic constrictive pericarditis is characterized by dense fibrous pericardial thickening. The prognosis depends on the underlying cause but is generally good in acute pericarditis, unless constriction occurs.

Causes
Common causes of this disease include:
- bacterial, fungal, or viral infection (infectious pericarditis)
- neoplasms (primary or metastatic from lungs, breasts, or other organs)
- high-dose radiation to the chest
- uremia
- hypersensitivity or autoimmune disease, such as acute rheumatic fever (most common cause of pericarditis in children), systemic lupus erythematosus, and rheumatoid arthritis
- postcardiac injury, such as myocardial infarction (MI), which later causes an autoimmune reaction (Dressler's syndrome) in the pericardium; trauma; or surgery that leaves the pericardium intact but causes blood to leak into the pericardial cavity
- drugs, such as hydralazine or procainamide
- idiopathic factors (most common in acute pericarditis).

Less common causes include aortic aneurysm with pericardial leakage and myxedema with cholesterol deposits in the pericardium.

Clinical presentation

Acute pericarditis typically produces a sharp and often sudden pain that usually starts over the sternum and radiates to the neck, shoulders, back, and arms. However, unlike the pain of MI, pericardial pain is often pleuritic, increasing with deep inspiration and decreasing when the patient sits up and leans forward, pulling the heart away from the diaphragmatic pleurae of the lungs.

Pericardial friction rub may have up to three components, corresponding to the timing of atrial systole, ventricular systole, and the rapid filling phase of ventricular diastole. Occasionally, it's heard only briefly or not at all. Nevertheless, its presence, together with other characteristic features, is diagnostic of acute pericarditis.

In addition, if acute pericarditis has caused very large pericardial effusions, the physical examination reveals:
- increased cardiac dullness
- diminished or absent apical impulse
- distant heart sounds.

In patients with chronic pericarditis, acute inflammation or effusions don't occur — only restricted cardiac filling.

Pericardial effusion, the major complication of acute pericarditis, may produce:
- effects of heart failure
- ill-defined substernal chest pain
- a feeling of fullness in the chest.

If fluid accumulates rapidly, cardiac tamponade may occur, resulting in:
- pallor
- clammy skin
- hypotension
- pulsus paradoxus
- neck vein distention
- cardiovascular collapse
- death.

Chronic constrictive pericarditis causes a gradual increase in systemic venous pressure and produces symptoms similar to those of chronic right-sided heart failure. Additionally, physical examination reveals:
- tachycardia
- jugular vein distention
- Kussmaul's sign
- pericardial knock in diastole.

Differential diagnoses

- Acute MI
- Pneumonia with pleurisy
- Pulmonary emboli
- Aortic dissection
- Pneumothorax
- Mediastinal emphysema
- Cholecystitis
- Pancreatitis
- Esophageal perforation, rupture, tear, or inflammation

Diagnosis

Because pericarditis commonly coexists with other conditions, diagnosis of acute pericarditis depends on typical clinical features and elimination of other possible causes.

Laboratory results reflect inflammation and may reveal its cause:
- normal or elevated white blood cell count, especially in infectious pericarditis
- elevated erythrocyte sedimentation rate
- slightly elevated cardiac enzyme levels with associated myocarditis
- culture of pericardial fluid obtained by open surgical drainage or cardiocentesis (sometimes enables identification of a causative organism in bacterial or fungal pericarditis)
- electrocardiogram showing the changes in acute pericarditis, including elevation of ST segments in the standard limb leads and most precordial leads without significant changes in QRS morphology that occur with MI, atrial ectopic rhythms such as atrial fibrillation and, in

pericardial effusion, diminished QRS voltage
■ echocardiography, which determines the presence of pericardial effusion, pericardial thickening, or diminished diastolic filling; left ventricular contraction is usually normal in constrictive pericarditis
■ chest X-ray, which shows a small pleural effusion and a "water bottle" cardiac silhouette in association with a large pericardial effusion; pericardial calcification is seen in 50% of patients with constrictive pericarditis.

Management
General
The goal of treatment is to relieve symptoms and manage underlying systemic disease. Treatment must also include management of other underlying disorders. Most cases of infectious pericarditis are viral, with treatment consisting mainly of bed rest.

In acute idiopathic pericarditis, post-MI pericarditis, and post-thoracotomy pericarditis, treatment consists of bed rest as long as fever and pain persist.

Medication
Nonsteroidal anti-inflammatory drugs to relieve pain and reduce inflammation include:
■ aspirin — 650 mg P.O. every 4 hours for 2 weeks
■ indomethacin — 25 to 50 mg P.O. every 6 to 8 hours for 2 weeks.

Corticosteroids produce rapid and effective relief; however, they must be used cautiously because episodes may recur when therapy is discontinued. Prednisone (60 mg P.O.) is given for 2 to 3 days, then quickly tapered.

If the case is bacterial, antibiotics specific for the causative agent are prescribed.

Surgical intervention
■ Cardiac tamponade may require pericardiocentesis.
■ Recurrent pericarditis may necessitate partial pericardiectomy (creating a window to allow fluid to drain into the pleural space). In constrictive pericarditis, total pericardiectomy to permit adequate filling and contraction of the heart may be necessary.

Referral
■ The patient may need to be referred to a cardiologist.

Follow-up
Follow-up in the office should occur in 2 weeks to evaluate cardiac status and the patient's symptomatology. A chest X-ray and electrocardiogram should be repeated in 4 weeks.

Patient teaching
■ Educate the patient about recognition of the return of symptoms because approximately 15% of patients have a recurrence within the first few months.

Complications
■ Pericardial tamponade
■ Recurrence
■ Noncompressive effusion
■ Chronic constrictive pericarditis

Special considerations
■ Anticoagulants are relatively contraindicated in acute pericarditis secondary to risk of pericardial tamponade or hemorrhage.

• • • • • • • • • • • •

RAYNAUD'S DISEASE

Raynaud's disease is one of several primary arteriospastic disorders characterized by episodic vasospasm in the small peripheral arteries and arterioles, precipitated by exposure to cold or stress. This condition occurs bilaterally and usually affects the hands or, less often, the feet.

AGE ALERT Raynaud's disease is most prevalent in females, particularly between puberty and age 40. It's a benign condition, requiring no specific treatment and causing no serious sequelae.

Raynaud's phenomenon — a condition often associated with several connective tissue disorders, such as scleroderma, systemic lupus erythematosus, or polymyositis — has a progressive course, leading to ischemia, gangrene, and amputation. Distinguishing between the two disorders is difficult because some patients who experience mild symptoms of Raynaud's disease for several years may later develop overt connective tissue disease — especially scleroderma.

Causes

Although the cause is unknown, several theories account for the reduced digital blood flow: intrinsic vascular wall hyperactivity to cold, increased vasomotor tone due to sympathetic stimulation, and antigen-antibody immune response (the most likely theory because abnormal immunologic test results accompany Raynaud's phenomenon).

Clinical presentation

After exposure to cold or stress, the skin on the fingers typically blanches and then becomes cyanotic before changing to red and before changing from cold to normal temperature. Numbness and tingling may also occur. These symptoms are relieved by warmth. In long-standing disease, trophic changes may occur, such as:
- sclerodactyly
- ulcerations
- chronic paronychia.

Although it's extremely uncommon, minimal cutaneous gangrene necessitates amputation of one or more phalanges.

Clinical criteria that establish Raynaud's disease include:
- skin color changes induced by cold or stress
- bilateral involvement
- absence of gangrene or, if present, minimal cutaneous gangrene
- normal arterial pulses
- a patient history of clinical symptoms of longer than 2 years' duration.

If tissue necrosis or ischemia is present in only one extremity, consider another underlying problem (such as scleroderma).

Differential diagnoses
- Thromboangiitis obliterans (Buerger's disease)
- Rheumatoid arthritis
- Progressive systemic sclerosis (scleroderma)
- Systemic lupus erythematosus
- Carpal tunnel syndrome
- Thoracic outlet syndrome
- Polycythemia
- Occupational injury (for example, from vibrating tools or masonry work)
- Drugs (beta-adrenergic blockers, clonidine, ergotamine, amphetamines, bromocriptine, bleomycin, vinblastine, cisplatin, or cyclosporine)

Diagnosis
- Laboratory tests, such as complete blood count, erythrocyte sedimentation rate, rheumatoid factor, antinuclear antibodies, immunoelectrophoresis, and esophageal motility studies, should be done to detect any underlying secondary causes.
- Cold stimulation test records temperature changes in the patient's fingers before and after submergence in an ice-

water bath. Digital blood pressure recording or examination of the arteries in the arm and palmar arch should precede this test to rule out arterial occlusion.

Management
General
Initially, treatment consists of avoiding cold, mechanical, or chemical injury; smoking cessation; and reassurance that symptoms are benign.

Medication
Because adverse drug effects, especially from vasodilators, may be more bothersome than the disease itself, the following drug therapy is reserved for unusually severe symptoms:
- nifedipine — 30 to 120 mg/day P.O.; may be needed only in the winter
- prazosin — 1 to 5 mg P.O. t.i.d.

Surgical intervention
When conservative treatment fails to prevent ischemic ulcers, sympathectomy (sympathetic ganglion blockade with a long-acting anesthetic) may be helpful; fewer than a quarter of patients require this procedure.

Referral
- Refer the patient to a specialist for any underlying disorders.

Follow-up
Follow-up is based on symptoms and exacerbations. Management of fingertip ulcers with rapid treatment for infection is important. Observe carefully for signs of associated illness, because Raynaud's may precede overt development by an average of 11 years.

Patient teaching
- Instruct the patient to avoid trauma to the fingertips or toes, avoid exposure to cold, and stop smoking.

Complications
- Gangrene
- Autoamputation of fingertips

••••••••••••

RHEUMATIC FEVER AND RHEUMATIC HEART DISEASE

Acute rheumatic fever is a systemic inflammatory disease of childhood, in many cases recurrent, that follows a group A beta-hemolytic streptococcal infection. Rheumatic heart disease refers to the cardiac manifestations of rheumatic fever and includes pancarditis (myocarditis, pericarditis, and endocarditis) during the early acute phase followed by chronic valvular disease. Long-term antibiotic therapy can minimize recurrence of rheumatic fever, reducing the risk of permanent cardiac damage and eventual valvular deformity. However, severe pancarditis occasionally produces fatal heart failure during the acute phase. Of the patients who survive this complication, about 20% die within 10 years. Approximately 1,800,000 people in the United States are afflicted with rheumatic fever and rheumatic heart disease. Although rheumatic fever tends to be familial, this may merely reflect contributing environmental factors. This disease strikes generally during cool, damp weather in the winter and early spring. In the United States, it's most common in the northern states.

AGE ALERT In lower socioeconomic groups, incidence of

rheumatic fever and rheumatic heart disease is highest in children between ages 5 and 15, probably as a result of malnutrition and crowded living conditions.

Causes

Rheumatic fever appears to be a hypersensitivity reaction to a group A beta-hemolytic streptococcal infection, in which antibodies manufactured to combat streptococci react and produce characteristic lesions at specific tissue sites, especially in the heart and joints. Because very few persons (0.3%) with streptococcal infections ever contract rheumatic fever, altered host resistance must be involved in its development or recurrence.

Clinical presentation

In 95% of patients, rheumatic fever characteristically follows a streptococcal infection that appeared a few days to 6 weeks earlier. The following signs and symptoms may occur:
- temperature of at least 100.4° F (38° C) occurs
- migratory joint pain or polyarthritis
- swelling, redness, and signs of effusion, which most commonly affects the knees, ankles, elbows, or hips
- skin lesions such as erythema marginatum
- firm, movable, nontender, subcutaneous nodules about 3 mm to 2 cm in diameter, usually near tendons or bony prominences of joints (especially the elbows, knuckles, wrists, and knees) and less often on the scalp and backs of the hands. These nodules persist for a few days to several weeks and, like erythema marginatum, often accompany carditis. Carditis is the most destructive effect of rheumatic fever and develops in up to 50% of patients.

Later, rheumatic fever may cause transient chorea, which develops up to 6 months after the original streptococcal infection. Mild chorea may produce hyperirritability, deterioration in handwriting, or inability to concentrate. Severe chorea causes purposeless, nonrepetitive, involuntary muscle spasms; poor muscle coordination; and weakness. Chorea always resolves without residual neurologic damage.

Severe rheumatic carditis may cause heart failure with dyspnea, right upper quadrant pain, tachycardia, tachypnea, a hacking nonproductive cough, edema, and significant mitral and aortic murmurs. The most common of such murmurs include:
- a systolic murmur of mitral insufficiency (high-pitched, blowing, holosystolic, loudest at apex, possibly radiating to the anterior axillary line)
- a midsystolic murmur due to stiffening and swelling of the mitral leaflet
- occasionally, a diastolic murmur of aortic insufficiency (low-pitched, rumbling, almost inaudible).

Valvular disease may eventually result in:
- chronic valvular stenosis
- mitral stenosis and insufficiency
- aortic insufficiency.

In children, mitral insufficiency remains the major sequela of rheumatic heart disease.

Differential diagnoses
- Lupus erythematosus
- Juvenile rheumatoid arthritis
- Infectious arthritis
- Viral myocarditis
- Innocent murmurs
- Tourette syndrome
- Kawasaki syndrome

Diagnosis

Diagnosis depends on recognition of one or more of the classic symptoms (carditis, rheumatic fever without carditis, polyarthritis, chorea, erythema marginatum, or subcutaneous nodules) and a detailed patient history. Laboratory data support the diagnosis:

- White blood cell count and erythrocyte sedimentation rate may be elevated (during the acute phase); blood studies show slight anemia due to suppressed erythropoiesis during inflammation.
- C-reactive protein is positive (especially during acute phase).
- Cardiac enzyme levels may be increased in severe carditis.
- Antistreptolysin O titer is elevated in 95% of patients within 2 months of onset.
- Electrocardiogram changes aren't diagnostic, but the PR interval is prolonged in 20% of patients.
- Chest X-rays show normal heart size (except with myocarditis, heart failure, or pericardial effusion).
- Echocardiography helps evaluate valvular damage, chamber size, and ventricular function.
- Cardiac catheterization evaluates valvular damage and left ventricular function in severe cardiac dysfunction.

Management
General
Effective management eradicates the streptococcal infection, relieves symptoms, and prevents recurrence, reducing the chance of permanent cardiac damage. Supportive treatment requires strict bed rest for about 5 weeks during the acute phase with active carditis, followed by a progressive increase in physical activity, depending on clinical and laboratory findings and the response to treatment.

Medication
Antibiotics (administered during the acute phase) may include:

- penicillin V — 1.2 million U I.M. for 1 dose for adults; 900,000 U I.M. for 1 dose for children weighing less than 60 lb (27 kg); 50,000 U/kg I.M. for 1 dose for children weighing more than 60 lb; 1.2 million U I.M. weekly for 5 years for prophylaxis
- erythromycin — 250 mg P.O. every 12 hours.

The following medications may also be used:
- aspirin — 60 mg/kg/day P.O.
- prednisone — 2 mg/kg/day P.O. for 2 weeks, then tapered over 2 weeks; used if carditis is present or salicylates fail to relieve pain and inflammation.

Surgical intervention
Severe mitral or aortic valvular dysfunction causing persistent heart failure requires corrective valvular surgery, including commissurotomy (separation of the adherent, thickened leaflets of the mitral valve), valvuloplasty (inflation of a balloon within a valve), or valve replacement (with a prosthetic valve). Corrective valvular surgery is rarely necessary before late adolescence.

Patient teaching
- Instruct the parents to watch for and report early signs of heart failure.
- Stress the need for bed rest during the acute phase.
- Warn patients and their parents to watch for and immediately report signs of recurrent streptococcal infection.
- Stress the importance of prolonged antibiotic therapy and follow-up care and the need for additional antibiotics during dental surgery. (See the prophylactic regimen in "Endocarditis," page 99.)

Complications
- Subsequent attacks of acute rheumatic fever secondary to streptococcal reinfection

- Carditis
- Mitral stenosis
- Heart failure

• • • • • • • • • • • •
THROMBOPHLEBITIS

Thrombophlebitis is an acute condition characterized by inflammation and thrombus formation. It occurs in deep (intermuscular or intramuscular) or superficial (subcutaneous) veins. Deep vein thrombophlebitis (DVT) affects small veins, such as the soleal venous sinuses, or large veins, such as the vena cava and the femoral, iliac, and subclavian veins, causing venous insufficiency. (See *Chronic venous insufficiency*.) This disorder is typically progressive, leading to pulmonary embolism, a potentially lethal complication. Superficial thrombophlebitis is usually self-limiting and seldom leads to pulmonary embolism. Thrombophlebitis often begins with localized inflammation alone (phlebitis), but such inflammation rapidly provokes thrombus formation. Rarely, venous thrombosis develops without associated inflammation of the vein (phlebothrombosis).

Thrombophlebitis occurs more frequently in women than in men.

AGE ALERT The incidence of thrombophlebitis increases after age 40 and triples with each additional 20 years. DVT is most common in adults over age 60 and occurs in approximately 2 of 1,000 people.

Causes and pathophysiology
A thrombus occurs when an alteration in the epithelial lining causes platelet aggregation and consequent fibrin entrapment of red and white blood cells and additional platelets. Thrombus formation is more rapid in areas where blood flow is slower, due to greater contact between platelet and thrombin accumulation. The rapidly expanding thrombus initiates a chemical inflammatory process in the vessel epithelium, which leads to fibrosis. The enlarging clot may occlude the vessel lumen partially or totally, or it may detach and embolize to lodge elsewhere in the systemic circulation.

DVT may be idiopathic, but it usually results from endothelial damage, accelerated blood clotting, and venous stasis. Predisposing factors are prolonged bed rest, trauma, surgery, hypercoagulable states, neoplasms, history of previous DVT, childbirth, and use of oral contraceptives, such as estrogens.

Causes of superficial thrombophlebitis include trauma, infection, I.V. drug abuse, and chemical irritation due to extensive use of the I.V. route for medications and diagnostic tests.

Clinical presentation
In both types of thrombophlebitis, clinical features vary with the site and length of the affected vein. Although DVT may occur asymptomatically, it may also produce the following:
- severe pain
- fever
- chills
- malaise
- swelling and cyanosis of the affected arm or leg.

Superficial thrombophlebitis produces visible and palpable signs along the length of the affected vein, such as:
- heat
- pain
- swelling
- rubor
- tenderness
- induration.

Varicose veins may also be present (see *Varicose veins*, page 130). Extensive vein involvement may cause lymphadenitis.

Differential diagnoses
DVT
- Cellulitis
- Ruptured synovial cyst (Baker's cyst)
- Lymphedema
- Extrinsic compression of the vein by tumor or enlarged lymph nodes
- Pulled, strained, or torn muscle
- Arterial occlusive disease

Superficial thrombophlebitis
- Cellulitis
- Erythema nodosa
- Cutaneous polyarteritis nodosa
- Sarcoid
- Kaposi's sarcoma

Diagnosis
Some patients display signs of inflammation and, possibly, a positive Homans' sign (pain on dorsiflexion of the foot) during physical examination; others are asymptomatic. Essential laboratory tests include:
- Duplex Doppler ultrasonography and impedance plethysmography, which make it possible to noninvasively examine the major veins (but not calf veins).
- Plethysmography shows decreased circulation distal to affected area; this test is more sensitive than ultrasound in detecting DVT.
- Phlebography, which shows filling defects and diverted blood flow, usually confirms the diagnosis.
- Contrast venography is the gold standard because it's most sensitive and specific.
- Diagnosis of superficial thrombophlebitis is based on physical examination.

Management
General
The goals of treatment are to control thrombus development, prevent complications, relieve pain, and prevent recur-

Chronic venous insufficiency

Chronic venous insufficiency results from the valvular destruction of deep vein thrombophlebitis, usually in the iliac and femoral veins and occasionally in the saphenous veins. It's often accompanied by incompetence of the communicating veins at the ankle, causing increased venous pressure and fluid migration into the interstitial tissue. Clinical effects include chronic swelling of the affected leg from edema, leading to tissue fibrosis, and induration; skin discoloration from extravasation of blood in subcutaneous tissue; and stasis ulcers around the ankle.

Treatment of small ulcers includes bed rest; elevation of the legs; warm, moist soaks; and antimicrobial therapy for infection. Treatment to counteract increased venous pressure, the result of reflux from the deep venous system to surface veins, may include compression dressings, such as a sponge rubber pressure dressing or a zinc gelatin boot (Unna's boot). This therapy begins after massive swelling subsides with leg elevation and bed rest.

Large stasis ulcers unresponsive to conservative treatment may require excision and skin grafting. Patient care includes daily inspection to assess healing. Other care measures are the same as those for varicose veins.

rence of the disorder. Symptomatic measures include bed rest, with elevation of the affected arm or leg; warm, moist soaks to the affected area; and analgesics.

Therapy for a patient with severe superficial thrombophlebitis may include an anti-inflammatory drug; antiembolism

Varicose veins

Varicose veins are dilated, tortuous veins that usually affect the subcutaneous leg veins — the saphenous veins and their branches. They can result from congenital weakness of the valves or venous wall; from diseases of the venous system, such as deep vein thrombophlebitis; from conditions that produce prolonged venostasis, such as pregnancy; or from occupations that necessitate standing for an extended period.

Varicose veins may be asymptomatic or produce mild to severe leg symptoms, including a feeling of heaviness; cramps at night; diffuse, dull aching after prolonged standing or walking; aching during menses; fatigability; palpable nodules; and, with deep-vein incompetency, orthostatic edema and stasis pigmentation of the calves and ankles.

TREATMENT

In mild to moderate varicose veins, antiembolism stockings or elastic bandages counteract pedal and ankle swelling by supporting the veins and improving circulation. An exercise program, such as walking, promotes muscular contraction and forces blood through the veins, thereby minimizing venous pooling. Severe varicose veins may necessitate stripping and ligation or, as an alternative to surgery, injection of a sclerosing agent into small affected vein segments.

Use the following measures to promote comfort and minimize worsening of varicosities:
- Discourage the patient from wearing constrictive clothing.
- Advise the patient to elevate his legs above heart level whenever possible and to avoid prolonged standing or sitting.

After stripping and ligation or after injection of a sclerosing agent:
- Order analgesics to relieve pain.
- Frequently check circulation in toes (color and temperature), and observe for bleeding.
- Watch for signs of complications, such as sensory loss in the leg (which could indicate saphenous nerve damage), calf pain (thrombophlebitis), and fever (infection).

stockings; warm, moist soaks; and elevation of the affected area.

After the acute episode of DVT subsides, the patient may resume activity while wearing antiembolism stockings applied before he gets out of bed.

Medication

These medications may be used to treat a patient with DVT:
- heparin — 80 U/kg bolus, then 18 U/kg/hour I.V. (Adjust based on activated partial thromboplastin time [aPTT] of approximately 1.5 times control. After some types of surgery, especially major abdominal or pelvic operations, prophylactic doses of anticoagulants may reduce the risk of DVT and pulmonary embolism. Low-molecular-weight heparins are effective in preventing DVT after general or orthopedic surgery.)
- warfarin — begin 1 to 3 days after starting heparin, in a single daily dose of 5 mg/day (Adjust based on the INR; aim for an INR of 2.0 to 3.0.)
- streptokinase — loading dose is 250,000 IU I.V. over 30 minutes, then I.V. infusion of 100,000 IU every hour for 72 hours, for lysis of acute, extensive DVT.

Therapy for a patient with severe superficial thrombophlebitis includes an anti-inflammatory drug such as indomethacin, 50 to 100 mg P.O. t.i.d.

Surgical intervention

Rarely, DVT may cause complete venous occlusion, which necessitates venous interruption through simple ligation to vein plication, or clipping. Embolectomy and insertion of a vena cava umbrella or filter may also be done.

Referral

■ Refer the patient to a vascular surgeon if appropriate.

Follow-up

A patient with DVT should be treated for 3 to 6 months after the first episode. Subsequent episodes necessitate treatment for 1 year. Significant bleeding, such as hematuria or GI bleeding, should be thoroughly investigated.

A patient with superficial thrombophlebitis should be monitored as symptoms dictate. Observe for secondary complications and repeat blood studies for fibrinolytic system, platelets, and factors.

Patient teaching

■ Instruct the patient to watch for signs and symptoms of bleeding. Encourage the patient to use an electric razor.
■ Tell the patient to avoid medications that contain aspirin.
■ Emphasize the importance of follow-up blood studies to monitor anticoagulant therapy.

Complications

■ Pulmonary embolism
■ Systemic embolism
■ Chronic venous insufficiency
■ Postphlebitic syndrome
■ Treatment-induced hemorrhage

■ Superficial thrombophlebitis can cause complications such as DVT

Special considerations

■ Avoid I.M. injections while the patient is receiving anticoagulation therapy. Periodically check stools and urine for occult blood.
■ Agents that may prolong or intensify the response to anticoagulants include alcohol, allopurinol, amiodarone, anabolic steroids, many antimicrobials, cimetidine, all nonsteroidal anti-inflammatory agents, tamoxifen, thyroid hormone, vitamin E, ranitidine, salicylates, and acetaminophen.
■ Agents that may diminish the effect of anticoagulants include antacids, barbiturates, carbamazepine, cholestyramine, diuretics, griseofulvin, rifampin, and oral contraceptives.

• • • • • • • • • • • •

VALVULAR HEART DISEASE

In valvular heart disease, three types of mechanical disruption can occur: stenosis, or narrowing, of the valve opening; incomplete closure of the valve; or prolapse of the valve. They can result from such disorders as endocarditis (most common), congenital defects, and inflammation, and they can lead to heart failure.

Valvular heart disease occurs in varying forms, as follows:
■ Mitral regurgitation — In this form, blood from the left ventricle flows back into the left atrium during systole, causing the atrium to enlarge to accommodate the backflow. As a result, the left ventricle also dilates to accommodate the increased volume of blood from the atrium and to compensate for diminishing cardiac output. Ventricular hypertrophy and increased end-diastolic pressure result in increased pulmonary artery pres-

sure, eventually leading to left- and right-sided heart failure.

■ Mitral stenosis — Narrowing of the valve by valvular abnormalities, fibrosis, or calcification obstructs blood flow from the left atrium to the left ventricle. Consequently, left atrial volume and pressure rise and the chamber dilates. Greater resistance to blood flow causes pulmonary hypertension, right ventricular hypertrophy, and right-sided heart failure. Also, inadequate filling of the left ventricle produces low cardiac output.

■ Mitral valve prolapse — One or both valve leaflets protrude into the left atrium. Mitral valve prolapse is the term used when the anatomic prolapse is accompanied by signs and symptoms unrelated to the valvular abnormality.

■ Aortic insufficiency — Blood flows back into the left ventricle during diastole, causing fluid overload in the ventricle, which dilates and hypertrophies. The excess volume causes fluid overload in the left atrium and, finally, the pulmonary system. Left-sided heart failure and pulmonary edema eventually result.

■ Aortic stenosis — Increased left ventricular pressure tries to overcome the resistance of the narrowed valvular opening. The added workload increases the demand for oxygen, whereas diminished cardiac output causes poor coronary artery perfusion, ischemia of the left ventricle, and left-sided heart failure.

■ Pulmonic insufficiency — Blood ejected into the pulmonary artery during systole flows back into the right ventricle during diastole, causing fluid overload in the ventricle, ventricular hypertrophy and, finally, right-sided heart failure.

■ Pulmonic stenosis — Obstructed right ventricular outflow causes right ventricular hypertrophy, eventually resulting in right-sided heart failure.

■ Tricuspid insufficiency — Blood flows back into the right atrium during systole, decreasing blood flow to the lungs and the left side of the heart. Cardiac output also lessens. Fluid overload in the right side of the heart can eventually lead to right-sided heart failure.

■ Tricuspid stenosis — Obstructed blood flow from the right atrium to the right ventricle causes the right atrium to dilate and hypertrophy. Eventually, this leads to right-sided heart failure and increases pressure in the vena cava.

Clinical presentation
Clinical presentation differs with valvular damage. (See *Valvular heart disease*.)

Differential diagnoses
The differential diagnosis varies depending on the type of valvular damage. A key to the assessment and identification of these types of valvular damage is identification of the corresponding heart murmurs.

Diagnosis
■ Two-dimensional echocardiography provides a clear picture of the valvular morphology.

■ Doppler echocardiography shows the flow gradient of the blood through the valve and gives an indication of diastolic function.

■ Chest X-ray is used to identify calcification, cardiomegaly, or venous congestion.

■ Cardiac catheterization is the best procedure available for obtaining information about the valve, determining the extent of valvular damage, calculating the ventricle ejection fraction, and identifying any coronary artery disease.

(Text continues on page 136.)

Valvular heart disease

CAUSES AND INCIDENCE	CLINICAL FEATURES	DIAGNOSTIC MEASURES
Aortic insufficiency ■ Results from rheumatic fever, syphilis, hypertension, endocarditis, or may be idiopathic ■ Associated with Marfan syndrome ■ Most common in males ■ Associated with ventricular septal defect, even after surgical closure	■ Dyspnea, cough, fatigue, palpitations, angina, syncope ■ Pulmonary venous congestion, heart failure, pulmonary edema (left-sided heart failure), "pulsating" nail beds (Quincke's sign) ■ Rapidly rising and collapsing pulses (pulsus biferiens), cardiac arrhythmias, wide pulse pressure in severe insufficiency ■ Auscultation reveals an S_3 and a diastolic blowing murmur at left sternal border. ■ Palpation and visualization of apical impulse in chronic disease	■ Cardiac catheterization: reduction in arterial diastolic pressures, aortic insufficiency, other valvular abnormalities, and increased left ventricular end-diastolic pressure ■ X-ray: left ventricular enlargement, pulmonary vein congestion ■ Echocardiography: left ventricular enlargement, alterations in mitral valve movement (indirect indication of aortic valve disease), and mitral thickening ■ Electrocardiography (ECG): sinus tachycardia, left ventricular hypertrophy, and left atrial hypertrophy in severe disease
Aortic stenosis ■ Results from congenital aortic bicuspid valve (associated with coarctation of the aorta), congenital stenosis of valve cusps, rheumatic fever, or atherosclerosis in elderly patients ■ Most common in males	■ Dyspnea on exertion, paroxysmal nocturnal dyspnea, fatigue, syncope, angina, palpitations ■ Pulmonary venous congestion, heart failure, pulmonary edema ■ Diminished carotid pulses, decreased cardiac output, cardiac arrhythmias; may have pulsus alternans ■ Auscultation reveals systolic murmur at base or in carotids and, possibly, S_4.	■ Cardiac catheterization: pressure gradient across valve (indicating obstruction), increased left ventricular end-diastolic pressures ■ X-ray: valvular calcification, left ventricular enlargement, and pulmonary venous congestion ■ Echocardiography: thickened aortic valve and left ventricular wall ■ ECG: left ventricular hypertrophy
Mitral insufficiency ■ Results from rheumatic fever, hypertrophic cardiomyopathy, mitral valve prolapse, myocardial infarction, severe left-sided heart failure, or ruptured chordae tendineae	■ Orthopnea, dyspnea, fatigue, angina, palpitations ■ Peripheral edema, jugular vein distention, hepatomegaly (right-sided heart failure) ■ Tachycardia, crackles, pulmonary edema ■ Auscultation reveals a holosystolic murmur at apex, possible split S_2, and an S_3.	■ Cardiac catheterization: mitral insufficiency with increased left ventricular end-diastolic volume and pressure, increased atrial pressure and pulmonary artery wedge pressure (PAWP); and decreased cardiac output ■ X-ray: left atrial and ventricular enlargement, pulmonary venous congestion

(continued)

Valvular heart disease *(continued)*

CAUSES AND INCIDENCE	CLINICAL FEATURES	DIAGNOSTIC MEASURES
Mitral insufficiency *(continued)* ■ Associated with other congenital anomalies, such as transposition of the great arteries ■ Rare in children without other congenital anomalies		■ Echocardiography: abnormal valve leaflet motion, left atrial enlargement ■ ECG: may show left atrial and ventricular hypertrophy, sinus tachycardia, and atrial fibrillation.
Mitral stenosis ■ Results from rheumatic fever (most common cause) ■ Most common in females ■ May be associated with other congenital anomalies	■ Dyspnea on exertion, paroxysmal nocturnal dyspnea, orthopnea, weakness, fatigue, palpitations ■ Peripheral edema, jugular vein distention, ascites, hepatomegaly (right-sided heart failure in severe pulmonary hypertension) ■ Crackles, cardiac arrhythmias (atrial fibrillation), signs of systemic emboli ■ Auscultation reveals a loud S_1 or opening snap and a diastolic murmur at the apex.	■ Cardiac catheterization: diastolic pressure gradient across valve; elevated left atrial pressure and PAWP ($>$ 15 mm Hg) with severe pulmonary hypertension and pulmonary artery pressures; elevated right-sided heart pressure; decreased cardiac output; and abnormal contraction of the left ventricle ■ X-ray: left atrial and ventricular enlargement, enlarged pulmonary arteries, and mitral valve calcification ■ Echocardiography: thickened mitral valve leaflets, left atrial enlargement ■ ECG: left atrial hypertrophy, atrial fibrillation, right ventricular hypertrophy, and right axis deviation
Mitral valve prolapse syndrome ■ Cause unknown. Researchers speculate that metabolic or neuroendocrine factors cause constellation of signs and symptoms. ■ Most commonly affects young women but may occur in both sexes and at all ages	■ May produce no signs ■ Chest pain, palpitations, headache, fatigue, exercise intolerance, dyspnea, light-headedness, syncope, mood swings, anxiety, panic attacks ■ Auscultation typically reveals a mobile, midsystolic click, with or without a mid-to-late systolic murmur.	■ Two-dimensional echocardiography: prolapse of mitral valve leaflets into left atrium ■ Color-flow Doppler studies: mitral insufficiency ■ Resting ECG: ST-segment changes, biphasic or inverted T-waves in leads II, III, or AV ■ Exercise ECG: evaluates chest pain and arrhythmias

Valvular heart disease *(continued)*

CAUSES AND INCIDENCE	CLINICAL FEATURES	DIAGNOSTIC MEASURES
Pulmonic insufficiency ■ May be congenital or may result from pulmonary hypertension ■ May rarely result from prolonged use of pressure monitoring catheter in the pulmonary artery	■ Dyspnea, weakness, fatigue, chest pain ■ Peripheral edema, jugular vein distention, hepatomegaly (right-sided heart failure) ■ Auscultation reveals diastolic murmur in pulmonic area.	■ Cardiac catheterization: pulmonic insufficiency, increased right ventricular pressure, and associated cardiac defects ■ X-ray: right ventricular and pulmonary arterial enlargement ■ ECG: right ventricular or right atrial enlargement
Pulmonic stenosis ■ Results from congenital stenosis of valve cusp or rheumatic heart disease (infrequent) ■ Associated with other congenital heart defects such as tetralogy of Fallot	■ Asymptomatic or symptomatic with dyspnea on exertion, fatigue, chest pain, syncope ■ May lead to peripheral edema, jugular vein distention, hepatomegaly (right-sided heart failure) ■ Auscultation reveals a systolic murmur at the left sternal border, a split S₂ with a delayed or absent pulmonic component.	■ Cardiac catheterization: increased right ventricular pressure, decreased pulmonary artery pressure, and abnormal valve orifice ■ ECG: may show right ventricular hypertrophy, right axis deviation, right atrial hypertrophy, and atrial fibrillation
Tricuspid insufficiency ■ Results from right-sided heart failure, rheumatic fever and, rarely, trauma and endocarditis ■ Associated with congenital disorders	■ Dyspnea and fatigue ■ May lead to peripheral edema, jugular vein distention, hepatomegaly, and ascites (right-sided heart failure) ■ Auscultation reveals possible S_3 and systolic murmur at lower left sternal border that increases with inspiration.	■ Right-sided heart catheterization: high atrial pressure, tricuspid insufficiency, decreased or normal cardiac output ■ X-ray: right atrial dilation, right ventricular enlargement ■ Echocardiography: shows systolic prolapse of tricuspid valve, right atrial enlargement ■ ECG: right atrial or right ventricular hypertrophy, atrial fibrillation
Tricuspid stenosis ■ Results from rheumatic fever ■ May be congenital ■ Associated with mitral or aortic valve disease ■ Most common in females	■ May be symptomatic with dyspnea, fatigue, syncope ■ Possibly peripheral edema, jugular vein distention, hepatomegaly, and ascites (right-sided heart failure) ■ Auscultation reveals diastolic murmur at lower left sternal border that increases with inspiration.	■ Cardiac catheterization: increased pressure gradient across valve, increased right atrial pressure, decreased cardiac output ■ X-ray: right atrial enlargement ■ Echocardiography: leaflet abnormality, right atrial enlargement ■ ECG: right atrial hypertrophy, right or left ventricular hypertrophy, and atrial fibrillation

Management
General
Therapy depends on the nature and severity of associated symptoms.

Medication
The following medications may be used to treat valvular heart disease:
- warfarin— 2 to 5 mg/day P.O. for 3 to 4 days; then dosage is based on a target INR of 2.0 to 3.0
- cefazolin—1 g I.M. or I.V. 30 to 60 minutes before surgery, then 0.5 to 1 g I.M. or I.V. 6 hours after procedure for 24 hours (for bacterial endocarditis prophylaxis).

Surgical intervention
If the patient has severe signs and symptoms that can't be managed medically, valve replacement or repair is indicated. Valvuloplasty is appropriate for certain patients with multiple sclerosis (without accompanied mitral regurgitation) and aortic stenosis.

Referral
- Refer the patient to a cardiologist and possibly a cardiothoracic surgeon if surgery is necessary.

Follow-up
Follow-up depends on the patient's condition. The patient should follow-up with the cardiologist.

Patient teaching
- Teach the patient about diet restrictions, medications, and the importance of consistent follow-up care.

Complications
Complications vary, depending on the valve involved. Some common complications for all valvular damage include:
- thromboembolism
- heart failure
- regurgitation
- arrhythmia.

Special considerations
- Watch closely for signs of heart failure or pulmonary edema and adverse effects of drug therapy.

• • • • • • • • • • • •

SELECTED REFERENCES

Apple, S., and Lindsay, J. *Principles & Practice of Interventional Cardiology*. Philadelphia: Lippincott Williams & Wilkins, 2000.

Auscultation Skills: Breath and Heart Sounds. Springhouse, Pa.: Springhouse Corp., 1999.

Beattie, S. "Cut the Risks for Cardiac Cath Patients," *RN* 62(1):50-55, January 1999.

Critical Care Nursing Made Incredibly Easy (CD-ROM). Springhouse, Pa.: Springhouse Corp., 2001.

Darovic, G.O., and Franklin, C.M. *Handbook of Hemodynamic Monitoring*. Philadelphia: W.B. Saunders Co., 1999.

Diepenbrock, N.H. *Quick Reference to Critical Care*. Philadelphia: Lippincott Williams & Wilkins, 1999.

ECG Cards, 3rd ed. Springhouse, Pa.: Springhouse Corp., 2000.

ECG Interpretation Made Incredibly Easy, 2nd ed. Springhouse, Pa.: Springhouse Corp., 2001.

Elkin, M.K., et al. *Nursing Interventions and Clinical Skills*, 2nd ed. St. Louis: Mosby–Year Book, Inc., 2000.

Goldman, L., and Bennett, J.C. *Cecil Textbook of Medicine*, 21st ed. Philadelphia: W.B. Saunders Co., 2000.

Guidelines for Cardiopulmonary Resuscitation and Emergency Cardiovascular Care. Dallas: American Heart Association, 2000.

Ignatavicius, D., et al. *Medical-Surgical Nursing Across the Health Care Continuum*, 3rd ed. Philadelphia: W.B. Saunders Co., 1999.

Kern, M.J. *The Cardiac Catheterization Handbook*, 3rd ed. St. Louis: Mosby–Year Book, Inc., 1999.

Lanken, P.N. *The Intensive Care Unit Manual*. Philadelphia: W.B. Saunders Co., 2001.

Lewis, A.M. "Cardiovascular Emergency!" *Nursing99* 29(6):49-51, June 1999.

Miracle, V.A., and Sims, J.M. "Making Sense of the 12-Lead ECG," *Nursing99* 29(7):34-39, July 1999.

Nursing Procedures, 3rd ed. Springhouse, Pa.: Springhouse Corp., 2000.

Rakel, R., ed. *Conn's Current Therapy*. Philadelphia: W.B. Saunders Co., 2001.

Savage, L.S., and Canody, C. "Life with a Left Ventricular Assist Device: The Patient's Perspective," *American Journal of Critical Care* 8(5):340-43, September 1999.

Singleton, J.K., et al. *Primary Care*. Philadelphia: Lippincott Williams & Wilkins, 1999.

Smeltzer, S.C., and Bare, B.G. *Brunner and Suddarth's Textbook of Medical-Surgical Nursing*, 9th ed. Philadelphia: Lippincott Williams & Wilkins, 2000.

Tierney, L.M., et al. *Current Medical Diagnosis and Treatment*, New York: Lange Medical Books/McGraw-Hill Book Co., 2001.

Turjanica, M.A. "Anatomy of a Code: How Do You Feel at the Start of a Code Blue?" *Nursing Management* 30(11):44-49, November 1999.

Hematologic disorders

The hematologic system consists of the blood and blood producing structures, especially the red bone marrow of the long bones and axial skeleton. The most important function of circulating blood is to transport oxygen and other vital elements to body tissues and return carbon dioxide and other waste products to the lungs, kidneys, and skin for expulsion. Blood also performs various defensive, protective, and regulatory functions in the body.

Blood disorders may result from increased or decreased cell production or cell destruction, intrinsic cell abnormalities, or dysfunction of plasma (the liquid portion of blood). Specific causes of blood disorders include trauma, chronic disease, surgery, malnutrition, drugs, toxins, radiation, and genetic and congenital defects that disrupt blood production and function.

ASSESSMENT

Because many signs and symptoms of hematologic disorders are nonspecific and systemic, such as malaise and light-headedness, assessment can be difficult. However, certain key findings may alert you to the possibility of a hematologic disorder. They include abnormal bleeding, petechiae, ecchymosis, fatigue, weakness, dyspnea with or without exertion, fever, lymphadenopathy, and joint and bone pain. Further assessment usually includes laboratory blood tests. (See *Tests for blood composition, production, and function.*)

Appearance and vital signs

Begin your assessment by observing the patient's physical appearance. Look for signs of acute illness, such as grimacing or profuse perspiration, and of chronic illness, such as emaciation and listlessness. Determine whether the patient's stated age and appearance agree. Chronic disease and nutritional deficiencies related to immune dysfunction can make a patient look older than he is.

Tests for blood composition, production, and function

OVERALL COMPOSITION
- Peripheral blood smear shows maturity and morphologic characteristics of blood elements and determines qualitative abnormalities.
- Complete blood count determines the actual number of blood elements in relation to volume and quantifies abnormalities.
- Bone marrow aspiration or biopsy allows the evaluation of hematopoiesis by showing blood elements and precursors and abnormal or malignant cells.

RED BLOOD CELL FUNCTION
- Hematocrit, or packed cell volume, measures the percentage of red blood cells (RBCs) per fluid volume of whole blood.
- Hemoglobin (Hb) level measures the amount (grams) of Hb per deciliter of blood, to determine oxygen-carrying capacity.
- Reticulocyte count assesses RBC production by determining concentration of this erythrocyte precursor.
- Schilling test determines the absorption of vitamin B_{12} (necessary for erythropoiesis) by measuring the excretion of radioactive vitamin B_{12} in the urine.
- Mean corpuscular volume describes RBCs in terms of size.
- Mean corpuscular Hb determines average amount of Hb per RBC.
- Mean corpuscular Hb concentration establishes average Hb concentration in 1 dl of packed RBCs.
- Sucrose hemolysis test assesses the susceptibility of RBCs to hemolyze with complement.
- Direct Coombs' test demonstrates the presence of immunoglobulin G (IgG) antibodies (such as antibodies to Rh factor) or complement on circulating RBCs.
- Indirect Coombs' test, a two-step test, detects the presence of IgG antibodies in the serum.
- Sideroblast test detects stainable iron (available for Hb synthesis) in normoblastic RBCs.
- Hb electrophoresis demonstrates abnormal Hb such as sickle cell.

HEMOSTASIS
- Platelet count determines the number of platelets.
- Bleeding time test (Ivy's test) assesses the capacity for platelets to stop bleeding in capillaries and small vessels.
- Prothrombin time (Quick's test and protime) assists in the evaluation of thrombin generation (extrinsic clotting mechanism).
- Partial thromboplastin time aids the evaluation of the adequacy of plasma-clotting factors (intrinsic clotting mechanism).
- Fibrin degradation products (fibrin split products) (FDPs) test the amount of clot breakdown products in serum.
- Thrombin time detects abnormalities in thrombin fibrinogen reaction.
- Fibrinogen level measures fibrinogen coagulation factor in plasma.
- D-dimer test determines if FDPs are from normal mechanisms or excessive fibrinolysis; it's commonly used to diagnose disseminated intravascular coagulation.

WHITE BLOOD CELL FUNCTION
- White blood cell (WBC) count differential establishes the quantity and ma-

(continued)

Tests for blood composition, production, and function (continued)

turity of WBC elements (neutrophils [called polymorphonuclear granulocytes or bands], basophils, eosinophils, lymphocytes, and monocytes).
■ Quantified CD4+/CD8+ T lymphocytes determines the helper-suppressor ratio important to immune function with human immunodeficiency virus infection.

PLASMA
■ Erythrocyte sedimentation rate measures the rate of RBCs settling from plasma and may reflect infection.
■ Electrophoresis of serum proteins determines the amount of various serum proteins (classified by mobility in response to an electrical field); it's commonly used to diagnose plasma cell myeloma.
■ Immunoelectrophoresis of serum proteins separates and classifies serum antibodies (immunoglobulins) through specific antisera.

Next, measure the patient's height and weight. Compare the findings with normal values for the patient's bone structure.

Observe the patient's posture, movements, and gait for abnormalities that could indicate joint, spinal, or neurologic changes caused by an immune disorder.

Assess his vital signs, noting especially whether they vary from his normal baseline measurements. Fever, with or without a chill, suggests infection. A subnormal temperature usually occurs with gram-negative infections. Other signs and symptoms of inflammation, such as redness, swelling, or tenderness, may accompany a fever. These effects may be absent if the patient has a white blood cell deficiency.

Assess the patient's pulse rate as well as respiratory rate and character. Note the heart rate. The heart may pump harder or faster to compensate for a decreased oxygen supply resulting from anemia or decreased blood volume from bleeding. This problem can cause tachycardia, palpitations, or arrhythmias. Check respirations for tachypnea. Mea-

sure blood pressure with the patient lying, sitting, and standing. Check for orthostatic hypotension as well as hypotension possibly caused by septicemia or hypovolemia.

Finally, assess your patient's level of consciousness, which may be impaired by hypoxia, fever or, possibly, an active intracranial hemorrhage. Be alert for critical changes that require immediate attention.

Inspecting related body structures

Pay special attention to the patient's skin and mucous membranes, fingernails, and eyes as well as to the spleen, liver and lymph nodes.

Skin and mucous membranes

Your patient's skin color directly reflects body fluid composition. Observe for pallor, cyanosis, or jaundice. Because normal skin colors vary widely, ask the patient if his present skin tone is normal. Decreased hemoglobin (Hb) content can cause pallor. Cyanosis, in turn, can result from excessive deoxygenated Hb in cutaneous blood vessels, a condition caused by hypoxia, which appears in some anemias. Check for erythema (redness), indicating a local inflammation, and plethora (red, florid complexion), which appears in polycythemia.

Focus on the skin over your patient's lymph nodes and note any color abnormalities. Nodes covered by red-streaked skin suggest a lymphatic disorder, including acute lymphadenitis. With lymphadenitis, also look for an obvious infection site. Also, note other infection signs, such as poor wound healing, wound drainage, induration (tissue hardening), or lesions. Pay close attention to sites of recent invasive procedures for evidence of wound healing.

When assessing the patient's mucous membranes and skin for jaundice, observe him in natural light, if possible. With dark-skinned patients, inspect the buccal mucosa, palms, and soles for a yellowish tinge. For an edematous patient, examine the inner forearm for jaundice. An elevated bilirubin level may appear secondary to increased erythrocyte hemolysis — either acquired or hereditary. *Note:* Excessive carrot or yellow vegetable intake may cause yellow skin but doesn't change sclera or mucous membrane color.

If you suspect a blood clotting abnormality, check the patient's skin for purpuric lesions. These vary in size and usually result from thrombocytopenia. With dark-skinned patients, check the oral mucosa or conjunctivae for petechiae or ecchymoses.

Check your patient's skin for dryness and coarseness, which can indicate iron deficiency anemia. Ask whether his skin itches. Itching (pruritus) can signal Hodgkin's disease, chronic lymphocytic leukemia, or polycythemia vera.

Inspect the mucous membranes, especially the gingivae. Bleeding, redness, swelling, or ulceration may indicate leukemia. A smooth tongue can signify vitamin B_{12} deficiency or iron deficiency anemia. An ulcerated tongue can signal leukemia or neutropenia or systemic lupus erythematosus (SLE). Fluffy, white patches scattered throughout the oral cavity indicate candidiasis, a fungal infection. Hairy leukoplakia, a lacy white plaque found typically on the buccal mucosa, appears with acquired immunodeficiency syndrome.

Fingernails

Note any abnormalities in the patient's nails. Longitudinal striation can indicate anemia. Koilonychia (spoon nail) characterizes iron deficiency anemia. The fingers may become clubbed; in this abnormality, the nail angle may change from 160 degrees to 180 degrees or more. Finger clubbing indicates chronic hypoxia.

Eyes

Inspect the color of the patient's conjunctivae (normally pink) and sclerae (normally white). Conjunctival pallor may accompany anemia. Yellowish sclerae may indicate an accumulation of bile pigment from excessive hemolysis. Retinal hemorrhages and exudates, seen with an ophthalmoscope, suggest severe anemia and thrombocytopenia. Also observe the eyelids for signs of infection or inflammation, such as swelling, redness, and lesions.

Spleen and liver

Inspect the abdominal area for enlargement, distention, and asymmetry, possibly indicating a tumor. The spleen and liver are further assessed while inspecting the GI system.

Percuss the spleen to estimate its size. On percussion, the spleen normally produces dullness in the left upper quadrant between the sixth and tenth ribs. Spleen enlargement (splenomegaly) may indicate polycythemia or hemolytic anemia.

Palpate the spleen to detect tenderness and confirm splenomegaly. The spleen must be enlarged to approximately three times normal size to be palpable. Splenic tenderness may result from infections or anemia.

Percussion of the liver can help you to estimate its size. Hepatomegaly (liver enlargement) is commonly associated with polycythemia or hemolytic anemia. Then palpate the liver to confirm enlargement and check the liver for tenderness.

Lymph nodes

The first step in regional lymph node assessment is inspecting areas where the patient reports "swollen glands" or "lumps" for color abnormalities and visible lymph node enlargement. Then inspect all other nodal regions. Proceed from head to toe to avoid missing regions. Normally, lymph nodes can't be seen.

Use the pads of your index and middle fingers to palpate the patient's superficial lymph nodes in the head and neck and in the axillary, epitrochlear, inguinal, and popliteal areas. Apply gentle pressure and rotary motion to feel the underlying nodes without obscuring them by pressing them into deeper soft tissues. Lymph nodes usually can't be felt in a healthy patient. Tenderness of sternal nodes may indicate anemia. (See *Palpating the lymph nodes*, pages 143 to 145.)

Assessing body systems

Hematologic disorders affect many body systems, each of which warrants inspection during a complete assessment.

Respiratory system

Observe the patient's respiratory rate, rhythm, and energy expenditure related to respiratory effort. Note the position he assumes to ease breathing. Exertional dyspnea, tachypnea, and orthopnea commonly accompany hypoxia.

Percuss the anterior, lateral, and posterior thorax, comparing one side with the other. A dull sound indicates consolidation, which may occur with pneumonia. Hyperresonance may result from trapped air, as in bronchial asthma.

Auscultate over the lungs to assess for adventitious (abnormal) sounds. Wheezing suggests asthma or an allergic response. Crackles may denote a respiratory infection such as pneumonia.

Cardiovascular system

Assess the pulse rate and rhythm for anemia-related tachycardia or other arrhythmias. Then palpate and auscultate the heart and vessels for other signs of blood disorders. First, palpate the point of maximal impulse (PMI), normally located in the fifth intercostal space at the midclavicular line. The PMI may be broadened, displaced, or less distinct because of ventricular enlargement, the body's compensatory mechanism for severe anemia.

Auscultate for heart sounds over the precordium. Normally, auscultation reveals only the first and second heart sounds (*lub-dub*). Any auscultated apical systolic murmurs may signify severe anemia; mitral, aortic, or pulmonary murmurs; sickle cell anemia; pericardial friction rub; endocarditis; or pericardial effusion, which occurs in about 50% of patients with SLE.

Inspect the patient's capillary refill, checking for delayed refill and pallor, which may indicate anemia. Palpate the peripheral pulses, which should be symmetrical and regular. Weak, irregular pulses also may indicate anemia.

GI system

With the patient lying down, auscultate the abdomen before palpation and per-

(Text continues on page 146.)

Palpating the lymph nodes

When assessing a patient for signs of an immune disorder, you need to palpate the superficial lymph nodes of the head, neck and axillary, epitrochlear, inguinal, and popliteal areas, using the pads of the index and middle fingers. Always palpate gently; begin with light pressure and gradually increase the pressure.

To palpate the submandibular, submental, anterior cervical, and occipital nodes, position your fingers as shown. Palpate over the mandibular surface and continue moving up and down the entire neck. Flex the head forward or to the side being examined. This relaxes the tissues and makes enlarged nodes more palpable. Reverse your hand position to palpate the opposite side.

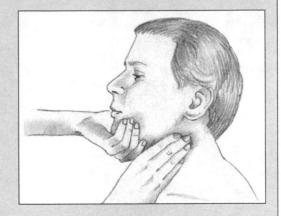

To palpate the preauricular, parotid, and mastoid nodes, position your fingers as shown.

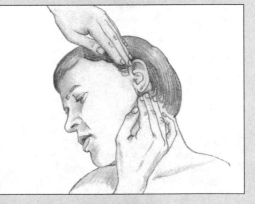

To palpate the posterior cervical nodes, place your fingertip pads along the anterior surface of the trapezius muscle as shown. Then move your fingertips toward the posterior surface of the sternocleidomastoid muscle.

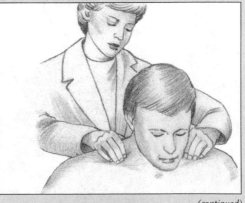

(continued)

Palpating the lymph nodes (continued)

To palpate the supraclavicular nodes, encourage the patient to relax so that the clavicles drop. To relax the soft tissues of the anterior neck, flex the patient's head slightly forward with your free hand. Then hook your left index finger over the clavicle lateral to the sternocleidomastoid muscle as shown. Rotate your fingers deeply into this area to feel these nodes.

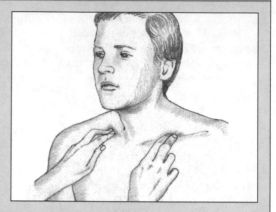

To palpate the axillary nodes, use your nondominant hand to support the patient's relaxed right arm and put your other hand as high in his right axilla as possible as shown. Then palpate the axillary nodes, gently pressing the soft tissues against the chest wall and the muscles surrounding the axilla (the pectorals, latissimus dorsi, subscapular, and anterior serratus). Repeat this procedure for the left axilla.

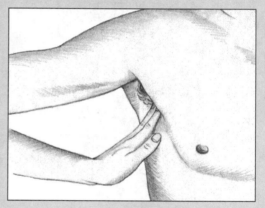

To palpate the epitrochlear lymph nodes, place your fingertips in the depression above and posterior to the medial area of the elbow as shown and palpate gently.

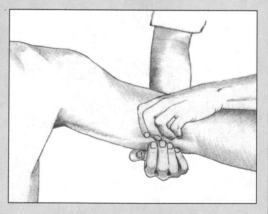

Palpating the lymph nodes (continued)

To palpate the inferior superficial inguinal (femoral) lymph nodes, gently press below the junction of the saphenous and femoral veins as shown.

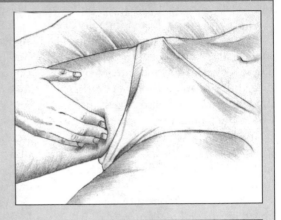

To palpate the superior superficial inguinal lymph nodes, press along the course of the saphenous veins as shown from the inguinal area to the abdomen.

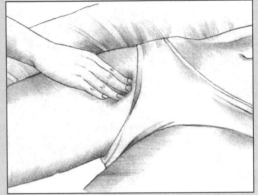

To palpate the popliteal nodes, press gently along the posterior muscles at the back of the knee as shown.

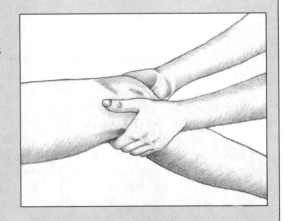

cussion to avoid altering bowel sounds. Listen for loud, high-pitched tinkling sounds, which herald the early stages of intestinal obstruction. Next, auscultate the liver and spleen. Listen carefully over both organs for friction rubs—grating sounds that fluctuate with respiration. These sounds usually indicate inflammation of the organ's peritoneal covering. Splenic friction rubs also suggest infarction and inflammation. Next, percuss the liver. Normally, the liver produces a dull sound over a span of 2½" to 4½" (6.5 to 11.5 cm). Hepatomegaly may accompany many immune disorders.

Palpate the abdomen to detect enlarged organs and tenderness. An enlarged liver that feels smooth and tender suggests hepatitis; one that feels hard and nodular suggests a neoplasm. Abdominal tenderness may result from infections.

Finally, inspect the anus, which should be pink and puckered without inflammation or breaks in the mucosal surface. Defer internal examination of the anus and rectal vault if you suspect or know that the patient has a low platelet count or granulocyte level.

Urinary system
Obtain a urine specimen and evaluate its color, clarity, and odor. Cloudy, malodorous urine may result from a urinary tract infection.

Nervous system
Evaluate the patient's level of consciousness (LOC) and mental status. Impaired neurologic function may occur secondary to hypoxia or fever. An anemic patient may not be able to concentrate or may become confused, especially if he's elderly. Hemorrhage also compromises oxygen supply to nerve tissues, resulting in similar symptoms. If bleeding occurs within the cranial vault, disorientation, progressive LOC, changes in motor and sensory capa-

bilities, changes in pupillary responses, and seizures may result.

Musculoskeletal system
Ask the patient to perform simple maneuvers, such as standing up, walking, and bending over. He should be able to do so effortlessly. Then test joint range of motion, particularly in the hand, wrist, and knee. Palpate the joints to assess for swelling, tenderness, and pain. If palpation reveals bone tenderness, the cause may be bone marrow hyperactivity, a compensatory mechanism for oxygen-carrying deficits prevalent in anemia. Bone tenderness may also result from a leukemic or immunoproliferative disorder such as plasma cell myeloma.

• • • • • • • • • • • •

ANEMIA, APLASTIC AND HYPOPLASTIC

Aplastic and hypoplastic anemias result from injury to or destruction of stem cells in the bone marrow or bone marrow matrix. The result is pancytopenia (anemia, granulocytopenia, and thrombocytopenia) and bone marrow hypoplasia. Although often used interchangeably with other terms for bone marrow failure, aplastic anemias properly refer to pancytopenia resulting from the decreased function of hypoplastic, fatty bone marrow.

Aplastic anemia affects men, women, and children of all ages and races. It's estimated that aplastic anemia affects 2 out of every 1 million people each year in the United States.

Aplastic and hypoplastic anemias generally produce fatal bleeding or infection. Mortality for patients with aplastic anemias with severe pancytopenia is 80% to 90%.

Causes and pathophysiology

Aplastic anemias usually develop when damaged or destroyed stem cells inhibit red blood cell (RBC) production. Less commonly, they develop when damaged bone marrow microvasculature creates an unfavorable environment for cell growth and maturation.

About one half of aplastic anemias result from the administration of drugs (antibiotics and anticonvulsants), use of toxic agents (such as benzene and chloramphenicol), or radiation. The rest may result from immunologic factors (unconfirmed), severe disease (especially hepatitis), or preleukemic and neoplastic infiltration of bone marrow.

Idiopathic anemias may be congenital and account for about 50% of confirmed cases. Two forms of idiopathic aplastic anemia have been identified: congenital hypoplastic anemia (Blackfan-Diamond anemia), which develops between age 2 and 3 months, and Fanconi's syndrome, which develops between birth and age 10.

In Fanconi's syndrome, chromosomal abnormalities are usually associated with multiple congenital anomalies, such as dwarfism and hypoplasia of the kidneys and spleen. When there's no consistent family or genetic history of aplastic anemia, such congenital abnormalities may result from an induced change in the development of the fetus.

Clinical presentation

Clinical features of aplastic anemias vary with the severity of pancytopenia but often develop insidiously. Signs and symptoms of anemia include:
- progressive weakness and fatigue
- shortness of breath
- headache
- pallor
- tachycardia
- heart failure.

Thrombocytopenia leads to ecchymosis, petechiae, hemorrhage, especially from the mucous membranes (nose, gums, rectum, and vagina) or into the retina or central nervous system. Neutropenia may lead to infection (fever, oral and rectal ulcers, and sore throat) but without the characteristic inflammation.

Differential diagnoses

- Myelodysplastic disorders
- Acute leukemia
- Hairy cell leukemia
- Disseminated infection
- Systemic lupus erythematosus
- Hypersplenism
- Other causes of pancytopenia

Diagnosis

Confirmation of aplastic anemia requires a series of laboratory tests:
- RBCs are usually normochromic and normocytic (although macrocytosis [larger-than-normal erythrocytes] and anisocytosis [excessive variation in erythrocyte size] may exist), with a total count of 1 million/µl or less. The absolute reticulocyte count is very low.
- Serum iron is elevated (unless bleeding occurs), but total iron-binding capacity is normal or slightly reduced. Hemosiderin is present, and tissue iron storage is visible microscopically.
- Platelet, white blood cell (WBC), and differential counts decrease.
- Coagulation tests are abnormal, reflecting decreased platelet count.
- Bone marrow aspiration from several sites may yield a "dry tap," and a biopsy shows severely hypocellular or aplastic marrow, with various amounts of fat, fibrous tissue, or gelatinous replacement; absence of tagged iron (because iron is deposited in the liver rather than in bone marrow) and megakaryocytes; and depression of erythroid elements.

Bone marrow transplantation

In bone marrow transplantation, usually 500 to 700 ml of marrow is aspirated from the pelvic bones of a human leukocyte antigen (HLA)–compatible donor (allogeneic) or of the recipient himself during complete remission (autologous). The aspirated marrow is filtered and then infused into the recipient in an attempt to repopulate the patient's marrow with normal cells. This procedure has effected long-term, healthy survival in about 50% of patients with severe aplastic anemia. Bone marrow transplantation may also be effective in patients with acute leukemia, certain immunodeficiency diseases, and solid tumor neoplasms.

Because bone marrow transplantation carries serious risks, it requires strict adherence to infection control and aseptic techniques. Explain to the patient that the success rate depends on the stage of the disease and an HLA-identical match.

TREATMENT
Assess the patient's understanding of bone marrow transplantation. If necessary, correct any misconceptions about this procedure and provide additional information as appropriate. Prepare the patient to expect an extended hospital stay. Explain that chemotherapy and possible radiation treatments are necessary to destroy cells that may cause the body to reject the transplanted tissue.

Various treatment protocols are used in bone marrow transplantation. For example, I.V. cyclophosphamide may be used with additional chemotherapeutic agents or total body irradiation and requires aggressive hydration to prevent hemorrhagic cystitis. Nausea and vomiting are controlled with an antiemetic, such as ondansetron, prochlorperazine, metoclopramide, or lorazepam, as needed. Allopurinol is used to prevent hyperuricemia resulting from tumor breakdown products.

Because alopecia is a common adverse effect of high-dose cyclophosphamide therapy, encourage the patient to choose a wig or scarf before treatment begins. Total body irradiation (in one dose or several daily doses) follows chemotherapy, inducing total marrow aplasia. Warn the patient that cataracts, GI disturbances, and sterility are possible adverse effects.

Management
General
Treatment is primarily inpatient. Identifiable causes must be eliminated and vigorous supportive measures must be provided, such as transfusions of packed RBCs, platelets, and experimental human antigen-matched leukocytes. Even after the cause is eliminated, recovery can take months.

Bone marrow transplantation is the treatment of choice for anemia due to severe aplasia and for patients who need constant RBC transfusions. (See *Bone marrow transplantation*.) Umbilical cord blood transplantation for treating patients with anemias is in the experimental stage.

Medication
Medications used to treat patients with aplastic and hypoplastic anemias include:
- prednisone — 5 to 60 mg/day P.O.; dosage individualized to stimulate erythroid production
- oxymetholone — 1 to 2 mg/kg/day P.O.

■ antithymocyte globulin—10 to 20 mg/kg diluted in 500 ml normal saline solution, I.V. over 4 to 6 hours for 8 to 14 days
■ cyclosporine—10 mg/kg P.O. initially, then taper to 5 to 10 mg/kg/day.

Referral
■ Any patient presenting with pancytopenia or suspected anemia needs an immediate referral to a hematologist-oncologist.

Follow-up
Follow-up requires close monitoring of all treatments by the collaborating specialist. Blood studies need to be monitored carefully in the patient who is receiving anemia-inducing drugs.

Patient teaching
■ Teach the patient with a low WBC count to take neutropenic precautions. Share this information with the patient's family members.
■ Teach the patient with a low platelet count what precautions must be taken to prevent bleeding.
■ Teach the patient to recognize signs of infection, and tell him to report them immediately.

Complications
■ Hemorrhage
■ Infection
■ Transfusion hepatitis
■ Heart failure
■ Complications due to therapy
■ Development of acute leukemia
■ Neoplasm

Special considerations
■ Encourage the patient who doesn't require hospitalization to continue his normal lifestyle, with appropriate restrictions (such as regular rest periods), until remission occurs.

■ People who work with the solvent benzene should be informed that 10 ppm is the highest safe environmental level and that a delayed reaction to benzene can develop.

• • • • • • • • • • • •
ANEMIA, FOLIC ACID DEFICIENCY

Folic acid deficiency anemia is a common, slowly progressive megaloblastic anemia. It's most prevalent in infants, adolescents, pregnant and lactating females, alcoholics, the elderly, and persons with malignant or intestinal diseases.

It's estimated that folic acid anemia affects 4 out of every 100,000 people in the United States.

Causes and pathophysiology
Folic acid deficiency anemia results from a deficiency or absence of folate, a vitamin that's essential for red blood cell (RBC) production and maturation. Causes include:
■ alcohol abuse (may suppress metabolic effects of folate)
■ poor diet (common in alcoholics, elderly people who live alone, and infants, especially those with infections or diarrhea)
■ impaired absorption (due to intestinal dysfunction from such disorders as celiac disease, tropical sprue, and regional jejunitis and from bowel resection)
■ bacteria competing for available folic acid
■ excessive cooking (can destroy a high percentage of folic acid in foods)
■ limited storage capacity in infants
■ prolonged drug therapy (with anticonvulsants and estrogens)

HEALTHY LIVING

Foods high in folic acid

Folic acid (pteroylglutamic acid or fo-lacin) is found in most body tissues, where it acts as a coenzyme in meta-bolic processes involving one carbon transfer. It's essential for the forma-tion and maturation of red blood cells and the synthesis of deoxyribo-nucleic acid.

Body stores of folic acid are rela-tively small (about 70 mg), and insuf-ficient daily folic acid intake (less than 50 mcg/day) usually induces folic acid deficiency within 4 months. Folic acid is plentiful in most well-balanced diets. However, because this vitamin is water-soluble and heat-labile, cooking easily destroys it. Also, approximately 20% of folic acid intake is excreted unabsorbed. Below is a list of foods high in folic acid.

FOOD	MCG/100 G
Asparagus spears	109
Beef liver	294
Broccoli spears	54
Collards (cooked)	102
Mushrooms	24
Oatmeal	33
Peanut butter	57
Red beans	180
Wheat germ	305

■ increased folic acid requirement during pregnancy, during rapid growth in infancy (common because of an increased sur-vival rate of preterm infants), during childhood and adolescence (because of a general use of folate-poor cow's milk), and in patients with neoplastic diseases and some skin diseases (chronic exfolia-tive dermatitis)

■ smoking (decreases vitamin C absorp-tion, which is necessary for folic acid ab-sorption).

Clinical presentation

Folic acid deficiency anemia gradually produces clinical features that are char-acteristic of other megaloblastic anemias but without the neurologic manifesta-tions. They include:

■ progressive fatigue
■ dyspnea
■ palpitations
■ weakness
■ glossitis
■ nausea
■ anorexia
■ headache
■ fainting
■ irritability
■ forgetfulness
■ pallor
■ slight jaundice
■ diarrhea
■ pica.

Folic acid deficiency anemia doesn't cause neurologic impairment unless it's associated with vitamin B_{12} deficiency, as in pernicious anemia.

Differential diagnoses

■ Pernicious anemia
■ Hemolytic anemia
■ Heart failure
■ Bowel disease
■ Thyroid dysfunction
■ Hodgkin's disease
■ Human immunodeficiency virus

Diagnosis

The Schilling test and a therapeutic trial of vitamin B_{12} injections are used to dis-tinguish between folic acid deficiency anemia and pernicious anemia. Significant findings include macrocytosis, a decreased reticulocyte count, low platelet count, and a RBC folate level less than 4 mg/ml. RBC folate is a more reliable indicator of folate deficiency because serum folate levels are dependent on dietary folate.

Management
General
The primary treatment modes for patients with folic acid deficiency anemia include dietary supplements and eliminating contributing causes. Many patients also respond favorably to a well-balanced diet. (See *Foods high in folic acid*.)

Medication
Medications used to treat patients with folic acid deficiency anemia include:
- folic acid—0.4 to 1 mg P.O., S.C., or I.M. daily
- hydroxocabalamin—30 mcg/day I.M. for 5 to 10 days; maintenance dose is 100 to 200 mcg I.M. once monthly.

If the patient has vitamin B_{12} and folate deficiencies, folic acid replenishment alone can aggravate neurologic dysfunction.

Referral
- Consult a hematologist if the patient isn't responding to folic acid or vitamin B_{12} injections. The patient may also need a nutrition consultation.

Follow-up
Follow-up blood work should be performed after therapy is completed. Consultation and collaboration with the hematologist is an integral part of follow-up.

Patient teaching
- Urge compliance with the prescribed course of therapy. Advise the patient not to stop taking the supplements when he begins to feel better.

- If the patient has glossitis, emphasize the importance of good oral hygiene. Suggest regular use of mild or diluted mouthwash and a soft toothbrush.

Complications
- In pregnancy, neural tube defects in the fetus
- Infertility
- Increased susceptibility to infection
- Heart failure

Special considerations
- If the patient has a severe deficiency, explain that diet only reinforces folic acid supplementation and isn't therapeutic by itself.

HEALTHY LIVING To prevent folic acid deficiency anemia, emphasize the importance of a well-balanced diet that's high in folic acid. Identify alcoholics with poor dietary habits and try to arrange for appropriate counseling.

• • • • • • • • • • • •

ANEMIA, IRON DEFICIENCY

In iron deficiency anemia, iron supplies are inadequate for optimal red blood cell (RBC) formation. The result is smaller (microcytic) cells with less color on staining. Body stores of iron, including plasma iron, decrease, as does transferrin, which binds with and transports iron. The depleted RBC mass, in turn, leads to decreased hemoglobin (Hb) concentration (hypochromia) and decreased oxygen-carrying capacity of the blood. (See *Absorption and storage of iron*, page 152.)

It's estimated that iron deficiency anemia, the most common form of anemia, occurs in 20% of women, 50% of pregnant women, and 3% of men. It's more prevalent among the lower socioeconomic population.

Absorption and storage of iron

Iron, which is essential to erythropoiesis, is abundant throughout the body. Two-thirds of total body iron is found in hemoglobin (Hb); the other third, mostly in the reticuloendothelial system (liver, spleen, and bone marrow), with small amounts in muscle, blood serum, and body cells.

Adequate dietary ingestion of iron and recirculation of iron released from disintegrating red cells maintain iron supplies. The duodenum and upper part of the small intestine absorb dietary iron. Such absorption depends on gastric acid content, the amount of reducing substances (for example, ascorbic acid) present in the alimentary canal, and dietary iron intake. If iron intake is deficient, the body gradually depletes its iron stores, causing decreased Hb levels and, eventually, symptoms of iron deficiency anemia.

Iron deficiency anemia is a common disease worldwide and affects 10% to 30% of the adult population of the United States.

Causes and pathophysiology

Iron deficiency anemia occurs most commonly in premenopausal women, infants (especially premature and low-birthweight infants), children, and adolescents (especially girls).

Iron deficiency anemia may result from:

- inadequate dietary intake of iron (less than 2 mg/day), as in prolonged, unsupplemented (not eating solid foods after age 6 months) breast- or bottle-feeding of infants and during periods of stress, such as rapid growth in children and adolescents

- iron malabsorption, as in chronic diarrhea, partial or total gastrectomy, and malabsorption syndromes such as celiac disease
- blood loss secondary to drug-induced GI bleeding (from anticoagulants, aspirin, and steroids) or due to heavy menses, hemorrhage from trauma, GI ulcers, cancer, or bleeding varices
- pregnancy, which diverts maternal iron to the fetus for erythropoiesis
- intravascular hemolysis-induced hemoglobinuria or paroxysmal nocturnal hemoglobinuria
- mechanical erythrocyte trauma caused by a prosthetic heart valve or vena cava filters.

Clinical presentation

Because of the gradual progression of iron deficiency anemia, many patients are initially asymptomatic. They tend to not seek medical treatment until anemia is severe.

At advanced stages, decreased Hb and the consequent decrease in the blood's oxygen-carrying capacity cause the patient to develop:

- dyspnea on exertion
- fatigue
- listlessness
- pallor
- inability to concentrate
- irritability
- headache
- susceptibility to infection.

Decreased oxygen perfusion causes the heart to compensate with increased cardiac output and tachycardia.

In chronic iron deficiency anemia, the following symptoms may occur:

- nails become spoon-shaped and brittle
- corners of the mouth crack
- tongue turns smooth
- dysphagia
- pica.

Associated neuromuscular effects include:
- vasomotor disturbances
- numbness and tingling of the extremities
- neuralgic pain.

Differential diagnoses
- Thalassemia
- Anemia of chronic disease

Diagnosis
Blood studies (serum iron, total iron-binding capacity, and ferritin levels) and stores in bone marrow may confirm iron deficiency anemia. However, the results of these tests can be misleading because of complicating factors, such as infection, pneumonia, blood transfusion, and iron supplements. Characteristic blood study results include:
- low Hb levels (males, less than 12 g/dl; females, less than 10 g/dl)
- low hematocrit (males, less than 47 ml/dl; females, less than 42 ml/dl)
- low serum iron levels, with high iron-binding capacity
- low serum ferritin levels
- low RBC count, with microcytic and hypochromic cells (in early stages, RBC count may be normal, except in infants and children)
- decreased mean corpuscular Hb in severe anemia.

Bone marrow studies reveal depleted or absent iron stores (done by staining) and normoblastic hyperplasia.

Management
General
The first priority of treatment is to determine the underlying cause of anemia. When this is determined, iron replacement therapy can begin.

Carefully assess a patient's drug history because certain drugs, such as pancreatic enzymes and vitamin E, may in-terfere with iron metabolism and absorption and because aspirin, steroids, and other drugs may cause GI bleeding.

Medication
Medications used in the treatment of iron deficiency anemia include:
- ferrous sulfate — 324 mg P.O. t.i.d., or a combination of iron and ascorbic acid to enhance iron absorption
- iron — 25 to 100 mg I.M.; Z-track method daily (see *How to inject iron solutions,* page 154).

Referral
- Provide a referral to a hematologist if the patient isn't responding to prescribed treatment.
- Provide a referral to an internist or gastroenterologist for evaluation of the cause of iron deficiency anemia (such as malignancies).

Follow-up
Evaluate serum iron levels and reticulocyte counts at 7- to 10-day intervals after treatment is initiated. Hb level and hematocrit should be evaluated monthly and an increase of at least 2 g/dl should be evident. Treatment should continue for 4 to 6 months after hematocrit returns to normal. To confirm that iron stores are adequate, serum ferritin levels should be also checked.

HEALTHY LIVING Health care providers can play a vital role in preventing iron deficiency anemia by encouraging families with deficient iron intake to eat meat, fish, or poultry; whole or enriched grain; and foods high in ascorbic acid.

Patient teaching
- Teach the patient the basics of a nutritionally balanced diet that includes red meat, green vegetables, eggs, whole wheat, iron-fortified bread, cereal, and

How to inject iron solutions

To inject iron solutions, use the Z-track technique to avoid subcutaneous (S.C.) irritation and discoloration.

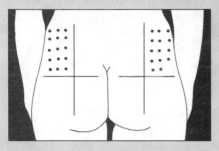

Choose a 19G to 20G 2″ to 3″ needle. After drawing up the solution, change to a fresh needle to avoid tracking the solution through to S.C. tissue. Draw 0.5 cc of air into the syringe as an "air lock."

Displace the skin and fat at the injection site (in upper outer quadrant of buttocks or the ventrogluteal site only) firmly to one side. Clean the area, and insert the needle. Aspirate to check for entry into a blood vessel. Inject the solution slowly, followed by the 0.5 cc of air in the syringe. Wait 10 seconds, then pull the needle straight out, and release tissues.

Apply direct pressure to the site, but don't massage it. Caution the patient against vigorous exercise for 15 to 30 minutes.

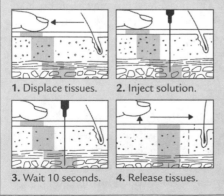

1. Displace tissues. **2.** Inject solution.

3. Wait 10 seconds. **4.** Release tissues.

milk. (No food in itself contains enough iron to treat iron deficiency anemia; an average-sized person with anemia would have to eat at least 10 lb [4.5 kg] of steak daily to receive therapeutic amounts of iron.)

■ Teach the patient that iron supplements should be taken on an empty stomach, or with orange juice, 1 hour before meals to obtain the most effective dose of iron. Food decreases iron delivery by 50%.

■ Advise the patient that milk or an antacid interferes with iron absorption but that vitamin C can increase absorption. Instruct the patient to drink liquid supplemental iron through a straw to prevent staining the teeth.

■ Tell the patient to report adverse reactions, such as nausea, vomiting, diarrhea, constipation, fever, and severe stomach pain, which may necessitate a dosage adjustment.

■ Review guidelines for managing anemia with the patient and family members.

■ Advise the patient that iron can cause black bowel movements.

■ Iron overdose is highly toxic. Keep supplements out of the reach of small children.

■ Emphasize a diet high in protein, iron-containing foods, and fiber to decrease the likelihood of constipation.

Complications

■ Preterm delivery, low birth weight, and learning deficits (if untreated during pregnancy)

■ Unidentified and hidden bleeding points, particularly bleeding malignancies

Special considerations

■ Emphasize the need for high-risk individuals—such as premature infants, children under age 2, and pregnant women—

to take prophylactic oral iron. (Children under age 2 should also receive supplemental cereals and formulas high in iron.)

• • • • • • • • • • •

ANEMIA, PERNICIOUS

Pernicious anemia is a megaloblastic anemia characterized by decreased gastric production of hydrochloric acid and a deficiency of intrinsic factor (IF), a substance normally secreted by the parietal cells of the gastric mucosa that's essential for vitamin B_{12} absorption. The resulting vitamin B_{12} deficiency causes serious neurologic, gastric, and intestinal abnormalities. Untreated pernicious anemia may lead to permanent neurologic disability and death.

Pernicious anemia primarily affects people of northern European ancestry; in the United States, it's most common in New England and the Great Lakes region because of ethnic concentrations. It's rare in children, Blacks, and Asians.

AGE ALERT Onset of pernicious anemia typically occurs between ages 50 and 60; incidence increases with age.

Causes and pathophysiology

Familial incidence of pernicious anemia suggests a genetic predisposition. A significantly higher incidence in patients with immunologically related diseases, such as thyroiditis, myxedema, and Graves' disease, supports a widely held theory that an inherited autoimmune response causes gastric mucosal atrophy and, therefore, deficiency of hydrochloric acid and IF.

Deficiency of IF impairs vitamin B_{12} absorption. The resulting vitamin B_{12} deficiency inhibits cell growth, particularly of red blood cells (RBCs), leading to insufficient and deformed RBCs with poor oxygen-carrying capacity. It also impairs myelin formation, causing neurologic damage. Iatrogenic induction can follow partial gastrectomy.

Clinical presentation

Characteristically, pernicious anemia has an insidious onset but eventually causes an unmistakable triad of symptoms:
- weakness
- sore tongue
- numbness and tingling in the extremities.

Other signs include:
- lips, gums, and tongue that appear markedly bloodless
- faintly jaundiced sclera
- pale to bright yellow skin.

GI signs include gastric mucosal atrophy and decreased hydrochloric acid production, which disturb digestion and lead to:
- nausea
- vomiting
- anorexia
- weight loss
- flatulence
- diarrhea
- constipation.

In addition, the patient may become highly susceptible to infection, especially of the genitourinary tract.

Gingival bleeding and tongue inflammation also may occur, hindering eating and intensifying anorexia.

Central nervous system (CNS) signs include nerve demyelination caused by vitamin B_{12} deficiency, which initially affects the peripheral nerves but gradually extends to the spinal cord. Also, neurologic effects of pernicious anemia may include neuritis, weakness in the extremities, peripheral numbness and paresthesia, disturbed position sense, lack of coordination, ataxia, impaired fine finger movement, positive Babinski's and Romberg's signs, light-headedness, optic muscle atrophy, loss of bowel and bladder control, impotence (in males), and altered vision (diplopia and blurred vision), taste, and hearing (tinnitus).

In addition, irritability, poor memory, headache, depression, and delirium are also symptoms, although some of these are temporary; irreversible CNS changes can occur if treatment is delayed.

Cardiovascular signs include increasingly fragile cell membranes, which induce widespread destruction of RBCs, resulting in low hemoglobin (Hb) levels. The impaired oxygen-carrying capacity of the blood secondary to lowered Hb leads to weakness, fatigue, and light-headedness. Other signs include compensatory increased cardiac output that results in palpitations, wide pulse pressure, dyspnea, orthopnea, tachycardia, premature beats and, eventually, heart failure.

Differential diagnoses
- Crohn's disease
- Alcoholism
- Folic acid deficiency
- Neurologic disorders without vitamin B_{12} deficiency
- Liver dysfunction
- Hemolysis or bleeding
- Hypothyroidism
- Myelodysplasia
- Tape worm infestation
- Drug effects

Diagnosis
A family history, typical ethnic heritage, and results of blood studies, bone marrow aspiration, gastric analysis, and the Schilling test establish the diagnosis of pernicious anemia. Laboratory screening must rule out other anemias that cause similar symptoms, such as folic acid deficiency anemia, because treatment differs.

Diagnosis must also rule out vitamin B_{12} deficiency resulting from malabsorption due to GI disorders, gastric surgery, radiation, or drug therapy.

Blood study results that suggest pernicious anemia include:
- decreased Hb level (4 to 5 g/dl) and RBC count
- increased mean corpuscular volume (greater than 120 μm^3) because larger-than-normal RBCs each contain increased amounts of Hb; also, an increased mean corpuscular Hb concentration
- possible low white blood cell and platelet counts and large, malformed platelets
- serum vitamin B_{12} assay level less than 0.1 mcg/ml
- elevated serum lactate dehydrogenase levels
- elevated serum iron level
- normal total iron binding capacity level
- elevated ferritin level.

Bone marrow aspiration reveals erythroid hyperplasia (crowded red bone marrow), with increased numbers of megaloblasts but few normally developing RBCs. Gastric analysis shows absence of free hydrochloric acid after histamine or pentagastrin injection.

The Schilling test is definitive for pernicious anemia. The patient receives a small oral dose (0.5 to 2.0 mcg) of radioactive vitamin B_{12} after fasting for 12 hours. A larger dose (1 mg) of nonradioactive vitamin B_{12} is given I.M. 2 hours later as a parenteral flush, and the radioactivity of a 24-hour urine specimen is measured. About 7% of the radioactive vitamin B_{12} dose is excreted in the first 24 hours; persons with pernicious anemia excrete less than 3%. (In pernicious anemia, the vitamin remains unabsorbed and is passed in the stool.) When the Schilling test is repeated with IF added, the test shows normal vitamin B_{12} excretion.

Important serologic findings may include IF antibodies and antiparietal cell antibodies.

Management
General
In addition to vitamin B_{12} replacement, therapeutic management of patients with pernicious anemia includes dietary measures, activity restrictions, and the prevention of infection and other complications. (See *Supportive management of patients with anemia*, page 158.)

Medication
Medications used to treat patients with pernicious anemia include:
- cyanocobalamin — 100 mcg/day I.M. or S.C. for 6 to 7 days, then once monthly S.C.
- ferrous sulfate — 324 mg P.O. t.i.d.
- folic acid — 0.4 to 1.0 mg/day P.O., S.C., or I.M.

Parenteral vitamin B_{12} replacement can reverse pernicious anemia, minimize complications, and possibly prevent permanent neurologic damage. An initial high dose of parenteral vitamin B_{12} (daily for 1 week, then weekly for 1 month) causes rapid RBC regeneration. Within 2 weeks, Hb levels should increase to normal and the patient's condition should markedly improve.

Because rapid cell regeneration increases the patient's iron and folate requirements, concomitant iron and folic acid replacement is necessary to prevent iron deficiency anemia. After the patient's condition improves, the vitamin B_{12} dosage can be decreased to maintenance levels and given monthly. Because such injections must be continued for the duration of the patient's life, patients should learn self-administration of vitamin B_{12}.

Referral
- The patient may need referral to a gastroenterologist for GI disturbances and to rule out malignancy.
- Referral to a radiologist may be needed for administration of the Schilling test.

Follow-up
Monthly follow-up is needed for vitamin B_{12} injections and regular laboratory evaluations. Endoscopy every 5 years is used to rule out gastric carcinoma.

Patient teaching
- Instruct the patient to eat a well-balanced diet, including foods high in vitamin B_{12} (meat, liver, fish, eggs, and milk).
- Warn the patient with a sensory deficit not to use a heating pad because it could cause burns.

Complications
- Hypokalemia (in the 1st week of treatment)
- CNS symptoms (may be permanent if the patient isn't treated within 6 months of the onset of symptoms)
- Gastric polyps
- Stomach cancer

Special considerations
- Stress that vitamin B_{12} replacement isn't a permanent cure and that these injections must be continued for the duration of the patient's life, even after symptoms subside.

HEALTHY LIVING To prevent pernicious anemia, emphasize the importance of vitamin B_{12} supplements to the patient who underwent extensive gastric resection or one who follows a strict vegetarian diet.

Supportive management of patients with anemia

Include these measures in the supportive management of a patient with anemia.

MEETING NUTRITIONAL NEEDS
- If the patient is fatigued, urge him to eat small, frequent meals throughout the day.
- If he has oral lesions, suggest soft, cool, bland foods.
- If he has dyspepsia, eliminate spicy foods from his diet and include milk and dairy products.
- If the patient is anorexic and irritable, encourage his family to bring his favorite foods from home (unless his diet is restricted) and to keep him company during meals, if possible.

SETTING LIMITS ON ACTIVITIES
- Assess the effect of a specific activity by monitoring the patient's pulse rate during the activity. If the pulse accelerates rapidly and the patient develops hypotension with hyperpnea, diaphoresis, light-headedness, palpitations, shortness of breath, or weakness, the activity is too strenuous.
- Tell the patient to pace activities and allow for frequent rest periods.

DECREASING SUSCEPTIBILITY TO INFECTION
- Use strict aseptic technique.
- Isolate the patient from infectious persons.
- Instruct the patient to avoid crowds and other sources of infection. Encourage him to practice good hand-washing technique.
- Stress the importance of receiving necessary immunizations and prompt medical treatment for any sign of infection.

PREPARING THE PATIENT FOR DIAGNOSTIC TESTING
- Explain erythropoiesis, the function of blood, and the purpose of diagnostic and therapeutic procedures.
- Tell the patient how he can participate in diagnostic testing. Give him an honest description of the pain or discomfort he'll probably experience.
- If possible, schedule all tests to avoid tiring the patient.

PREVENTING COMPLICATIONS
- Observe for signs of bleeding that may exacerbate anemia. Check stool for occult bleeding. Assess for ecchymoses, gingival bleeding, and hematuria.
- If blood transfusions are needed for severe anemia (hemoglobin level less than 5 g/dl), give washed red blood cells in partial exchange if evidence of pump failure is present. Carefully monitor for signs of circulatory overload or transfusion reaction.
- Warn the patient to move about or change positions slowly to minimize dizziness induced by cerebral hypoxia.

• • • • • • • • • • • •

ANEMIA, SICKLE CELL

Sickle cell anemia is a congenital hemolytic anemia that occurs primarily, but not exclusively, in the black population. It results from a defective hemoglobin (Hb) molecule (Hb S) that causes red blood cells (RBCs) to roughen and become sickle-shaped. Such cells impair circulation, resulting in chronic ill health (fatigue, dyspnea on exertion, and swollen joints), periodic crises, long-term complications, and premature death.

Sickle cell anemia is most common in Africans of tropical descent and in people of African descent; about 1 in 10 blacks carry the abnormal gene. If two such carriers have offspring, there is a 1 in 4 chance (25%) that each child will have the disease. Overall, 1 in every 400 to 600 black children has sickle cell anemia.

This disease also occurs in the populations of Puerto Rico, Turkey, India, the Middle East, and the Mediterranean, among others. The defective Hb gene may have persisted in areas where malaria is endemic because the heterozygous sickle cell trait provides resistance to malaria and is actually beneficial.

Penicillin prophylaxis can decrease morbidity and mortality from bacterial infections. Half of such patients die by their early twenties; few live to middle age.

Causes and pathophysiology

Sickle cell anemia results from homozygous inheritance of the Hb S gene, which causes the substitution of the amino acid valine for glutamic acid in the beta-hemoglobin chain. Heterozygous inheritance of this gene results in sickle cell trait, usually an asymptomatic condition. (See *Sickle cell trait*.)

Sickle cell trait

Sickle cell trait is a relatively benign condition that results from heterozygous inheritance of the abnormal hemoglobin (Hb) S-producing gene. Like sickle cell anemia, this condition is most common in blacks. The sickle cell trait never progresses to sickle cell anemia.

In persons with sickle cell trait (known as carriers), 20% to 40% of their total Hb is Hb S; the rest is normal. Such persons usually have no symptoms. They have normal Hb levels and hematocrit and can expect a normal life span. Nevertheless, they must avoid situations that provoke hypoxia, which can occasionally cause a sickling crisis similar to that in sickle cell anemia.

Genetic counseling is essential for sickle cell carriers. If two sickle cell carriers reproduce, each of their children has a 25% chance of inheriting sickle cell anemia.

The abnormal Hb S found in RBCs of patients with sickle cell anemia becomes insoluble whenever hypoxia occurs. As a result, these RBCs become rigid, rough, and elongated, forming a crescent, or sickle, shape. Such sickling can produce hemolysis (cell destruction). (See *Comparing normal and sickled red blood cells*, page 160.)

In addition, these altered cells tend to pile up in capillaries and smaller blood vessels, making the blood more viscous. Normal circulation is impaired, causing pain, tissue infarctions, and swelling. Such blockage causes anoxic changes that lead to further sickling and obstruction.

Comparing normal and sickled red blood cells

When a person with sickle cell anemia develops hypoxia, the abnormal hemoglobin S found in the red blood cells (RBCs) becomes insoluble. This causes the RBCs to become rigid, rough, and elongated, forming the characteristic sickle shape.

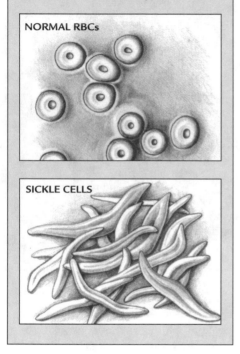

NORMAL RBCs

SICKLE CELLS

Clinical presentation

Characteristically, sickle cell anemia produces the following clinical effects:
- tachycardia
- cardiomegaly
- systolic and diastolic murmurs
- pulmonary infarctions (which may result in cor pulmonale)
- chronic fatigue
- unexplained dyspnea or dyspnea on exertion
- hepatomegaly
- jaundice
- pallor

- joint swelling
- aching bones
- chest pains
- ischemic leg ulcers (especially around the ankles)

- increased susceptibility to infection.

Such signs and symptoms usually don't develop until after age 6 months because large amounts of fetal Hb protect infants for the first few months after birth. Low socioeconomic status and related problems, such as poor nutrition and education, may delay diagnosis and supportive treatment.

Infection, stress, dehydration, and conditions that provoke hypoxia — strenuous exercise, high altitude, unpressurized aircraft, cold, and vasoconstrictive drugs — may all provoke periodic crises. Four types of crises can occur: painful, aplastic, acute sequestration, or hemolytic.

In painful crisis

Also called a vaso-occlusive crisis or infarctive crisis, painful crisis is the most common crisis and is the hallmark of this disease. It usually appears periodically after age 5.

A painful crisis results from blood vessel obstruction by rigid, tangled sickle cells, which causes tissue anoxia and possible necrosis. It's characterized by:
- severe abdominal, thoracic, muscular, or bone pain
- possibly increased jaundice
- dark urine
- low-grade fever.

Autosplenectomy, in which splenic damage and scarring is so extensive that the spleen shrinks and becomes impalpable, occurs in patients with long-term disease. This can lead to increased susceptibility to *Streptococcus pneumoniae* sepsis, which can be fatal if not promptly treated.

After the crisis subsides (in 4 days to several weeks), infection may develop, causing such signs and symptoms as lethargy, sleepiness, fever, and apathy.

In aplastic crisis

Aplastic crisis (also called megaloblastic crisis) results from bone marrow depression and is associated with infection, usually viral. It's characterized by:
- pallor
- lethargy
- sleepiness
- dyspnea
- possible coma
- markedly decreased bone marrow activity
- RBC hemolysis.

In acute sequestration crisis

In infants between ages 8 months and 2 years, an acute sequestration crisis can cause sudden massive entrapment of RBCs in the spleen and liver. This rare crisis causes lethargy and pallor; if untreated, it commonly progresses to hypovolemic shock and death.

In hemolytic crisis

Hemolytic crisis is quite rare, usually occurring in patients who have glucose-6-phosphate dehydrogenase deficiency with sickle cell anemia. It probably results from complications of sickle cell anemia, such as infection, rather than from the disorder itself.

Hemolytic crisis causes liver congestion and hepatomegaly as a result of degenerative changes. It worsens chronic jaundice, although increased jaundice doesn't always point to a hemolytic crisis.

Indicators of crisis

Suspect any type of crisis described above in a sickle cell anemia patient with these signs and symptoms:

- pale lips, tongue, palms, or nail beds
- lethargy
- listlessness
- sleepiness, with difficulty awakening
- irritability
- severe pain
- temperature over 104° F (40° C), or a fever of 100° F (37.8° C) that persists for 2 days.

Long-term complications

Sickle cell anemia also causes long-term complications. Typically, such a child is small for his age and puberty is delayed. (However, fertility isn't impaired). If he reaches adulthood, his body build tends to be spiderlike — narrow shoulders and hips, long extremities, curved spine, barrel chest, and elongated skull.

Premature death commonly results from infection or repeated occlusion of small blood vessels and consequent infarction or necrosis of major organs.

Differential diagnoses

- Anemia and other hemoglobinopathies
- Infection or other causes of acute pain in joints, bones, and abdomen (similar to painful crisis)
- Vaso-occlusive, hemolytic, or aplastic crisis
- Retinal detachment
- Cerebrovascular accident (CVA)
- Severe infection
- Dehydration

Diagnosis

A family history and typical clinical features suggest sickle cell anemia:
- Hb electrophoresis showing Hb S or other hemoglobinopathies can confirm the diagnosis. Electrophoresis should be done on umbilical cord blood samples at birth to provide sickle cell disease screening for all neonates at risk.
- Additional laboratory studies show a low RBC count, elevated white blood

Inheritance patterns in sickle cell anemia

When both parents are carriers of the sickle cell trait, each child has a 25% chance of developing sickle cell anemia, a 25% chance of being a normal noncarrier, and a 50% chance of being a carrier of the sickle cell trait.

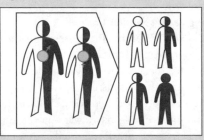

When one parent has sickle cell anemia and one is normal, all offspring are carriers of the sickle cell trait.

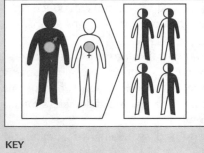

KEY

☐ Normal, noncarrier

▮ Normal, carrier of sickle cell trait

■ Sickle cell anemia (affected with sickle cell disease)

cell and platelet counts, decreased erythrocyte sedimentation rate, increased serum iron level, decreased RBC survival, and reticulocytosis. Hb level may be low or normal.

Management
General
If the patient's Hb level drops suddenly or if his condition deteriorates rapidly, a transfusion of packed RBCs is needed. In an acute sequestration crisis, treatment may include sedation, administration of analgesics, blood transfusion, oxygen administration, and large amounts of oral and I.V. fluids. Hospitalization is required for most crises and complications.

Medication
A good antisickling agent isn't yet available; the most commonly used drug, sodium cyanate, has many adverse effects.

To prevent painful crises give hydroxyurea 15 mg/kg/day P.O. may be increased every 12 weeks until maximum tolerated dose or 35 mg/kg/day.

To treat pain with sickle cell anemia give:
- ibuprofen — 400 mg P.O. q.i.d. for mild pain
- morphine — 2 to 10 mg I.V. infusion every hour p.r.n.

Referral
- The patient requires a hematology consultation.
- The patient and family members may require psychiatric counseling to cope with the effects of this illness. Also, support groups such as the Sickle Cell Association of America may be helpful.
- Refer the parents of a child with sickle cell anemia for genetic counseling to answer their questions about the risk to future children. Recommend screening of other family members to determine if they're heterozygote carriers. (See *Inheritance patterns in sickle cell anemia*.)

CLINICAL CAUTION A woman with sickle cell anemia may be a poor obstetric risk and her use of oral contraceptives is risky. Refer her to birth control counseling with a gynecologist.

Follow-up
Monitoring of the patient may take place in a primary care office with intermittent

follow-up by the specialist. Any crisis should be immediately referred to the specialist for treatment. If infection occurs, blood and urine cultures, chest X-ray, complete blood count, and reticulocyte testing should be done.

Patient teaching
■ Instruct all parents and patients to report signs and symptoms of infection.

During remission
■ Advise the patient to avoid tight clothing that restricts circulation.
■ Warn against strenuous exercise, vasoconstricting medication, cold temperatures (including drinking large amounts of ice water and swimming), unpressurized aircrafts, high altitudes, and other conditions that provoke hypoxia.
■ Stress the need to increase fluid intake to prevent dehydration resulting from the impaired ability to concentrate urine. Tell the parents to encourage such a child to drink more fluids, especially in the summer, by offering milk shakes, ice pops, and eggnog.

Complications
■ Bone infarct
■ Aseptic necrosis of the femoral head
■ CVAs with neurologic sequelae
■ Chronic leg ulcers
■ Cardiac enlargement
■ Hematuria
■ Retinopathy
■ Infections, with increased risk of sepsis
■ Prolonged priapism
■ Dehydration
■ Neuropathy

Special considerations
■ Stress the importance of normal childhood immunizations, meticulous wound care, good oral hygiene, regular dental checkups, and a balanced diet as safeguards against infection.

■ Encourage normal mental and social development in the child by warning the parents against being overprotective. Although the child must avoid strenuous exercise, he can enjoy most everyday activities.

• • • • • • • • • • • •

ANEMIA, SIDEROBLASTIC

Sideroblastic anemias, a group of heterogeneous disorders, produce a common defect: failure to use iron in hemoglobin (Hb) synthesis, despite the availability of adequate iron stores. These anemias may be hereditary, acquired, or idiopathic; the acquired form, in turn, can be primary or secondary.

Hereditary sideroblastic anemia commonly responds to treatment with pyridoxine. Correction of the secondary acquired form depends on the causative disorder; the primary acquired (idiopathic) form, however, resists treatment and is usually fatal within 10 years after the onset of complications or a concomitant disease.

Causes and pathophysiology
Hereditary sideroblastic anemia appears to be transmitted by X-linked inheritance, occurring mostly in young males; females are carriers and usually show no signs of this disorder.

The acquired form may be secondary to ingestion of or exposure to toxins, such as alcohol and lead, or to drugs, such as isoniazid and chloramphenicol. It can also occur as a complication of other diseases, such as rheumatoid arthritis, lupus erythematosus, multiple myeloma, tuberculosis, and severe infections.

The primary acquired form, known as refractory anemia with ringed sideroblasts, is most common among elderly patients. It's often associated with throm-

Ringed sideroblast

Electron microscopy shows large iron deposits in the mitochondria that surround the nucleus, forming the characteristic ringed sideroblast shown below.

bocytopenia or leukopenia as part of a myelodysplastic syndrome.

In sideroblastic anemia, normoblasts fail to use iron to synthesize Hb. As a result, iron is deposited in the mitochondria of normoblasts, which are then called ringed sideroblasts. (See *Ringed sideroblast*.)

Clinical presentation

Sideroblastic anemia usually produces nonspecific clinical effects, which may exist for several years before being identified. Such effects include:

- anorexia
- fatigue
- weakness
- dizziness
- pale skin and mucous membranes
- occasionally enlarged lymph nodes.

Heart and liver failure may develop from excessive iron accumulation in these organs, causing:

- dyspnea
- exertional angina
- slight jaundice
- hepatosplenomegaly.

Hereditary sideroblastic anemia is associated with increased GI absorption of iron, causing signs of hemosiderosis. Additional signs and symptoms in secondary sideroblastic anemia depend on the underlying cause.

Differential diagnoses

- Leukemia
- Thalassemia
- Idiopathic thrombocytopenic purpura

Diagnosis

Ringed sideroblasts on microscopic examination of bone marrow aspirate stained with Prussian blue or alizarin red dye confirm the diagnosis.

Microscopic examination of blood shows hypochromic or normochromic, and slightly macrocytic, erythrocytes. Red blood cell (RBC) precursors may be megaloblastic, with anisocytosis (abnormal variation in RBC size) and poikilocytosis (abnormal variation in RBC shape).

Unlike iron deficiency anemia, sideroblastic anemia decreases Hb and increases serum iron and transferrin levels. In turn, faulty Hb production increases urobilinogen and bilirubin levels. Platelet and leukocyte levels remain normal, but thrombocytopenia or leukopenia occasionally occurs.

Management
General

The underlying cause determines the type of treatment. An elderly patient is less likely to improve and more likely to develop serious complications. Carefully crossmatched transfusions can be initiated as an effective palliative measure that provide needed Hb for a patient with the primary acquired form of sideroblastic anemia. However, this form is essentially resistant to treatment and commonly leads to death from acute leukemia or respiratory or cardiac complications. The acquired secondary form of sideroblastic anemia generally subsides after the causative drug or toxin is removed or the underlying condition is adequately treated.

Medication
Medications used to treat sideroblastic anemia include:
- pyridoxine — 100 to 200 mg/day P.O.; may reverse anemia in hereditary, acquired, and idiopathic anemia
- folic acid — 0.4 to 1 mg P.O., S.C., or I.M. daily; may be beneficial when concomitant megablastic nuclear changes in RBC precursors are present
- deferoxamine mesylate — 20 to 50 mg/kg S.C. over 8 to 10 hours (via pump) 3 to 5 nights per week
- ascorbic acid — 250 to 500 mg/day P.O.; increases iron excretion and is given with desferrioxamine.

Referral
- The patient should be referred to a hematologist-oncologist for treatment.
- The patient should be referred for genetic counseling.
- Identify patients who abuse alcohol, and refer them for appropriate therapy.

Follow-up
The patient should follow up with the specialist and be monitored for appropriate laboratory results.

Patient teaching
- Teach the patient the importance of continuing prescribed therapy, even after he begins to feel better.

Complications
- Hemorrhage
- Infection
- Fatigue

Special considerations
- If phlebotomy must be repeated frequently, encourage the patient to follow a high-protein diet to help replace the protein lost during phlebotomy.
- Always inquire about the possibility of exposure to lead in the home (especially for children) or on the job.

• • • • • • • • • • •
HEMOPHILIA

Hemophilia is a hereditary bleeding disorder resulting from a deficiency of specific clotting factors. Hemophilia A (classic hemophilia), which affects more than 80% of all patients with hemophilia, results from a deficiency of factor VIII; hemophilia B (Christmas disease), which affects 15% of hemophiliac patients, results from a deficiency of factor IX.

Hemophilia is the most common X-linked genetic disease, occurring in about 1.25 in 10,000 live male births. Hemophilia A is five times more common than hemophilia B.

The severity and prognosis of bleeding disorders vary with the degree of deficiency and the site of bleeding. The overall prognosis is best in mild hemophilia, which doesn't cause spontaneous bleeding and joint deformities. Advances in treatment have greatly improved the prognosis, and many hemophiliacs live normal life spans. Surgical procedures can be done safely at special treatment centers for hemophiliac patients under the guidance of a hematologist.

Causes and pathophysiology

Hemophilias A and B are inherited as X-linked recessive traits. This means that a female carrier has a 50% chance of transmitting the gene to each daughter, who would then be a carrier, and a 50% chance of transmitting the gene to each son, who would be born with hemophilia.

Hemophilia causes abnormal bleeding because of a specific clotting factor malfunction. After a person with hemophilia forms a platelet plug at a bleeding site, clotting factor deficiency impairs the capacity to form a stable fibrin clot.

Clinical presentation

Hemophilia produces abnormal bleeding, which may be mild, moderate, or severe, depending on the degree of factor deficiency.

The mild form of hemophilia frequently goes undiagnosed until adulthood because the patient with a mild deficiency doesn't bleed spontaneously after minor trauma but has prolonged bleeding if challenged by major trauma or surgery. Postoperative bleeding continues as a slow ooze or ceases and starts again up to 8 days after surgery.

Moderate hemophilia causes signs and symptoms similar to those of severe hemophilia but produces only occasional spontaneous bleeding episodes.

Severe hemophilia causes spontaneous bleeding. The first sign of severe hemophilia usually is excessive bleeding after circumcision. Later, spontaneous bleeding or severe bleeding after minor trauma may produce large subcutaneous and deep intramuscular hematomas.

Bleeding into joints and muscles may cause:

- pain
- swelling
- extreme tenderness
- permanent deformity.

Bleeding near peripheral nerves may cause:

- peripheral neuropathies
- pain
- paresthesia
- muscle atrophy.

If bleeding impairs blood flow through a major vessel, it can cause ischemia and gangrene. Pharyngeal, lingual, intracardiac, intracerebral, and intracranial bleeding may lead to shock and death.

Differential diagnoses

- Von Willebrand's disease
- Vitamin K deficiency
- Platelet disorders

Diagnosis

A history of prolonged bleeding after trauma or surgery (including dental extractions) or episodes of spontaneous bleeding into muscles or joints usually indicates some defect in the hemostatic mechanism.

Specific coagulation factor assays can be used to diagnose the type and severity of hemophilia. A family history may be used to help diagnose hemophilia, but 20% of all patients have no family history of the disease.

Characteristic findings in hemophilia A include:

- factor VIII assay 0% to 30% of normal
- prolonged activated partial thromboplastin time
- normal platelet count and function, bleeding time, and prothrombin time.

Characteristics of hemophilia B include:

- deficient factor IX
- baseline coagulation results similar to those in hemophilia A, with normal factor VIII.

In hemophilia A or B, the degree of factor deficiency determines the severity:
- In mild hemophilia, factor levels are 5% to 40% of normal.
- In moderate hemophilia, factor levels are 1% to 5% of normal.
- In severe hemophilia, factor levels are less than 1% of normal.

Management
General
Hemophilia isn't curable, but treatment can prevent crippling deformities and prolong life expectancy. Correct treatment quickly stops bleeding by increasing plasma levels of the deficient clotting factor. This helps to prevent disabling deformities due to repeated bleeding into muscles and joints. Treatment varies according to the type of hemophilia. (See *Factor replacement products*.)

Medication
Medications used to treat patients with hemophilia include:
- cryoprecipitate antihemophilic factor (AHF), lyophilized AHF, or both—given in I.V. doses large enough to increase clotting factor levels to more than 25% of normal; permits normal hemostasis (in hemophilia A)
- factor IX concentrate—1 unit/kg I.V. to raise levels 1% during bleeding episodes
- aminocaproic acid—initially 5 g P.O. or slow I.V. infusion, then 1 to 1.25 g hourly until bleeding is controlled (maximum dose is 30 g/24 hours).

Surgical intervention
The hemophilic patient requires replacement of the deficient factor before and after surgery. Such replacement may be necessary even for minor surgery such as a dental extraction.

Factor replacement products

The following agents are used to replace a specific clotting factor.

CRYOPRECIPITATE
- Contains factor VIII (70 to 100 U/bag); doesn't contain factor IX
- Can be stored frozen up to 12 months but must be used within 6 hours after it thaws
- Given through a blood filter; compatible with normal saline solution only
- No longer treatment of choice

LYOPHILIZED FACTOR VIII OR IX
- Freeze-dried
- Can be stored for up to 2 years at about 36° to 46° F (2.2° to 7.8° C); up to 6 months at room temperature not exceeding 88° F (31.1° C)
- Labeled with exact units of factor VIII or IX contained in vial (200 to 1,500 U of factor VIII or IX per vial; 20 to 40 ml after reconstitution with diluent)
- No blood filter needed; usually given by slow I.V. push through a butterfly infusion set

FRESH FROZEN PLASMA
- Contains approximately 0.75 U/ml of factor VIII and approximately 1 U/ml of factor IX; not practical for most hemophiliacs because a large volume is needed to increase factors to hemostatic levels
- Can be stored frozen for up to 12 months but must be used within 2 hours after it thaws
- Given through a blood filter; compatible with normal saline solution only

Managing hemophilia

The following guidelines can help parents care for their child with hemophilia.

■ Instruct parents to report injuries immediately, even if they're minor, but especially after an injury to the head, neck, or abdomen. Such injuries may require special blood factor replacement. Also, advise them to report any potential dental extractions or necessary surgery.

■ Stress the importance of regular, careful toothbrushing with a soft-bristled toothbrush to prevent the need for dental surgery.

■ Teach parents to be alert for signs of severe internal bleeding, such as severe pain or swelling in a joint or muscle, stiffness, decreased joint movement, severe abdominal pain, blood in urine, black tarry stools, and severe headache.

■ Advise the parents that the child is at risk for hepatitis from blood components. Early signs and symptoms — headache, fever, decreased appetite, nausea, vomiting, abdominal tenderness, and pain over the liver — may appear 3 weeks to 6 months after treatment with blood components. Discuss with parents the possibility of hepatitis vaccination.

■ Instruct the parents to make sure their child wears a medical identification bracelet at all times.

■ Teach the parents never to give their child aspirin, which can aggravate the bleeding tendency. Advise them to give acetaminophen instead.

■ Instruct the parents to protect their child from injury but to avoid unnecessary restrictions that impair his normal development. For example, they can sew padded patches into the knees and elbows of a toddler's clothing to protect

these joints during falls. They should forbid an older child to participate in contact sports, such as football, but can encourage him to swim or play golf.

■ Teach the parents to elevate and apply cold compresses or ice bags to an injured area and to apply light pressure to a bleeding site. To prevent recurrence of bleeding, advise the parents to restrict the child's activity for 48 hours after bleeding is under control.

■ If the parents have been trained to administer blood factor components at home to avoid frequent hospitalization, make sure they know proper venipuncture and infusion techniques and they don't delay treatment during bleeding episodes.

■ Instruct the parents to keep blood factor concentrate and infusion equipment on hand at all times, even on vacation.

■ Emphasize the importance of having the child keep routine medical appointments at the local hemophilia center.

■ Daughters of hemophiliacs should undergo genetic screening to determine if they're hemophilia carriers. Affected males should undergo counseling as well. If they mate with a noncarrier, all of their daughters will be carriers; if they mate with a carrier, each male or female child has a 25% chance of being affected.

■ For more information, refer parents to the National Hemophilia Foundation.

Referral
- The patient should have a consultation with a hematologist.
- The patient and family members may be referred for counseling to deal with this illness. Support groups such as the National Hemophilia Foundation may be helpful.
- Refer the patient and family members for genetic counseling to understand how the disease is inherited, and discuss prenatal testing.

Follow-up
The patient should be evaluated every 6 to 12 months for blood studies and a musculoskeletal evaluation.

Patient teaching
- Teach the patient how to avoid trauma, manage minor bleeding, and recognize bleeding that requires immediate medical intervention. (See *Managing hemophilia.*)

Complications
- Hemorrhage
- Hepatitis
- Human immunodeficiency virus
- Chronic liver disease

Special considerations
- During bleeding episodes, give deficient clotting factor or plasma as needed. The body uses up AHF in 48 to 72 hours, so repeat infusions as needed until bleeding stops.

• • • • • • • • • • • •

IDIOPATHIC THROMBOCYTOPENIC PURPURA

Idiopathic thrombocytopenic purpura (ITP) is thrombocytopenia that results from immunologic platelet destruction. ITP may be acute (postviral thrombocytopenia) or chronic (Werlhof's disease, purpura hemorrhagica, essential thrombocytopenia, and autoimmune thrombocytopenia).

The prognosis for acute ITP is excellent; nearly four out of five patients recover without treatment. The prognosis for chronic ITP is good; remissions lasting weeks or years are common, especially among women.

AGE ALERT Acute ITP usually affects children between ages 2 and 6; chronic ITP mainly affects adults under age 50, especially women between ages 20 and 40.

Causes and pathophysiology
ITP may be an autoimmune disorder; antibodies that reduce the survival time of platelets are found in nearly all patients. The spleen probably helps to remove platelets changed by the antibody. Acute ITP usually follows a viral infection, such as rubella or chickenpox, and can follow immunization with a live virus vaccine. Chronic ITP seldom follows infection and is often linked to immunologic disorders such as systemic lupus erythematosus (SLE). It's also linked to drug reactions.

Clinical presentation
Clinical features of ITP common to all forms of thrombocytopenia include:
- petechiae
- ecchymoses
- mucosal bleeding from the mouth, nose, or GI tract.

Hemorrhage is a rare physical finding. Purpuric lesions may occur in vital organs, such as the lungs, kidneys, or brain, and may be fatal.

In acute ITP, which commonly occurs in children, onset is usually sudden and without warning, causing the following:

- easy bruising
- epistaxis
- bleeding gums.
  Onset of chronic ITP is insidious.

Differential diagnoses

- Acute leukemia
- SLE
- Lymphoma
- Drug-induced thrombocytopenia
- Infections
- Decreased marrow production; malignancy, drugs, viruses, and megaloblastic anemia
- Alcohol induced
- Disseminated intravascular coagulation
- Thrombocytopenia secondary to sepsis
- Myelodysplastic syndrome
- Hemolytic uremic syndrome
- Posttransfusion

Diagnosis

A platelet count of 5,000 µl to 75,000 µl and prolonged bleeding time suggest ITP. Platelet size and morphologic appearance may be abnormal. Anemia may be present if bleeding has occurred.

As in thrombocytopenia, bone marrow studies show an abundance of megakaryocytes and a shortened circulating platelet survival time (hours or days). Occasionally, platelet antibodies may be found in vitro, but this diagnosis is usually inferred from platelet survival data and the absence of an underlying disease.

Management

General

Acute ITP may be allowed to run its course without intervention or may be treated with medication or surgery.

Medication

Medications used in the treatment of patients with ITP include:

- prednisone—for acute ITP, 1 to 2 mg/kg/day P.O. for 4 weeks, and then taper; for chronic ITP, 60 mg/day P.O. for 4 to 6 weeks, then taper
- immune globulin (IGIV)—1 to 2 g/kg I.V. infusion as a single dose or 400 mg/kg/day for 5 days
- $Rh_o(D)$ immune globulin—50 mcg/kg I.V. infusion as a single dose or in two divided doses over 2 days then 25 to 60 mcg/kg I.V. p.r.n.
- azathioprine—2 mg/kg/day P.O. for 1 to 6 months.

Surgical intervention

Patients who fail to respond within 1 to 4 months or who need high steroid dosage are candidates for splenectomy, which has an 85% success rate. Pneumococcal vaccine must be administered at least 2 weeks before surgery.

Referral

- Patients with ITP should be referred to a hematologist.

Follow-up

Platelet counts should be measured daily to weekly, with regular hemostasis evaluation.

Patient teaching

- Instruct the patient to restrict activity.
- Urge the patient to avoid taking aspirin, ibuprofen, indomethacin, and phenylbutazone.
- Teach the patient how to identify bleeding problems and measures to control it or treat it.
- Teach the patient to observe for petechiae, ecchymoses, and other signs of recurrence.

Complications

- Intracranial hemorrhage
- Severe blood loss

- Corticosteroid adverse effects
- Pneumococcal infections (if patient must have splenectomy)

Special considerations

- If the patient must undergo splenectomy, administer the pneumococcal vaccine.
- Monitor patients receiving immunosuppressive therapy for signs of bone marrow depression, infection, mucositis, GI ulcers, and severe diarrhea or vomiting.
- Children with platelet counts greater than 30,000 µl don't require treatment if they're asymptomatic. Treat adults with platelet counts of 20,000 µl or platelet counts of 50,000 µl with symptoms or risks of bleeding, such as hypertension and peptic ulcers.

• • • • • • • • • • • •

THALASSEMIA

Thalassemia, a hereditary group of hemolytic anemias, is characterized by defective synthesis in the polypeptide chains necessary for hemoglobin production. Red blood cell (RBC) synthesis is also impaired. Thalassemia is most common in persons of Mediterranean ancestry (especially Italian and Greek), but it also occurs in blacks and persons from southern China, Southeast Asia, and India.

It's estimated that 2 million people in the United States are carriers of the genetic trait for thalassemia.

Beta-thalassemia is the most common form of this disorder, resulting from defective beta polypeptide chain synthesis. It occurs in three clinical forms: thalassemia major, intermedia, and minor. The severity of the resulting anemia depends on whether the patient is homozygous or heterozygous for the thalassemic trait.

The prognoses for patients with beta-thalassemia vary. Patients with thalassemia major seldom survive to adulthood; children with thalassemia intermedia develop normally into adulthood, although puberty is usually delayed; persons with thalassemia minor can expect a normal life span.

Causes and pathophysiology

Thalassemia major and intermedia result from homozygous inheritance of the partially dominant autosomal gene for this trait. Thalassemia minor results from heterozygous inheritance of the same gene.

In all these disorders, total or partial deficiency of beta polypeptide chain production impairs hemoglobin synthesis (Hb) and results in continual production of fetal Hb (Hb F), lasting even past the neonatal period.

Clinical presentation

The three clinical forms of thalassemia have different signs and symptoms. In thalassemia major (also known as Cooley's anemia, Mediterranean disease, and erythroblastic anemia), the infant is well at birth but develops:

- severe anemia
- bone abnormalities
- failure to thrive
- life-threatening complications. (See *Skull abnormality in thalassemia major,* page 172.)

Often, the first signs of thalassemia major are pallor and yellow skin and sclera in infants ages 3 to 6 months. Later clinical features, in addition to severe anemia, include:

- splenomegaly or hepatomegaly, with abdominal enlargement
- frequent infections
- bleeding tendencies (especially toward epistaxis)
- anorexia.

Skull abnormality in thalassemia major

The X-ray image below shows a characteristic skull abnormality in thalassemia major: diploetic fibers extending from the internal lamina.

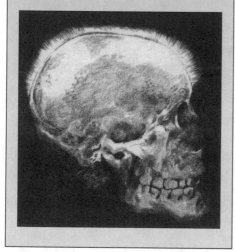

Children with thalassemia major commonly have small bodies and large heads and may also be mentally retarded. Infants may have mongoloid features because bone marrow hyperactivity thickens the bone at the base of the nose. As these children grow older, they become susceptible to pathologic fractures as a result of expansion of the marrow cavities with thinning of the long bones.

They're also subject to cardiac arrhythmias, heart failure, and other complications that result from iron deposits in the heart and in other tissues from repeated blood transfusions.

The condition thalassemia intermedia encompasses moderate thalassemic disorders in homozygotes. Patients show these signs:

- degree of anemia
- jaundice
- splenomegaly

- possibly, signs of hemosiderosis due to increased intestinal absorption of iron.

Thalassemia minor may cause mild anemia but usually produces no symptoms and is often overlooked. The prognosis for this form is excellent.

Differential diagnoses
- Iron deficiency
- Other hemoglobinopathies
- Other hemolytic anemia

Diagnosis
In thalassemia major
- Laboratory results show lowered RBC count and Hb level, microcytosis, and elevated reticulocyte, bilirubin, and urinary and fecal urobilinogen levels.
- A low serum folate level indicates increased folate utilization by the hypertrophied bone marrow.
- A peripheral blood smear reveals target cells, microcytes, pale nucleated RBCs, and marked anisocytosis.
- X-rays of the skull and long bones show thinning and widening of the marrow space because of overactive bone marrow. The bones of the skull and vertebrae may appear granular; long bones may show areas of osteoporosis. The phalanges may also be deformed (rectangular or biconvex).
- Quantitative Hb studies show a significant increase in Hb F and a slight increase in Hb A_2. Diagnosis must rule out iron deficiency anemia, which also produces hypochromia (slightly reduced Hb) and microcytic (notably small) RBCs.

In thalassemia intermedia
- Laboratory results show hypochromia and microcytic RBCs, but the anemia is less severe than that in thalassemia major.

In thalassemia minor
- Laboratory results show hypochromia and microcytic RBCs. Quantitative Hb

studies show a significant increase in Hb A$_2$ levels and a moderate increase in Hb F levels.

Management
General
Therapy for patients with thalassemia major is essentially supportive. Patients with thalassemia intermedia and thalassemia minor generally don't require treatment but should follow a low iron diet. Transfusions of packed RBCs increase Hb levels but must be used judiciously to minimize iron overload.

Medication
Medications used to treat patients with thalassemia include:
- deferoxamine mesylate — 20 to 50 mg/kg S.C. over 8 to 10 hours (via pump) 3 to 5 nights per week
- ascorbic acid — 250 to 500 mg/day P.O.; increases iron excretion and is given with desferrioxamine.

Iron supplements are contraindicated for patients with all forms of thalassemia.

Surgical intervention
Splenectomy is used for patients with hypersplenism that requires markedly increased transfusions; surgery is usually deferred until after age 4. Bone marrow transplantation is available for selected patients with a matched sibling or unrelated donor. This cures the disease but is associated with significant mortality and morbidity.

Referral
- The patient should have a hematology consultation for thalassemia major or thalassemia intermedia.
- Refer the patient for genetic counseling.

Follow-up
Follow-up for patients with thalassemia major and intermedia should be with the consulting specialist because these require lifelong monitoring. Thalassemia minor can be monitored regularly by the nurse practitioner, with the consulting specialist if any changes are detected.

Patient teaching
- Stress the importance of good nutrition, meticulous wound care, periodic dental checkups, and other measures to prevent infection.
- Teach parents to watch for signs of hepatitis and iron overload, complications that are always possible with frequent transfusions.
- Teach the patient and family about foods that contain low iron, such as turkey, chicken, fish, and fruit.

Complications
- Chronic hemolysis
- Infections after splenectomy
- Infections from blood transfusions
- Intercurrent infections
- Jaundice
- Leg ulcers
- Cholelithiasis
- Pathologic fractures
- Impaired growth rate
- Delayed or absent puberty
- Hemolytic anemia
- Splenomegaly
- Cardiac disease from iron overload

Special considerations
- Discuss with the parents of a young patient various options for healthy physical and creative outlets.
- A child with thalassemia major must avoid strenuous athletic activity because of increased oxygen demand and the tendency toward pathologic fractures, but he may participate in less stressful activities.

■ Be sure to tell patients with thalassemia minor that the condition is benign.

• • • • • • • • • • • •

THROMBOCYTOPENIA

Thrombocytopenia is characterized by a deficiency of circulating platelets. Because platelets play a vital role in coagulation, this disease poses a serious threat to hemostasis and is the most common cause of hemorrhagic disorders.

Thrombocytopenia affects women more than men and is more common in children than adults. In children, treatment isn't usually necessary and occurs most often after a viral infection. The incidence overall is 1 in 10,000 people.

The prognosis is excellent for a patient with drug-induced thrombocytopenia if the offending drug is withdrawn; in such cases, recovery may be immediate. In other cases, the prognosis depends on the patient's response to treatment for the cause.

Causes and pathophysiology

Thrombocytopenia may be congenital or acquired; the acquired form is more common. In either case, it usually results from:
■ decreased or defective production of platelets in the marrow (such as occurs in leukemia, aplastic anemia, or toxicity with certain drugs)
■ increased destruction outside the marrow caused by an underlying disorder (such as cirrhosis of the liver, disseminated intravascular coagulation, or severe infection)
■ less commonly, sequestration (hypersplenism, hypothermia) or platelet loss.

Acquired thrombocytopenia may result from the use of certain drugs, such as nonsteroidal anti-inflammatory agents, sulfonamides, histamine blockers, alkyl-

ating agents, or antibiotic chemotherapeutic agents.

An idiopathic form of thrombocytopenia commonly occurs in children. A transient form may follow viral infections (Epstein-Barr virus or infectious mononucleosis). (See *Causes of decreased circulating platelets*.)

Clinical presentation

Thrombocytopenia typically produces a sudden onset of petechiae or ecchymoses in the skin or bleeding into any mucous membrane. Nearly all patients are otherwise asymptomatic, although some may complain of malaise, fatigue, and general weakness.

In adults, large blood-filled bullae characteristically appear in the mouth. In severe thrombocytopenia, hemorrhage may lead to tachycardia, shortness of breath, loss of consciousness, and death. (See *What happens in thrombocytopenia*, pages 176 and 177.)

Differential diagnoses
■ Idiopathic thrombocytopenic purpura
■ Bone marrow suppression from malignancy
■ Connective tissue disorders
■ Human immunodeficiency virus

Diagnosis

To diagnose thrombocytopenia, look for the following laboratory test results:
■ Coagulation tests reveal a decreased platelet count (in adults, less than $100,000/mm^3$), prolonged bleeding time, and normal prothrombin time and partial thromboplastin time.
■ If increased destruction of platelets is causing thrombocytopenia, bone marrow studies reveal a greater number of megakaryocytes (platelet precursors) and shortened platelet survival (several hours or days rather than the usual 7 to 10 days).

Causes of decreased circulating platelets

Thrombocytopenia usually results from insufficient production or increased peripheral destruction of platelets. Less commonly, it results from sequestration or platelet loss.

DIMINISHED OR DEFECTIVE PLATELET PRODUCTION
Congenital
- Wiskott-Aldrich syndrome
- Maternal ingestion of thiazides
- Neonatal rubella

Acquired
- Aplastic anemia
- Marrow infiltration (acute and chronic leukemias and tumor)
- Nutritional deficiency (vitamin B_{12} and folic acid)
- Myelosuppressive agents
- Drugs that directly influence platelet production (thiazides, alcohol, and hormones)
- Radiation
- Viral infections (measles and dengue)

INCREASED PERIPHERAL PLATELET DESTRUCTION
Congenital
- Nonimmune (prematurity, erythroblastosis fetalis, and infection)

- Immune (drug sensitivity, maternal idiopathic thrombocytopenic purpura [ITP])

Acquired
- Nonimmune (infection, disseminated intravascular coagulation, and thrombotic thrombocytopenic purpura)
- Immune (drug-induced, especially with quinine and quinidine; posttransfusion purpura; acute and chronic ITP; sepsis; and alcohol)
- Invasive lines and devices
- Intra-aortic balloon pump
- Prosthetic heart valves
- Heparin

PLATELET SEQUESTRATION
- Hypersplenism
- Hypothermia

PLATELET LOSS
- Hemorrhage
- Extracorporeal perfusion

Management
General
Effective treatment varies with the underlying cause and may include corticosteroids or immune globulin to increase platelet production. When possible, treatment consists of correcting the underlying cause or, in drug-induced thrombocytopenia, removing the offending agents. Platelet transfusions are helpful in thrombocytopenia only in treating complications of severe hemorrhage.

Medication
Medications used to treat patients with thrombocytopenia include:
- prednisone — 5 to 60 mg/day P.O.; dosage is highly individualized
- gamimune N — 400 mg/kg 5% dextrose solution I.V. infusion for 5 days
- sandoglobulin — 400 mg/kg I.V. infusion for 2 to 5 days
- $Rh_0(D)$ immune globulin — 50 mcg/kg I.V. infusion; blood product that achieves a temporary elevation in platelets that lasts approximately 1 month.

(*Text continues on page 178.*)

What happens in thrombocytopenia

Thrombocytopenia is the most common cause of bleeding disorders and is characterized by a severe decrease in platelets. This platelet decrease can result from hematologic malignancy, radiation or drug therapy, idiopathic causes, blood transfusions, disseminated intravascular coagulation, or splenomegaly. Excessive hemorrhaging can lead to shock if interventions are delayed. This chart shows how these conditions and treatments develop into thrombocytopenic hemorrhage.

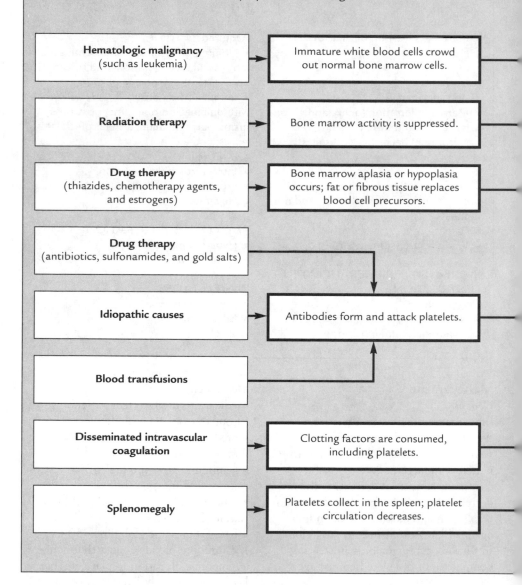

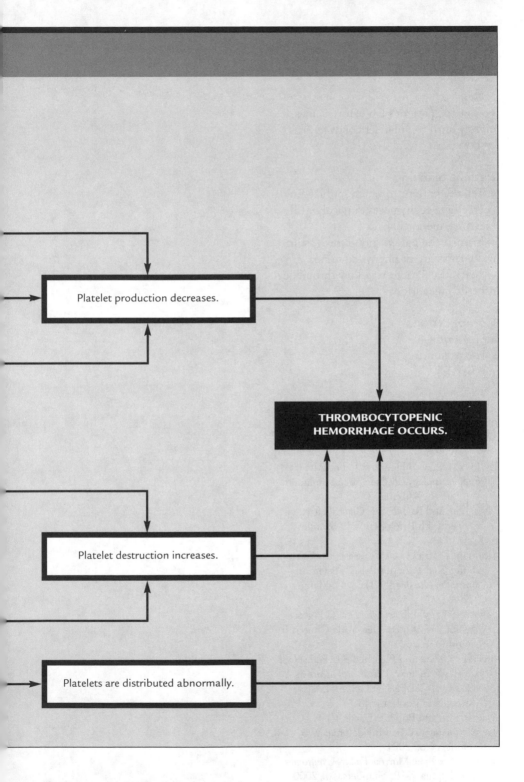

Referral
■ Refer the patient to a hematologist-oncologist for treatment.

Follow-up
Follow the patient's laboratory values closely until the platelet count returns to normal.

Patient teaching
■ Tell the patient to watch for bleeding (petechiae, ecchymoses, surgical or GI bleeding, menorrhagia).
■ Instruct the patient not to take aspirin, indomethacin, or phenylbutazone.
■ Teach the patient to follow thrombocytopenic precautions.

Complications
■ Hemorrhage
■ Heart failure
■ Anemia

• • • • • • • • • • • •

SELECTED REFERENCES

Bullock, B.L., and Henze, R.L. *Focus on Pathophysiology*. Philadelphia: Lippincott Williams & Wilkins, 2000.

Carr, J.H., and Rodak, B.F. *Clinical Hematology Atlas*. Philadelphia: W.B. Saunders Co., 1999.

Gorman, K. "Sickle Cell Disease: Do You Doubt Your Patient's Pain?" *American Journal of Nursing* 99(3):38-43, March 1999.

Lewis, S.M., et al. *Dacie and Lewis's Practical Hematology*, 9th ed. New York: Churchill Livingstone, 2001.

McCance, K.L., and Heuther, S.E. *Pathophysiology: The Biological Basis for Disease in Adults and Children*, 3rd ed. St. Louis: Mosby—Year Book, Inc., 1997.

Rakel, R.E., and Bope, E.T., eds. *Conn's Current Therapy 2001*. Philadelphia: W.B. Saunders Co., 2001.

Yound, N.S. *Bone Marrow Failure Syndromes*. Philadelphia: W.B. Saunders Co., 2000.

Renal and urologic disorders

The kidneys and other structures of the urinary system produce and eliminate urine, retaining useful materials and excreting foreign or excessive materials and waste in the process. Through this basic function, the kidneys profoundly affect other body systems and the patient's overall health. Assessing the renal and urologic system can uncover clues to possible problems in any body system.

• • • • • • • • • • • •
ASSESSMENT

Begin the physical examination by documenting baseline vital signs and weighing the patient. Comparing subsequent weight measurements with this baseline may reveal a developing problem, such as dehydration or fluid retention. A thorough assessment of the urinary system includes examining related body systems in addition to using inspection, auscultation, percussion, and palpation techniques. (For some common abnormal assessment findings, see *Interpreting renal and urologic assessment findings*, pages 180 and 181.)

Physical examination
Ask the patient to urinate into a specimen cup. Assess the sample for color, odor, and clarity. Give the patient a gown and drapes, ask him to undress, and proceed with a systematic physical examination.

Inspection
Urinary system inspection includes examination of the abdomen and urethral meatus.

Abdomen
Help the patient assume a supine position with his arms relaxed at his sides. Make sure he's comfortable and draped appropriately. Expose the patient's abdomen from the xiphoid process to the symphysis pubis, and inspect the abdomen for gross enlargements or fullness by comparing the left and right sides, noting any asymmetrical areas. In a nor-

Interpreting renal and urologic assessment findings

After completing your assessment, you're ready to form a diagnostic impression of the patient's condition. This chart will help you form such an impression by grouping significant signs and symptoms, related findings you may discover during the health history and physical assessment, and the possible cause indicated by a cluster of these findings.

KEY SIGNS AND SYMPTOMS	RELATED FINDINGS	POSSIBLE CAUSE
■ Oliguria possibly progressing to anuria ■ Hematuria or smoke- or coffee-colored urine	■ Poststreptococcal throat or skin infection ■ Systemic lupus erythematosus, vasculitis, or scleroderma ■ Pregnancy ■ Elevated blood pressure ■ Periorbital edema progressing to dependent edema ■ Ascites ■ Pleural effusion	Acute glomerulo-nephritis
■ Oliguria ■ Dark, smoke-colored urine ■ Anorexia and vomiting	■ Crush injury or illness associated with shock such as burns ■ Muscle necrosis ■ Exposure to nephrotoxic agent such as lead ■ I.V. pyelography using dye injection ■ Recent aminoglycoside therapy ■ Oliguria progressing to anuria ■ Dyspnea ■ Bibasilar crackles ■ Dependent edema	Acute tubular necrosis
■ Proteinuria, hematuria, vomiting, pruritus (patient may be asymptomatic until advanced disease stage)	■ Primary renal disorder, such as membranoproliferative glomerulonephritis or focal glomerular sclerosis ■ Elevated blood pressure ■ Ascites and dependent edema ■ Dyspnea ■ Bibasilar crackles	Chronic glomerulonephritis
■ Urinary frequency and urgency ■ Burning sensation on urination ■ Nocturia, cloudy hematuria, dysuria ■ Low back or flank pain	■ Recurrent urinary tract infection ■ Recent chemotherapy or systemic antibiotic therapy ■ Recent vigorous sexual activity ■ Suprapubic pain on palpation ■ Fever ■ Inflamed perineal area	Cystitis

Interpreting renal and urologic assessment findings *(continued)*

KEY SIGNS AND SYMPTOMS	RELATED FINDINGS	POSSIBLE CAUSE
▪ Severe radiating pain from costovertebral angle to flank, suprapubic region, and external genitalia ▪ Nausea and vomiting ▪ Hematuria	▪ Strenuous physical activity in hot environment ▪ Previous renal calculi ▪ Recent kidney infection ▪ Fever and chills ▪ Poor skin turgor, concentrated urine, and dry mucous membranes	Nephrolithiasis
▪ Abdominal or flank pain ▪ Gross hematuria	▪ Youth (especially younger than age 7) ▪ Congenital anomalies ▪ Firm, smooth, palpable abdominal mass in enlarged abdomen ▪ Fever ▪ Elevated blood pressure ▪ Urine retention	Wilms' tumor

mal adult, the abdomen is smooth, flat or scaphoid (concave), and symmetrical. Note any scars, lesions, bruises, or discolorations.

Extremely prominent veins may accompany other vascular signs associated with renal dysfunction, such as hypertension and renal artery bruits. Distention, skin tightness and glistening, and striae (streaks or linear scars caused by rapidly developing skin tension) may signal fluid retention. If you suspect ascites, perform a fluid wave test. Ascites may suggest nephrotic syndrome.

Urethral meatus
Help the patient feel more at ease during your inspection by examining the urethral meatus last and by explaining beforehand how you'll assess this area. Be sure to wear gloves.

Urethral meatus inspection may reveal several abnormalities. In a male patient, a meatus deviating from the normal central location may represent a congenital defect. In any patient, inflammation and discharge may signal urethral

infection. Ulceration usually indicates a sexually transmitted disease.

In the male, the penis can be palpated for tenderness or induration. Induration may suggest urethral stricture. Palpation may be omitted in a young, asymptomatic male patient.

Auscultation
Auscultate the renal arteries in the left and right upper abdominal quadrants by pressing the stethoscope bell lightly against the abdomen and telling the patient to exhale deeply. Begin auscultating at the midline and work to the left. Then return to the midline and work to the right. Systolic bruits (whooshing sounds) or other unusual sounds are potentially significant abnormalities. For example, in a patient with hypertension, systolic bruits suggest renal artery stenosis.

Percussion
After auscultating the renal arteries, percuss the patient's kidneys to detect any tenderness or pain, and percuss the bladder to evaluate its position and contents. Abnormal kidney percussion findings in-

Palpating the urinary organs

In the normal adult, the kidneys usually can't be palpated because they're located deep within the abdomen. However, they may be palpable in a thin patient or in one with reduced abdominal muscle mass. (Because the right kidney is slightly lower than the left, it may be easier to palpate.) Keep in mind that both kidneys descend with deep inhalation.

If palpable, the bladder normally feels firm and relatively smooth. However, remember that an adult's bladder may not be palpable.

Using bimanual manipulation, begin on the patient's right side and proceed as follows.

KIDNEY PALPATION

1. Help the patient to a normal supine position and expose the abdomen from the xiphoid process to the symphysis pubis. Standing at the right side, place your left hand under the back, midway between the lower costal margin and the iliac crest.

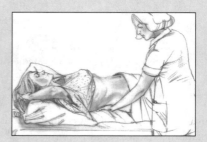

2. Next, place your right hand on the patient's abdomen, directly above your left hand. Angle this hand slightly toward the costal margin. To palpate the right lower edge of the right kidney, press your right fingertips about ½" (1.3 cm) above the right iliac crest at the midinguinal line; press your fingertips upward into the right costovertebral angle.

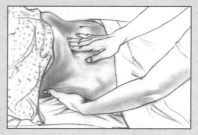

3. Instruct the patient to inhale deeply so that the lower portion of the right kidney can move down between your hands. If it does, note its shape and size. Normally, it feels smooth, solid, and firm, yet elastic. Ask the patient if palpation causes tenderness. (*Note:* avoid using excessive pressure to palpate the kidney because this may cause intense pain.)

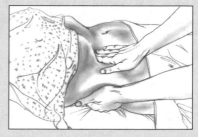

4. To assess the left kidney, move to the patient's left side and position your hands as described above, but with this change: Place your right hand 2" (5.1 cm) above the iliac crest. Then apply pressure with both hands as the patient inhales. If the left kidney can be palpated, compare it with the right kidney; it should be the same size.

BLADDER PALPATION

Before palpating the bladder, make sure the patient has voided. Then locate the edge of the bladder by pressing deeply in the midline about 1″ to 2″ (2.5 to 5 cm) above the symphysis pubis. As the bladder is palpated, note its size and location and check for lumps, masses, and tenderness. The bladder normally feels firm and relatively smooth. During deep palpation, the patient may report the urge to urinate — a normal response.

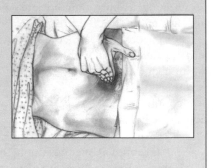

clude tenderness and pain, suggesting glomerulonephritis or glomerulonephrosis. A dull sound heard on percussion in a patient who has just urinated may indicate urine retention, reflecting bladder dysfunction or infection.

Palpation

Next, palpate the kidneys and bladder. (See *Palpating the urinary organs.*) Through palpation, you can detect lumps, masses, or tenderness. To achieve optimal results, have the patient relax his abdomen by taking deep breaths through his mouth. Abnormal kidney and bladder palpation findings may signify various problems that require further investigation to confirm.

• • • • • • • • • • • •

BENIGN PROSTATIC HYPERPLASIA

Most men over age 50 have some prostatic enlargement. In benign prostatic hyperplasia (BPH), also known as benign prostatic hypertrophy, the prostate gland enlarges sufficiently to compress the urethra and cause some overt urinary obstruction. Depending on the size of the enlarged prostate, age and health of the patient, and extent of obstruction, BPH is treated symptomatically or surgically.

Causes

Evidence suggests a link between BPH and hormonal activity. As men age, the production of androgenic hormones decreases, causing an imbalance in androgen and estrogen levels and high levels of dihydrotestosterone, the main prostatic intracellular androgen. Other causes include neoplasm, arteriosclerosis, inflammation, and metabolic or nutritional disturbances.

Whatever the cause, BPH begins with changes in periurethral glandular tissue. As the prostate enlarges, it may extend into the bladder and obstruct urinary outflow by compressing or distorting the prostatic urethra. BPH may also cause a pouch to form in the bladder that retains urine when the rest of the bladder empties. This retained urine may lead to calculus formation or cystitis.

Clinical presentation

Clinical features of BPH depend on the extent of prostatic enlargement and the lobes affected. Characteristically, the condition starts with a group of signs and symptoms known as prostatism, such as:

- reduced urinary stream caliber and force
- urinary hesitancy
- difficulty starting micturition (resulting in straining, feeling of incomplete voiding, and an interrupted stream).

As the obstruction increases, it causes:
- frequent urination with nocturia
- dribbling
- urine retention
- incontinence
- possibly hematuria.

Physical examination indicates a visible midline mass above the symphysis pubis that represents an incompletely emptied bladder; rectal palpation discloses an enlarged prostate. Examination may reveal secondary anemia and, possibly, renal insufficiency secondary to obstruction.

As BPH worsens, complete urinary obstruction may follow infection or the use of decongestants, tranquilizers, alcohol, antidepressants, or anticholinergics.

Differential diagnoses
- Bladder calculi
- Urethral stricture
- Bladder neck constriction
- Cancer
- Urinary tract infection (UTI)
- Neurologic disorders

Diagnosis
Clinical features and a rectal examination are usually sufficient for a diagnosis. Other findings help to confirm it:
- Excretory urography may indicate urinary tract obstruction, hydronephrosis, calculi or tumors, and filling and emptying defects in the bladder.
- Elevated blood urea nitrogen and serum creatinine levels suggest renal dysfunction.

- Urinalysis and urine cultures show hematuria, pyuria and, when the bacterial count exceeds 100,000/µl, UTI.
- Serum prostate-specific antigen analysis is optional unless the physical findings on rectal examination raise suspicions of prostate cancer.

When symptoms are severe, a cystourethroscopy is definitive, but this test is performed only immediately before surgery to help determine the best procedure. It can show prostate enlargement, bladder wall changes, and a raised bladder.

The American Urologic Association has developed an index to classify the severity of symptoms and to guide treatment planning. (See *American Urological Association symptom index for BPH*.)

Management
General
Conservative therapy includes prostate massages, sitz baths, fluid restriction for bladder distention, and antimicrobials for infection. Regular ejaculation may help relieve prostatic congestion.

Medication
Alpha$_1$-adrenergic blockers improve urine flow rates by relieving bladder outlet obstruction by preventing contractions of the prostatic capsule and bladder neck. Medications and dosages used in the treatment of patients with BPH include:
- terazosin — initially 1 mg P.O. h.s., increased to 2, 5, or 10 mg/day to desired response
- doxazosin — initially 1 mg/day P.O., may be increased to 2 mg, then 4 mg or 8 mg; adjust every 1 to 2 weeks
- tamsulosin — 0.4 mg/day P.O., may increase to 0.8 mg/day after 2 to 4 weeks, if needed.

American Urological Association symptom index for BPH

When assessing your patient for benign prostatic hyperplasia (BPH), use the following questions to determine the severity of his urinary symptoms. To calculate the symptom score index, take the number to each answer and add them up. A symptom score index of 0 to 8 indicates periodic reevaluation; 9 to 12 indicates potential treatment; 13 to 16 indicates initiation of therapy; and 17 to 35 indicates treatment according to the severity of the symptoms.

QUESTIONS TO BE ANSWERED	NOT AT ALL	LESS THAN 1 TIME IN 5	LESS THAN HALF THE TIME	ABOUT HALF THE TIME	MORE THAN HALF THE TIME	ALMOST ALWAYS
	(None)	(1 time)	(2 times)	(3 times)	(4 times)	(5 times)
Over the past month, how often have you had a sensation of not emptying your bladder completely after you finish urinating?	0	1	2	3	4	5
Over the past month, how often have you had to urinate again less than 2 hours after you finished urinating?	0	1	2	3	4	5
Over the past month, how often have you found you stopped and started again several times when you urinated?	0	1	2	3	4	5
Over the past month, how often have you found it difficult to postpone urination?	0	1	2	3	4	5
Over the past month, how often have you had a weak urinary stream?	0	1	2	3	4	5
Over the past month, how often have you had to push or strain to begin urination?	0	1	2	3	4	5
Over the past month, how many times did you most typically get up to urinate from the time you went to bed at night until the time you got up in the morning?	0	1	2	3	4	5

Adapted from Barry, M.J., et al. "The American Urological Association Symptom Index for Benign Prostatic Hyperplasia," *J Urol* 148(5):1549-1557, November 1992, with permission of the publisher.

Surgical intervention

Surgery is the only effective therapy to relieve acute urine retention, hydronephrosis, severe hematuria, recurrent UTIs, and other intolerable symptoms. A transurethral resection may be performed if the prostate weighs less than 2 oz (56.7 g). In this procedure, a resectoscope removes tissue with a wire loop and electric current. In high-risk patients, continuous drainage with an indwelling urinary catheter alleviates urine retention.

The following procedures involve open surgical removal:
■ suprapubic (transvesical) resection — most common and useful when prostatic enlargement remains within the bladder
■ retropubic (extravesical) resection — allows direct visualization; potency and continence are usually maintained.

Balloon dilatation of the prostate is still being investigated. Balloon dilatation or balloon urethroplasty involves passing a flexible balloon catheter guided by fluoroscope into the urethra at the level of the prostate. The balloon is inflated for a short period of time to distend the prostatic urethra.

Referral

■ Refer the patient to a urologist for surgical intervention, urinary retention, recurrent or persistent UTI, recurrent prostatic bleeding, or changes in the kidney, ureter, or bladder caused by obstruction, abnormal urinary flow, or bladder calculi.

Follow-up

The patient should be seen frequently (every 2 weeks) until stable, then urinalysis and serum creatinine should be checked every 6 months. The patient should be reassessed yearly.

Patient teaching

■ Make sure the patient understands the advantages and risks of each treatment option.
■ Teach the patient how to monitor symptom progression.
■ Instruct the patient to report any abrupt changes.
■ After surgery, reinforce prescribed limits on activity. Warn the patient against lifting, strenuous exercise, and long automobile rides because these activities increase bleeding tendencies. Restrict sexual activities for at least several weeks.

Complications

■ Infection
■ Renal insufficiency
■ Hemorrhage
■ Shock

• • • • • • • • • • • •

CONGENITAL ANOMALIES OF THE URETER, BLADDER, AND URETHRA

Congenital anomalies of the ureter, bladder, and urethra are among the most common birth defects, occurring in about 5% of all births. The most common malformations include duplicated ureter, retrocaval ureter, ectopic orifice of the ureter, stricture or stenosis of the ureter, ureterocele, exstrophy of the bladder, congenital bladder diverticulum, hypospadias, and epispadias. (See *Congenital urologic anomalies*, pages 187 to 189.)

Causes

The causes of congenital anomalies of the ureter, bladder, and urethra are unknown.

Congenital urologic anomalies

ANOMALY	PATHOPHYSIOLOGY	CLINICAL FEATURES	DIAGNOSIS AND TREATMENT
Duplicated ureter			
	■ Most common ureteral anomaly ■ *Complete* — a double collecting system with two separate pelves, each with its own ureter and orifice ■ *Incomplete (Y type)* — two separate ureters joining before entering bladder	■ Persistent or recurrent infection ■ Frequency, urgency, or burning on urination ■ Diminished urine output ■ Flank pain, fever, and chills	■ Excretory urography ■ Voiding cystoscopy ■ Cystourethrography ■ Retrograde pyelography ■ Surgery for obstruction, reflux, or severe renal damage
Retrocaval ureter (preureteral vena cava)			
	■ Right ureter passing behind the inferior vena cava before entering the bladder; compression of the ureter between the vena cava and the spine, causing dilation and elongation of the pelvis; hydroureter, hydronephrosis; fibrosis and stenosis of ureter in the compressed area ■ Relatively uncommon; higher incidence in males	■ Right flank pain ■ Recurrent urinary tract infection (UTI) ■ Renal calculi ■ Hematuria	■ Excretory urography, demonstrating superior ureteral enlargement with spiral appearance ■ Surgical resection and anastomosis of ureter with renal pelvis, or reimplantation into bladder
Ectopic orifice of ureter			
	■ Ureters single or duplicated in females, ureteral orifice usually inserts in urethra or vaginal vestibule, beyond external urethral sphincter; in males, in prostatic urethra, or in seminal vesicles or vas deferens	■ Symptoms rare, when ureteral orifice opens between trigone and bladder neck ■ Obstruction, reflux, and incontinence (dribbling) in 50% of females ■ In males, flank pain, frequency, and urgency	■ Excretory urography ■ Urethroscopy and vaginoscopy ■ Voiding cystourethrography ■ Resection and ureteral reimplantation into bladder for incontinence

(continued)

Congenital urologic anomalies *(continued)*

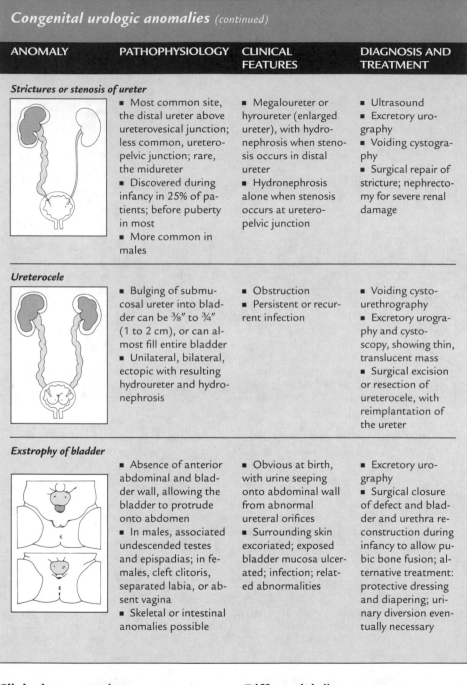

ANOMALY	PATHOPHYSIOLOGY	CLINICAL FEATURES	DIAGNOSIS AND TREATMENT
Strictures or stenosis of ureter	▪ Most common site, the distal ureter above ureterovesical junction; less common, ureteropelvic junction; rare, the midureter ▪ Discovered during infancy in 25% of patients; before puberty in most ▪ More common in males	▪ Megaloureter or hyroureter (enlarged ureter), with hydronephrosis when stenosis occurs in distal ureter ▪ Hydronephrosis alone when stenosis occurs at ureteropelvic junction	▪ Ultrasound ▪ Excretory urography ▪ Voiding cystography ▪ Surgical repair of stricture; nephrectomy for severe renal damage
Ureterocele	▪ Bulging of submucosal ureter into bladder can be ⅜″ to ¾″ (1 to 2 cm), or can almost fill entire bladder ▪ Unilateral, bilateral, ectopic with resulting hydroureter and hydronephrosis	▪ Obstruction ▪ Persistent or recurrent infection	▪ Voiding cystourethrography ▪ Excretory urography and cystoscopy, showing thin, translucent mass ▪ Surgical excision or resection of ureterocele, with reimplantation of the ureter
Exstrophy of bladder	▪ Absence of anterior abdominal and bladder wall, allowing the bladder to protrude onto abdomen ▪ In males, associated undescended testes and epispadias; in females, cleft clitoris, separated labia, or absent vagina ▪ Skeletal or intestinal anomalies possible	▪ Obvious at birth, with urine seeping onto abdominal wall from abnormal ureteral orifices ▪ Surrounding skin excoriated; exposed bladder mucosa ulcerated; infection; related abnormalities	▪ Excretory urography ▪ Surgical closure of defect and bladder and urethra reconstruction during infancy to allow pubic bone fusion; alternative treatment: protective dressing and diapering; urinary diversion eventually necessary

Clinical presentation

Some congenital abnormalities are obvious at birth; others aren't apparent and are recognized only after they produce symptoms.

Differential diagnoses

▪ Renal failure
▪ Urinary tract infection

Congenital urologic anomalies *(continued)*

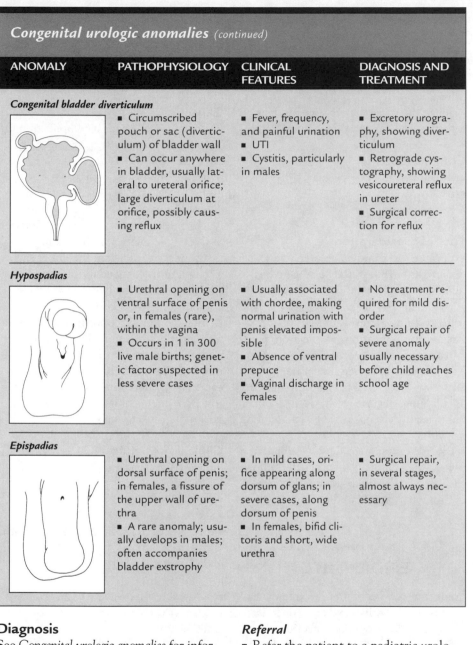

ANOMALY	PATHOPHYSIOLOGY	CLINICAL FEATURES	DIAGNOSIS AND TREATMENT
Congenital bladder diverticulum	■ Circumscribed pouch or sac (diverticulum) of bladder wall ■ Can occur anywhere in bladder, usually lateral to ureteral orifice; large diverticulum at orifice, possibly causing reflux	■ Fever, frequency, and painful urination ■ UTI ■ Cystitis, particularly in males	■ Excretory urography, showing diverticulum ■ Retrograde cystography, showing vesicoureteral reflux in ureter ■ Surgical correction for reflux
Hypospadias	■ Urethral opening on ventral surface of penis or, in females (rare), within the vagina ■ Occurs in 1 in 300 live male births; genetic factor suspected in less severe cases	■ Usually associated with chordee, making normal urination with penis elevated impossible ■ Absence of ventral prepuce ■ Vaginal discharge in females	■ No treatment required for mild disorder ■ Surgical repair of severe anomaly usually necessary before child reaches school age
Epispadias	■ Urethral opening on dorsal surface of penis; in females, a fissure of the upper wall of urethra ■ A rare anomaly; usually develops in males; often accompanies bladder exstrophy	■ In mild cases, orifice appearing along dorsum of glans; in severe cases, along dorsum of penis ■ In females, bifid clitoris and short, wide urethra	■ Surgical repair, in several stages, almost always necessary

Diagnosis

See *Congenital urologic anomalies* for information about diagnosing congenital anomalies of the ureter, bladder, and urethra.

Management

General

See *Congenital urologic anomalies* for information about treating congenital anomalies of the ureter, bladder, and urethra.

Referral

■ Refer the patient to a pediatric urologist.
■ Refer the family for genetic counseling, if appropriate.

Follow-up

The patient should be seen according to the specialist's recommendations.

Patient teaching

- Instruct parents in specific care measures for the anomaly involved.
- Tell parents to observe the child's urinary function by evaluating diapers and urination.
- Teach the parents to observe for signs of infection and to report them immediately.

Complications

- Infection
- Obstruction
- Renal failure

Special considerations

- Because these anomalies aren't always obvious at birth, carefully evaluate the neonate's urogenital function. Discuss with parents the amount and color of urine, voiding pattern, strength of stream, and indications of infection, such as fever and urine odor. Tell parents to watch for these signs at home. In all children, watch for signs of obstruction, such as dribbling, oliguria or anuria, abdominal mass, hypertension, fever, bacteriuria, or pyuria.
- Provide reassurance and emotional support to the parents. When possible, allow them to participate in their child's care to promote normal bonding.

• • • • • • • • • • • •

EPIDIDYMITIS

Epididymitis, infection of the epididymis, the testicle's cordlike excretory duct, is one of the most common infections of the male reproductive tract. It usually affects adults and is rare before puberty. Epididymitis may spread to the testicle itself, causing orchitis; bilateral epididymitis can cause sterility. (See *Understanding orchitis*.)

Epididymitis is the most common cause of acute scrotal pain in post pubertal males (patients may have a history of sexual activity). Sexually transmitted epididymitis is usually associated with urethritis. In the United States, the incidence of epididymitis is less than 1 in 1,000 males per year.

Causes

Epididymitis is usually a complication of pyogenic bacterial infection of the urinary tract (urethritis or prostatitis). The pyogenic organisms, such as staphylococci, *Escherichia coli*, streptococci, *Chlamydia trachomatis*, and *Neisseria gonorrhoeae*, reach the epididymis through the lumen of the vas deferens. Rarely, epididymitis is secondary to a distant infection, such as pharyngitis or tuberculosis, that spreads through the lymphatics or, less commonly, the bloodstream. Other causes include trauma, gonorrhea, syphilis, or a chlamydial infection. Trauma may reactivate a dormant infection or initiate a new one. Epididymitis may be a complication of prostatectomy and may also result from chemical irritation by extravasation of urine through the vas deferens.

Clinical presentation

The key signs and symptoms of epididymitis are:

- pain
- extreme tenderness
- swelling in the groin and scrotum with erythema
- high fever
- malaise
- a characteristic waddle in an attempt to protect the groin and scrotum during walking.

An acute hydrocele may also result from inflammation. Testicular pain is unilateral, accompanied by dysuria and urethral discharge. Fever occurs in approximately 50% of patients.

Differential diagnoses

- Testicular torsion
- Testicular trauma

- Testicular tumor
- Hydrocele
- Spermatocele
- Varicocele
- Mumps orchitis

Diagnosis

Clinical features suggest epididymitis, but the diagnosis is made with the aid of laboratory tests:

- urinalysis showing increased white blood cell (WBC) count indicates infection
- urine culture and sensitivity tests may identify causative organism
- serum WBC count is more than 10,000/µl in infection.

Scrotal ultrasonography may help differentiate acute epididymitis from other conditions such as testicular torsion, which is a surgical emergency.

Management

General

The goal of treatment is to reduce pain and swelling and to combat infection. Therapy must begin immediately, especially in the patient with bilateral epididymitis because sterility is always a threat. During the acute phase, treatment consists of bed rest, scrotal elevation with towel rolls or adhesive strapping, broad-spectrum antibiotics, and analgesics. An ice bag applied to the area may reduce swelling and relieve pain (heat is contraindicated because it could damage germinal cells, which are viable only at or below normal body temperature). When pain and swelling subside and allow walking, an athletic supporter may prevent pain.

Medication

Medications used to treat patients with sexually transmitted epididymitis include:

- doxycycline — 100 mg P.O. b.i.d. for 7 to 10 days; and ceftriaxone — 250 mg

---

Understanding orchitis

Orchitis, infection of the testicles, is a serious complication of epididymitis. This infection may also result from mumps (which may also lead to sterility) and, less often, from another systemic infection, testicular torsion, or severe trauma. Its typical effects include unilateral or bilateral tenderness, sudden onset of pain, and swelling of the scrotum and testicles. The affected testicle may be red. Nausea and vomiting also occur. Sudden cessation of pain indicates testicular ischemia, which may result in permanent damage to one or both testicles.

Treatment consists of immediate antibiotic therapy or, in mumps orchitis, diethylstilbestrol, which may relieve pain, swelling, and fever. Severe orchitis may require surgery to incise and drain the hydrocele and to improve testicular circulation. Other treatment is similar to that for epididymitis. To prevent mumps orchitis, stress the need for prepubertal males to receive the mumps vaccine (or gamma globulin injection after contracting mumps).

I.M. as a single dose for gonococcal or chlamydial infection

- ofloxacin — 300 mg P.O. b.i.d. for 10 days for an enteric organism or for those allergic to tetracycline or cephalosporins.

Occasionally, corticosteroids may be prescribed to help counteract inflammation, but their use is controversial.

Surgical intervention

In an older patient undergoing open prostatectomy, bilateral vasectomy may be necessary to prevent epididymitis as a postoperative complication; however, antibiotic therapy alone may prevent it. When epididymitis is refractory to antibiotic therapy, epididymectomy under local anesthetic is necessary.

Referral
■ A urologist should be consulted if surgical intervention is warranted.

Follow-up
A repeat urine culture should be done after treatment.

Patient teaching
■ Emphasize the importance of completing the prescribed antibiotic therapy, even after signs and symptoms subside.
■ If the patient faces the possibility of sterility, suggest supportive counseling as necessary.

Complications
■ Sterility
■ Recurrent epididymitis
■ Fournier's gangrene

Special considerations
■ Watch closely for abscess formation (localized, hot, red, tender area) or extension of infection into the testes.

• • • • • • • • • • • •

PROSTATITIS

Prostatitis, inflammation of the prostate gland, may be acute or chronic. Acute prostatitis most often results from gram-negative bacteria and is easy to recognize and treat. However, chronic prostatitis, the most common cause of recurrent urinary tract infections (UTIs) in men, is less easy to recognize.

As many as 35% of men over age 50 have chronic prostatitis.

Causes
About 80% of bacterial prostatitis cases result from infection by *Escherichia coli;* the rest, from infection by *Klebsiella, Enterobacter, Proteus, Pseudomonas, Streptococcus,* or *Staphylococcus.* These organisms probably spread to the prostate by the bloodstream or from ascending urethral infection, invasion of rectal bacteria through the lymphatic system, reflux of infected bladder urine into prostate ducts or, less commonly, infrequent or excessive sexual intercourse or such procedures as cystoscopy or catheterization. Chronic prostatitis usually results from bacterial invasion from the urethra. Nonbacterial prostatitis results from infections by *Trichomonas vaginalis,* chlamydia species, *Ureaplasma urealyticum,* or mycoplasma.

Clinical presentation
Acute prostatitis begins with these signs and symptoms:
■ fever
■ chills
■ low back pain
■ myalgia
■ perineal fullness
■ arthralgia
■ urinary frequency and urgency
■ dysuria
■ nocturia
■ urinary obstruction
■ perineal pain
■ suprapubic pain.

The urine may appear cloudy. When palpated rectally, the prostate is tender, indurated, swollen, firm, and warm.

Chronic bacterial prostatitis sometimes produces no symptoms but usually elicits the same urinary symptoms as the acute form but to a lesser degree. UTI is a common complication. Other possible signs include:
■ painful ejaculation
■ hemospermia
■ persistent urethral discharge
■ sexual dysfunction
■ perineal, inguinal, or suprapubic pain.

Prostate examination may be non-specific or reveal a tender or boggy prostate.

Differential diagnoses

- Acute or chronic bacterial prostatitis
- Acute pyelonephritis
- Acute epididymitis
- Acute diverticulitis
- Prostate cancer
- Bladder cancer
- Urethral stricture

Diagnosis

Characteristic rectal examination findings suggest prostatitis. In many cases, a urine culture can identify the causative infectious organism. A firm diagnosis depends on a comparison of urine cultures of specimens obtained by the Meares and Stamey technique. This test requires four specimens: one collected when the patient starts voiding (voided bladder one [VB1]); another midstream (VB2); another after the patient stops voiding and the doctor massages the prostate to produce secretions (expressed prostate secretions); and a final voided specimen (VB3). A significant increase in colony count in the prostatic specimens confirms prostatitis.

Management
General
Acute bacterial prostatitis
Symptomatic treatment including bed rest and sitz baths for 20 to 30 minutes two to three times daily may be helpful. Hydration may be necessary. The patient with acute bacterial prostatitis may require hospitalization for parenteral antibiotics. If test results and clinical response are favorable, parenteral therapy continues for 48 hours to 1 week; then an oral agent is substituted for 30 more days.

Chronic bacterial prostatitis
In symptomatic chronic prostatitis, regular massage of the prostate is most effective. Regular ejaculation may help promote drainage of prostatic secretions.

Nonbacterial prostatitis
For patients with nonbacterial prostatitis, prostate massage and frequent participation in sexual activity may be helpful.

Medication
Medications used in the treatment of patients with acute bacterial prostatitis include:
- co-trimoxazole — 8 to 10 mg/kg/day (based on trimethoprim component) I.V. in divided doses every 6 to 12 hours or 1 DS tablet P.O. b.i.d. until cultures are available, then for 2 to 4 weeks
- gentamicin — 3 mg/kg/day I.V. in divided doses every 8 hours
- ampicillin — 1 to 12 g/day I.V. in divided doses every 4 to 6 hours
- norfloxacin — 400 mg tablets P.O. every 12 hours for 28 days.

Medications used in the treatment of patients with chronic bacterial prostatitis include:
- co-trimoxazole — 160/800 mg P.O. b.i.d.; or norfloxacin — 400 mg P.O. b.i.d. for 1 to 3 months
- ciprofloxacin — 500 mg P.O. b.i.d. for 1 to 2 months.

Medications used in the treatment of patients with nonbacterial prostatitis include:
- doxycycline — 100 mg P.O. b.i.d. for 2 weeks
- erythromycin — 500 mg P.O. q.i.d. for 2 weeks

Anticholinergics and analgesics may help relieve nonbacterial prostatitis symptoms. Alpha-adrenergic blockers and muscle relaxants may relieve prostatodynia.

Surgical intervention

If drug therapy isn't successful, treatment may include transurethral resection of the prostate, which requires removal of all infected tissue. However, this procedure isn't usually performed on young adults because it can cause retrograde ejaculation and sterility. Total prostatectomy is curative but may cause impotence and incontinence.

Referral

■ Refer the patient with a severe case of acute bacterial prostatitis to a urologist. Hospitalization may be needed.

Follow-up

Urine cultures should be repeated monthly until negative.

Patient teaching

■ Emphasize the need for strict adherence to the prescribed drug regimen. Instruct the patient to drink at least eight glasses of water per day. Have him report adverse drug reactions.
■ Teach the patient how to use a sitz bath.
■ Tell the patient to use condoms during sexual intercourse to avoid reinfection.
■ Tell the patient with acute bacterial prostatitis to avoid anal intercourse.

Complications

■ Sepsis
■ Abscess
■ Urine retention

Special considerations

■ The prostate should be palpated gently because excessive manipulation can cause bacteremia.

• • • • • • • • • • • •

PYELONEPHRITIS, ACUTE

Acute pyelonephritis (also known as acute infective tubulointerstitial nephritis) is the sudden inflammation caused by bacteria that primarily affect the interstitial area and the renal pelvis or, less often, the renal tubules. It's one of the most common renal diseases affecting more than 250,000 people in the United States each year. With treatment and continued follow-up care, the prognosis is good, and extensive permanent damage is rare.

Causes

Acute pyelonephritis results from bacterial infection of the kidneys. Infecting bacteria usually are normal intestinal and fecal flora that grow readily in urine. The most common causative organism is *Escherichia coli*, but *Proteus, Pseudomonas, Staphylococcus aureus*, and *Enterococcus faecalis* (formerly *Streptococcus faecalis*) also cause this infection.

Typically, the infection spreads from the bladder to the ureters, then to the kidneys, as in vesicoureteral reflux. Vesicoureteral reflux may result from congenital weakness at the junction of the ureter and the bladder. Bacteria refluxed to intrarenal tissues may create colonies of infection within 24 to 48 hours. Infection may also result from instrumentation (such as catheterization, cystoscopy, or urologic surgery), from a hematogenic infection (as in septicemia or endocarditis), or possibly from lymphatic infection.

Pyelonephritis may also result from an inability to empty the bladder (for example, in patients with neurogenic bladder), urinary stasis, or urinary obstruction due to tumors, strictures, or benign prostatic hyperplasia.

Pyelonephritis occurs more often in females, probably because of a shorter urethra and the proximity of the urinary meatus to the vagina and the rectum—both conditions allow bacteria to reach the bladder more easily—and a lack of the antibacterial prostatic secretions produced in the male. Incidence increases with age and is higher in the following groups:

- *sexually active women*—Intercourse increases the risk of bacterial contamination.
- *pregnant women*—About 5% develop asymptomatic bacteriuria; if untreated, about 40% develop pyelonephritis.
- *diabetics*—Neurogenic bladder causes incomplete emptying and urinary stasis; glycosuria may support bacterial growth in the urine.
- *patients with other renal diseases*—Compromised renal function aggravates susceptibility.
- *homosexual males*—Increased risk of urinary tract infection (UTI) secondary to lifestyle affects this population.

Clinical presentation
Typical clinical features include:
- urgency, frequency, and burning during urination
- dysuria
- nocturia
- hematuria (usually microscopic but may be gross)
- cloudy urine
- urine with an ammonia-like or fishy odor
- a temperature of 102° F (38.9° C) or higher
- shaking chills
- flank pain
- anorexia
- headache
- malaise
- costovertebral angle tenderness
- general fatigue.

These signs and symptoms characteristically develop rapidly over a few hours or a few days. Although these symptoms may disappear within days, even without treatment, residual bacterial infection is likely and can cause symptoms to recur later.

Elderly patients may exhibit GI or pulmonary symptoms rather than the usual febrile responses to pyelonephritis.

In children younger than 2 years, fever, vomiting, nonspecific abdominal complaints, or failure to thrive may be the only signs or symptoms of acute pyelonephritis.

Differential diagnoses
Males
- Gonococcal and nongonococcal urethritis
- Prostatitis
- Epididymitis
- Benign prostatic hypertrophy

Females
- Interstitial cystitis
- Urethral syndrome
- Vulvovaginitis
- Vaginitis
- Urinary calculi
- Bladder outlet obstruction

Diagnosis
Diagnosis requires urinalysis and culture. Typical findings include:
- *pyuria (pus in urine)*—Urine sediment reveals the presence of leukocytes singly, in clumps, and in casts and, possibly, a few red blood cells.
- *significant bacteriuria*—Urine culture reveals more than 100,000 organisms/µl of urine.
- *low specific gravity and osmolality*—These findings result from a temporarily decreased ability to concentrate urine.
- *slightly alkaline urine pH*—This finding signifies a kidney disorder.
- *proteinuria, glycosuria, and ketonuria*—These conditions are less common.

A computed tomography (CT) scan also helps in the evaluation of acute

Chronic pyelonephritis

Chronic pyelonephritis is a persistent kidney inflammation that can scar the kidneys and may lead to chronic renal failure. Its etiology may be bacterial, metastatic, or urogenous. This disease is most common in patients who are predisposed to recurrent acute pyelonephritis, such as those with urinary obstructions or vesicoureteral reflux.

Patients with chronic pyelonephritis may have a childhood history of unexplained fevers or bed-wetting. Clinical effects may include flank pain, anemia, low urine specific gravity, proteinuria, leukocytes in urine and, especially in late stages, hypertension. Uremia rarely develops from chronic pyelonephritis unless structural abnormalities exist in the excretory system. Bacteriuria may be intermittent. When no bacteria are found in the urine, diagnosis depends on excretory urography (the renal pelvis may appear small and flattened) and renal biopsy.

Effective treatment of chronic pyelonephritis requires control of hypertension, elimination of the existing obstruction (when possible), and long-term antimicrobial therapy.

pyelonephritis. A kidney-ureter-bladder CT scan may reveal calculi, tumors, or cysts in the kidneys and urinary tract. Excretory urography may show asymmetrical kidneys.

Management
General
Treatment is focused on antibiotic therapy appropriate to the specific infecting organism after identification by urine culture and sensitivity studies.

Medication
Symptoms may disappear after several days of antibiotic therapy. Although urine usually becomes sterile within 48 to 72 hours, the course of such therapy is 10 to 14 days.

Antibiotic treatment is dependent on the organism identified through urine cultures. Some common antibiotics used to treat acute pyelonephritis are discussed here.

Broad spectrum
- ampicillin—adults, 500 mg P.O. every 6 hours; children weighing less than 44 lb (20 kg), 100 mg/kg/day P.O. in four divided doses

For enterococcus or staphylococcus infections
- penicillin G potassium—adults, 1.6 to 3.2 million U P.O. daily in four divided doses; children younger than age 12, 25,000 to 100,000 U/kg P.O. daily in four divided doses

For enterococcus infections
- vancomycin—adults, 125 to 500 mg P.O. every 6 hours; children, 40 mg/kg P.O. in four divided doses

For Escherichia coli infections and proteus infections
- sulfisoxazole—adults, 2 to 4 g P.O. initially, then 4 to 8 g/day in four to six doses; children over age 2 months, 75 mg/kg/day P.O. initially, then 150 mg/kg/day P.O. in four divided doses

In antibiotic therapy, symptoms may disappear after several days. Although urine usually becomes sterile within 48 to 72 hours, the course of such therapy is 10 to 14 days.

Surgical intervention
For patients with infection from obstruction or vesicoureteral reflux, antibiotics may be less effective; surgery may be nec-

essary to relieve the obstruction or correct the anomaly. Patients at high risk for recurring urinary tract and kidney infections, such as those with prolonged use of an indwelling urinary catheter or maintenance antibiotic therapy, require long-term follow-up. Recurrent episodes of acute pyelonephritis can eventually result in chronic pyelonephritis. (See *Chronic pyelonephritis*.)

Referral

■ Consider making a urology referral for women with upper tract infections, recurrent multiple infections, and infections with unusual organisms. Refer all males to urologists, except young healthy males who don't have recurrent infections.

Follow-up

Repeat urine culture 1 week after drug therapy stops, then periodically for the next year to detect residual or recurring infection.

Patient teaching

■ Tell the patient to avoid having a full bladder.
■ Advise the patient to increase fluid intake at the first sign of infection.
■ Stress the need to complete the prescribed antibiotic therapy, even after symptoms subside.
■ Instruct females to prevent bacterial contamination by wiping the perineum from front to back after defecation.
■ Advise routine checkups for a patient with a history of UTIs. Teach the patient to recognize signs and symptoms of infection, such as cloudy urine, burning on urination, and urinary urgency and frequency, especially when accompanied by a low-grade fever.

Complications

■ Septic shock
■ Chronic renal insufficiency

• • • • • • • • • • • •

RENAL CALCULI

Renal calculi (commonly called kidney stones) may form anywhere in the urinary tract but usually develop in the renal pelvis or in the calyces of the kidneys. Among Americans, renal calculi develop in 1 in 1,000 people, are three times more common in men (especially those ages 30 to 50) than in women, and are rare in blacks and children. They're prevalent in certain geographic areas such as the southeastern United States (stone belt), possibly because a hot climate fosters dehydration or because of regional dietary habits.

Twenty percent of patients require admission to a health care facility for treatment while 80% to 85% of patients will pass kidney stones spontaneously.

Causes

Calculi formation follows precipitation of substances normally dissolved in the urine (calcium oxalate, calcium phosphate, magnesium ammonium phosphate or, occasionally, urate or cystine). The natural sequence of stone development includes urine saturation, urine supersaturation, formation of crystalline materials, crystal nucleation, aggregation, retention of crystals by the urothelium, and continual growth of the stone. (See *How urine pH affects calculi formation*, page 198.)

Renal calculi vary in size and may be solitary or multiple. They may remain in the renal pelvis or enter the ureter and may damage renal parenchyma; large calculi cause pressure necrosis. In some sites, calculi cause obstruction, with resultant hydronephrosis, and tend to recur.

Although the exact cause of renal calculi is unknown, predisposing factors include:

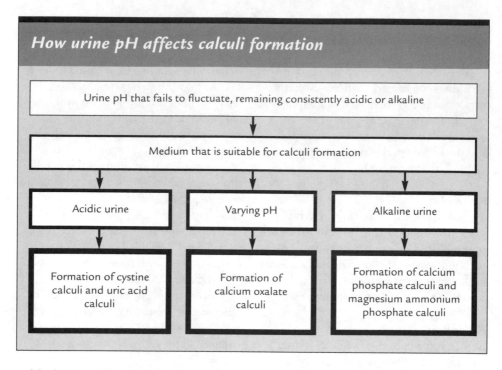

How urine pH affects calculi formation

Urine pH that fails to fluctuate, remaining consistently acidic or alkaline

↓

Medium that is suitable for calculi formation

↓

| Acidic urine | Varying pH | Alkaline urine |

↓ ↓ ↓

| Formation of cystine calculi and uric acid calculi | Formation of calcium oxalate calculi | Formation of calcium phosphate calculi and magnesium ammonium phosphate calculi |

- *dehydration* — Decreased urine production concentrates calculi-forming substances.
- *infection* — Infected, damaged tissue serves as a site for calculi development; pH changes provide a favorable medium for calculi formation (especially for magnesium ammonium phosphate or calcium phosphate calculi); or infected calculi (usually magnesium ammonium phosphate or staghorn calculi) may develop if bacteria are the nuclei in calculi formation. Infections may promote destruction of the renal parenchyma.
- *obstruction* — Urinary stasis (as in immobility from a spinal cord injury) allows calculis constituents to collect and adhere, forming calculi. Obstruction also promotes infection, which, in turn, compounds the obstruction.
- *metabolic factors* — Factors that may predispose patients to renal calculi include hyperparathyroidism, renal tubular acidosis, elevated uric acid (usually with gout), a defective metabolism of oxalate, a genetic defect in metabolism of cystine,

and excessive intake of vitamin D or dietary calcium.
- *medication* — Calculi formation is a possible adverse effect of some medication, such as acetazolamide, antacids, ascorbic acid, hydrochlorothiazide, and indinavir.

Clinical presentation
Clinical effects vary with the size, location, and etiology of calculi. Pain, the key symptom, usually results from obstruction; large, rough calculi occlude the opening to the ureter and increase the frequency and force of peristaltic contractions. The pain of classic renal colic travels from the costovertebral angle to the flank, then to the suprapubic region and external genitalia. The intensity of this pain fluctuates and may be excruciating at its peak. If calculi are in the renal pelvis and calyces, pain may be more constant and dull. Back pain (from calculi that produce an obstruction within a kidney) and severe abdominal pain (from calculi traveling down a ureter) may also

occur. Nausea and vomiting usually accompany severe pain. (See *Types of renal calculi.*)

Other associated signs include:
- fever
- chills
- hematuria (when calculi abrade a ureter)
- abdominal distention
- pyuria
- rarely, anuria (from bilateral obstruction, or unilateral obstruction in the patient with one kidney).

Differential diagnoses
- Gastroenteritis
- Salpingitis
- Ovarian cysts
- Peptic ulcer disease
- Aortic abdominal aneurysm
- Acute appendicitis
- Incarcerated inguinal hernia
- Diverticular disease
- Biliary stones
- Bowel obstruction

Diagnosis
Diagnosis is based on the clinical picture and these tests:
- A computed tomography scan is highly sensitive for identifying hydronephrosis and detecting small renal and urethral stones.
- Excretory urography may be used to diagnose obstruction by a urinary calculus and to determine the size and location of calculi.
- Kidney-ureter-bladder X-rays reveal most renal calculi.
- Stone analysis shows mineral content.
- Kidney ultrasonography is an easily performed, noninvasive, nontoxic test to detect obstructive changes such as hydronephrosis.
- Urine culture of midstream sample may indicate urinary tract infection.
- Urinalysis may be normal or show increased specific gravity and acid or alka-

Types of renal calculi

Multiple small calculi may vary in size; they may remain in the renal pelvis or pass down the ureter.

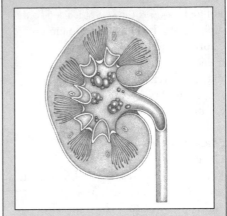

A staghorn calculus (a cast of the calyceal and pelvic collecting system) may form from a stone that stays in the kidney.

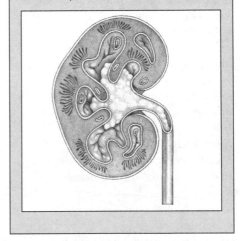

line pH suitable for different types of stone formation. Other urinalysis findings include hematuria (gross or microscopic), crystals (urate, calcium, or cystine), casts, and pyuria with or without bacteria and white blood cells.
- A 24-hour urine collection is evaluated for calcium oxalate, phosphorus, and uric acid excretion levels.

- A complete blood count with differential is used to exclude infection.
- Serial blood calcium and phosphorus levels are used to detect hyperparathyroidism and show an increased calcium level in proportion to normal serum protein.
- The blood protein level is used to determine the level of free calcium unbound to protein.
- Blood chloride and bicarbonate levels may show renal tubular acidosis.
- Increased blood uric acid levels may indicate gout as the cause.

Management
General
Because 90% of renal calculi are smaller than 5 mm in diameter, treatment usually consists of measures to promote their natural passage. Along with vigorous hydration, such treatment includes antimicrobial therapy (varying with the cultured organism) for infection, analgesics such as meperidine for pain, and diuretics to prevent urinary stasis and further calculi formation (thiazides decrease calcium excretion into the urine). Prophylaxis to prevent calculi formation includes a low-calcium, low-protein, and low-sodium diet for absorptive hypercalciuria.

Medication
Medications used in the treatment of patients with renal calculi include:
- allopurinol — 200 to 300 mg/day P.O. for uric acid calculi
- ascorbic acid — 4 to 12 g/day P.O. in divided doses to acidify the urine
- sodium bicarbonate — 325 mg to 2 g P.O. up to q.i.d. to help prevent stone formation
- penicillamine — adults, 250 mg to 1 g P.O. a.c. to help prevent cystine stone formation; children, 30 mg/kg/day in four divided doses.

Surgical intervention
Parathyroidectomy may be necessary for hyperparathyroidism. Calculi too large for natural passage may require surgical removal. When a calculus is in the ureter, a cystoscope may be inserted through the urethra and the calculus manipulated with catheters or retrieval instruments. Extraction of calculi from other areas (kidney calyx and renal pelvis) may necessitate a flank or lower abdominal approach. Percutaneous ultrasonic lithotripsy and extracorporeal shock wave lithotripsy shatter the calculus into fragments for removal by suction or natural passage.

Referral
- The patient may need referral to a urologist for both medical and surgical treatment if symptoms last more than 2 weeks or if obstruction is suspected.

Follow-up
Stone analysis should be done if retrieved, and treatment planned according to the composition of the stone. Obtain creatinine levels weekly to evaluate kidney function until the stone is passed. Abdominal films should be obtained weekly to monitor the progress of the stone.

Patient teaching
- To facilitate spontaneous passage, encourage the patient to walk, if possible. Also promote sufficient intake of fluids to maintain a urine output of 3 to 4 L/day (urine should be very dilute and colorless).
- To help acidify urine, tell the patient to drink fruit juices, especially cranberry juice.
- Stress the importance of a proper diet and compliance with the drug therapy. For example, if the patient's stone is caused by a hyperuricemic condition, ad-

vise the patient or caregiver about avoiding foods that are high in purine.

Complications
- Kidney failure
- Obstruction
- Hydronephrosis

• • • • • • • • • • • •

RENAL FAILURE, ACUTE

Acute renal failure is the sudden interruption of kidney function due to obstruction, reduced circulation, or renal parenchymal disease. It usually occurs in approximately 5% of hospitalized patients. Acute renal failure is usually reversible with medical treatment; otherwise, it may progress to end-stage renal disease, uremic syndrome, and death.

Causes
The causes of acute renal failure are classified as prerenal, intrinsic (or parenchymal), and postrenal. Prerenal failure is associated with diminished blood flow to the kidneys, possibly resulting from hypovolemia, shock, embolism, blood loss, sepsis, pooling of fluid due to ascites or burns, or from cardiovascular disorders, such as heart failure, arrhythmias, and tamponade. Prerenal acute renal failure doesn't result in structural kidney damage.

Intrinsic renal failure results from damage to the kidneys themselves, usually due to acute tubular necrosis, but possibly due to acute poststreptococcal glomerulonephritis, systemic lupus erythematosus, periarteritis nodosa, vasculitis, sickle-cell disease, bilateral renal vein thrombosis, nephrotoxins, ischemia, renal myeloma, and acute pyelonephritis. Intrinsic renal failure can result from prolonged prerenal acute renal failure resulting in acute tubular necrosis.

Postrenal failure results from bilateral obstruction of urinary outflow. Its multiple causes include kidney stones, blood clots, papillae from papillary necrosis, tumors, benign prostatic hyperplasia, strictures, and urethral edema from catheterization.

Acute renal failure can also be classified—depending on the amount of urine that is produced—as anuric, oliguric, or nonoliguric.

Clinical presentation
Acute renal failure is a critical illness. Its early signs are oliguria, azotemia and, rarely, anuria. Electrolyte imbalance, metabolic acidosis, and other severe effects follow. As the patient becomes increasingly uremic and renal dysfunction disrupts other body systems, look for these signs and symptoms:
- GI—anorexia, nausea, vomiting, diarrhea or constipation, stomatitis, bleeding, hematemesis, dry mucous membranes, and uremic breath
- *central nervous system*—headache, drowsiness, irritability, confusion, peripheral neuropathy, seizures, and coma
- *cutaneous*—dryness, pruritus, pallor, purpura and, rarely, uremic frost
- *cardiovascular*—early in the disease, hypotension; later, hypertension, arrhythmias, fluid overload, heart failure, systemic edema, anemia, and altered clotting mechanisms
- *respiratory*—pulmonary edema, Kussmaul's respirations.

Fever and chills indicate infection, a common complication.

Differential diagnoses
- Prerenal failure
- Intrarenal failure
- Postrenal failure
- Chronic renal failure

Diagnosis

The patient's history may include a disorder that can cause renal failure. Risk factors for developing acute renal failure include chronic renal insufficiency, chronic renal failure, liver disease, diabetes mellitus, vesicular disease, and advanced age.

Blood test results indicating intrinsic acute renal failure include:

- elevated blood urea nitrogen (BUN)
- elevated serum creatinine
- elevated potassium levels
- low blood pH
- low bicarbonate level
- low hematocrit and hemoglobin levels.

Urine specimens show casts, cellular debris, decreased specific gravity and, in glomerular diseases, proteinuria and urine osmolality close to serum osmolality. The urine sodium level is less than 20 mEq/L if oliguria is due to decreased perfusion; more than 40 mEq/L if due to an intrinsic problem.

Other studies include:

- renal ultrasonography
- kidney-ureter-bladder X-rays.

Excretory urography, renal scan, and nephrotomography should be used cautiously.

Management

General

Supportive measures include a diet high in calories and low in protein, sodium, and potassium, with supplemental vitamins and restricted fluids. Meticulous electrolyte monitoring is essential to detect hyperkalemia. If hyperkalemia occurs, acute therapy may include dialysis, hypertonic glucose and insulin infusions, and sodium bicarbonate — all administered I.V. — and sodium polystyrene sulfonate, by mouth or by enema, to remove potassium from the body.

If measures fail to control uremic symptoms, hemodialysis or peritoneal dialysis may be necessary. Continuous arteriovenous hemodiafiltration and continuous venovenous hemodiafiltration are alternative hemodialysis techniques for treating patients with acute renal failure, generally used when intermittent dialysis fails to control hypervolemia or uremia or when peritoneal dialysis isn't possible.

Medication

Medications used in the treatment of patients with acute renal failure include:

- furosemide — 20 to 100 mg I.V. every 6 hours
- calcium gluconate — 10 ml of 10% solution I.V. infusion; given for hyperkalemia
- sodium polystyrene — adults, 15 g daily to q.i.d. mixed with 100 ml of 20% sorbitol P.O., 30 to 50 g in 50 ml of 70% sorbitol, and 150 ml of tap water P.R. q.i.d. for hyperkalemia; children, 1 g/kg/dose
- sodium bicarbonate — dosage dependent on laboratory values; given for acidosis.

Referral

- Patients with acute renal failure should be immediately referred to the emergency department.
- A nephrologist should be consulted because of the high mortality rate (5% to 80%) associated with acute renal failure.

Follow-up

The patient's laboratory values (BUN and creatinine and potassium) should be monitored post recovery; the level of renal function recovered is used to determine the frequency of monitoring.

Patient teaching

- Instruct the patient to follow a high-calorie, low-protein, low-sodium, and low-potassium diet with vitamin supplements.

■ If the patient requires dialysis, explain what equipment is used during treatments and the monitoring that's involved with any type of dialysis.
■ Explain the importance of fluid restriction and the need for daily weight measurements.

Complications
■ Arrhythmias
■ Heart failure
■ Death
■ Sepsis
■ Seizures
■ Hypotension
■ Hyperkalemia
■ Edema

Special considerations
■ When replacing blood components, don't use whole blood if the patient is prone to heart failure and can't tolerate extra fluid volume. Packed red cells are given to deliver the necessary blood components without added volume.

• • • • • • • • • • • •

RENAL FAILURE, CHRONIC

Chronic renal failure is usually the end result of a gradually progressive loss of renal function; occasionally, it's the result of a rapidly progressive disease with sudden onset. Few symptoms develop until more than 75% of glomerular filtration is lost; then the remaining normal parenchyma deteriorates progressively and symptoms worsen as renal function decreases.

The highest incidence of chronic renal failure occurs in patients with diabetes, followed by those with hypertension and those with glomerulonephritis. Males are affected more than females, with the highest incidence of end-stage renal disease occurring in patients ages

45 to 64. The prevalence of patients being treated for end-stage renal disease is 1 per 1,000 in the United States. Incidence overall is 3 patients per 1,000.

If this condition continues unchecked, uremic toxins accumulate and produce potentially fatal physiologic changes in all major organ systems. If the patient can tolerate it, maintenance dialysis or kidney transplantation can sustain life.

Causes
Chronic renal failure may result from:
■ chronic glomerular disease such as glomerulonephritis
■ chronic infections, such as chronic pyelonephritis or tuberculosis
■ congenital anomalies such as polycystic kidneys
■ vascular diseases, such as renal nephrosclerosis or hypertension
■ obstructive processes such as calculi
■ collagen diseases such as systemic lupus erythematosus
■ nephrotoxic agents such as long-term aminoglycoside therapy
■ endocrine diseases such as diabetic neuropathy.

These conditions gradually destroy the nephrons and eventually cause irreversible renal failure. Similarly, acute renal failure that fails to respond to treatment becomes chronic renal failure. This syndrome may progress through the following stages:
■ reduced renal reserve (creatinine clearance glomerular filtration rate [GFR] is 40 to 70 ml/minute)
■ renal insufficiency (GFR 20 to 40 ml/minute)
■ renal failure (GFR 10 to 20 ml/minute)
■ end-stage renal disease (GFR less than 10 ml/minute).

Clinical presentation
Chronic renal failure produces major changes in all body systems:

■ *renal and urologic*—Initially, salt-wasting and consequent hyponatremia produce hypotension, dry mouth, loss of skin turgor, listlessness, fatigue, and nausea; later, somnolence and confusion develop. As the number of functioning nephrons decreases, so does the kidneys' capacity to excrete sodium, resulting in salt retention and overload. Accumulation of potassium causes muscle irritability, then muscle weakness as the potassium level continues to increase. Fluid overload and metabolic acidosis also occur. Urinary output decreases; the urine is very dilute and contains casts and crystals.

■ *cardiovascular*—Renal failure leads to hypertension, arrhythmias (including life-threatening ventricular tachycardia or fibrillation), cardiomyopathy, uremic pericarditis, pericardial effusion with possible cardiac tamponade, heart failure, and peripheral edema.

■ *respiratory*—Pulmonary changes include reduced pulmonary macrophage activity with increased susceptibility to infection, pulmonary edema, pleuritic pain, pleural friction rub and effusions, uremic pleuritis and uremic lung (or uremic pneumonitis), dyspnea due to heart failure, and Kussmaul's respirations as a result of acidosis.

■ *GI*—Inflammation and ulceration of the GI mucosa cause stomatitis, gum ulceration and bleeding and, possibly, parotitis, esophagitis, gastritis, duodenal ulcers, lesions on the small and large bowel, uremic colitis, pancreatitis, and proctitis. Other GI symptoms include a metallic taste in the mouth, uremic fetor (ammonia smell to breath), anorexia, nausea, and vomiting.

■ *cutaneous*—Typically, the skin is pallid, yellowish bronze, dry, and scaly. Other cutaneous signs and symptoms include severe itching; purpura; ecchymoses; petechiae; uremic frost (most often in criti-

cally ill or terminal patients); thin, brittle fingernails with characteristic lines; and dry, brittle hair that may change color and fall out easily.

■ *neurologic*—Restless leg syndrome, one of the first signs of peripheral neuropathy, causes pain, burning, and itching in the legs and feet, which may be relieved by voluntarily shaking, moving, or rocking them. Eventually, this condition progresses to paresthesia and motor nerve dysfunction (usually bilateral footdrop) unless dialysis is initiated. Other signs and symptoms include muscle cramping and twitching, shortened memory and attention span, apathy, drowsiness, irritability, confusion, coma, and seizures. Electroencephalogram changes indicate metabolic encephalopathy.

■ *endocrine*—Common endocrine abnormalities include stunted growth patterns in children (even with elevated growth hormone levels), infertility and decreased libido in both sexes, amenorrhea and cessation of menses in women, impotence and decreased sperm production in men, increased aldosterone secretion (related to increased renin production), and impaired carbohydrate metabolism (with increased blood glucose levels similar to diabetes mellitus).

■ *hematopoietic*—Anemia, decreased red blood cell survival time, blood loss from dialysis and GI bleeding, mild thrombocytopenia, and platelet defects occur. Other problems include increased bleeding and clotting disorders demonstrated by purpura, hemorrhage from body orifices, easy bruising, ecchymoses, and petechiae.

■ *skeletal*—Calcium-phosphorus imbalance and consequent parathyroid hormone imbalances cause muscle and bone pain, skeletal demineralization, pathologic fractures, and calcifications in the brain, eyes, gums, joints, myocardium, and blood vessels. Arterial calcification may produce coronary artery disease. In children, renal osteodystrophy (renal rickets) may develop.

Differential diagnoses
- Glomerulonephritis
- Polycystic kidney disease
- Nephrotoxic drugs
- Diabetic nephropathy
- Hypertensive nephrosclerosis

Diagnosis
A diagnosis of chronic renal failure is based on the clinical assessment, a history of chronic progressive debilitation, and the gradual deterioration of renal function as determined by creatinine clearance tests. The following laboratory findings also aid in diagnosis:
- Blood studies show elevated blood urea nitrogen, serum creatinine, and potassium levels; decreased arterial pH and bicarbonate; and low hemoglobin level and hematocrit.
- Urine specific gravity becomes fixed at 1.010; urinalysis may show proteinuria, glycosuria, erythrocytes, leukocytes, and casts, depending on the etiology.
- X-ray studies include kidney-ureter-bladder films, excretory urography, nephrotomography, renal scan, and renal arteriography.
- Kidney biopsy is useful in diagnosing glomerulonephritis.

Management
General
The goal of conservative treatment is to correct specific symptoms. A low-protein diet reduces the production of end products of protein metabolism that the kidneys can't excrete. (A patient receiving continuous peritoneal dialysis should have a high-protein diet.) A high-calorie diet prevents ketoacidosis and the negative nitrogen balance that results in catabolism and tissue atrophy and restricts

sodium and potassium. Fluid balance must be maintained.

Treatment may also include regular stool analysis (guaiac test) to detect occult blood and, as needed, cleansing enemas to remove blood from the GI tract.

Blood gas measurements may indicate acidosis; intensive dialysis and thoracentesis can relieve pulmonary edema and pleural effusions.

Hemodialysis or peritoneal dialysis (particularly continuous ambulatory peritoneal dialysis and continuous cyclic peritoneal dialysis) can help control most manifestations of end-stage renal disease; altering dialyzing bath fluids can correct fluid and electrolyte disturbances. (See *Comparing peritoneal dialysis and hemodialysis*, page 206, and *Continuous ambulatory peritoneal dialysis*, page 207.) Anemia, peripheral neuropathy, cardiopulmonary and GI complications, sexual dysfunction, and skeletal defects may persist. Kidney transplantation may eventually be the treatment of choice for some patients with end-stage renal disease.

Children require more dialysis in relation to their body weight than adults do because their metabolic rates and, therefore food intake, are higher.

Severe anemia requires infusion of fresh frozen packed cells or washed packed cells. However, transfusions relieve anemia only temporarily.

Medication
Medications used in the treatment of patients with chronic renal failure include:
- furosemide — 20 to 80 mg/day P.O.
- digoxin — 0.0625 to 0.25 mg/day P.O.
- atenolol — 25 to 50 mg/day P.O.
- metoclopramide hydrochloride — 10 mg P.O. a.c.
- famotidine — 20 mg P.O. h.s.

(*Text continues on page 208.*)

Comparing peritoneal dialysis and hemodialysis

TYPE	ADVANTAGES	DISADVANTAGES	POSSIBLE COMPLICATIONS
Peritoneal dialysis	■ Can be performed immediately ■ Requires less complex equipment and less specialized personnel than hemodialysis ■ Requires small amounts of heparin or none at all ■ No blood loss; minimal cardiovascular stress ■ Can be performed by patient anywhere (continuous ambulatory peritoneal dialysis), without assistance and with minimal patient teaching ■ Allows patient independence without long interruptions in daily activities ■ Lower cost	■ Contraindicated within 72 hours of abdominal surgery ■ Requires 48 to 72 hours for significant response to treatment ■ Severe protein loss necessitates high-protein diet (up to 100 g/day) ■ High risk of peritonitis; possible scarring with repeated bouts, preventing further treatments with peritoneal dialysis ■ Urea clearance less than with hemodialysis (60%)	■ Bacterial or chemical peritonitis ■ Pain (abdominal, low back, and shoulder) ■ Shortness of breath, or dyspnea ■ Atelectasis and pneumonia ■ Severe loss of protein into the dialysis solution in the abdominal cavity (10 to 20 g/day) ■ Fluid overload ■ Excessive fluid loss ■ Constipation ■ Catheter site inflammation, infection, or leakage
Hemodialysis	■ Takes only 3 to 5 hours per treatment ■ Faster results in an acute situation ■ Total number of hours of maintenance treatment that's only half that of peritoneal dialysis ■ In an acute situation, can use an I.V. route without a surgical access route	■ Requires surgical creation of a vascular access between circulation and dialysis machine ■ Requires complex water treatment, dialysis equipment, and highly trained personnel ■ Requires administration of larger amounts of heparin ■ Confines patient to special treatment unit	■ Septicemia ■ Air emboli ■ Rapid fluid and electrolyte imbalance (disequilibrium syndrome) ■ Hemolytic anemia ■ Metastatic calcification ■ Increased risk of hepatitis ■ Hypotension or hypertension ■ Itching ■ Pain (generalized or in chest) ■ Heparin overdose, possibly causing hemorrhage ■ Leg cramps ■ Nausea and vomiting ■ Headache

Continuous ambulatory peritoneal dialysis

Continuous ambulatory peritoneal dialysis is a useful alternative to hemodialysis in patients with renal failure. Using the peritoneum as a dialysis membrane, it allows almost uninterrupted exchange of dialysis solution. With this method, four to six exchanges of fresh dialysis solution are infused each day. The approximate dwell-time for the daytime ex-changes is 5 hours; for the overnight exchange, the dwell-time is 8 to 10 hours. After each dwell-time, the patient removes the dialyzing solution by gravity drainage. This form of dialysis offers the unique advantages of a simple, easily taught procedure and patient independence from a special treatment center.

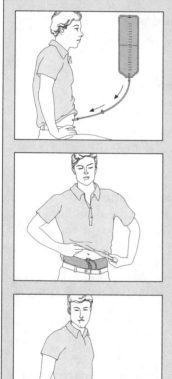

In this procedure, a Tenckhoff catheter is surgically implanted in the abdomen, just below the umbilicus. A bag of dialysis solution is aseptically attached to the tube, and the fluid is allowed to flow into the peritoneal cavity (this takes about 10 minutes).

The dialyzing fluid remains in the peritoneal cavity for 4 to 6 hours. During this time, the bag may be rolled up and placed under a shirt or blouse, and the patient can go about normal activities while dialysis takes place.

The fluid is then drained out of the peritoneal cavity through gravity flow by unrolling the bag and suspending it below the pelvis (drainage takes about 20 minutes). After the fluid drains, the patient aseptically connects a new bag of dialyzing solution and fills the peritoneal cavity again. He repeats this procedure four to six times per day.

- methylcellulose—0.45 to 3 g/day P.O.; or docusate sodium, 50 to 200 mg/day P.O.
- diphenhydramine—25 to 50 mg P.O. t.i.d.
- ferrous sulfate—324 mg P.O. t.i.d.
- folic acid—0.4 to 1 mg/day P.O., S.C. or I.M.
- epoetin alfa—50 to 100 units/kg I.V. infusion 3 times weekly; maintenance dose is individualized
- calcium gluconate—10 ml of 10% solution
- sodium polystyrene—15 g mixed with 100 ml of 20% sorbitol P.O.; 50 g in 30 to 50 ml of 70% sorbitol and 150 ml of tap water P.R.

Surgical intervention
Cardiac tamponade resulting from pericardial effusion may necessitate emergency pericardial tap or surgery.

Referral
- Refer the patient to a nephrologist.
- Refer the patient and his family to appropriate counseling agencies for help in coping with chronic renal failure.
- Refer the patient to a nutritionist if he's having difficulty following the prescribed dietary restrictions.

Follow-up
Laboratory values should be checked monthly, then every 3 months if the patient is stable. If the patient is on dialysis, laboratory values are checked as ordered by the nephrologist.

Patient teaching
- Teach the patient the importance of good skin care. Glycerin-containing soaps shouldn't be used because they cause skin drying.
- Encourage the intake of high-calorie foods. Instruct the outpatient to avoid high-sodium and high-potassium foods.

Encourage adherence to fluid and protein restrictions. To prevent constipation, stress the need for exercise and sufficient dietary fiber.
- If the patient is on hemodialysis, be sure that he understands how to protect and care for the arteriovenous shunt, fistula, or other vascular access.
- Tell the patient to withhold the 6 a.m. (or morning) doses of antihypertensive medication on the mornings of dialysis.
- Instruct the anemic patient to conserve energy and rest frequently.

Complications
- Anemia
- Infection
- Uremia
- Hypothyroidism
- Seizures
- Infertility
- Refractory ascites
- Dialysis dementia
- Protein wasting

Special considerations
- Assess for signs of pericarditis, such as a pericardial friction rub and chest pain. Also, watch for the disappearance of friction rub, with a decrease of 15 to 20 mm Hg in blood pressure during inspiration (paradoxical pulse), an early sign of pericardial tamponade.

• • • • • • • • • • • •

TESTICULAR TORSION

Testicular torsion is an abnormal twisting of the spermatic cord due to the rotation of a testis or the mesorchium (a fold in the area between the testis and epididymis), which causes strangulation and, if untreated, eventual infarction of the testis. This condition is almost always (90%) unilateral.

AGE ALERT Testicular torsion is most common between ages 12 and 18, but it can occur at any age. The prognosis is good with early detection and prompt treatment.

Causes

Normally, the tunica vaginalis envelops the testis and attaches to the epididymis and spermatic cord. In intravaginal torsion (the most common type of testicular torsion in adolescents), testicular twisting may result from an abnormality of the tunica, in which the testis is abnormally positioned, or from a narrowing of the mesentery support. In extravaginal torsion (most common in neonates), loose attachment of the tunica vaginalis to the scrotal lining causes spermatic cord rotation above the testis. A sudden forceful contraction of the cremaster muscle may precipitate this condition. (See *Extravaginal torsion*.)

Clinical presentation

Torsion produces excruciating pain in the affected testis or iliac fossa. In some cases, there is minimal swelling and little or no pain. Nausea and vomiting occurs in 50% of patients.

Differential diagnoses

- Epididymitis
- Orchitis
- Incarcerated inguinal hernia
- Vasculitis
- Tumor
- Idiopathic scrotal edema

Diagnosis

Physical examination reveals tense, tender swelling in the scrotum or inguinal canal and hyperemia of the overlying skin. Doppler ultrasonography helps to distinguish testicular torsion from a strangulated hernia, undescended testes, or epididymitis.

Extravaginal torsion

In extravaginal torsion, rotation of the spermatic cord above the testis causes strangulation and, eventually, infarction of the testis.

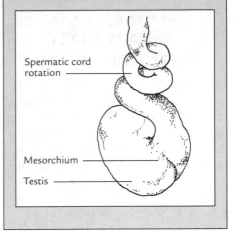

Spermatic cord rotation

Mesorchium

Testis

Management

General

Treatment consists of immediate surgical repair.

Surgical intervention

Surgical repair involves orchiopexy (fixation of a viable testis to the scrotum) or orchiectomy (excision of a nonviable testis). As with ovarian torsion in the female, preserving the organ is the preferred option.

Referral

- Refer the patient to a surgeon for treatment.

Follow-up

- The patient will be seen by the surgeon for follow-up.

Patient teaching

- Instruct the patient to use an ice bag to reduce edema.

- Tell the patient to protect the wound from contamination.

Complications
- Infection
- Infertility

• • • • • • • • • • •

URINARY TRACT INFECTION, LOWER

Cystitis and urethritis, the two forms of lower urinary tract infection (UTI), are nearly 10 times more common in women than in men and affect approximately 10% to 20% of all women at least once. Lower UTI is also a prevalent bacterial disease in children; girls are most commonly affected. In men and children, lower UTI is commonly related to anatomic or physiologic abnormalities and require close evaluation. UTI often responds readily to treatment, but recurrence and resistant bacterial flare-ups during therapy are possible.

Lower UTIs can be considered uncomplicated or complicated. Uncomplicated UTI is characterized by signs of bladder irritation, frequency, urgency, dysuria, and occasionally, hematuria. Complicated UTI results from underlying urologic or gynecologic abnormalities, pathogen resistance, underlying disease, or the presence of an indwelling urinary catheter.

Causes
Most lower UTIs result from ascending infection by a single, gram-negative, enteric bacteria, such as *Escherichia coli*, *Klebsiella*, *Proteus*, *Enterobacter*, *Pseudomonas*, or *Serratia*. However, in a patient with neurogenic bladder, an indwelling urinary catheter, or a fistula between the intestine and bladder, lower UTI may result from simultaneous infection with multiple pathogens. Recent studies suggest that infection results from a breakdown in local defense mechanisms in the bladder that allow bacteria to invade the bladder mucosa and multiply. These bacteria can't be readily eliminated by normal micturition.

Bacterial flare-up during treatment is generally caused by the pathogenic organism's resistance to the prescribed antimicrobial therapy. The presence of even a small number (less than 10,000/μl) of bacteria in a midstream urine sample obtained during treatment casts doubt on the effectiveness of treatment.

In 99% of patients, recurrent lower UTI results from reinfection by the same organism or from some new pathogen; in the remaining 1%, recurrence reflects persistent infection, usually from renal calculi, chronic bacterial prostatitis, or a structural anomaly that may become a source of infection.

The high incidence of lower UTI among women may result from the shortness of the female urethra (1¼" to 2" [3.2 cm to 5.1 cm]), which predisposes women to infection caused by bacteria from the vagina, perineum, or rectum or from a sexual partner. Men are less vulnerable because their urethras are longer (7¾" [19.7 cm]) and their prostatic fluid serves as an antibacterial shield. In both men and women, infection usually ascends from the urethra to the bladder.

As a person ages, his bladder muscles weaken, which may result in incomplete bladder emptying and chronic urine retention, factors that predispose the older person to bladder infections.

Clinical presentation
Lower UTI usually produces:
- urgency
- urinary frequency
- dysuria
- cramps or spasms of the bladder

- itching
- burning during urination
- nocturia
- urethral discharge in males.

Inflammation of the bladder wall also causes hematuria and fever. Other common features include:
- lower back pain
- malaise
- nausea
- vomiting
- abdominal pain or tenderness over the bladder area
- chills
- flank pain.

Differential diagnoses
- Acute infections
- Chronic infections
- Structural abnormalities
- Renal calculi
- Prostate enlargement
- Intrarenal or prerenal abscess

Diagnosis
Characteristic clinical features and a microscopic urinalysis showing red blood cells and more than 10 white blood cells per high-power field suggest lower UTI. A clean-catch midstream urine specimen revealing a bacterial count greater than 100,000/µl confirms the diagnosis.

Lower bacterial counts don't necessarily rule out infection, especially if the patient voids frequently, because bacteria require 30 to 45 minutes to reproduce in urine. Careful midstream, clean-catch collection is preferred to catheterization, which can reinfect the bladder with urethral bacteria.

Sensitivity testing is used to determine the appropriate therapeutic antimicrobial agent. If the patient history and physical examination findings warrant, a blood test or a stained smear of the discharge rules out venereal disease. Voiding cystourethrography or excretory urogra-

phy may be used to detect congenital anomalies that predispose the patient to recurrent UTI.

Management
General
The primary treatment for most UTIs is antibiotic therapy. The patient should also increase fluid intake and avoid coffee, alcohol, and spicy food. A heating pad may help relieve pain.

Medication
Antibiotics used to treat patients with UTIs may include:
- co-trimoxazole — adults, one DS tablet P.O. b.i.d. for 3 to 14 days depending on severity; children, 8 mg/kg/day (based on TMP dose) P.O. in two divided doses for 3 to 14 days
- ciprofloxacin — 250 mg P.O. b.i.d. for 3 to 14 days depending on the severity
- amoxicillin/clavulanate — adults, 500 mg P.O. every 12 hours for 10 to 14 days; children, 20 to 40 mg/kg/day (based on amoxicillin dose) P.O. in two or three divided doses for 7 to 10 days
- phenazopyridine — adults, 200 mg/dose P.O. t.i.d. p.c. to relieve dysuria; children, 12 mg/kg/day in three divided doses for 2 days.

Surgical intervention
Recurrent infections due to infected renal calculi, chronic prostatitis, or structural abnormality may necessitate surgery; prostatitis also requires long-term antibiotic therapy.

Referral
- Refer a patient with frequent or recurring UTI to a urologist.
- Patients who are acutely ill or have symptoms of obstruction or sepsis should be referred to the hospital for immediate treatment.

Follow-up

If the UTI is the first occurrence for the patient and symptoms resolve with treatment, no follow-up is necessary. If recurrent infection or symptoms persist, repeat the urinalysis and culture.

Patient teaching

▪ Explain the nature and purpose of antimicrobial therapy. Emphasize the importance of completing the prescribed course of therapy or, with long-term prophylaxis, of adhering strictly to the ordered dosage.

▪ Urge the patient to drink plenty of water (at least eight glasses a day). Stress the need to maintain a consistent fluid intake of about 2 qt/day (1.9 L/day). More or less than this amount may alter the effect of the prescribed antimicrobial. Fruit juices, especially cranberry juice, and oral doses of vitamin C may help to acidify the urine and enhance the action of the medication.

▪ Tell the patient to watch for GI disturbances from antimicrobial therapy. Nitrofurantoin macrocrystals, taken with milk or a meal, prevent such distress. If therapy includes phenazopyridine, warn the patient that this drug commonly turns urine red-orange.

▪ To prevent recurrent lower UTI, teach the female patient to carefully wipe the perineum from front to back and to clean it thoroughly with soap and water after defecation. Advise an infection-prone woman to void immediately after sexual intercourse. Also stress the need to completely empty the bladder. To prevent recurrent infections in men, urge prompt treatment of predisposing conditions such as chronic prostatitis.

Complications

▪ Recurrent infections
▪ Pyelonephritis

Special considerations

▪ A child with a proven UTI should receive a workup to exclude an abnormality of the urinary tract that would predispose him to renal damage.

▪ Fluoroquinolones aren't used for children because of possible adverse effects on developing cartilage.

• • • • • • • • • • •

SELECTED REFERENCES

Diagnostics: An A-to-Z Nursing Guide to Laboratory Tests & Diagnostic Procedures. Springhouse, Pa.: Springhouse Corp., 2001.

Dillon, J.J. "Continuous Renal Replacement Therapy or Hemodialysis for Acute Renal Failure?" *International Journal of Artificial Organs* 22(3):125-27, March 1999.

Diseases, 3rd ed. Springhouse, Pa.: Springhouse Corp., 2001.

Fauci, A.S., et al. *Harrison's Principles of Internal Medicine,* 15th ed. New York: McGraw-Hill Book Co., 2001.

Humes, H. "Limiting Acute Renal Failure," *Hospital Practice* 34(1):31-38, 41-42, 47-48, January 1999.

Ignatavicius, D.D., et al., eds. *Medical-Surgical Nursing Across the Health Care Continuum,* 3rd ed. Philadelphia: W.B. Saunders Co., 1999.

Kluth, D.C., and Rees, A.J. "New Approaches to Modify Glomerular Inflammation," *Journal of Nephrology* 12(2):66-75, March/April 1999.

Neurologic disorders

The neurologic system coordinates and organizes the functions of all body systems. This intricate communication network has three main divisions:
- central nervous system (CNS), the control center, which is made up of the brain and the spinal cord
- peripheral nervous system, which includes motor and sensory nerves that connect the CNS to remote body parts and relay and receive messages from them
- autonomic nervous system (part of the peripheral nervous system), which regulates involuntary functioning of internal organs.

• • • • • • • • • • • •

ASSESSMENT

Assessment, the first step of the nursing process, is critical in neurologic disorders. You can identify neurologic problems while performing a complete assessment or while investigating a complaint. You can evaluate overall neurologic function and detect abnormalities as you assess mental status, cranial nerves, sensorimotor function, and reflexes.

Physical examination
A complete neurologic assessment provides information about five categories of neurologic function: cerebral function (including level of consciousness [LOC], mental status, and language), cranial nerves, motor system and cerebellar functions, sensory system, and reflexes. Complex and time-consuming, this assessment can take 2 to 3 hours to complete.

Usually, you'll perform a neurologic screening assessment. This type of assessment evaluates some of the key indicators of neurologic function and helps identify areas of dysfunction. A neurologic screening assessment usually includes evaluation of LOC, selected cranial nerve assessment, and motor and sensory screening. If a screening assessment reveals areas of neurologic dysfunction, you must evaluate those areas in more detail.

Finally, you may have to perform a brief neurologic assessment, called a neuro check. This will enable you to make rapid, repeated evaluations of several key indicators of nervous system status: LOC, pupil size and response, verbal responsiveness, extremity strength and movement, and vital signs. After you've estab-

Documenting neurologic assessment

When documenting assessment findings, you will, of course, always describe the patient's response to the stimulus. However, don't forget to document the stimulus used to elicit the response.

Many clinicians use subjective terms to describe level of arousal. However, learn to describe it objectively. For example, describe a lethargic patient's responses this way: "Awakened when called loudly, then immediately fell asleep."

A patient's response will vary depending on the stimulus used, but if you describe the behavior in concrete terms, your documentation will give a more accurate, useful picture of the patient's condition.

lished baseline values, regularly reevaluating these key indicators reveals trends in a patient's neurologic function and helps detect transient changes that can be warning signs of problems.

Always begin with an assessment of cerebral function, including LOC. Because the brain's neurons are extremely sensitive to changes in their internal environment, cerebral dysfunction usually serves as the earliest sign of a developing CNS disorder.

Cerebral function

Basic assessment of cerebral function includes LOC, communication and, briefly, mental status. Further assessment includes formal evaluation of language skills and a complete mental status evaluation.

Level of consciousness

To assess the patient's consciousness, you'll need to evaluate his level of arousal or wakefulness and orientation to person, place, and time.

Assess the patient's degree of wakefulness. Decreased arousal commonly precedes disorientation.

Begin by quietly observing the patient's behavior. If the patient is sleeping, try to arouse him by speaking his name in a normal tone of voice. If he doesn't respond, try to arouse him starting with a minimal stimulus, increasing its intensity as necessary.

Next, note the type and intensity of stimulus required to elicit a response. Compare the findings with results of previous assessments. Note any trends or factors that could affect patient responsiveness such as administration of CNS depressant medication. (See *Documenting neurologic assessment*.)

To assess orientation, always ask open-ended questions, which require the patient to provide more than a yes-or-no answer. Test orientation to time by asking the patient the time of day, day of the week, date (month and year), and season. If mental status becomes impaired, orientation to time usually vanishes before orientation to place and person.

To minimize the subjectivity of LOC assessment and to establish a greater degree of reliability, you may use the Glasgow Coma Scale. (See *Using the Glasgow Coma Scale*.)

Communication

Assess the patient's ability to comprehend speech, writing, numbers, and gestures. Language skills include learning and recalling words, using grammar, and structuring message content logically. Speech involves neuromuscular actions of the mouth, tongue, and oropharynx.

During the interview and physical assessment, observe the patient when you ask a question. Note the quality of the patient's speech, the appropriateness of

Using the Glasgow Coma Scale

Originally designed to help predict a patient's survival and recovery after a head injury, the Glasgow Coma Scale assesses level of consciousness (LOC). It minimizes the use of subjective impressions to evaluate LOC by testing and scoring three observations: eye response, motor response, and response to verbal stimuli.

Each response receives a point value. If the patient is alert, can follow simple commands, and is completely oriented to person, place, and time, his score will total 15 points. If the patient is comatose, his score will total 7 or less. A score of 3, the lowest possible score, indicates deep coma and a poor prognosis.

Many hospitals display the Glasgow Coma Scale on neurologic flowsheets to show changes in the patient's LOC over time.

OBSERVATION	RESPONSE ELICITED	SCORE
Eye response	Opens spontaneously	4
	Opens to verbal command	3
	Opens to pain	2
	No response	1
Motor response	Reacts to verbal command	6
	Reacts to painful stimuli:	
	– Identifies localized pain	5
	– Flexes and withdraws	4
	– Assumes flexor posture	3
	– Assumes extensor posture	2
	No response	1
Verbal response	Is oriented and converses	5
	Is disoriented, but converses	4
	Uses inappropriate words	3
	Makes incomprehensible sounds	2
	No response	1

his responses, the words he chooses, his articulation, and his understanding and execution of verbal commands. Increasing language difficulties may indicate deteriorating neurologic status, warranting further evaluation and doctor notification.

Impaired language function occurs in dysphasia or aphasia. Speech problems include articulation difficulties and slurred speech, which may result from facial muscle paralysis.

Evaluation of the extent and characteristics of the patient's language deficits is usually performed by a speech pathologist. This may help pinpoint the site of a CNS lesion.

Mental status

A complete mental status examination provides information about the patient's cognitive, psychological, and intellectual skills. It's usually only performed on a chronically disoriented patient or a pa-

Mental status screening questions

As part of a neurologic screening assessment, ask the following questions to help identify patients with disordered thought processes. An incorrect answer to any question may indicate the need for a complete mental status examination.

QUESTION	FUNCTION SCREENED
What's your name?	Orientation to person
What's today's date?	Orientation to time
What year is it?	Orientation to time
Where are you now?	Orientation to place
How old are you?	Memory
Where were you born?	Remote memory
What did you have for breakfast?	Recent memory
Who is the U.S. president?	General knowledge
Can you count backwards from 20 to 1?	Attention and calculation skills
Why are you here?	Judgment

tient with suspected mental status deficits after prescreening.

To identify the need for more in-depth evaluation, you may perform an abbreviated version of the complete mental status examination. The brief mental status screening proves useful if a patient's responses to interview questions seem unreliable or indicate a possible disturbance of memory or cognitive processes. (See *Mental status screening questions.*)

Cranial nerves

Cranial nerve assessment provides valuable information about the condition of the CNS, particularly the brain stem. Because of their anatomic locations, some cranial nerves are more vulnerable to the effects of increasing intracranial pressure (ICP). Therefore, a neurologic screening assessment of the cranial nerves focuses on these key nerves: the optic (II), oculomotor (III), trochlear (IV), and abducens (VI) nerves. Evaluate the other nerves only if the patient's history or symptoms indicate a potential cranial nerve disorder or when performing a complete nervous system assessment. (See *When cranial nerves function normally* and *Evaluating brain stem function,* page 218.)

Motor function

This portion of the assessment evaluates the motor function of the cerebral cortex, cerebellum, spinal cord, and the muscles.

A screening assessment always includes examination of the patient's muscle strength (including size and symmetry), arm and leg movement, and gait.

Patients who need a complete neurologic examination or who display a motor deficit during the screening assessment may undergo a complete motor system assessment. When performing a complete assessment, proceed from head to toe, assessing all muscles of the major joints. Then assess the patient's gait and cerebellar functions.

Remain alert for any involuntary movement of the limbs, trunk, or face.

When cranial nerves function normally

OLFACTORY (CN I)
- The patient can identify a variety of smells.

OPTIC (CN II)
- The patient has visual acuity and full visual fields.
- Funduscopic examination reveals no pathology.

OCULOMOTOR (CN III), TROCHLEAR (CN IV), AND ABDUCENS (CN VI)
- The patient follows up to six cardinal positions of gaze.
- The pupils are unremarkable.
- The patient exhibits no nystagmus and no ptosis.

TRIGEMINAL (CN V)
- The patient clenches teeth with firm bilateral pressure.
- The patient has no lateral jaw deviation with mouth open.
- The patient feels a cotton wisp touched to forehead, cheek, and chin.
- The patient differentiates sharp and dull sensations on face.
- The patient blinks when cotton is touched to each cornea.

FACIAL (CN VII)
- The patient has facial symmetry.
- The patient can raise eyebrows symmetrically and grimace.

- The patient can shut eyes tightly.
- The patient can identify sweet and sour on anterior tongue.

ACOUSTIC (CN VIII)
- The patient can hear a whisper at 1' to 2' (0.3 to 0.6 m).
- The patient can hear a watch tick at 1" to 2" (2.5 to 5 cm). (The patient doesn't lateralize the Weber test.)
- The patient can hear AC better than BC in Rinne test.

GLOSSOPHARYNGEAL (CN IX) AND VAGUS (CN X)
- The patient speaks and swallows without hoarseness.
- The palate and uvula rise symmetrically when patient says "ah."
- The patient has a bilateral gag reflex.

SPINAL ACCESSORY (CN XI)
- The patient demonstrates resistance to head turning and can shrug against resistance.

HYPOGLOSSAL (CN XII)
- The patient can stick tongue out, move it from side to side, and push it strongly against resistance.

Determine whether the movement is proximal or distal and whether it occurs during sleep. Further assess any involuntary movements for rhythm or repetition.

Muscle tone and cerebellar function
Muscle tone represents the muscles' resistance to passive stretching. To test muscle tone, move the patient's extremities through passive range-of-motion exercises, progressing from the fingers, wrist, elbow, and shoulder to the ankle, knee, and hip. To evaluate cerebellar function, test the patient's balance and coordination. (See *Assessing cerebellar function*, page 220.)

Evaluating brain stem function

In an unconscious patient, you can assess brain stem function by testing for the oculocephalic (doll's eyes) reflex and the oculovestibular reflex. If the patient has a cervical spine injury, expect to use the oculovestibular reflex test as an alternative. The oculovestibular reflex test may also be used to determine the status of the vestibular portion of CN VIII.

OCULOCEPHALIC REFLEX

Before beginning, examine the patient's cervical spine. Don't perform this procedure if you suspect a cervical spine injury.

■ If the patient has no cervical spine injury, place both hands on either side of his head and use your thumbs to hold open his eyelids gently.

■ While watching the patient's eyes, briskly rotate his head from side to side, or briskly flex and extend his neck.

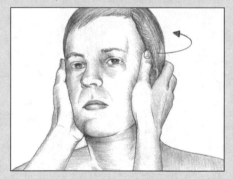

■ Observe how the patient's eyes move in relation to head movement. In a normal response, which indicates an intact brain stem, the eyes appear to move opposite to the movement of the head. For example, if the neck flexes, the eyes appear to look upward. If the neck extends, the eyes gaze downward. In an abnormal (doll's eyes) response, the eyes appear to move passively in the same direction as the head, indicating the absence of an oculocephalic reflex. This suggests a deep coma or severe brain stem damage at the level of the pons or midbrain.

OCULOVESTIBULAR REFLEX

To assess the oculovestibular reflex, first determine that the patient has an intact tympanic membrane and a clear external ear canal.

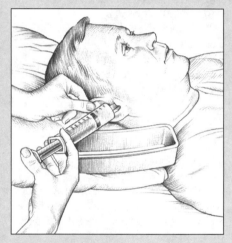

■ Elevate the head of the bed 30 degrees.

■ Using a large syringe with a small catheter on the tip, slowly irrigate the external auditory canal with 20 to 200 ml of cold water or ice water.

■ During irrigation, watch the patient's eye movements. In a patient with an intact oculovestibular reflex, the eyes will show nystagmus and will dart away from the stimulated ear. In a normal, conscious individual, as little as 10 ml of ice water will produce such a response and may also cause nausea. In a comatose patient with an intact brain stem, the eyes tonically deviate toward the stimulated ear. Absence of eye movement suggests a brain stem lesion.

Sensory system

The sensory system portion of the assessment evaluates how well the sensory receptors detect a stimulus, how well the afferent nerves carry sensory nerve impulses to the spinal cord, and the ability of the sensory tracts in the spinal cord to carry sensory messages to the brain. You'll also assess the sensory, interpretive, and integrative functions of the cerebral cortex.

Basic screening usually consists of evaluating light-touch sensation in all extremities and comparing arms and legs for symmetry of sensation.

Because the sensory system becomes fatigued with repeated stimulation, complete sensory system testing in all dermatomes tends to give unreliable results. A few screening procedures can usually reveal any dysfunctions.

Before beginning, ask the patient about any areas of numbness or unusual sensations. Such areas require special attention. Compare sensations on both sides of the patient's body in the upper arm, back of the hand, thigh, lower leg, and top of the foot. Be alert for complaints of numbness, tingling, or unusual sensations that accompany the tactile stimulus. Also note the degree of stimulation required to evoke a response. A light, brief touch should be sufficient.

If a localized deficit appears or the patient complains of localized numbness or an unpleasant sensation (dysesthesia), perform a complete sensory assessment. Also perform a complete neurologic assessment for a patient with motor or reflex abnormalities or trophic skin changes, such as ulceration, atrophy, or absent sweating. (See *Assessing the sensory system,* pages 221 and 222.)

Reflexes

Assessment of deep tendon and superficial reflexes provides information about the integrity of the sensory receptor organ and evaluates how well afferent nerves relay sensory messages to the spinal cord. It also evaluates how well the spinal cord or brain stem segment mediates the reflex, the lower motor neurons transmit messages to the muscles, and the muscles respond to the motor message. It's usually reserved for a complete neurologic assessment.

You'll also indirectly glean information about the presence or absence of inhibiting brain messages. These messages travel along the corticospinal tract to modify reflex strength.

Reflexes fall into one of three groups: deep tendon reflexes, superficial reflexes, and pathologic superficial reflexes. (See *Assessing the reflexes,* pages 223 and 224.)

Vital signs

The CNS, primarily by way of the brain stem and autonomic nervous system, controls the body's vital functions: heart rate and rhythm; respiratory rate, depth, and pattern; blood pressure; and body temperature. Note that changes in vital signs — temperature, pulse rate, respiration, and blood pressure — usually aren't early indicators of CNS deterioration.

Temperature

Damage to the hypothalamus or upper brain stem can impair the body's ability to maintain a constant temperature, resulting in profound hypothermia (temperature below 94° F [34.4° C]) or hyperthermia (temperature above 106° F [41.1° C]). Such damage can result from petechial hemorrhages in the hypothalamus or brain stem, trauma, or destructive lesions.

Pulse rate

The autonomic nervous system controls heart rate and rhythm, so pressure on the brain stem and cranial nerves slows the pulse rate by stimulating the vagus nerve.

(*Text continues on page 222.*)

Assessing cerebellar function

To evaluate cerebellar function, you'll test the patient's balance and coordination while he performs heel-and-toe walking, the Romberg test, point-to-point movements, and rapid skilled movements.

HEEL-AND-TOE WALKING

Ask the patient to walk heel-and-toe and observe his balance. Although he may be slightly unsteady, he should be able to maintain his balance while walking forward.

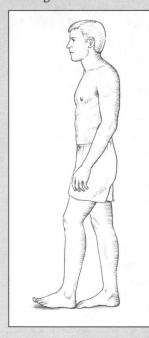

ther side of him so that you can support him if he sways to one side. Note whether he loses his balance or sways. If he falls to one side, the Romberg test is positive.

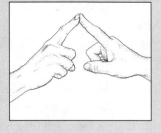

finger to another position and ask him to repeat the maneuver. Have him increase his speed gradually as you repeat the test. Then test his other hand.

RAPID SKILLED MOVEMENTS

Ask the patient to touch the thumb of his right hand to his right index finger and then to each of his remaining fingers. Then instruct him to increase his speed. Observe his movements for smoothness and accuracy. Repeat the test on his left hand.

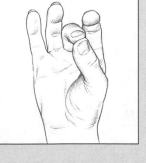

ROMBERG TEST

Ask the patient to stand with his feet together, his eyes open, and his arms at his side. Observe his balance, and then ask him to close his eyes. Hold your outstretched arms on ei-

POINT-TO-POINT MOVEMENTS

Have the patient sit about 2′ (0.6 m) away from you. Hold your index finger up, and ask him to touch the tip of his index finger to the tip of yours and then touch his nose. Next, move your

Assessing the sensory system

Further evaluate the patient's sensory function by assessing for two-point discrimination, temperature sensation, sense of position (proprioception), and point localization. Also assess number identification, superficial pain, response to vibration, extinction, and the patient's ability to recognize objects by the sense of touch (stereognosis). Perform all sensory testing with the patient's eyes closed.

TWO-POINT DISCRIMINATION
Alternately touch one or two sharp objects to the patient's skin. First assess whether he can feel one or two points; then assess the smallest distance between the two points at which he can still discriminate the presence of two points. Acuity varies in different body areas. On the finger pads, an area rich in tactile sensory receptors, the average distance necessary for two-point discrimination is less than 5 mm (less than ¼″). On the back, however, two-point discrimination requires a much wider distance.

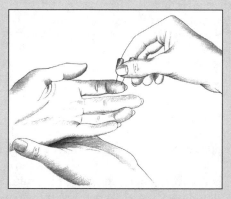

TEMPERATURE SENSATION
First fill two test tubes with water: one with hot and the other with cold. Alternately touch the patient's skin with the hot and cold tubes, and ask him to differentiate between them. Test and compare distal and proximal portions of all extremities.

SENSE OF POSITION
Grasp the sides of the patient's great toe between your thumb and forefinger. Move the toe upward or downward, asking the patient to describe the position. Repeat on the other foot, and then perform the same technique on the patient's fingers.

If the patient exhibits an impaired sense of position, proceed to the next joint on the extremity and repeat the procedure. On the leg, progress from the ankle to the knee; on the arm, go from the wrist to the elbow.

POINT LOCALIZATION
Have the patient close both eyes while you briefly touch a point on his skin. Ask him to open his eyes and point to the place just touched. He should be able to identify the spot.

NUMBER IDENTIFICATION
Trace a number on the patient's palm with an object such as the blunt end of a pencil. He should be able to identify the number.

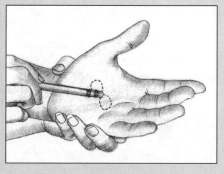

(continued)

Assessing the sensory system (continued)

SUPERFICIAL PAIN

Lightly touch — but don't puncture — the patient's skin using a sharp object such as a sterile needle. Occasionally alternate sharp and blunt ends. (Remember to discard the sharp object safely after use, and never use the same object on another patient.)

Ask the patient to identify the sensation as sharp or dull. Test and compare the distal and proximal portions of all extremities. If he displays abnormal pain sensation, test for temperature sensation.

RESPONSE TO VIBRATION

Tap a low-pitched tuning fork (preferably 128 cycles/second) on the heel of your hand; then firmly place the base of the tuning fork on an interphalangeal joint (any of the patient's fingers or his great toe).

Ask the patient to describe the sensation, differentiating between pressure and vibration, and then to state when the feeling stops. Proceed from distal to proximal areas.

If the patient has intact distal vibration sensation, further testing is unnecessary. However, if he suffers from an absence of distal vibration sensation, test the next most proximal bony prominence. When assessing the leg, progress from the medial malleolus to the patella, the anterior superior iliac spine, and the spinous process of the vertebra. For the arm, progress from the wrist to the elbow to the shoulder.

EXTINCTION

Touch two corresponding parts on the patient (such as the forearms just above the wrist) simultaneously. Ask him to describe the location of the touch. He should sense the touch in both locations.

STEREOGNOSIS

Place a familiar object, such as a key, pencil, or paper clip, in the patient's hand and ask him to identify the object by feel — which he should be able to do.

Bradycardia occurs in the later stages of increasing ICP and usually accompanies rising systolic blood pressure and widening pulse pressure. The patient commonly has a bounding pulse. Cervical spinal cord injuries can also cause bradycardia.

In a patient with acutely increased ICP or a brain injury, tachycardia signals decompensation (a condition in which the body has exhausted its compensatory measures for managing ICP), which rapidly leads to death.

Respiration

Respiratory centers in the medulla and pons control the rate, depth, and pattern of respiration. Neurologic dysfunction, particularly when it involves the brain stem or both cerebral hemispheres, commonly alters respirations. Assessment of respiration provides valuable information about a CNS lesion's site and severity.

One of the first signs of a cerebral or upper brain stem disorder is Cheyne-Stokes respiration. However, it may occur normally in an elderly patient during sleep, probably the result of generalized brain atrophy from aging.

(*Text continues on page 225.*)

Assessing the reflexes

Use the following procedures for testing each deep tendon, superficial, and pathologic superficial reflex. Reflex assessment helps to evaluate the intactness of specific cervical (C), thoracic (T), lumbar (L), and sacral (S) spinal segments. These segments are listed parenthetically after the appropriate reflex.

DEEP TENDON REFLEXES

The deep tendon reflexes include the patient's biceps, triceps, brachioradialis, quadriceps, and Achilles reflexes.

Biceps reflex (C5, C6)
Have the patient partially flex one arm at the elbow, with the palm facing down. Place your thumb or finger over the biceps tendon. Then tap lightly over your finger with the reflex hammer. An impulse from the tapping should travel to the biceps tendon and cause brisk elbow flexion that's visible and palpable.

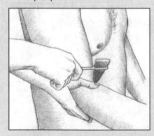

Triceps reflex (C7, C8)
Have the patient partially flex one arm at the elbow, with the palm facing the body. Support the arm and pull it slightly across the patient's chest. Using a direct blow with the re-flex hammer, tap the triceps tendon at its insertion (about 1″ to 2″ [2.5 to 5 cm] above the elbow on the olecranon process of the ulnar bone). Normally, this action causes brisk extension of the elbow, with visible and palpable contraction of the triceps muscle.

Brachioradialis (supinator) reflex (C5, C6)
Position the patient with one arm flexed at the elbow, palm down, and resting in the lap or, if he's lying down, against the abdomen. Then tap the styloid process of the radius with the reflex hammer, about 1″ to 2″ above the wrist. Normally, this action causes elbow flexion, forearm supination, and finger and hand flexion.

Quadriceps (knee-jerk or patellar) reflex (L2, L3, L4).
Have the patient sit with one knee flexed and the lower leg dangling over the side of the examination table, or place him in the supine position. (For the supine patient, place your hand under his knee, slightly raising and flexing it.) Then tap the patellar tendon with the reflex hammer. The patient's knee should extend and the quadriceps should contract.

Achilles (ankle-jerk) reflex (S1, S2)
First, position the patient with his knee bent and his ankle dorsiflexed. For best results, have him sit with his legs dangling over the side of the examination table. Then tap the Achilles tendon, which should cause plantar flexion followed by muscle relaxation.

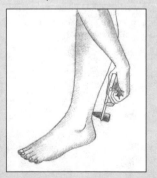

SUPERFICIAL REFLEXES

The superficial reflexes include the pharyngeal, abdominal, and cremasteric reflexes as well as the anal

(continued)

Assessing the reflexes *(continued)*

and bulbocavernosus reflexes. Assess the last two reflexes, known as the perineal reflexes, only in patients with suspected sacral spinal cord or sacral spinal nerve disorders.

Pharyngeal reflex (CN IX, CN X)
Have the patient open his mouth wide. Then touch the posterior wall of the pharynx with a tongue blade. Normally, this will cause the patient to gag.

Abdominal reflex (T8, T9, T10)
Use a fingernail or the tip of the handle of the reflex hammer to stroke one side, and then the opposite side, of the patient's abdomen above the umbilicus. Repeat on the lower abdomen. Normally, the abdominal muscles contract and the umbilicus deviates toward the stimulated side.

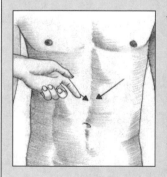

Cremasteric reflex (L1, L2)
In a male patient, use a tongue blade to scratch the inner aspect of each thigh gently. This should cause elevation of the testicles.

Anal reflex (S3, S4, S5)
Gently scratch the skin at the side of the anus with a blunt instrument, such as a tongue blade or a gloved finger. Look for puckering of the anus, a normal response.

Bulbocavernosus reflex (S3, S4)
In a male patient, apply direct pressure over the bulbocavernous muscle behind the scrotum and gently pinch the foreskin or glans. This action should cause the bulbocavernous muscle to contract.

PATHOLOGIC SUPERFICIAL REFLEXES
The pathologic superficial reflexes include the grasp, sucking, snout, and Babinski's reflexes. They indicate central nervous system damage.

Grasp reflex
Stimulate the palm of the patient's hand with your fingers. (Because a lack of inhibition by the brain can cause the patient to squeeze tightly, avoid finger injury or pain by crossing your middle and index fingers before placing them in his palm.) In a positive grasp reflex, the patient's hand will grasp yours upon stimulation, indicating frontal lobe damage, bilateral thalamic degeneration, or cerebral degeneration or atrophy.

Sucking reflex
Stimulate the patient's lips with a mouth swab. A sucking movement on stimulation can indicate cerebral degeneration.

Snout reflex
Gently percuss the oral area with your fingers. This action may make the patient's lips pucker, indicating cerebral degeneration or late-stage dementia.

Babinski's reflex
Stroke the lateral aspect of the sole of the patient's foot. A positive Babinski reflex occurs when the toes dorsiflex and fan out, indicating upper motor neuron disease.

Spinal cord damage above C7 weakens or paralyzes the respiratory muscles, causing varying degrees of respiratory impairment.

Blood pressure
Pressor receptors in the medulla oblongata of the brain stem constantly monitor blood pressure. In a patient with no history of hypertension, rising systolic blood pressure may signal rising ICP. If ICP continues to rise, pulse pressure widens as systolic pressure climbs and diastolic pressure remains stable or falls. In the late stages of acutely elevated ICP, blood pressure plummets as cerebral perfusion fails, resulting in the patient's death.

Although rare, hypotension accompanying a brain injury is an ominous sign. In addition, cervical spinal cord injuries may interrupt sympathetic nervous system pathways, causing peripheral vasodilation and hypotension.

• • • • • • • • • • • •

ALZHEIMER'S DISEASE

Alzheimer's disease, also called primary degenerative dementia, accounts for more than half of all dementias. This disease isn't found exclusively in the elder population. Its onset begins in middle age in 1% to 10% of cases. Because this is a primary progressive dementia, the prognosis for a patient with this disease is poor.

Causes and pathophysiology
The cause of Alzheimer's disease is unknown; however, it's thought that several factors are implicated in this disease. These include neurochemical factors, such as deficiencies in the neurotransmitter acetylcholine, somatostatin, substance P, and norepinephrine; environ-mental factors; and genetic immunologic factors. Genetic studies show that an autosomal dominant form of Alzheimer's disease is associated with early onset and early death. A family history of Alzheimer's disease and the presence of Down syndrome are two established risk factors.

The brain tissue of patients with Alzheimer's disease has three hallmark features: neurofibrillary tangles, neuritic plaques, and granulovascular degeneration. Examination of the brain after death also finds that it's atrophic, commonly weighing less than 1,000 g, compared with a normal brain weight of about 1,380 g.

Clinical presentation
Onset is insidious. Initially, the patient undergoes almost imperceptible changes, such as:
- forgetfulness
- recent memory loss
- difficulty learning
- remembering new information
- deterioration in personal hygiene and appearance
- inability to concentrate.

Gradually, tasks that require abstract thinking and activities that require judgment become more difficult. Progressive difficulty in communication and severe deterioration in memory, language, and motor function result in a loss of coordination and an inability to write or speak. Personality changes (restlessness, irritability) and nocturnal awakenings are common.

Patients also exhibit:
- loss of eye contact
- a fearful look
- wringing of the hands
- other signs of anxiety.

When a patient with Alzheimer's disease is overwhelmed with anxiety, he

Organic brain syndrome

Although many behavioral disturbances are clearly linked to organic brain dysfunction, the clinical syndromes associated with this type of impairment are sometimes hard to detect. Why? Because they aren't always determined by the affected area of the brain or even by the extent of tissue damage. Instead, the way the patient's personality interacts with the brain injury determines the specific clinical effects. General symptoms commonly include impairment of orientation, memory, and intellectual and emotional function. These primary cognitive deficits help to distinguish organic brain syndromes from neurosis and depression.

DIAGNOSIS
Diagnosis of an organic brain syndrome depends on a detailed history of the onset of cognitive and behavioral disturbances; a complete neurologic assessment; and such tests as EEGs, computed tomography scans, brain X-rays, cerebrospinal fluid analyses, and psychological studies. Organic brain syndromes are classified by etiology and specific clinical effects. Causes include infection, brain trauma, nutritional deficiency, cerebrovascular disease, degenerative disease, tumor, toxins, and metabolic or endocrine disorders.

TREATMENT
Effective treatment requires correction of the underlying cause. Special considerations may include reality orientation, emotional support for the patient and family, a safe environment, mat therapy for an agitated or aggressive patient, and referral for psychological counseling.

becomes dysfunctional, acutely confused, agitated, compulsive, or fearful.

Eventually, the patient becomes disoriented, and emotional lability and physical and intellectual disability progress. The patient becomes susceptible to infection and accidents. Usually, death results from infection.

Differential diagnoses
- Head trauma
- Tumor
- Depression
- Epilepsy
- Toxin exposure
- Demyelinating disease

Diagnosis
Early diagnosis of Alzheimer's disease is difficult because the patient's signs and symptoms are subtle. (See *Organic brain syndrome.*) Diagnosis relies on an accurate history from a reliable family member, mental status and neurologic examinations, and psychometric testing. A positron emission tomography scan measures the metabolic activity of the cerebral cortex and may help in early diagnosis. An EEG and a computed tomography scan may help in later diagnosis. Currently, the disease is diagnosed by exclusion; that is, tests are performed to rule out other disorders. The presence of Alzheimer's disease can't be confirmed until death, when pathologic findings are revealed during an autopsy. Cognitive function can be determined by performing the Folstein Mini-Mental Status Examination.

Management

General

Overall care focuses on supporting the patient's remaining abilities and compensating for those he has lost.

Medication

If depression seems to exacerbate the patient's dementia, an antidepressant, such as fluoxetine (20 to 80 mg/day P.O.) is given.

To treat memory deficits, anticholinesterase agents are given; they include:
- tacrine — 10 to 40 mg P.O. q.i.d.
- donepezil — 5 to 10 mg/day P.O.
- rivastigmine tartrate — 1.5 mg b.i.d., increase by 3 mg/day every 2 weeks.

To decrease symptoms of psychosis, an antipsychotic such as haloperidol (0.5 to 5 mg P.O. b.i.d. to t.i.d.) may be given.

Antioxidant therapy, such as with 1,000 IU vitamin E b.i.d. P.O., is currently under study for its delaying effect on the disease and its symptoms.

Estrogen replacement therapy appears to slow progression of disease, or possibly prevent it.

Referral

- If additional care that the family can't provide is required, refer the patient to a home health agency.
- Refer the patient and family to a support group, such as the National Alzheimer's Association
- Refer the family to social service and community resources for legal and financial advice and support.

Follow-up

The patient should be seen as often as necessary to monitor drug use and assess mental status. Serial mental status testing should be done. Any coexisting medical conditions need to be monitored.

Patient teaching

- Teach the family to provide the patient with a safe environment.
- Encourage the patient to exercise to help maintain mobility.

Complications

- Hostile, uncontrollable behavior
- Depression
- Injury
- Caregiver burnout

Special considerations

- Establish an effective communication system with the patient and family to help them adjust to the patient's altered cognitive abilities
- Advise the family to establish durable power of attorney and advance directives as early as possible.

• • • • • • • • • • • •

AMYOTROPHIC LATERAL SCLEROSIS

Amyotrophic lateral sclerosis (ALS), also known as Lou Gehrig disease, is the most common of the motor neuron diseases that cause muscle atrophy. (See *Motor neuron disease*, page 228.) Other motor neuron diseases include progressive muscular atrophy and progressive bulbar palsy. More than 30,000 Americans have ALS; about 5,000 new cases are diagnosed each year, with men affected three times more commonly than women.

AGE ALERT Onset occurs between ages 40 and 70. A chronic, progressively debilitating disease, ALS may be fatal in less than 1 year or continue for 10 years or more, depending on the muscles it affects.

Motor neuron disease

In its final stages, motor neuron disease affects both upper and lower motor neuron cells. However, the site of initial cell damage varies according to the specific disease:
- progressive bulbar palsy — degeneration of upper motor neurons in the medulla oblongata
- progressive muscular atrophy — degeneration of lower motor neurons in the spinal cord
- amyotrophic lateral sclerosis — degeneration of upper motor neurons in the medulla oblongata and lower motor neurons in the spinal cord.

Causes
The exact cause of ALS is unknown, but about 5% to 10% of cases have a genetic component. In these patients, it's an autosomal dominant trait.

ALS may result from:
- heredity
- a slow-acting virus
- nutritional deficiency related to a disturbance in enzyme metabolism
- metabolic interference in nucleic acid production by the nerve fibers
- autoimmune disorders that affect immune complexes in the renal glomerulus and basement membrane.

Clinical presentation
Patients with ALS develop fasciculations, accompanied by muscle weakness most commonly of the hands, arms, and legs. Other signs include:
- impaired speech
- difficulty chewing, swallowing, and breathing (if brain stem is affected)
- choking and excessive drooling (occasionally).

Mental deterioration doesn't occur, but patients may become depressed as a reaction to the disease. Precipitating factors for acute deterioration include any severe stress, such as a myocardial infarction, trauma, viral infections, and physical exhaustion.

Differential diagnoses
- Multiple sclerosis
- Spinal cord neoplasm
- Central nervous system syphilis
- Polyarteritis
- Syringomyelia
- Myasthenia gravis
- Progressive muscular dystrophy
- Progressive cerebrovascular accidents

Diagnosis
Characteristic clinical features indicate a combination of upper and lower motor neuron involvement without sensory impairment. Electromyography and muscle biopsy help determine the presence of nerve, rather than muscle, disease. The protein content of cerebrospinal fluid is increased in one-third of patients, but this finding alone doesn't confirm ALS.

Management
General
Management aims to control symptoms and provide emotional, psychological, and physical support.

Medication
Riluzole (50 mg P.O. every 12 hours on an empty stomach) may increase quality of life and survival.

Referral
- Refer the patient to a neurologist.
- Refer the patient to a rehabilitation program designed to maintain independence as long as possible.
- Refer the patient to a home health care agency for a visiting nurse to oversee the

patient's status, to provide support, and to teach the family about the illness.
■ Patients and family members should be referred to local support groups such as the ALS Association.

Follow-up
Initially, the patient should be seen every 3 months. Visits should be increased as necessary for symptomatic treatment.

Patient teaching
■ Depending on the patient's muscular capacity, teach the family to assist with bathing, personal hygiene, and wheelchair to bed transfers.
■ Teach the patient to establish a regular bowel and bladder routine.
■ To help the patient handle increased accumulation of secretions and dysphagia, teach him to suction himself. He should have a suction machine handy at home to reduce fear of choking.

Complications
■ Infection
■ Pressure ulcers
■ Aspiration pneumonia
■ Injury
■ Pulmonary emboli

Special considerations
■ Remember that mental status remains intact while progressive physical degeneration takes place, so the patient acutely perceives every change. This threatens the patient's relationships, career, income, muscle coordination, sexuality, and energy.
■ A discussion of directives regarding health care decisions should be instituted before the patient can't communicate his wishes. Prepare the patient and family members for his eventual death, and encourage the start of the grieving process.

BELL'S PALSY

Bell's palsy is a disease of the seventh cranial nerve (facial) that produces unilateral or bilateral facial weakness or paralysis. Onset is rapid. In 80% to 90% of patients, it subsides spontaneously, with complete recovery in 1 to 8 weeks; however, recovery may be delayed in elderly patients. If recovery is partial, contractures may develop on the paralyzed side of the face. Bell's palsy may recur on the same or opposite side of the face.

AGE ALERT Although it affects all age-groups, it occurs most commonly in people under age 60.

Causes
Bell's palsy blocks the seventh cranial nerve, which is responsible for motor innervation of the muscles of the face. The conduction block is due to an inflammatory reaction around the nerve (usually at the internal auditory meatus), which is commonly associated with infections and can result from hemorrhage, tumor, meningitis, or local trauma.

Clinical presentation
Bell's palsy usually produces:
■ unilateral facial weakness
■ aching pain around the angle of the jaw or behind the ear
■ mouth droops on weak side (causing drooling from the corner of his mouth)
■ taste perception (distorted over the affected anterior portion of the tongue)
■ ability to close the eye on the weak side is markedly impaired
■ Bell's phenomenon (upward roll of the affected eye when attempting to close, along with excessive tearing).

Although Bell's phenomenon occurs in normal people, it isn't apparent because the eyelids close completely and

Recognizing unilateral Bell's palsy

Bell's palsy usually causes a unilateral facial paralysis. This produces a distorted appearance with an inability to wrinkle the forehead, close the eyelid, smile, show the teeth, or puff out the cheek.

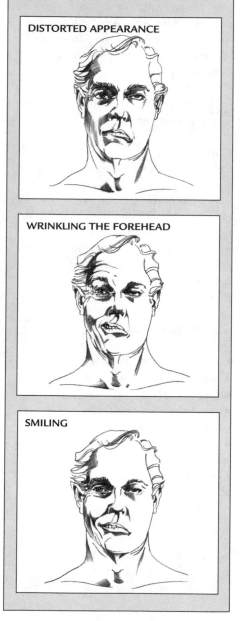

DISTORTED APPEARANCE

WRINKLING THE FOREHEAD

SMILING

cover the upward eye roll. In Bell's palsy, incomplete eye closure makes this upward eye roll obvious. Other symptoms may include loss of taste and ringing in the ear.

Differential diagnoses
- Cerebrovascular accident
- Transient ischemic attack
- Brain tumor
- Guillain-Barré syndrome

Diagnosis
Diagnosis is based on clinical presentation, such as distorted facial appearance and inability to raise the eyebrow, close the eyelid, smile, show the teeth, or puff out the cheek. (See *Recognizing unilateral Bell's palsy.*) After 10 days, electromyography helps predict the level of expected recovery by distinguishing temporary conduction defects from a pathologic interruption of nerve fibers.

Management
Medication
To reduce facial nerve edema and improve nerve conduction and blood flow, give the oral corticosteroid prednisone (60 to 80 mg/day P.O. for 5 days, then taper over the next 5 days). After the 14th day of prednisone therapy, electrotherapy may help prevent atrophy of facial muscles.

If Bell's palsy is caused by herpes zoster, administer the antiviral agent acyclovir (800 mg P.O. five times per day for 7 to 10 days).

For neuritic pain, give phenytoin (200 to 600 mg/day in divided doses).

Referral
- Refer the patient to a neurologist.
- The patient may be referred to a physical therapist.
- Refer the patient to an ophthalmologist if corneal abrasion occurs.

Follow-up
The patient should be rechecked monthly for up to 1 year.

Patient teaching
- Teach the patient about adverse steroid effects, especially GI distress and fluid retention. If GI distress is troublesome, a concomitant antacid usually provides relief. If the patient has diabetes, prednisone must be used with caution, and serum glucose levels should be monitored frequently.
- To reduce pain, teach the patient to apply moist heat to the affected side of the face, taking care not to burn the skin.
- To help maintain muscle tone, teach the patient to massage his face with a gentle upward motion two to three times daily for 5 to 10 minutes. When he's ready for active exercises, teach him to exercise by grimacing in front of a mirror.
- Advise the patient to protect his eye by covering it with an eye patch, especially when outdoors. Tell him to keep warm and avoid exposure to dust and wind. When exposure is unavoidable, instruct him to cover his face.

Complications
- Corneal abrasion
- Infection (masked by steroid use)
- Poor functional recovery

•••••••••••••

CEREBRAL PALSY

The most common cause of crippling in children, cerebral palsy (CP) is a group of neuromuscular disorders resulting from prenatal, perinatal, or postnatal central nervous system damage. Although nonprogressive, these disorders may become more obvious as an affected infant grows older. Three major types of CP occur — spastic, athetoid, and ataxic — sometimes in mixed forms. Motor impairment may be minimal (sometimes apparent only during physical activities such as running) or severely disabling. Associated defects, such as seizures, speech disorders, and mental retardation, are common. The prognosis varies; in cases of mild impairment, proper treatment may make a near-normal life possible.

CP occurs in an estimated 7,000 live births every year. Incidence is highest in premature infants (anoxia plays the greatest role in contributing to CP) and in infants who are small for their gestational age. CP is slightly more common in males than in females. CP occurs more commonly in whites than other races.

Causes
Cerebral anorexia, hemorrhage, or other damage may cause cerebral palsy. For other common causes see *Causes of cerebral palsy*, page 232.

Clinical presentation
All forms of CP have similar clinical features, although certain differences do occur. A patient may present with one of the following types of CP:
- Spastic CP is the most common type, affecting about 70% of CP patients. It's characterized by hyperactive deep tendon reflexes, increased stretch reflexes, rapid alternating muscle contraction and relaxation, muscle weakness, underdevelopment of affected limbs, muscle contraction in response to manipulation, and a tendency to contractures. Typically, a child with spastic CP walks on his toes with a scissors gait, crossing one foot in front of the other.
- Athetoid CP, which affects about 20% of CP patients, is characterized by involuntary movements — grimacing, wormlike writhing, dystonia, and sharp jerks — impair voluntary movement. Usually, these involuntary movements affect the

Causes of cerebral palsy

Conditions that result in cerebral anoxia, hemorrhage, or other damage are probably responsible for cerebral palsy (CP):

- *Prenatal conditions that may increase risk of CP*—maternal infection (especially rubella), maternal drug ingestion, radiation, anoxia, toxemia, maternal diabetes, abnormal placental attachment, malnutrition, and isoimmunization
- *Perinatal and birth difficulties that increase the risk of CP*—forceps delivery, breech presentation, placenta previa, abruptio placentae, metabolic or electrolyte disturbances, abnormal maternal vital signs from general or spinal anesthetic, prolapsed cord with delay in delivery of head, premature birth, prolonged or unusually rapid labor, and multiple birth (especially infants born last in a multiple birth)
- *Infection or trauma during infancy*—poisoning, severe kernicterus resulting from erythroblastosis fetalis, brain infection, head trauma, prolonged anoxia, brain tumor, cerebral circulatory anomalies causing blood vessel rupture, and systemic disease resulting in cerebral thrombosis or embolus.

arms more severely than the legs; involuntary facial movements may make speech difficult. These athetoid movements become more severe during stress, decrease with relaxation, and disappear entirely during sleep.

- Ataxic CP accounts for about 10% of CP patients. Its characteristics include disturbed balance, incoordination (especially of the arms), hypoactive reflexes, nystagmus, muscle weakness, tremor, lack of leg movement during infancy, and a wide gait as the child begins to walk. Ataxia makes sudden or fine movements almost impossible.

Some children with CP display a combination of these clinical features. In most, impaired motor function makes eating, especially swallowing, difficult and retards growth and development. Up to 40% of these children are mentally retarded, about 25% have seizure disorders, and about 80% have impaired speech. Many also have dental abnormalities, vision and hearing defects, and reading disabilities.

Differential diagnoses
- Muscle disease

Diagnosis
Early diagnosis is essential for effective treatment and requires precise neurologic assessment and careful clinical observation during infancy. Suspect CP whenever an infant:

- has difficulty sucking or keeping the nipple or food in his mouth.
- seldom moves voluntarily or has arm or leg tremors with voluntary movement.
- crosses his legs when lifted from behind rather than pulling them up or "bicycling" as with a normal infant.
- has legs that are difficult to separate, making diaper changing difficult.
- persistently uses only one hand or, as he gets older, uses hands well but not legs.

Infants at particular risk include those with low birth weight, low Apgar scores at 5 minutes, seizures, and metabolic disturbances. However, all infants should have a screening test for CP as a regular part of their 6-month checkup.

Management
General
CP can't be cured, but proper treatment can help affected children reach their full potential within the limitations set by this disorder. Such treatment requires a comprehensive and cooperative effort involving doctors, nurses, teachers, psychologists, the child's family, and occupational, physical, and speech therapists. Home care is commonly possible. Treatment usually includes interventions that encourage optimum development:
- Braces or splints and special appliances, such as adapted eating utensils and a low toilet seat with arms, help these children perform activities independently.
- An artificial urinary sphincter may be indicated for the incontinent child who can use the hand controls.
- Range-of-motion exercises minimize contractures.

Children with milder forms of CP should attend a regular school; severely afflicted children may need special classes.

Medication
Medications used to control seizures include:
- phenytoin—adults, 300 to 600 mg/day P.O.; children, 5 mg/kg P.O. divided b.i.d. to t.i.d to a maximum 300 mg/day
- phenobarbital—adults, 60 to 200 mg/day P.O.; children, 3 to 6 mg/kg/day P.O. divided in two doses.

A muscle relaxant may also be given; for example, diazepam (adults, 2 to 10 mg P.O. b.i.d. to q.i.d.; children older than age 5, 5 to 10 mg I.M. or I.V. every 3 to 4 hours; children younger than age 5, 1 to 2 mg I.M. or I.V. every 3 to 4 hours p.r.n.).

Surgical intervention
- Orthopedic surgery may be indicated to correct contractures.

- Neurosurgery may be required to decrease muscle spasticity

Referral
- Refer the patient to an orthopedic surgeon if contractures occur.
- Refer the patient to a neurologist if seizures occur.
- A referral for physical therapy will be needed to help maintain muscle tone and function.
- Refer the family for psychological counseling if needed.
- To help the patient and family cope with the illness, refer them to local support groups such as the United Cerebral Palsy Association.

Patient teaching
- Teach the family to provide a high-calorie diet that's adequate enough to meet the child's high energy needs.
- During meals, tell the family to maintain a quiet, unhurried atmosphere with as few distractions as possible. The child should be encouraged to feed himself and may need special utensils and a chair with a solid footrest. Teach him to place food far back in his mouth to facilitate swallowing. Tell them to encourage the child to chew food thoroughly, drink through a straw, and suck on lollipops to develop the muscle control needed to minimize drooling.
- Tell the family to allow the child to wash and dress independently, assisting only as needed. The child may need clothing modifications.

Complications
- Permanent disability
- Contractures

Special considerations
- Speak slowly and distinctly. Encourage the child to ask for things he wants. Listen patiently and don't rush him.

- Perform all assessments in an unhurried manner; otherwise, muscle spasticity may increase.
- Encourage the parents to set realistic individual goals.
- Stress the child's need to develop peer relationships; warn the parents against being overprotective.
- Identify and deal with family stress. The parents may feel unreasonable guilt about their child's handicap and may need psychological counseling.

• • • • • • • • • • • •

CEREBROVASCULAR ACCIDENT

A cerebrovascular accident (CVA), commonly known as a "brain attack" or stroke, is a sudden impairment of cerebral circulation in one or more of the blood vessels supplying the brain. A CVA interrupts or diminishes oxygen supply and commonly causes serious damage or necrosis in brain tissues. Eighty percent of CVAs are caused by cerebral ischemia and 20% result from hemorrhage. The sooner circulation returns to normal after a CVA, the better chances are for complete recovery. However, about 50% of those who survive a CVA remain permanently disabled and experience a recurrence within weeks, months, or years.

CVA is the third most common cause of death in the United States today and the most common cause of neurologic disability. It strikes 500,000 people each year, half of whom die.

Causes and pathophysiology

CVA results from obstruction of a blood vessel, typically in extracerebral vessels but occasionally in intracerebral vessels. Factors that increase the risk of CVA include history of transient ischemic attacks (TIAs), atherosclerosis, hypertension, kidney disease, arrhythmias (specifically atrial fibrillation), electrocardiogram changes, rheumatic heart disease, diabetes mellitus, postural hypotension, cardiac or myocardial enlargement, high serum triglyceride levels, lack of exercise, use of oral contraceptives, cigarette smoking, and family history of CVA. (See *Transient ischemic attack*.)

The major causes of CVA are thrombosis, embolism, and hemorrhage. Thrombosis is the most common cause of ischemic CVA in middle-aged and elderly people who have a higher incidence of atherosclerosis, diabetes, and hypertension. Thrombosis causes ischemia in brain tissue supplied by the affected vessel as well as congestion and edema; the latter may produce more clinical effects than thrombosis itself, but these symptoms subside with the edema. Thrombosis may develop while the patient sleeps or shortly after he awakens; it can also occur during surgery or after a myocardial infarction. The risk increases with obesity, smoking, or the use of oral contraceptives. Cocaine-induced ischemic stroke is now being seen in younger patients.

Embolism, the second most common cause of ischemic CVA, is an occlusion of a blood vessel caused by a fragmented clot, a tumor, fat, bacteria, or air. It can occur at any age, especially among patients with a history of rheumatic heart disease, endocarditis, posttraumatic valvular disease, myocardial fibrillation and other cardiac arrhythmias, or after open-heart surgery. It usually develops rapidly — in 10 to 20 seconds — and without warning. When an embolus reaches the cerebral vasculature, it cuts off circulation by lodging in a narrow portion of an artery, most commonly the middle cerebral artery, causing necrosis and edema. If the embolus is septic and infection extends beyond the vessel wall, encephalitis or an abscess may develop.

Transient ischemic attack

A transient ischemic attack (TIA) is a recurrent episode of neurologic deficit, lasting from seconds to hours, that clears within 12 to 24 hours. It's usually considered a warning sign of an impending thrombotic cerebrovascular accident (CVA). In fact, TIAs have been reported in 50% to 80% of patients who have had a cerebral infarction from such thrombosis. The age of onset varies. Incidence rises dramatically after age 50 and is highest among blacks and men.

CAUSES
In TIA, microemboli released from a thrombus probably temporarily interrupt blood flow, especially in the small distal branches of the arterial tree in the brain. Small spasms in those arterioles may impair blood flow and also precede TIA. Predisposing factors are the same as for thrombotic CVAs. The most distinctive characteristics of TIAs are the transient duration of neurologic deficits and complete return of normal function. The symptoms of TIA easily correlate with the location of the affected artery. These symptoms include double vision, speech deficits (slurring or thickness), unilateral blindness, staggering or uncoordinated gait, unilateral weakness or numbness, falling because of weakness in the legs, and dizziness.

TREATMENT
During an active TIA, treatment aims to prevent a completed stroke and consists of aspirin or anticoagulants to minimize the risk of thrombosis. After or between attacks, preventive treatment includes carotid endarterectomy or cerebral microvascular bypass.

Hemorrhage, the third most common cause of CVA, may, like embolism, occur suddenly, at any age, and affects more women than men. Hemorrhage results from chronic hypertension or aneurysms, which cause sudden rupture of a cerebral artery, thereby diminishing blood supply to the area served by the artery. In addition, blood accumulates deep within the brain, further compressing neural tissue and causing even greater damage.

CVAs are classified according to their course of progression. The least severe is the TIA, or "little stroke," which results from a temporary interruption of blood flow, most commonly in the carotid and vertebrobasilar arteries. A progressive stroke, or stroke-in-evolution (thrombus-in-evolution), begins with slight neurologic deficit and worsens in a day or two. In a completed stroke, neurologic deficits are maximal at onset.

Clinical presentation
Clinical features of CVA vary with the artery affected (and, consequently, the portion of the brain it supplies), the severity of damage, and the extent of collateral circulation that develops to help the brain compensate for decreased blood supply. If the CVA occurs in the left hemisphere, it produces symptoms on the right side; if it develops in the right hemisphere, symptoms are on the left side. However, a CVA that causes cranial nerve damage produces signs of cranial nerve dysfunction on the same side as the hemorrhage.

Symptoms are usually classified according to the artery affected:
■ middle cerebral artery—aphasia, dysphasia, visual field cuts, and hemiparesis

on affected side (more severe in the face and arm than in the leg)

- carotid artery — weakness, paralysis, numbness, sensory changes, and visual disturbances on affected side; altered level of consciousness; bruits; headaches; aphasia; and ptosis
- vertebrobasilar artery — weakness on affected side, numbness around lips and mouth, visual field cuts, diplopia, poor coordination, dysphagia, slurred speech, dizziness, amnesia, and ataxia
- anterior cerebral artery — confusion, weakness, and numbness (especially in the leg) on affected side; incontinence; loss of coordination; impaired motor and sensory functions; and personality changes
- posterior cerebral arteries — visual field cuts, sensory impairment, dyslexia, coma, and cortical blindness; typically, paralysis is absent.

Symptoms can also be classified as premonitory, generalized, and focal. Premonitory symptoms, such as drowsiness, dizziness, headache, and mental confusion, are rare. Generalized symptoms, such as headache, vomiting, mental impairment, seizures, coma, nuchal rigidity, fever, and disorientation, are typical. Focal symptoms, such as sensory and reflex changes, reflect the site of hemorrhage or infarct and may worsen.

Differential diagnoses

- Brain tumor
- Trauma
- Hyperglycemia, hypoglycemia
- Seizure
- Subdural hematoma
- Aneurysm

Diagnosis

Diagnosis of CVA is based on observation of clinical features, a history of risk factors, and the results of diagnostic tests:

- Computed tomography scanning shows evidence of hemorrhagic stroke immediately but may not show evidence of thrombotic infarction for 48 to 72 hours.
- Magnetic resonance imaging may help identify ischemic or infarcted areas and cerebral swelling.
- Brain scan shows ischemic areas but may not be positive for up to 2 weeks after the CVA.
- Lumbar puncture reveals bloody cerebrospinal fluid in hemorrhagic stroke.
- Ophthalmoscopy may show signs of hypertension and atherosclerotic changes in retinal arteries.
- Angiography outlines blood vessels and pinpoints occlusion or the rupture site.
- EEG helps to localize the damaged area.
- Carotid Doppler study should be done if a carotid bruit is present.

Other baseline laboratory studies include urinalysis, coagulation studies, complete blood count, serum osmolality, and electrolyte, glucose, triglyceride, creatinine, and blood urea nitrogen levels.

Management

General

During the acute phase, efforts focus on survival needs and prevention of further complications. Effective care emphasizes continuing neurologic assessment, support of respiration, continuous monitoring of vital signs, careful positioning to prevent aspiration and contractures, management of GI problems, and careful monitoring of fluid, electrolyte, and nutritional status. Patient care must also include measures to prevent complications such as infection.

Medication

These medications may be used in treating CVA:

- clopidogrel bisulfate — 75 mg/day P.O.; may be more effective than aspirin in preventing CVA and reducing risk of recurrence.
- tissue plasminogen activator (tPa) (follow protocol) — has been used successfully in clot dissolution when administered within 3 hours of the onset of symptoms.
- phenytoin — 300 to 600 mg/day P.O.
- phenobarbital — 60 to 200 mg/day P.O.
- docusate sodium — 50 to 500 mg/day P.O.
- dexamethasone — initially 10 mg I.V., then 4 to 6 mg I.V. infusion or I.M. every 4 to 6 hours then tapered over 5 to 7 days to decrease cerebral edema
- codeine — 15 to 60 mg P.O., S.C., I.V., or I.M. every 4 to 6 hours p.r.n.

Surgical intervention

Surgery performed to improve cerebral circulation for patients with thrombotic or embolic CVA includes endarterectomy (removal of atherosclerotic plaques from the inner arterial wall) and microvascular bypass (surgical anastomosis of an extracranial vessel to an intracranial vessel).

Referral

- Refer the patient immediately to a hospital if he's having symptoms of CVA.
- The patient may need a referral to a neurosurgeon or neurologist, depending on the type of CVA.
- Depending on the severity of the CVA, the patient may need referrals for physical, occupational, and speech therapy.
- A social worker should be consulted regarding care of the patient.
- Psychological counseling may be needed for the patient and family to cope with the illness.
- Refer the patient to local support groups such as the American Heart Association.

Follow-up

The patient should be seen frequently after discharge from the hospital. The frequency of visits will be related to the severity of the CVA. The patient may be seen 1 week after discharge, then every 2 to 3 weeks, then monthly, then every 3 months.

Patient teaching

- Explore the family's and patient's abilities to cope with this life-altering illness. Focus on what they want and can participate in, and support all their efforts. Enlist aid when appropriate.
- The patient may fail to recognize that he has a paralyzed side (called unilateral neglect) and must be taught to inspect that side of his body for injury and protect it from harm.
- If speech therapy is indicated, encourage the patient to begin as soon as possible and follow through with the speech pathologist's suggestions. Teach the family about aspiration pneumonia and how to prevent it.
- Teach the patient or his family about premonitory signs of a CVA, such as severe headache, drowsiness, confusion, and dizziness. Emphasize the importance of regular follow-up visits.
- If aspirin has been prescribed to minimize the risk of embolic stroke, tell the patient to watch for possible GI bleeding. Make sure the patient and family realize that acetaminophen isn't a substitute for aspirin.

Complications

- Depression
- Disability
- Death
- Muscle atrophy

Special considerations
• Provide psychological support. Set realistic short-term goals. Involve the patient's family in his care when possible, and explain his deficits and strengths.

To help prevent CVA:
• Stress the need to control diseases, such as diabetes and hypertension.
• Teach all patients (especially those at high risk) the importance of following a low-cholesterol, low-salt diet; watching their weight; increasing activity; avoiding smoking and prolonged bed rest; and minimizing stress.

• • • • • • • • • • • •

DOWN SYNDROME

The first disorder attributed to a chromosome aberration, Down syndrome (trisomy 21) characteristically produces mental retardation, dysmorphic facial features, and other distinctive physical abnormalities. It's commonly associated with congenital heart defects (in approximately 60% of patients) and other abnormalities.

Life expectancy for patients with Down syndrome has increased significantly because of improved treatment for related complications (heart defects, respiratory and other infections, acute leukemia). Nevertheless, up to 44% of such patients who have congenital heart defects die before age 1.

Causes
Down syndrome usually results from trisomy 21, a spontaneous chromosomal abnormality in which chromosome 21 has three copies instead of the normal two because of faulty meiosis (nondisjunction) of the ovum or, sometimes, the sperm. This results in a karyotype of 47 chromosomes instead of the normal 46.

In about 4% of patients, Down syndrome results from an unbalanced translocation in which the long arm of chromosome 21 breaks and attaches to another chromosome. The disorder may also be due to chromosomal mosaicism with two cell lines — one with a normal number of chromosomes (46) and one with 47 (an extra chromosome 21).

AGE ALERT Down syndrome occurs in 1 in 650 to 700 live births, but the incidence increases with advanced parental age, especially when the mother is age 34 or older at delivery or the father is older than age 42. At age 20, a woman has about 1 chance in 2,000 of having a child with Down syndrome; by age 49, she has 1 chance in 12. However, if a woman has had one child with Down syndrome, the risk of recurrence is 1% to 2% unless the trisomy results from translocation.

Clinical presentation
The physical signs of Down syndrome (especially hypotonia) as well as some dysmorphic facial features and heart defects may be apparent at birth. The degree of mental retardation may not become apparent until the infant grows older. People with Down syndrome typically have craniofacial anomalies, such as:
• slanting, almond-shaped eyes with epicanthic folds
• flat face
• protruding tongue
• small mouth and chin
• single transverse palmar crease (simian crease)
• small white spots (Brushfield's spots) on the iris
• strabismus
• small skull
• flat bridge across the nose
• slow dental development (with abnormal or absent teeth)

- small ears
- short neck
- cataracts.

Other physical effects may include dry, sensitive skin with decreased elasticity; umbilical hernia; short stature; short extremities, with broad, flat, and squarish hands and feet; clinodactyly (small little finger that curves inward); a wide space between the first and second toe; and abnormal fingerprints and footprints. Hypotonic limb muscles impair reflex development, posture, coordination, and balance.

Congenital heart disease (septal defects or pulmonary or aortic stenosis), duodenal atresia, megacolon, and pelvic bone abnormalities are common. The incidence of leukemia and thyroid disorders may be increased. Frequent upper respiratory infections can be a serious problem. Genitalia may be poorly developed and puberty delayed. Females may menstruate and be fertile. Males are infertile with low serum testosterone levels; many have undescended testicles.

Down syndrome patients may have an IQ between 30 and 70; however, social performance is usually beyond that expected for mental age. The level of intellectual function depends greatly on the environment and the amount of early stimulation received in addition to the IQ.

Differential diagnoses
- Hypotonia with minor familial anomalies (depressed nasal bridge)

Diagnosis
Physical findings at birth, especially hypotonia, may suggest this diagnosis, but no physical feature is diagnostic in itself.

A karyotype showing the specific chromosomal abnormality provides a definitive diagnosis. Amniocentesis allows prenatal diagnosis and is recommended for pregnant women over age 34, even if the family history is negative. Amniocentesis is also recommended for a pregnant woman of any age when either she or the father carries a translocated chromosome.

Management
General
Down syndrome has no known cure. Most patients with Down syndrome are now cared for at home and attend special education classes. As adults, some may work in a sheltered workshop or live in a group home facility.

Medication
Antibiotic therapy for recurrent infection may include:
- ampicillin—adults, 250 to 500 mg P.O. every 6 hours; children weighing less than 88 lb (40 kg), 25 to 100 mg/kg/day P.O. in four divided doses
- penicillin G potassium—adults, 1.6 to 3.2 million U P.O. in divided doses every 6 hours; children younger than age 12, 25,000 to 100,000 U/kg P.O. in divided doses every 6 hours.

Surgical intervention
Surgery may be done to correct heart defects and other related congenital abnormalities. Plastic surgery is occasionally done to correct the characteristic facial traits, especially the protruding tongue. Benefits beyond improved appearance may include improved speech, reduced susceptibility to dental caries, and fewer orthodontic problems later.

Referral
- Refer the parents and older siblings for genetic and psychological counseling, as appropriate, to help them evaluate future reproductive risks. Discuss options for prenatal testing.

■ Refer the parents to national or local Down syndrome organizations and support groups.

Follow-up

Initially, one to two visits are recommended for counseling and teaching. Then the patient should be seen for yearly checkups, or more often if illness occurs or cardiac status changes.

Patient teaching

■ Teach the parents the importance of a balanced diet for their child. Stress the need for patience while feeding the child, who may have difficulty sucking and may be less demanding and seem less eager to eat than normal babies.
■ Emphasize the importance of adequate exercise and maximal environmental stimulation; refer the parents for infant stimulation classes, which may begin in the early months of life.

Complications

■ Congenital heart disease
■ Bowel obstruction
■ Thyroid disease

Special considerations

■ Establish a trusting relationship with the parents, and encourage communication during the difficult period soon after diagnosis. Recognize signs of grieving.
■ Encourage the parents to hold and nurture their child.
■ Help the parents set realistic goals for their child. Explain that, although the child's mental development may seem normal at first, they shouldn't view this early development as a sign of future progress. By the time he's 1 year old, the child's development may begin to lag behind that of other children.

ENCEPHALITIS

Encephalitis is a severe inflammation of the brain, usually caused by a mosquito-borne or, in some areas, a tick-borne virus. However, transmission by means other than arthropod bites may occur through ingestion of infected goat's milk and accidental injection or inhalation of the virus. Eastern equine encephalitis may produce permanent neurologic damage and is commonly fatal.

In encephalitis, intense lymphocytic infiltration of brain tissues and the leptomeninges causes cerebral edema, degeneration of the brain's ganglion cells, and diffuse nerve cell destruction.

Causes

Encephalitis generally results from infection with arboviruses specific to rural areas. However, in urban areas, it's most commonly caused by enteroviruses (coxsackievirus, poliovirus, and echovirus). Other causes include herpesvirus, mumps virus, human immunodeficiency virus, adenoviruses, and demyelinating diseases after measles, varicella, rubella, or vaccination.

Between World War I and the Depression, a type of encephalitis known as lethargic encephalitis, von Economo's disease, or sleeping sickness occurred with some regularity. The causative virus was never clearly identified, and the disease is rare today. Even so, the term sleeping sickness persists and is commonly mistakenly used to describe other types of encephalitis.

Clinical presentation

All viral forms of encephalitis have similar clinical features, although certain differences do occur. Usually, the acute illness begins with:
■ sudden onset of fever

- headache
- vomiting.

It progresses to include additional signs and symptoms, such as:
- meningeal irritation (stiff neck and back)
- neuronal damage (drowsiness, coma, paralysis, seizures, ataxia, tremors, nausea, vomiting, and organic psychoses).

After the acute phase of the illness, coma may persist for days or weeks.

The severity of arbovirus encephalitis may range from subclinical to rapidly fatal necrotizing disease. Herpes encephalitis also produces signs and symptoms that vary from subclinical to acute and commonly fatal fulminating disease. Associated effects include disturbances of taste or smell.

Differential diagnoses
- Bacterial infection
- Trauma
- Intracranial hemorrhage
- Thromboembolism
- Rocky Mountain spotted fever
- Syphilis
- Hypoglycemia

Diagnosis
During an encephalitis epidemic, diagnosis is readily made on clinical findings and patient history. However, sporadic cases are difficult to distinguish from other febrile illnesses, such as gastroenteritis or meningitis. When possible, identification of the virus in cerebrospinal fluid (CSF) or blood confirms the diagnosis. The common viruses that also cause herpes, measles, and mumps are easier to identify than arboviruses. Arboviruses and herpes viruses can be isolated by inoculating young mice with a specimen taken from the patient. In herpes encephalitis, serologic studies may show rising titers of complement-fixing antibodies.

In all forms of encephalitis, CSF pressure is elevated and, despite inflammation, the fluid is commonly clear. White blood cell and protein levels in the CSF are slightly elevated, but the glucose level remains normal. An EEG reveals abnormalities. Occasionally, a computed tomography scan may be ordered to rule out cerebral hematoma.

Management
The antiviral agent acyclovir is effective only against herpes encephalitis. Treatment of all other forms of encephalitis is entirely supportive, such as adequate fluid and electrolyte intake to prevent dehydration and antibiotics for an associated infection such as pneumonia. Isolation is unnecessary.

Medication
For herpes virus infections, give acyclovir (adults, 5 mg/kg I.V. infusion over 1 hour every 8 hours for 7 to 14 days; children younger than age 12, 250 mg/m^2 I.V. infusion over 1 hour every 8 hours for 7 days).

For seizures, give phenytoin (adults, 300 to 600 mg/day P.O.; children, 5 mg/kg/day P.O. divided in two to three doses; maximum 300 mg/day).

To reduce cerebral inflammation and edema, give:
- dexamethasone — 10 mg I.V. initially, then 4 to 6 mg every 6 hours until symptoms subside; then taper off
- furosemide — 20 to 40 mg/day I.V. or P.O.
- mannitol — 1.5 to 2 g/kg as a 15% to 20% I.V. solution over 30 to 60 minutes.

To relieve headache and reduce fever, give:
- aspirin — 325 to 650 mg P.O. every 4 hours p.r.n.
- acetaminophen — 325 to 650 mg P.O. every 4 hours p.r.n.

Sedatives are given for restlessness.

Referral
- If a neurologic deficit is severe and appears permanent, refer the patient to a rehabilitation program as soon as the acute phase has passed.
- If intracranial pressure monitoring is needed, refer to a neurosurgeon.

Follow-up
The patient should be seen as needed after discharge depending on the severity of the illness.

Patient teaching
- Reassure the patient and his family that behavior changes caused by encephalitis usually disappear.

Complications
- Diminished neurologic function
- Seizures
- Death

Special considerations
- Because the course of this disorder can be fast and fatal, provide information to the family regarding expected and potential outcomes.

• • • • • • • • • • • •

EPILEPSY

Epilepsy, also called seizure disorder, is a condition of the brain marked by a susceptibility to recurrent seizures — paroxysmal events associated with abnormal electrical discharges of neurons in the brain. Epilepsy affects 1% to 2% of the population. However, 80% of patients have good seizure control if they strictly adhere to the prescribed treatment regimen.

Causes
In about half of epilepsy cases, the cause is unknown. However, possible causes of epilepsy include:

- birth trauma (inadequate oxygen supply to the brain, blood incompatibility, or hemorrhage)
- perinatal infection
- anoxia (after respiratory or cardiac arrest)
- infectious diseases (meningitis, encephalitis, or brain abscess)
- ingestion of toxins (mercury, lead, or carbon monoxide)
- tumors of the brain
- inherited disorders or degenerative disease, such as phenylketonuria or tuberous sclerosis
- head injury or trauma
- metabolic disorders, such as hypoglycemia or hypoparathyroidism
- cerebrovascular accident (hemorrhage, thrombosis, or embolism).

Alcohol and drug withdrawal (especially Demerol) can cause nonepileptic seizures.

Clinical presentation
The hallmarks of epilepsy are recurring seizures, which can be classified as partial or generalized (some patients may be affected by more than one type):

- Partial seizures arise from a localized area of the brain, causing specific symptoms. In some patients, partial seizure activity may spread to the entire brain, causing a generalized seizure. Partial seizures include simple partial (jacksonian) and complex partial (psychomotor or temporal lobe) seizures.
- Simple partial motor-type seizures begin as localized motor seizures characterized by a spread of abnormal activity to adjacent areas of the brain. They typically produce a stiffening or jerking in one extremity, accompanied by a tingling sensation in the same area. For example, they may start in the thumb and spread to the entire hand and arm. The patient seldom loses consciousness, although the

seizure may progress to a generalized seizure.

- Simple partial sensory-type seizures involve perceptual distortion, which can include hallucinations.
- Complex partial seizure symptoms vary but usually include purposeless behavior. The patient experiences an aura immediately before the seizure. An aura represents the beginning of abnormal electrical discharges within a focal area of the brain and may include a pungent smell, GI distress (nausea or indigestion), a rising or sinking feeling in the stomach, a dreamy feeling, an unusual taste, or a visual disturbance. Overt signs of a complex partial seizure include a glassy stare, picking at one's clothes, aimless wandering, lip-smacking or chewing motions, and unintelligible speech; these signs may last for just a few seconds or for as long as 20 minutes. Mental confusion may last several minutes after the seizure; as a result, an observer may mistakenly suspect intoxication with alcohol or drugs or psychosis.
- Generalized seizures, as the term suggests, cause a generalized electrical abnormality within the brain and include several distinct types:
- Absence (petit mal) seizures occur most commonly in children, although they may affect adults as well. They usually begin with a brief change in level of consciousness, indicated by blinking or rolling of the eyes, a blank stare, and slight mouth movements. There is little or no tonic-clonic movement. The patient retains his posture and continues preseizure activity without difficulty. Typically, each seizure lasts from 1 to 10 seconds. If not properly treated, seizures can recur as often as 100 times per day. An absence seizure may progress to generalized tonic-clonic seizures.
- Myoclonic seizures are characterized by brief, involuntary muscular jerks of the body or extremities, which may occur in a rhythmic fashion and may precede generalized tonic-clonic seizures by months or years.
- Generalized tonic-clonic (grand mal) seizures typically begin with a loud cry, precipitated by air rushing from the lungs through the vocal cords. The patient then falls to the ground, losing consciousness. The body stiffens (tonic phase) and then alternates between episodes of muscular spasm and relaxation (clonic phase). Tongue-biting, incontinence, labored breathing, apnea, and subsequent cyanosis may also occur. The seizure stops in 2 to 5 minutes, when abnormal electrical conduction of the neurons is completed. The patient then regains consciousness but is somewhat confused and may have difficulty talking. If he can talk, he may complain of drowsiness, fatigue, headache, muscle soreness, and arm or leg weakness. He may fall into deep sleep after the seizure. These seizures may start as facial seizures and spread to become generalized.
- Akinetic seizures are characterized by a general loss of postural tone (the patient falls in a flaccid state) and a temporary loss of consciousness. They occur in young children and are sometimes called a "drop attack" because it causes the child to fall.

Status epilepticus is a continuous seizure state that can occur in all seizure types. The most life-threatening example is generalized tonic-clonic status epilepticus, a continuous generalized tonic-clonic seizure without intervening return of consciousness. Status epilepticus is accompanied by respiratory distress. It can result from abrupt withdrawal of anticonvulsant medication, hypoxic encephalopathy, acute head trauma, metabolic encephalopathy, or septicemia secondary to encephalitis or meningitis.

Differential diagnoses

Infancy
- Birth injury
- Acute infection

Childhood
- Febrile seizure
- Acute infection
- Trauma

Adolescent
- Trauma
- Drug and alcohol related
- Arteriovenous malformation

Adult
- Trauma
- Drug and alcohol related
- Tumor
- Idiopathic

Diagnosis

Clinically, the diagnosis of epilepsy is based on the occurrence of one or more seizures and proof or the assumption that the condition that led to them is still present.

Diagnostic information is obtained from the patient's history and description of seizure activity and from family history, physical and neurologic examinations, and computed tomography scanning or magnetic resonance imaging. These scans offer density readings of the brain and may indicate abnormalities in internal structures. Paroxysmal abnormalities on the EEG confirm the diagnosis by providing evidence of the continuing tendency to have seizures. A negative EEG doesn't rule out epilepsy because the paroxysmal abnormalities occur intermittently. Other tests may include serum glucose and calcium studies, skull X-rays, lumbar puncture, brain scan, and cerebral angiography.

Management

General

The primary goals of the health care professional and family members caring for a patient having a seizure are protection from injury, protection from aspiration, and observation of the seizure activity. Generalized tonic-clonic seizures may necessitate first aid.

Medication

Antiseizure medications specific to the type of seizure include:
- phenytoin — adults, 100 mg P.O. t.i.d; children, 5 mg/kg/day P.O.
- carbamazepine — children ages 6 to 12, 200 to 800 mg/day P.O.; adults and children older than age 12, 400 to 1,200 mg/day
- phenobarbital — adults, 60 to 200 mg/day; children, 3 to 6 mg/kg/day P.O.
- primidone — adults and children older than age 8, 100 to 125 mg P.O. h.s. initially with increasing doses until maintenance of 1 g/day, if needed; children younger than age 8, 50 mg P.O. h.s. initially with increasing doses until maintenance of 10 to 25 mg/kg/day; administered individually for generalized tonic-clonic seizures and complex partial seizures.

The following medications are given for absence seizures:
- valproic acid — 15 to 60 mg/kg/day P.O.
- clonazepam — adults, 1.5 to 20 mg/day P.O. in divided doses; children weighing less than 66 lb (30 kg), 0.01 to 0.03 mg/kg/day p.r.n. in divided doses
- ethosuximide — 20 mg/kg/day.

These medications are given for emergency treatment:
- diazepam — adults, 5 to 10 mg I.V. or I.M. repeated every 10 to 15 minutes to maximum dose of 30 mg; children age 5 and older, 1 mg I.V. every 2 to 5 minutes up to maximum of 10 mg; children

younger than age 5, 0.2 to 0.5 mg I.V. slowly every 2 to 5 minutes up to maximum of 5 mg

- lorazepam — 0.05 to 0.1 mg/kg I.V.
- dextrose 50% I.V. — when seizures are secondary to hypoglycemia
- thiamine — 100 mg I.V. in chronic alcoholism or withdrawal.

If the patient is already taking an anticonvulsant, serum levels should be checked and medication administered according to results. A patient taking anticonvulsant medication requires monitoring for toxic signs, such as nystagmus, ataxia, lethargy, dizziness, drowsiness, slurred speech, irritability, nausea, and vomiting.

Surgical intervention
If drug therapy fails, treatment may include surgical removal of a demonstrated focal lesion to attempt to stop seizures. Also, correction of an underlying disorder (such as a brain tumor) may help to stop seizures.

Referral
- Refer the patient to a neurologist if he experiences seizures.
- Psychological counseling may be needed to cope with the diagnosis of a seizure disorder.
- Refer the patient to the Epilepsy Foundation of America for general information and support
- Refer the patient to the state motor vehicle department for information about a driver's license.

Follow-up
The patient should have regular monitoring of anticonvulsant medication levels, initially every 2 weeks, then monthly based on therapeutic levels attained. The patient should also be monitored for adverse reactions.

Patient teaching
- Because drug therapy is the treatment of choice for most people with epilepsy, information about medication is invaluable.
- Stress the need for compliance with the prescribed drug schedule. Reinforce dosage instructions and stress the importance of taking medication regularly, at scheduled times. Caution the patient to monitor the quantity of medication he has so he doesn't run out of it.
- Teach the patient about possible adverse effects — drowsiness, lethargy, hyperactivity, confusion, and visual and sleep disturbances — all of which indicate the need for dosage adjustment. Phenytoin therapy may lead to hyperplasia of the gums, which may be relieved by conscientious oral hygiene. Instruct the patient to immediately report adverse reactions.
- Emphasize the importance of having anticonvulsant blood levels checked at regular intervals, even if the seizures are under control.
- Warn the patient against drinking alcoholic beverages.

Complications
- Injury
- Drug toxicity
- Status epilepticus

Special considerations
- One key to support is a true understanding of the nature of epilepsy and the misconceptions that surround it. Encourage the patient and family to express their feelings about the patient's condition. Answer their questions, and help them cope by dispelling some of the myths about epilepsy, such as the myth that epilepsy is contagious. Assure them that epilepsy is controllable for most patients who follow a prescribed regimen of

medication and that most patients maintain a normal lifestyle.

- A patient may potentially be weaned off medication if he's seizure-free for 2 years and has a normal EEG and a normal neurologic examination.

• • • • • • • • • • • •
GUILLAIN-BARRÉ SYNDROME

Guillain-Barré syndrome is an acute, rapidly progressive, and potentially fatal form of polyneuritis that causes muscle weakness and mild distal sensory loss. This syndrome affects both sexes equally. Recovery is spontaneous and complete in about 95% of patients, although mild motor or reflex deficits in the feet and legs may persist. The prognosis is best when symptoms clear between 15 and 20 days after onset.

AGE ALERT Also called infectious polyneuritis, Landry-Guillain-Barré syndrome, and acute idiopathic polyneuritis, this syndrome can occur at any age but is most common between ages 30 and 50.

Causes
The precise cause of Guillain-Barré syndrome is unknown, but it may be a cell-mediated immunologic attack on peripheral nerves in response to a virus. The major pathologic effect is segmental demyelination of the peripheral nerves. Because this syndrome causes inflammation and degenerative changes in both the posterior (sensory) and anterior (motor) nerve roots, signs of sensory and motor losses occur simultaneously.

Clinical presentation
About 50% of patients with Guillain-Barré syndrome have a history of minor febrile illness (10 to 14 days before onset), usually an upper respiratory tract infection or, less commonly, gastroenteritis. When infection precedes the onset of Guillain-Barré syndrome, signs of infection subside before neurologic features appear. Other possible precipitating factors include surgery, rabies or swine influenza vaccination, viral illness, Hodgkin's or other malignant disease, and lupus erythematosus.

Symmetrical muscle weakness, the major neurologic sign, usually appears in the legs first (ascending type) and then extends to the arms and facial nerves in 24 to 72 hours. Sometimes, muscle weakness develops in the arms first (descending type) or in the arms and legs simultaneously. (See *Testing for thoracic sensation*.) In milder forms of this disease, muscle weakness may affect only the cranial nerves or may not occur at all.

Another common neurologic sign is paresthesia, which sometimes precedes muscle weakness but tends to vanish quickly. However, some patients with this disorder never develop this symptom. Other clinical features may include:
- facial diplegia (possibly with ophthalmoplegia)
- dysphagia or dysarthria
- weakness of the muscles supplied by cranial nerve XI.

Muscle weakness develops so quickly that muscle atrophy doesn't occur, but hypotonia and areflexia do. Stiffness and pain in the form of a severe "charley horse" commonly occur.

The clinical course of Guillain-Barré syndrome is divided into three phases. The initial phase begins when the first definitive symptom appears and ends 1 to 3 weeks later, when no further deterioration manifests. The plateau phase lasts several days to 2 weeks and is followed by the recovery phase, which is believed to coincide with remyelination and axonal process regrowth. The recovery phase extends over 4 to 6 months; patients with severe disease may take up to 2 years to recover, and recovery may not be complete.

Differential diagnoses
- Myasthenia gravis
- Multiple sclerosis
- Cerebrovascular accident
- Spinal cord syndromes

Diagnosis
A history of preceding febrile illness (usually a respiratory tract infection) and typical clinical features suggest Guillain-Barré syndrome.

Several days after onset of signs and symptoms, cerebrospinal fluid (CSF) protein levels begin to rise, peaking in 4 to 6 weeks, probably due to widespread inflammatory disease of the nerve roots. CSF white blood cell count remains normal but, in severe disease, CSF pressure may rise above normal. Probably because of predisposing infection, a complete blood count shows leukocytosis and a shift to immature forms early in the illness, but blood studies soon return to normal. Electromyography may show repeated firing of the same motor unit instead of widespread sectional stimulation. Nerve conduction velocities are slowed soon after paralysis develops. Diagnosis must rule out similar diseases such as acute poliomyelitis.

Management
General
There's no cure for Guillain-Barré syndrome. Treatment is primarily supportive, consisting of endotracheal intubation or tracheotomy if the patient has difficulty clearing secretions as well as preventing complications and reducing disability. Plasmapheresis is commonly used during the initial phase but offers no benefit if begun 2 weeks after onset.

Testing for thoracic sensation

When Guillain-Barré syndrome progresses rapidly, test for ascending sensory loss by touching the patient or pressing his skin lightly with a pin every hour. Move systematically from the iliac crest (T12) to the scapula (T6), occasionally substituting the blunt end of the pin to test the patient's ability to discriminate between sharp and dull.

Mark the level of diminished sensation to measure any change. If diminished sensation ascends to T8 or higher, the patient's intercostal muscle function (and consequently respiratory function) will probably be impaired. As Guillain-Barré syndrome subsides, sensory and motor weakness descends to the lower thoracic segments, heralding a return of intercostal and extremity muscle function.

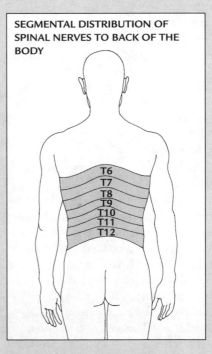

SEGMENTAL DISTRIBUTION OF SPINAL NERVES TO BACK OF THE BODY

T6
T7
T8
T9
T10
T11
T12

KEY: **T**= thoracic segments

Medication

To lessen the progression of the disease, give prednisone (5 to 60 mg/day P.O.); dosage is highly individualized. If prednisone produces no noticeable improvement after 7 days, discontinue the drug.

To lessen the immune system attack on the nerves, give immune globulin (IGIV) therapy (0.4 gm/kg/day I.V. over 5 days).

Referral

■ Refer the patient to a hospital at initial onset or if respiratory difficulty occurs. A pulmonologist may be needed to manage respiratory care.
■ The patient will need physical therapy and rehabilitation.
■ If Guillain-Barré syndrome is mild, then home health care is recommended for careful, frequent monitoring. If the patient is recovering from Guillain-Barré syndrome, then home care will be needed during the recovery phase.
■ Refer the patient and family for psychological counseling or local support if they're having difficulty coping with the illness. The Guillain-Barré Syndrome Foundation International provides education and support for patients and their families.

Patient teaching

■ Teach the family to perform passive range-of-motion exercises within the patient's pain limits. (Although this disease doesn't produce pain, exercising little-used muscles will.) Remember that the proximal muscle group of the thighs, shoulders, and trunk will be the most tender and will cause the most pain with passive movement and turning. When the patient's condition stabilizes, change to gentle stretching and active assistance exercises.
■ Teach the family to prevent aspiration, test the gag reflex, and elevate the head of the bed before giving the patient anything to eat. If the gag reflex is absent, give nasogastric feedings until this reflex returns.
■ Tell the family to inspect the patient's legs regularly for signs of thrombophlebitis (localized pain, tenderness, erythema, edema, and positive Homans' sign), a common complication of Guillain-Barré syndrome. To prevent thrombophlebitis, have them apply antiembolism stockings and give prophylactic anticoagulants, as they are prescribed.
■ Tell the family to watch for urine retention. Tell them to encourage adequate fluid intake of 2 qt [2 L]/day, unless contraindicated. Because the abdominal muscles are weak, the patient may need manual pressure on the bladder (Credé's method) before he can urinate. If the patient can't urinate at all, tell the family to contact the nurse practitioner.
■ To prevent and relieve constipation, have the family offer prune juice and a high-bulk diet. If necessary, alternate-day or daily suppositories (glycerin or bisacodyl) or enemas should be given.

Complications

■ Respiratory failure
■ Paralysis
■ Aspiration
■ Cardiac arrhythmias
■ Ileus
■ Injury
■ Depression
■ Sepsis
■ Joint contractures
■ Deep vein thrombosis

Special considerations

■ Monitoring the patient for escalation of symptoms is of special concern. Watch for ascending sensory loss, which precedes motor loss.

••••••••••••

HEADACHE

The most common patient complaint, headache usually occurs as a symptom of an underlying disorder. Ninety percent of all headaches are known as primary headache syndromes and aren't related to structural or organic problems. Ten percent of headaches are due to underlying intracranial, systemic, or psychological disorders. Migraine headaches, probably the most intensively studied, are throbbing, vascular headaches that usually begin to appear in childhood or adolescence and recur throughout adulthood. Affecting up to 10% of Americans, they're more common in females and have a strong familial incidence.

Causes

Most chronic headaches result from tension (muscle contraction), which may be caused by emotional stress, fatigue, menstruation, or environmental stimuli (noise, crowds, or bright lights). Other possible causes include glaucoma; inflammation of the eyes or mucosa of the nasal or paranasal sinuses; diseases of the scalp, teeth, extracranial arteries, or external or middle ear; muscle spasms of the face, neck, or shoulders; and cervical arthritis. In addition, headaches may be caused by vasodilators (nitrates, alcohol, and histamine), systemic disease, hypoxia, hypertension, head trauma and tumor, intracranial bleeding, abscess, or aneurysm.

The cause of migraine headache is unknown, but it's associated with constriction and dilation of intracranial and extracranial arteries. Certain biochemical abnormalities are thought to occur during a migraine attack. These include local leakage of a vasodilator polypeptide called neurokinin through the dilated arteries and a decrease in the plasma level of serotonin.

Headache pain may emanate from the pain-sensitive structures of the skin, scalp, muscles, arteries, and veins; cranial nerves V, VII, IX, and X; or cervical nerves 1, 2, and 3. Intracranial mechanisms of headaches include traction or displacement of arteries, venous sinuses, or venous tributaries and inflammation or direct pressure on the cranial nerves with afferent pain fibers.

Clinical presentation

Initially, migraine headaches usually produce unilateral, pulsating pain, which later becomes more generalized. (See *Clinical features of migraine headaches,* page 250.) They're commonly preceded by:
- scintillating scotoma
- hemianopsia
- unilateral paresthesia
- speech disorders.

The patient may experience:
- irritability
- anorexia
- nausea
- vomiting
- photophobia
- odor sensitivity
- chills
- diaphoresis
- diarrhea.

Muscle contraction and traction-inflammatory vascular headaches produce a dull, persistent ache, tender spots on the head and neck, and a feeling of tightness around the head, with a characteristic "hatband" distribution. The pain is commonly severe and unrelenting. If caused by intracranial bleeding, these headaches may result in such neurologic deficits as paresthesia and muscle weakness; narcotics may fail to relieve pain in these cases. If caused by a tumor, pain is most severe when the patient awakens.

Clinical features of migraine headaches

TYPE	SIGNS AND SYMPTOMS
Common migraine (most prevalent) Usually occurs on weekends and holidays	■ Prodromal symptoms (fatigue, nausea, vomiting, and fluid imbalance) preceding headache by about 1 day ■ Sensitivity to light and noise (most prominent feature) ■ Headache pain (unilateral or bilateral, aching or throbbing)
Classic migraine Usually occurs in compulsive personalities and within families	■ Prodromal symptoms, including visual disturbances, such as zigzag lines and bright lights (most common), sensory disturbances (tingling of face, lips, and hands), or motor disturbances (staggering gait) ■ Recurrent and periodic headaches
Hemiplegic and ophthalmoplegic migraine (rare) Usually occurs in young adults	■ Severe, unilateral pain ■ Extraocular muscle palsies (involving third cranial nerve) and ptosis ■ With repeated headaches, possible permanent third cranial nerve injury ■ In hemiplegic migraine, neurologic deficits (hemiparesis, hemiplegia) possibly persisting after headache subsides
Basilar artery migraine Occurs in young women before their menstrual periods	■ Prodromal symptoms, usually including partial vision loss followed by vertigo; ataxia; dysarthria; tinnitus; and, sometimes, tingling of fingers and toes, lasting from several minutes to almost 1 hour ■ Headache pain, severe occipital throbbing, vomiting

Differential diagnoses

■ Meningitis
■ Brain tumor
■ Sleep apnea
■ Fever
■ Hemorrhage
■ Aneurysm

Diagnosis

Diagnosis requires a history of recurrent headaches and physical examination of the head and neck. Such examination includes percussion, auscultation for bruits, inspection for signs of infection, and palpation for defects, crepitus, or tender spots (especially after trauma). Firm diagnosis also requires a complete neurologic examination, assessment for other systemic diseases such as hypertension, and a psychosocial evaluation when such factors are suspected.

Diagnostic tests include cervical spine and sinus X-rays, EEG, computed tomography scanning—performed before lumbar puncture to rule out increased intracranial pressure (ICP)—or magnetic resonance imaging. A lumbar puncture isn't done if there's evidence of increased ICP or if a brain tumor is suspected because rapidly reducing pressure by removing spinal fluid can cause brain herniation.

Management
General
Measures include identification and elimination of causative factors and, possibly, psychotherapy for headaches caused by emotional stress. Headaches seldom require hospitalization unless caused by a serious disorder. In that case, care is directed to the underlying problem.

Medication
Analgesics may provide symptomatic relief; examples include:
■ aspirin — 325 to 650 mg P.O. every 4 to 6 hours p.r.n.
■ codeine — 15 to 60 mg P.O. every 4 to 6 hours p.r.n.

Muscle relaxants, such as cyclobenzaprine (10 mg P.O. t.i.d.), may be used for chronic tension headaches.

An effective treatment for migraine headaches alone or with caffeine may include:
■ ergotamine — initially, 2 mg P.O. or S.L., then 1 to 2 mg P.O. every 30 minutes to a maximum of 6 mg in 24 hours; for cluster headaches, 1 to 2 mg P.O. h.s. for 10 to 14 days. (Remember that this medication can't be taken by pregnant women because it stimulates uterine contractions.)
■ sumatriptan — 25 to 100 mg P.O. with a second dose of up to 100 mg in 2 hours.

Medications that can help prevent migraine headaches include:
■ propranolol — initially 80 mg/day P.O. in divided doses; maintenance dose of 160 to 240 mg/day, in divided doses, t.i.d. or q.i.d.
■ clonidine — 0.05 to 0.15 mg/day P.O. in divided doses

■ amitriptyline — 50 to 100 mg/day.

To prevent nausea and vomiting, give metoclopramide (10 mg P.O. up to q.i.d.); it works best when taken early in the course of an attack.

Referral
■ Refer the patient to a doctor if treatment is unsuccessful.
■ The patient may need to be referred for psychological counseling if the headaches are caused by stress.

Follow-up
Initially, the patient should be seen frequently (every 2 weeks) to monitor medication control. After headaches are controlled, the patient should be seen every 3 to 4 months.

Patient teaching
■ Instruct the patient to take the prescribed medication at the onset of migraine symptoms, to prevent dehydration by drinking plenty of fluids after nausea and vomiting subside, and to use other headache relief measures.
■ When a headache occurs, advise the patient to lie down in a dark, quiet room (if possible) and to place ice packs on his forehead or a cold cloth over his eyes.

Complications
■ Misdiagnosis
■ Status migraines
■ Drug dependency
■ Disruption of lifestyle

Special considerations
■ Obtain a complete patient history: duration and location of the headache; time of day it usually begins; nature of the pain; concurrence with other symptoms such as blurred vision; precipitating factors, such as tension, menstruation, loud noises, menopause, or alcohol use; med-

ication taken, such as oral contraceptives; or prolonged fasting. Exacerbating factors can also be assessed through ongoing observation of the patient's personality, habits, activities of daily living, family relationships, coping mechanisms, and relaxation activities. Using the history as a guide, help the patient avoid exacerbating factors.

■ If possible, avoid repeated use of narcotics.

• • • • • • • • • • • •

HUNTINGTON'S DISEASE

Also called Huntington's chorea, hereditary chorea, chronic progressive chorea, or adult chorea, Huntington's disease is a hereditary disease in which degeneration in the cerebral cortex and basal ganglia causes chronic progressive chorea and mental deterioration, ending in dementia.

AGE ALERT Huntington's disease usually strikes people between ages 25 and 55 (the average age is 35); however, 2% of cases occur in children, and 5% of cases occur as late as age 60. Death from suicide, heart failure, or pneumonia usually results 10 to 15 years after onset. Genetic testing is now available for people with a family history of the disease.

Causes
Huntington's disease is transmitted as an autosomal dominant trait; either sex can transmit and inherit it. Each child of a parent with this disease has a 50% chance of inheriting it, but a child who doesn't inherit Huntington's disease can't pass it on to his own children. Because of its hereditary transmission, Huntington's disease is prevalent in areas where affected families have lived for several generations.

Clinical presentation
Onset is insidious. The patient eventually becomes totally dependent — emotionally and physically — through the loss of musculoskeletal control, and he develops progressively severe choreic movements. Such movements are rapid, commonly violent, and purposeless. Initially, they're unilateral and more prominent in the face and arms than in the legs, progressing from mild fidgeting to grimacing, tongue smacking, dysarthria (indistinct speech), athetoid movements (especially of the hands) related to emotional state, and torticollis.

Ultimately, the patient with Huntington's disease develops progressive dementia, although the dementia doesn't always progress at the same rate as the chorea. Dementia can be mild at first, but eventually it causes severe disruption of the patient's personality. Personality changes include:
■ obstinacy
■ carelessness
■ untidiness
■ moodiness
■ apathy
■ inappropriate behavior
■ loss of memory and concentration
■ paranoia.

Differential diagnoses
■ Movement disorders, including Wilson's disease, systemic lupus erythematosus, encephalitis, drug-induced, hyperthyroidism, and Parkinson's disease
■ Dementia
■ Emotional disorder
■ Alcoholism

Diagnosis
Huntington's disease can be detected by positron emission tomography and deoxyribonucleic acid analysis. Diagnosis is based on a characteristic clinical history:

progressive chorea and dementia, onset in early middle age (35 to 40), and confirmation of a genetic link. Computed tomography scanning and magnetic resonance imaging demonstrate brain atrophy. Molecular genetics may detect the gene for Huntington's disease in people at risk while they're still asymptomatic.

Management
General
Because Huntington's disease has no known cure, treatment is supportive, protective, and symptomatic. Institutionalization is commonly necessary because of mental deterioration, which can't be halted or managed by drugs.

Medication
Tranquilizers as well as one of the following agents help control choreic movements and alleviate discomfort and depression, making the patient easier to manage:
- chlorpromazine — 30 to 75 mg/day P.O. in divided doses
- haloperidol — 0.5 to 5 mg P.O. b.i.d. to t.i.d.
- imipramine — 75 to 100 mg/day P.O. in divided doses.

However, tranquilizers increase patient rigidity. To control choreic movements without rigidity, prescribe choline (1.5 to 3.5 g/day P.O.).

Referral
- Refer the patient and family to a genetic counselor.
- Psychological counseling or a local support group may be needed to cope with the illness.
- Refer the patient and family to the Huntington's Disease Association for education and support.

Follow-up
The patient should be monitored for personality changes and treatment ordered accordingly.

Patient teaching
- Teach the family to participate in the patient's care. Teach them about the disease, and listen to their concerns and special problems. Keep in mind the patient's dysarthria, and allow him extra time to express himself, thereby decreasing frustration.

CLINICAL CAUTION Instruct the family to stay alert for possible suicide attempts. Tell them to control the patient's environment to protect him from suicide or other self-inflicted injury.

Complications
- Personality changes
- Subdural hematoma
- Dementia
- Choking
- Death

• • • • • • • • • • •
MENINGITIS

In meningitis, the brain and the spinal cord meninges become inflamed, usually as a result of a viral or, less commonly, a bacterial infection. Such inflammation may involve all three meningeal membranes — the dura mater, the arachnoid, and the pia mater. The prognosis is good and complications are rare if the disease is recognized early and the infecting organism responds to antibiotics; however, mortality in untreated meningitis is 70% to 100%. The prognosis is worse for infants and elderly patients, particularly if antibiotic therapy isn't started within hours of the onset of symptoms.

Aseptic meningitis

Aseptic meningitis is a benign syndrome characterized by headache, fever, vomiting, and meningeal symptoms. It results from some form of viral infection, including enteroviruses (most common), arboviruses, herpes simplex virus, mumps virus, or lymphocytic choriomeningitis virus.

Aseptic meningitis begins suddenly with a fever up to 104° F (40° C), alterations in consciousness (drowsiness, confusion, stupor), and neck or spine stiffness, which is slight at first. (The patient experiences such stiffness when bending forward.) Other signs and symptoms include headaches, nausea, vomiting, abdominal pain, poorly defined chest pain, and sore throat.

Patient history of recent illness and knowledge of seasonal epidemics are essential in differentiating among the many forms of aseptic meningitis. Negative bacteriologic cultures, cerebrospinal fluid (CSF) analysis showing pleocytosis, and increased protein levels suggest the diagnosis. Isolation of the virus from CSF confirms it.

Treatment is supportive, including bed rest, maintenance of fluid and electrolyte balance, analgesics for pain, and exercises to combat residual weakness. Isolation isn't necessary. Careful handling of excretions and good hand-washing technique prevent the spread of the disease.

Causes

Meningitis is almost always a complication of another bacterial infection — bacteremia (especially from pneumonia, empyema, osteomyelitis, or endocarditis), sinusitis, otitis media, encephalitis, myelitis, or brain abscess — usually caused by *Neisseria meningitidis*, *Haemophilus influenzae* (in children and young adults), or *Streptococcus pneumoniae* (in adults). Meningitis may also follow a skull fracture, penetrating head wound, lumbar puncture, or ventricular shunting procedures. Aseptic meningitis may result from a virus or other organism. (See *Aseptic meningitis*.) Sometimes, no causative organism can be found. Meningitis commonly begins as an inflammation of the pia-arachnoid, which may progress to congestion of adjacent tissues and destruction of some nerve cells.

Clinical presentation

The cardinal signs of meningitis include:
- infection (fever, chills, and malaise)
- increased intracranial pressure (ICP) (headache, vomiting and, rarely, papilledema).

Signs of meningeal irritation include:
- nuchal rigidity
- positive Brudzinski's and Kernig's signs
- exaggerated and symmetrical deep tendon reflexes
- opisthotonos (spasm in which the back and extremities arch backward so that the body rests on the head and heels).

Other manifestations of meningitis are irritability; sinus arrhythmias; photophobia, diplopia, and other visual problems; and delirium, deep stupor, and coma. (See *Two signs of meningitis*.)

An infant may not show clinical signs of infection but may be fretful and refuse to eat. Such an infant may vomit a great deal, leading to dehydration; this prevents a bulging fontanel and thus masks this important sign of increased ICP. As the illness progresses, twitching, seizures (in 30% of infants), or coma may develop. Most older children have the same symptoms as adults. In subacute meningitis, the onset may be insidious.

Two signs of meningitis

BRUDZINSKI'S SIGN
Place the patient in a dorsal recumbent position, put your hands behind her neck, and bend it forward. Pain and resistance may indicate meningeal inflammation, neck injury, or arthritis. If the patient also flexes the hips and knees in response to this manipulation, chances are she has meningitis.

KERNIG'S SIGN
Place the patient in a supine position. Flex her leg at the hip and knee and then straighten the knee. Pain or resistance points to meningitis.

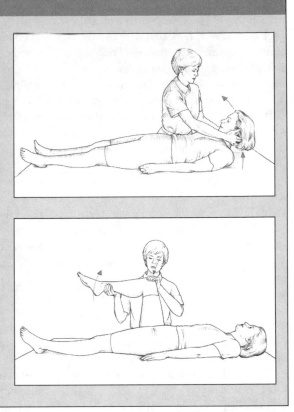

Differential diagnoses
- Sepsis
- Seizures
- Bacteremia

Diagnosis
A lumbar puncture showing typical cerebrospinal fluid (CSF) findings, when accompanied by positive Brudzinski's and Kernig's signs, usually establishes a diagnosis. The following tests can uncover the primary sites of infection: cultures of blood, urine, and nose and throat secretions; chest X-ray; electrocardiogram; and a physical examination, with special attention to skin, ears, and sinuses. Lumbar puncture usually indicates elevated CSF pressure, from obstructed outflow at the arachnoid villi. The fluid may appear cloudy or milky white, depending on the number of white blood cells present. CSF protein levels tend to be high; glucose levels may be low. (In subacute meningitis, CSF findings may vary.) CSF culture and sensitivity tests usually identify the infecting organism, unless it's a virus. Leukocytosis and serum electrolyte abnormalities are also common. Computed tomography scanning can rule out cerebral hematoma, hemorrhage, or tumor.

Management
General
Treatment of meningitis includes vigorous supportive care. Supportive measures include bed rest, hypothermia, and measures to prevent dehydration. The room is kept darkened and quiet because any increase in sensory stimulation may cause a seizure. Isolation is necessary if nasal cultures are positive. Appropriate therapy for any coexisting conditions, such as endocarditis or pneumonia, is included as well.

Medication
Usually, I.V. antibiotics are given for at least 2 weeks and are followed by oral antibiotics, such as:
- ceftriaxone — 2 g every 12 hours I.M. or I.V.
- cefotaxime — 3 to 8 g I.M. or I.V. daily in divided doses
- vancomycin — 15 mg/kg I.V. every 12 hours alone or in combination with rifampin (600 mg/day P.O. or I.V.); may be used if resistant strains of bacteria are found
- penicillin V — 125 to 500 mg P.O. every 6 hours following a full course of I.V. therapy
- ampicillin — 250 to 500 mg P.O. every 6 hours following a full course of I.V. therapy.

Dexamethasone (initially, 10 mg I.V., then 4 to 6 mg every 6 hours, then tapered down) has been shown to be effective as adjunctive therapy in the treatment of meningitis caused by *H. influenzae* type B and in pneumococcal meningitis if given before the first dose of antibiotic. It has also been shown to reduce the incidence of deafness, a common complication of meningitis.

To control arrhythmias, give digoxin (0.125 to .25 mg P.O. or I.V.).

To decrease cerebral edema, give mannitol (1.5 to 2 g/kg as a 15% to 20% I.V. solution over 30 to 60 minutes).

The anticonvulsant phenytoin (100 mg I.V. or P.O. every 8 hours) can also be given.

To relieve headache and fever, give:
- aspirin — 325 to 650 mg every 4 to 6 hours p.r.n.
- acetaminophen — 325 to 650 mg every 4 to 6 hours p.r.n.

To prevent meningitis, prophylactic antibiotics are sometimes used after ventricular shunting procedures, skull fracture, or penetrating head wounds, but their use is controversial.

Referral
- The patient should be sent to the hospital immediately.
- If a severe neurologic deficit appears permanent, refer the patient to a rehabilitation program as soon as the acute phase of this illness has passed.

Follow-up
The patient should be seen 1 week after discharge from the hospital and then every 3 months.

Patient teaching
- To help prevent development of meningitis, teach patients with chronic sinusitis or other chronic infections the importance of proper medical treatment. Teach strict sterile technique to patients with head wounds or skull fractures.

Complications
- Seizures
- Subdural effusions
- Sensorineural hearing loss
- Learning deficits
- Death

MULTIPLE SCLEROSIS

Multiple sclerosis (MS) is a progressive disease caused by demyelination of the white matter of the brain and spinal cord. (See *Demyelination in multiple sclerosis,* page 258.) In this disease, sporadic patches of demyelination throughout the central nervous system induce widely disseminated and varied neurologic dysfunction. Characterized by exacerbations and remissions, MS is a major cause of chronic disability in young adults.

The prognosis varies. MS may progress rapidly, disabling some patients by early adulthood or causing death within months of onset. However, 70% of patients lead active, productive lives with prolonged remissions. The course of the disease is estimated to be 12 to 25 years.

AGE ALERT MS usually begins between ages 20 and 40 (the average age of onset is age 27). It affects three women for every two men and five Whites for every one Black. A family history of MS and living in a cold, damp climate increase the risk.

Causes

The exact cause of MS is unknown, but current theories suggest a slow-acting or latent viral infection and an autoimmune response. Other theories suggest that environmental and genetic factors may also be linked to MS. Emotional stress, overwork, fatigue, pregnancy, and acute respiratory tract infections have been known to precede the onset of this illness.

Clinical presentation

Clinical findings in MS depend on the extent and site of myelin destruction, the extent of remyelination, and the adequacy of subsequent restored synaptic transmission.

Signs and symptoms in MS may be transient, or they may last for hours or weeks. They may wax and wane with no predictable pattern, vary from day to day, and be bizarre and difficult for the patient to describe.

In most patients, visual problems and sensory impairment, such as numbness and tingling sensations (paresthesia), are the first signs that something may be wrong. Other characteristic changes include:
- ocular disturbances — optic neuritis, diplopia, ophthalmoplegia, blurred vision, and nystagmus
- muscle dysfunction — weakness, paralysis ranging from monoplegia to quadriplegia, spasticity, hyperreflexia, intention tremor, and gait ataxia
- urinary disturbances — incontinence, frequency, urgency, and frequent infections
- emotional lability — characteristic mood swings, irritability, euphoria, and depression.

Associated signs and symptoms include poorly articulated or scanning speech and dysphagia. Clinical effects may be so mild that the patient is unaware of them or so bizarre that he appears hysterical.

Differential diagnoses
- Amyotrophic lateral sclerosis
- Cerebellar tumors
- Small cerebral infarcts
- Ruptured intervertebral disc
- Spinal cord tumors
- Sarcoidosis
- Syphilis
- Systemic lupus erythematosus

Diagnosis

A misdiagnosis of psychiatric problems is common. Because early symptoms may be mild, years may elapse between onset of the first signs and the diagnosis, which

Demyelination in multiple sclerosis

In this illustration, a transverse section of cervical spine shows partial loss of myelin, characteristic of multiple sclerosis. This degenerative process is called demyelination.

As shown on the right, the loss of myelin is nearly complete. Clinical features of multiple sclerosis depend on the extent of demyelination.

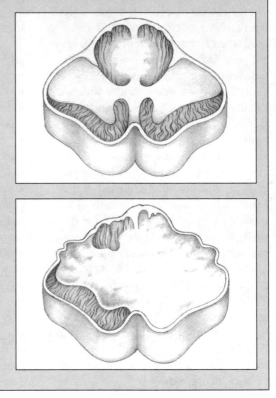

typically requires evidence of multiple neurologic attacks and characteristic remissions and exacerbations. Magnetic resonance imaging may detect MS lesions; however, diagnosis still remains difficult. Periodic testing and close observation of the patient are necessary, perhaps for years, depending on the course of the disease.

Abnormal EEG findings occur in one-third of patients. Lumbar puncture shows elevated gamma globulin fraction of immunoglobulin G but normal total cerebrospinal fluid (CSF) protein levels. Elevated CSF gamma globulin is significant only when serum gamma globulin

levels are normal because it reflects hyperactivity of the immune system due to chronic demyelination. Oligoclonal bands of immunoglobulin can be detected when gamma globulin in CSF is examined by electrophoresis, and these bands are present in most patients, even when the percentage of gamma globulin in CSF is normal. In addition, the white blood cell count in CSF may rise.

Management
General
The goal of treatment is to shorten exacerbations and relieve neurologic deficits so that the patient can resume a normal

lifestyle. During acute exacerbations, supportive measures, include bed rest, comfort measures, such as massages, prevention of fatigue, prevention of pressure ulcers, bowel and bladder training (if necessary), administration of antibiotics for bladder infections, physical therapy, and counseling.

Medication
The following medications are used to reduce the associated edema of the myelin sheath during exacerbations:
- corticotropin — 80 to 120 U I.M. daily for 2 to 3 weeks
- prednisone — 200 mg/day P.O. for 7 days, then 80 mg P.O. every other day for 1 month
- dexamethasone — 10 mg I.V. initially, then 4 to 6 mg every 6 hours and then tapered down.

Corticotropin and corticosteroids may relieve symptoms and hasten remission but don't prevent future exacerbations.

Numerous other drugs are used with corticotropin and corticosteroids. To mitigate mood swings, give chlordiazepoxide (5 to 10 mg P.O. t.i.d. to q.i.d.).

To relieve spasticity, give:
- baclofen — initially 5 mg P.O. t.i.d. for 3 days, then 10 mg P.O. t.i.d. for 3 days up to maximum of 80 mg/day
- dantrolene — 25 mg/day P.O. increased gradually up to maximum of 400 mg/day.

To relieve urine retention and minimize frequency and urgency, give:
- bethanechol — 10 to 50 mg P.O. t.i.d. to q.i.d.
- oxybutynin — 5 mg P.O. b.i.d. to q.i.d.

To relieve fatigue, give:
- amantadine — 200 mg/day P.O.
- fluoxetine — 20 to 80 mg/day.

To treat ataxia, beta-adrenergic blockers, anticonvulsants, and benzodiazepines are used; examples include:

- propranolol — 40 mg P.O. b.i.d.
- gabapentin — 300 mg/day P.O. to t.i.d.
- clonazepam — 0.25 to 0.5 mg/day P.O.

To reduce the frequency of exacerbation for ambulatory patients with relapsing-remitting MS, give:
- interferon beta-1b — 8 million IU S.C. every other day
- interferon beta-1a — 30 mcg I.M. once a week.

Immunosuppressants, such as cyclophosphamide (40 to 50 mg/kg I.V. in divided doses over 2 to 5 days or 1 to 5 mg/kg/day P.O.) may suppress the immune response.

Referral
- For education and support, refer the patient to the National Multiple Sclerosis Society.
- Refer the patient to a neurologist for treatment.
- The patient may need a referral for physical and occupational therapy.
- The patient and family may need psychological counseling in order to cope with having MS.

Follow-up
The patient will need to be monitored according to the progression of the disease.

Patient teaching
- Educate the patient and family concerning the chronic course of MS. Emphasize the need to avoid stress, infections, and fatigue and to maintain independence by developing new ways of performing daily activities. Be sure to tell the patient to avoid exposure to infections.
- Teach the family to assist with physical therapy. Increase patient comfort with massages and relaxing baths. Make sure the bath water isn't too hot because it may temporarily intensify otherwise sub-

tle symptoms. Teach the family to assist with active, resistive, and stretching exercises to maintain muscle tone and joint mobility, decrease spasticity, improve coordination, and boost morale.

■ Stress to the patient the importance of eating a nutritious, well-balanced diet that contains sufficient roughage and adequate fluids to prevent constipation.

■ Encourage the family and patient to establish a daily routine to maintain optimal functioning. Activity level is regulated by tolerance level. Encourage regular rest periods to prevent fatigue and daily physical exercise.

■ Inform the patient that exacerbations are unpredictable, necessitating physical and emotional adjustments in lifestyle.

Complications
■ Emotional lability
■ Paraplegia
■ Urinary tract infection
■ Delirium
■ Coma

Special considerations
■ Watch for adverse drug effects. For instance, dantrolene may cause muscle weakness and decreased muscle tone.

• • • • • • • • • • • •

MYASTHENIA GRAVIS

Myasthenia gravis produces sporadic but progressive weakness and abnormal fatigability of striated (skeletal) muscles, exacerbated by exercise and repeated movement but improved by anticholinesterase drugs. Usually, this disorder affects muscles innervated by the cranial nerves (face, lips, tongue, neck, and throat), but it can affect any muscle group. Myasthenia gravis follows an unpredictable course of recurring exacerbations and periodic

remissions. There's no known cure. Drug treatment has improved prognosis and allows patients to lead relatively normal lives except during exacerbations. When the disease involves the respiratory system, it may be life-threatening.

Myasthenia gravis affects 1 in 25,000 people at any age. About 20% of infants born to myasthenic mothers have transient (or occasionally persistent) myasthenia. This disease may coexist with immunologic and thyroid disorders; about 15% of myasthenic patients have thymomas. Remissions occur in about 25% of patients.

AGE ALERT Incidence of myasthenia gravis peaks between ages 20 and 40. It's three times more common in women than men, but after age 40 the incidence is similar.

Causes
Myasthenia gravis causes a failure in the transmission of nerve impulses at the neuromuscular junction. Theoretically, such impairment may result from an autoimmune response, ineffective acetylcholine release, or inadequate muscle fiber response to acetylcholine. (See *Impaired transmission in myasthenia gravis*.)

Clinical presentation
The dominant symptoms of myasthenia gravis are skeletal muscle weakness and fatigability. Ocular motor disturbances are the initial symptoms in two-thirds of all myasthenia gravis patients. In the early stages, easy fatigability of certain muscles may appear with no other findings. Later, it may be severe enough to cause paralysis. Typically, myasthenic muscles are strongest in the morning but weaken throughout the day, especially after exercise. Short rest periods temporarily restore muscle function. Muscle weakness is progressive; more and more muscles be-

Impaired transmission in myasthenia gravis

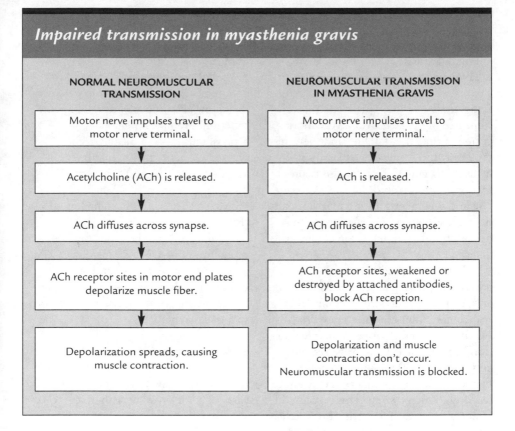

NORMAL NEUROMUSCULAR TRANSMISSION	NEUROMUSCULAR TRANSMISSION IN MYASTHENIA GRAVIS
Motor nerve impulses travel to motor nerve terminal.	Motor nerve impulses travel to motor nerve terminal.
Acetylcholine (ACh) is released.	ACh is released.
ACh diffuses across synapse.	ACh diffuses across synapse.
ACh receptor sites in motor end plates depolarize muscle fiber.	ACh receptor sites, weakened or destroyed by attached antibodies, block ACh reception.
Depolarization spreads, causing muscle contraction.	Depolarization and muscle contraction don't occur. Neuromuscular transmission is blocked.

come weak, and eventually some muscles may lose function entirely. Resulting symptoms depend on the muscle group affected; they become more intense during menses and after emotional stress, prolonged exposure to sunlight or cold, or infections.

Onset may be sudden or insidious. Initial signs may include:
- weak eye closure
- ptosis
- diplopia.

Patients with myasthenia gravis usually have blank and expressionless faces and nasal vocal tones. They experience frequent nasal regurgitation of fluids and have difficulty chewing and swallowing. Because of this, they often worry about choking. Their eyelids droop (ptosis),

and they may have to tilt their heads back to see. Their neck muscles may become too weak to support their heads without bobbing.

In patients with weakened respiratory muscles, decreased tidal volume and vital capacity make breathing difficult and predispose them to pneumonia and other respiratory tract infections. Respiratory muscle weakness (myasthenic crisis) may be severe enough to require an emergency airway and mechanical ventilation.

Differential diagnoses
- Horner's syndrome
- Bell's palsy
- Multiple sclerosis
- Cerebrovascular accident
- Transient ischemic attacks

- Brain tumor
- Cerebral aneurysm
- Brain abscess
- Thyroid disease
- Thymoma

Diagnosis

Repeated muscle use over a very short period of time that fatigues and then improves with rest suggests a diagnosis of myasthenia gravis. Tests for this neurologic condition record the effect of exercise and subsequent rest on muscle weakness. Electromyography, with repeated neural stimulation, may help confirm the diagnosis.

The classic proof of myasthenia gravis is improved muscle function after an I.V. injection of edrophonium or neostigmine (anticholinesterase drugs).

In myasthenic patients, muscle function improves within 30 to 60 seconds and lasts up to 30 minutes. Long-standing ocular muscle dysfunction may fail to respond to such testing. This test can differentiate a myasthenic crisis from a cholinergic crisis (caused by acetylcholine overactivity at the neuromuscular junction). The acetylcholine receptor antibody titer may be elevated in generalized myasthenia.

Management
General

Treatment is symptomatic. Plasmapheresis is used in severe myasthenic exacerbation. Acute exacerbations that cause severe respiratory distress necessitate emergency treatment. Endotracheal intubation, positive-pressure ventilation, and vigorous suctioning to remove secretions usually produce improvement in a few days. Because anticholinesterase drugs aren't effective in myasthenic crisis, they're stopped until respiratory function improves. Myasthenic crisis requires immediate hospitalization and vigorous respiratory support.

Medication

Anticholinesterase drugs are used to counteract fatigue and muscle weakness and allow about 80% of normal muscle function; examples include:
- neostigmine — 45 mg/day P.O. increased gradually to 150 mg/day
- pyridostigmine — 60 to 180 mg P.O. b.i.d. to t.i.d. up to 1,500 mg/day. However, these drugs become less effective as the disease worsens.

Additional medications include:
- prednisone — 60 to 80 mg/day P.O., tapered to 35 mg every other day
- cyclophosphamide — 40 to 50 mg/kg I.V. in divided doses over 2 to 5 days or 1 to 5 mg/kg/day P.O.

Surgical intervention

Patients with thymomas require thymectomy, which may cause remission in some cases of adult-onset myasthenia.

Referral

- Refer the patient to a neurologist for treatment.
- For myasthenia crisis, refer the patient to the hospital immediately.
- For more information and support, refer the patient to the Myasthenia Gravis Foundation.

Follow-up

The patient should be monitored for any exacerbations, or as decided by the neurologist.

Patient teaching

- To prevent relapses, tell the patient to adhere closely to the ordered drug administration schedule.
- Teach the patient to plan exercise, meals, patient care, and activities to

make the most of energy peaks. For example, the patient should take his medication 20 to 30 minutes before meals to facilitate chewing or swallowing.

▪ Emphasize that periodic remissions, exacerbations, and day-to-day fluctuations are common.

▪ Teach the patient how to recognize adverse effects and signs of toxicity of anticholinesterase drugs (headaches, weakness, sweating, abdominal cramps, nausea, vomiting, diarrhea, excessive salivation, and bronchospasm) and corticosteroids (euphoria, insomnia, edema, and increased appetite).

▪ Warn the patient to avoid strenuous exercise, stress, infection, and needless exposure to the sun or cold. All of these may worsen signs and symptoms. Wearing an eye patch or glasses with one frosted lens may help the patient with diplopia.

Complications
▪ Acute respiratory arrest
▪ Aspiration
▪ Chronic respiratory failure

Special considerations
▪ Careful baseline assessment, early recognition and treatment of potential crises, supportive measures, and thorough patient teaching can minimize exacerbations and complications. Continuity of care is essential.

CLINICAL CAUTION Signs of an impending crisis include increased muscle weakness, respiratory distress, and difficulty in talking or chewing.

• • • • • • • • • • • •

NEURITIS, PERIPHERAL

Peripheral neuritis (also called multiple neuritis, peripheral neuropathy, and polyneuritis) is the degeneration of peripheral nerves supplying mainly the distal muscles of the extremities. It results in muscle weakness with sensory loss and atrophy and decreased or absent deep tendon reflexes. This syndrome is associated with a noninflammatory degeneration of the axon and myelin sheaths, chiefly affecting the distal muscles of the extremities. Because onset is usually insidious, patients may compensate by overusing unaffected muscles. In patients with severe infection or those with chronic alcohol intoxication, onset is rapid. If the cause can be identified and eliminated, the prognosis is good.

AGE ALERT Although peripheral neuritis can occur at any age, incidence is highest in men between ages 30 and 50.

Causes
Causes of peripheral neuritis include:
▪ chronic intoxication (ethyl alcohol, arsenic, lead, carbon disulfide, benzene, phosphorus, and sulfonamides)
▪ infectious diseases (meningitis, diphtheria, syphilis, tuberculosis, pneumonia, mumps, and Guillain-Barré syndrome)
▪ metabolic and inflammatory disorders (gout, diabetes mellitus, rheumatoid arthritis, polyarteritis nodosa, sarcoidosis and systemic lupus erythematosus)
▪ nutritive diseases (beriberi and other vitamin deficiencies and cachectic states).

Clinical presentation
The clinical effects of peripheral neuritis develop slowly, and the disease usually affects the motor and sensory nerve fibers. Neuritis typically produces:
▪ flaccid paralysis
▪ wasting
▪ loss of reflexes
▪ pain of varying intensity
▪ loss of ability to perceive vibratory sensations

- paresthesia, hyperesthesia, anesthesia in the hands and feet
- diminished or absent deep tendon reflexes
- atrophied muscles (that are tender or hypersensitive to pressure or palpation)
- footdrop.

Cutaneous manifestations include glossy red skin and decreased sweating. Patients commonly have a history of clumsiness and may complain of frequent vague sensations.

Differential diagnoses
- Multiple sclerosis
- Depression

Diagnosis
Patient history and physical examination delineate characteristic distribution of motor and sensory deficits. Electromyography may show a delayed action potential if this condition impairs motor nerve function.

Management
General
Effective treatment of peripheral neuritis consists of supportive measures to relieve pain, adequate bed rest, and physical therapy, as needed. Spinal cord stimulation has been found to be beneficial for neuropathy pain and parenthesis. Most importantly, however, the underlying cause must be identified and corrected. For instance, it's essential to identify and remove the toxic agent, correct nutritional and vitamin deficiencies (the patient needs a high-calorie diet rich in vitamins, especially B complex), and counsel the patient to avoid alcohol.

Medication
Medications used to treat peripheral neuritis include:

- gabapentin — up to 1,800 mg/day P.O. in divided doses
- amitriptyline — 50 to 150 mg h.s. P.O.
- nortriptyline — 25 mg P.O. t.i.d. to q.i.d. up to 150 mg/day
- propoxyphene — 65 to 100 mg P.O. every 4 hours p.r.n.

Referral
- The patient should be referred to a neurologist for treatment.
- The patient may need a referral to a pain management team for adequate control of pain.
- The patient may need psychological counseling to cope with the illness.
- The patient should be referred for physical or occupational therapy.

Patient teaching
- Instruct the patient to rest and refrain from using the affected extremity.
- Tell the patient to use a foot cradle to decrease pressure on his heels.
- Instruct the patient that the use of devices supplied by the physical therapist, such as splints and braces, will help prevent contractures.

Complications
- Footdrop
- Injury
- Narcotic dependency
- Alteration in lifestyle

• • • • • • • • • • • •

PARKINSON'S DISEASE

Named for James Parkinson, the English doctor who wrote the first accurate description of the disease in 1817, Parkinson's disease characteristically produces progressive muscle rigidity, akinesia, involuntary tremor, and dementia. Death may result from aspiration pneumonia or an infection. Parkinson's disease, also called parkinsonism, paralysis agitans, and shaking palsy, is one of the most common crippling diseases in the United States. According to current statistics, Parkinson's disease strikes 1% of people over age 65. It's rarely seen before age 40. It occurs in men and women, with men being slightly more affected. Because of increased longevity, this amounts to roughly 50,000 new cases diagnosed annually in the United States alone.

Causes

Although the cause of Parkinson's disease is unknown, study of the extrapyramidal brain nuclei (corpus striatum, globus pallidus, and substantia nigra) has established that a dopamine deficiency prevents affected brain cells from performing their normal inhibitory function within the central nervous system.

Clinical presentation

The cardinal symptoms of Parkinson's disease are muscle rigidity and akinesia and an insidious resting tremor that begins in the fingers (unilateral pill-rolling tremor), increases during stress or anxiety, and decreases with purposeful movement and sleep. Muscle rigidity results in resistance to passive muscle stretching, which may be uniform (lead-pipe rigidity) or jerky (cogwheel rigidity). Akinesia causes:

- difficulty walking (gait lacks normal parallel motion and may be retropulsive or propulsive)
- high-pitched, monotone voice
- drooling
- masklike facial expression
- loss of posture control (the patient walks with body bent forward)
- dysarthria, dysphagia, or both.

Occasionally, akinesia may also cause oculogyric crises (eyes are fixed up-ward, with involuntary tonic movements) or blepharospasm (eyelids are completely closed). Parkinson's disease itself doesn't impair the intellect, but a coexisting disorder, such as arteriosclerosis, may do so.

Differential diagnoses

- Involutional depression
- Cerebral arteriosclerosis
- Intracranial tumors
- Wilson's disease
- Phenothiazine or other drug toxicity

Diagnosis

Generally, laboratory data are of little value in identifying Parkinson's disease; consequently, diagnosis is based on the patient's age, history, and characteristic clinical picture. Conclusive diagnosis is possible only after ruling out other causes of symptoms. A positron emission tomography scan may help confirm Parkinson's disease but currently this testing is expensive and not routinely used.

Management
General

Because there's no cure for Parkinson's disease, the primary goal of treatment is to relieve symptoms and keep the patient functional as long as possible. Treatment consists of drugs, physical therapy, and stereotactic neurosurgery (in severe disease states that are unresponsive to drugs). Individually planned physical therapy complements drug treatment and neurosurgery to maintain normal muscle tone and function. Appropriate physical therapy includes both active and passive range-of-motion exercises, routine daily activities, walking, and baths and massage to help relax muscles.

Medication

Medications used in the treatment of Parkinson's disease may include:

- carbidopa-levodopa — 1 tablet of 25 mg carbidopa and 100 mg/day of levodopa P.O. t.i.d., increasing 1 tablet or every other day to a maximum of 8 tablets
- pergolide — 0.05 mg/day P.O. for the first 2 days, then increasing to 0.1 to 0.15 mg every third day over 12 days given in three divided doses
- pramipexole — 0.375 to 4.5 mg/day P.O. in three divided doses
- trihexyphenidyl — 1 mg P.O. initially, then increasing daily to 6 to 10 mg/day in three divided doses
- benztropine — 0.5 to 6 mg/day P.O. or I.M.
- amantadine — 100 mg to 200 mg/day P.O.
- tolcapone — 100 to 200 mg P.O. t.i.d
- selegiline — 5 mg P.O. b.i.d.

CLINICAL CAUTION Medication for Parkinson's disease needs to be used in combination. The timing of the medication is important and must be adjusted according to the patient's symptoms and response to treatment.

Surgical intervention

Stereotactic neurosurgery or the controversial experimental treatment called fetal cell transplantation can be used to treat Parkinson's disease. When drug therapy fails, stereotactic neurosurgery, such as subthalamotomy and pallidotomy, may be an alternative. In these procedures, electrical coagulation, freezing, radioactivity, or ultrasound destroys the ventrolateral nucleus of the thalamus to prevent involuntary movement. This is most effective in young, otherwise healthy people with unilateral tremor or muscle rigidity. Neurosurgery can only relieve symptoms.

In fetal cell transplantation, fetal brain tissue is injected into the patient's brain. If the injected cells grow within the recipient's brain, they will allow the brain to process dopamine, thereby either halting or reversing disease progression.

Referral

- Refer the patient and family to the National Parkinson Foundation or the United Parkinson Foundation for information and support.
- The patient and family may need psychological counseling to help cope with this illness.
- The patient may require physical or occupational therapy to maintain functional muscle tone.

Follow-up

The patient should be seen frequently when drug therapy is initiated (every 2 weeks); otherwise the patient may be seen monthly if stable.

Patient teaching

- Encourage independence. Teach the patient with excessive tremor that he may achieve partial control of his body by sitting on a chair and using its arms to steady himself. Advise the patient to change position slowly and dangle his legs before getting out of bed.
- Teach the patient and family how to overcome problems related to eating and elimination. Tell him to establish a regular bowel routine by encouraging him to drink at least 2 qt (2 L) of liquids daily and eat high-fiber foods. He may need an elevated toilet seat to assist him from a standing to a sitting position.

Complications

- Depression
- Injury

- Aspiration pneumonia
- Dementia

Special considerations
- Effectively caring for the patient with Parkinson's disease requires careful monitoring of drug treatment, emphasis on teaching self-reliance, and generous psychological support.
- Establish long- and short-term treatment goals, and be aware of the patient's need for intellectual stimulation and diversion.

• • • • • • • • • • • •

REYE'S SYNDROME

Reye's syndrome is an acute childhood illness that causes fatty infiltration of the liver with concurrent hyperammonemia, encephalopathy, and increased intracranial pressure (ICP). In addition, fatty infiltration of the kidneys, brain, and myocardium may occur. Reye's syndrome affects children from infancy to adolescence and occurs equally in boys and girls.

Prognosis depends on the severity of central nervous system depression. Until recently, mortality was as high as 90%. Today, ICP monitoring and, consequently, early treatment of increased ICP, along with other treatment measures, have cut mortality to about 20%. Death is usually a result of cerebral edema or respiratory arrest. Comatose patients who survive may have residual brain damage.

Causes
Reye's syndrome typically begins within 1 to 3 days of an acute viral infection, such as an upper respiratory tract infection, type B influenza, or varicella (chickenpox). Incidence commonly rises during influenza outbreaks and may be linked to aspirin use. For this reason, use of aspirin for children under age 15 isn't recommended.

In Reye's syndrome, damaged hepatic mitochondria disrupt the urea cycle, which normally changes ammonia to urea for its excretion from the body. This results in hyperammonemia, hypoglycemia, and an increase in serum short-chain fatty acids, leading to encephalopathy. Simultaneously, fatty infiltration occurs in renal tubular cells, neuronal tissue, and muscle tissue, including the heart.

Clinical presentation
The severity of the child's signs and symptoms varies with the degree of encephalopathy and cerebral edema. In any case, Reye's syndrome develops in five stages. After the initial viral infection, a brief recovery period follows when the child doesn't seem seriously ill. A few days later, he develops intractable vomiting; lethargy; rapidly changing mental status (mild to severe agitation, confusion, irritability, and delirium); rising blood pressure, respiratory rate, and pulse rate; and hyperactive reflexes.

Reye's syndrome commonly progresses to coma. As coma deepens, seizures develop, followed by decreased tendon reflexes and, frequently, respiratory failure.

Increased ICP, a serious complication, is now considered the result of an increased cerebral blood volume causing intracranial hypertension. Such swelling may develop as a result of acidosis, increased cerebral metabolic rate, and an impaired autoregulatory mechanism.

Differential diagnoses
- Drug poisoning
- Hepatic coma
- Encephalitis

Stages of treatment for Reye's syndrome

SIGNS AND SYMPTOMS	BASELINE TREATMENT	BASELINE INTERVENTION
Stage I Vomiting, lethargy, hepatic dysfunction	■ To decrease intracranial pressure (ICP) and brain edema, give I.V. fluids at 2/3 maintenance. Also give an osmotic diuretic (mannitol 1.5 to 2 g/kg as a 15% to 20% I.V. solution over 30 to 60 minutes) or furosemide (10 to 40 mg I.V.). ■ To treat hypoprothrombinemia, give vitamin K (2.5 to 10 mg orally, subcutaneously, or I.M.); if vitamin K is unsuccessful, give fresh frozen plasma. ■ Monitor serum ammonia and blood glucose levels and plasma osmolality every 4 to 8 hours to check progress.	■ Monitor vital signs and check level of consciousness for increasing lethargy. ■ Monitor fluid intake and output to prevent fluid overload. Maintain urine output at 1.0 ml/kg/hour; plasma osmolality, 290 mOsm; and blood glucose, 150 mg/ml. (Goal: Keep glucose level high, osmolality normal to high, and ammonia level low.) Also restrict protein.
Stage II Hyperventilation, delirium, hepatic dysfunction, hyperactive reflexes	■ Continue baseline treatment.	■ Maintain seizure precautions. ■ Note any signs of coma that require invasive, supportive therapy such as intubation. ■ Keep head of bed at 30-degree angle.
Stage III Coma, hyperventilation, decorticate rigidity, hepatic dysfunction	■ Continue baseline and seizure treatment. ■ Monitor ICP with a subarachnoid screw or other invasive device. ■ Provide endotracheal intubation and mechanical ventilation to control partial pressure of arterial carbon dioxide ($PaCO_2$) levels. A paralyzing agent, such as pancuronium (0.04 to 0.1 mg/kg I.V. every 30 to 60 minutes as needed), may help maintain ventilation. ■ Give mannitol I.V. (1.5 to 2 g/kg as a 15% to 20% I.V. solution over 30 to 60 minutes).	■ Monitor ICP (should be less than 20 mm Hg before suctioning) or give a barbiturate I.V. ■ When ventilating the patient, maintain $PaCO_2$ between 25 and 30 mm Hg and partial pressure of arterial oxygen between 80 and 100 mm Hg. ■ Closely monitor cardiovascular status with a pulmonary artery catheter or central venous pressure line.

Stages of treatment for Reye's syndrome *(continued)*

SIGNS AND SYMPTOMS	BASELINE TREATMENT	BASELINE INTERVENTION
Stage IV Deepening coma; decerebrate rigidity; large, fixed pupils; minimal hepatic dysfunction	■ Continue baseline and supportive care. ■ If all previous measures fail, some pediatric centers use barbiturate coma, decompressive craniotomy, hypothermia, or exchange transfusion.	■ Check the patient for loss of reflexes and signs of flaccidity. ■ Give the family the extra support they need, considering their child's poor prognosis.
Stage V Seizures, loss of deep tendon reflexes, flaccidity, respiratory arrest, ammonia level greater than 300 mg/dl	■ Continue baseline and supportive care.	■ Help the family to face the patient's impending death.

Diagnosis

A history of a recent viral disorder with typical clinical features strongly suggests Reye's syndrome. An increased serum ammonia level, abnormal clotting studies, and hepatic dysfunction confirm it. Testing serum salicylate level rules out aspirin use. Absence of jaundice despite increased liver aminotransferase levels rules out acute hepatic failure and hepatic encephalopathy.

Abnormal test results may include:
■ liver function studies—aspartate aminotransferase and alanine aminotransferase elevated to twice normal levels; bilirubin level usually normal
■ liver biopsy—fatty droplets uniformly distributed throughout cells
■ cerebrospinal fluid (CSF) analysis—white blood cell count less than 10/µl; with coma, increased CSF pressure
■ coagulation studies—prothrombin time and partial thromboplastin time prolonged

■ blood values—serum ammonia levels elevated; serum glucose levels normal or, in 15% of cases, low; serum fatty acid and lactate levels increased.

Management

For treatment guidelines, see *Stages of treatment for Reye's syndrome*.

Referral

■ The patient may require hospitalization.
■ Refer the family for psychological counseling as needed.
■ For more information and support, refer the parents to the National Reye's Syndrome Foundation.

Follow-up

Medical follow-up will depend on the residual effects of the illness.

Patient teaching

- Advise parents to give nonsalicylate analgesics and antipyretics such as acetaminophen.

Complications

- Respiratory failure
- Cerebral edema
- Death

• • • • • • • • • • • •

TRIGEMINAL NEURALGIA

Trigeminal neuralgia, also called tic douloureux, is a painful disorder of one or more branches of the fifth cranial (trigeminal) nerve that produces paroxysmal attacks of excruciating facial pain precipitated by stimulation of a trigger zone. It occurs on the right side of the face more commonly than the left. Trigeminal neuralgia can subside spontaneously, and remissions may last from several months to years.

AGE ALERT Trigeminal neuralgia occurs more commonly in women than men over age 40.

Causes

Although the cause remains undetermined, trigeminal neuralgia may reflect an afferent reflex in the brain stem or in the sensory root of the trigeminal nerve. Such neuralgia may also be related to compression of the nerve root by posterior fossa tumors, middle fossa tumors, or vascular lesions (subclinical aneurysm), although such lesions usually produce simultaneous loss of sensation. Occasionally, trigeminal neuralgia is a manifestation of multiple sclerosis or herpes zoster. Whatever the cause, the pain of trigeminal neuralgia is probably produced by an interaction or short-circuiting of touch and pain fibers.

Clinical presentation

Typically, the patient reports a searing or burning pain that:

- occurs in lightning-like jabs
- lasts from 1 to 15 minutes (usually 1 to 2 minutes)
- occurs in an area innervated by one of the divisions of the trigeminal nerve (primarily the superior mandibular or maxillary division)
- rarely affects more than one division and seldom the first division (ophthalmic) or both sides of the face.

Pain affects the second (maxillary) and third (mandibular) divisions of the trigeminal nerve equally. (See *Trigeminal nerve function and distribution.*)

These attacks characteristically follow stimulation of a trigger zone, usually by a light touch to a hypersensitive area, such as the tip of the nose, cheeks, or gums. Although attacks can occur at any time, they may follow a draft of air, exposure to heat or cold, eating, smiling, talking, or drinking hot or cold beverages. The frequency of attacks varies greatly, from many times per day to several times per month or year. Between attacks, most patients are free from pain, although some have a constant, dull ache. No patient is ever free from the fear of the next attack.

Differential diagnoses

- Tumor
- Dental abscess
- Herpes zoster
- Dystonia
- Migraine headache

Diagnosis

The patient's pain history is the basis for diagnosis because trigeminal neuralgia produces no objective clinical or pathologic changes. Physical examination shows no impairment of sensory or motor function; indeed, sensory impairment implies a space-occupying lesion as the cause of pain.

Observation during the examination shows the patient favoring (splinting) the affected area. To ward off a painful attack, the patient often holds his face immobile when talking. He may also leave the affected side of his face unwashed and unshaven or protect it with a coat or shawl. When asked where the pain occurs, he points to—but never touches—the affected area. Witnessing a typical attack helps to confirm diagnosis. Rarely, a tumor in the posterior fossa can produce pain that is clinically indistinguishable from trigeminal neuralgia. Skull X-rays, computed tomography scanning, and magnetic resonance imaging rule out sinus or tooth infections and tumors. If the patient has trigeminal neuralgia, these test results are normal.

Management
General
Treatment focuses on management of pain. Observe and record the characteristics of each attack, including the patient's protective mechanisms.

Medication
To temporarily relieve or prevent pain, these agents may be effective:
- carbamazepine — 200 to 1,200 mg/day P.O. in divided doses
- phenytoin — 200 to 600 mg/day P.O. in divided doses.

Surgical intervention
When these medical measures fail or attacks become increasingly frequent or severe, neurosurgical procedures may provide permanent relief. The preferred procedure is percutaneous electrocoagulation of nerve rootlets under local anesthetic. New treatments include a percutaneous

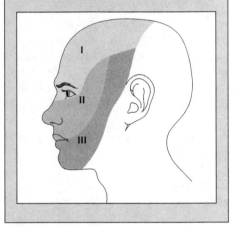

Trigeminal nerve function and distribution

FUNCTION
- Motor: chewing movements
- Sensory: sensations of face, scalp, and teeth (mouth and nasal chamber)

DISTRIBUTION
I ophthalmic
II maxillary
III mandibular

radio frequency procedure, which causes partial root destruction and relieves pain, and microsurgery for vascular decompression of the trigeminal nerve.

Referral
- Refer the patient to a neurologist if medication isn't effective.

Follow-up
For the first 3 months of carbamazepine therapy, complete blood count and liver function should be monitored weekly, then monthly thereafter

Patient teaching
- Warn the patient to immediately report fever, sore throat, mouth ulcers, easy

bruising, or petechial or purpuric hemor-rhage because these may signal thrombo-cytopenia or aplastic anemia and may re-quire discontinuation of drug therapy.
▪ After resection of the first branch of the trigeminal nerve, tell the patient to avoid rubbing his eyes and using aerosol spray. Advise him to wear glasses or gog-gles outdoors and to blink often.
▪ After surgery to sever the second or third branch, tell the patient to avoid hot foods and drinks, which could burn his mouth, and to chew carefully to avoid biting the inside of his mouth. It may be necessary for the patient to eat pureed food, possibly through a straw. Advise him to place food in the unaffected side of his mouth when chewing, to brush his teeth and rinse his mouth often, and to see the dentist twice per year to detect cavities because he won't experience pain from cavities in the area of the sev-ered nerve.

Complications
▪ Adverse effects of medication

Special considerations
▪ Provide emotional support, and en-courage the patient to express his fear and anxiety. Promote independence through self-care and maximum physical activity. Reinforce natural avoidance of stimulation (air, heat, and cold) of trigger zones (lips, cheeks, and gums).

• • • • • • • • • • • •

SELECTED REFERENCES

Diagnostics: An A-to-Z Nursing Guide to Labo-ratory Tests & Diagnostic Procedures. Springhouse, Pa.: Springhouse Corp., 2001.

Diseases, 3rd ed. Springhouse, Pa.: Spring-house Corp., 2001.

Fauci, A.S., et al. *Harrison's Principles of Inter-nal Medicine Companion Handbook*, 15th ed. New York: McGraw-Hill Book Co., 2001.

Ignatavicius, D.D., et al., eds. *Medical-Surgical Nursing Across the Health Care Continuum*, 3rd ed., Philadelphia: W.B. Saunders Co., 1999.

Kingsley, R.E. *Concise Text of Neuroscience*, 2nd ed. Philadelphia: Lippincott Williams & Wilkins, 1999.

Simon, R.P., et al. *Clinical Neurology*, 4th ed. Stamford, Conn.: Appelton & Lange, 1999.

Musculoskeletal disorders

Be prepared to call on the full range of your nursing skills when providing musculoskeletal care. Fractures, dislocations, and other musculoskeletal injuries are some of the most common problems you'll see. Osteoarthritis and other disorders commonly debilitate the muscles, bones, and joints of elderly patients. This chapter will help you refine the many clinical skills needed for this diverse patient population.

• • • • • • • • • • • •

ASSESSMENT

When the patient's health history or physical findings suggest musculoskeletal involvement, you'll need to perform a complete assessment of this system, beginning with a thorough history.

Evaluate the patient's body symmetry, posture, gait, and muscle and joint function as well as his general appearance. You may need to check neurovascular status, including motion, sensation, and circulation. Because joint or bone pain symptoms commonly indicate a sys-

temic disease, the patient may require a complete physical examination.

Physical examination
Perform a head-to-toe assessment, simultaneously evaluating muscle and joint function of each body area in turn. You'll need to observe the patient's posture, gait, and coordination and inspect and palpate his muscles, joints, and bones.

Preparing for the examination
Gather the necessary equipment, including a tape measure and a goniometer or protractor for measuring angles. Position the examination table to allow full range of motion (ROM) for the patient and easy access for the assessment.

Observing posture, gait, and coordination
Assessment begins the instant you see the patient. Observe muscle strength, facial muscle movement, body symmetry, and obvious physical or functional deformities or abnormalities.

Assess the patient's overall body symmetry as he moves. Note marked dissimilarities in side-to-side size, shape, and motion.

Posture

Evaluating posture includes inspecting spinal curvature and knee positioning.

To assess the spine, instruct the patient to stand as straight as possible. Standing to the patient's side, back, and front, respectively, inspect the spine for alignment and the shoulders, iliac crests, and scapulae for symmetry of position and height. Then have the patient bend forward at the waist, with his arms relaxed and dangling. Standing behind him, inspect the straightness of the spine, noting flank and thorax position and symmetry. Normally, convex curvature characterizes the thoracic spine and concave curvature characterizes the lumbar spine in a standing patient.

Other normal findings include a midline spine without lateral curvatures, a concave lumbar curvature that changes to a convex curvature in the flexed position, and iliac crests, shoulders, and scapulae at the same horizontal level.

To assess knee positioning, have the patient stand with his feet together. Note the relation of one knee to the other. They should be bilaterally symmetrical and located at the same height in a forward-facing position. Normally, the knees are less than 1″ (2.5 cm) apart and the medial malleoli (ankle bones) are less than 1⅛″ (3 cm) apart.

Gait

Direct the patient to walk away, turn around, and walk back. Observe and evaluate his posture, movement (such as pace and length of stride), foot position, coordination, and balance. During the stance phase, the foot on the floor should flatten completely and be able to bear the weight of the body. As the patient pushes off, the toes should be flexed. In the swing phase, the foot in midswing should clear the floor and pass the opposite leg in its stance phase. When the swing phase ends, he should be able to control the swing as it stops, as the foot again contacts the floor.

Other normal findings include smooth, coordinated movements, the head leading the body when turning, and erect posture with approximately 2″ to 4″ (5 to 10 cm) of space between the feet. Be sure to remain close to an elderly or infirm patient and be ready to help if he should stumble or start to fall.

Coordination

Evaluate how well a patient's muscles produce movement. Coordination results when neuromuscular integrity provides the ability to make voluntary and productive movements.

Assess gross motor skills by having the patient perform any body action involving the muscles and joints in natural directional movements, such as lifting the arm to the side or other ROM exercises. Assess fine motor coordination by asking him to pick up a small object.

Inspecting and palpating muscles

Expect to perform inspection and palpation simultaneously during the musculoskeletal assessment. You'll evaluate muscle tone, mass, and strength. Palpate the muscles gently, never forcing movement when the patient reports pain or when you feel resistance. Watch his face and body language for signs of discomfort; a patient may suffer silently.

Tone and mass

Assess muscle tone by palpating a muscle at rest and during passive ROM. Palpate a muscle at rest from the muscle attachment at the bone to the edge of the muscle. Normally, a relaxed muscle should feel soft, pliable, and nontender; a contracted muscle should be firm.

Muscle mass is the actual size of a muscle. Assessment of muscle mass usually involves measuring the circumference of the thigh, calf, and upper arm. When measuring, establish landmarks to ensure measurement at the same location on each area.

Strength and joint ROM

Assessing joint ROM tests the joint function; assessing muscle strength against resistance tests the function of the muscles. (See *Assessing muscle strength and joint range of motion*, pages 276 to 283).

Inspecting and palpating joints and bones

Expect to measure the patient's height and the length of the extremities (arms and legs), and evaluate joint and bone characteristics and joint ROM.

Never force joint movement if you feel resistance or if the patient complains of pain. General deviations from normal include pain, swelling, stiffness, deformities, altered ROM, crepitation (a grating sound or sensation accompanying joint movement), ankylosis (joint fusion or fixation), and contracture (muscle shortening).

Length of the extremities

Place the patient on a flat surface in the supine position with his arms and legs fully extended and his shoulders and hips adducted. Measure each arm from the acromial process to the tip of the middle finger. Measure each leg from the anterior superior iliac spine to the medial malleolus with the tape crossing at the medial side of the knee.

Cervical spine

Inspect the cervical spine from behind, from the side, and from the front of the

patient as he sits or stands. Observe the alignment of the head with the body. The nose should be in line with the midsternum and extend beyond the shoulders when viewed from the side. The head should align with the shoulders. Normally, the seventh cervical and first thoracic vertebrae appear more prominent than the others.

Clavicles

Inspect and palpate the length of the clavicles, including the sternoclavicular and acromioclavicular joints. Normal findings include firm, smooth, and continuous bones.

Scapulae

To inspect and palpate the scapulae, sit directly behind the patient as he sits with his shoulders thrust backward. Normally, the scapulae are located over thoracic ribs two through seven. Check for an equal distance from the medial scapular edges to the midspinal line.

Ribs

After assessing the scapulae, inspect the ribs for visual abnormalities and palpate the surfaces of the ribs. Normal findings include firm, smooth, continuous bones.

Shoulders

Palpate the moving joints for crepitus. Inspect the skin overlying the shoulder joints for erythema, masses, or swelling.

Next, palpate the acromioclavicular joint and the area over the greater humeral tuberosity. Ask the patient to hold his arm at his side; then have him move his arm across his chest (adduction). Next, place your thumb on the anterior portion of the patient's shoulder joint and your fingers on the posterior portion of the joint. Ask the patient to abduct his arm, and palpate the shoulder joint as he does so.

(*Text continues on page 283.*)

Assessing muscle strength and joint range of motion

To evaluate muscle strength, have the patient perform active range-of-motion (ROM) movements as you apply resistance. Normally, the patient can move joints a certain distance (measured in degrees) and can easily resist pressure applied against movement. If the muscle group is weak, lessen the resistance to permit a more accurate assessment. Note that strength is normally symmetrical.

To assess joint ROM, ask the patient to move specific joints through normal ROM. If he can't do so, perform passive ROM. Use a goniometer to measure the angle achieved.

On the following pages, you'll find descriptions and diagrams of tests for muscle strength and ROM, including the expected degree of motion for each joint tested.

GRADING MUSCLE STRENGTH

When evaluating muscle strength, use the scale below. Column 1 describes the possible muscle response and its significance. Column 2 grades the response.

MUSCLE RESPONSE AND SIGNIFICANCE	GRADE RATING
No visible or palpable contraction ■ Paralysis	0
Slightly palpable contraction ■ Paresis, severe weakness	1
Passive ROM maneuvers when gravity is removed ■ Paresis, moderate weakness	2
Active ROM against gravity alone or against light resistance ■ Mild weakness	3 to 4
Active ROM against full resistance ■ Normal	5

CERVICAL SPINE AND NECK
Muscle strength

To assess muscles responsible for flexion of the cervical spine, place your hand on the patient's forehead, applying pressure. Ask him to bend his head forward and touch his chin to his chest. (Perform this maneuver only after cervical spine injury has been ruled out.)

To assess muscles responsible for cervical spine rotation, place your hand along the jaw. Ask the patient to push laterally against your hand while you attempt to prevent movement. At the same time, palpate the sternocleidomastoid on the opposite side. Repeat on the other side.

To assess muscles responsible for extension of the cervical spine, apply pressure with your hand on the patient's occipital bone. Ask him to bend his head backward as far as possible.

Assessing muscle strength and joint range of motion (continued)

Range of motion

Ask the patient to flex his neck, at tempting to touch his chin to his chest, and to extend his neck, bending his head backward.

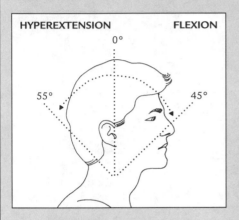

Next, ask him to bend laterally, touching his ears to his shoulders.

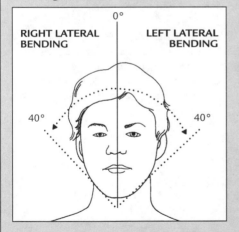

Then ask him to rotate his head from side to side (as shown at top right).

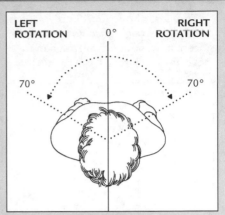

SHOULDER

Muscle strength

Test the trapezius muscles (of the shoulder and upper back) simultaneously. Ask the patient to shrug his shoulders freely, then again as you press down on them.

Range of motion

Observe and measure ROM as the patient demonstrates forward flexion, with the arms straight in front, and backward extension, with the arms straight and extended backward.

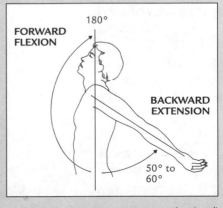

(continued)

ssing muscle strength and joint range of motion *(continued)*

To assess abduction, ask the patient to raise his straightened arm out to the side; to assess adduction, ask him to move his straightened arm to midline.

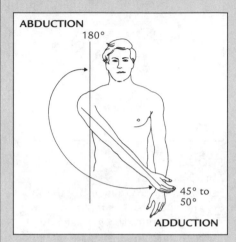

ABDUCTION
180°

45° to 50°

ADDUCTION

To assess external rotation, ask the patient to abduct his arm with his elbow bent, placing his hand behind his head.

To assess internal rotation, ask the patient to abduct his arm with his elbow bent, placing his hand behind the small of his back.

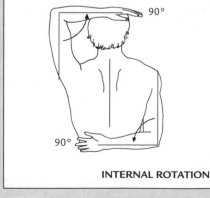

EXTERNAL ROTATION
90°

90°

INTERNAL ROTATION

UPPER ARM AND ELBOW
Muscle strength
To test triceps strength, try to flex the patient's arm while she tries to extend it (as shown below).

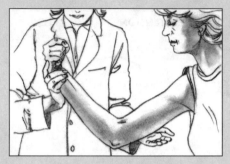

To assess biceps strength, try to pull the patient's flexed arm into extension while she resists.

To test deltoid strength, push down on the patient's arm (abducted to 90 degrees) while she resists.

Range of motion
Ask the patient to sit or stand. Then assess flexion by having him bend his arm and attempt to touch his shoulder. To assess extension, ask him to straighten his arm.

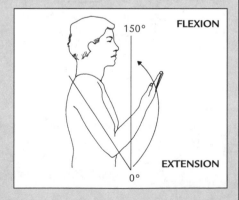

150° **FLEXION**

EXTENSION
0°

Assessing muscle strength and joint range of motion (continued)

Assess pronation by holding the patient's elbow in a flexed position while he rotates the arm until the palm faces the floor.

Assess supination by holding the patient's elbow in a flexed position while he rotates the arm until the palm faces upward.

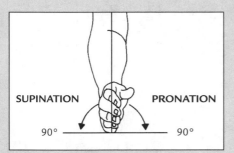

WRIST AND HAND
Muscle strength
Test muscle strength and movement of both hands simultaneously by having the patient squeeze the first two fingers of your hand, make a fist, resist your efforts to straighten a flexed wrist, and resist your efforts to flex a straightened wrist. (Normally, the dominant hand may be slightly stronger.)

Range of motion
To assess flexion, ask the patient to bend his wrist downward; assess extension by having him straighten his wrist.

To assess hyperextension or dorsiflexion, ask him to bend his wrist upward.

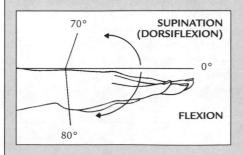

To assess the metacarpophalangeal joints, ask the patient to hyperextend (dorsiflex), extend (straighten), and flex (make a fist) the fingers.

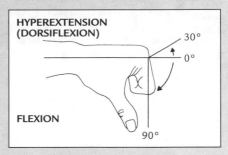

Assess radial deviation by asking the patient to move his hand toward the radial side; assess ulnar deviation by asking him to move his hand toward the ulnar side.

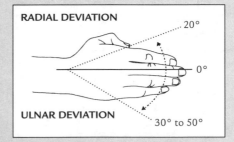

Also ask the patient to straighten the fingers, then spread them (abduct) and bring them together (adduct). Abduction should be 20 degrees between fingers; adduction, the fingers touch.

To assess palmar adduction, ask the patient to bring the thumb to the index finger; assess palmar abduction by asking the patient to move the thumb away from the palm. Assess opposition by having the patient touch the thumb to each fingertip.

(continued)

Assessing muscle strength and joint range of motion *(continued)*

THORACIC AND LUMBAR SPINE
Range of motion
Assess rotation by first stabilizing the patient's pelvis, then ask him to rotate the upper body from side to side.

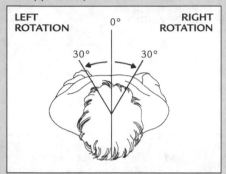

With the patient standing, observe and evaluate spinal ROM as he demonstrates hyperextension by bending backward from the waist and flexion by bending to touch the floor with the knees slightly bent.

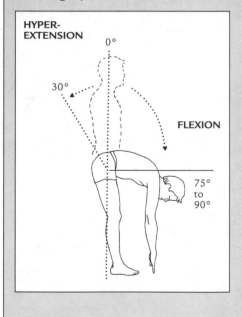

Ask the patient to bend to each side (lateral bending).

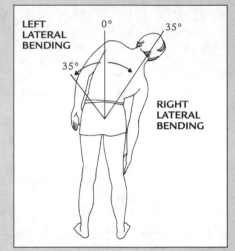

HIP AND PELVIS
Muscle strength
With the patient lying down (in a prone and, later, supine position) and then sitting, evaluate muscle strength and palpate muscles as you carry out these tests.

To assess hip extensors, ask the prone patient to hyperextend her leg backward (toward the ceiling) as you try to push her leg downward.

To assess hip flexors, ask the patient to sit and raise her knee to her chest as you apply downward pressure proximal to the knee.

To assess hip abductors, ask the side-lying patient to move her straightened leg away from midline as you try to push it toward midline.

To assess hip adductors, ask the side-lying patient to move her leg toward midline as you try to pull it away from midline (as shown at the top of the next page).

Assessing muscle strength and joint range of motion (continued)

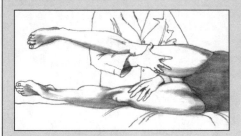

Range of motion

With the patient prone or standing, observe and evaluate ROM as the patient demonstrates flexion by bending the knee to the chest with the back straight. *Caution:* Don't perform this movement without the surgeon's permission on a patient who has undergone total hip replacement because the motion can cause the prosthesis to dislocate.

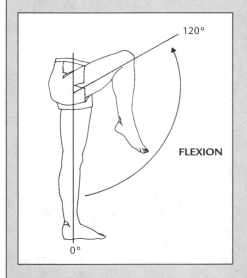

Evaluate extension by asking the patient to straighten his knee, and hyperextension by asking him to extend his leg backward with his knee straight. *Note:* This motion can be performed with the patient prone or standing.

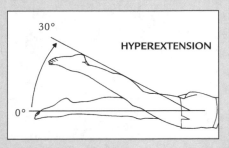

To assess abduction, have the patient move his straightened leg away from midline; assess adduction by having him move his straightened leg toward the opposite leg. *Caution:* This motion can displace a hip prosthesis.

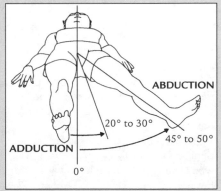

Finally, assess internal and external rotation by asking the patient to bend his knee and turn the leg inward and outward, respectively (as shown at top of the next page).

(continued)

Assessing muscle strength and joint range of motion (continued)

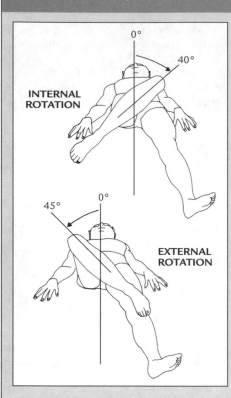

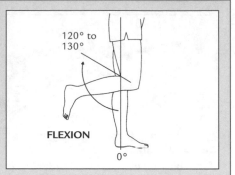

KNEE
Muscle strength
To assess knee extensors, ask the patient to sit or lie in a supine position and extend his leg as you attempt to flex it.

To assess knee flexors, ask the patient to sit or lie in a supine position while you try to extend his leg as he flexes his knee.

Range of motion
With the patient sitting or standing, observe and measure ROM as the patient demonstrates extension by straightening his leg at the knee. With the patient standing, have him demonstrate flexion by bending his leg at the knee and bringing his foot up to touch his buttock.

ANKLE AND FOOT
Muscle strength
To assess dorsiflexion of the ankle joint, apply pressure with your hand to the dorsal surface of the patient's foot as he attempts to bend his foot up.

To assess plantar flexion, apply pressure with your hand to the plantar surface of the patient's foot as he attempts to bend his foot down.

To assess inversion, apply pressure with your hand to the medial surface of the patient's first metatarsal bone as he attempts to move his toes inward. Assess eversion by placing your hand on the lateral surface of the 5th metatarsal bone and applying pressure as he attempts to move his toes outward.

Range of motion
Ask the patient who is sitting, lying, or standing to demonstrate plantar flexion by bending his foot downward and dorsiflexion by bending his foot upward.

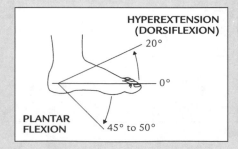

Assessing muscle strength and joint range of motion (continued)

Then ask him to invert his foot by pointing the toes and turning the foot inward and to evert the foot by pointing the toes and turning the foot outward.

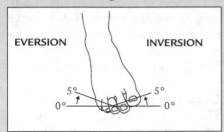

To assess forefoot adduction and abduction, stabilize the patient's heel while he turns his forefoot inward and outward, respectively.

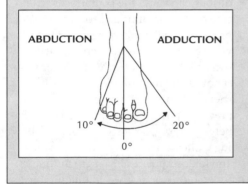

TOES
Muscle strength
To assess flexion, apply pressure with your finger to the plantar surface of the patient's toes as he attempts to bend his toes downward.

To assess extension, apply pressure with your finger to the dorsal surface of the patient's toes as he attempts to point his toes upward.

Range of motion
To assess the metatarsophalangeal joints, ask the patient to extend (straighten) and flex (curl) the toes. Then ask him to hyperextend his toes by straightening and pointing them upward.

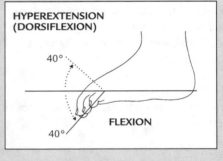

Now stand behind the patient. With your fingertips placed over the greater humeral tuberosity, instruct him to rotate his shoulder internally by moving the arm behind the back. This allows you to palpate a portion of the musculotendinous rotator cuff as well as the bony structures of the shoulder joint.

Elbows
Inspect joint contour and the skin over each elbow. Palpate the elbows at rest and during movement.

Wrists
Inspect the wrists for masses, erythema, skeletal deformities, and swelling. Palpate the wrist at rest and during movement by gently grasping it between your thumb and fingers.

Fingers and thumbs
On each hand, inspect the fingers and thumb for nodules, erythema, spacing, length, and skeletal deformities. Palpate fingers and thumb at rest and during movement.

Thoracic and lumbar spine

You'll need to palpate the length of the spine for tenderness and vertebral alignment. To check for tenderness, percuss each spinous process with the ulnar side of your fist.

Note whether the patient can move with full ROM, while maintaining balance, smoothness, and coordination.

Hips and pelvis

Inspect and palpate over the bony prominences: iliac crests, symphysis pubis, anterior spine, ischial tuberosities, and greater trochanters. Palpate the hip at rest and during movement.

Knees

Inspect the knees with the patient seated. Palpate the knee at rest and during movement. Inspect and palpate the popliteal spaces. Knee movements should be smooth. Palpate the joint line. If pain is elicited, you may be exacerbating a torn meniscus.

Ankles and feet

Inspect and palpate the ankles and feet at rest and during movement.

Toes

The patient may be sitting or lying in a supine position for toe assessment. Inspect all toe surfaces. Palpate toes at rest and during movement.

• • • • • • • • • • • •

CARPAL TUNNEL SYNDROME

Carpal tunnel syndrome, a form of repetitive stress injury, is the most common of the nerve entrapment syndromes. It results from compression of the median nerve at the wrist, within the carpal tunnel. This compression neuropathy causes sensory and motor changes in the median distribution of the hand.

AGE ALERT Carpal tunnel injury usually occurs in women between ages 30 and 60 and poses a serious occupational health problem.

Assembly-line workers and packers and people who repeatedly use poorly designed tools are most likely to develop this disorder. Any strenuous use of the hands — sustained grasping, twisting, or flexing — aggravates this condition.

Causes and pathophysiology

The carpal tunnel is formed by the carpal bones and the transverse carpal ligament. Inflammation or fibrosis of the tendon sheaths that pass through the carpal tunnel commonly causes edema and compression of the median nerve. Many conditions can cause the contents or structure of the carpal tunnel to swell and press the median nerve against the transverse carpal ligament. Such conditions include rheumatoid arthritis, flexor tenosynovitis (commonly associated with rheumatic disease), nerve compression, pregnancy, renal failure, menopause, diabetes mellitus, acromegaly, edema following Colles' fracture, hypothyroidism, amyloidosis, myxedema, benign tumors, tuberculosis, and other granulomatous diseases. Another source of damage to the median nerve is dislocation or acute sprain of the wrist.

Clinical presentation

The patient with carpal tunnel syndrome usually exhibits:

- weakness, pain, burning, numbness, or tingling in one or both hands
- paresthesia that affects the thumb, forefinger, middle finger, and half of the fourth finger
- inability to clench his hand into a fist
- atrophic nails
- dry and shiny skin

- symptoms are typically worse at night and in the morning.

The pain may spread to the forearm and, in severe cases, as far as the shoulder. The patient can usually relieve such pain by shaking or rubbing his hands vigorously or dangling his arms at his side. (See *The carpal tunnel*.)

Differential diagnoses
- Generalized peripheral neuropathy
- Brachial plexus lesion

Diagnosis
Physical examination reveals decreased sensation to light touch or pinpricks in the affected fingers. Thenar muscle atrophy occurs in about half of all cases of carpal tunnel syndrome, but it's usually a late sign. The patient exhibits a positive Tinel's sign (tingling over the median nerve on light percussion) and responds positively to Phalen's maneuver (holding the forearms vertically and allowing both hands to drop into complete flexion at the wrists for 1 minute reproduces symptoms of carpal tunnel syndrome). A compression test supports this diagnosis: A blood pressure cuff inflated above systolic pressure on the forearm for 1 to 2 minutes provokes pain and paresthesia along the distribution of the median nerve.

Electromyography detects a median nerve motor conduction delay of more than 5 milliseconds. Other laboratory tests may identify underlying disease.

Management
General
Conservative treatment should be tried first, including resting the hands by splinting the wrist in neutral extension for 1 to 2 weeks. If a definite link has been established between the patient's occupation and the development of repetitive stress injury, he may have to seek other work. Effective treatment may

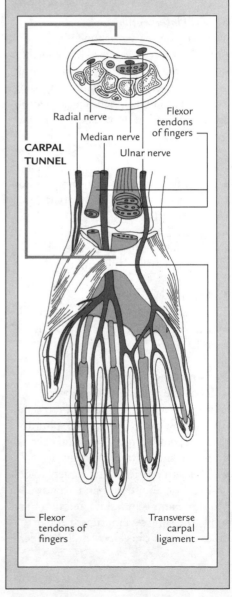

The carpal tunnel

The carpal tunnel is clearly visible in this palmar view and cross section of a right hand. Note the median nerve, flexor tendons of fingers, and blood vessels passing through the tunnel on their way from the forearm to the hand.

Radial nerve

Flexor tendons of fingers

Median nerve

CARPAL TUNNEL

Ulnar nerve

Flexor tendons of fingers

Transverse carpal ligament

also require correction of an underlying disorder.

Medication

Ibuprofen (300 to 800 mg P.O. t.i.d. to q.i.d.) may provide symptomatic relief.

Injecting the carpal tunnel with 5 to 75 mg of hydrocortisone every 2 to 3 weeks may provide significant but temporary relief.

Surgical intervention

When conservative treatment fails, the only alternative is surgical decompression of the nerve by resecting the entire transverse carpal tunnel ligament or by using endoscopic surgical techniques. Neurolysis (freeing of the nerve fibers) may also be necessary.

Referral

▪ Refer the patient to an orthopedic surgeon or neurosurgeon if conservative treatment fails.
▪ Suggest occupational counseling for the patient who has to change jobs because of repetitive stress injury.

Follow-up

The effectiveness of treatment should be monitored initially every 2 weeks then monthly.

Patient teaching

▪ Teach the patient how to apply a splint. Tell him not to make it too tight. Show him how to remove the splint to perform gentle range-of-motion exercises, which should be done daily.
▪ Advise the patient after surgery to occasionally exercise his hands in warm water. If the arm is in a sling, tell him to remove the sling several times per day to do exercises for his elbow and shoulder.

Complications

▪ Permanent disability
▪ Postoperative infection

• • • • • • • • • • • •

CLUBFOOT

Clubfoot, or talipes, is the most common congenital disorder of the lower extremities. It's marked primarily by a deformed talus and shortened Achilles tendon, which give the foot a characteristic club-like appearance. In talipes equinovarus, the foot points downward (equinus) and turns inward (varus), whereas the front of the foot curls toward the heel (forefoot adduction).

Clubfoot, which has an incidence of approximately 1 per 1,000 live births, usually occurs bilaterally and is twice as common in boys than in girls. It may be associated with other birth defects, such as myelomeningocele, spina bifida, and arthrogryposis. Clubfoot is correctable with prompt treatment.

Causes

A combination of genetic and environmental factors in utero appears to cause clubfoot. Heredity is a definite factor in some cases, although the mechanism of transmission is undetermined. If a child is born with clubfoot, his sibling has a 1 in 35 chance of being born with the same anomaly. Children of a parent with clubfoot have 1 in 10 chance. In children without a family history of clubfoot, this anomaly seems linked to arrested development during the 9th and 10th weeks of embryonic life, when the feet are formed. Researchers also suspect muscle abnormalities, leading to variations in length and tendon insertions, as possible causes of clubfoot.

Clinical presentation

Talipes equinovarus varies greatly in severity. Deformity may be so extreme that the toes touch the inside of the ankle, or it may be only vaguely apparent. In every case, these conditions are found:
- deformed talus
- shortened Achilles tendon
- shortened and flattened calcaneus.

Depending on the degree of the varus deformity, these conditions may be found:
- shortened and underdeveloped calf muscles
- soft-tissue contractures at the site of deformity
- foot is tight and resists manual efforts to push it into normal position.

Clubfoot is painless, except in elderly, arthritic patients. In older children, clubfoot may be secondary to paralysis, poliomyelitis, or cerebral palsy, in which case treatment must include management of the underlying disease.

Differential diagnoses
- True clubfoot
- Apparent clubfoot

Diagnosis

Early diagnosis of clubfoot is usually no problem because the deformity is obvious. In subtle deformity, however, true clubfoot must be distinguished from apparent clubfoot (metatarsus varus or pigeon-toed). Apparent clubfoot results when a fetus maintains a position in utero that gives his feet a clubfoot appearance at birth. This can usually be corrected manually. Another form of apparent clubfoot is inversion of the feet, resulting from the peroneal type of progressive muscular atrophy and progressive muscular dystrophy. In true clubfoot, X-rays show superimposition of the talus and the calcaneus and a ladderlike appearance of the metatarsals. (See *Recognizing clubfoot*, page 288.)

Management
General

The primary concern is recognition of clubfoot as early as possible, preferably in newborn infants.

Treatment for clubfoot is performed in three stages: correcting the deformity, maintaining the correction until the foot regains normal muscle balance, and observing the foot closely for several years to prevent the deformity from recurring. In neonates with true clubfoot, corrective treatment should begin at once. An infant's foot contains large amounts of cartilage; the muscles, ligaments, and tendons are supple. The ideal time to begin treatment is during the first few days and weeks of life, when the foot is most malleable.

Clubfoot deformities are usually corrected in sequential order. Several therapeutic methods have been tested and found effective in correcting clubfoot. In all patients, the first procedure should be simple manipulation and casting, whereby the foot is gently manipulated into a partially corrected position and held in place by a cast for several days or weeks. (The skin should be painted with a nonirritating adhesive liquid beforehand to prevent the cast from slipping.) After the cast is removed, the foot is manipulated into an even better position and casted again. This procedure is repeated as many times as necessary. In some cases, the shape of the cast can be transformed through a series of wedging maneuvers instead of changing the cast each time.

After correction of clubfoot, proper foot alignment should be maintained through exercise, night splints, and orthopedic shoes. With manipulating and casting, correction usually takes about 3

Recognizing clubfoot

Clubfoot may have various names, depending on the orientation of the deformity, as shown in the illustrations.

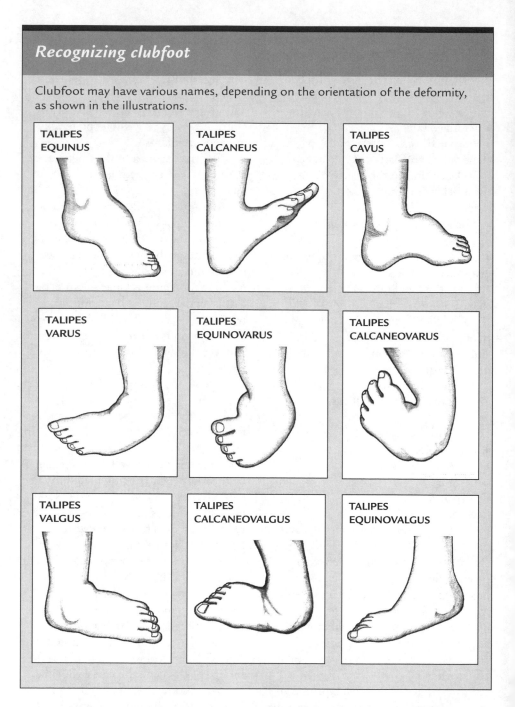

TALIPES EQUINUS

TALIPES CALCANEUS

TALIPES CAVUS

TALIPES VARUS

TALIPES EQUINOVARUS

TALIPES CALCANEOVARUS

TALIPES VALGUS

TALIPES CALCANEOVALGUS

TALIPES EQUINOVALGUS

months. The Denis Browne splint, a device that consists of two padded, metal footplates connected by a flat, horizontal bar, is sometimes used as a follow-up measure to help promote bilateral correction and strengthen the foot muscles.

Surgical intervention

Resistant clubfoot may require surgery. Older children, for example, with recurrent or neglected clubfoot usually need surgery. Tenotomy, tendon transfer, stripping of the plantar fascia, and capsulotomy are some of the surgical procedures that may be used. In severe cases, bone surgery (wedge resections, osteotomy, or astragalectomy) may be appropriate. After surgery, a cast is applied to preserve the correction. Clubfoot that's severe enough to require surgery is rarely totally correctable; however, surgery can usually ameliorate the deformity.

Referral

- Refer the patient to an orthopedic surgeon for treatment.
- The patient may need physical therapy.

Follow-up

The patient's progress should be evaluated as per the orthopedic surgeon and follow-up based on rate of recovery.

Patient teaching

- Stress to parents the importance of prompt treatment. Make sure they understand that clubfoot demands immediate therapy and orthopedic supervision until growth is completed.
- If the child is old enough to walk, caution parents not to let the foot part of the cast get soft and thin from wear. If it does, much of the correction may be lost.
- Explain to the older child and his parents that surgery can improve clubfoot with good function but can't totally correct it; the affected calf muscle will remain slightly underdeveloped.
- Emphasize the need for long-term orthopedic care to maintain correction. Teach parents the prescribed exercises that the child can do at home. Urge them to make the child wear the corrective shoes ordered and the splints during naps and at night. Make sure they understand that treatment for clubfoot continues during the entire growth period. Permanently correcting this defect takes time and patience.

Complications
- Residual deformity

Special considerations
- Look for any exaggerated attitudes in an infant's feet. Make sure you recognize the difference between true clubfoot and apparent clubfoot. Don't use excessive force in trying to manipulate a clubfoot. The foot with apparent clubfoot moves easily.

• • • • • • • • • • • •

DYSPLASIA OF THE HIP, DEVELOPMENTAL

Developmental dysplasia of the hip (DDH), an abnormality of the hip joint that's present from birth, is the most common disorder affecting hip joints of children under age 3. DDH can be unilateral or bilateral. This abnormality occurs in three forms of varying severity: unstable hip dysplasia, in which the hip is positioned normally but can be dislocated by manipulation; subluxation or incomplete dislocation, in which the femoral head rides on the edge of the acetabulum; and complete dislocation, in which the femoral head is totally outside the acetabulum.

Developmental hip subluxation or dislocation can cause abnormal acetabular development and permanent disability. About 85% of affected infants are females.

Causes

Experts are uncertain about the causes of DDH, but they know it's more likely to occur in the following circumstances:

■ Dislocation is 10 times more common after breech delivery (malpositioning in utero) than after cephalic delivery.

■ The condition is more common among large neonates and twins.

■ DDH occurs most commonly in members of the Navaho tribe, the Lapps of Scandinavia, and northern Italians.

Clinical presentation

Clinical effects of hip dysplasia vary with age. In newborns, dysplasia doesn't cause gross deformity or pain. However, in complete dysplasia, the hip rides above the acetabulum, causing the level of the knees to be uneven. As the child grows older and begins to walk, the abduction on the dislocated side is limited. Uncorrected bilateral dysplasia may cause him to sway from side to side, a condition known as "duck waddle"; unilateral dysplasia may produce a limp. If corrective treatment isn't begun until after age 2, DDH may cause degenerative hip changes, lordosis, joint malformation, and soft-tissue damage.

Differential diagnoses

■ Congenital subluxation of the hip
■ Congenital dislocation of the hip

Diagnosis

Several observations during physical examination of the relaxed child strongly suggest DDH. First, place the child on his back, and inspect the folds of skin over his thighs. Usually, a child in this position has an equal number of thigh folds on each side, but a child with subluxation or dislocation may have an extra fold on the affected side (this extra fold is also apparent when the child lies prone). Next, with the child lying prone, check

for alignment of the buttock fold. In a child with dysplasia, the buttock fold on the affected side is higher. In addition, abduction of the affected hip is restricted. (See *Complete dysplasia of the hip*.)

A positive Ortolani's sign confirms DDH. To elicit Ortolani's sign, place the infant on his back, with his hip flexed and in abduction. Adducting the hip while pressing the femur downward will dislocate the hip. Then abducting the hip while moving the femur upward will move the femoral head over the acetabular rim. If you hear a click or feel a jerk as the femoral head moves, the test is positive. This sign indicates subluxation in an infant younger than 1 month and subluxation or complete dislocation in an older infant.

A positive Trendelenburg's sign also confirms DDH. To elicit Trendelenburg's sign, have the child rest his weight on the side of the dislocation and lift his other knee. His pelvis drops on the normal side because of weak abductor muscles in the affected hip. However, when the child stands with his weight on the normal side and lifts the other knee, the pelvis remains horizontal.

X-rays show the location of the femur head and a shallow acetabulum; they can also be used to monitor the progress of the disease or treatment. Sonography and magnetic resonance imaging may also be used to assess reduction.

Management

General

The earlier the infant receives treatment, the better his chances are for normal development. Treatment varies with the patient's age. In infants younger than 3 months, treatment includes gentle manipulation to reduce the dislocation, followed by holding the hips in a flexed and abducted position with a splint-brace or harness to maintain the reduction. The infant must wear this apparatus continuously for 2 to 3 months and then use a night splint for another month so the joint capsule can tighten and stabilize in correct alignment.

If treatment doesn't begin until after age 3 months, it may include bilateral skin traction (in infants) or skeletal traction (in children who have started walking) in an attempt to reduce the dislocation by gradually abducting the hips. In Bryant's traction, or divarication traction, both extremities are placed in traction, even if only one is affected, to help maintain immobilization. This type of traction is used in children who are younger than 3 years and weigh less than 35 lb (16 kg). The length of treatment is 2 to 3 weeks.

Surgical intervention

If traction fails, gentle closed reduction under general anesthesia can further abduct the hips; the child is then placed in a hip spica cast for 4 to 6 months. If closed treatment fails, open reduction, followed by immobilization in a hip spica cast for an average of 6 months, or osteotomy may be considered.

In the child aged 2 to 5 years, treatment is difficult and includes skeletal traction and subcutaneous adductor tenotomy. Treatment begun after age 5 rarely restores satisfactory hip function.

Referral

- The patient may need to be referred to an orthopedic surgeon for cast placement and hip abduction.
- If necessary, refer the child and parents to a child-life specialist to ensure continued developmental progress.

Follow-up

The patient should follow up with the orthopedic physician in order to assess successful treatment.

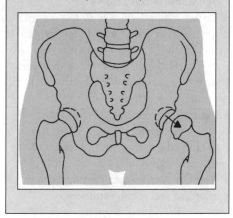

Complete dysplasia of the hip

In complete dislocation, the femoral head is totally displaced outside the acetabulum (see arrow).

Patient teaching

- Teach parents how to correctly splint or brace the patient's hips, as ordered. Stress the need for frequent checkups.
- During the child's first few days in a cast or splint-brace, he may be prone to irritability due to the unaccustomed restricted movement. Encourage his parents to stay with him as much as possible and to calm and reassure him.
- Instruct parents to remove braces and splints while bathing the infant but to replace them immediately afterward. Stress good hygiene; parents should bathe and change the child frequently and wash his perineum with warm water and soap at each diaper change.
- Tell parents to watch for signs that the child is outgrowing the cast (cyanosis, cool extremities, or pain).
- The patient in Bryant's traction may be cared for at home if the parents are taught traction application and maintenance.

Complications
- Reduced hip function
- Inability to reduce dislocation
- Degenerative hip changes
- Joint malformation

Special considerations
- Listen sympathetically to the parents' expressions of anxiety and fear. Explain possible causes of developmental hip dislocation, and give reassurance that early, prompt treatment will probably result in complete correction.
- Assure parents that the child will adjust to this restriction and return to normal sleeping, eating, and playing behavior in a few days.
- Tell the parents that treatment may be prolonged and requires patience.

• • • • • • • • • • • • •

EPICONDYLITIS

Lateral epicondylitis of the elbow (tennis elbow) is inflammation of the extensor tendons of the forearm. Medial epicondylitis (golfer's elbow) is inflammation at the origin of the flexor muscles of the wrist.

Causes
Epicondylitis probably begins as a partial tear and is common among tennis players or persons whose activities require a forceful grasp, wrist extension against resistance, or frequent rotation of the forearm. Untreated epicondylitis may become disabling as adherent fibers form between the tendons and the elbow capsule.

Clinical presentation
The patient's initial symptom is elbow pain that gradually worsens and often radiates to the forearm and back of the hand whenever he grasps an object or twists his elbow.

Other associated signs and symptoms include:
- tenderness over the involved lateral or medial epicondyle or over the head of the radius
- weak grasp
- local heat
- swelling
- restricted range of motion.

Differential diagnoses
- Trauma to elbow
- Fracture of elbow

Diagnosis
Because X-rays are almost always negative, diagnosis typically depends on clinical signs and symptoms and a patient history of playing tennis or engaging in similar activities. The pain can be reproduced by wrist extension and supination with lateral involvement or by flexion and pronation with medial epicondyle involvement. A "tennis elbow strap" has helped many patients. This strap, which is wrapped snugly around the forearm approximately 1″ (2.5 cm) below the epicondyle, helps relieve the strain on affected forearm muscles and tendons.

Management
General
Supportive treatment includes an immobilizing splint from the distal forearm to the elbow, which generally relieves pain in 2 to 3 weeks; heat therapy, such as warm compresses, short wave diathermy, and ultrasound (alone or in combination with diathermy); and physical therapy, such as manipulation and massage to detach the tendon from the chronically inflamed periosteum.

Medication
Medications used to treat epicondylitis may include:

- prednisolone — 2 to 30 mg, injected into affected joint
- lidocaine 1% — 0.5 to 1 ml, injected into affected joint
- ibuprofen — 300 to 800 mg P.O. t.i.d. to q.i.d.

Surgical intervention
If supportive measures prove ineffective, surgical release of the tendon at the epicondyle may be necessary.

Referral
- The patient may need to be referred to an orthopedic surgeon.
- The patient may need physical therapy.

Follow-up
The patient should be monitored until symptoms subside.

Patient teaching
- Instruct the patient to rest the elbow until inflammation subsides.
- Instruct the patient to follow the prescribed exercise program. For example, he may stretch his arm and flex his wrist to the maximum, then press the back of his hand against a wall until he can feel a pull in his forearm; he should hold this position for 1 minute.
- Advise the patient to warm up for 15 to 20 minutes before beginning any sports activity.
- Urge the patient to wear an elastic support or splint during any activity that stresses the forearm or elbow.

Complications
- Tendon rupture
- Permanent disability of elbow

Special considerations
- Tell the patient to check his equipment. For example, a tennis racquet may not be the right size or weight. Also changing surfaces may help to reduce stress.

FIBROMYALGIA SYNDROME

A diffuse pain syndrome, fibromyalgia syndrome (FMS, previously called fibrositis) is one of the most common causes of chronic musculoskeletal pain; it's observed in up to 15% of patients seen in general rheumatology practice and 5% of general medicine clinic patients. Symptoms of FMS include diffuse musculoskeletal pain, daily fatigue, and sleep disturbances. Multiple tender points in specific areas on examination is the characteristic feature. Women are affected more commonly than men. It may occur as a primary disorder or in association with an underlying disease, such as systemic lupus erythematosus, rheumatoid arthritis, osteoarthritis, and sleep apnea syndromes.

AGE ALERT FMS can affect all age-groups; its peak incidence is between ages 20 and 60.

FMS has also been reported in children, who tend to have more diffuse pain and sleep disturbances than adult patients. Children may have fewer tender points, and many patients improve over 2 to 3 years.

Causes
The cause of FMS is unknown, but there are many theories regarding its pathophysiology. Although the pain is located primarily in muscle areas, no distinct abnormalities have been documented on microscopic evaluation of biopsies of tender points when compared with normal muscle. Other theories suggest decreased blood flow to muscle tissue (due to poor muscle aerobic conditioning versus other physiologic abnormalities); decreased blood flow in the thalamus and caudate nucleus, leading to a lowering of the pain threshold; endocrine dysfunction, such as abnormal pituitary-adrenal axis respons-

Tender points of fibromyalgia

The patient with fibromyalgia syndrome may complain of specific areas of tenderness, as indicated in the illustrations.

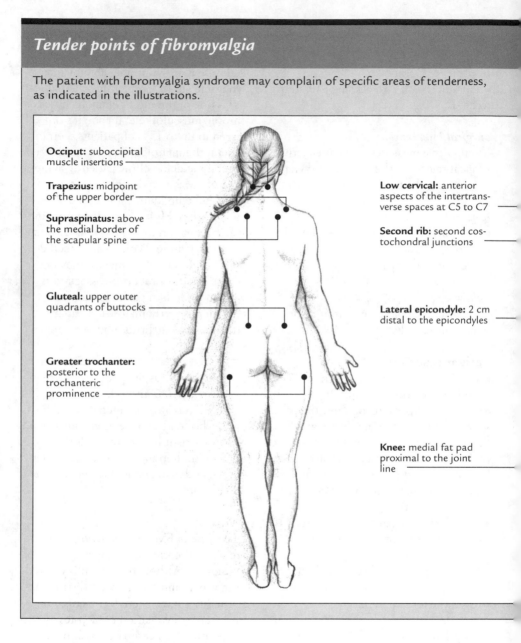

Occiput: suboccipital muscle insertions

Trapezius: midpoint of the upper border

Supraspinatus: above the medial border of the scapular spine

Gluteal: upper outer quadrants of buttocks

Greater trochanter: posterior to the trochanteric prominence

Low cervical: anterior aspects of the intertransverse spaces at C5 to C7

Second rib: second costochondral junctions

Lateral epicondyle: 2 cm distal to the epicondyles

Knee: medial fat pad proximal to the joint line

es; and abnormal levels of the neurotransmitter serotonin in brain centers, which affect pain and sleep. Abnormal functioning of other pain-processing pathways may also be involved. Considering overlap of symptoms with other pain syndromes, such as chronic fatigue syndrome, raises the question of an asso-

ciation with an infection, such as with parvovirus B19. Human immunodeficiency virus infection and Lyme disease have also been associated with FMS.

It's possible that the development of FMS is multifactorial and is influenced by stress (physical and mental), physical conditioning, and quality of sleep as well

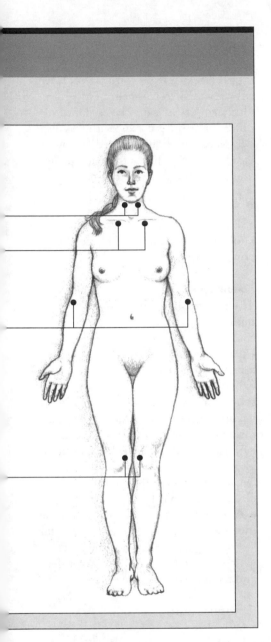

lower back, and proximal limbs. It can involve all four body quadrants — bilateral upper trunk and arms and bilateral lower trunk and legs. Other signs and symptoms include:
- pain is commonly worse in the morning, accompanied by stiffness
- pain that varies from day to day (may be exacerbated by stress, lack of sleep, weather changes, and inactivity).
- sleep disturbance.

Other clinical features associated with FMS include:
- irritable bowel syndrome
- tension headaches
- "puffy hands" (sensation of hand swelling, especially in the morning)
- paresthesia.

Differential diagnoses
- Muscle strain
- Temporal arteritis
- Muscle disease
- Chronic fatigue syndrome
- Tendinitis

Diagnosis
Diagnostic testing for FMS (not associated with an underlying disease) usually doesn't reveal significant abnormalities. For example, an examination of joints doesn't reveal synovitis or significant swelling; a neurologic examination is normal; and no laboratory or radiologic abnormalities are common in FMS patients. Tenderness can be elicited by applying a moderate amount of pressure to specific locations. (See *Tender points of fibromyalgia.*) Although this examination can be fairly subjective, many FMS patients with true tender points wince or withdraw when pressure is applied to a tender point. Pressure can also be applied to nontender control points, such as the midforehead, distal forearm, and midanterior thigh, to assess for conversion reactions (psychogenic rheumatism), in

as by neuroendocrine, psychiatric and, possibly, hormonal factors (due to the female predominance).

Clinical presentation
The primary symptom of FMS is a diffuse, dull, aching pain that's typically concentrated across the neck, shoulders,

which patients hurt everywhere, or for other psychosomatic illnesses.

Overall, the diagnosis of FMS is made in a patient with characteristic symptoms and multiple tender points on examination and after ruling out other illnesses that can cause similar features.

Management
General
The most important aspect of FMS management is patient education. Patients must understand that although FMS pain can be severe and is commonly chronic, this syndrome is common and doesn't lead to deforming or life-threatening complications.

A regular, low-impact aerobic exercise program can be effective in improving muscle conditioning, energy levels, and an overall sense of well-being. The patient may also benefit from physical therapy, the injection of tender points with steroids or lidocaine, massage therapy, and ultrasound treatments for particularly problem areas. A few studies have shown that acupuncture and phototherapy are also beneficial.

Medication
Drug therapy is typically used to improve the patient's quality of sleep and for pain control. Tricyclic antidepressants may improve sleep but produce anticholinergic adverse effects and daytime drowsiness; examples include:
- amitriptyline — 50 to 150 mg P.O. h.s. p.r.n.
- nortriptyline — 75 to 150 mg/day P.O.

Hypnotic agents, such as diazepam (2 to 10 mg P.O. b.i.d. to t.i.d.), are less useful overall because they generally don't prevent the frequent awakenings through the night.

The combination of a tricyclic antidepressant at bedtime with a serotonin uptake inhibitor such as fluoxetine (20 to 80 mg/ day) during the day may also be useful.

Nonsteroidal anti-inflammatory drugs (NSAIDs) and corticosteroids typically aren't effective against FMS pain, although NSAIDs may be used if tendinitis or arthritis coexist with this disorder. Narcotics should be used only with extreme caution to control pain, preferably under the guidance of a pain clinic.

Referral
- The patient may need a referral for psychological counseling to help cope with chronic pain.

Follow-up
The patient should be seen in 3 to 6 months.

Patient teaching
- Explain to the patient that she may experience increased muscle pain when starting a new exercise program. If this occurs, suggest that she decrease the duration or intensity of the exercise. Encourage the patient not to stop exercising altogether, unless otherwise indicated, because even a limited amount of exercise each day may be beneficial.
- Advise the patient whose drug regimen includes a tricyclic antidepressant to take the dose 1 to 2 hours before bedtime, which may improve its benefits for sleep and reduce morning drowsiness.

Complications
- Work loss
- Disability
- Drug loss

Special considerations
- FMS shouldn't be confused with chronic myofascial pain, which is characterized by unilateral and commonly focal or regional pain (as opposed to FMS, in which the pain is bilateral and diffuse), minimal fa-

tigue or stiffness, and few focal tender points (commonly distinguished as trigger points) that may produce a radiating pain along a muscle group or tendon (unlike in FMS, where tender points aren't usually associated with radiating pain along a muscle group or tendon).

• • • • • • • • • • • •

GOUT

Gout, also called gouty arthritis, is a metabolic disease marked by urate deposits, which cause painfully arthritic joints. It can strike any joint but favors those in the feet and legs. Gout follows an intermittent course and commonly leaves patients totally free from symptoms for years between attacks. It can cause chronic disability or incapacitation and, rarely, severe hypertension and progressive renal disease. The prognosis is good with treatment.

AGE ALERT Primary gout usually occurs in men older than age 30 and in postmenopausal women; secondary gout occurs in elderly patients.

Causes

Although the exact cause of primary gout remains unknown, it appears to be linked to a genetic defect in purine metabolism, which causes elevated blood levels of uric acid (hyperuricemia) due to overproduction of uric acid, retention of uric acid, or both. In secondary gout, which develops during the course of another disease (such as obesity, diabetes mellitus, hypertension, sickle cell anemia, and renal disease), hyperuricemia results from the breakdown of nucleic acids. Myeloproliferative and lymphoproliferative diseases, psoriasis, and hemolytic anemia are the most common causes. Secondary gout can also follow drug therapy, especially with hydrochlorothiazide or pyrazinamide,

both of which interfere with urate excretion. Other medications that impair the tubular excretion of urate, such as low-dose salicylates and cyclosporine, can also cause hyperuricemia. Increased concentration of uric acid leads to urate deposits (tophi) in joints or tissues and consequent local necrosis or fibrosis.

Clinical presentation

Gout develops in four stages: asymptomatic, acute, intercritical, and chronic.
- Asymptomatic gout causes serum urate levels to rise but produces no symptoms. As the disease progresses, it may cause hypertension or nephrolithiasis accompanied by severe back pain.
- Acute gout strikes suddenly and peaks quickly. Although it generally involves only one or a few joints, this initial attack is extremely painful. Affected joints are hot, tender, and inflamed and appear dusky-red or cyanotic. The metatarsophalangeal joint of the great toe usually becomes inflamed first (podagra), followed by the instep, ankle, heel, knee, or wrist joints. Sometimes a low-grade fever is present. Mild acute attacks commonly subside quickly but tend to recur at irregular intervals. Severe attacks may persist for days or weeks. (See *Sydenham's description of gout*, page 298.)
- Intercritical gout produces periods that are symptom-free intervals between gout attacks. After the initial attack, most patients have a second attack within 6 months to 2 years, but in some the second attack doesn't occur for 5 to 10 years. Delayed attacks are more common in untreated patients and tend to be longer and more severe than initial attacks. Such attacks are also polyarticular, invariably affecting joints in the feet and legs, and are sometimes accompanied by fever. A migratory attack sequentially strikes various joints and the Achilles tendon and is

Sydenham's description of gout

For clarity and vividness, few passages in medical literature can rival the following classic description of an acute gout attack written by Thomas Sydenham, the famous 17th-century British doctor who suffered from gout for 34 years:

"The victim goes to bed and sleeps in good health. About two o'clock in the morning he is awakened by a severe pain in the great toe; more rarely in the heel, ankle, or instep. This pain is like that of a dislocation, and yet the parts feel as if cold water were poured over them. Then follow chills and shivers, and a little fever. The pain, which was at first moderate, becomes more intense. With its intensity the chills and shivers increase. After a time this comes to its height, accommodating itself to the bones and ligaments of the tarsus and metatarsus. Now it's a violent stretching and tearing of the ligaments — now it's a gnawing pain and now a pressure and tightening. So exquisite and lively meanwhile is the feeling of the part affected, that it cannot bear the weight of bedclothes nor the jar of a person walking in the room. The night is passed in torture, sleeplessness, turning of the part affected, and perpetual change of posture; the tossing about of the body being as incessant as the pain of the tortured joint, and being worse as the fit comes on. Hence the vain effort by change of posture, both in the body and the limb affected, to obtain an abatement of the pain."

From *The Works of Thomas Sydenham,* translated by R.G. Latham. Vol. II, p. 214. London: Sydenham Society, 1850.

associated with either subdeltoid or olecranon bursitis.

■ Chronic polyarticular gout eventually sets in. This final, unremitting stage of the disease is marked by persistent painful polyarthritis, with large, subcutaneous tophi in cartilage, synovial membranes, tendons, and soft tissue. Tophi form in fingers, hands, knees, feet, ulnar sides of the forearms, helix of the ear, Achilles tendons and, rarely, internal organs, such as the kidneys and myocardium. (See *Gouty deposits.*) The skin over the tophus may ulcerate and release a chalky, white exudate or pus. Chronic inflammation and tophaceous deposits precipitate secondary joint degeneration, with eventual erosions, deformity, and disability. Kidney involvement, with associated tubular damage, leads to chronic renal dysfunction. Hypertension and albuminuria occur in some patients; urolithiasis is common.

Differential diagnoses
■ Infectious arthritis
■ Cellulitis
■ Pseudogout
■ Lyme disease

Diagnosis
The presence of monosodium urate monohydrate crystals in synovial fluid taken from an inflamed joint or tophus establishes the diagnosis.

Aspiration of synovial fluid (arthrocentesis) or of tophaceous material reveals needlelike intracellular crystals of sodium urate. Although hyperuricemia isn't specifically diagnostic of gout, serum uric acid is above normal. Urinary uric acid is usually higher in secondary gout than in primary gout. In acute attacks, erythrocyte sedimentation rate and white blood cell (WBC) count are usually elevated, and WBC count shifts to the left.

Initially, X-rays are normal. However, in chronic gout, X-rays show "punched out" erosions, sometimes with periosteal overgrowth. Outward displacement of the overhanging margin from the bone contour characterizes gout. X-rays rarely show tophi. (See *Understanding pseudogout*, page 300.)

Management
General
Correct management seeks to terminate an acute attack, reduce hyperuricemia, and prevent recurrence, complications, and the formation of kidney stones. Treatment for the patient with acute gout consists of bed rest; immobilization and protection of the inflamed, painful joints; and local application of heat or cold, whichever one works for the patient. Treatment for chronic gout aims to decrease serum uric acid level through the use of medication and diet. Adjunctive therapy emphasizes a few dietary restrictions, primarily the avoidance of alcohol and purine-rich foods. Obese patients should try to lose weight because obesity puts additional stress on painful joints.

Medication
The following medications may be used to treat gout:
- ibuprofen — 300 to 800 mg P.O. t.i.d. to q.i.d.
- indomethacin — 50 mg P.O. t.i.d.
- allopurinol — 200 to 600 mg/day P.O.
- probenecid — 250 mg P.O. b.i.d. for 1 week then 500 mg P.O. b.i.d to a maximum of 2 g/day
- sulfinpyrazone — 200 to 400 mg P.O. b.i.d.
- colchicine — initially 0.5 to 1.3 mg P.O. followed by 0.5 to 0.65 mg P.O. every 1 to 2 hours; maximum daily dose is 4 mg P.O.

Gouty deposits

The final stage of gout is marked by painful polyarthritis, with large, subcutaneous, tophaceous deposits in cartilage, synovial membranes, tendons, and soft tissue. The skin over the tophus is shiny, thin, and taut.

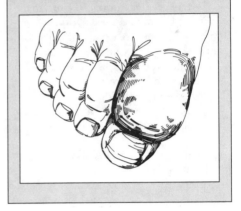

For resistant inflammation or joint aspiration, the following agents may be required:
- corticotropin — 40 to 80 U/day I.M.
- prednisone — 5 to 60 mg/day P.O.; dosage is highly individualized.

An intra-articular corticosteroid injection may be needed.

Surgical intervention
In some cases, surgery may be necessary to improve joint function or correct deformities. Tophi must be excised and drained if they become infected or ulcerated. They can also be excised to prevent ulceration, improve the patient's appearance, or make it easier for him to wear shoes or gloves.

Referral
- The patient may need to be referred to an orthopedic surgeon if surgery is required.

Understanding pseudogout

Also known as calcium pyrophosphate disease or CPPD, pseudogout results when calcium pyrophosphate crystals collect in periarticular joint structures.

SIGNS AND SYMPTOMS

Like true gout, pseudogout causes sudden joint pain and swelling, most commonly of the knee, wrist, and ankle or other peripheral joints.

Pseudogout attacks are self-limiting and triggered by stress, trauma, surgery, severe dieting, thiazide therapy, or alcohol abuse. Associated symptoms resemble those of rheumatoid arthritis.

ESTABLISHING A DIAGNOSIS

Diagnosis of pseudogout hinges on joint aspiration and synovial biopsy to detect calcium pyrophosphate crystals. X-rays show calcium deposits in the fibrocartilage and linear markings along the bone ends. Blood tests may detect an underlying endocrine or metabolic disorder.

RELIEF FOR PRESSURE AND INFLAMMATION

Management of pseudogout may include aspirating the joint to relieve pressure; instilling corticosteroids and administering analgesics, salicylates, phenylbutazone, or other nonsteroidal anti-inflammatory drugs to treat inflammation; and, if appropriate, treating the underlying disorder. Without treatment, pseudogout leads to permanent joint damage in about half of those it affects, most of whom are older adults.

Follow-up

The effectiveness of treatment should be assessed within 48 to 72 hours after initiation, then in 1 week, and then in 1 month. Blood studies (complete blood count, renal and hepatic panels) and urinalysis should be checked initially after treatment starts, then every 3 to 6 months.

Patient teaching

- Urge the patient to drink plenty of fluids (up to 64 oz [2 L] per day) to prevent the formation of kidney stones. When forcing fluids, record intake and output accurately. Be sure to monitor serum uric acid levels regularly. Alkalinize urine with sodium bicarbonate or other agent, if ordered.
- Make sure the patient understands the importance of checking serum uric acid levels periodically. Tell him to avoid high-purine foods, such as anchovies, liver, sardines, kidneys, sweetbreads, lentils, and alcoholic beverages—especially beer and wine—which raise the urate level. Explain the principles of a gradual weight reduction diet to obese patients. Such a diet features foods containing moderate amounts of protein and very little fat.
- Advise the patient receiving allopurinol, probenecid, and other drugs to immediately report any adverse effects, such as drowsiness, dizziness, nausea, vomiting, urinary frequency, or dermatitis. Warn the patient taking probenecid or sulfinpyrazone to avoid aspirin or any other salicylate. Their combined effect causes urate retention.
- Inform the patient that long-term colchicine therapy is essential during the first 3 to 6 months of treatment with uricosuric drugs or allopurinol.

Complications

- Renal calculi
- Uric acid neuropathy
- Deformed joints

Special considerations

■ Watch for acute gout attacks 24 to 96 hours after surgery. Even minor surgery can precipitate an attack. Before and after surgery, administer colchicine, as ordered, to help prevent gout attacks.

• • • • • • • • • • • •

HERNIATED DISK

Herniated disk, also called ruptured or slipped disk and herniated nucleus pulposus, occurs when all or part of the nucleus pulposus — the soft, gelatinous, central portion of an intervertebral disk — is forced through the disk's weakened or torn outer ring (anulus fibrosus). When this happens, the extruded disk may impinge on spinal nerve roots as they exit from the spinal canal or on the spinal cord itself, resulting in back pain and other signs of nerve root irritation. Herniated disk usually occurs in adults (mostly men) under age 45.

Causes

Herniated disks may result from severe trauma or strain or may be related to intervertebral joint degeneration. In elderly patients, whose disks have begun to degenerate, minor trauma may cause herniation. Ninety percent of herniation occurs in the lumbar and lumbosacral, 8% in the cervical, and 1% to 2% in the thoracic regions of the spine. Patients with a congenitally small lumbar spinal canal or with osteophyte formation on the vertebrae may be more susceptible to nerve root compression by a herniated disk and are more likely to have neurologic symptoms.

Clinical presentation

The overriding symptom of lumbar herniated disk is severe lower back pain that radiates to the buttocks, legs, and feet, usually unilaterally. When herniation follows trauma, the pain may begin suddenly, subside in a few days, and then recur at shorter intervals and with progressive intensity. Sciatic pain follows, beginning as a dull pain in the buttocks. Valsalva's maneuver, coughing, sneezing, or bending intensifies the pain, which is commonly accompanied by muscle spasms. Herniated disk may also cause sensory and motor loss in the area innervated by the compressed spinal nerve root and, in later stages, weakness and atrophy of leg muscles.

Differential diagnoses

■ Compression fracture
■ Vertebral fracture
■ Primary tumor
■ Malingering

Diagnosis

Obtaining a careful patient history is vital because the events that intensify disk pain are diagnostically significant. The straight-leg–raising test and its variants are perhaps the best tests for herniated disk.

X-rays of the spine are essential to rule out other abnormalities but may not diagnose herniated disk because marked disk prolapse can be present despite a normal X-ray. A thorough check of the patient's peripheral vascular status — including posterior tibial and dorsalis pedis pulses and skin temperature of extremities — helps rule out ischemic disease, another cause of leg pain or numbness. After physical examination and X-rays, myelography, computed tomography scanning, and magnetic resonance imaging (MRI) provide the most specific diagnostic information, showing spinal canal compression by herniated disk material. MRI is the method of choice to confirm the diagnosis and determine the exact level of herniation.

Management
General
Unless neurologic impairment progresses rapidly, treatment is initially conservative and consists of several weeks of bed rest (possibly with pelvic traction), administration of heat applications, nonsteroidal anti-inflammatory drugs, and an exercise program. Physical therapy may be used to reduce pain. Herniated disk requires supportive care, careful patient teaching, and strong emotional support to help the patient cope with the discomfort and frustration of chronic lower back pain.

Medication
Epidural corticosteroids, short-term oral corticosteroids, or nerve root blocks, may be used to decrease pain.

Muscle relaxants, such as the following agents, may relieve associated muscle spasms:
- diazepam — 2 to 10 mg P.O. b.i.d. to q.i.d.
- methocarbamol — 1 to 1.5 g P.O. q.i.d.
- cyclobenzaprine — 20 to 60 mg/day P.O.

Injection of chymopapain pKat (2,000 to 4,000 U) into the herniated disk produces a loss of water and proteoglycans from the disk, thereby reducing both the disk's size and the pressure in the nerve root.

Surgical intervention
A herniated disk that fails to respond to conservative treatment may require surgery. The most common procedure, laminectomy, involves excision of a portion of the lamina and removal of the protruding disk. If laminectomy doesn't alleviate pain and disability, a spinal fusion may be necessary to overcome segmental instability. Laminectomy and spinal fusion are sometimes performed concurrently to stabilize the spine. Microdiskectomy can also be used to remove fragments of nucleus pulposus.

Referral
- The patient may need to be referred to an orthopedic surgeon or neurosurgeon, if surgery is necessary.
- The patient may need psychological counseling to help cope with chronic pain.

Follow-up
The patient should be monitored every 2 weeks until full recovery occurs.

Patient teaching
- Teach the patient to use antiembolism stockings, and encourage the patient to move his legs, as allowed.
- Advise the patient to drink plenty of fluids to prevent renal stasis, and remind him to cough, deep-breathe, and use an incentive spirometer to preclude pulmonary complications.
- Teach the patient who has undergone spinal fusion how to wear a brace. Assist with toe-pointing exercises and straight-leg–raising. Teach proper body mechanics — bending at the knees and hips (never at the waist), standing straight, and carrying objects close to the body. Advise the patient to lie down when tired and to sleep on his side (never on his abdomen) on an extra-firm mattress or a bed board. Urge maintenance of proper weight to prevent lordosis caused by obesity.
- Tell the patient who must receive a muscle relaxant of possible adverse effects, especially drowsiness. Warn him to avoid activities that require alertness until he has built up a tolerance to the drug's sedative effects.

Complications
- Limited movement
- Alteration in lifestyle and work
- Footdrop
- Chronic lower back pain
- Depression

Special considerations
- During conservative treatment, watch for any deterioration in neurologic status, which may indicate an urgent need for surgery.
- If the patient requires chemonucleolysis, make sure he isn't allergic to meat tenderizers (chymopapain is a similar substance). Such an allergy contraindicates the use of this enzyme, which can produce severe anaphylaxis in a sensitive patient.

• • • • • • • • • • • •

KYPHOSIS

Kyphosis, also called humpback, is an anteroposterior curving of the spine that causes a bowing of the back, commonly at the thoracic, but sometimes at the thoracolumbar or sacral, level. The normal spine displays some convexity, but excessive thoracic kyphosis is pathologic. Kyphosis occurs in children and adults.

Causes
Congenital kyphosis is rare but usually severe, with resultant cosmetic deformity and reduced pulmonary function.

Adolescent kyphosis (Scheuermann's disease, juvenile kyphosis, vertebral epiphysitis), the most common form of this disorder, may result from growth retardation or a vascular disturbance in the vertebral epiphysis (usually at the thoracic level) during periods of rapid growth or from congenital deficiency in the thickness of the vertebral plates. Other causes include infection, inflammation, aseptic necrosis, and disk degeneration. The subsequent stress of weight bearing on the compromised vertebrae may result in the thoracic hump commonly seen in adolescents with kyphosis. Symptomatic adolescent kyphosis is more prevalent in girls than in boys and occurs most commonly between ages 12 and 16.

Adult kyphosis (adult humpback) may result from aging and associated degeneration of intervertebral disks, atrophy, and osteoporotic collapse of the vertebrae; from endocrine disorders, such as hyperparathyroidism and Cushing's disease; and from prolonged steroid therapy. Adult kyphosis may also result from conditions, such as arthritis, Paget's disease, polio, compression fracture of the thoracic vertebrae, metastatic tumor, plasma cell myeloma, or tuberculosis. In children and adults, kyphosis may also result from poor posture. (See *Identifying kyphosis*, page 304.)

Disk lesions called Schmorl's nodes may develop in anteroposterior curving of the spine and are localized protrusions of nuclear material through the cartilage plates and into the spongy bone of the vertebral bodies. If the anterior portions of the cartilage are destroyed, bridges of new bone may transverse the intervertebral space, causing ankylosis.

Clinical presentation
Development of adolescent kyphosis is usually insidious, commonly occurring after a history of excessive sports activity, and may be asymptomatic except for the obvious curving of the back (sometimes more than 90 degrees). In some adolescents, kyphosis may produce:
- mild pain at the apex of the curve (about 50% of patients)

Identifying kyphosis

If the patient has a pronounced kyphosis, the thoracic curve is abnormally rounded, as shown here.

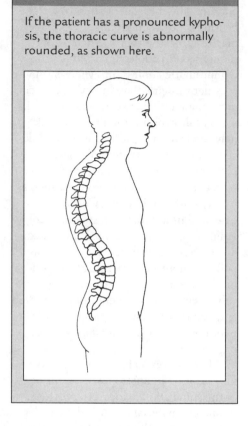

- fatigue
- tenderness or stiffness in the involved area or along the entire spine
- prominent vertebral spinous processes at the lower dorsal and upper lumbar levels
- compensatory increased lumbar lordosis
- hamstring tightness.

Rarely, kyphosis may cause:
- neurologic damage
- spastic paraparesis secondary to spinal cord compression
- herniated nucleus pulposus.

In the adolescent and adult forms of kyphosis that aren't due to poor posture alone, the spine won't straighten when the patient assumes a recumbent position.

Adult kyphosis produces a characteristic humpback appearance, possibly associated with pain, weakness of the back, and generalized fatigue. Unlike the adolescent form, adult kyphosis rarely produces local tenderness, except in osteoporosis with a recent compression fracture.

Differential diagnoses
- Osteoporosis
- Compression fracture
- Herniated disc
- Neoplastic disease
- Infection

Diagnosis

Physical examination reveals curvature of the thoracic spine in varying degrees of severity. X-rays may show vertebral wedging, Schmorl's nodes, irregular end plates, and possibly mild scoliosis of 10 to 20 degrees. Adolescent kyphosis must be distinguished from tuberculosis and other inflammatory or neoplastic diseases that cause vertebral collapse; the severe pain, bone destruction, or systemic symptoms associated with these diseases help rule out a diagnosis of kyphosis. Other sites of bone disease, primary sites of malignancy, and infection must also be evaluated, possibly through vertebral biopsy.

Management
General

Effective management of kyphosis necessitates first-rate supportive care for patients in traction or a brace, skillful patient teaching, and sensitive emotional support. For kyphosis caused by poor posture alone, treatment may consist of therapeutic exercises, bed rest on a firm mattress (with or without traction), and a brace to straighten the kyphotic curve until spinal growth is complete. Corrective exercises include pelvic tilt to decrease lumbar lordosis, hamstring stretch to overcome muscle contractures, and thoracic hyperextension to flatten the kyphotic curve. These exercises may be performed in or out of the brace. Lateral X-rays taken every 4 months evaluate correction. Gradual weaning from the brace can begin after maximum correction of the kyphotic curve and after vertebral wedging has decreased and the spine has reached full skeletal maturity. Loss of correction indicates that weaning from the brace has been too rapid, and time out of the brace is decreased accordingly.

Treatment for adolescent and adult kyphosis also includes appropriate measures for the underlying cause and, possibly, spinal arthrodesis for the relief of symptoms.

Surgical intervention

Although rarely necessary, surgery may be recommended when kyphosis causes neurologic damage, a spinal curve greater than 60 degrees, or intractable and disabling back pain in a patient with full skeletal maturity. Preoperative measures may include halo traction. Corrective surgery includes a posterior spinal fusion with spinal instrumentation, iliac bone grafting, and plaster immobilization. Anterior spinal fusion followed by immobilization in plaster may be necessary when kyphosis produces a spinal curve greater than 70 degrees.

Referral

- The patient may need a referral to an orthopedic surgeon if surgery is necessary.
- The patient may need psychological counseling to cope with chronic pain.

Follow-up

Monitoring will depend on the degree of kyphosis and the method of correction.

Patient teaching

- Teach the patient with adolescent kyphosis caused by poor posture alone the prescribed therapeutic exercises and the fundamentals of good posture. Suggest bed rest when pain is severe. Encourage the use of a firm mattress, preferably with a bed board. If the patient needs a brace, explain its purpose and teach him how and when to wear it.
- Teach good skin care. Tell the patient not to use lotions, ointments, or powders where the brace contacts the skin. Warn him that only a health care professional should adjust the brace.

Complications

- Spinal deformity
- Depression
- Chronic pain

• • • • • • • • • • • •

MUSCULAR DYSTROPHY

Muscular dystrophy is actually a group of congenital disorders characterized by progressive symmetrical wasting of skeletal muscles without neural or sensory defects. Paradoxically, these wasted muscles tend to enlarge because of connective tissue and fat deposits, giving an erroneous impression of muscle strength. The four main types of muscular dystrophy are Duchenne's dystrophy (pseudohypetrophic), which accounts for 50% of all cases; Becker type muscular dystrophy (benign pseudohypertrophic); facioscapulohumeral muscular dystrophy (Landouzy-Dejerine dystrophy); and limb-girdle muscular dystrophy.

Duchenne's and Becker's muscular dystrophies affect males almost exclusively. The incidence of Duchenne's muscular dystrophy is 13 to 33 per 100,000 males; Becker's muscular dystrophy occurs in about 1 to 3 per 100,000 males. Facioscapulohumeral and limb-girdle dystrophies affect both sexes about equally.

The prognosis varies. Duchenne's muscular dystrophy generally strikes during early childhood and usually results in death by age 20. Patients with Becker's muscular dystrophy typically live into their 40s. Facioscapulohumeral and limb-girdle dystrophies usually don't shorten life.

Causes

Muscular dystrophy is caused by various genetic mechanisms. Duchenne's and Becker's muscular dystrophies are X-linked recessive disorders. Both result from defects in the gene coding for the muscle protein dystrophin; the gene has been mapped to the Xp21 locus.

Facioscapulohumeral dystrophy is an autosomal dominant disorder. Limb-girdle dystrophy is usually autosomal recessive.

Clinical presentation

Although all four types of muscular dystrophy cause progressive muscular deterioration, the degree of severity and age of onset vary.

■ Duchenne's muscular dystrophy begins insidiously, between ages 3 and 5. Initially, it affects leg and pelvic muscles but eventually spreads to the involuntary muscles. Muscle weakness produces a waddling gait, toe-walking, and lordosis. Children with this disorder have difficulty climbing stairs, fall down often, can't run properly, and their scapulae flare out (or "wing") when they raise their arms. Calf muscles especially become enlarged and firm. Muscle deterioration progresses rapidly, and contractures develop. Some have abrupt intermittent oscillations of the irises in response to light (Gowers' sign). Usually, these children are confined to wheelchairs by between ages 9

and 12. Late in the disease, progressive weakening of cardiac muscle causes complications. Death commonly results from sudden heart failure, respiratory failure, or infection.

■ Becker's muscular dystrophy produces signs and symptoms that resemble those of Duchenne's muscular dystrophy, but they progress more slowly. Although symptoms start around age 5, the patient can still walk well beyond age 15, and sometimes into his 40s.

■ Facioscapulohumeral dystrophy is a slowly progressive and relatively benign form of muscular dystrophy that commonly occurs before age 10 but may develop during early adolescence. Initially, it weakens the muscles of the face, shoulders, and upper arms but eventually spreads to all voluntary muscles, producing a pendulous lower lip and absence of the nasolabial fold. Early symptoms include inability to pucker the mouth or whistle, abnormal facial movements, and absence of facial movements when laughing or crying. Other signs consist of diffuse facial flattening that leads to a masklike expression, winging of the scapulae, inability to raise the arms above the head and, in infants, the inability to suckle.

■ Limb-girdle dystrophy follows a similarly slow course and commonly causes only slight disability. Usually, it begins between ages 6 and 10; less commonly, in early adulthood. Muscle weakness first appears in the upper arm and pelvic muscles. Other symptoms include winging of the scapulae, lordosis with abdominal protrusion, waddling gait, poor balance, and inability to raise the arms.

Differential diagnoses

■ Spinal muscular atrophy
■ Chromosomal disorders
■ Encephalitis
■ Myasthenia gravis

Diagnosis

Diagnosis depends on typical clinical findings, family history, and diagnostic test findings. If another family member has muscular dystrophy, its clinical characteristics can indicate the type of dystrophy the patient has and how he may be affected.

Electromyography typically demonstrates short, weak bursts of electrical activity or high-frequency, repetitive waxing and waning discharges in affected muscles. Muscle biopsy shows variations in the size of muscle fibers and, in later stages, shows fat and connective tissue deposits; dystrophin is absent in Duchenne's dystrophy and diminished in Becker's dystrophy. Serum creatine kinase is markedly elevated in Duchenne's, but only moderately elevated in Becker's and facioscapulohumeral dystrophies.

Immunologic and molecular biological assays now available in specialized medical centers facilitate accurate prenatal and postnatal diagnosis of Duchenne's and Becker's muscular dystrophies and are replacing muscle biopsy and elevated serum creatine kinase levels in diagnosing these dystrophies. These assays can also help to identify carriers.

Management
General

To date, scientists have found that no treatment stops the progressive muscle impairment of muscular dystrophy. Orthopedic appliances and physical therapy help to maintain muscle strength and mobility.

Medication

Prednisone (adults, 5 to 60 mg/day P.O.; children, 0.14 mg/kg/day P.O. in divided doses) improves muscle strength in patients with Duchenne's dystrophy.

Surgical intervention

Surgery to correct contractures can help preserve the patient's mobility and independence.

Referral

- Refer the patient for physical therapy.
- The patient may need to be referred to an orthopedic surgeon if surgery is necessary.
- The patient may need psychological counseling in order to cope with the illness.
- If necessary, refer adult patients for sexual counseling.
- Refer those who must acquire new job skills for vocational rehabilitation. (Contact the Department of Labor and Industry in your state for more information.)
- For information on social services and financial assistance, refer these patients and their families to the Muscular Dystrophy Association.
- Refer family members for genetic counseling.

Follow-up

Monitoring will be determined by the patient's age and progression of the disease.

Patient teaching

- When respiratory involvement occurs in Duchenne's muscular dystrophy, encourage coughing, deep-breathing exercises, and diaphragmatic breathing. Teach parents how to recognize early signs of respiratory complications.
- Teach active and passive range-of-motion exercises to preserve joint mobility and prevent muscle atrophy.
- Advise the patient to avoid long periods of bed rest and inactivity; if necessary, limit television viewing and other sedentary activities.
- Tell the patient to have an adequate fluid intake, increase dietary bulk, and

take a stool softener. The patient is prone to obesity due to reduced physical activity; help him and his family plan a low-calorie, high-protein, high-fiber diet.

Complications
- Depression
- Cardiac arrhythmias
- Respiratory failure
- Dysphagia
- Seizures

Special considerations
- Always allow the patient plenty of time to perform even simple physical tasks because he's likely to be slow and awkward.
- Encourage communication between family members to help them deal with the emotional strain this disorder produces. Provide emotional support to help the patient cope with continual changes in body image.
- Help the child with Duchenne's muscular dystrophy maintain peer relationships and realize his intellectual potential by encouraging his parents to keep him in a regular school as long as possible.

• • • • • • • • • • • •

OSGOOD-SCHLATTER DISEASE

Osgood-Schlatter disease, also called osteochondrosis, is a painful, incomplete separation of the epiphysis of the tibial tubercle from the tibial shaft. It's most common in active adolescent boys, generally affecting one or both knees. Severe disease may cause permanent tubercle enlargement.

Causes
Osgood-Schlatter disease probably results from trauma before the complete fusion of the epiphysis to the main bone has oc-

curred (between ages 10 and 15). Such trauma may be a single violent action or repeated knee flexion against a tight quadriceps muscle. Other causes include locally deficient blood supply and genetic factors.

Clinical presentation
The patient complains of constant aching and pain and tenderness below the kneecap, which worsens during any activity that causes forceful contraction of the patellar tendon on the tubercle, such as ascending or descending stairs, running, jumping, or forced flexion. The pain may be associated with some obvious soft-tissue swelling and localized heat and tenderness.

Differential diagnoses
- Patellar tendinitis
- Stress fracture of the proximal tibia
- Proximal tibia neoplasm
- Osteomyelitis of the proximal tibia

Diagnosis
Physical examination supports the diagnosis. The examiner forces the tibia into internal rotation while slowly extending the patient's knee from 90 degrees of flexion; at about 30 degrees, flexion produces pain that subsides immediately with external rotation of the tibia.

X-rays may be normal or show epiphyseal separation and soft-tissue swelling for up to 6 months after onset; eventually, they may show bone fragmentation. Bone scan may show increased uptake in the area of the tibial tuberosity—even greater than the typical increased uptake in the normal epiphysis of the unaffected side.

Management
General
Osteochondrosis is usually self-limiting, and conservative treatment designed to

reduce pain and decrease stress to the affected knee is usually adequate. The patient should avoid strenuous exercises that involve the knee and apply ice frequently after exercise for pain. Rest and quadriceps strengthening, hip extension, adductor strengthening, and hamstring and quadriceps stretching exercises are recommended. Knee immobilization in extension for 6 to 8 weeks may be necessary.

Medication
The following medications may reduce pain in Osgood-Schlatter disease:
- ibuprofen—200 to 800 mg P.O. every 4 to 6 hours p.r.n.
- acetaminophen—325 to 650 mg P.O. every 4 to 6 hours p.r.n.

Surgical intervention
Rarely, conservative measures fail, and surgery may be necessary. Such surgery includes removal or fixation of the epiphysis or drilling holes through the tubercle to the main bone to form channels for rapid revascularization.

Referral
- The patient may need to be referred to an orthopedic surgeon if surgery is necessary.

Follow-up
The patient should be monitored according to effectiveness of treatment and the occurrence of disability.

Patient teaching
- Teach the proper use of crutches. Tell the patient to protect the injured knee with padding and to avoid trauma and repeated flexion (running, contact sports).

Complications
- Patellar tendon avulsion

- Patellofemoral degenerative arthritis
- Alteration in lifestyle

Special considerations
- Monitor for muscle atrophy.
- Give reassurance and emotional support because disruption of normal activities is difficult for an active teenager. Emphasize that restrictions are temporary.

• • • • • • • • • • • •

OSTEOARTHRITIS

Osteoarthritis, the most common form of arthritis, is a chronic disease that causes deterioration of the joint cartilage and formation of reactive new bone at the margins and subchondral areas of the joints. This degeneration results from a breakdown of chondrocytes, most commonly in the distal interphalangeal and proximal interphalangeal joints, but also in the hip and knee joints. Primary osteoarthritis is strongly associated with aging, which predisposes the patient to cartilage degeneration.

Osteoarthritis is widespread, occurring equally in both sexes. Disability depends on the site and severity of involvement and can range from minor limitation of the dexterity of the fingers to severe disability in persons with hip or knee involvement. The rate of progression varies, and joints may remain stable for years in an early stage of deterioration.

AGE ALERT The earliest symptoms of osteoarthritis typically begin after age 40 and may progress with advancing age.

Causes
Studies indicate that osteoarthritis is acquired and probably results from a combination of metabolic, genetic,

What happens in osteoarthritis

The characteristic breakdown of articular cartilage is a gradual response to aging or to predisposing factors, such as joint abnormalities or traumatic injury.

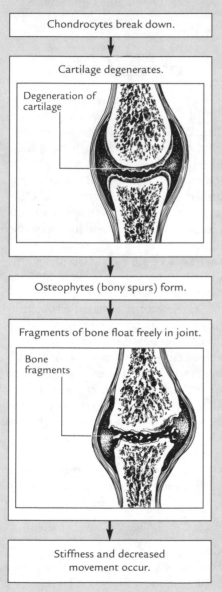

Chondrocytes break down.

Cartilage degenerates.

Degeneration of cartilage

Osteophytes (bony spurs) form.

Fragments of bone float freely in joint.

Bone fragments

Stiffness and decreased movement occur.

chemical, and mechanical factors. Secondary osteoarthritis usually follows an identifiable predisposing event—most commonly trauma, congenital deformity, or obesity—and leads to degenerative changes.

Clinical presentation

The most common symptom of osteoarthritis is a deep, aching joint pain, particularly after exercise or weight bearing, that's usually relieved by rest. Other symptoms include:

- stiffness in the morning and after exercise (relieved by rest)
- aching during changes in weather
- grating of the joint during motion
- altered gait contractures
- limited movement.

These symptoms increase with poor posture, obesity, and stress to the affected joint.

Osteoarthritis of the interphalangeal joints produces irreversible joint changes and node formation. The nodes eventually become red, swollen, and tender, causing numbness and loss of dexterity. (See *What happens in osteoarthritis*.)

Differential diagnoses

- Osteoporosis
- Rheumatoid arthritis
- Gout
- Malignancy
- Vasculitis

Diagnosis

A thorough physical examination confirms typical symptoms, and absence of systemic symptoms rules out an inflammatory joint disorder. X-rays of the affected joint help confirm diagnosis of osteoarthritis but may be normal in the early stages. X-rays may require many views and typically show:

- narrowing of joint space or margin

■ cystlike bony deposits in joint space and margins and sclerosis of the subchondral space
■ joint deformity due to degeneration or articular damage
■ bony growths at weight-bearing areas
■ fusion of joints.

No laboratory test is specific for osteoarthritis. (See *Digital joint deformities*.)

Management

General

The goal of treatment is to relieve pain, maintain or improve mobility, and minimize disability. Effective treatment also reduces stress by supporting or stabilizing the joint with crutches, braces, a cane, a walker, a cervical collar, or traction. Other supportive measures include massage, moist heat, paraffin dips for hands, protective techniques for preventing undue stress on the joints, and adequate rest (particularly after activity). Occasionally, exercise may be indicated if the knees are affected.

Medication

The following medications may be used to treat osteoarthritis:
■ aspirin — 325 to 650 mg P.O. every 4 hours or other nonnarcotic analgesics; maximum 6 g/day
■ ibuprofen — 300 to 800 mg P.O. t.i.d. to q.i.d., or other nonsteroidal anti-inflammatory drugs (NSAIDs).

Intra-articular injections of corticosteroids given every 4 to 6 months may delay the development of nodes in the hands.

Surgical intervention

Surgical treatment is reserved for patients who have severe disability or uncontrollable pain; examples include:

Digital joint deformities

Osteoarthritis of the interphalangeal joints produces irreversible changes in the distal joints (Heberden's nodes, as shown bottom left) and the proximal joints (Bouchard's nodes, as shown bottom right). Initially painless, these nodes gradually progress to or suddenly flare up as redness, swelling, tenderness, and impaired sensation and dexterity.

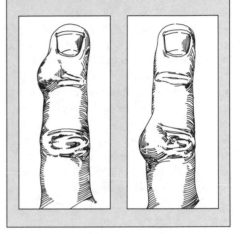

■ arthroplasty (partial or total) — replacement of the deteriorated part of a joint with a prosthetic appliance
■ arthrodesis — surgical fusion of bones, used primarily in the spine (laminectomy)
■ osteoplasty — scraping and lavage of deteriorated bone from a joint
■ osteotomy — change in the alignment of bone to relieve stress by excision of wedge of bone or cutting of bone.

Referral

■ The patient may need to be referred to an orthopedic surgeon if surgery is necessary.
■ The patient may need a referral for physical therapy.

Follow-up
The patient should be monitored at regular intervals (3 to 6 months) for functional status and pain control. If the patient is frequently using NSAIDs or aspirin, periodic complete blood counts, renal function tests, and stool for occult blood should be performed.

Patient teaching
- Tell the patient to get adequate rest, particularly after activity. Plan rest periods during the day, and provide for adequate sleep at night. Moderation is the key — teach the patient to pace daily activities.
- Encourage the patient to perform gentle, isometric range-of-motion exercises.
- Teach the patient to take medication exactly as prescribed, and report adverse effects immediately.
- Advise the patient to avoid overexertion. He should take care to stand and walk correctly, to minimize weight-bearing activities, and to be especially careful when stooping or picking up objects.
- Instruct the patient to wear proper-fitting, supportive shoes and to keep the heels from becoming worn down.
- Advise the patient to install safety devices at home such as guard rails in the bathroom.

Complications
- Chronic pain
- Deformity of joint
- Alteration in lifestyle

Special considerations
- Provide emotional support and reassurance to help the patient cope with limited mobility.
- Explain that osteoarthritis isn't a systemic disease.

OSTEOMYELITIS

Osteomyelitis is a pyogenic bone infection that may be chronic or acute. It commonly results from a combination of local trauma — usually quite trivial but resulting in hematoma formation — and an acute infection originating elsewhere in the body. Although osteomyelitis typically remains localized, it can spread through the bone to the marrow, cortex, and periosteum. Acute osteomyelitis is usually a blood-borne disease, which most commonly affects rapidly growing children. Chronic osteomyelitis, which is rare, is characterized by multiple draining sinus tracts and metastatic lesions.

Osteomyelitis occurs more commonly in children (especially boys) than in adults — usually as a complication of an acute localized infection. The most common sites in children are the lower end of the femur and the upper end of the tibia, humerus, and radius. The most common sites in adults are the pelvis and vertebrae, generally as a result of contamination associated with surgery or trauma. Other common sites are sternoclavicular, sacroiliac, and symphysis pubis. The incidence of chronic and acute osteomyelitis is declining, except in drug abusers. With prompt treatment, the prognosis for acute osteomyelitis is very good; for chronic osteomyelitis, which is more prevalent in adults, the prognosis is still poor.

Causes and pathophysiology
Virtually any pathogenic bacteria can cause osteomyelitis under the right circumstances. The most common pyogenic organism in osteomyelitis is *Staphylococcus aureus;* others include *Streptococcus pyogenes, Pneumococcus, Pseudomonas aeruginosa, Escherichia coli,* and *Proteus*

vulgaris. Typically, these organisms find a culture site in a hematoma from recent trauma or in a weakened area, such as the site of local infection (for example, furunculosis), and spread directly to bone. As the organisms grow and form pus within the bone, tension builds within the rigid medullary cavity, forcing pus through the haversian canals. This forms a subperiosteal abscess that deprives the bone of its blood supply and may eventually cause necrosis. In turn, necrosis stimulates the periosteum to create new bone (involucrum); the old bone (sequestrum) detaches and works its way out through an abscess or the sinuses. By the time sequestrum forms, osteomyelitis is chronic.

Clinical presentation

Onset of acute osteomyelitis is usually rapid, with sudden pain accompanied by tenderness, heat, swelling, and restricted movement of the affected area. Associated systemic symptoms may include:

- tachycardia
- sudden fever
- nausea
- malaise.

Generally, the clinical features of chronic and acute osteomyelitis are the same, except that a chronic infection can persist intermittently for years, flaring up spontaneously after minor trauma. Sometimes, however, the only symptom of chronic infection is the persistent drainage of pus from an old pocket in a sinus tract.

Differential diagnoses

- Cellulitis
- Tumor
- Gout
- Systemic infection
- Neuropathic bone disease

Diagnosis

Patient history, physical examination, and blood tests help to confirm osteomyelitis:

- White blood cell count shows leukocytosis.
- Erythrocyte sedimentation rate or C-reactive protein is usually elevated but nonspecific in acute cases.
- Blood cultures identify the causative organism in about 50% of cases.
- Magnetic resonance imaging is best for detecting spinal infection.
- Computed tomography scanning is best for visualizing islands of dead bone.

X-rays may not show bone involvement until the disease has been active for some time, usually 2 to 3 weeks. Bone scans can detect early infection. Diagnosis must rule out poliomyelitis, rheumatic fever, myositis, and bone fractures. The gold standard for diagnosing osteomyelitis is histopathologic and microscopic examination of bone.

Management

General

Treatment for acute osteomyelitis should begin before definitive diagnosis: immobilization of the affected bone by plaster cast, traction, or bed rest; and supportive measures, such as analgesics and I.V. fluids, along with medication. Some centers use hyperbaric oxygen to increase the activity of naturally occurring leukocytes. Free-tissue transfers and local muscle flaps are also used to fill in dead space and increase blood supply.

Medication

Large doses of I.V. antibiotics are given after blood cultures are taken:

- nafcillin — 2 g every 4 hours
- cefazolin — 1 to 2 g every 8 hours
- vancomycin — 1 to 1.5 g every 12 hours.

Antibiotic therapy to control infection may include administration of systemic antibiotics; intracavitary instillation of antibiotics through closed-system continuous irrigation with low intermittent suction; limited irrigation with blood drainage system with suction (Hemovac); or local application of packed, wet, antibiotic-soaked dressings.

For pain management, give:
- ibuprofen — 300 to 800 mg P.O. t.i.d. to q.i.d.
- propoxyphene hydrochloride — 65 mg P.O. every 4 hours p.r.n.
- morphine — 2 to 4 mg I.V. every 2 to 4 hours.

Surgical intervention

Early surgical drainage to relieve pressure buildup and sequestrum formation should be done.

If an abscess forms, treatment includes incision and drainage, followed by a culture of the drained fluid. In addition to these therapies, chronic osteomyelitis usually requires surgery to remove dead bone (sequestrectomy) and to promote drainage (saucerization). Prognosis is poor even after surgery. Patients are commonly in great pain and require prolonged hospitalization. Resistant chronic osteomyelitis in an arm or leg may necessitate amputation.

Referral

- Refer the patient to the hospital for administration of an I.V. antibiotic.
- The patient may need a referral to an orthopedic surgeon if surgery is necessary.
- The patient may need psychological counseling to cope with the outcome of the illness (such as amputation).

Follow-up

The patient should be monitored posthospitalization initially after 1 week, then every 2 to 3 weeks until condition is resolved.

Patient teaching

- Teach the patient how to protect and clean the wound and, most importantly, how to recognize signs of recurring infection (increased temperature, redness, localized heat, and swelling). Stress the need for follow-up examinations. Instruct the patient to seek prompt treatment for possible sources of recurrence — blisters, boils, styes, and impetigo.

Complications

- Sepsis
- Amputation
- Fracture
- Abscess
- Depression

• • • • • • • • • • • •

OSTEOPOROSIS

Osteoporosis is a metabolic bone disorder in which the rate of bone resorption accelerates while the rate of bone formation slows down, causing a loss of bone mass. Bones affected by this disease lose calcium and phosphate salts and thus become porous, brittle, and abnormally vulnerable to fractures. Osteoporosis may be primary or secondary to an underlying disease. Primary osteoporosis is also called postmenopausal osteoporosis because it most commonly develops in postmenopausal women.

Causes

The cause of primary osteoporosis is unknown; however, a mild but prolonged negative calcium balance, resulting from an inadequate dietary intake of calcium, may be an important contributing factor, as may declining gonadal or adrenal function, faulty protein metabolism due to estrogen deficiency, and a sedentary lifestyle. There are many causes of secondary osteoporosis, including prolonged therapy with steroids or heparin, total immobilization or disuse of a bone (as with hemiplegia, for example), alcoholism, malnutrition, malabsorption, scurvy, lactose intolerance, hyperthyroidism, osteogenesis imperfecta, and Sudeck's atrophy (localized to hands and feet, with recurring attacks).

Clinical presentation

Osteoporosis is usually discovered when an elderly person bends to lift something, hears a snapping sound, and then feels a sudden pain in the lower back. Vertebral collapse, causing a backache with pain that radiates around the trunk, is the most common presenting feature. Any movement or jarring aggravates the backache.

In another common pattern, osteoporosis can develop insidiously, exhibiting:
- increasing deformity
- kyphosis
- loss of height
- spontaneous wedge fractures
- pathologic fractures of the neck or femur
- Colles' fractures after a minor fall
- hip fractures become increasingly common.

Osteoporosis, commonly affecting older people, is a major risk factor in vertebral compression fractures and hip fractures.

Osteoporosis primarily affects the weight-bearing vertebrae. Only when the condition is advanced or severe, as in Cushing's syndrome or hyperthyroidism, do comparable changes occur in the skull, ribs, and long bones.

Differential diagnoses
- Multiple myeloma
- Other neoplasia
- Osteomalacia
- Osteogenesis imperfecta tardia
- Skeletal hyperparathyroidism
- Hyperthyroidism

Diagnosis

Initial evaluation attempts to identify the specific cause of osteoporosis through the patient history.

Other diagnostic tests used may include:
- X-rays show typical degeneration in the lower thoracic and lumbar vertebrae. Early changes include increased width of intervertebral spaces and vertical striations of vertebral bodies. Late changes include cortical plate fractures, vertebral compression, wedge and crush fractures, and fractures at the ends of long bones. Loss of bone mineral becomes evident in later stages.
- Dual- or single-photon absorptiometry measures bone mass of the extremities, hips, and spine.
- Blood studies should include calcium, phosphorus, alkaline phosphatase, renal function, and liver function. Tests to rule out other pathogens include complete blood count and immunoglobulin, thyroid-stimulating hormone, parathyroid hormone, urinary cortisol, and serum testosterone levels.
- Bone biopsy shows thin, porous, but otherwise normal-looking bone.

Management
General

Treatment aims to prevent additional fractures and control pain. A physical therapy program, emphasizing gentle exercise and activity, is an important part of the treatment. Weakened vertebrae should be supported, usually with a back brace. The incidence of primary osteoporosis may be reduced through adequate intake of dietary calcium and regular exercise. Hormonal and fluoride treatments may also offer some preventive benefit. Secondary osteoporosis can be prevented through effective treatment of the underlying disease as well as corticosteroid therapy, early mobilization after surgery or trauma, decreased alcohol consumption, careful observation for signs of malabsorption, and prompt treatment of hyperthyroidism.

Medication
The following medications may be used to treat osteoporosis:
- estrogen — 0.625 mg/day P.O. in cyclic regimen (3 weeks on and 1 week off)
- alendronate — 10 mg/day P.O.
- calcium supplement with vitamin D — 1,200 mg/day P.O.
- calcitonin (salmon) — 100 IU/day I.M. or S.C. or 200 IU/day intranasally.
- risedronate sodium — 5 mg/day P.O
- raloxifene — 60 mg/day P.O.

Surgical intervention
Surgery can correct pathologic fractures of the femur by open reduction and internal fixation. Colles' fracture requires reduction with plaster immobilization for 4 to 10 weeks.

Referral
- Refer the patient to an orthopedic surgeon if fracture occurs.
- Refer the patient to a physical therapist.

Follow-up
The patient should be evaluated in 1 month and then every 3 to 6 months. The patient should have an annual bone mineral density test.

Patient teaching
- If possible, tell the patient to walk several times daily. As appropriate, encourage the patient to perform active exercises. Make sure the patient regularly attends scheduled physical therapy sessions.
- Explain to the patient's family how easily an osteoporotic patient's bones can fracture.
- Make sure the patient and family clearly understand the prescribed drug regimen. Tell them how to recognize significant adverse effects and to report them immediately.
- The patient should report any new pain sites immediately, especially after trauma, no matter how slight.
- Advise the patient to sleep on a firm mattress and avoid excessive bed rest. Make sure she knows how to wear her back brace.
- Teach the patient good body mechanics — to stoop before lifting anything and to avoid twisting movements and prolonged bending.
- Instruct the female patient taking estrogen in the proper technique for breast self-examination. Emphasize the need for regular gynecologic examinations. Tell her to report abnormal bleeding promptly.

Complications
- Fracture
- Chronic pain
- Depression
- Alteration in lifestyle

• • • • • • • • • • • • •

PAGET'S DISEASE

Paget's disease, also called osteitis deformans, is a slowly progressive metabolic bone disease characterized by an initial phase of excessive bone resorption (osteoclastic phase), followed by a reactive phase of excessive abnormal bone formation (osteoblastic phase). The new bone structure, which is chaotic, fragile, and weak, causes painful deformities of both external contour and internal structure. Paget's disease usually localizes in one or more areas of the skeleton (most commonly the lower torso), but occasionally skeletal deformity is widely distributed. It can be fatal, particularly when it's associated with heart failure (widespread disease creates a continuous need for high cardiac output), bone sarcoma, or giant-cell tumors.

AGE ALERT In the United States, Paget's disease affects approximately 2.5 million people over age 40 (mostly men).

Causes
Although its exact cause is unknown, one theory holds that early viral infection (possibly with mumps virus) causes a dormant skeletal infection that erupts many years later as Paget's disease. In 5% of the patients, the involved bone will undergo malignant changes.

Clinical presentation
Clinical effects of Paget's disease vary. Early stages may be asymptomatic, but when pain does develop, it's usually severe and persistent and may coexist with impaired movement resulting from impingement of abnormal bone on the spinal cord or sensory nerve root. Such pain intensifies with weight bearing.

The patient with skull involvement shows characteristic cranial enlargement over frontal and occipital areas (hat size may increase) and may complain of headaches. Other deformities include:
- kyphosis
- barrel-shaped chest
- asymmetrical bowing of the tibia and femur, which commonly reduces height

- pagetic sites are warm and tender and are susceptible to pathologic fractures after minor trauma.

Pagetic fractures heal slowly and commonly incompletely.

Differential diagnoses
- Kyphosis
- Malignancy
- Osteoporosis

Diagnosis
X-rays taken before overt symptoms develop show increased bone expansion and density. A bone scan clearly shows early pagetic lesions. Computed tomography scanning or magnetic resonance imaging shows extra bony extension if sarcomatous degeneration occurs. Bone biopsy reveals characteristic mosaic pattern.

Other laboratory findings include:
- anemia
- elevated serum alkaline phosphatase levels (an index of osteoblastic activity and bone formation)
- elevated 24-hour urine levels for hydroxyproline (amino acid excreted by kidneys and an index of osteoclastic hyperactivity).

Increasing use of routine chemistry screens is making early diagnosis more common. Serum osteocalcin and N-telopeptide are usually increased.

Management
Medication
Primary treatment consists of drug therapy and includes:
- calcitonin (salmon) — 100 IU/day S.C. or I.M. initially, then 50 to 100 IU every other day or three times per week
- etidronate — 5 to 10 mg/kg/day P.O., not to exceed 6 months of therapy
- alendronate — 40 mg/day P.O. for 6 months

- plicamycin — 15 to 25 mcg/kg/day I.V. over 4 to 6 hours for 3 to 4 days
- aspirin — 325 to 650 mg every 4 to 6 hours p.r.n.
- acetaminophen — 325 to 650 mg every 4 to 6 hours p.r.n.
- ibuprofen — 300 to 800 mg t.i.d. to q.i.d.

Surgical intervention
Patients may need surgery to reduce or prevent pathologic fractures, correct secondary deformities, and relieve neurologic impairment. To decrease the risk of excessive bleeding from hypervascular bone, drug therapy with calcitonin and etidronate or plicamycin must precede surgery. Joint replacement is difficult because bonding material (methyl methacrylate) doesn't set properly on pagetic bone.

Referral
- The patient may need referral to an orthopedic surgeon if surgery is required.
- The patient may require psychological counseling in order to cope with the illness.
- The patient may need to be referred for physical therapy.
- Help the patient and family make use of community support resources, such as a visiting nurse or home health agency. For more information, refer them to the Paget's Disease Foundation.

Follow-up
The patient should be followed depending on effectiveness of treatment and progression of disease. Serum calcium and alkaline phosphatase levels should be monitored.

Patient teaching
- To help the patient adjust to the changes in lifestyle imposed by this disease, teach him how to pace activities and, if necessary, how to use assistive devices. Encourage him to follow a recommended exercise program, avoiding immobilization and excessive activity. Suggest a firm mattress or a bed board to minimize spinal deformities.
- Warn against imprudent use of analgesics because diminished sensitivity to pain resulting from analgesic use may make the patient unaware of new fractures.
- To prevent falls at home, advise removal of throw rugs and other obstacles.
- Tell the patient who is receiving etidronate to take this medication with fruit juice 2 hours before or after meals (milk or other high-calcium fluids impair absorption), to divide the daily dosage to minimize adverse effects, and to watch for and report stomach cramps, diarrhea, fractures, and new or increased bone pain.

Complications
- Chronic pain
- Depression
- Alteration in lifestyle
- Blindness
- Hearing loss with tinnitus and vertigo
- Hypertension
- Renal calculi
- Hypercalcemia
- Gout
- Heart failure
- Change in gout

• • • • • • • • • • • •

SCOLIOSIS

Scoliosis is a lateral curvature of the spine that may occur in the thoracic, lumbar, or thoracolumbar spinal segment. The curve may be convex to the right (more common in thoracic curves) or to the left (more common in lumbar curves). Rotation of the vertebral column around its axis occurs and may cause rib cage deformity. Scoliosis is commonly associated with kyphosis (humpback) and lordosis (swayback).

Causes

Scoliosis may be functional or structural. Functional (postural) scoliosis usually results from poor posture or a discrepancy in leg lengths rather than from a fixed deformity of the spinal column; it corrects when the patient bends toward the convex side. Structural scoliosis results from a deformity of the vertebral bodies, and it doesn't correct when the patient bends to the side. Structural scoliosis may be:

■ congenital — usually related to a congenital defect, such as wedge vertebrae, fused ribs or vertebrae, or hemivertebrae; may result from trauma to zygote or embryo

■ paralytic or musculoskeletal — develops several months after asymmetrical paralysis of the trunk muscles due to polio, cerebral palsy, or muscular dystrophy

■ idiopathic (the most common form) — may be transmitted as an autosomal dominant or multifactoral trait. This form appears in a previously straight spine during the growing years. Brain stem dysfunction, possibly due to a lesion of the posterior columns or the inner ear, may be the cause.

Idiopathic scoliosis can be classified as infantile, which affects mostly male infants between birth and age 3 and causes left thoracic and right lumbar curves; juvenile, which affects both sexes between ages 4 and 10 and causes varying types of curvature; or adolescent, which generally affects females between age 10 and achievement of skeletal maturity and causes varying types of curvature.

Clinical presentation

The most common curve in functional or structural scoliosis arises in the thoracic segment, with convexity to the right, and compensatory curves (S curves) in the cervical segment above and the lumbar segment below, both with convexity to the left. (See *Cobb method for measuring angle of curvature*, page 320.) As the spine curves laterally, compensatory curves develop to maintain body balance and mark the deformity. Scoliosis rarely produces subjective symptoms until it's well established; when symptoms do occur, they include:

■ backache
■ fatigue
■ dyspnea.

Because many teenagers are shy about their bodies, their parents suspect that something is wrong only after they notice uneven hemlines, pant legs that appear unequal in length, or subtle physical signs such as one hip appearing higher than the other.

Differential diagnoses

■ Kyphosis
■ Poor posture

Diagnosis

Anterior, posterior, and lateral spinal X-rays, taken with the patient standing upright and bending, confirm scoliosis and determine the degree of curvature (Cobb method) and flexibility of the spine.

A scoliometer can also be used to measure the angle of trunk rotation. Physical examination reveals unequal shoulder heights, elbow levels, and heights of the iliac crests. Muscles on the convex side of the curve may be rounded; those on the concave side, flattened, producing asymmetry of paraspinal muscles.

Cobb method for measuring angle of curvature

The Cobb method measures the angle of curvature in scoliosis. The top vertebra in the curve (T6 in the illustration) is the uppermost vertebra whose upper face tilts toward the curve's concave side. The bottom vertebra in the curve (T12) is the lowest vertebra whose lower face tilts toward the curve's concave side. The angle at which perpendicular lines drawn from the upper face of the top vertebra and the lower face of the bottom vertebra intersect is the angle of the curve.

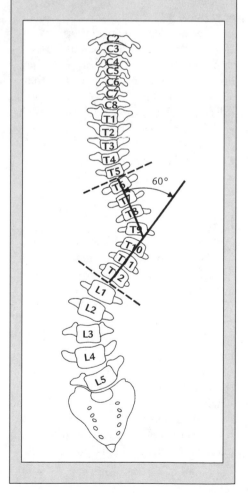

Management
General

Only two treatments effectively treat scoliosis: spinal bracing and surgery. If monitored closely, a properly constructed and fitted brace can successfully halt progression of a curve in approximately 70% of cooperative patients. Most braces should be worn over a long T-shirt or similar article of clothing for 23 hours per day. However, mild curvatures may require less. Exercises must be done daily in and out of the brace to maintain muscle strength. Patients should be seen for follow-up and brace adjustment every 3 months. Radiographs should be repeated at 6-month intervals. As the skeleton matures, as seen radiographically, brace wear should be gradually decreased until it's worn only at night until the spine has fully matured. Electric stimulation of muscle with long-term follow-up is being used as a treatment for scoliosis in a large number of children. It may prove to be an effective alternative to bracing.

Surgical intervention

The primary indications for surgery are:
- relentless curve progression
- significant curve progression despite bracing
- inability to wean patient from brace
- significant pain
- progressive thoracic lordosis
- progressive loss of pulmonary function
- emotional or psychiatric problems with bracing
- severe cosmetic changes in upper torso.

Surgery corrects lateral curvature by posterior spinal fusion and internal stabilization with a Harrington rod. A distraction rod on the concave side of the curve straightens the spine and provides an internal splint. A Cotrel-Dubousset rod may also be used. An alternative procedure, anterior spinal fusion with Dwyer or Zielke instrumentation, corrects curvature with vertebral staples and an anterior stabilizing cable. Some spinal fusions may require postoperative immobilization in a brace.

Referral
- Refer the patient to an orthotist for brace fitting.
- The patient may need to be referred to an orthopedic surgeon for surgery.
- The patient may need psychological counseling in order to cope with treatment of the disorder.

Follow-up
The patient should be monitored for correction of the disorder. Postoperatively, periodic checkups are required for several months to monitor stability of the correction.

Patient teaching
- Explain to the patient what a brace does and how to care for it (how to check the screws for tightness and pad the uprights to prevent excessive wear on clothing). Suggest that loose-fitting, oversized clothes be worn for greater comfort.
- Tell the patient to wear the brace 23 hours per day and to remove it only for bathing and exercise. While he's still adjusting to the brace, tell him to lie down and rest several times per day.
- To prevent skin breakdown, advise the patient not to use lotions, ointments, or powders on areas where the brace contacts the skin. Tell him to keep the skin dry and clean and to wear a snug T-shirt under the brace.
- Advise the patient to increase activities gradually and avoid vigorous sports. Emphasize the importance of conscientiously performing prescribed exercises. Recommend swimming during the hour

Cast syndrome

Cast syndrome is a serious complication that sometimes follows spinal surgery and application of a body cast. Characterized by nausea, abdominal pressure, and vague abdominal pain, cast syndrome probably results from hyperextension of the spine. Hyperextension of the spine accentuates lumbar lordosis, compressing the third portion of the duodenum between the superior mesenteric artery anteriorly and the aorta and vertebral column posteriorly. High intestinal obstruction produces nausea, vomiting, and ischemic infarction of the mesentery.

After removal of the cast, treatment includes gastric decompression and I.V. fluids, with nothing by mouth. Antiemetics should be given sparingly because they may mask symptoms of cast syndrome, which, if untreated, may be fatal.

Teach patients who are discharged in body jackets, localizer casts, or high hip spica casts how to recognize cast syndrome, which may manifest several weeks or months after application of the cast.

out of the brace, but strongly warn against diving.
- Instruct the patient to turn his whole body, instead of just his head, when looking to the side. To make reading easier, tell him to hold the book so he can look straight ahead at it instead of down. If he finds this difficult, help him obtain prism glasses.

Complications
- Permanent deformity
- Depression

- Pulmonary insufficiency
- Back pain
- Degenerative arthritis of the spine
- Disk disease
- Sciatica

Special considerations
- Watch for skin breakdown and signs of cast syndrome. Teach the patient how to recognize these signs. (See *Cast syndrome*, page 321.)
- If you work in a school, screen children routinely for scoliosis during physical examinations.

• • • • • • • • • • • •

SEPTIC ARTHRITIS

Septic, or infectious, arthritis is a medical emergency that occurs when bacterial invasion of a joint causes inflammation of the synovial lining, effusion and pyogenesis, and destruction of bone and cartilage. Septic arthritis can lead to ankylosis and even fatal septicemia. However, prompt antibiotic therapy and joint aspiration or drainage cures most patients.

Causes
In most cases of septic arthritis, bacteria spread from a primary site of infection — usually in adjacent bone or soft tissue — through the bloodstream to the joint. Common infecting organisms in children are gram-positive cocci and *Staphylococcus aureus*, *Streptococcus pyogenes*, and *Streptococcus pneumoniae*; less commonly, two strains of gram-negative cocci — *Neisseria gonorrhoeae* and *Haemophilus influenzae*; and various gram-negative bacilli — *Escherichia coli*, *Salmonella*, and *Pseudomonas*, for example. Adults are usually infected by *N. gonorrhoeae*, *S. aureus*, streptococci and, rarely, gram-negative bacilli.

Various factors can predispose a person to septic arthritis. Any concurrent bacterial infection (of the genitourinary or the upper respiratory tract, for example) or serious chronic illness (such as malignancy, renal failure, rheumatoid arthritis, systemic lupus erythematosus, diabetes, or cirrhosis) heightens susceptibility. Consequently, alcoholics and elderly persons run a higher risk of developing septic arthritis. Of course, diseases that depress the immune system and immunosuppressive therapy increase susceptibility. I.V. drug abuse (by heroin addicts, for example) can also cause septic arthritis. Other predisposing factors include recent articular trauma, joint surgery, intra-articular injections, and local joint abnormalities.

Clinical presentation
Acute septic arthritis begins abruptly, causing intense pain, inflammation, and swelling of the affected joint and low-grade fever. It usually affects a single joint. It most commonly develops in the large joints but can strike any joint, including the spine and small peripheral joints. Systemic signs of inflammation may not appear in some patients. Migratory polyarthritis sometimes precedes localization of the infection. If the bacteria invade the hip, pain may occur in the groin, upper thigh, or buttock or may be referred to the knee.

Differential diagnoses
- Gout
- Pseudogout
- Rheumatoid arthritis

Diagnosis
Identifying the causative organism in a Gram stain or culture of synovial fluid or a biopsy of synovial membrane confirms septic arthritis. When the synovial fluid culture is negative, a positive blood cul-

ture may confirm the diagnosis. Two sets of positive cultures and Gram stain smears of skin exudates, sputum, urethral discharge, stools, urine, or nasopharyngeal discharge also confirm septic arthritis.

Joint fluid analysis shows gross pus or watery, cloudy fluid of decreased viscosity, usually with 50,000/µl or more white blood cells, primarily neutrophils. Synovial fluid glucose is usually more than 40 mg/dl. (See *Other types of arthritis*, page 324.)

X-rays can show typical changes as early as 1 week after initial infection — distention of joint capsules, for example, followed by narrowing of joint space (indicating cartilage damage) and erosions of bone (joint destruction).

White blood cell count may be elevated, with many polymorphonuclear cells; erythrocyte sedimentation rate is increased.

Lactic assay can distinguish septic arthritis from nonseptic arthritis.

Radioisotope joint scan for less accessible joints (such as spinal articulations) may help detect infection or inflammation, but this test must be combined with other tests to confirm diagnosis.

Management
General
Treatment of septic arthritis requires monitoring of progress by frequent analysis of joint fluid cultures, synovial fluid leukocyte counts, and glucose determinations. Bioassays or bactericidal assays of synovial fluid and bioassays of blood may confirm clearing of the infection. The affected joint can be immobilized with a splint or put into traction until the patient can tolerate movement.

Medication
In children, usual initial treatment is either a combination of nafcillin (25 to 100 mg/kg/day I.M. or I.V. in divided doses) or oxacillin (50 to 200 mg/kg/day

I.M. or I.V. in divided doses) and cefotaxime (50 to 180 mg/kg/day I.M. or I.V. in divided doses) or ceftriaxone (50 to 75 mg/kg/day I.M. or I.V.).

Adults with a gram-negative stain may be treated with:
- ceftriaxone — 1 to 2 g I.M. or I.V. q.d. in divided doses every 12 hours
- cefotaxime — 1 g I.V. every 8 hours
- ceftizoxime — 1 g I.V. every 8 hours

Adults with a gram-positive stain may be treated with:
- nafcillin — 2 g I.V. every 4 hours
- oxacillin — 2 g I.V. every 4 hours.

For pain, give:
- codeine — 15 to 60 mg P.O. every 4 to 6 hours p.r.n.
- propoxyphene — 65 mg P.O. every 4 hours p.r.n.

Aspirin causes a misleading reduction in swelling, hindering accurate monitoring of progress.

Surgical intervention
Needle aspiration (arthrocentesis), done under sterile conditions to remove grossly purulent joint fluid, should be repeated daily until fluid appears normal. If a large quantity of fluid is aspirated or the leukocyte count remains elevated, open surgical drainage (usually arthrotomy with lavage of the joint) may be necessary to treat resistant infection or chronic septic arthritis.

Late reconstructive surgery is warranted only for severe joint damage and only after all signs of active infection have disappeared, which usually takes several months. Recommended procedures include arthroplasty and joint fusion. Prosthetic replacement remains controversial because it may exacerbate the infection, but it has helped patients with damaged femoral heads or acetabulums.

Other types of arthritis

INTERMITTENT HYDRARTHROSIS

Characterized by regular, recurrent joint effusions, intermittent hydrarthrosis is a rare, benign condition that most commonly affects the knee. The patient may have difficulty moving the affected joint but have no other arthritic symptoms. The cause of intermittent hydrarthrosis is unknown; onset is usually at or soon after puberty and may be linked to familial tendencies, allergies, or menstruation. No effective treatment exists.

TRAUMATIC ARTHRITIS

Blunt, penetrating, or repeated trauma or forced inappropriate motion of a joint or ligament causes traumatic arthritis. Clinical effects may include swelling, pain, tenderness, joint instability, and internal bleeding. Treatment includes analgesics, nonsteroidal anti-inflammatory drugs, application of cold followed by heat and, if needed, compression dressings, splinting, joint aspiration, casting, or possibly surgery.

SCHÖNLEIN-HENOCH PURPURA

A vasculitic syndrome, Schönlein-Henoch purpura is marked by palpable purpura, abdominal pain, and arthralgia that most commonly affects the knees and ankles, producing swollen, warm, and tender joints without joint erosion or deformity. Renal involvement is also common. Most patients have microscopic hematuria and proteinuria 4 to 8 weeks after onset. Incidence is highest in children and young adults, occurring most commonly in the spring after a respiratory infection. Treatment may include corticosteroids.

HEMOPHILIC ARTHROSIS

Transient or permanent joint changes are a result of hemophilic arthrosis. Commonly precipitated by trauma, hemophilic arthrosis usually arises between ages 1 and 5 and tends to recur until about age 10. It usually affects only one joint at a time — most commonly the knee, elbow, or ankle — and tends to recur in the same joint. Initially, the patient may feel only mild discomfort; later, he may experience warmth, swelling, tenderness, and severe pain with adjacent muscle spasm that leads to flexion of the extremity.

Mild hemophilic arthrosis may cause only limited stiffness that subsides within a few days. In prolonged bleeding, however, symptoms may subside after weeks or months or not at all. Severe hemophilic arthrosis may be accompanied by fever and leukocytosis; severe, prolonged, or repeated bleeding may lead to chronic hemophilic joint disease.

Effective treatment includes I.V. infusion of the deficient clotting factor, bed rest with the affected extremity elevated, application of ice packs, analgesics, and joint aspiration. Physical therapy includes progressive range-of-motion and muscle-strengthening exercises to restore motion and to prevent contractures and muscle atrophy.

Referral
▪ The patient may need a referral to a surgeon or orthopedic surgeon if aspiration or reconstructive surgery is necessary.

▪ Refer the patient for psychological counseling is he's having trouble coping with the illness.

Follow-up
The patient should be seen within 1 week after discharge from the hospital, then within 1 month to assess the effectiveness of the antibiotics.

Patient teaching
▪ Tell the patient to check splints or traction regularly. Tell him to keep the joint in proper alignment, but to avoid prolonged immobilization. Have the family start passive range-of-motion exercises immediately and progress to active exercises as soon as the patient can move the affected joint and put weight on it.
▪ Discuss all prescribed medications with the patient. Explain why therapy must be carefully monitored.

Complications
▪ Chronic pain
▪ Depression
▪ Limited joint movement
▪ Osteomyelitis
▪ Sepsis
▪ Death

Special considerations
▪ Be especially aware of the prolonged use of narcotics in the older adult. Narcotics can impair mental status and may contribute to falls and other accidents.

• • • • • • • • • • • • •

TENDINITIS AND BURSITIS

Tendinitis is a painful inflammation of tendons and of tendon–muscle attachments to bone, usually in the shoulder rotator cuff, hip, Achilles tendon, or hamstring. Bursitis is a painful inflammation of one or more of the bursae — closed sacs lubricated with small amounts of synovial fluid that facilitate the motion of muscles and tendons over bony promi-

nences. Bursitis usually occurs in the subdeltoid, olecranon, trochanteric, calcaneal, or prepatellar bursae.

Causes
Tendinitis commonly results from overuse (such as strain during sports activity), another musculoskeletal disorder (rheumatic diseases, congenital defects), postural misalignment, abnormal body development, or hypermobility.

Bursitis usually occurs in middle age from recurring trauma that stresses or pressures a joint or from an inflammatory joint disease (rheumatoid arthritis, gout). Chronic bursitis follows attacks of acute bursitis or repeated trauma and infection. Septic bursitis may result from wound infection or from bacterial invasion of skin over the bursa.

Clinical presentation
The patient with tendinitis of the shoulder complains of restricted shoulder movement, especially abduction, and localized pain, which is most severe at night and commonly interferes with sleep. The pain extends from the acromion (the shoulder's highest point) to the deltoid muscle insertion, predominantly in the so-called painful arc — that is, when the patient abducts his arm between 50 and 130 degrees. Fluid accumulation causes swelling. In calcific tendinitis, calcium deposits in the tendon cause proximal weakness and, if calcium erodes into adjacent bursae, acute calcific bursitis.

In bursitis, fluid accumulation in the bursae causes irritation, inflammation, sudden or gradual pain, and limited movement. Other symptoms vary according to the affected site. Subdeltoid bursitis impairs arm abduction, prepatellar bursitis (housemaid's knee) produces pain when the patient climbs stairs, and hip bursitis makes crossing the legs painful.

Differential diagnoses
- Arthritis
- Stress fracture
- Compartment syndrome
- Avulsion of the tendon

Diagnosis

In tendinitis, X-rays may be normal at first but later show bony fragments, osteophyte sclerosis, or calcium deposits. Arthrography is usually normal, with occasional small irregularities on the undersurface of the tendon. Computed tomography scanning and magnetic resonance imaging (MRI) have replaced X-ray and even arthrography of the shoulder as diagnostic tools. An MRI will usually identify tears, partial tears, inflammation, or tumor but can't reveal irregularities of the tendon sheath itself. Diagnosis of tendinitis must rule out other causes of shoulder pain, such as myocardial infarction, cervical spondylosis, and tendon tear or rupture. Significantly, in tendinitis, heat aggravates shoulder pain; in other painful joint disorders, heat usually provides relief.

Localized pain and inflammation and a history of unusual strain or injury 2 to 3 days before the onset of pain are the bases for diagnosing bursitis. During the early stages, X-rays are usually normal, except in calcific bursitis, where X-rays may show calcium deposits.

Management
General

Treatment to relieve pain includes resting the joint (by immobilization with a sling, splint, or cast), systemic analgesics, application of cold or heat, ultrasound, or local injection of an anesthetic and corticosteroids to reduce inflammation. Supplementary treatment includes fluid removal by aspiration and heat therapy; for calcific tendinitis, ice packs, physical therapy, ultrasonography, or hydrotherapy generally helps maintain or regain range of motion. It may be necessary to delay treatment until the acute attack is over to ensure maximum patient compliance. Long-term control of chronic bursitis and tendinitis may require changes in the patient's lifestyle to prevent recurring joint irritation.

Medication

The following medications may be used to treat tendinitis or bursitis:
- ibuprofen — 300 to 800 mg P.O. t.i.d. or q.i.d.
- naproxen — 250 to 500 mg b.i.d. P.O.
- indomethacin — 75 to 150 mg/day P.O. in divided doses
- oxaprozin — 1,200 mg/day P.O.

The following medications may also be given for pain:
- propoxyphene — 65 mg P.O. every 4 hours p.r.n.
- codeine — 15 to 60 mg P.O. every 4 hours p.r.n.
- acetaminophen with codeine — 1 to 2 tablets every 4 to 6 hours p.r.n.
- lidocaine 1% — 0.5 to 1 ml injected into affected joint
- prednisolone — 2 to 30 mg injected into affected joint.

Surgical intervention

Rarely, calcific tendinitis requires surgical removal of calcium deposits.

Referral
- The patient may need to be referred for physical therapy.
- The patient may need to be referred to an orthopedist for steroid injection.

Follow-up

The patient should be monitored in the 1st week of treatment and then in 2 weeks.

Patient teaching
- Advise the patient to perform strengthening exercises and avoid activities that aggravate the joint.
- The patient should be reminded to wear a triangular sling during the first few days of an attack of subdeltoid bursitis or tendinitis to support the arm and protect the shoulder, particularly at night. Demonstrate how to wear the sling so it won't put too much weight on the shoulder. Show the patient's family how to pin the sling or how to tie a square knot that will lie flat on the back of the patient's neck. To protect the shoulder during sleep, a splint may be worn instead of a sling. Instruct the patient to remove the splint during the day.
- Advise the patient to maintain joint mobility and prevent muscle atrophy by performing exercises or physical therapy when he's free from pain.

Complications
- Alteration in lifestyle
- Tendon rupture
- Avulsion fracture

• • • • • • • • • • • •

SELECTED REFERENCES

Beers, M., et al. *Merck Manual Diagnosis and Therapy*. Whitehouse Station, N.J.: Merck and Co., Inc., 1999.

Brinker, M. *Fundamentals of Orthopaedics*. Philadelphia: W.B. Saunders, 1999.

Evans, R. *Illustrated Orthopedic Physical Assessment, 2nd ed.* St. Louis: Mosby–Year Book, Inc., 2001.

Schoen, D. *Adult Orthopaedic Nursing*. Philadelphia: Lippincott Williams & Wilkins, 1999.

Suddarth's Textbook of Medical-Surgical Nursing, 9th ed. Philadelphia: Lippincott Williams & Wilkins, 1999.

Respiratory disorders

The respiratory system consists of the lungs and related structures, including the nose, pharynx, larynx, trachea, and bronchi. The primary functions of the respiratory system are to maintain the exchange of oxygen and carbon dioxide in the lungs and tissues and to regulate acid-base balance. Any change in this system affects every other body system. Furthermore, changes in other body systems may also reduce the lungs' ability to provide oxygen.

• • • • • • • • • • •

ASSESSMENT

Because the body depends on the respiratory system to survive, respiratory assessment is a critical nursing responsibility. A thorough assessment allows you to evaluate obvious and subtle respiratory changes. Respiratory assessment begins with a complete physical examination, including inspection, palpation, percussion, and auscultation techniques.

Physical examination

Begin your assessment of the patient's respiratory system by inspecting the skin. A dusky or bluish skin tint (cyanosis) may indicate decreased oxygen content in the arterial blood. (See *Effects of chronic ineffective gas exchange*, pages 330 and 331.)

It's important to distinguish central cyanosis from peripheral cyanosis. Central cyanosis results from hypoxemia and affects all body organs. It may appear in patients with right-to-left cardiac shunting or a pulmonary disease such as chronic bronchitis that causes hypoxemia. Cyanosis appears on the skin; on the mucous membranes of the mouth, lips, and conjunctivae; or in other highly vascular areas, such as the earlobes and nail beds.

Peripheral cyanosis results from vasoconstriction, vascular occlusion, or reduced cardiac output. Commonly seen in patients exposed to cold, it appears in the nail beds, nose, ears, and fingers; it doesn't affect the mucous membranes.

In dark-skinned patients, inspect the oral mucous membranes and lips. If a dark-skinned patient has central cyanosis, these areas will appear ashen, rather than blue. Facial skin may appear pale gray, or ashen, in a cyanotic black-skinned patient and yellowish brown in a cyanotic brown-skinned patient.

Next, assess the patient's nail beds and toes for abnormal enlargement. This condition, called *clubbing,* results from chronic tissue hypoxia. Nail thinning, accompanied by an abnormal alteration of the angle of the finger and toe bases, distinguishes clubbing.

Preparing for respiratory assessment

After obtaining an overall picture of the patient's oxygenation, begin your assessment of the respiratory system. You'll need a stethoscope with a diaphragm, a felt-tipped marking pen, a ruler, and a tape measure.

Have the patient sit in a position that allows access to the anterior and posterior thorax. Make sure the patient isn't cold because shivering may alter breathing patterns.

If the patient can't sit up, use the supine semi-Fowler position to assess the anterior chest wall and the side-lying position to assess the posterior thorax. Keep in mind that these positions may distort some findings; for example, they may not allow optimal lung expansion.

When performing the assessment, you may find it easier to inspect, palpate, percuss, and auscultate the anterior chest before the posterior chest.

Inspection

Assess respiratory function by inspecting the patient's breathing and the anterior and posterior thorax, noting any abnormal findings. Determine the rate, rhythm, and quality of the patient's respirations; inspect the patient's chest configuration and symmetry, skin condition, and accessory muscle use; also check for nasal flar-

ing. (See *Recognizing common chest deformities,* page 332.)

Respiration

Count the number of respirations (each composed of an inspiration and an expiration) for 1 full minute. For a patient with periodic or irregular breathing, monitor the respirations for more than 1 minute to accurately determine the rate. Assess the duration of any periods without spontaneous respiration (apnea), and note abnormal respiratory patterns, such as tachypnea and bradypnea. (See *Assessing abnormal breath sounds,* page 333.)

Assess the quality of respiration by observing the type and depth of breathing. Also assess the method of ventilation by having the patient lie supine to expose the chest and abdominal walls. Patients with chronic obstructive pulmonary disease (COPD) may exhibit pursed-lip breathing, which prevents small airway collapse during exhalation. Forced inspiration or expiration may alter assessment findings; therefore, ask the patient to breathe normally.

Note the depth of breathing, assessing for shallow chest wall expansion (hypopnea) or unusually deep chest wall expansion (hyperpnea). Use your judgment to assess the depth of breathing, but be sure to use the terms *hypopnea* or *hyperpnea* — not *hypoventilation* or *hyperventilation.* Detecting hypoventilation or hyperventilation requires a measurement of partial pressure of carbon dioxide in arterial blood.

Anterior thorax

Inspect the thorax for structural deformities such as a concave or convex curvature of the anterior chest wall over the sternum. Inspect between and around the ribs for visible sinking of soft tissues (retractions). Assess the patient's respiratory

Effects of chronic ineffective gas exchange

Prolonged hypoxemia and hypercapnia, as seen in patients with chronic respiratory disorders, eventually take their toll on other vital systems.

CARDIOVASCULAR EFFECTS

Respiratory neuromuscular disorders, lung disease, and pulmonary vascular disease can produce acute or chronic enlargement of the right ventricle (cor pulmonale). Cor pulmonale is usually chronic, occurring secondary to chronic obstructive disease. Acute cor pulmonale may develop from massive pulmonary embolism, from acute pulmonary infection, or from another condition that worsens hypoxemia.

Cor pulmonale may result from widespread destruction of lung tissue or pulmonary capillaries, increased pulmonary vascular resistance, shunting of unoxygenated blood, or pulmonary vasoconstriction and pulmonary artery hypertension. Pulmonary hypertension leads to right ventricular dilation and hypertrophy, followed by right-sided heart failure, reduced cardiac output, and shock.

NEUROLOGIC EFFECTS

Severe hypercapnia dulls the medullary respiratory center, forcing peripheral chemoreceptors in the aortic and carotid bodies to direct respiration. Because these receptors respond to low partial pressure of arterial oxygen (PaO_2), oxygen therapy must be strictly controlled in accordance with blood gas analysis.

RENAL EFFECTS

Sustained hypercapnia causes renal retention of bicarbonate ions, sodium, and water, leading to fluid overload. Sustained hypoxemia stimulates the kidneys to release erythropoietic factor into the blood. This factor causes a plasma transport protein to yield erythropoietin, the compound that spurs red blood cell (RBC) production and increases hematocrit.

MUSCULOSKELETAL EFFECTS

When PaO_2 is low, an increase in pulmonary vasculature in response to chronic hypoxemia may cause pulmonary osteoarthropathy, also called secondary hypertrophic osteoarthropathy. This condition shows up as bone and tissue changes in the extremities, such as arthralgia, clubbing, and proliferation of subperiosteal tissues in long bones.

HEMATOPOIETIC EFFECTS

Chronic hypoxemia commonly causes an increase in the number of RBCs, which makes embolism and thrombosis more likely and increases the heart's workload.

---

pattern for symmetry. Look for abnormalities in skin color or alterations in muscle tone.

Initially, inspect the chest wall to identify the shape of the thoracic cage. In an adult, the thorax should have a greater diameter laterally (from side to side) than anteroposteriorly (from front to back).

Note the angle between the ribs and the sternum at the point immediately above the xiphoid process. This angle, called the *costal angle*, should be less than 90 degrees in an adult; it widens if the

PROLONGED HYPOXEMIA AND HYPERCAPNIA

Cardiovascular effects
- Pulmonary capillary vasoconstriction
- Increased pulmonary vascular resistance
- Pulmonary hypertension
- Shunting of unoxygenated blood
- Cor pulmonale

Neurologic effects
- Dulling of medullary respiratory center
- Respiration stimulated by aortic and carotid bodies

Renal effects
- Release of erythropoietin
- Increased retention of bicarbonate ions, sodium, and water
- Fluid overload

Musculoskeletal effects
- Pulmonary osteoarthropathy (arthralgia, digital clubbing, proliferation of subperiosteal tissues in long bones)
- Increased myoglobin in muscles

Hematopoietic effects
- Polycythemia
- Increased risk of embolism and thrombosis

chest wall is chronically expanded, as in increased anteroposterior diameter (barrel chest).

To inspect the anterior chest for symmetry of movement, have the patient lie supine. Stand at the foot of the bed and carefully observe the patient's deep breathing for equal expansion of the chest wall. Watch for the abnormal collapse of part of the chest wall during inspiration along with an abnormal expansion of the same area during expiration (paradoxical movement). Paradoxical

(*Text continues on page 334.*)

Recognizing common chest deformities

Inspect the patient's anterior chest for deviations in size or shape. Normally, the anteroposterior diameter is one-half the lateral diameter. The illustrations below depict three common deformities. The signs, associated conditions, and characteristics typical of each are described. For each deformity, a cross-sectional view is given to compare the anteroposterior and lateral diameters of the normal chest with those of the deformed chest (as indicated by the dotted line).

DEFORMITY	SIGNS AND ASSOCIATED CONDITIONS	CHARACTERISTICS
Funnel chest (pectus excavatum) Anteroposterior diameter Lateral diameter	▪ Postural disorders such as forward displacement of the neck and shoulders ▪ Upper thoracic kyphosis ▪ Protuberant abdomen ▪ Functional heart murmur	▪ Sinking or funnel-shaped depression of the lower sternum ▪ Diminished anteroposterior chest diameter ▪ Slightly increased lateral diameter
Pigeon chest (pectus carinatum) Anteroposterior diameter Lateral diameter	▪ Functional cardiovascular or respiratory disorders	▪ Projection of sternum beyond the frontal plane of abdomen, with projection greatest at the xiphoid process or at or near the center of the sternum ▪ Increased anteroposterior diameter ▪ Greatly decreased lateral diameter at the front of the chest
Barrel chest Anteroposterior diameter Lateral diameter	▪ Chronic respiratory disorders ▪ Increasing dyspnea ▪ Chronic cough ▪ Wheezing	▪ Enlarged anteroposterior and lateral chest dimensions; chest appears barrel-shaped ▪ Prominent accessory muscles ▪ Prominent sternal angle ▪ Thoracic kyphosis

Assessing abnormal breath sounds

The table below may be used as a guide to the descriptions, locations, and causes of the most common abnormal breath sounds.

TYPE	DESCRIPTION	LOCATION	CAUSE
Crackles	Light crackling, popping, nonmusical sound, like hairs being rubbed together; further classified by pitch: high, medium, or low	Anywhere; heard in lung bases initially, usually during inspiration; also in dependent lung portions of bedridden patients; aren't abnormal if clear with coughing	Air passing through moisture, especially in small airways and alveoli, with pulmonary edema; also, alveoli "popping open" in atelectasis
Wheezes	Whistling sound; described as sonorous, moaning, musical, sibilant and rumbling, or groaning	Anywhere; heard during inspiration or expiration; if clear with coughing, may originate in the larger upper airways	Fluid or secretions in the large airways or in airways narrowed by mucus, bronchospasm, or tumor
Rhonchi	Gurgling sound	Central airways; heard during inspiration and expiration	Air passing through fluid-filled airways, as in upper respiratory tract infection
Pleural friction rub	Superficial squeaking or grating sound, like pieces of sandpaper or leather being rubbed together	Lateral lung field; heard during inspiration and expiration (with patient in upright position)	Inflamed parietal and visceral pleural linings rubbing together
Grunting	Grunting noise	Central airways; heard during expiration in children	Physiological retention of air in lungs to prevent alveolar collapse
Stridor	Crowing noise	Larynx or trachea; heard during inspiration	Forced movement of air through edematous upper airway; in adults, laryngoedema, as in allergic reaction or smoke inhalation, and laryngospasm, as in tetany

movement indicates a loss of normal chest wall function.

Next, check for accessory muscle use during respiration by observing the sternocleidomastoid, scalene, and trapezius muscles in the shoulders and neck. During normal inspiration and expiration, the diaphragm and external intercostal muscles alone should easily maintain the breathing process. Hypertrophy of any of the accessory muscles may indicate frequent use, especially if found in an elderly patient, but may be normal in a well-conditioned athlete. Observe the position the patient assumes to breathe. A patient who depends on accessory muscles may assume a "tripod position," resting the arms on the knees or on the sides of a chair.

Observe the patient's skin on the anterior chest for unusual color, lumps, or lesions, and note the locations of any abnormalities.

Posterior thorax

To inspect the posterior chest, observe the patient's breathing again. If he can't sit in a backless chair or lean forward against a supporting structure, have him lie in a lateral position; remember, however, that this may distort your findings.

Assess the posterior chest wall for the same characteristics as the anterior one: chest structure, respiratory pattern, symmetry of expansion, skin color and muscle tone, and accessory muscle use.

Palpation

By carefully palpating the trachea and the anterior and posterior thorax, you can detect structural and skin abnormalities, areas of pain, and chest asymmetry.

Trachea and anterior thorax

First, palpate the trachea for position. Observe the patient to determine whether he uses accessory neck muscles to breathe.

Next, palpate the suprasternal notch. In most patients, the arch of the aorta lies close to the surface just behind the suprasternal notch. Use your fingertips to gently evaluate the strength and regularity of the patient's aortic pulsations.

Then palpate the thorax to assess the skin and underlying structures. Gentle palpation shouldn't be painful, so assess complaints of pain for localization, radiation, and severity. Be especially careful to palpate areas that looked abnormal during inspection. If necessary, support the patient during the procedure with one hand while using your other hand to palpate one side at a time, continuing to compare sides. Note unusual findings, such as masses, crepitus, skin irregularities, or painful areas.

If the patient complains of chest pain, attempt to determine the cause by palpating the anterior chest. Palpation doesn't worsen pain caused by cardiac or pulmonary disorders, such as angina and pleurisy.

Next, palpate the costal angle. The area around the xiphoid process contains many nerve endings, so be gentle to avoid causing pain. If a patient frequently uses the internal intercostal muscles to breathe, these muscles will eventually pull the chest cavity upward and outward. If this has occurred, the costal angle will be greater than the normal 90 degrees.

Posterior thorax

Palpate the posterior thorax in a similar manner, using the palmar surface of the fingertips of one or both hands. Identify bony structures, such as the vertebrae and scapulae.

To determine the location of an abnormality, identify the first thoracic vertebra (with the patient's head tipped forward) and count the number of spinous processes from this landmark to the abnormal finding. Use this reference point for documentation. Also, identify the inferior scapular tips and medial borders of both bones to define the margins of the upper and lower lung lobes posteriorly. Locate and describe all abnormalities in relation to these landmarks.

Tactile fremitus

Because sound travels more easily through solid structures than through air, assessing for tactile fremitus (the palpation of vocalizations) informs you about the contents of the lungs. (See *Palpating for tactile fremitus.*)

The patient's vocalization should produce vibrations of equal intensity on both sides of the chest. Normally, vibrations should occur in the upper chest, close to the bronchi, and then decrease and finally disappear toward the periphery of the lungs.

Conditions that restrict air movement, such as pneumonia, pleural effusion, and COPD with overinflated lungs, decrease tactile fremitus. Conditions that consolidate tissue or fluid in a portion of the pleural area, such as a lung tumor and pulmonary fibrosis, increase tactile fremitus. A grating feeling may signify a pleural friction rub.

Percussion

Percussion helps you to determine the boundaries of the lungs and how much gas, liquid, or solid exists in them. It can be used to assess structures as deep as 1¾″ to 3″ (4.5 to 7.5 cm). Perform percussion in a quiet environment, and proceed systematically, percussing the anterior, lateral, and posterior chest over the inter-

Palpating for tactile fremitus

Follow the procedure described below to assess for tactile fremitus.
1. Place your open palm flat against the patient's chest without touching the chest with your fingers.

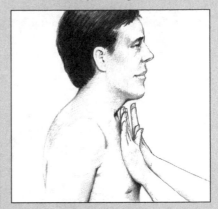

2. Ask the patient to repeat a resonant phrase like "99" as you systematically move your hands over his chest from the central airways to the lung periphery and back. Always proceed in a systematic manner from the top of the suprascapular, interscapular, infrascapular, and hypochondriac areas (areas found from the fifth to tenth intercostal spaces to the right and left of the midline).
3. Repeat this procedure on the posterior thorax. You should feel vibrations of equal intensity on either side of the chest. Fremitus usually occurs in the upper chest, close to the bronchi, and feels strongest at the second intercostal space on either side of the sternum. Little or no fremitus should occur in the lower chest. The intensity of the vibrations varies according to the thickness and structure of the patient's chest wall as well as the patient's voice intensity and pitch.

Percussing the thorax

When percussing a patient's thorax, always use mediate percussion and follow the same sequence, comparing sound variations from one side with the other. This helps to ensure consistency and prevents you from overlooking important findings. Auscultation follows the same sequence as percussion.

To percuss the anterior thorax, place your fingers over the lung apices in the supraclavicular area. Then proceed downward, moving from side to side at 1½" to 2" (4- to 5-cm) intervals as shown on the left.

To percuss the lateral thorax, start at the axilla and move down the side of the rib cage, percussing between the ribs, as shown in the middle.

To percuss the posterior thorax, progress in a zigzag fashion from the suprascapular to the interscapular to the infrascapular areas, avoiding the spinal column and the scapulae, as shown on the right.

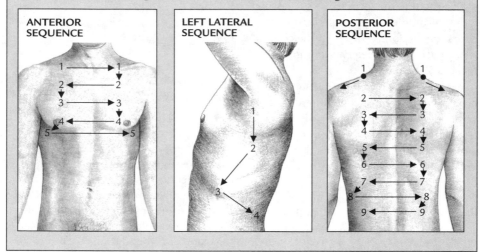

ANTERIOR SEQUENCE

LEFT LATERAL SEQUENCE

POSTERIOR SEQUENCE

costal spaces. (See *Percussing the thorax.*) Avoid percussing over bones, which yields no useful information. Percussion over a healthy lung elicits a resonant sound (hollow and loud, with a low pitch and long duration).

To percuss the anterior chest, have the patient sit facing forward, hands resting at the side of the body. Following the anterior percussion sequence, percuss and compare sound variations from one side with the other. Anterior chest percussion should produce resonance from below the clavicle to the fifth intercostal space

on the right (where dullness occurs close to the liver) and to the third intercostal space on the left (where dullness occurs near the heart).

Next, percuss the lateral chest to obtain information about the left upper and lower lobes and about the right upper, middle, and lower lobes. The patient's left arm should be positioned on his head. Repeat the same sequence on the right side. Lateral chest percussion should produce resonance to the sixth or eighth intercostal space.

Finally, percuss the posterior thorax according to the percussion sequence. Posterior percussion should sound resonant to the level of T10.

Auscultation

Auscultate the anterior, lateral, and posterior thorax to detect normal and abnormal breath sounds. To auscultate the thorax of an adult, first warm the stethoscope between your hands, and then place the diaphragm of the stethoscope directly on the patient's skin.

If the patient has significant hair growth over the area to be auscultated, wet the hair to decrease sound blurring. Instruct the patient to take deep breaths through the mouth, and caution him against breathing too deeply or too rapidly to prevent light-headedness or dizziness.

During auscultation, first identify normal breath sounds, and then assess and identify abnormal sounds. Specific breath sounds occur normally only in certain locations; therefore, the same sound heard anywhere else in the lung field is an important abnormality requiring appropriate documentation.

Anterior and lateral thorax

Systematically auscultate the anterior and lateral thorax for normal as well as abnormal breath sounds, following the same sequence used for percussion. Begin at the upper lobes, and move from side to side and down. Have the patient breathe slowly and deeply with an open mouth.

Auscultate a point on one side of the chest, and then auscultate the same point on the other side of the chest, comparing findings. Always assess one full breath at each point.

To assess the right middle lung lobe, auscultate for breath sounds laterally at the level of the fourth to the sixth intercostal spaces, following the lateral auscultation sequence, which is the same as the lateral percussion sequence. The right middle lobe is a common site of aspiration pneumonia, so it requires special attention.

Normal breath sounds include tracheal, bronchial, bronchovesicular, and vesicular sounds. Tracheal sounds, which are harsh and discontinuous, are heard equally during inspiration and expiration. Bronchial sounds, high-pitched and discontinuous, are prolonged during expiration. Bronchovesicular sounds, which are medium-pitched and continuous, are equally audible during inspiration and expiration. Vesicular sounds, which are low-pitched and continuous, are prolonged during inspiration. (See *Normal breath sounds*, page 338.)

Classify normal and abnormal breath sounds according to location, intensity (amplitude), characteristic sound, pitch (tone), and duration during the inspiratory and expiratory phases. When assessing duration, time the inspiratory and expiratory phases to determine the ratio.

For the last step in auscultation, identify the inspiratory and expiratory phase of normal and abnormal breath sounds. Also determine whether the sound occurs during inspiration, expiration, or both.

Posterior thorax

Auscultate the posterior thorax in the same pattern as the percussion sequence. During auscultation, remain aware of the patient's breathing pattern. Have the patient sit with arms folded and head bent forward.

In a normal adult, bronchovesicular breath sounds (the sound of air moving through the bronchial airways) should occur over the interscapular area; vesicular breath sounds (the sound of air moving

Normal breath sounds

The illustrations here depict the locations of the various breath sounds.

Tracheal sounds result from air passing through the glottis. They're heard best over the trachea as harsh, discontinuous sounds. The ratio of inspiration to expiration is 1:1.

Bronchial sounds result from high rates of turbulent airflow through the large bronchi. They're loud, high-pitched, hollow, harsh, or coarse sounds heard over the manubrium. The inspiration to expiration ratio is 2:3.

Bronchovesicular sounds result from transitional airflow moving through the branches and convergences of the smaller bronchi and bronchioles. These soft, breezy sounds are pitched about two notes lower than bronchial sounds. Anteriorly, they're heard near the mainstem bronchi in the first and second intercostal spaces; posteriorly, between the scapulae. The inspiration to expiration ratio is 1:1.

Vesicular sounds result from laminar airflow moving through the alveolar ducts and alveoli at low flow rates. They're heard best in the periphery of the lungs but are inaudible over the scapulae. These soft, swishy, breezy sounds are about two notes lower than bronchovesicular sounds. Their inspiration to expiration ratio is 3:1.

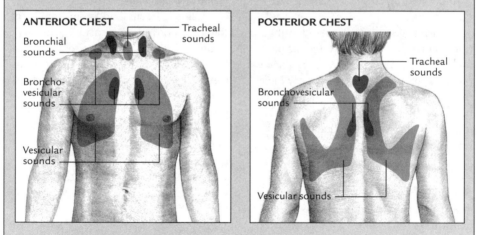

through the alveoli) should occur in the suprascapular and infrascapular areas. Note any absent, decreased, or adventitious breath sounds. For example, bronchovesicular sounds auscultated in the periphery of the lungs are adventitious. Crackles and rhonchi (gurgles) are also adventitious; if you hear them, instruct the patient to cough, and then listen again.

Diaphragmatic excursion
This technique allows you to evaluate your patient's diaphragm movement. (See *Measuring diaphragmatic excursion.*) Normal diaphragmatic excursion is 1¼" to 2¼" (3 to 5.5 cm). Failure of the diaphragm to contract downward may indicate paralysis or muscle flattening, a condition that results from COPD.

Measuring diaphragmatic excursion

Follow the procedure described here to measure the extent of diaphragmatic excursion (the distance that the diaphragm travels between inhalation and exhalation).

■ First instruct the patient to take a deep breath and hold it while you percuss down the right side of the posterior thorax. Begin at the lower border of the scapula and continue until the percussion note changes from resonance to dullness, which identifies the location of the diaphragm. Using a washable, felt-tipped pen, mark this point with a small line.

■ Now instruct the patient to take a few normal breaths. Then ask him to exhale completely and hold it while you percuss again to locate the point where the resonant sounds become dull. Mark this point with a small line.

■ Repeat this entire procedure on the left side of the posterior thorax. Keep in mind that the diaphragm usually sits slightly higher on the right side than on

the left because of the position of the liver.

■ Next, using a tape measure or ruler, measure the distance between the two marks on each side of the posterior thorax, as shown here. The distance between these two marks reflects diaphragmatic excursion.

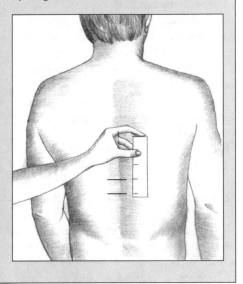

Voice resonance

To assess voice resonance, instruct the patient to say "99." As he speaks, auscultate in the usual sequence. The voice normally sounds muffled and indistinct during auscultation; the sound is loudest medially and softest in the lung periphery. However, conditions producing lung tissue consolidation cause bronchophony, which is the greater resonance that allows you to hear "99" clearly during auscultation.

To test increased resonance further, ask the patient to repeat the letter *e*, which should sound muffled and indistinct on auscultation. If the letter sounds

like *a* and the voice sounds nasal or bleating, the patient is exhibiting egophony, another indication of consolidation.

To perform another test for increased resonance, ask the patient to whisper the words "one-two-three." On auscultation, these words should be barely audible. If the words sound distinct and understandable, you have heard whispered pectoriloquy, which suggests lung tissue consolidation from such conditions as a lung tumor, pneumonia, or pulmonary fibrosis.

• • • • • • • • • • • •

ATELECTASIS

Atelectasis is an incomplete expansion of lobules (clusters of alveoli) or lung segments, which can lead to partial or complete lung collapse. Because parts of the lung are unavailable for gas exchange, unoxygenated blood passes through these areas unchanged, causing hypoxemia. Atelectasis may be chronic or acute. Many patients undergoing upper abdominal or thoracic surgery experience atelectasis to some degree. Once lung tissue is reexpanded for optimal gas exchange, prognosis is good unless residual damage has occurred.

Causes and pathophysiology

Atelectasis commonly results from bronchial occlusion by mucus plugs. It's a problem in many patients with chronic obstructive pulmonary disease, bronchiectasis, cystic fibrosis, and postgeneral anesthesia and in those who smoke heavily (smoking increases mucus production and damages cilia). Atelectasis also results from occlusion by foreign bodies, bronchogenic carcinoma, and inflammatory lung disease.

Other causes include respiratory distress syndrome of the neonate (hyaline membrane disease), oxygen toxicity, and pulmonary edema, in which alveolar surfactant changes increase surface tension and permit complete alveolar deflation.

External compression, which inhibits full lung expansion, or any condition that makes deep breathing painful, may also cause atelectasis. Such compression or pain may result from upper abdominal surgical incisions, rib fractures, pleuritic chest pain, tight dressings around the chest, stab wounds, impalement accidents, car accidents in which the driver slams into the steering column, or obesity (which elevates the diaphragm and reduces tidal volume).

Prolonged immobility may also cause atelectasis by producing preferential ventilation of one area of the lung over another. Mechanical ventilation using constant small tidal volumes without intermittent deep breaths may also result in atelectasis. Central nervous system depression (as in drug overdose) eliminates periodic sighing and is a predisposing factor of progressive atelectasis.

Clinical presentation

Clinical effects vary with the severity and degree of hypoxemia and any underlying disease but generally include some degree of dyspnea. Atelectasis of a small area of the lung may produce only minimal symptoms that subside without specific treatment. However, massive collapse can produce:

- severe dyspnea
- anxiety
- cyanosis
- diaphoresis
- peripheral circulatory collapse
- tachycardia
- substernal or intercostal retraction.

Also, atelectasis may result in compensatory hyperinflation of unaffected areas of the lung, mediastinal shift to the affected side, and elevation of the ipsilateral hemidiaphragm.

Differential diagnoses

- Pneumothorax
- Hemothorax
- Acute asthma
- Adult respiratory distress syndrome
- Pneumonia
- Pulmonary neoplasms

Diagnosis

Diagnosis requires an accurate patient history, a physical examination, and a chest X-ray. Auscultation reveals diminished or bronchial breath sounds. When much of the lung is collapsed, percussion reveals dullness. However, extensive areas of "microatelectasis" may exist without abnormalities on the chest X-ray. In widespread atelectasis, the chest X-ray shows characteristic horizontal lines in the lower lung zones. With segmental or lobar collapse, characteristic dense shadows often associated with hyperinflation of neighboring lung zones are also apparent. If the cause is unknown, diagnostic procedures may include bronchoscopy to rule out an obstructing neoplasm or a foreign body.

Management
General
Treatment includes incentive spirometry, frequent coughing, and deep-breathing exercises. If atelectasis is secondary to mucus plugging, mucolytics, chest percussion, and postural drainage may be used. If these measures fail, bronchoscopy may be helpful in removing secretions. Humidity and bronchodilators can improve mucociliary clearance and dilate airways; they're sometimes used with a nebulizer. Postoperative thoracic and abdominal surgery patients require analgesics to facilitate deep breathing, which minimizes the risk of atelectasis.

Surgical intervention
Atelectasis secondary to an obstructing neoplasm may require surgery or radiation therapy.

Referral
■ If the patient's atelectasis is severe, he should be referred to a hospital for admission and treatment.
■ Encourage the patient to stop smoking and to lose weight as needed. Refer him to appropriate support groups for help.

Follow-up
Initially, the patient should be seen within 48 hours, then in 1 week. If the patient's condition improves, he should be seen monthly until the atelectasis is resolved, as shown by chest X-ray.

Patient teaching
■ To prevent atelectasis, teach preoperative patients to cough and deep-breathe effectively.
■ Teach the patient to use an incentive spirometer to encourage deep inspiration through positive reinforcement. Encourage him to use it every 1 to 2 hours.
■ Teach the family how to perform postural drainage and chest percussion.

Complications
■ Infection
■ Hypoxia

Special considerations
■ Provide reassurance and emotional support; the patient will probably be frightened by his limited breathing capacity.

• • • • • • • • • • • •

B.O.O.P., IDIOPATHIC

Idiopathic bronchiolitis obliterans with organizing pneumonia (BOOP), also known as cryptogenic organizing pneumonia, is one of several types of bronchiolitis obliterans. *Bronchiolitis obliterans* is a generic term used to describe an inflammatory disease of the small airways. *Organizing pneumonia* refers to unresolved pneumonia in which inflammatory alveolar exudate persists and eventually undergoes fibrosis.

AGE ALERT Most patients with BOOP are between 50 and 60 years old.

Incidence is equally divided between men and women. A history of smoking doesn't seem to increase the risk of developing BOOP.

Causes

BOOP has no known cause. However, other forms of bronchiolitis obliterans and organizing pneumonia may be associated with specific diseases or situations, such as bone marrow, heart, or heart-lung transplantation; collagen vascular diseases, such as rheumatoid arthritis and systemic lupus erythematosus; inflammatory diseases, such as Crohn's disease, ulcerative colitis, and polyarteritis nodosa; bacterial, viral, or mycoplasmal respiratory infections; inhalation of toxic gases; and drug therapy with amiodarone, bleomycin, penicillamine, or lomustine.

Clinical presentation

The presenting symptoms of BOOP are usually subacute, with a flulike syndrome of:
- fever
- persistent and nonproductive cough
- dyspnea (especially with exertion)
- malaise
- anorexia
- weight loss lasting for several weeks to several months.

Physical assessment findings may reveal dry crackles as the only abnormality. Less common signs and symptoms include a productive cough, hemoptysis, chest pain, generalized aching, and night sweats.

Differential diagnoses
- Tuberculosis
- Sarcoidosis
- Neoplasm
- Histoplasmosis
- Usual interstitial pneumonitis

Diagnosis

Diagnosis begins with a thorough patient history meant to exclude any known cause of bronchiolitis obliterans or diseases with a pathology that includes an organizing pneumonia pattern. It may also include these tests:
- Chest X-rays usually show patchy, diffuse airspace opacities with a ground-glass appearance that may migrate from one location to another. High-resolution computed tomography scans show areas of consolidation. Except for the migrating opacities, these findings are nonspecific and present in many other respiratory disorders.
- Pulmonary function tests may be normal or show reduced capacities. The diffusing capacity for carbon monoxide is generally low.
- Arterial blood gas analysis usually shows mild to moderate hypoxemia at rest, which worsens with exercise.
- Blood tests reveal an increased erythrocyte sedimentation rate, increased C-reactive protein level, increased white blood cell count with a somewhat increased proportion of neutrophils, and a minor rise in eosinophils. Immunoglobulin G (IgG) and IgM levels are normal or slightly increased, and IgE level is normal.
- Bronchoscopy reveals normal or slightly inflamed airways. Bronchoalveolar lavage fluid obtained during bronchoscopy shows a moderate elevation in lymphocytes and, sometimes, elevated neutrophil and eosinophil levels. Foamy-looking alveolar macrophages may also be found.

Lung biopsy, thoracoscopy, or bronchoscopy is required to confirm the diagnosis of BOOP. Pathologic changes in lung tissue include plugs of connective tissue in the lumen of the bronchioles, alveolar ducts, and alveolar spaces.

These changes may occur in other types of bronchiolitis and in other diseases that cause organizing pneumonia. They also differentiate BOOP from constrictive bronchiolitis (characterized by inflammation and fibrosis that surround and may narrow or completely obliterate the bronchiolar airways). Although the pathologic findings in proliferative and constrictive bronchiolitis are different from those in BOOP, the causes and presentations may overlap. Any known cause of bronchiolitis obliterans or organizing pneumonia must be ruled out before the diagnosis of BOOP is made.

Management
General
Oxygen is used to correct hypoxemia. The patient may need either no oxygen or a small amount of oxygen at rest and a greater amount when he exercises.

Other treatments vary, depending on the patient's symptoms, and may include inhaled bronchodilators, cough suppressants, and bronchial hygiene therapies.

Medication
Corticosteroids are the current treatment for BOOP, although the ideal dosage and duration of treatment remain topics of discussion. In most cases, treatment begins with 1 mg/kg/day of prednisone for at least several days to several weeks; the dosage is then gradually reduced over several months to a year, depending on the patient's response. Relapse is common when corticosteroids are tapered off or stopped. This usually can be reversed when steroids are increased or resumed. Occasionally, a patient may need to continue corticosteroids indefinitely. BOOP is very responsive to treatment and usually can be completely reversed with corticosteroid therapy.

Immunosuppressive-cytotoxic drugs, such as cyclophosphamide (1 to 5 mg/kg/day P.O.), have been used in the few cases of intolerance or unresponsiveness.

Referral
- The patient may need to be referred to a pulmonologist for treatment.
- If the patient needs oxygen at home, ensure continuity of care by making appropriate referrals to discharge planners, respiratory care practitioners, and home equipment vendors.

Follow-up
The patient should initially be seen weekly and then monitored according to recovery and relapse episodes. The patient should be monitored for adverse effects of medication.

Patient teaching
- Teach the patient and family about the adverse effects of the medications prescribed, emphasizing which reactions they should report.
- Teach measures that may help prevent complications related to treatment, such as infection control and improved nutrition.
- Teach breathing, relaxation, and energy conservation techniques to help the patient manage symptoms.

Complications
- Bronchiectasis
- Death

Special considerations
- BOOP was first described in 1901, but confusing terminology and pathology that overlapped other diseases of the small airways kept it from being sufficiently recognized until the mid-1980s. Since then, BOOP has been diagnosed with increasing frequency, although the

various pathologies and classifications of bronchiolitis obliterans are still debated.
- Explain the diagnosis to the patient and his family. This uncommon diagnosis may cause confusion and anxiety.

• • • • • • • • • • •

BRONCHITIS, CHRONIC

Chronic bronchitis is marked by excessive production of tracheobronchial mucus that is sufficient to cause a cough for at least 3 months each year for 2 consecutive years.

The severity of the disease is linked to the amount of pollutants inhaled. A respiratory tract infection typically exacerbates the cough and related signs and symptoms. However, few patients with chronic bronchitis develop significant airway obstruction. Women have a higher incidence of this disorder.

AGE ALERT Bronchitis occurs more frequently in people over age 45.

Causes and pathophysiology

Cigarette smoking is the most common cause of chronic bronchitis. Some studies suggest a genetic predisposition to the disease as well.

The disease is directly correlated to heavy pollution and is more prevalent in people exposed to organic or inorganic dusts and to noxious gases. Children of parents who smoke are at higher risk for respiratory tract infections, which can lead to chronic bronchitis.

Chronic bronchitis results in hypertrophy and hyperplasia of the bronchial mucous glands, increased goblet cells, ciliary damage, squamous metaplasia of the columnar epithelium, and chronic leukocytic and lymphocytic infiltration of bronchial walls. Additional effects include

widespread inflammation, airway narrowing, and mucus within the airways—all of which produce resistance in the small airways and, in turn, a severe ventilation-perfusion imbalance. (See *Understanding chronic bronchitis*.)

Clinical presentation

The patient's history typically reflects a long-time smoker who has frequent upper respiratory tract infections. Usually, the patient seeks treatment for a productive cough and exertional dyspnea. He may describe his cough as initially prevalent in the winter months but gradually becoming a year-round problem with increasingly severe episodes. He also typically reports progressively worsening dyspnea that takes increasingly longer to subside.

Other signs and symptoms include:
- productive cough
- cyanosis
- use of accessory respiratory muscles for breathing (a "blue bloater")
- tachypnea
- substantial weight gain
- pedal edema
- neck vein distention
- wheezing
- prolonged expiratory time
- rhonchi.

Differential diagnoses

- Asthma
- Chronic obstructive pulmonary disease
- Emphysema
- Bronchiolitis
- Laryngotracheobronchitis
- Pertussis
- Pneumonia
- Sinusitis
- Influenza
- Cystic fibrosis

Diagnosis

To diagnose chronic bronchitis, look for these results:

- Chest X-rays may show hyperinflation and increased bronchovascular markings.
- Pulmonary function tests demonstrate increased residual volume, decreased vital capacity and forced expiratory flow, and normal static compliance and diffusing capacity.
- Arterial blood gas analysis displays decreased partial pressure of arterial oxygen and normal or increased partial pressure of arterial carbon dioxide.
- Sputum culture may reveal many microorganisms and neutrophils.
- Electrocardiography may reveal atrial arrhythmias, peaked P waves in leads II, III, and aV_F and, occasionally, right ventricular hypertrophy.

Management

General

The most effective treatment is for the patient to stop smoking and to avoid air pollutants as much as possible. Adequate fluid intake is essential, and chest physiotherapy may be needed to mobilize secretions. Oxygen may be necessary to treat a patient with hypoxia.

Medication

Antibiotics can be used to treat patients with recurring infections:

- erythromycin — adults, 250 to 500 mg P.O. every 6 hours; children, 30 to 50 mg/kg/day P.O. in divided doses
- clarithromycin — adults, 250 to 500 mg P.O. every 12 hours; children, 7.5 mg/kg/day P.O. divided every 12 hours.
- azithromycin — adults, Z-pak 500 mg P.O. the 1st day, then 250 mg for the next 4 days.

Bronchodilators may also be used:

- albuterol inhaler — one to two inhalations every 4 to 6 hours

Understanding chronic bronchitis

In chronic bronchitis, irritants inhaled for a prolonged period inflame the tracheobronchial tree. The inflammation leads to increased mucus production and a narrowed or blocked airway.

As inflammation continues, the mucus-producing goblet cells undergo hypertrophy, as do the ciliated epithelial cells that line the respiratory tract. Hypersecretion from the goblet cells blocks the free movement of the cilia, which normally sweep dust, irritants, and mucus from the airways. As a result, the airway stays blocked, and mucus and debris accumulate in the respiratory tract.

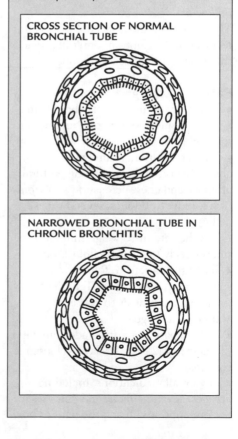

CROSS SECTION OF NORMAL BRONCHIAL TUBE

NARROWED BRONCHIAL TUBE IN CHRONIC BRONCHITIS

- ipratropium — one to two inhalations q.i.d.

Additional medication may include:
- prednisone — 5 to 60 mg P.O. per day; dosage must be individualized
- furosemide — 20 to 40 mg P.O. per day
- guaifenesin with dextromethorphan — adults, 5 to 10 ml P.O. every 4 hours as necessary; children ages 2 to 6, 2.5 ml P.O. every 4 hours; children ages 6 to 12, 5 ml P.O. every 4 hours.

Referral
- Refer the patient to a pulmonologist if recurrences are severe.
- Refer the patient and family members to appropriate support services.
- Refer the patient to a stop-smoking program or counseling, if appropriate.

Follow-up
The patient should be seen 2 weeks after recurrence. If symptoms don't improve, the patient should be seen sooner.

Patient teaching
- Tell the patient to report changes in baseline respiratory function and to note sputum quality and quantity.
- Teach the patient's family to perform chest physiotherapy, including postural drainage and chest percussion and vibration for involved lobes, several times daily.
- Tell the patient to weigh himself three times weekly to evaluate fluid status.
- Teach the patient to follow a high-calorie, protein-rich diet. Tell him to eat small, frequent meals to conserve energy and prevent fatigue.
- Tell the patient to drink adequate fluids (at least 3 qt [2.8 L] per day) to loosen secretions.
- Review all medications, including dosages, adverse effects, and purposes for the prescriptions. Teach the patient how

to use an inhaler. Advise him to report adverse reactions immediately.
- Warn the patient that exposure to blasts of cold air may precipitate bronchospasm. Instruct the patient to avoid cold, windy weather or to cover his mouth and nose with a scarf or mask if going outside is essential.

Complications
- Cor pulmonale
- Pulmonary hypertension
- Right ventricular hypertrophy
- Acute respiratory failure

Special considerations
- If the patient smokes, encourage him to stop.

• • • • • • • • • • • •

CHRONIC OBSTRUCTIVE PULMONARY DISEASE

Chronic obstructive pulmonary disease (COPD) is a chronic airway obstruction due to emphysema, chronic bronchitis, asthma, or any combination of these disorders. (See *Types of chronic obstructive pulmonary disease*, pages 348 to 351, and *Three types of emphysema*, page 352.) Usually, more than one of these underlying conditions coexist; in most cases, bronchitis and emphysema occur together.

COPD is the most common chronic lung disease, affecting an estimated 32 million Americans; it's the fourth leading cause of death in the United States. Two-thirds of those affected are male and one-third are female, probably because (until recently) men were more likely to smoke heavily. It doesn't always produce symptoms and causes only minimal disability in many patients. COPD tends to worsen with time; quick identification reduces mortality.

Causes

Predisposing factors include cigarette smoking, recurrent or chronic respiratory infections, air pollution, occupational exposure to chemicals, and allergies. Smoking is by far the most important of these factors; it impairs ciliary action and macrophage function, inflames airways, increases mucus production, destroys alveolar septa, and causes peribronchiolar fibrosis. Early inflammatory changes may reverse if the patient stops smoking before lung destruction is extensive. Familial and hereditary factors (such as deficiency of alpha$_1$-antitrypsin) also may predispose a person to COPD.

Clinical presentation

The typical patient is a long-term cigarette smoker who has no symptoms until middle age. The patient's ability to exercise or do strenuous work gradually starts to decline, and he begins to develop a productive cough. These signs are subtle at first but become more pronounced as the patient gets older and the disease progresses. Signs of COPD include:

- productive cough
- cyanosis
- increased erythema
- wheezing
- dyspnea on minimal exertion
- frequent respiratory infections
- intermittent or continuous hypoxemia
- grossly abnormal pulmonary function studies.

Advanced COPD may cause severe dyspnea, overwhelming disability, cor pulmonale, severe respiratory failure, and death.

Differential diagnoses

- Asthma
- Pneumonia
- COPD: emphysema
- COPD: chronic bronchitis

- Pulmonic valve stenosis
- Heart failure
- Pulmonary edema

Diagnosis

Diagnostic tests may vary according to the type of COPD. Basic testing includes:

- arterial blood gas analysis to identify hypoxia and CO_2 retention
- serum electrolyte studies to identify sodium retention and hypokalemia
- complete blood count to identify polycythemia
- pulmonary function tests to identify decreased forced expiratory volume and forced vital capacity and increased total lung capacity and residual volume.

Management

General

Treatment is designed to relieve symptoms and prevent complications. Because most COPD patients receive outpatient treatment, they need comprehensive patient teaching to help them comply with therapy and to understand the nature of this chronic, progressive disease. Oxygen in low concentration may be needed.

Medication

Most patients are treated with medication given by metered-dose inhaler, such as:

- albuterol (beta-agonist bronchodilator) — 5 mg/ml solution for nebulizer
- ipratropium (anticholinergic bronchodilator) — adults, one to two inhalations q.i.d.; children, 125 to 250 mcg nebulizer treatment every 4 to 6 hours
- beclomethasone (corticosteroid) — adults, two inhalations q.i.d.; children, one to two inhalations t.i.d. to q.i.d.; or triamcinolone — adults, two inhalations q.i.d.; children, one to two inhalations t.i.d. to q.i.d.

(*Text continues on page 350.*)

Types of chronic obstructive pulmonary disease

DISEASE	CAUSES AND PATHOPHYSIOLOGY	CLINICAL FEATURES
Emphysema ■ Abnormal, irreversible enlargement of air spaces distal to terminal bronchioles due to destruction of alveolar walls, resulting in decreased elastic recoil properties of lungs ■ Most common cause of death from respiratory disease in the United States	■ Cigarette smoking and alpha$_1$-antitrypsin deficiency ■ Recurrent inflammation associated with release of proteolytic enzymes from cells in lungs, causing bronchiolar and alveolar wall damage and, ultimately, destruction; loss of lung supporting structure, resulting in decreased elastic recoil and airway collapse on expiration; destruction of alveolar walls, decreasing surface area for gas exchange	■ Insidious onset, with dyspnea the predominant symptom ■ *Other signs and symptoms of long-term disease:* anorexia, weight loss, malaise, barrel chest, use of accessory muscles of respiration, prolonged expiratory period with grunting, pursed-lip breathing, and tachypnea ■ *Complications:* recurrent respiratory tract infections, cor pulmonale, and respiratory failure
Chronic bronchitis ■ Excessive mucus production with productive cough for at least 3 months a year for 2 successive years ■ No development of significant airway obstruction in most patients with chronic bronchitis	■ Severity of disease related to amount and duration of smoking; respiratory infection exacerbates symptoms ■ Hypertrophy and hyperplasia of bronchial mucous glands, increased goblet cells, damage to cilia, squamous metaplasia of columnar epithelium, and chronic leukocytic and lymphocytic infiltration of bronchial walls ■ Widespread inflammation, distortion, narrowing of airways, and mucus in the airways, producing resistance in small airways and causing severe ventilation-perfusion imbalance	■ Insidious onset, with productive cough and exertional dyspnea predominant symptoms ■ *Other signs:* colds associated with increased sputum production and worsening dyspnea, which take progressively longer to resolve; copious sputum (gray, white, or yellow); weight gain due to edema; cyanosis; tachypnea; wheezing; and prolonged expiratory time and use of accessory muscles of respiration

CONFIRMING DIAGNOSTIC MEASURES

- *Physical examination:* hyperresonance on percussion, decreased breath sounds, expiratory prolongation, and quiet heart sounds
- *Chest X-ray:* in advanced disease, flattened diaphragm, reduced vascular markings at lung periphery, overaeration of lungs, vertical heart, enlarged anteroposterior chest diameter, and large retrosternal air space
- *Pulmonary function tests:* increased residual volume, total lung capacity, and compliance; decreased vital capacity, diffusing capacity, and expiratory volumes
- *Arterial blood gas analysis:* reduced partial pressure of arterial oxygen (PaO_2) with normal partial pressure of arterial carbon dioxide ($PaCO_2$) until late in disease
- *ECG:* tall, symmetrical P waves in leads II, III, and aV_F vertical QRS axis; signs of right ventricular hypertrophy late in disease
- *CBC:* increased hemoglobin late in disease when persistent severe hypoxia is present

MANAGEMENT

- Oxygen at low-flow settings to treat hypoxia
- Avoidance of smoking and air pollutants
- Breathing techniques to control dyspnea
- Treatment only slightly helpful for emphysema component of chronic obstructive pulmonary disease
- Lung volume reduction surgery for selected patients

- *Physical examination:* rhonchi and wheezes on auscultation, prolonged expiration, neck vein distention, and pedal edema
- *Chest X-ray:* hyperinflation and increased bronchovascular markings
- *Pulmonary function tests:* increased residual volume, decreased vital capacity and forced expiratory volumes, and normal static compliance and diffusing capacity
- *Arterial blood gas analysis:* decreased PaO_2, normal or increased $PaCO_2$
- *ECG:* trial arrhythmias; peaked P waves in leads II, III, and aV_F; and, occasionally, right ventricular hypertrophy

- *Antibiotics for infections (erythromycin:* adults: 250 to 500 mg P.O. q.i.d.; children: 30 to 50 mg/kg/day P.O. in divided doses)
- Avoidance of smoking and air pollutants
- Bronchodilators (albuterol: 5 mg/ml solution for nebulizer) to relieve bronchospasm and facilitate mucociliary clearance
- Adequate fluid intake and chest physiotherapy to mobilize secretions
- Ultrasonic or mechanical nebulizer treatments to loosen secretions and aid in mobilization
- Occasionally, corticosteroids (methylprednisolone: 4 to 48 mg/day P.O.)
- Diuretics (furosemide: 20 to 40 mg/day P.O.) for edema
- Oxygen for hypoxemia

(continued)

Types of cardiac obstructive pulmonary disease (continued)

DISEASE	CAUSES AND PATHOPHYSIOLOGY	CLINICAL FEATURES
Asthma ■ Increased bronchial reactivity to a variety of stimuli; produces episodic bronchospasm and airway obstruction in conjunction with airway inflammation ■ Asthma with onset in adulthood — often without distinct allergies; asthma with onset in childhood — often associated with definite allergens; status asthmaticus — acute asthma attack with severe bronchospasm that fails to clear with bronchodilator therapy ■ More than half of asthmatic children become asymptomatic as adults; more than half of asthmatics with onset after age 15 have persistent disease, with occasional severe attacks	■ Allergy (family tendency and seasonal occurrence); allergic reaction resulting in the release of mast cell vasoactive and bronchospastic mediators ■ Precipitating events include upper airway infection, exercise, anxiety and, rarely, coughing or laughing ■ Paroxysmal airway obstruction (associated with nasal polyps in response to aspirin or indomethacin ingestion) ■ Airway obstruction from spasm of bronchial smooth muscle narrowing airways; inflammatory edema of the bronchial wall and inspissation of tenacious mucoid secretions (particularly in status asthmaticus)	■ History of intermittent attacks of dyspnea and wheezing ■ Mild wheezing progresses to severe dyspnea, audible wheezing, chest tightness (a feeling of not being able to breathe), and cough producing thick mucus. ■ *Other signs and symptoms:* prolonged expiration, intercostal and supraclavicular retraction on inspiration, accessory muscle use during respiration; flaring nostrils, tachypnea, tachycardia, perspiration, and flushing; and eczema and allergic rhinitis (hay fever) ■ Respiratory failure in patients with status asthmaticus (unless treated promptly) ■ Nocturnal flare-ups

Antibiotics may be given to treat respiratory infections:

■ erythromycin — adults, 250 to 500 mg P.O. every 6 hours; children, 30 to 50 mg/kg/day P.O. in divided doses

■ azithromycin — adults, Z-pak 500 mg P.O. 1st day, then 250 mg for next 4 days; children, 10 mg/kg P.O. 1st day, then 5 mg/kg/day P.O. days 2 through 5.

Surgical intervention

Lung volume reduction surgery is a new procedure for carefully selected patients primarily with emphysema. Nonfunctional parts of the lung (diseased tissue that provides little ventilation or perfusion) are surgically removed. Removal allows more functional lung tissue to expand and the diaphragm to return to its normally elevated position.

CONFIRMING DIAGNOSTIC MEASURES

- *Physical examination:* usually normal between attacks; auscultation revealing rhonchi and wheezing throughout lung fields on expiration and, at times, inspiration; absent or diminished breath sounds during severe obstruction; loud bilateral wheezing, possibly grossly audible; hyperinflated chest
- *Chest X-ray:* hyperinflated lungs with air trapping during attack; normal during remission
- *Sputum culture:* presence of Curschmann's spirals (casts of airways), Charcot-Leyden crystals, and eosinophils
- *Pulmonary function tests:* during attacks, decreased forced expiratory volumes that improve significantly after inhaled bronchodilator; increased residual volume and, occasionally, total lung capacity; may be normal between attacks
- *Arterial blood gas analysis:* decreased PaO_2; decreased, normal, or increased $PaCO_2$ (in severe attack)
- *ECG:* sinus tachycardia during an attack; severe attack possibly producing signs of cor pulmonale (right axis deviation and peaked P wave) that resolve after the attack
- *Skin tests:* possible identification of allergens

MANAGEMENT

- Aerosol containing beta-adrenergic blockers, such as albuterol (5 mg/ml solution for nebulizer); also oral beta-adrenergic blockers (terbutaline: adults, 2.5 to 5 mg P.O. every 6 hours three times per day; children, 2 mg P.O. every 6 hours three times per day) and oral methylxanthines (theophylline: adults, 3 mg/kg every 8 hours; children, 3 to 4 mg/kg every 6 hours); most patients require inhaled, oral, or I.V. corticosteroids
- Emergency treatment: oxygen therapy, corticosteroids (hydrocortisone: 100 to 500 mg I.V.), bronchodilators (S.C. epinephrine: 0.1 to 0.5 ml of 1:1000), and inhaled agents (metaproterenol: two to three inhalations; albuterol: 5 mg/ml solution; ipratropium: adults, one or two inhalations; children, 125 to 250 mcg nebulizer solution)
- Monitor for deteriorating respiratory status and note sputum characteristics; provide adequate fluid intake and oxygen as ordered
- *Prevention:* Tell the patient to avoid possible triggers and to use inhaled corticosteroids, antihistamines, decongestants, cromolyn powder by inhalation, and oral or aerosol bronchodilators; explain the influence of stress and anxiety and frequent association with exercise (especially running), cold air, and nocturnal flare-ups
- Help the patient identify triggers and teach him how to a use metered-dose inhaler and a peak flow meter

Referral

- The patient with severe disease may need a referral to a pulmonologist.
- Refer the patient to a home health agency, if needed.
- For additional information and support, refer the patient and family members to the American Lung Association.
- Refer the patient to a local pulmonary rehabilitation program.

Follow-up

The patient should be seen initially every 2 weeks for evaluation of treatment. Thereafter, monitor according to the severity of the disorder.

Patient teaching

- To help mobilize secretions, teach the patient how to cough effectively. If the patient with copious secretions has diffi-

Three types of emphysema

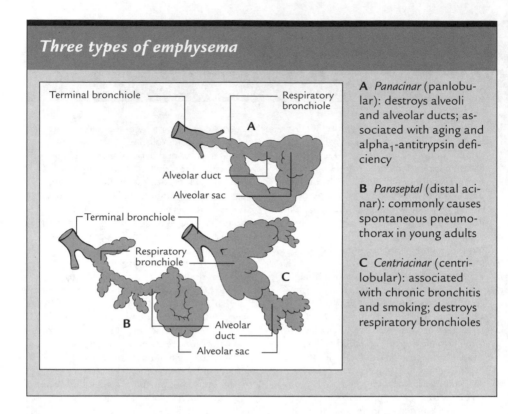

Terminal bronchiole

Respiratory bronchiole

A

Alveolar duct

Alveolar sac

Terminal bronchiole

Respiratory bronchiole

C

B

Alveolar duct

Alveolar sac

A *Panacinar* (panlobular): destroys alveoli and alveolar ducts; associated with aging and alpha$_1$-antitrypsin deficiency

B *Paraseptal* (distal acinar): commonly causes spontaneous pneumothorax in young adults

C *Centriacinar* (centrilobular): associated with chronic bronchitis and smoking; destroys respiratory bronchioles

culty mobilizing secretions, teach his family how to perform postural drainage and chest physiotherapy. If secretions are thick, urge the patient to drink 12 to 15 glasses of fluid per day. A home humidifier may be beneficial, particularly in the winter.

■ Help the patient and family members adjust their lifestyles to accommodate the limitations imposed by this debilitating chronic disease. Instruct the patient to allow for daily rest periods and to exercise daily as his physician directs.

■ Emphasize the importance of a balanced diet. Because the patient may tire easily when eating, suggest frequent, small meals and have him consider using oxygen, administered by nasal cannula, during meals.

■ To strengthen the muscles of respiration, teach the patient to take slow, deep breaths and to exhale through pursed lips.

■ Explain to the patient and family members that excessive oxygen therapy may eliminate the hypoxic respiratory drive.

■ Urge the patient to stop smoking. Provide smoking-cessation counseling or referral to a program. Tell him to avoid other respiratory irritants, such as secondhand smoke, aerosol spray products, and outdoor air pollution. An air conditioner with an air filter in his home may be helpful.

■ Teach the patient and his family how to recognize early signs of infection; warn the patient to avoid contact with people with respiratory infections. Encourage good oral hygiene to help prevent infection. Pneumococcal vaccination and annual influenza vaccinations are important preventive measures.

Complications
- Infection
- Cor pulmonale
- Pulmonary hypertension
- Polycythemia
- Respiratory failure

• • • • • • • • • • • •
CROUP

Croup is a severe inflammation and an obstruction of the upper airway, occurring as acute laryngotracheobronchitis (most common), laryngitis, and acute spasmodic laryngitis; it must always be distinguished from epiglottiditis. Croup is a childhood disease that affects more boys than girls and usually occurs during the winter. Up to 15% of patients have a strong family history of croup. Recovery is usually complete.

AGE ALERT Croup typically affects children between ages 3 months and 3 years.

Causes
Croup usually results from a viral infection. Parainfluenza viruses cause two-thirds of such infections; adenoviruses, respiratory syncytial virus (RSV), influenza and measles viruses, and bacteria (pertussis, diphtheria, and mycoplasma) account for the rest.

Clinical presentation
The onset of croup usually follows an upper respiratory tract infection. Clinical features include:
- inspiratory stridor
- hoarse or muffled vocal sounds
- varying degrees of laryngeal obstruction
- respiratory distress
- characteristic sharp, barking, seal-like cough.

These signs may last for only a few hours or may persist for 1 to 2 days. As it progresses, croup causes inflammatory edema and, possibly, spasm, which can obstruct the upper airway and severely compromise ventilation. (See *How croup affects the upper airway*, page 354.)

Each form of croup has the following additional characteristics:
- In *laryngotracheobronchitis*, the symptoms seem to worsen at night. Inflammation causes edema of the bronchi and bronchioles as well as increasingly difficult expiration that frightens the child. Other characteristic features include fever, diffusely decreased breath sounds, expiratory rhonchi, and scattered crackles.
- *Laryngitis*, which results from vocal cord edema, is usually mild and produces no respiratory distress except in infants. Early signs and symptoms include a sore throat and cough, which may progress to marked hoarseness, suprasternal and intercostal retractions, inspiratory stridor, dyspnea, diminished breath sounds, restlessness and, in later stages, severe dyspnea and exhaustion.
- *Acute spasmodic laryngitis* affects children between ages 1 and 3, particularly those with allergies and a family history of croup. It typically begins with mild to moderate hoarseness and nasal discharge, followed by the characteristic cough and noisy inspiration that commonly wakes the child at night, labored breathing with retractions, rapid pulse, and clammy skin. The child understandably becomes anxious, which may lead to increasing dyspnea and transient cyanosis. These severe symptoms diminish after several hours but reappear in a milder form on the next one or two nights.

Differential diagnoses
- Epiglottiditis

How croup affects the upper airway

In croup, inflammatory swelling and spasms constrict the larynx, thereby reducing airflow. This cross-sectional drawing (from chin to chest) shows the upper airway changes caused by croup. Inflammatory changes almost completely obstruct the larynx (which includes the epiglottis) and significantly narrow the trachea.

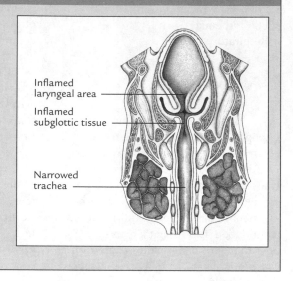

Inflamed laryngeal area

Inflamed subglottic tissue

Narrowed trachea

- Upper respiratory infection
- Laryngitis

Diagnosis

The clinical picture is very characteristic, so the diagnosis should be suspected immediately. When bacterial infection is the cause, throat cultures may identify the organisms and their sensitivity to antibiotics as well as rule out diphtheria. On a posterior-anterior chest X-ray, narrowing of the upper airway ("steeple sign") may be apparent. Laryngoscopy may reveal inflammation and obstruction in epiglottal and laryngeal areas. In evaluating the patient, assess for foreign body obstruction (a common cause of croup-like cough in young children) as well as masses and cysts.

Management

General

For most children with croup, home care with rest, cool humidification during sleep, and antipyretics such as aceta-

minophen relieve symptoms. However, respiratory distress that's severe or interferes with oral hydration necessitates hospitalization and parenteral fluid replacement to prevent dehydration. Oxygen therapy also may be required.

Medication

If bacterial infection is the cause, antibiotic therapy is necessary. Inhaled racemic epinephrine and corticosteroids may be used to alleviate respiratory distress.

Referral

- Refer the patient to the hospital emergency department if he's in respiratory distress.

Follow-up

If not hospitalized, the patient should be seen in 24 hours to assess respiratory status and then 1 week after discharge.

Patient teaching
- Tell family members to keep the child as quiet as possible but to avoid sedation because it can depress respiration. If the patient is an infant, instruct family members to position him in an infant seat or prop him up with a pillow; place an older child in Fowler's position.
- Instruct the parents how to carry out effective home care. Suggest the use of a cool humidifier (vaporizer). To relieve croupy spells, tell parents to carry the child into the bathroom, shut the door, and turn on the hot water. Breathing in warm, moist air quickly eases an acute spell of croup.
- Warn parents that ear infections and pneumonia are complications of croup and may appear about 5 days after recovery. Stress the importance of immediately reporting earache, productive cough, high fever, or increased shortness of breath.

Complications
- Respiratory distress
- Dehydration
- Ear infection
- Pneumonia

Special considerations
- Isolate patients suspected of having RSV and parainfluenza infections, if possible.

• • • • • • • • • • • •

CYSTIC FIBROSIS

Cystic fibrosis is a generalized dysfunction of the exocrine glands that affects multiple organ systems. It's transmitted as an autosomal recessive trait and is the most common fatal genetic disease in white children. In the United States, the incidence of cystic fibrosis is highest in Whites of northern European ancestry (1 in 2,500 live births) and lowest in Blacks (1 in 17,000 live births), Native Americans, and people of Asian ancestry. The disease occurs equally in both sexes.

Cystic fibrosis is a chronic disease. With improvements in treatment over the past decade, the average life expectancy has risen from age 16 to age 28 and older.

Causes and pathophysiology
The gene responsible for cystic fibrosis encodes a protein that involves chloride transport across epithelial membranes; over 100 specific mutations of the gene are known. (See *Cystic fibrosis transmission risk*, page 356.)

The symptoms of cystic fibrosis are due to increased viscosity of bronchial, pancreatic, and other mucous gland secretions and consequent obstruction of glandular ducts. Cystic fibrosis accounts for almost all cases of pancreatic enzyme deficiency in children.

Clinical presentation
The clinical effects of cystic fibrosis may become apparent soon after birth or take years to develop. They include the following major aberrations in sweat gland, respiratory, and GI function:
- Sweat gland dysfunction is the most consistent abnormality. Increased concentrations of sodium and chloride in the sweat lead to hyponatremia and hypochloremia and can eventually induce fatal shock and arrhythmias, especially in hot weather.
- Respiratory signs reflect obstructive changes in the lungs — wheezy respirations; a dry, nonproductive paroxysmal cough; dyspnea; and tachypnea. These changes stem from thick, tenacious secretions in the bronchioles and alveoli and eventually lead to severe atelectasis and

Cystic fibrosis transmission risk

The probability that a relative of a person with cystic fibrosis or a person with no family history will carry the cystic fibrosis gene is shown below.

GENETIC PROFILE	CARRIER CHANCE
Relative of affected person	
Brother or sister	2 in 3 (67%)
Niece or nephew	1 in 2 (50%)
Aunt or uncle	1 in 3 (33%)
First cousin	1 in 4 (25%)
No known family history	
Whites	1 in 25 (4%)
Blacks	1 in 65 (1.5%)
Asians	1 in 150 (0.67%)

emphysema. A child with cystic fibrosis has a barrel chest and exhibits cyanosis and clubbing of the fingers and toes. The child suffers recurring bronchitis and pneumonia as well as associated nasal polyps and sinusitis. Death typically results from pneumonia, emphysema, or atelectasis.

- The GI effects of cystic fibrosis occur mainly in the intestines, pancreas, and liver. One early sign is meconium ileus; the neonate with cystic fibrosis doesn't excrete meconium, a dark green mucilaginous material found in the intestine at birth. He develops symptoms of intestinal obstruction, such as abdominal distention, vomiting, constipation, dehydration, and electrolyte imbalance.

Eventually, obstruction of the pancreatic ducts and resulting deficiency of trypsin, amylase, and lipase prevent the conversion and absorption of fat and protein in the GI tract. The undigested food is then excreted in frequent, bulky, foul-smelling, pale stools with a high fat content. This malabsorption induces poor weight gain, poor growth, ravenous appetite, distended abdomen, thin extremities, and sallow skin with poor turgor. The inability to absorb fats results in a deficiency of fat-soluble vitamins (A, D, E, and K), leading to clotting problems, retarded bone growth, and delayed sexual development. Males may experience azoospermia and sterility; females may experience secondary amenorrhea but can reproduce. A common complication in infants and children is rectal prolapse secondary to malnutrition and wasting of perirectal supporting tissues.

In the pancreas, fibrotic tissue, multiple cysts, thick mucus, and eventually fat replace the acini (small, saclike swellings normally found in this gland), producing signs of pancreatic insufficiency — insufficient insulin production, abnormal glucose tolerance, and glycosuria. About 15% of patients have adequate pancreatic exocrine function for normal digestion and, therefore, have a better prognosis. Biliary obstruction and fibrosis may prolong neonatal jaundice. In some patients, cirrhosis and portal hypertension may lead to esophageal varices, episodes of hematemesis and, occasionally, hepatomegaly.

Differential diagnoses

- Atelectasis
- Bronchiectasis
- Pneumonia
- Malignancies

Diagnosis

The diagnostic indications of cystic fibrosis include:

- Sweat test is a definitive diagnostic study for cystic fibrosis. The result shows sodium and chloride concentrations greater than 50 mEq/L.
- Chest X-rays show hyperinflation, bronchiectasis, mucus plugs, cysts, and focal atelectasis.
- Stool specimen analysis, indicating the absence of trypsin, suggests pancreatic insufficiency.

The following test results may support the diagnosis:

- Arterial blood gas analysis shows hypoxemia.
- Deoxyribonucleic acid testing can now locate the presence of the Delta F 508 deletion (found in about 70% of cystic fibrosis patients, although the disease can cause more than 100 other mutations). It allows prenatal diagnosis in families with a previously affected child.
- Pulmonary function tests reveal decreased vital capacity, elevated residual volume due to air entrapments, and decreased forced expiratory volume in 1 second. This test is used if pulmonary exacerbation already exists.
- Sputum culture reveals organisms that cystic fibrosis patients typically and chronically colonize, such as *Staphylococcus* and *Pseudomonas*.
- Serum albumin measurement helps assess nutritional status.
- Electrolyte analysis assesses hydration status.

Management

General

The goal of treatment is to help the child lead as normal a life as possible. The type of treatment depends on the organ systems involved. Management of pulmonary dysfunction includes chest physiotherapy, postural drainage, and breathing exercises several times daily to remove secretions from lungs. Antihistamines are contraindicated because they have a drying effect on mucous membranes, making expectoration of mucus difficult or impossible.

To combat electrolyte losses in sweat, the patient's food is generously salted and, in hot weather, sodium supplements are administered. The patient needs to maintain a diet that is low in fat but high in protein and calories and that provides supplements of water-miscible, fat-soluble vitamins (A, D, E, and K).

Medication

The following medications may be given to treat cystic fibrosis:

- pancrelipase (given with meals and snacks) — adults, 4,000 to 48,000 U P.O.; children ages 7 to 12, 4,000 to 12,000 U P.O.; children ages 1 to 6, 4,000 to 8,000 U P.O.
- dornase alfa — one ampule (2.5 mg) inhaled daily
- tobramycin (aerosolized) — 300 mg inhaled b.i.d.; 28 days on and 28 days off
- albuterol — one to two inhalations every 4 to 6 hours
- acetylcysteine — 6 to 10 ml of 10% solution every 2 to 3 hours.

Surgical intervention

Lung transplant is done in some patients to reduce the effects of the disease.

Referral

- Refer family members to social services for support measures.

■ For more information and sources of support, refer the patient to the Cystic Fibrosis Foundation.
■ Refer patients or the parents of an affected child for genetic counseling.

Follow-up
The patient should be seen at least three times per year.

Patient teaching
■ Teach the patient and family about maintaining a diet low in fat and high in sodium, protein, and calories. Emphasize the importance of adequate hydration.
■ Teach the patient and family how to perform chest physiotherapy, including postural drainage and chest percussion and vibration.

Complications
■ Atelectasis
■ Pneumothorax
■ Infection
■ Right-sided heart failure
■ Pulmonary hypertension
■ Intestinal obstructions
■ Malnutrition

Special considerations
■ Clinical trials of aerosol gene therapy show promise in reducing pulmonary symptoms.
■ The genetic defect responsible for cystic fibrosis has also been identified in individuals experiencing some forms of unexplained pancreatitis.

• • • • • • • • • • • •
EPIGLOTTIDITIS

Epiglottiditis is an acute inflammation of the supraglottic region of the oropharynx with inflammation of the epiglottis and aryepiglottic folds that tends to cause airway obstruction. It typically strikes children between ages 2 and 8 but may also affect adults. Epiglottiditis is a critical emergency that may prove fatal in 8% to 12% of victims unless it's recognized and treated promptly. It affects approximately 1 out of every 10,000 people.

Causes
Epiglottiditis usually results from infection with *Haemophilus influenzae* type B and, rarely, pneumococci and streptococci. Since the advent of the Hib vaccine, epiglottiditis is becoming rare.

Clinical presentation
Laryngeal obstruction results from inflammation and edema of the epiglottis. Accompanying signs and symptoms include:
■ high fever
■ stridor
■ sore throat
■ dysphagia
■ irritability
■ restlessness
■ drooling.
    To relieve severe respiratory distress, the child with epiglottiditis may lean forward with his mouth open, tongue protruding, with nostrils flaring as he tries to breathe. He may develop inspiratory retractions, rhonchi, and lethargy. The barking cough of croup is notably absent.
CLINICAL CAUTION Epiglottiditis is usually preceded by an upper respiratory infection and may rapidly progress to complete upper airway obstruction within 2 to 5 hours.

Differential diagnoses
■ Anaphylaxis
■ Angioedema
■ Anxiety
■ Croup
■ Foreign body ingestion
■ Pharyngitis
■ Sepsis

Diagnosis

In acute epiglottiditis, throat examination reveals a large, edematous, bright red epiglottis. Such examination should follow lateral neck X-rays and, generally, shouldn't be performed if the suspected obstruction is great. Make sure a laryngoscope and endotracheal tubes are available because a tongue blade can cause sudden complete airway obstruction. Trained personnel (such as an anesthesiologist) should be on hand during the throat examination to secure an emergency airway. On the lateral soft tissue X-ray of the neck, a large, thick, but indistinct ("thumbprint") epiglottis will be seen.

Management

General

A child with acute epiglottiditis and airway obstruction requires emergency hospitalization; he may need emergency endotracheal intubation or a tracheotomy with subsequent monitoring in an intensive care unit. Respiratory distress that interferes with swallowing necessitates parenteral fluid administration to prevent dehydration.

Medication

A patient with acute epiglottiditis should always receive a 10-day course of parenteral antibiotics such as cefotaxime (80 to 160 mg/kg/day I.V. in divided doses).

Referral

- The patient should be referred to a hospital if epiglottiditis is suspected.

Follow-up

The patient should be monitored in the hospital with airway support at the bedside. After discharge, the patient should be seen in 1 week.

Patient teaching

- Teach the patient and family members about emergency interventions that may be needed and the medication necessary for recovery.
- Emphasize to the family members the need to keep the patient quiet and calm.

Complications

- Pneumonia
- Meningitis
- Pericarditis
- Respiratory failure
- Death

Special considerations

- If a tracheotomy is necessary, reassure the patient and family members that the tracheotomy is a short-term intervention (usually from 4 to 7 days).

• • • • • • • • • • • •

PLEURISY

Pleurisy, also known as pleuritis, is an inflammation of the visceral and parietal pleurae that line the inside of the thoracic cage and envelop the lungs.

Causes

Pleurisy develops as a complication of pneumonia, tuberculosis, viruses, systemic lupus erythematosus, rheumatoid arthritis, uremia, Dressler's syndrome, certain cancers, pulmonary infarction, and chest trauma.

Pleuritic pain is caused by the inflammation or irritation of sensory nerve endings in the parietal pleura. As the lungs inflate and deflate, the visceral pleura covering the lungs moves against the fixed parietal pleura lining the pleural space, causing pain. This disorder usually begins suddenly. Recovery is dependent on the cause of the disorder.

Clinical presentation
Sharp, stabbing pain that increases with deep breathing may be so severe that it limits movement on the affected side. Dyspnea also occurs. Other symptoms vary according to the underlying pathologic process.

Differential diagnoses
- Pneumonia
- Atelectasis
- Bronchiectasis
- Metastatic lung disease
- Sepsis
- Empyema

Diagnosis
Auscultation of the chest reveals a characteristic pleural friction rub (a coarse, creaky sound heard during late inspiration and early expiration) directly over the area of pleural inflammation. Palpation over the affected area may reveal coarse vibration.

Management
General
Treatment usually focuses on relieving symptoms. Pleurisy with pleural effusion calls for thoracentesis as both a therapeutic and a diagnostic measure.

Medication
Medication used in the treatment of a patient with pleurisy may include:
- ibuprofen — 300 to 600 mg P.O. q.i.d.
- codeine — 30 to 60 mg P.O. every 8 hours as necessary
- intercostal nerve block of two or three intercostal nerves for severe pain.

Referral
- The patient may need a referral to a physician if a thoracentesis is required.

Follow-up
The patient should be seen 1 to 2 weeks after treatment, depending on the underlying cause of the illness.

Patient teaching
- Stress the importance of bed rest, and plan your care to allow the patient as much uninterrupted rest as possible.
- Encourage the patient to cough. Tell him to apply firm pressure at the site of the pain during coughing exercises to minimize pain.

Complications
- Impaired respiratory function
- Pulmonary fibrosis

• • • • • • • • • • • •
PNEUMOCYSTIS CARINII PNEUMONIA

Because of its association with human immunodeficiency virus (HIV) infection, *Pneumocystis carinii* pneumonia (PCP), an opportunistic infection, has increased in incidence since the 1980s. Before the advent of PCP prophylaxis, this disease was the first clue in about 60% of patients with HIV infection.

PCP was the leading cause of death in these patients. Prophylactic co-trimoxazole therapy in patients with HIV and low immune function has prevented PCP from higher mortality. Disseminated infection doesn't occur.

PCP also is associated with other immunocompromising conditions, including organ transplantation, leukemia, lymphoma, and steroid use.

Causes
P. carinii, the cause of PCP, usually is classified as a protozoan, although some investigators consider it more closely re-

lated to fungi. The organism exists as a saprophyte in the lungs of humans and various animals. *P. carinii* is part of the normal flora in most healthy people but becomes an aggressive pathogen in the immunocompromised patient. Impaired cell-mediated (T-cell) immunity is thought to be more important than impaired humoral (B-cell) immunity in predisposing the patient to PCP, but the immune defects involved are poorly understood. *P. carinii* becomes activated in immunocompromised patients when the CD4+ T-cell count falls below 200/µl.

P. carinii invades the lungs bilaterally and multiplies extracellularly. As the infestation grows, alveoli fill with organisms and exudate, impairing gas exchange. The alveoli hypertrophy and thicken progressively, eventually leading to extensive consolidation.

The primary transmission route seems to be air, although the organism is already present in most people. The incubation period probably lasts for 4 to 8 weeks.

Clinical presentation

The patient typically has a history of an immunocompromising condition (such as HIV infection, leukemia, or lymphoma) or procedure (such as organ transplantation).

PCP begins insidiously with increasing shortness of breath and a nonproductive cough. Other signs and symptoms include:

- anorexia
- generalized fatigue
- weight loss
- tachypnea
- dyspnea
- accessory muscle use for breathing
- crackles (in about one-third of patients)
- marked pallor

- decreased breath sounds (in advanced pneumonia).

The patient may have hypoxemia and hypercapnia without exhibiting significant symptoms; he may, however, have a low-grade, intermittent fever. Cyanosis may appear with acute illness; pulmonary consolidation develops later.

Differential diagnoses

- Viral or bacterial pneumonia
- Tuberculosis
- *Mycobacterium avium-intracellulare*

Diagnosis

Histologic studies confirm *P. carinii*. In all patients, fiber-optic bronchoscopy is the most commonly used study to confirm PCP. Invasive procedures, such as transbronchial biopsy and open-lung biopsy, are performed less commonly.

In patients with HIV infection, initial examination of a first-morning sputum specimen (induced by inhaling an ultrasonically dispersed saline mist) may be sufficient; however, this technique usually is ineffective in patients not infected with HIV.

Other diagnostic indications of PCP include:

- Chest X-rays show approximately 75% of the slowly progressing, fluffy infiltrates and, occasionally, nodular lesions or a spontaneous pneumothorax, but these findings must be differentiated from findings in other types of pneumonia or adult respiratory distress syndrome.
- Gallium scan may show increased uptake over the lungs even when the chest X-ray appears relatively normal.
- Arterial blood gas analysis detects hypoxia and an increased A-a gradient.
- CD4+ T-cell count is less than 200.
- Serum low-density lipoprotein level is elevated.

Management

General

Supportive measures, such as oxygen therapy, mechanical ventilation, adequate nutrition, and fluid balance, are important adjunctive therapies.

Medication

The dosages for prophylaxis of PCP include:

- pentamidine isethionate — 3 to 4 mg/kg/day I.V. or I.M. for 14 to 21 days
- diphenhydramine — 25 to 50 mg P.O. q.i.d. for adverse effects of medication.

For treatment of PCP give co-trimoxazole: adults and children, trimethoprim (15 to 20 mg/kg) and sulfamethoxazole (75 to 100 mg/kg) P.O. daily in 3 to 4 divided doses for 14 to 21 days.

Experimental treatments include:

- dapsone — 100 mg/day P.O. with trimethoprim 20 mg/kg/day in three divided doses for 21 days
- clindamycin — 300 to 450 mg P.O. q.i.d. with primaquine 15 to 30 mg P.O. daily
- trimetrexate — 45 mg/m²/day I.V. for 21 days with leucovorin 20 mg/m² I.V. or P.O.

Referral

- The patient may need referral to a hospital for treatment.
- Consider referring the patient to a pulmonologist.
- Because this infection is usually associated with acquired immunodeficiency syndrome (AIDS), provide the patient with information about resources and support organizations for patients with AIDS or HIV.

Follow-up

The patient should be seen every 2 weeks until his condition is stable.

Patient teaching

- Encourage the patient to ambulate and perform deep-breathing exercises and incentive spirometry to facilitate effective gas exchange.
- Encourage the patient to eat a high-calorie, protein-rich diet. Tell him to eat small, frequent meals if he can't tolerate large amounts of food.
- Instruct the patient in energy conservation measures.
- Instruct the patient about the medication regimen, especially about the adverse effects.

Complications

- Respiratory failure
- Pneumothorax
- Extrapulmonary pneumocystis

Special considerations

- Implement standard precautions to prevent contagion.

• • • • • • • • • • • •

PNEUMONIA

Pneumonia is an acute infection of the lung parenchyma that commonly impairs gas exchange. The prognosis is generally good for people who have normal lungs and adequate host defenses before the onset of pneumonia; however, pneumonia is the fifth leading cause of death in the United States and the leading cause of death from infection.

AGE ALERT There's an increased risk of pneumonia in people over age 60 or under age 2.

Causes

Pneumonia can be classified in several ways (see *Types of pneumonia*):

- Microbiologic etiology — Pneumonia can be viral, bacterial, fungal, protozoan,

(*Text continues on page 366.*)

Types of pneumonia

TYPE	SIGNS AND SYMPTOMS	DIAGNOSIS	TREATMENT
Viral			
Influenza (prognosis poor even with treatment; 50% mortality)	■ Cough (initially nonproductive; later, purulent sputum), marked cyanosis, dyspnea, high fever, chills, substernal pain and discomfort, moist crackles, frontal headache, and myalgia ■ Death, resulting from cardiopulmonary collapse	■ *Chest X-ray:* diffuse bilateral bronchopneumonia radiating from hilus ■ *White blood cell (WBC) count:* normal to slightly elevated ■ *Sputum smears:* no specific organisms	■ *Supportive:* for respiratory failure, endotracheal intubation and ventilator assistance; for fever, hypothermia blanket or antipyretics; and for influenza A, amantadine (200 mg P.O. daily) or rimantadine (100 mg P.O. b.i.d.)
Adenovirus (insidious onset; generally affects young adults)	■ Sore throat, fever, cough, chills, malaise, small amounts of mucoid sputum, retrosternal chest pain, anorexia, rhinitis, adenopathy, scattered crackles, and rhonchi	■ *Chest X-ray:* patchy distribution of pneumonia, more severe than indicated by physical examination ■ *WBC count:* normal to slightly elevated	■ For symptoms only ■ Mortality low; usually clears with no residual effects
Respiratory syncytial virus (most prevalent in infants and children)	■ Listlessness, irritability, tachypnea with retraction of intercostal muscles, wheezing, slight sputum production, fine moist crackles, fever, severe malaise, and possibly cough or croup	■ *Chest X-ray:* patchy bilateral consolidation ■ *WBC count:* normal to slightly elevated	■ *Supportive:* humidified air, oxygen, antimicrobials (commonly given until viral etiology confirmed), and aerosolized ribavirin (20 mg/ml mist for 12 to 18 hours/day for 3 to 7 days) ■ Complete recovery in 1 to 3 weeks
Measles (rubeola)	■ Fever, dyspnea, cough, small amounts of sputum, coryza, rash, and cervical adenopathy	■ *Chest X-ray:* reticular infiltrates, sometimes with hilar lymph node enlargement ■ *Lung tissue specimen:* characteristic giant cells	■ *Supportive:* bed rest, adequate hydration, and antimicrobials; assisted ventilation, if necessary
Chicken pox (varicella) (uncommon in children, but present in 30% of adults with varicella)	■ Cough, dyspnea, cyanosis, tachypnea, pleuritic chest pain, hemoptysis, and rhonchi 1 to 6 days after onset of rash	■ *Chest X-ray:* shows more extensive pneumonia than indicated by physical examination and bilateral, patchy, diffuse, nodular infiltrates	■ *Supportive:* adequate hydration, oxygen therapy in critically ill patients

(continued)

Types of pneumonia *(continued)*

TYPE	SIGNS AND SYMPTOMS	DIAGNOSIS	TREATMENT
Viral *(continued)*			
Chicken pox *(continued)*		■ *Sputum analysis:* predominant mononuclear cells and characteristic intranuclear inclusion bodies, with characteristic skin rash, confirming diagnosis	■ *Therapy with acyclovir I.V.:* acyclovir (adults and children older than age 12, 10 mg/kg every 8 hours for 7 days; children younger than age 12, 500 mg/m² I.V. every 8 hours for 7 to 10 days).
Cytomegalovirus	■ Difficult to distinguish from other nonbacterial pneumonias ■ Fever, cough, shaking chills, dyspnea, cyanosis, weakness, and diffuse crackles ■ Occurs in neonates as devastating multisystemic infection; in normal adults, resembles mononucleosis; in immunocompromised hosts, varies from clinically inapparent to devastating infection	■ *Chest X-ray:* in early stages, variable patchy infiltrates; later, bilateral, nodular, and more predominant in lower lobes ■ *Percutaneous aspiration of lung tissue, transbronchial biopsy, or open lung biopsy:* microscopic examination showing typical intranuclear and cytoplasmic inclusions; can culture the virus from lung tissue	■ Generally, benign and self-limiting in mononucleosis-like form ■ *Supportive:* adequate hydration and nutrition, oxygen therapy, and bed rest ■ In immunosuppressed patients, disease is more severe and may be fatal; ganciclovir (5 mg/kg I.V. every 12 hours for 14 to 21 days) or foscarnet (60 mg/kg I.V. every 8 hours for 14 to 21 days) treatment warranted
Bacterial			
Streptococcus (Streptococcus pneumoniae)	■ Sudden onset of a single, shaking chill and sustained temperature of 102° to 104° F (38.9° to 40° C); commonly preceded by upper respiratory tract infection	■ *Chest X-ray:* areas of consolidation, commonly lobar ■ *WBC count:* elevated ■ *Sputum culture:* may show gram-positive *S. pneumoniae;* this organism not always recovered	■ *Antimicrobial therapy:* penicillin G (1.6 to 3.2 million U P.O. daily in divided doses) for 7 to 10 days, beginning after culture specimen is obtained, but without waiting for results
Klebsiella	■ Fever and recurrent chills; cough producing rusty, bloody, viscous sputum (currant jelly); cyanosis of lips and nail beds due to hypoxemia; and shallow, grunting respirations	■ *Chest X-ray:* typically, but not always, consolidation in the upper lobe that causes bulging of fissures ■ *WBC count:* elevated	■ *Antimicrobial therapy:* an aminoglycoside and a cephalosporin

Types of pneumonia *(continued)*

TYPE	SIGNS AND SYMPTOMS	DIAGNOSIS	TREATMENT
Bacterial *(continued)*			
Klebsiella *(continued)*	▪ Common in patients with chronic alcoholism, pulmonary disease, diabetes, or those at risk for aspiration	▪ *Sputum culture and Gram stain:* may show gram-negative cocci *Klebsiella*	
Staphylococcus	▪ Temperature of 102° to 104° F (38.9° to 40° C), recurrent shaking chills, bloody sputum, dyspnea, tachypnea, and hypoxemia ▪ Should be suspected with viral illness, such as influenza or measles, and in patients with cystic fibrosis	▪ *Chest X-ray:* multiple abscesses and infiltrates; high incidence of empyema ▪ *WBC count:* elevated ▪ *Sputum culture and Gram stain:* may show gram-positive staphylococci	▪ *Antimicrobial therapy:* nafcillin (250 to 500 mg P.O. every 4 to 6 hours) or oxacillin (500 mg to 1 g P.O. every 4 to 6 hours) for 14 days if staphylococci are penicillinase-producing ▪ *Supportive:* chest tube drainage
Protozoan			
Pneumocystis carinii	▪ Occurs in immunocompromised persons ▪ Dyspnea and nonproductive cough ▪ Anorexia, weight loss, and fatigue ▪ Low-grade fever	▪ *Fiber-optic bronchoscopy:* obtains specimens for histologic studies ▪ *Chest X-ray:* nonspecific infiltrates, nodular lesions, or spontaneous pneumothorax	▪ *Antimicrobial therapy:* co-trimoxazole, adults and children, trimethoprim (15 to 20 mg/kg) and sulfamethoxazole (75 to 100 mg/kg P.O. daily in 3 to 4 divided doses for 14 to 21 days) or pentamidine (3 to 4 mg/kg I.V. or I.M. daily for 14 to 21 days) ▪ *Supportive:* oxygen and improved nutrition
Aspiration			
Results from vomiting and aspiration of gastric or oropharyngeal contents into trachea and lungs	▪ Possible noncardiogenic pulmonary edema following damage to respiratory epithelium from contact with stomach acid ▪ Crackles, dyspnea, cyanosis, hypotension, and tachycardia ▪ Possible subacute pneumonia with cavity formation, or possible lung abscess if foreign body is present	▪ *Chest X-ray:* locates areas of infiltrates, which suggest diagnosis	▪ *Antimicrobial therapy:* penicillin G (1.2 to 24 million U I.V. or I.M. daily in divided doses) or clindamycin (300 to 600 mg I.M. or I.V. every 6 to 12 hours) ▪ *Supportive:* oxygen therapy, suctioning, coughing, deep breathing, and adequate hydration

mycobacterial, mycoplasmal, or rickett-sial in origin.

■ Location—Bronchopneumonia in-volves distal airways and alveoli; lobular pneumonia, part of a lobe; and lobar pneumonia, an entire lobe.

■ Type—Primary pneumonia results from inhalation or aspiration of a path-ogen; it includes pneumococcal and viral pneumonia. Secondary pneumonia may follow initial lung damage from a noxious chemical or other insult (superinfection) or may result from hematogenous spread of bacteria from a distant focus.

Predisposing factors for bacterial and viral pneumonia include chronic illness and debilitation, cancer (particularly lung cancer), abdominal and thoracic surgery, atelectasis, common colds or other viral respiratory infections, such as acquired immunodeficiency syndrome, chronic res-piratory disease (chronic obstructive pul-monary disease [COPD], asthma, bron-chiectasis, and cystic fibrosis), influenza, smoking, malnutrition, alcoholism, sickle cell disease, tracheostomy, exposure to noxious gases, aspiration, and immuno-suppressive therapy.

Predisposing factors for aspiration pneumonia include old age, debilitation, artificial airway use, nasogastric tube feedings, impaired gag reflex, poor oral hygiene, and decreased level of con-sciousness.

Clinical presentation
The five cardinal signs and symptoms of early bacterial pneumonia are:
■ coughing
■ sputum production
■ pleuritic chest pain
■ shaking chills
■ fever over 102° F (38.9° C).

Physical signs and symptoms vary widely, ranging from diffuse, fine crackles to signs of localized or extensive consoli-dation and pleural effusion. Abdominal

pain, fatigue, and sore throat are also fre-quent complaints.

Differential diagnoses
■ Pleurisy
■ Pleuritis
■ Pleural effusion
■ Pulmonary abscess
■ Neoplasm
■ Sepsis
■ Asthma
■ Bronchitis
■ Heart failure
■ Tuberculosis
■ COPD

Diagnosis
Clinical features, chest X-ray showing in-filtrates, and sputum culture demonstrat-ing acute inflammatory cells support this diagnosis. Positive blood cultures in pa-tients with pulmonary infiltrates strongly suggest pneumonia produced by the or-ganisms isolated from the blood cultures. Pleural effusions, if present, should be tapped and fluid analyzed for evidence of infection in the pleural space. Occasion-ally, a transtracheal aspirate of tracheo-bronchial secretions or bronchoscopy with brushings or washings may be done to obtain material for a smear and cul-ture. The patient's response to antimicro-bial therapy also provides important evi-dence of the presence of pneumonia.

Management
General
Therapy should be reevaluated early in the course of treatment. Supportive mea-sures include humidified oxygen therapy for hypoxemia, mechanical ventilation for respiratory failure, a high-calorie diet and adequate fluid intake, bed rest, and an analgesic to relieve pleuritic chest pain. Patients with severe pneumonia on mechanical ventilation may require posi-

tive end-expiratory pressure to facilitate adequate oxygenation.

Medication
The following medications may be used to treat pneumonia:
- antimicrobial therapy—varies with causative agent
- acetaminophen—325 to 650 mg P.O. every 4 hours to reduce fever.

Referral
- If pneumonia is resistant to treatment, refer the patient to a pulmonologist or specialist in infectious disease.
- If the patient develops respiratory distress, immediately refer him to the hospital for treatment.
- For more information, refer the patient and family members to the American Lung Association.

Follow-up
The patient should be contacted in the first 24 to 48 hours after treatment is initiated, then in 2 to 3 weeks. A repeat chest X-ray should be done in 4 to 6 weeks.

Patient teaching
- Teach the patient how to cough and perform deep-breathing exercises to clear secretions; encourage him to do so often.
- Tell the patient to eat a high-calorie, high-protein diet consisting of soft, easy-to-eat foods. Tell him to limit the use of milk products as they may increase sputum production.
- Tell the family to provide a quiet, calm environment for the patient, with frequent rest periods.

Complications
- Empyema
- Pulmonary abscess
- Sepsis
- Adult respiratory distress syndrome
- Death
- Lung abscess
- Respiratory failure

Special considerations
- To prevent pneumonia, advise the patient to avoid using antibiotics indiscriminately during minor viral infections because their use may result in upper airway colonization with antibiotic-resistant bacteria. If the patient then develops pneumonia, the organisms producing the pneumonia may require treatment with more toxic antibiotics.

HEALTHY LIVING Encourage annual influenza vaccination and Pneumovax for high-risk patients, such as those with COPD, chronic heart disease, or sickle cell disease.

• • • • • • • • • • • •

PNEUMOTHORAX

Pneumothorax is an accumulation of air in the pleural space. The amount of air trapped in the intrapleural space determines the degree of lung collapse. A pneumothorax may be classified as either spontaneous, traumatic, or tension. In a tension pneumothorax, the air in the pleural space is under higher pressure than air in adjacent lung and vascular structures. Without prompt treatment, a tension or a large pneumothorax results in fatal pulmonary and circulatory impairment.

Causes and pathophysiology
Spontaneous pneumothorax usually occurs in otherwise healthy adults ages 20 to 40. It may be caused by air leakage from ruptured congenital blebs adjacent to the visceral pleural surface, near the apex of the lung. It may also result from

an emphysematous bulla that ruptures during exercise or coughing or from tubercular, pneumocystic, or malignant lesions that erode into the pleural space. In tall, thin, marfanoid-appearing patients, spontaneous pneumothorax has been reported frequently. Spontaneous pneumothorax may also occur in interstitial lung disease, such as eosinophilic granuloma or lymphangiomyomatosis. Smoking is also a factor. Spontaneous pneumothorax is 22 times more likely to occur in male smokers and 9 times more likely to occur in female smokers. Approximately 7 out of 100,000 men per year suffer from spontaneous pneumothorax compared with 1 out of 100,0000 women.

Traumatic pneumothorax may result from the insertion of a central venous line, thoracic surgery, or a penetrating chest injury such as a gunshot or knife wound. It may follow a transbronchial biopsy, or it may also occur during thoracentesis or a closed pleural biopsy. When traumatic pneumothorax follows a penetrating chest injury, it frequently coexists with hemothorax (blood in the pleural space). Traumatic pneumothorax occurs in 40% to 50% of patients with chest trauma.

In tension pneumothorax, positive pleural pressure develops as a result of any of the causes of traumatic pneumothorax. When air enters the pleural space through a tear in lung tissue and is unable to leave by the same vent, each inspiration traps air in the pleural space, resulting in positive pleural pressure. This in turn causes collapse of the ipsilateral lung and marked impairment of venous return, which can severely compromise cardiac output and may cause a mediastinal shift. Decreased filling of the great veins of the chest results in diminished cardiac output and lowered blood pressure. Tension pneumothorax is a compli-

cation of idiopathic spontaneous pneumothorax in approximately 1% to 2% of cases.

Pneumothorax can also be classified as open or closed. In open pneumothorax (usually the result of trauma), air flows between the pleural space and the outside of the body. In closed pneumothorax, air reaches the pleural space directly from the lung.

Clinical presentation

The cardinal features of pneumothorax are:

- sudden, sharp, pleuritic pain (exacerbated by movement of the chest, breathing, and coughing), usually on the affected side
- asymmetrical chest wall movement
- shortness of breath while at rest.

Additional signs and symptoms of tension pneumothorax are weak and rapid pulse, pallor, neck vein distention, and anxiety. Tension pneumothorax produces the most severe respiratory symptoms; a spontaneous pneumothorax that releases only a small amount of air into the pleural space may cause no symptoms. In a nontension pneumothorax, severity of symptoms is usually related to the size of the pneumothorax and the degree of preexisting respiratory disease.

Differential diagnoses

- Pleurisy
- Myocardial infarction
- Pericarditis
- Pulmonary embolism
- Dissecting abdominal aneurysm

Diagnosis

Sudden, sharp chest pain and shortness of breath suggest pneumothorax. Chest X-ray to confirm the diagnosis shows air in the pleural space and, possibly, mediastinal shift.

In the absence of a definitive chest X-ray, the physical examination may reveal:

- on inspection, overexpansion and rigidity of the affected chest side; in tension pneumothorax, neck vein distention with hypotension and tachycardia
- on palpation, crackling beneath the skin, indicating subcutaneous emphysema (air in tissue) and decreased vocal fremitus
- on percussion, hyperresonance on the affected side
- on auscultation, decreased or absent breath sounds over the collapsed lung.

If the pneumothorax is significant, arterial blood gas findings include pH less than 7.35, partial pressure of arterial oxygen less than 80 mm Hg, and partial pressure of arterial carbon dioxide greater than 45 mm Hg.

Management
General
Treatment is conservative for spontaneous pneumothorax in which no signs of increased pleural pressure (indicating tension pneumothorax) appear, lung collapse is less than 30%, and the patient shows no signs of dyspnea or other indications of physiologic compromise. Such treatment consists of bed rest; careful monitoring of blood pressure and pulse and respiratory rates; oxygen administration; and, possibly, needle aspiration of air with a large-bore needle attached to a syringe. If more than 30% of the lung is collapsed, treatment to reexpand the lung includes placing a thoracostomy tube in the second or third intercostal space in the midclavicular line (or in the fifth or sixth intercostal space in the midaxillary line), connected to an underwater seal or to low suction pressures.

Surgical intervention
- Recurring spontaneous pneumothorax requires thoracotomy and pleurectomy; these procedures prevent recurrence by causing the lung to adhere to the parietal pleura.
- Traumatic and tension pneumothoraces require chest tube drainage; traumatic pneumothorax may also require thoracotomy and pleurectomy.

Referral
- Refer the patient to the hospital for treatment if insertion of a chest tube is necessary.
- Refer the patient to a pulmonologist if the condition is recurrent.

Follow-up
The patient should be seen within 1 week after discharge. If treated as an outpatient, he should be reevaluated within 48 hours.

Patient teaching
- Urge the patient to control coughing and gasping during thoracotomy. However, after the chest tube is in place, encourage him to cough and breathe deeply (at least once per hour) to facilitate lung expansion.
- Tell the patient to stop smoking to reduce the chance of recurrent pneumothorax.

Complications
- Tension pneumothorax
- Recurrent pneumothorax
- Reexpansion pulmonary edema
- Shock
- Death

Special considerations
- Participation in diving or flying should be evaluated because of the increased air pressure involved with these activities.

• • • • • • • • • • • •
PULMONARY EMBOLISM

Pulmonary embolism is an obstruction of the pulmonary arterial bed by any embolic material (blood clot, fat, bone, air, amniotic fluid, or tissue). It's the most common pulmonary complication in hospitalized patients, striking an estimated 6 million adults each year in the United States and resulting in 50,000 deaths annually. Although pulmonary infarction that results from embolism may be so mild as to be asymptomatic, massive embolism (more than 50% obstruction of pulmonary arterial circulation) and the accompanying infarction can be rapidly fatal.

Causes and pathophysiology
Pulmonary embolism generally results from dislodged thrombi originating in the leg veins. More than half of such thrombi arise in the deep veins of the legs. Other less common sources of thrombi are the pelvic veins, renal veins, hepatic vein, right side of the heart, and upper extremities. Such thrombus formation results directly from vascular wall damage, venostasis, or hypercoagulability of the blood. Trauma, clot dissolution, sudden muscle spasm, intravascular pressure changes, or a change in peripheral blood flow can cause the thrombus to loosen or fragmentize. Then the thrombus — now called an embolus — floats to the heart's right side and enters the lung through the pulmonary artery. There, the embolus may dissolve, continue to fragmentize, or grow.

By occluding the pulmonary artery, the embolus prevents alveoli from producing enough surfactant to maintain alveolar integrity. As a result, alveoli collapse and atelectasis develops. If the embolus enlarges, it may clog most or all of the pulmonary vessels and cause death.

Rarely, the emboli contain air, fat, bacteria, amniotic fluid, talc (from drugs intended for oral administration, which are injected intravenously by addicts), or tumor cells.

Predisposing factors for pulmonary embolism include long-term immobility, chronic pulmonary disease, heart failure or atrial fibrillation, thrombophlebitis, polycythemia vera, thrombocytosis, autoimmune hemolytic anemia, sickle cell disease, varicose veins, recent surgery, advanced age, pregnancy, lower extremity fractures or surgery, burns, obesity, vascular injury, cancer, I.V. drug abuse, or oral contraceptives.

Clinical presentation
Total occlusion of the main pulmonary artery is rapidly fatal; smaller or fragmented emboli produce symptoms that vary with the size, number, and location of the emboli. Usually, the first symptom of pulmonary embolism is dyspnea, which may be accompanied by anginal or pleuritic chest pain. Other clinical features include:
- tachycardia
- productive cough (sputum may be blood-tinged)
- low-grade fever
- pleural effusion.

Less common signs include:
- massive hemoptysis
- splinting of the chest
- leg edema
- cyanosis, syncope, and distended neck veins (with a large embolus).

In addition, pulmonary embolism may cause dullness on chest percussion on the affected side, pleural friction rub, ventricular gallop, and signs of circulatory collapse (weak, rapid pulse and hypotension) and signs of hypoxia (restlessness and anxiety).

Differential diagnoses

- Myocardial infarction
- Rib fractures
- Pericarditis
- Gastritis
- Pleuritis
- Pneumonia
- Heart failure
- Pleural effusion

Diagnosis

The patient history should reveal any predisposing conditions for pulmonary embolism. A triad of deep venous thrombosis (DVT) formation is stasis, endothelial injury, and hypercoagulability. A positive Homans' sign indicates DVT. Risk factors include long car or plane trips, cancer, pregnancy, hypercoagulability, prior DVTs, and pulmonary emboli.

Other diagnostic indications include:

- Chest X-ray helps to rule out other pulmonary diseases; areas of atelectasis, elevated diaphragm and pleural effusion, prominent pulmonary artery and, occasionally, the characteristic wedge-shaped infiltrate suggestive of pulmonary infarction or focal oligemia of blood vessels are apparent.
- Ventilation perfusion scan shows perfusion defects in areas beyond occluded vessels; however, it doesn't rule out microemboli.
- Pulmonary angiography is the most definitive test but requires a skilled angiographer and radiologic equipment; it also poses some risk to the patient. Its use depends on the uncertainty of the diagnosis and the need to avoid unnecessary anticoagulant therapy in high-risk patients.
- Electrocardiography (ECG) helps to distinguish pulmonary embolism from myocardial infarction. In extensive embolism, ECG may show right axis deviation; right bundle-branch block; tall,

peaked P waves; ST-segment depression and T-wave inversion depression (indicative of right-sided heart strain); and supraventricular tachyarrhythmias. A pattern sometimes observed is S_1, Q_3, T_3 (S wave in lead I, Q wave in lead III, and inverted T wave in lead III).

- Auscultation occasionally reveals a right ventricular S_3 gallop and increased intensity of a pulmonic component of S_2. Also, crackles and a pleural rub may be heard at the site of embolism.
- Arterial blood gas measurements showing decreased partial pressure of arterial oxygen and partial pressure of arterial carbon dioxide are characteristic but don't always occur.

If pleural effusion is present, thoracentesis may rule out empyema, which indicates pneumonia.

Management

General

Treatment is designed to maintain adequate cardiovascular and pulmonary function during resolution of the obstruction and to prevent recurrence of embolic episodes. Most emboli resolve within 10 to 14 days. Oxygen therapy should be administered as needed.

Medication

The following medications may be used in the treatment of pulmonary emboli:

- heparin — initially 5,000 to 10,000 U I.V. push, then by continuous I.V. infusion; monitored by coagulation studies (partial thromboplastin time) every 4 hours
- urokinase — 4,400 IU/kg I.V. given over 10 minutes, then 4,400 IU/kg hourly for 12 hours
- streptokinase — 250,000 IU I.V. over 30 minutes, then 100,000 IU I.V. hourly for 24 to 72 hours
- alteplase — 100 mg I.V. over 2 hours

- dopamine — titrated to a maximum of 20 mcg/kg/minute for hypotension caused by pulmonary embolism
- antibiotics (organism specific) — to treat septic emboli.

Surgical intervention

Surgery is performed on patients who can't take anticoagulants, have recurrent emboli during anticoagulant therapy, or have been treated with thrombolytic agents or pulmonary thromboendarterectomy. This procedure (which shouldn't be performed without angiographic evidence of pulmonary embolism) consists of vena caval ligation, plication, or insertion of a device (umbrella filter) to filter blood returning to the heart and lungs. Pulmonary embolectomy often has dismal outcomes.

Referral

- Refer the patient to the hospital for immediate treatment.

Follow-up

The patient should be followed for anticoagulation therapy, with monitoring of International Normalized Ratio on a monthly basis so long as therapy is in effect (minimum of 3 months).

Patient teaching

- Instruct the patient to maintain adequate nutrition and fluid balance to promote healing.
- Tell the patient to report frequent pleuritic chest pain, so that analgesics can be prescribed.
- Warn the patient not to cross his legs; this promotes thrombus formation.
- Most patients need treatment with an oral anticoagulant (warfarin) for 3 to 6 months after a pulmonary embolism. Advise such patients to watch for signs of bleeding (bloody stools, blood in urine, and large ecchymoses), to take the pre-

scribed medication exactly as ordered, not to change dosages, and to avoid taking any additional medication (even for headaches or colds). Stress the importance of follow-up laboratory tests (prothrombin time) to monitor anticoagulant therapy.

- Tell the patient to discontinue smoking, or oral contraceptives, if appropriate

Complications

- Pulmonary infarction
- Acute respiratory failure
- Death
- Acute cor pulmonale

Special considerations

- Low-molecular-weight heparin may be given to prevent pulmonary embolism in high-risk patients.

• • • • • • • • • • • •

SARCOIDOSIS

Sarcoidosis is a multisystem, granulomatous disorder that characteristically produces lymphadenopathy, pulmonary infiltration, and skeletal, liver, eye, or skin lesions. In the United States, sarcoidosis occurs predominantly among blacks, affecting twice as many women as men. Acute sarcoidosis usually resolves within 2 years. Chronic, progressive sarcoidosis, which is uncommon, is associated with pulmonary fibrosis and progressive pulmonary disability.

AGE ALERT Sarcoidosis occurs most often in young adults ages 20 to 40.

Causes

The cause of sarcoidosis is unknown, but the following factors may play a role:

- hypersensitivity response (possibly from T-cell imbalance) to such agents as atypical mycobacteria, fungi, and pine pollen

- genetic predisposition (suggested by a slightly higher incidence of sarcoidosis within the same family)
- chemicals, such as zirconium and beryllium, that can lead to illnesses resembling sarcoidosis, suggesting an extrinsic cause for this disease.

Clinical presentation
Initial symptoms of sarcoidosis include arthralgia (in the wrists, ankles, and elbows), fatigue, malaise, and weight loss.

Other clinical features vary according to the extent and location of the fibrosis:
- respiratory — breathlessness, cough (usually nonproductive), substernal pain; complications in advanced pulmonary disease include pulmonary hypertension and cor pulmonale
- cutaneous — erythema nodosum, subcutaneous skin nodules with maculopapular eruptions, and extensive nasal mucosal lesions
- ophthalmic — anterior uveitis (common), glaucoma, and blindness (rare)
- lymphatic — bilateral hilar and right paratracheal lymphadenopathy and splenomegaly
- musculoskeletal — muscle weakness, polyarthralgia, pain, and punched-out lesions on phalanges
- hepatic — granulomatous hepatitis, usually asymptomatic
- genitourinary — hypercalciuria
- cardiovascular — arrhythmias (premature beats, bundle-branch or complete heart block) and, rarely, cardiomyopathy
- central nervous system (CNS) — cranial or peripheral nerve palsies, basilar meningitis, seizures, and pituitary and hypothalamic lesions producing diabetes insipidus.

Differential diagnoses
- Tuberculosis
- Berylliosis
- Lymphoma

Diagnosis
Typical clinical features with appropriate laboratory data and X-ray findings suggest sarcoidosis. A positive Kveim-Stilzbach skin test supports the diagnosis. In this test, the patient receives an intradermal injection of an antigen prepared from human sarcoidal spleen or lymph nodes from patients with sarcoidosis. If the patient has active sarcoidosis, granuloma develops at the injection site in 2 to 6 weeks. This reaction is considered positive when a biopsy of the skin at the injection site shows discrete epithelioid cell granuloma.

Tests showing other relevant findings include:
- chest X-ray — bilateral hilar and right paratracheal adenopathy with or without diffuse interstitial infiltrates; occasionally large nodular lesions are present in lung parenchyma
- lymph node, skin, or lung biopsy — noncaseating granulomas with negative cultures for mycobacteria and fungi
- other laboratory data — rarely, increased serum calcium, mild anemia, leukocytosis, and hyperglobulinemia
- pulmonary function tests — decreased total lung capacity and compliance, and decreased diffusing capacity
- arterial blood gas analysis — decreased arterial oxygen tension.

Negative tuberculin skin test, fungal serologies, and sputum cultures for mycobacteria and fungi as well as negative biopsy cultures help rule out infection.

Management
General
Asymptomatic sarcoidosis requires no treatment. However, sarcoidosis that causes ocular, respiratory, CNS, cardiac, or systemic signs (such as fever and weight loss) requires treatment with systemic or topical steroids, as does sarcoidosis that produces hypercalcemia or

destructive skin lesions. Such therapy is usually continued for 1 to 2 years, but some patients may need lifelong therapy. Other measures include a low-calcium diet and avoidance of direct exposure to sunlight in patients with hypercalcemia.

Medication
The following medications may be used to treat sarcoidosis:
- prednisone — 5 to 60 mg P.O. daily; dose is highly individualized
- hydrocortisone cream — applied to skin lesions q.i.d.

Referral
- Refer the patient with failing vision to community support and resource groups and to the American Foundation for the Blind, if necessary.

Follow-up
- Monitor the patients on prednisone every month for possible adverse effects.
- If the patient is stable, monitor every 3 months for 2 years after diagnosis.

Patient teaching
- Tell the patient to follow a nutritious, high-calorie diet and to drink plenty of fluids. If the patient has hypercalcemia, suggest a low-calcium diet. Instruct the patient to check his weight regularly to detect changes.
- Stress the need to comply with the prescribed steroid therapy and to undergo regular follow-up examinations and treatment.

Complications
- Chronic disease
- Serious involvement of other organs
- Pneumothorax
- Pulmonary embolus
- Cor pulmonale

TUBERCULOSIS

Tuberculosis (TB) is an acute or chronic infection caused by *Mycobacterium tuberculosis*. It's characterized by pulmonary infiltrates, formation of granulomas with caseation, fibrosis, and cavitation. People who live in crowded, poorly ventilated conditions and those who are immunocompromised are most likely to become infected.

The incidence of TB has increased in the United States secondary to homelessness, drug abuse, and human immunodeficiency virus (HIV) infection. TB resurged in the United States with the HIV epidemic of 1985. Globally, tuberculosis is the leading infectious cause of morbidity and mortality, generating 8 to 10 million new cases each year and 2 million deaths. Two-thirds of the cases are in minority populations in urban settings. Twice as many men are affected than women. The World Health Organization predicts that between the years 2000 and 2020 there will be 1 billion cases of TB.

In 1991, the Centers for Disease Control and Prevention (CDC) reported multidrug-resistant strains of M. *tuberculosis*; these strains produced fatal disease in immunocompromised patients, as well as exposed health care providers. The CDC has revised its management and exposed prophylaxis guidelines and suggested uses for the bacillus Calmette-Guérin (BCG) vaccine. For patients with strains that are resistant to two or more of the major antitubercular agents, mortality is 50%.

 AGE ALERT The most prevalent age-group for TB is ages 25 to 44.

Causes and pathophysiology

After exposure to M. *tuberculosis*, a person may develop active TB or a latent infection. The latent infection is more common; 10% to 30% progress to active disease. Skin test conversion and identification of Ghon's complex on chest X-ray are the only means of identifying latent infection. Those with latent infection are asymptomatic and noncontagious.

Although the primary infection site is the lung (80%), mycobacteria can exist in other parts of the body. (In immunocompromised patients, extrapulmonary sites are common.) The host's immune system usually controls the tubercle bacillus by killing it or walling it up in a tiny nodule (tubercle). The bacillus may lie dormant within the tubercle for years and later reactivate and spread. A number of factors increase the risk of infection reactivation, including gastrectomy, uncontrolled diabetes mellitus, Hodgkin's disease, leukemia, silicosis, acquired immunodeficiency syndrome, and treatment with corticosteroids or immunosuppressants.

Transmission is by droplet nuclei produced when infected persons cough or sneeze. One cough can have 3,000 infective droplets. If an inhaled tubercle bacillus settles in an alveolus, infection occurs, with alveolocapillary dilation and endothelial cell swelling. Alveolitis results, with replication of tubercle bacilli and influx of polymorphonuclear leukocytes. These organisms spread through the lymph system to the circulatory system and then throughout the body.

Cell-mediated immunity to the mycobacteria, which develops 3 to 6 weeks later, usually contains the infection and arrests the disease. If the infection reactivates, the body's response characteristically leads to caseation (the conversion of necrotic tissue to a cheeselike material). The caseum may localize, undergo fibrosis, or excavate and form cavities, the walls of which are studded with multiplying tubercle bacilli. If this happens, infected caseous debris may spread throughout the lungs by the tracheobronchial tree. Sites of extrapulmonary TB include the pleurae, meninges, joints, lymph nodes, peritoneum, genitourinary tract, and bowel.

Clinical presentation

After an incubation period of 4 to 8 weeks, TB is usually asymptomatic in primary infection but may produce nonspecific signs and symptoms, such as:

- fatigue
- weakness
- anorexia
- weight loss
- night sweats
- low-grade fever.

Auscultation discloses crepitant crackles, bronchial breath sounds, wheezing, and whispered pectoriloquy. Chest percussion discloses dullness over the affected area, indicating consolidation or pleural fluid.

Fever and night sweats, the typical hallmarks of TB, may not be present in an elderly patient, who instead may exhibit a change in activity or weight. Assess older patients carefully.

In reactivation, symptoms may include a cough that produces mucopurulent sputum, occasional hemoptysis, and chest pains.

Differential diagnoses

- Pneumonia (another source)
- Fungal infection
- Pleural effusion
- Malignancy
- Lymphoma

Diagnosis

Diagnostic tests include chest X-rays, a tuberculin skin test, and sputum smears and cultures to identify M. *tuberculosis*. The diagnosis must be precise because several other diseases (such as lung cancer, lung abscess, pneumoconiosis, and bronchiectasis) may mimic tuberculosis.

The following procedures aid diagnosis:

- Chest X-ray shows nodular lesions, patchy infiltrates (mainly in upper lobes), cavity formation, scar tissue, and calcium deposits; however, it may not be able to distinguish active from inactive TB.
- Tuberculin skin test detects TB infection. Intermediate-strength purified protein derivative or 5 tuberculin units (0.1 ml) are injected intracutaneously on the forearm. The test results are read in 48 to 72 hours; a positive reaction (induration of 5 to 15 mm or more, depending on risk factors) develops 2 to 10 weeks after infection in both active and inactive TB. However, severely immunosuppressed patients may never develop a positive reaction.
- Stains and cultures (of sputum, cerebrospinal fluid, urine, drainage from abscess, or pleural fluid) show heat-sensitive, nonmotile, aerobic, acid-fast bacilli. Patients who are positive for TB and unaware of their HIV status should undergo HIV testing.

Management

Medication

To avoid drug-resistant organisms, treatment must consist of four medications until drug susceptibility becomes known from laboratory data. A 6-month course would include:

- isoniazid — 5 mg/kg/day, up to 300 mg/day P.O.
- rifampin — 600 mg/day P.O.
- pyrazinamide — 15 to 30 mg/kg/day P.O.
- ethambutol — 15 mg/kg/day P.O.

If sputum smears convert and symptoms resolve, the final 4 months of treatment include:

- isoniazid — 300 mg/day P.O.
- rifampin — 600 mg/day P.O.

In multidrug-resistant TB, administer an injectable anti-TB aminoglycoside such as amikacin — 15 mg/kg/day divided every 8 to 12 hours I.M. or I.V.

Administer with a fluoroquinolone such as ciprofloxacin — 750 mg P.O. or 400 mg I.V. every 12 hours.

Also have the patient take isoniazid, rifampin, pyrazinamide, and ethambutol, and either cycloserine (250 mg P.O. every 12 hours for 2 weeks then dose is adjusted according to blood levels) or ethionamide (0.5 to 1 g/day P.O. in divided doses).

Referral

- Refer the patient to a TB specialist if there is no improvement in 3 months.
- Refer the patient to the U.S. Department of Health and Human Services for assistance (provides treatment at no cost).
- Refer the patient and family members to local support groups such as the American Lung Association.

Follow-up

The patient should be seen monthly during treatment. Sputum should be cultured monthly and chest X-rays should be obtained at least every 3 months.

Patient teaching

- Teach the infectious patient to cough and sneeze into tissues and to dispose of all secretions properly.
- Remind the patient to get plenty of rest. Stress the importance of eating balanced meals to promote recovery. If the patient is anorexic, urge him to eat small meals frequently. Tell him to record his weight weekly.

- Teach the patient to watch for adverse effects from medication and warn him to report these immediately. Emphasize the importance of regular follow-up examinations. Instruct the patient and his family members about the signs and symptoms of recurring TB. Stress the need to follow long-term treatment faithfully.
- Emphasize the importance of taking the medications daily as prescribed. The patient may also elect to enroll in a supervised administration program to avoid the development of drug-resistant organisms.

Complications
- Cavity lesions
- Transmission of disease to others
- Drug resistance

Special considerations
- Initiate acid-fast bacillus (AFB) isolation precautions immediately for all patients suspected or confirmed to have TB. AFB isolation precautions include the use of a private room with negative pressure in relation to surrounding areas and a minimum of six air exchanges per hour (air exhausted should be exhausted directly to the outside). Continue AFB isolation until there is clinical evidence of reduced infectiousness (substantially decreased cough, lower number of organisms on sequential sputum smears).

• • • • • • • • • • • •

SELECTED REFERENCES

Auscultation Skills: Breath and Heart Sounds. Springhouse, Pa.: Springhouse Corp., 1999.

Bartlett, J.G. *Management of Respiratory Tract Infections,* 3rd ed. Philadelphia: Lippincott Williams & Wilkins, 2001.

Blank-Reid, C., and Reid, P. "Taking the Tension Out of Traumatic Pneumothoraxes," *Nursing99* 29(4):41-46, April 1999.

Elkin, M.K., et al. *Nursing Interventions and Clinical Skills,* 2nd ed. St. Louis: Mosby–Year Book, Inc., 2000.

Fauci, A.S., et al., eds. *Harrison's Principles of Internal Medicine,* 15th ed. New York: McGraw-Hill Book Co., 2001.

Grenvik, A., et al. *Textbook of Critical Care,* 4th ed. Philadelphia: W.B. Saunders Co., 2000.

Ignatavicius, D., et al. *Medical-Surgical Nursing across the Health Care Continuum,* 3rd ed. Philadelphia: W.B. Saunders Co., 1999.

Jett, J.R., et al., eds. *The 2000 Yearbook of Pulmonary Disease.* St. Louis: Mosby–Year Book, Inc., 2000.

Nursing Procedures, 3rd ed. Springhouse, Pa.: Springhouse Corp., 2000.

Shortall, S.P., and Perkins, L.A. "Interpreting the Ins and Outs of Pulmonary Function Tests," *Nursing99* 29(12):41-46, December 1999.

Singleton, J.K., et al. *Primary Care.* Philadelphia: Lippincott Williams & Wilkins, 1999.

Smeltzer, S.C., and Bare, B.G. *Brunner and Suddarth's Textbook of Medical-Surgical Nursing,* 9th ed. Philadelphia: Lippincott Williams & Wilkins, 2000.

Gastrointestinal disorders

The GI system consists of the alimentary canal or GI tract (the oral cavity, pharynx, esophagus, stomach, and small and large intestines) and the accessory glands and organs (the salivary glands, liver, gall bladder, bile ducts, and pancreas). As the site of the body's digestive processes, the GI system has the critical task of extracting from food the essential nutrients that fuel the cells of the brain, heart, lungs, and other organs and tissues. GI function also profoundly affects the quality of life by its impact on overall health.

• • • • • • • • • • • •

ASSESSMENT

GI signs and symptoms can have many baffling causes. To help sort out significant symptoms, you first need to collect a thorough patient history. Next, conduct a complete physical examination using inspection, auscultation, palpation, and percussion.

Physical assessment

Physical assessment of the GI system usually includes evaluation of the mouth, abdomen, liver, and rectum. To perform a thorough abdominal and rectal assessment, gather the following equipment: gloves, stethoscope, flashlight, measuring tape, felt-tip pen, and a gown and drapes to cover the patient.

Assessing the oral cavity

Start by assessing the oral structures. Structural problems or disorders such as those listed here may affect GI functioning. Here's what to look for when assessing the oral structures:
- mouth — asymmetry, motility, or malocclusion
- lips — abnormal color, lesions, nodules, vesicles, or fissures
- teeth — caries; missing, broken, or displaced teeth; dental appliances (such as dentures or braces)
- gums — recession, redness, pallor, hypertrophy, ulcers, or bleeding
- tongue — deviation to one side, tremors, redness, swelling, ulcers, lesions, or abnormal coatings

Identifying abdominal landmarks

To aid accurate abdominal assessment and documentation of findings, you can mentally divide the patient's abdomen into regions; the quadrant method is easiest and most commonly used. Divide the abdomen into four equal regions by imagining two perpendicular lines that cross above the umbilicus, as depicted below.

RIGHT UPPER QUADRANT (RUQ)
- Liver and gallbladder
- Pylorus
- Duodenum
- Head of pancreas
- Hepatic flexure of colon
- Portions of ascending and transverse colon

LEFT UPPER QUADRANT (LUQ)
- Left liver lobe
- Stomach
- Body of pancreas
- Splenic flexure of colon
- Portions of transverse and descending colon

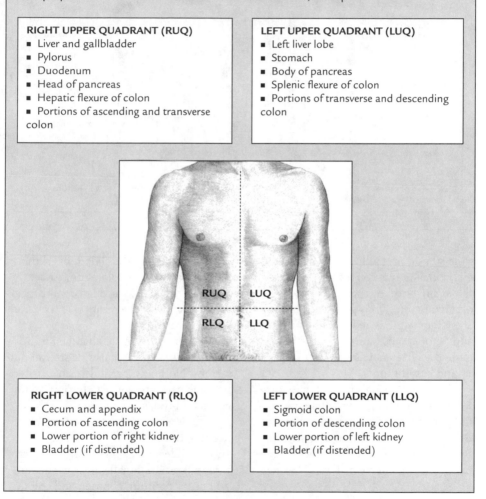

RIGHT LOWER QUADRANT (RLQ)
- Cecum and appendix
- Portion of ascending colon
- Lower portion of right kidney
- Bladder (if distended)

LEFT LOWER QUADRANT (LLQ)
- Sigmoid colon
- Portion of descending colon
- Lower portion of left kidney
- Bladder (if distended)

- buccal mucosa—pallor, redness, swelling, ulcers, lesions, or leukoplakia (a disease marked by white, thickened patches that may tend to fissure)
- hard and soft palates—redness, lesions, patches, petechiae, or pallor
- pharynx—uvular deviation, tonsil abnormalities, lesions, ulcers, plaques, exudate, or unusual mouth odor (such as fruity or fetid).

Assessing the abdomen
Mentally divide the patient's abdomen into four regions, or quadrants. (See *Identifying abdominal landmarks*.) Then, when assessing the abdomen, perform the four

Identifying areas of referred pain

Pain may occur relatively near its source or distant from it. Use these illustrations to help you identify the areas and causes of referred pain.

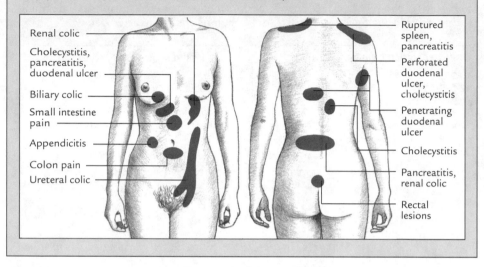

Renal colic

Cholecystitis, pancreatitis, duodenal ulcer

Biliary colic

Small intestine pain

Appendicitis

Colon pain

Ureteral colic

Ruptured spleen, pancreatitis

Perforated duodenal ulcer, cholecystitis

Penetrating duodenal ulcer

Cholecystitis

Pancreatitis, renal colic

Rectal lesions

basic steps in the following sequence: inspection, auscultation, percussion, and palpation. Unlike other body systems, in which auscultation is performed last, the GI system requires abdominal auscultation before percussion and palpation because the latter can alter intestinal activity and bowel sounds.

When assessing a patient with abdominal pain, always auscultate, percuss, and palpate the painful quadrant last. Otherwise, the patient might tense up, making further assessment difficult. (See *Identifying areas of referred pain.*)

Inspection

Begin by inspecting the patient's entire abdomen, noting overall contour and skin integrity, appearance of the umbilicus, and any visible pulsations. Note any distention or irregular contours for further assessment.

Next, inspect the abdominal skin. Look for areas of discoloration, striae, rashes or other lesions, dilated veins, and scars. Document the location and character of these findings.

Observe the entire abdomen for movement from peristalsis or arterial pulsations. Normally, peristalsis isn't visible. In some patients, aortic pulsations may be seen in the epigastric area.

To detect umbilical or incisional hernias, have the patient raise his head and shoulders while remaining in a supine position. Finally, inspect the umbilicus for position, contour, and color.

Auscultation

Auscultation provides information on bowel motility and the underlying vessels and organs. To auscultate for bowel sounds, lightly press the stethoscope diaphragm on the abdominal skin in all four quadrants. Normally, air and fluid moving through the bowel by peristalsis create soft, bubbling sounds with no regular pattern, often mixed with soft clicks and gurgles, every 5 to 15 seconds. Rapid, high-pitched, loud, and gurgling bowel sounds are hyperactive and may occur normally in a hungry patient. Sounds occurring at a rate of one every minute or longer are hypoactive and normally occur after bowel surgery or when the colon is filled with feces.

Before reporting absent bowel sounds, be sure the patient has an empty bladder. Audible bowel sounds may be initiated by gently pressing on the abdominal surface or by having the patient eat or drink something.

Next, use the bell of the stethoscope to auscultate for vascular sounds. Normally, you should detect no vascular sounds. Note any bruit, venous hum, or friction rub.

Percussion
Abdominal percussion helps determine the size and location of abdominal organs and detects excessive accumulation of fluid and air. Percuss in all four quadrants, keeping approximate organ locations in mind as you progress. Percuss the abdomen systematically, starting with the right upper quadrant and moving clockwise. If a patient complains of pain in a particular quadrant, percuss that quadrant last. Percussion sounds vary, depending on the density of underlying structures. The predominant abdominal percussion sound is tympany, created by percussing over an air-filled stomach or intestine. Dull sounds normally occur over the liver, the spleen, a lower intestine filled with feces, and a bladder filled with urine.

Note: Keep in mind that abdominal percussion or palpation is contraindicated in patients with suspected abdominal

aortic aneurysm or those who have received abdominal organ transplants. It should be performed cautiously in patients with suspected appendicitis.

If the patient's abdomen is distended, assess its progression by taking serial measurements of abdominal girth.

Palpation
Palpation elicits useful clues about the character of the abdominal wall, organs, any masses, and abdominal pain. Commonly used techniques include light palpation, deep palpation, and ballottement.

To perform light palpation, gently press your fingertips about ½" to ¾" (1.5 to 2 cm) into the abdominal wall. The light touch helps relax the patient.

To perform deep palpation, press the fingertips of both hands about 1½" (4 cm) into the abdominal wall. Move your hands in a slightly circular fashion so that the abdominal wall moves over the underlying structures. If you detect a mass on light or deep palpation, note its location, size, shape, consistency, type of border, degree of tenderness, presence of pulsations, and degree of mobility. Deep palpation may evoke rebound tenderness when you suddenly withdraw your fingertips, a possible sign of peritoneal inflammation. (See *Eliciting abdominal pain,* page 382.)

■ **CLINICAL CAUTION** Don't palpate a pulsating midline mass; it may be a dissecting aneurysm, which can rupture under the pressure of palpation.

Ballottement involves lightly tapping or bouncing your fingertips against the abdominal wall. This technique helps elicit abdominal muscle resistance or guarding that can be missed with deep palpation, or it may detect the movement or bounce of a freely movable mass. Your fingers should also bounce at the

Eliciting abdominal pain

Rebound tenderness and the iliopsoas and obturator signs can indicate appendicitis or peritonitis. You can elicit the following signs of abdominal pain.

REBOUND TENDERNESS

Position the patient supine with his knees flexed to relax the abdominal muscles. Place your hands gently on the right lower quadrant at McBurney's point — located about midway between the umbilicus and the anterior superior iliac spine.

Slowly and deeply dip your fingers into the area; then release the pressure in a quick, smooth motion. Pain on release — rebound tenderness — is a positive sign. The pain may radiate to the umbilicus. *Caution:* To minimize the risk of rupturing an inflamed appendix don't repeat this maneuver.

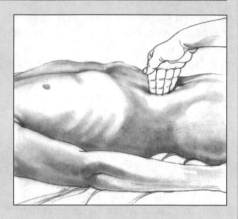

ILIOPSOAS SIGN

Position the patient supine with his legs straight. Instruct him to raise his right leg upward as you exert slight pressure with your hand.

Repeat the maneuver with the left leg. When testing either leg, increased abdominal pain is a positive result, indicating irritation of the psoas muscle.

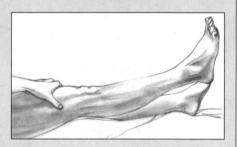

OBTURATOR SIGN

Position the patient supine with his right leg flexed 90 degrees at the hip and knee. Hold the leg just above the knee and at the ankle; then rotate the leg laterally and medially. Pain in the hypogastric region is a positive sign, indicating irritation of the obturator muscle.

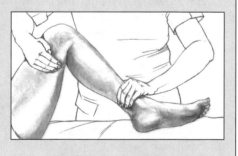

underlying dense liver tissue in the right upper quadrant. If the patient has ascites, use deep ballottement by pushing your fingertips deeply inward in a rapid motion; then quickly release the pressure, maintaining fingertip contact with the abdominal wall. You should feel the movement of an underlying organ or a movable mass toward your fingertips.

Assessing the liver

You can estimate the size and position of the liver through percussion and palpation.

Percussion

Use fist percussion (or blunt percussion) to detect tenderness, a common symptom of gallbladder or liver disease or inflammation. To perform this maneuver, place one hand flat over the patient's lower right rib cage along the midclavicular line, then strike the back of this hand with your other hand clenched in a fist. Discomfort and muscle guarding indicate tenderness. *Note:* Use this maneuver only on a patient with unconfirmed but suspected inflammation or hepatomegaly, and defer it until the end of the abdominal assessment. If the patient complains of discomfort during the assessment, particularly over the spleen, don't perform this maneuver.

Palpation

Usually, palpating the liver in an adult is impossible. If palpable, the liver border usually feels smooth and firm, with a rounded, regular edge. A palpable liver may indicate hepatomegaly; it also may occur in an extremely thin patient or in the following variations:

■ A low diaphragm, as occurs in emphysema, displaces a normal-sized liver downward.
■ In a normal variation known as Riedel's lobe, the right lobe is elongated down toward the right lower quadrant and is palpable below the right costal margin.

Assessing the rectum

Usually, a routine rectal examination is done only for patients over age 40. You may also perform it for a patient of any age with a history of bowel elimination changes or anal area discomfort and for an adult male of any age with a urinary problem. As a rule, perform the rectal examination at the end of the physical assessment.

Inspection

To begin, ask an ambulatory patient to stand with his toes pointed inward and bend his body forward over the examination table. If the knee-chest position in bed isn't suitable for an ill, elderly, or pregnant patient, position such a patient in left lateral Sims' position, with the knees drawn up and the buttocks near the edge of the bed or examination table.

Spread the patient's buttocks to expose the anus and surrounding area. Inspect for breaks in the skin, fissures, discharge, inflammation, lesions, scars, rectal prolapse, skin tags, and external hemorrhoids. Ask the patient to strain as though defecating to make internal hemorrhoids, polyps, rectal prolapse, and fissures visible.

Palpation

Next, palpate the external rectum. Put on a glove and apply lubricant to your index finger. As the patient strains again, palpate for any anal outpouchings or bulges, nodules, or tenderness. Then palpate the internal rectum. Before beginning, explain to the patient what you'll be doing. Have the patient breathe through the mouth and relax. When the anal sphincter is relaxed, gently insert your finger approximately 2½" to 4" (6.5 to 10 cm), angling it toward the umbilicus. *Note:* Don't attempt to force entry through a constricted anal sphincter. Once you've inserted your finger, rotate it systematically to palpate all aspects of the rectal wall for nodules, tenderness, irregularities, and fecal impaction. The rectal wall should feel smooth and soft. In a female patient, try to feel the posterior side of the uterus through the anterior rectal wall. In a male patient, assess the prostate gland when palpating the anterior rectal wall; the prostate should feel firm and smooth.

With your finger fully inserted, ask the patient to bear down again; this may cause lesions higher in the rectum to move down to a palpable level. To assess anal sphincter competence, ask the patient to tighten the anal muscles around your finger. Finally, withdraw your finger and examine it for blood, mucus, or stool. If stool appears, note its color and test a sample for occult blood.

Ongoing assessment

Whenever a patient reports a GI complaint, reassessment is needed. For example, if the nature and location of the pain is changed, more extensive involvement or a new disorder may be indicated. Reassure the patient that ongoing assessment doesn't necessarily mean he has a significant health problem.

• • • • • • • • • • • •

ANAL FISSURE

Anal fissure is a laceration or crack in the lining of the anus that extends to the circular muscle. Posterior fissure, the most common type, is equally prevalent in males and females. Anterior fissure, the rarer type, is 10 times more common in females. The prognosis is very good, especially with fissurectomy and good anal hygiene.

An estimated 235,000 new cases of anal fissure occur yearly in the United States. Of those cases, 40% become chronic.

Causes

Posterior fissure results from passage of large, hard stools that stretch the lining beyond its limits. Anterior fissure usually results from strain on the perineum during childbirth and, rarely, from scar stenosis. Occasionally, anal fissure is secondary to proctitis, anal tuberculosis, or carcinoma.

Clinical presentation

Onset of an acute anal fissure is characterized by tearing, cutting, or burning pain during or immediately after a bowel movement. A few drops of blood may streak toilet paper or underclothes. Painful anal sphincter spasms result from ulceration of a "sentinel pile" (swelling at the lower end of the fissure). A fissure may heal spontaneously and completely or it may partially heal and break open again. Chronic fissure produces scar tissue that hampers normal bowel evacuation.

Differential diagnoses

- Hemorrhoids

Diagnosis

An anoscopy showing a longitudinal tear and typical clinical features helps to establish the diagnosis. Digital examination that elicits pain and bleeding supports the diagnosis. Gentle traction on perianal skin can create enough eversion to visualize a fissure directly.

Management
General

Treatment varies according to the severity of the tear. For superficial fissures without hemorrhoids, forcible digital dilatation of the anal sphincter under local anesthesia stretches the lower portion of the sphincter to allow easier passage of stool. Patients with anal fissures should follow a low-residue diet and drink plenty of fluid. Sitz baths may be used for relief of pain and to keep the affected area clean.

Medication

The following medication may be used to treat anal fissures:

■ docuate sodium — 50 to 500 mg/day P.O.

■ nitroglycerin ointment — applied locally (phase III trial stage for analgesic and healing effects).

Surgical intervention

For complicated fissures, treatment includes surgical excision of tissue, adjacent skin, and mucosal tags and division of internal sphincter muscle from external.

Referral

■ Refer the patient to a surgeon, if necessary.

■ Refer the patient to the American Society of Colon and Rectal Surgeons for more information.

Follow-up

The patient should be monitored according to the severity of the tear.

Patient teaching

■ Teach the patient about hot sitz baths, warm soaks, and local anesthetic ointment to relieve pain.

■ Tell the patient that a low-residue diet, adequate fluid intake, and stool softeners may help prevent straining during defecation.

Complications

■ Infection

■ Difficult bowel evacuation

Special considerations

■ Control diarrhea with diphenoxylate or other antidiarrheals.

•••••••••••••

ANORECTAL ABSCESS AND FISTULA

Anorectal abscess is a localized collection of pus due to an inflammation of the soft tissue near the rectum or anus. Inflammation may produce an anal fistula — an abnormal opening in the anal skin — that may communicate with the rectum. Anorectal abscess is four times more common in men than in women. In 50% of patients, the abscesses will develop into anal fistulas. Superficial abscesses aren't uncommon in infants wearing diapers who have a history of anal fissure. Prompt treatment provides relief and permits good outcomes.

Causes

The inflammatory process that leads to an abscess may begin with an abrasion or tear in the lining of the anal canal, rectum, or perianal skin, and subsequent infection by *Escherichia coli*, staphylococci, or streptococci. Trauma may result from injections for treatment of internal hemorrhoids, enema-tip abrasions, puncture wounds from ingested eggshells or fish bones, or insertion of foreign objects. Other preexisting lesions include infected anal fissure, infections from the anal crypt through the anal gland, ruptured anal hematoma, prolapsed thrombosed internal hemorrhoids, and septic lesions in the pelvis, such as acute appendicitis, acute salpingitis, and diverticulitis. Systemic illnesses that can cause abscesses include ulcerative colitis and Crohn's disease. Many abscesses develop without preexisting lesions.

As the abscess produces more pus, a fistula may form in the soft tissue beneath the muscle fibers of the sphincters (especially the external sphincter), usually extending into the perianal skin. The internal (primary) opening of the abscess or fistula is usually near the anal glands and crypts; the external (secondary) opening, in the perianal skin.

Clinical presentation

Characteristics are throbbing pain and tenderness at the site of the abscess. A hard, painful lump develops on one side, preventing comfortable sitting.

Differential diagnoses

- Ulcerative colitis
- Crohn's disease
- Pilonidal abscess
- Carcinoma
- Rectal polyps

Diagnosis

Anorectal abscess is detectable on physical examination:

- Perianal abscess (80% of patients) is a red, tender, localized, oval swelling close to the anus. Sitting or coughing increases pain, and pus may drain from the abscess. Digital examination reveals no abnormalities.
- Ischiorectal abscess (15% of patients) involves the entire perianal region on the affected side of the anus. It's tender but may not produce drainage. Digital examination reveals a tender induration bulging into the anal canal.
- Submucous or high intermuscular abscess (5% of patients) may produce a dull, aching pain in the rectum, tenderness and, occasionally, induration. Digital examination reveals a smooth swelling of the upper part of the anal canal or lower rectum.
- Pelvirectal abscess (rare) produces fever, malaise, and myalgia but no local anal or external rectal signs or pain. Digital examination reveals a tender mass high in the pelvis, perhaps extending into one of the ischiorectal fossae.

If the abscess drains by forming a fistula, the pain usually subsides and the major signs become pruritic drainage and subsequent perianal irritation. The external opening of a fistula generally appears as a pink or red elevated, discharging sinus or ulcer on the skin near the anus. Depending on the severity of infection, the patient may have chills, fever, nausea, vomiting, and malaise. Digital examination may reveal a palpable indurated tract and a drop or two of pus on palpation. The internal opening may be palpated as a depression or ulcer in the midline anteriorly or at the dentate line posteriorly. Examination with a probe may require an anesthetic. Sigmoidoscopy, barium studies, and colonoscopy may be done to rule out other conditions.

Management

General

Treatment for a patient with anorectal abscess and fistula may involve the use of antibiotics, analgesics, and stool softeners. Sitz baths may be used to assist with localization of the abscess to permit drainage. Surgery also may be needed to facilitate drainage.

Medication

Antibiotics may be initiated; examples include:

- ciprofloxacin — 500 mg P.O. every 12 hours
- cephalexin — 250 mg to 1 g P.O. every 6 hours.

Analgesics may be needed; examples include:

- ibuprofen — 300 to 800 mg P.O. q.i.d.
- codeine — 30 to 60 mg P.O. q.i.d.

Stool softeners, such as docusate sodium (50 to 500 mg/day P.O.), may be beneficial.

Surgical intervention

Anorectal abscesses require surgical incision under caudal anesthesia to promote drainage. Fistulas require a fistulotomy—removal of the fistula and associated granulation tissue—under caudal anesthesia. If the fistula tract is epithelialized, treatment requires fistulectomy—removal of the fistulous tract—followed by the insertion of drains, which remain in place for 48 hours.

Referral
- Refer the patient to a surgeon for treatment.
- Refer the patient to the American Society of Colon and Rectal Surgeons for more information.

Follow-up
The patient should be monitored for wound healing weekly initially, then every 2 to 3 weeks until the site is healed, possibly up to 12 weeks.

Patient teaching
- Stress the importance of perianal cleanliness.

Complications
- Incontinence
- Infection

Special considerations
- Proper healing of the wound should progress from the inside out. Healing should be complete in 4 to 5 weeks for perianal fistulas; in 12 to 16 weeks for deeper wounds.

• • • • • • • • • • • •
APPENDICITIS

Appendicitis, the most common major surgical disease, is an inflammation of the vermiform appendix due to an obstruction. Appendicitis can occur at any age and affects both sexes equally but, between puberty and age 25, it's more prevalent in men. Appendicitis is invariably fatal if untreated; however, since the advent of antibiotics, the incidence of and death rate due to appendicitis have declined.

Causes
Appendicitis probably results from an obstruction of the appendiceal lumen caused by a fecal mass, stricture, barium ingestion, or viral infection. This obstruction sets off an inflammatory process that can lead to infection, thrombosis, necrosis, and perforation. If the appendix ruptures or perforates, the infected contents spill into the abdominal cavity, causing peritonitis, the most common and most perilous complication of appendicitis.

Clinical presentation
Typically, appendicitis begins with generalized or localized abdominal pain in the right upper abdomen, followed by anorexia, nausea, and vomiting (rarely profuse). Other signs and symptoms include:
- localized pain in the right lower abdomen (McBurney's point)
- abdominal "boardlike" rigidity
- retractive respirations
- increasing tenderness
- increasingly severe abdominal spasms
- rebound tenderness (rebound tenderness on the opposite side of the abdomen suggests peritoneal inflammation).

Later signs and symptoms include constipation or diarrhea, slight fever, and tachycardia. The patient may walk bent over or lie with his right knee flexed to reduce pain.

CLINICAL CAUTION Sudden cessation of abdominal pain indicates perforation or infarction of the appendix.

Differential diagnoses
- Gastritis
- Gastroenteritis
- Ileitis
- Colitis
- Pancreatitis
- Renal colic
- Bladder infection
- Ovarian cyst
- Uterine disease

Diagnosis
Diagnosis of appendicitis is based on physical findings and characteristic clinical symptoms. Supportive findings include a temperature of 99° to 102° F (37.2° to 38.9° C) and a moderately elevated white blood cell count (12,000 to 15,000/µl), with increased immature cells.

In older patients, be aware of vague signs and symptoms, such as mild pain or fever, and leukocytes with a shift to the left on differential.

Management
General
Appendicitis necessitates surgical intervention. If peritonitis develops, treatment involves GI intubation, parenteral replacement of fluids and electrolytes, and administration of antibiotics.

Medication
Postoperatively, the patient may require analgesics, such as:
- morphine — 2 to 4 mg I.V. every 2 to 4 hours p.r.n. or patient-controlled analgesia
- percocet — 1 to 2 tablets every 3 to 4 hours p.r.n.

Surgical intervention
Appendectomy is the only effective treatment. Laparoscopic appendectomy decreases the patient's recovery time and hospital stay.

Referral
- Refer the patient to the hospital and a surgeon.

Follow-up
The patient should be monitored for postoperative complications and wound healing.

Patient teaching
- Encourage the patient to cough and deep-breathe postoperatively to prevent atelectasis.
- Teach the patient proper wound care and how to recognize signs of infection.

Complications
- Peritonitis from perforation
- Gangrene
- Abscess formation

• • • • • • • • • • • •

CHOLELITHIASIS AND RELATED DISORDERS

Cholelithiasis is characterized by stones or calculi (gallstones) in the gallbladder that result from changes in bile components. Diseases of the gallbladder and biliary tract are common and, in many cases, painful conditions that usually require surgery and may be life threatening. They're generally associated with deposition of calculi and inflammation. (See *Common sites of calculus formation.*)

Cholelithiasis is the fifth leading cause of hospitalization among adults and accounts for 90% of all gallbladder and duct diseases. The prognosis is usually good with treatment unless infection occurs, in which case prognosis depends on its severity and response to antibiotics.

Causes and pathophysiology
Gallstones are composed of cholesterol, calcium bilirubinate, or a mixture of cho-

Common sites of calculus formation

This illustration shows sites where calculi typically collect. Stones vary in size; small stones may travel.

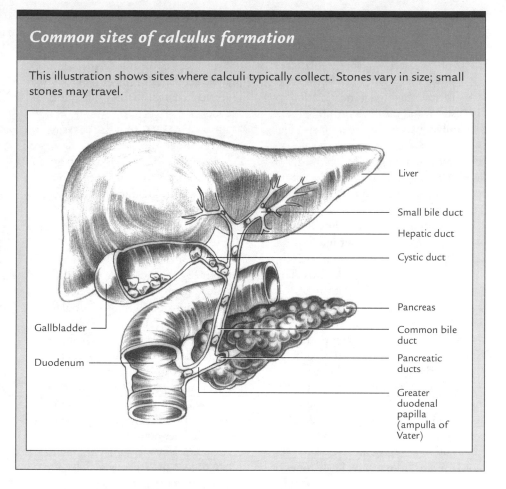

Liver

Small bile duct

Hepatic duct

Cystic duct

Pancreas

Common bile duct

Pancreatic ducts

Greater duodenal papilla (ampulla of Vater)

Gallbladder

Duodenum

lesterol and bilirubin pigment. They arise during periods of sluggishness in the gallbladder due to pregnancy, oral contraceptive use, diabetes mellitus, celiac disease, cirrhosis of the liver, or pancreatitis.

One out of 10 patients with gallstones develops choledocholithiasis, or gallstones in the common bile duct (sometimes called common duct stones). This occurs when stones passed out of the gallbladder lodge in the hepatic and common bile ducts and obstruct the flow of bile into the duodenum. Prognosis is good unless infection occurs.

Cholangitis, infection of the bile duct, is commonly associated with choledocholithiasis and may follow percuta-

neous transhepatic cholangiography or occlusion of endoscopic stents. Predisposing factors may include bacterial or metabolic alteration of bile acids. Widespread inflammation can cause fibrosis and stenosis of the common bile duct. The prognosis for a patient with this rare condition is poor without stenting or surgery.

Cholecystitis, an acute or a chronic inflammation of the gallbladder, is usually associated with a gallstone impacted in the cystic duct, causing painful distention of the gallbladder. Cholecystitis accounts for 10% to 25% of patients requiring gallbladder surgery. The acute form is most common during middle age; the chronic form occurs most commonly among elderly patients. The prognosis is good with treatment.

Cholesterolosis, polyps or crystal deposits of cholesterol in the gallbladder's submucosa, may result from bile secretions containing high concentrations of cholesterol and insufficient bile salts. The polyps may be localized or speckle the entire gallbladder. Cholesterolosis, the most common pseudotumor, isn't related to widespread inflammation of the mucosa or the lining of the gallbladder. The prognosis is good with surgery.

Biliary cirrhosis, ascending infection of the biliary system, sometimes follows viral destruction of liver and duct cells, but the primary cause is unknown. This condition usually leads to obstructive jaundice and involves the portal and periportal spaces of the liver. It's nine times more common among women ages 40 to 60 than among men. The prognosis is poor without liver transplantation.

Gallstone ileus results from a gallstone lodging at the terminal ileum; it's more common in elderly patients. The prognosis is good with surgery.

Postcholecystectomy syndrome commonly results from residual gallstones or stricture of the common bile duct. It occurs in 1% to 5% of patients whose gallbladders have been surgically removed and may produce right upper quadrant abdominal pain, biliary colic, fatty food intolerance, dyspepsia, and indigestion. The prognosis is good with selected radiologic procedures, endoscopic procedures, or surgery.

Acalculous cholecystitis is more common in critically ill patients, accounting for about 5% of cholecystitis cases. It may result from primary infection with such organisms as *Salmonella typhi, Escherichia coli,* or *Clostridium* or from obstruction of the cystic duct due to lymphadenopathy or a tumor. It appears that

ischemia, usually related to a low cardiac output, also has a role in the pathophysiology of this disease. Signs and symptoms of acalculous cholecystitis include unexplained sepsis, right upper quadrant pain, fever, leukocytosis, and a palpable gallbladder.

AGE ALERT In most cases, gallbladder and bile duct diseases occur during middle age. Between ages 20 and 50, they're six times more common in women, but incidence in men and women becomes equal after age 50. Incidence increases with each succeeding decade.

Each of these disorders produces its own set of complications. Cholelithiasis may lead to any of the disorders associated with gallstone formation: cholangitis, cholecystitis, choledocholithiasis, and gallstone ileus. Cholecystitis can progress to gallbladder complications, such as empyema, hydrops or mucocele, or gangrene. Gangrene can lead to perforation, resulting in peritonitis, fistula formation, pancreatitis, limy bile, and porcelain gallbladder. Other complications include chronic cholecystitis and cholangitis.

Choledocholithiasis may lead to cholangitis, obstructive jaundice, pancreatitis, and secondary biliary cirrhosis. Cholangitis, especially in the suppurative form, can progress to septic shock and death. Gallstone ileus can cause bowel obstruction, which can lead to intestinal perforation, peritonitis, septicemia, secondary infection, and septic shock.

Clinical presentation
Although gallbladder disease may produce no symptoms, acute cholelithiasis, acute cholecystitis, choledocholithiasis, and cholesterolosis produce the symptoms of a classic gallbladder attack. Attacks commonly follow meals rich in fats or may occur at night, suddenly waking

the patient. They begin with acute abdominal pain in the right upper quadrant that may radiate to the back, between the shoulders, or to the front of the chest; the pain may be so severe that the patient seeks emergency department care. Other possible features include:

- recurring fat intolerance
- biliary colic
- belching
- flatulence
- indigestion
- diaphoresis
- nausea
- vomiting
- chills
- low-grade fever
- jaundice (if a stone obstructs the common bile duct)
- clay-colored stools (with choledocholithiasis).

Clinical features of cholangitis include an increase in eosinophils, jaundice, abdominal pain, high fever, and chills; biliary cirrhosis may produce jaundice, related itching, weakness, fatigue, slight weight loss, and abdominal pain. Gallstone ileus produces signs and symptoms of small bowel obstruction, including nausea, vomiting, abdominal distention, and absent bowel sounds (if the bowel is completely obstructed). Its most telling symptom is intermittent recurrence of colicky pain over several days.

Differential diagnoses
- Myocardial infarction
- Angina
- Pancreatitis
- Pancreatic head cancer
- Pneumonia
- Peptic ulcer
- Hiatal hernia
- Esophagitis
- Gastritis

Diagnosis

Initially, serial cardiac enzyme testing and electrocardiogram should be done to rule out myocardial infarction.

Echography and X-rays detect gallstones. Other tests may include:
- Ultrasound reflects stones in the gallbladder with 96% accuracy.
- Percutaneous transhepatic cholangiography, done under fluoroscopic control, distinguishes between gallbladder or bile duct disease and cancer of the pancreatic head in patients with jaundice.
- Endoscopic retrograde cholangiopancreatography visualizes the biliary tree after insertion of an endoscope down the esophagus into the duodenum, cannulation of the common bile and pancreatic ducts, and injection of contrast medium.
- Hida scan of the gallbladder detects obstruction of the cystic duct.
- Computed tomography scan, although not used routinely, helps to distinguish between obstructive and nonobstructive jaundice.
- Flat plate of the abdomen identifies calcified, but not cholesterol, stones with 15% accuracy.
- Oral cholecystography shows stones in the gallbladder and biliary duct obstruction.

Elevated icteric index, total bilirubin, urine bilirubin, and alkaline phosphatase support the diagnosis. White blood cell count is slightly elevated during a cholecystitis attack.

Management
General
Treatment includes a low-fat diet to prevent attacks. During an acute attack, a nasogastric tube may be inserted; an I.V. line may be used for I.V. fluid administration. A nonsurgical treatment for choledocholithiasis involves placement of a catheter through the percutaneous tran-

shepatic cholangiographic route. This procedure can be performed endoscopically.

Medication

Medications may include:
- ursodiol — 8 to 10 mg/kg/day b.i.d. to t.i.d. for up to 2 years for oral dissolution of stones
- vitamin K — 10 mg/day S.C.
- morphine — 2 to 4 mg I.V. p.r.n.
- ibuprofen — 200 to 400 mg P.O. q.i.d.
- cefazolin — 250 mg to 1.5 g I.V. every 6 to 8 hours.

Surgical intervention

Surgery, usually elective, is the treatment of choice for gallbladder and bile duct diseases and may include open or laparoscopic cholecystectomy, cholecystectomy with operative cholangiography, and possibly exploration of the common bile duct.

Referral

- The patient may need referral to a surgeon.

Follow-up

If the patient undergoes surgery, monitor for postoperative complications and adequate wound healing after 1 week, then in 2 to 3 weeks. If the patient is treated medically with oral dissolution agents, monitor liver enzymes, cholesterol levels, and gall bladder ultrasound every 6 months.

Patient teaching

- Teach the patient to deep-breathe, cough, expectorate, and perform leg exercises that are necessary after surgery. Also teach splinting, repositioning, and ambulation techniques.

- Teach patients who will be discharged with a T tube how to perform dressing changes and routine skin care.
- Advise the patient against heavy lifting or straining for 6 weeks. Urge him to walk daily.
- Tell him that food restrictions are unnecessary unless he has an intolerance to a specific food or some underlying condition that requires such restriction.
- Instruct the patient to report pain that lasts more than 24 hours and any signs or symptoms of jaundice, anorexia, nausea or vomiting, fever, or tenderness in the abdominal area because these may indicate a biliary tract injury from cholestectomy, which requires immediate attention.

Complications

- Gallstone pancreatitis
- Acute cholecystitis
- Obstructive jaundice
- Liver abscess
- Peritonitis

Special considerations

Patients undergoing laparoscopic cholecystectomy may be discharged the same day or within 24 hours after surgery. These patients should have minimal pain, be able to tolerate a regular diet within 24 hours after surgery, and be able to return to normal activity within a few days to a week.

• • • • • • • • • • • •

CIRRHOSIS AND FIBROSIS

Cirrhosis is a chronic hepatic disease characterized by diffuse destruction and fibrotic regeneration of hepatic cells. As necrotic tissue yields to fibrosis, this disease alters liver structure and normal vasculature, impairs blood and lymph flow and, ultimately, causes hepatic insufficiency. It's twice as common in men as in women, and it's especially prevalent among malnourished, chronic alcoholics over age 50. Mortality is high: Many patients die within 5 years of onset. The prognosis is better in noncirrhotic forms of hepatic fibrosis, which cause minimal hepatic dysfunction and don't destroy liver cells.

Causes

The following clinical types of cirrhosis reflect its diverse etiology:

- Portal, nutritional, or alcoholic (Laën-nec's) cirrhosis, the most common type, occurs in 30% to 50% of cirrhotic patients, up to 90% of whom have a history of alcoholism. Liver damage results from malnutrition, especially of dietary protein, and chronic alcohol ingestion. Fibrous tissue forms in portal areas and around central veins.
- Biliary cirrhosis (15% to 20% of patients) results from injury or prolonged obstruction.
- Postnecrotic (posthepatitic) cirrhosis (10% to 30% of patients) stems from various types of hepatitis.
- Pigment cirrhosis (5% to 10% of patients) may result from disorders such as hemochromatosis.
- Cardiac cirrhosis (rare) refers to liver damage caused by right-sided heart failure.
- Idiopathic cirrhosis (about 10% of patients) has no known cause.

Noncirrhotic fibrosis may result from schistosomiasis or congenital hepatic fibrosis or may be idiopathic.

Clinical presentation

Clinical manifestations of cirrhosis and fibrosis are similar for all types, regardless of cause. Early indications are vague but usually include GI signs and symptoms (anorexia, indigestion, nausea, vomiting, constipation, or diarrhea) and dull abdominal ache. Major and late signs and symptoms develop as a result of hepatic insufficiency and portal hypertension and include:

- respiratory—pleural effusion, limited thoracic expansion due to abdominal ascites, interfering with efficient gas exchange and leading to hypoxia
- central nervous system—progressive signs or symptoms of hepatic encephalopathy, including lethargy, mental changes, slurred speech, asterixis (flapping tremor), peripheral neuritis, paranoia, hallucinations, extreme obtundation, and coma
- hematologic—bleeding tendencies (nosebleeds, easy bruising, and bleeding gums) and anemia
- endocrine—testicular atrophy, menstrual irregularities, gynecomastia, and loss of chest and axillary hair
- skin—severe pruritus, extreme dryness, poor tissue turgor, abnormal pigmentation, spider angiomas, palmar erythema, and possibly jaundice
- hepatic—jaundice, hepatomegaly, ascites, edema of the legs, hepatic encephalopathy, and hepatorenal syndrome with full-fledged cirrhosis
- miscellaneous—musty breath, enlarged superficial abdominal veins, muscle atrophy, pain in the right upper abdominal quadrant that worsens when the patient sits up or leans forward, palpable liver or spleen, and temperature of 101° to 103° F (38.3° to 39.4° C). Bleeding from esophageal varices results from portal hypertension. (See *Portal hypertension and esophageal varices*, page 394.)

Differential diagnoses

A differential diagnosis depends on the clinical presentation:

Portal hypertension and esophageal varices

Portal hypertension — elevated pressure in the portal vein — occurs when blood flow meets increased resistance. The disorder is a common result of cirrhosis but may also stem from mechanical obstruction and occlusion of the hepatic veins (Budd-Chiari syndrome). As portal pressure increases, blood backs up into the spleen and flows through collateral channels to the venous system, bypassing the liver. Consequently, portal hypertension produces splenomegaly with thrombocytopenia, dilated collateral veins (esophageal varices, hemorrhoids, or prominent abdominal veins), and ascites.

In many patients, the first sign of portal hypertension is bleeding from esophageal varices, which are dilated tortuous veins in the submucosa of the lower esophagus. Bleeding esophageal varices commonly cause massive hematemesis, requiring emergency treatment to control hemorrhage and prevent hypovolemic shock.

DIAGNOSIS AND TREATMENT
The following procedures are used to diagnose and correct esophageal varices:
- Endoscopy identifies the ruptured varix as the bleeding site and excludes other potential sources in the upper GI tract.
- Angiography aids diagnosis but is less precise than endoscopy.

- Vasopressin infused into the superior mesenteric artery may temporarily stop bleeding. When angiography is unavailable, vasopressin may be infused by I.V. drip, diluted with 5% dextrose in water (except in patients with coronary vascular disease), but this route is usually less effective.
- A Minnesota or Sengstaken-Blakemore tube may be used to control hemorrhage by applying pressure on the bleeding site. Iced saline lavage through the tube may help control bleeding.

The use of vasopressin or a Minnesota or Sengstaken-Blakemore tube is a temporary measure, especially in a patient with a severely deteriorated liver. Fresh blood and fresh frozen plasma, if available, are preferred for blood transfusions to replace clotting factors. Treatment with lactulose promotes elimination of old blood from the GI tract, which combats excessive production and accumulation of ammonia.

Appropriate surgical bypass procedures include portosystemic anastomosis, splenorenal shunt, and mesocaval shunt. A portacaval or a mesocaval shunt decreases pressure within the liver and reduces ascites, plasma loss, and risk of hemorrhage by directing blood from the liver into collateral vessels. Emergency shunts carry a mortality of 25% to 50%.

- Encephalopathy may be due to drugs, renal failure, or cardiopulmonary disease.
- Ascites may be due to pancreatitis, heart failure, malignancy, or thyroid disease.
- Hemoptysis may be due to upper GI bleeding, esophageal varices, or a Mallory-Weiss syndrome.

Diagnosis
Liver biopsy, the definitive test for cirrhosis, is used to detect destruction and fibrosis of hepatic tissue.

Liver scan shows abnormal thickening and a liver mass. Cholecystography and cholangiography visualize the gallbladder and the biliary duct system, respectively; splenoportal venography visualizes the portal venous system. Percuta-

Clinical evidence suggests that the portosystemic bypass doesn't prolong the patient's survival time; however, he will eventually die of hepatic coma rather than of hemorrhage.

PATIENT CARE

Care for the patient who has portal hypertension with esophageal varices focuses on careful monitoring for signs and symptoms of hemorrhage and subsequent hypotension, compromised oxygen supply, and altered level of consciousness:

- Monitor vital signs, urine output, and central venous pressure to determine fluid volume status.
- Assess level of consciousness often.
- Provide emotional support and reassurance in the wake of massive GI bleeding, which is always a frightening experience.
- Keep the patient as quiet and comfortable as possible, but remember that tolerance of sedatives and tranquilizers may be decreased because of liver damage.
- Carefully monitor the patient with a Minnesota or Sengstaken-Blakemore tube in place for persistent bleeding in gastric drainage.

neous transhepatic cholangiography differentiates extrahepatic from intrahepatic obstructive jaundice and discloses hepatic pathology and the presence of gallstones.

The following laboratory findings are characteristic of cirrhosis:

- decreased white blood cell count, hemoglobin level, hematocrit, albumin, serum electrolytes (sodium, potassium, chloride, and magnesium), and cholinesterase
- elevated levels of globulin, serum ammonia, total bilirubin, alkaline phosphatase, serum aspartate aminotransferase, serum alanine aminotransferase, and lactate dehydrogenase and increased thymol turbidity
- anemia, neutropenia, and thrombocytopenia, characterized by prolonged prothrombin and partial thromboplastin times
- deficiencies of folic acid, iron, and vitamins A, B_{12}, C, and K
- positive tests for galactose tolerance and urine bilirubin
- fecal urobilinogen levels greater than 280 mg/24 hours
- urine urobilinogen levels greater than 1.16 mg/24 hours.

Management

General

Treatment goals are to remove or alleviate the underlying cause of cirrhosis or fibrosis, prevent further liver damage, and prevent or treat complications. The patient may benefit from a high-calorie and moderate-protein to high-protein diet, but developing hepatic encephalopathy mandates restricted protein intake. In addition, sodium is usually restricted to 200 to 500 mg/day, and fluids are restricted to 1 L to 1.5 L/day.

If the patient's condition continues to deteriorate, tube feedings or total parenteral nutrition may be necessary. Supplemental vitamins — A, B complex, D, and K — may also be needed to compensate for the liver's inability to store these nutrients; vitamin B_{12}, folic acid, and thiamine may be necessitated by deficiency anemia. Rest, moderate exercise, and avoidance of exposure to infections and toxic agents are essential. Paracentesis and infusions of salt-poor albumin may alleviate ascites.

Circulation in portal hypertension

As portal vein pressure increases, blood backs up into the spleen and flows through collateral channels to the venous system, bypassing the liver and resulting in esophageal varices.

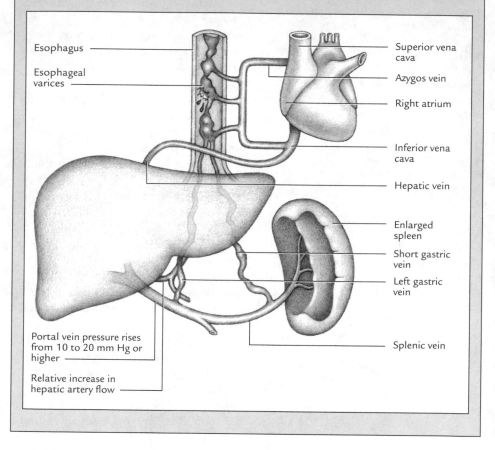

Esophagus
Esophageal varices
Superior vena cava
Azygos vein
Right atrium
Inferior vena cava
Hepatic vein
Enlarged spleen
Short gastric vein
Left gastric vein
Portal vein pressure rises from 10 to 20 mm Hg or higher
Relative increase in hepatic artery flow
Splenic vein

Medication

Drug therapy requires special caution because the cirrhotic liver can't detoxify harmful substances efficiently. Alcohol is prohibited; sedatives should be avoided or prescribed with great care.

When absolutely necessary, the following medications may be used:
- metoclopramide — 10 mg I.V. or I.M. every 4 to 6 hours p.r.n.
- trimethobenzamide — 250 mg P.O. t.i.d. or 200 mg I.M. or P.R. t.i.d. to q.i.d.

- vasopressin — 0.2 to 0.4 U/min I.V. by continuous infusion
- propranolol — initially 40 mg/day P.O., then increasing 20 to 40 mg/day to an average of 70 mg/day to decrease baseline heart rate by 25%
- furosemide — 40 to 160 mg/day I.V. or P.O. to reduce edema
- spironolactone — 100 to 400 mg/day P.O. for ascites
- lactulose — 15 to 30 ml/day P.O. for encephalopathy or high ammonia levels.

Surgical intervention

Surgical procedures include sclerotherapy, ligation of varices, splenectomy, esophagogastric resection, and splenorenal or portacaval anastomosis to relieve portal hypertension. (See *Circulation in portal hypertension.*) Programs for preventing cirrhosis usually emphasize alcohol avoidance.

Referral

- Refer the patient to a gastroenterologist.
- The patient may need to be referred to a surgeon if surgery is indicated.
- Refer the patient to Alcoholics Anonymous, if necessary.

Follow-up

The patient may be seen yearly if stable. Liver function testing should be done yearly— more frequently if the patient is symptomatic.

Patient teaching

- Tell the patient to check skin, gums, stools, and vomitus regularly for bleeding. Warn the patient against taking nonsteroidal anti-inflammatory drugs, straining during bowel movements, and blowing his nose or sneezing too vigorously. Suggest using an electric razor and soft toothbrush.
- Instruct family members to observe the patient closely for signs of behavioral or personality changes. Report increasing stupor, lethargy, hallucinations, or neuromuscular dysfunction.
- Tell the patient that rest and good nutrition will conserve energy and decrease metabolic demands on the liver. Urge him to eat frequent small meals. Stress the need to avoid infections and abstain from alcohol.
- Tell the patient to monitor weight for indications of fluid weight gain.

Complications

- Ascites
- Hepatic encephalopathy
- Jaundice
- Bleeding esophageal varices
- Liver failure
- Renal failure

• • • • • • • • • • • •

CORROSIVE ESOPHAGITIS AND STRICTURE

Corrosive esophagitis is inflammation and damage to the esophagus after ingestion of a caustic chemical. Similar to a burn, this injury may be temporary or may lead to permanent stricture (narrowing or stenosis) of the esophagus that's correctable only through surgery. Severe injury can quickly lead to esophageal perforation, mediastinitis, and death from infection, shock, and massive hemorrhage (due to aortic perforation).

Causes

The most common chemical injury to the esophagus follows the ingestion of lye or other strong alkalies; ingestion of strong acids is less common. The type and amount of chemical ingested determine the severity and location of the damage. In children, household chemical ingestion is accidental; in adults, it's usually a suicide attempt or gesture. The chemical may damage only the mucosa or submucosa or it may damage all layers of the esophagus.

Esophageal tissue damage occurs in three phases: the acute phase, consisting of edema and inflammation; the latent phase, with ulceration, exudation, and tissue sloughing; and the chronic phase, in which there's diffuse scarring.

Clinical presentation

Effects vary from none at all to intense pain in the mouth and anterior chest, marked salivation, inability to swallow, and tachypnea. Bloody vomitus containing pieces of esophageal tissue signals severe damage. Signs of esophageal perforation and mediastinitis, especially crepitation, indicate destruction of the entire esophagus. Inability to speak implies laryngeal damage.

The acute phase subsides in 3 to 4 days, enabling the patient to eat again. Fever suggests secondary infection. Symptoms of dysphagia return if stricture develops, usually within weeks; rarely, stricture is delayed and develops several years after the injury.

Differential diagnoses

- Foreign body ingestion
- Gastritis
- Peptic ulcer disease
- Angina
- Myocardial infarction

Diagnosis

A history of chemical ingestion and physical examination revealing oropharyngeal burns (including white membranes and edema of the soft palate and uvula) usually confirm the diagnosis.

The type and amount of the chemical ingested must be identified; this may be done by examining the container of the ingested material or by calling a poison control center.

Two procedures are helpful in evaluating the severity of the injury:
- Endoscopy (in the first 24 hours after ingestion) delineates the extent and location of the esophageal injury and assesses depth of the burn. This procedure may also be performed a week after ingestion to assess stricture development.
- Barium swallow (1 week after ingestion and every 3 weeks thereafter) may identify segmental spasm or fistula but doesn't always show mucosal injury.

Management

General

Conservative treatment of corrosive esophagitis and stricture includes monitoring the victim's condition, early endoscopy, and administering appropriate medications. Supportive treatment includes I.V. therapy to replace fluids or total parenteral nutrition while the patient can't swallow, gradually progressing to clear liquids and a soft diet.

Medication

The following medications may be used to treat corrosive esophagitis and stricture:
- prednisone — 5 to 60 mg/day P.O. in single or divided doses
- ampicillin — 250 to 500 mg P.O. every 6 hours or 1 to 12 g/day I.M. or I.V. in divided doses every 4 to 6 hours.

Surgical intervention

Treatment may also include bougienage, a procedure in which a slender, flexible, cylindrical instrument called a bougie is passed into the esophagus to dilate it and minimize stricture. Bougienage may be used immediately and then regularly to maintain a patent lumen and prevent stricture; other times it may be delayed for a week to avoid the risk of esophageal perforation.

Surgery is necessary immediately for esophageal perforation or later to correct stricture untreatable with bougienage. Corrective surgery may involve transplanting a piece of the colon to the damaged esophagus. However, even after surgery, stricture may recur at the site of the anastomosis.

Referral
- Refer the patient to a gastroenterologist for treatment.
- Refer the patient for psychological counseling if the ingestion of corrosive materials was intentional.

Follow-up
The patient should be seen as needed to maintain a patent esophageal lumen. An endoscopy may need to be repeated in 6 to 12 weeks if the patient develops dysphagia.

Patient teaching
- Teach the patient or family about potential corrosive chemicals in the household.
- Encourage the patient to follow a soft diet until the esophagus is fully healed. Instruct him to report any difficulty swallowing.

Complications
- Esophageal perforation
- Esophageal bleeding
- Barrett esophagus
- Squamous cell carcinoma
- Weight loss and malnutrition

• • • • • • • • • • • •

CROHN'S DISEASE

Crohn's disease, also known as regional enteritis and granulomatous colitis, is an inflammation of any part of the GI tract (usually the proximal portion of the colon or, less commonly, the terminal ileum) that extends through all layers of the intestinal wall. It may also involve regional lymph nodes and the mesentery. Crohn's disease occurs in an estimated 1.2 to 15 cases per 100,000 people in the United States. Patients with relatives

who have Crohn's disease are 10 times more likely to develop the disease.

AGE ALERT Crohn's disease may affect a person of any age but is most prevalent in people between ages 15 and 30 and ages 60 and 80.

Causes
The exact cause of Crohn's disease is unknown; possible causes include allergies and other immune disorders and infection, although no infecting organism has been isolated. Several factors also implicate a genetic cause: Crohn's disease sometimes occurs in monozygotic twins, and up to 5% of those with the disease have one or more affected relatives. However, no simple pattern of mendelian inheritance has been identified. Whatever the cause of Crohn's disease, lacteal blockage in the intestinal wall leads to edema and, eventually, to inflammation, ulceration, stenosis, and possibly the development of abscesses and fistulas.

Clinical presentation
Clinical effects may be mild and nonspecific, initially; they vary according to the location and extent of the lesion. Bleeding may occur and, although usually mild, may be massive. Bloody stools may also occur. Acute inflammatory signs and symptoms mimic appendicitis and include:
- steady, colicky pain in the right lower quadrant
- cramping
- tenderness
- flatulence
- nausea
- fever
- diarrhea.

Chronic symptoms, which are typical of the disease, are persistent and less severe; they include diarrhea (four to six stools a day) with pain in the right lower

The "string sign"

In Crohn's disease, the characteristic "string sign" (marked narrowing of the bowel), resulting from inflammatory disease and scarring, strengthens the diagnosis.

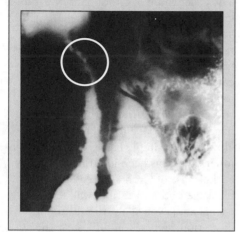

abdominal quadrant, steatorrhea (excess fat in feces), marked weight loss and, rarely, clubbing of fingers. The patient may complain of weakness and fatigue.

Differential diagnoses
- Ulcerative colitis
- Irritable bowel syndrome
- Colorectal cancer
- Infection
- Drug reaction
- Ischemic colitis

Diagnosis
Laboratory findings commonly indicate:
- increased white blood cell count
- increased erythrocyte sedimentation rate
- decreased hemoglobin level
- hypokalemia
- hypocalcemia
- hypomagnesemia.

Barium enema showing the "string sign" (segments of stricture separated by normal bowel) supports this diagnosis. (See *The "string sign."*) Sigmoidoscopy and colonoscopy may show patchy areas of inflammation, thus helping to rule out ulcerative colitis. Biopsy is required for a definitive diagnosis.

Management
General
Treatment is symptomatic. In debilitated patients, therapy includes total parenteral nutrition to maintain nutritional status while resting the bowel. Effective treatment requires important changes in lifestyle: physical rest, restricted fiber diet (no fruit or vegetables), and elimination of dairy products for lactose intolerance.

Medication
Drug therapy may include:
- azathioprine — 1 to 3 mg/kg P.O. or I.V. daily
- sulfasalazine — 3 to 4 mg P.O. in divided doses
- olsalazine — 500 mg P.O. b.i.d.
- metronidazole — 7.5 mg/kg I.V. or P.O. every 6 hours; effective in some patients
- opium tincture — 0.6 ml P.O. q.i.d.
- diphenoxylate — 5 mg P.O. q.i.d.
- infliximab — 5 mg/kg single I.V. infusion; decreases inflammation in the intestinal lining.

Surgical intervention
Surgery may be necessary to correct bowel perforation, massive hemorrhage, fistulas, or acute intestinal obstruction. Colectomy with ileostomy is necessary in many patients with extensive disease of the large intestine and rectum.

Referral
- Refer the patient to a gastroenterologist.

- Refer the patient to a surgeon, if necessary.
- The patient and family members may need referrals for psychological counseling to cope with this disorder.
- Refer the patient and family members to the Crohn's & Colitis Foundation of America for information and support.

Follow-up
The patient should be seen every 3 to 6 months when stable, or according to the specialist's recommendation.

Patient teaching
- If the patient requires surgery, teach stoma care.
- Tell the family members what to expect in the course of this illness.
- Teach the patient the adverse effects of any medication.

Complications
- Malnutrition
- Colon perforation
- Malignancy
- Fistula
- Depression
- Intestinal obstruction
- Perianal and perirectal abscesses and fistulas

• • • • • • • • • • • • •

DIVERTICULAR DISEASE

In diverticular disease, bulging pouches (diverticula) in the GI wall push the mucosal lining through the surrounding muscle. The most common site for diverticula is in the sigmoid colon, but they may develop anywhere, from the proximal end of the pharynx to the anus. Other typical sites are the duodenum, near the pancreatic border or the ampulla of Vater, and the jejunum. Diverticular disease of the stomach is rare and is commonly a precursor of peptic or neoplastic disease. Diverticular disease of the ileum (Meckel's diverticulum) is the most common congenital anomaly of the GI tract. (See *Meckel's diverticulum*, page 402.)

Diverticular disease has two clinical forms. In diverticulosis, diverticula are present but don't cause symptoms. In diverticulitis, diverticula are inflamed and may cause potentially fatal obstruction, infection, or hemorrhage. Diverticular disease is most prevalent in men over age 40. Five percent to 10% of cases occur in people over age 50, and 50% of cases occur in people over age 70.

Causes and pathophysiology
Diverticula probably result from high intraluminal pressure on areas of weakness in the GI wall, where blood vessels enter. Diet may also be a contributing factor because insufficient fiber reduces fecal residue, narrows the bowel lumen, and leads to higher intra-abdominal pressure during defecation. The prevalence of diverticulosis in Western industrialized nations, where processing removes much of the roughage from foods, supports this theory.

In diverticulitis, retained undigested food mixed with bacteria accumulates in the diverticular sac, forming a hard mass (fecalith). This substance cuts off the blood supply to the thin walls of the sac, making them more susceptible to attack by colonic bacteria. Inflammation follows, possibly leading to perforation, abscess, peritonitis, obstruction, or hemorrhage. Occasionally, the inflamed colon segment produces a fistula by adhering to the bladder or other organs.

Clinical presentation
The major forms of diverticular disease (diverticulosis and mild, severe, or

Meckel's diverticulum

In Meckel's diverticulum, a congenital abnormality—a blind tube, like the appendix—opens into the distal ileum near the ileocecal valve. The lining of the diverticulum is gastric mucosa. This disorder results from failure of the intra-abdominal portion of the yolk sac to close completely during fetal development. It occurs in 2% of the population, mostly in males.

COMPLICATIONS

Uncomplicated Meckel's diverticulum produces no symptoms, but complications cause abdominal pain, especially around the umbilicus, and dark red melena or hematochezia. This disorder can lead to peptic ulceration, perforation, and peritonitis and sometimes resembles acute appendicitis.

Meckel's diverticulum can cause bowel obstruction when a fibrous band that connects the diverticulum to the abdominal wall, the mesentery, or other structures, snares a loop of the intestine. This can cause intussusception into the diverticulum or volvulus near the diverticular attachment to the back of the umbilicus or other intra-abdominal structure. Meckel's diverticulum should be considered in cases of GI obstruction or hemorrhage, especially when routine GI X-rays are negative.

TREATMENT

Treatment consists of surgical resection of the inflamed bowel and antibiotic therapy if infection is present.

chronic diverticulitis) produce the following characteristic signs and symptoms:

- Diverticulosis usually produces no symptoms, but can cause recurrent left lower quadrant pain, which is commonly accompanied by alternating constipation and diarrhea and is relieved by defecation or the passage of flatus. Symptoms resemble irritable bowel syndrome and suggest that both disorders may coexist.
- Mild diverticulitis produces moderate left lower abdominal pain, mild nausea, gas, irregular bowel habits, low-grade fever, and leukocytosis.
- In severe diverticulitis, the diverticula can rupture and produce abscesses or peritonitis, which occurs in up to 20% of such patients. Signs and symptoms of rupture include abdominal rigidity and left lower quadrant pain. Peritonitis fol-

lows the release of fecal material from the rupture site and causes signs of sepsis and shock. Rupture of a diverticulum near a vessel can cause microscopic or massive hemorrhage, depending on the vessel's size.

- Chronic diverticulitis can cause fibrosis and adhesions that narrow the bowel's lumen and lead to bowel obstruction. Signs and symptoms of incomplete obstruction are constipation, ribbonlike stools, intermittent diarrhea, and abdominal distention. Increasing obstruction causes abdominal rigidity and pain, diminishing or absent bowel sounds, nausea, and vomiting.

Differential diagnoses

- Irritable bowel syndrome
- Appendicitis
- Tumor

- Crohn's disease
- Ulcerative colitis
- Gastroenteritis

Diagnosis

In many cases, diverticular disease produces no symptoms and is found during an upper GI series performed as part of a differential diagnosis. Upper GI series confirms or rules out diverticulosis of the esophagus and upper bowel; barium enema confirms or rules out diverticulosis of the lower bowel. Barium-filled diverticula can be single, multiple, or clustered like grapes and may have a wide or narrow mouth. Barium outlines but doesn't fill diverticula blocked by impacted feces. In patients with acute diverticulitis, a barium enema requires caution because it can rupture the bowel. If irritable bowel syndrome accompanies diverticular disease, X-rays may reveal colonic spasm.

Biopsy results can be used to rule out cancer; however, a colonoscopic biopsy isn't recommended during acute diverticular disease because of the strenuous bowel preparation it requires. Blood studies may show an elevated erythrocyte sedimentation rate in diverticulitis, especially if the diverticula are infected.

Management

General

Asymptomatic diverticulosis generally doesn't necessitate treatment. Intestinal diverticulosis with pain, mild GI distress, constipation, or difficult defecation may respond to a liquid or bland diet, stool softeners, and occasional doses of mineral oil. These measures relieve symptoms, minimize irritation, and lessen the risk of progression to diverticulitis. After pain subsides, patients also benefit from a high-residue diet and bulk-forming medication such as psyllium.

The goals of treatment for patients with mild diverticulitis without signs of perforation are to prevent constipation and combat infection. Treatment may include bed rest, a liquid diet, and medication. The patient would gradually incorporate fiber-rich foods and fiber supplements into his diet.

Patients who hemorrhage need blood replacement and careful monitoring of fluid and electrolyte balance; bleeding usually stops spontaneously. If it continues, angiography may be performed to guide catheter placement for infusing vasopressin into the bleeding vessel.

Medication

Medications used in the treatment of patients with diverticular disease may include:

- docusate sodium — 50 to 500 mg/day P.O.
- amoxicillin — 250 to 500 mg P.O. every 8 hours for 7 days
- meperidine — 50 to 150 mg P.O. every 3 to 4 hours p.r.n.
- propantheline — 15 mg P.O. a.c. and 30 mg P.O. h.s.

Surgical intervention

Diverticulitis that's refractory to medical treatment necessitates colon resection to remove the involved segment. Perforation, peritonitis, obstruction, or fistula that accompanies diverticulitis may necessitate a temporary colostomy to drain abscesses and rest the colon, later followed by reanastomosis, 6 weeks to 3 months after the initial surgery.

Referral

- Refer the patient to a gastroenterologist.
- If needed, refer the patient to a surgeon.

- If dietary issues arise, refer the patient to a nutritionist.

Follow-up
If the patient is stable, see him yearly. If the patient is being treated with antibiotics, see him in 1 week.

Patient teaching
- Make sure the patient understands the importance of dietary fiber and the harmful effects of constipation and straining during bowel movements. Encourage increased intake of foods high in indigestible fiber, including fresh fruits and vegetables, whole grain bread, and wheat or bran cereals. Warn that a high-fiber diet may temporarily cause flatulence and discomfort.
- Advise the patient to relieve constipation with stool softeners or bulk-forming cathartics. Caution against taking bulk-forming cathartics without plenty of water; if swallowed dry, they may absorb enough moisture in the mouth and throat to swell and obstruct the esophagus or trachea.
- Teach ostomy care as needed.

Complications
- Perforation
- Bowel obstruction
- Fistula
- Hemorrhage

• • • • • • • • • • • •
GASTRITIS

Gastritis, an inflammation of the gastric mucosa, may be acute or chronic. Acute gastritis produces mucosal reddening, edema, hemorrhage, and erosion. Chronic gastritis is common among elderly patients and people with pernicious anemia. It commonly occurs as chronic atrophic gastritis, in which all stomach mucosal layers are inflamed, with reduced numbers of chief and parietal cells. Gastritis occurs in 2 out of every 10,000 people in the United States and may affect more people over age 60. The prognosis is good with treatment.

Causes
Acute gastritis has various causes, including:
- chronic ingestion of (or an allergic reaction to) irritating foods or beverages, such as hot peppers or alcohol
- drugs such as aspirin and other nonsteroidal anti-inflammatory drugs (in large doses), cytotoxic agents, caffeine, corticosteroids, antimetabolites, phenylbutazone, and indomethacin
- ingestion of poisons, especially DDT, ammonia, mercury, carbon tetrachloride, and corrosive substances
- endotoxins released from infecting bacteria, such as staphylococci, *Escherichia coli*, or salmonella.

Acute gastritis leading to stress ulcers also may develop in acute illnesses, especially when the patient has had major traumatic injuries; burns; severe infection; hepatic, renal, or respiratory failure; or major surgery.

Chronic gastritis is sometimes associated with peptic ulcer disease or gastrostomy, both of which cause chronic reflux of pancreatic secretions, bile, and bile acids from the duodenum into the stomach. Recurring exposure to irritating substances, such as drugs, alcohol, cigarette smoke, or environmental agents, can also lead to chronic gastritis. Chronic gastritis sometimes occurs with pernicious anemia, renal disease, or diabetes mellitus. Pernicious anemia is often associated with atrophic gastritis, a chronic inflammation of the stomach resulting from degeneration of the gastric mucosa. In pernicious anemia, the stomach can no longer secrete intrinsic factor, which is needed for vitamin B_{12} absorption.

Bacterial infection with *Helicobacter pylori* is a common cause of nonerosive chronic gastritis.

Clinical presentation
After exposure to the offending substance, the patient with acute gastritis typically reports rapid onset of signs and symptoms that last from a few hours to a few days, such as:
- epigastric discomfort
- indigestion
- cramping
- anorexia
- nausea
- vomiting
- hematemesis.

The patient with chronic gastritis may describe similar symptoms or have only mild epigastric discomfort, or complaints may be vague, such as an intolerance for spicy or fatty foods or slight pain relieved by eating. The patient with chronic atrophic gastritis may be asymptomatic.

Differential diagnoses
- Gastric cancer
- Peptic ulcer disease
- Food poisoning

Diagnosis
Gastroscopy (with biopsy) confirms gastritis when done before lesions heal (usually within 24 hours). This test is contraindicated after ingestion of a corrosive agent.

Laboratory analyses can detect occult blood in vomitus or stools (or both) if the patient has gastric bleeding. Hemoglobin levels and hematocrit are decreased if the patient has developed anemia from bleeding.

Management
General
Treatment for gastritis focuses on eliminating the cause. Until healing occurs, oxygen needs, blood volume, and fluid and electrolyte balance must be monitored. Simply avoiding aspirin and spicy foods may relieve chronic gastritis.

Medication
Medication used in the treatment for gastritis depends on the cause of the disorder.

For bacterial gastritis
- Antibiotics (specific for cultured organism)

In case of ingested poison
- Antidote to neutralize the poison

For gastric secretions
- cimetidine — 300 mg P.O. every 6 hours

For pernicious anemia
- Vitamin B_{12} — 100 to 200 mcg I.M. monthly

For H. pylori infection
- amoxicillin — 1 g P.O. b.i.d. for 2 weeks
- bismuth — 30 ml P.O. q.i.d. for 2 weeks
- metronidazole — 250 to 500 mg P.O. to q.i.d.

Surgical intervention
Vagotomy and pyloroplasty have been used with limited success when conservative treatments fail. Rarely, partial or total gastrectomy may be required.

Referral
- Refer the patient to a gastroenterologist if treatment fails.
- The patient may need referral to a surgeon.

• If the patient smokes, refer him to a smoking cessation program.

Follow-up
The patient should be seen 2 and 4 weeks after treatment is initiated. If treatment isn't effective, a repeat gastroscopy may be needed.

Patient teaching
• Tell the patient to eat small, frequent meals to reduce irritating gastric secretions. Review the patient's normal diet and eliminate foods that cause gastric upset. Tell the patient to avoid alcohol, caffeine, and irritating foods such as spicy or highly seasoned foods.
• Urge the patient to seek immediate attention for recurring symptoms, such as hematemesis, nausea, or vomiting.
• Urge the patient to take prophylactic medications as ordered. To reduce gastric irritation, advise the patient to take steroids with milk, food, or antacids. Instruct him to take antacids between meals and at bedtime and to avoid aspirin-containing compounds.

Complications
• Ulcer
• Bleeding
• Gastric cancer

• • • • • • • • • • • •
GASTROENTERITIS

Gastroenteritis is a self-limiting disorder characterized by diarrhea, nausea, vomiting, and acute or chronic abdominal cramping. It's also called intestinal flu, traveler's diarrhea, viral enteritis, or food poisoning. Gastroenteritis can occur in a person of any age and is a major cause of morbidity and mortality in underdeveloped nations. In the United States, gastroenteritis ranks second to the common cold as a leading cause of lost work time and fifth as the leading cause of death among young children. It also can be life-threatening in elderly or debilitated people.

Causes
Gastroenteritis has many possible causes:
• bacteria (responsible for acute food poisoning), such as *Staphylococcus aureus*, *Salmonella*, *Shigella*, *Clostridium botulinum*, *C. perfringens*, *Escherichia coli*
• amebae, especially *Entamoeba histolytica*
• parasites, such as *Ascaris*, *Enterobius*, and *Trichinella spiralis*
• viruses (may be responsible for traveler's diarrhea), such as adenoviruses, echoviruses, or coxsackieviruses
• ingestion of toxins, including plants or toadstools
• drug reactions, for example, to antibiotics
• enzyme deficiencies
• food allergens.
    The bowel reacts to any of these enterotoxins with hypermotility, producing severe diarrhea and secondary depletion of intracellular fluid. Chronic gastroenteritis is usually the result of another GI disorder such as ulcerative colitis.

Clinical presentation
Clinical manifestations vary depending on the pathologic organism and the level of GI tract involved. Gastroenteritis in adults is usually an acute, self-limiting, nonfatal disease that produces:
• diarrhea
• abdominal discomfort (ranging from cramping to pain)
• nausea
• vomiting
• fever
• malaise
• borborygmi.

In children, elderly patients, and debilitated people, gastroenteritis produces the same symptoms, but intolerance to electrolyte and fluid losses leads to a higher mortality in such patients.

Differential diagnoses
- Ulcerative colitis
- Irritable bowel syndrome

Diagnosis
Patient history can aid the diagnosis of gastroenteritis. Stool culture (by direct rectal swab) or blood culture is used to identify causative bacteria or parasites.

Management
General
Treatment is usually supportive and consists of bed rest, nutritional support, and increased fluid intake. When gastroenteritis is severe or affects a young child or an elderly or a debilitated person, treatment may include hospitalization, specific antimicrobials, and I.V. fluid and electrolyte replacement.

Medication
Medications used in the treatment of a patient with gastroenteritis may include:
- bismuth — 30 ml P.O. q.i.d.
- prochlorperazine — 5 to 10 mg P.O. q.i.d., or 5 to 10 mg I.M. every 3 to 4 hours or 25 mg P.R. b.i.d. for nausea and vomiting.

Referral
- If the patient's clinical picture doesn't improve, refer him to a gastroenterologist.
- Severe dehydration may necessitate hospitalization.

Follow-up
The patient should be reevaluated within 48 hours.

Patient teaching
- If the patient can eat, tell him to replace lost fluids and electrolytes with broth, ginger ale, lemonade, or a commercially prepared electrolyte solution as tolerated. Warn the patient to avoid milk and milk products, which may provoke recurrence.
- Teach good hygiene to prevent recurrence. Instruct patients to cook foods — especially pork — thoroughly; refrigerate perishable foods, such as milk, mayonnaise, potato salad, and cream-filled pastry; always wash hands with warm water and soap before handling food, especially after using the bathroom; clean utensils thoroughly; avoid drinking water or eating raw fruit or vegetables when visiting a foreign country; and eliminate flies and roaches in the home.

Complications
- Dehydration
- Fluid and electrolyte imbalance

Special considerations
- If food poisoning is the likely cause of gastroenteritis, contact public health authorities so they can interview patients and food handlers, and take samples of the suspected contaminated food.

• • • • • • • • • • • •

GASTROESOPHAGEAL REFLUX

Gastroesophageal reflux, also called gastroesophageal reflux disease (GERD), is the backflow of gastric or duodenal contents, or both, into the esophagus and past the lower esophageal sphincter (LES) without associated belching or vomiting. Reflux may cause symptoms or pathologic changes. Persistent reflux can cause reflux esophagitis (an inflammation of the esophageal mucosa). The prognosis varies with the underlying cause.

The U.S. Department of Health and Human Services estimates that 7 million Americans are afflicted with GERD. It affects all ethnic groups and people of every socioeconomic class.

AGE ALERT Although GERD may affect people of all ages, incidence dramatically increases in people over age 40. More than 50% of patients with GERD are between ages 45 and 64.

Causes

The function of the LES—a high-pressure area in the lower esophagus, just above the stomach—is to prevent gastric contents from backing up into the esophagus. Normally, the LES creates pressure, closing the lower end of the esophagus and relaxing after each swallow to allow food into the stomach. Reflux occurs when LES pressure is deficient or when pressure in the stomach exceeds LES pressure. (See *Factors that decrease lower esophageal sphincter pressure.*)

Studies have shown that a person with symptomatic reflux can't swallow often enough to create sufficient peristaltic amplitude to clear gastric acid from the lower esophagus. This results in prolonged periods of acidity in the esophagus when reflux occurs.

Predisposing factors include:
- pyloric surgery (alteration or removal of the pylorus), which allows reflux of bile or pancreatic juice
- long-term NG intubation (more than 4 or 5 days)
- any agent that decreases LES pressure, such as food, alcohol, and cigarettes; anticholinergics (atropine, belladonna, and propantheline); or other drugs (morphine, diazepam, calcium channel blockers, and meperidine)
- hiatal hernia with incompetent sphincter
- any condition or position that increases intra-abdominal pressure, such as straining, bending, or coughing.

Clinical presentation

GERD doesn't always cause symptoms, and in patients showing clinical effects, confirmation of physiologic reflux may not always be possible. The most common feature of GERD is pyrosis, which may become more severe with vigorous exercise, bending, or lying down, and may be relieved by antacids or sitting upright. The pain of esophageal spasm resulting from reflux esophagitis tends to be chronic and may mimic angina pectoris, radiating to the neck, jaws, and arms.

Other symptoms include:
- odynophagia, which may be followed by a dull substernal ache from severe, long-term reflux
- dysphagia from esophageal spasm, stricture, or esophagitis
- bleeding (bright red or dark brown)
- nocturnal regurgitation that wakens the patient with coughing, choking, and a mouthful of saliva (rare).

Reflux may be associated with hiatal hernia. Direct hiatal hernia becomes clinically significant only when reflux is confirmed.

Pulmonary symptoms result from reflux of gastric contents into the throat and subsequent aspiration; they include chronic pulmonary disease or nocturnal wheezing, bronchitis, asthma, morning hoarseness, and cough. In children, other signs consist of failure to thrive and forceful vomiting from esophageal irritation. Such vomiting sometimes causes aspiration pneumonia.

Differential diagnoses
- Angina pectoris
- Reflux esophagitis
- Motility disorder
- Peptic ulcer disease

Diagnosis
After a careful history and physical examination, tests to confirm GERD include barium swallow fluoroscopy, esophageal pH probe, esophageal manometry, and esophagoscopy. In children, barium esophagography under fluoroscopic control can show reflux.

Recurrent reflux after age 6 weeks is abnormal. An acid perfusion (Bernstein) test can show that reflux is the cause of symptoms. Finally, endoscopy and biopsy allow visualization and confirmation of any pathologic changes in the mucosa.

Management
General
Effective management begins by teaching the patient to avoid factors that decrease lower esophageal sphincter pressure or cause esophageal irritation. The patient should eat a low-fat, high-fiber diet and avoid caffeine, tobacco, and carbonated beverages. He shouldn't eat 2 hours before going to bed, avoid tight clothing, elevate the head of the bed 6″ to 8″ (15 to 20.5 cm), and maintain a normal body weight.

If possible, NG intubation shouldn't be continued for more than 4 to 5 days because the tube interferes with sphincter integrity and allows reflux, especially when the patient lies flat.

Positional therapy is especially useful in infants and children who experience GERD without complications.

Medication
Medications used in the treatment of a patient with GERD may include:

> ### Factors that decrease lower esophageal sphincter pressure
>
> - Fat
> - Whole milk
> - Orange juice
> - Tomatoes
> - Antiflatulent (simethicone)
> - Chocolate
> - High-dose ethanol
> - Cigarette smoking
> - Lying on right or left side
> - Sitting

- metoclopramide — 10 to 15 mg P.O. q.i.d. p.r.n. 30 minutes a.c. and h.s.
- famotidine — 20 to 40 mg P.O. b.i.d. for up to 12 weeks.

Surgical intervention
Surgery may be necessary to control severe and refractory symptoms, such as pulmonary aspiration, hemorrhage, obstruction, severe pain, perforation, incompetent LES, or associated hiatal hernia. Surgical procedures that create an artificial closure at the gastroesophageal junction include Belsey Mark IV operation (to invaginate the esophagus into the stomach) and Nissen procedures (to create a gastric wraparound with or without fixation). The Nissen fundoplication procedure can now be performed laparoscopically. Also, vagotomy or pyloroplasty may be combined with an antireflux regimen to modify gastric contents.

Referral
- The patient may need referral to a gastroenterologist if treatment is unsuccessful.

Follow-up

The patient should be seen 2 weeks after treatment is initiated and then after 8 weeks.

Patient teaching

■ Teach the patient what causes reflux, how to avoid reflux with an antireflux regimen (medication, diet, and positional therapy), and what symptoms to watch for and report.

■ Advise the patient to sit upright, particularly after meals, and to eat small, frequent meals. Tell him to avoid highly seasoned food, acidic juices, alcoholic drinks, bedtime snacks, and foods high in fat or carbohydrates, which reduce LES pressure. He should eat meals at least 2 to 3 hours before lying down.

Complications

■ Aspiration
■ Peptic stricture
■ Loss of dental enamel
■ Barrett's esophagus

• • • • • • • • • • • •

HEMORRHOIDS

Hemorrhoids are varicosities in the superior or inferior hemorrhoidal venous plexus. Dilation and enlargement of the superior plexus produce internal hemorrhoids; dilation and enlargement of the inferior plexus produce external hemorrhoids that may protrude from the rectum. (See *Types of hemorrhoids.*) Hemorrhoids occur in both sexes.

AGE ALERT Incidence of hemorrhoids is usually highest in people between ages 20 and 50. Approximately 50% of the U.S. population have hemorrhoids by age 50.

Causes

Hemorrhoids probably result from increased venous pressure in the hemorrhoidal plexus. Predisposing factors include occupations that require prolonged standing or sitting; straining due to constipation, diarrhea, coughing, sneezing, or vomiting; heart failure; hepatic disease, such as cirrhosis, amebic abscesses, or hepatitis; alcoholism; anorectal infections; loss of muscle tone due to old age, rectal surgery, or episiotomy; anal intercourse; and pregnancy.

Clinical presentation

Although hemorrhoids may be asymptomatic, they characteristically cause painless, intermittent bleeding, which occurs on defecation. Bright red blood appears on the stool or on toilet paper because of injury of the fragile mucosa covering the hemorrhoid. These first-degree hemorrhoids may itch because of poor anal hygiene. When second-degree hemorrhoids prolapse, they're usually painless and spontaneously return to the anal canal following defecation. Third-degree hemorrhoids cause constant discomfort and prolapse in response to any increase in intra-abdominal pressure. They must be manually reduced. Thrombosis of external hemorrhoids produces sudden rectal pain and a subcutaneous, large, firm lump that the patient can feel. If hemorrhoids cause severe or recurrent bleeding, they may lead to secondary anemia with significant pallor, fatigue, and weakness; however, such systemic complications are rare.

Differential diagnoses

■ Prolapse of the rectal mucosa
■ Anal tags
■ Rectal or anal neoplasia

Diagnosis

Physical examination confirms external hemorrhoids. Proctoscopy confirms internal hemorrhoids and rules out rectal polyps.

Management

General

Treatment depends on the type and severity of the hemorrhoid and the patient's overall condition. Generally, treatment includes measures to ease pain, combat swelling and congestion, and regulate bowel habits. Patients can relieve constipation by increasing the amount of raw vegetables, fruit, and whole grain cereal in the diet or by using stool softeners. Venous congestion can be prevented by avoiding prolonged sitting on the toilet; local swelling and pain can be decreased with local anesthetic agents (lotions, creams, or suppositories), astringents, or cold compresses, followed by warm sitz baths or thermal packs. Rarely, the patient with chronic, profuse bleeding may require blood transfusion. Other nonsurgical treatments are injection of a sclerosing solution to produce scar tissue that decreases prolapse, manual reduction, and hemorrhoid ligation or laser ablation.

Medication

Medications used to treat a patient with hemorrhoids may include:

- docusate sodium—50 to 500 mg/day P.O.
- benzocaine cream—topically q.i.d. for analgesia
- hydrocortisone cream—topically q.i.d. for pruritus or bleeding.

Surgical intervention

Hemorrhoidectomy, the most effective treatment, is necessary for patients with

Types of hemorrhoids

Covered by mucosa, internal hemorrhoids bulge into the rectal lumen and may prolapse during defecation. Covered by skin, external hemorrhoids protrude from the rectum and are more likely to thrombose than internal hemorrhoids. The illustrations below show frontal and cross-sectional views.

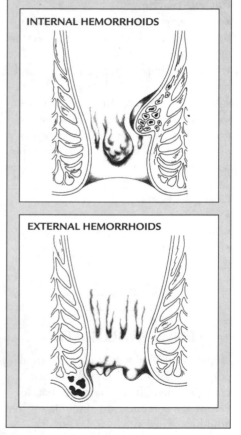

INTERNAL HEMORRHOIDS

EXTERNAL HEMORRHOIDS

severe bleeding, intolerable pain and pruritus, and large prolapse. This procedure is contraindicated in patients with blood dyscrasias (acute leukemia, aplastic anemia, or hemophilia) or GI carcinoma, and during the first trimester of pregnancy.

Referral
▪ Refer the patient to a surgeon if other treatments fail.

Follow-up
The patient should be seen 2 weeks after treatment is initiated and then as needed.

Patient teaching
▪ After surgery, tell the patient to keep the wound site clean to prevent infection and irritation.
▪ Stress the importance of regular bowel habits and good anal hygiene.
▪ Warn the patient against using stool-softening medication soon after hemorrhoidectomy because a firm stool acts as a dilator to prevent anal stricture from the scar tissue.

Complications
▪ Infection
▪ Incontinence
▪ Thrombosis

• • • • • • • • • • • •

HEPATIC ENCEPHALOPATHY

Hepatic encephalopathy, also known as portosystemic encephalopathy or hepatic coma, is a neurologic syndrome that develops as a complication of fulminant liver failure or chronic liver disease. It's most common in patients with cirrhosis; this syndrome is due primarily to ammonia intoxication of the brain. It may be acute and self-limiting or chronic and progressive. Treatment requires correction of the precipitating cause and reduction of blood ammonia levels. In advanced stages, the prognosis is extremely poor despite vigorous treatment. Hepatic encephalopathy occurs in 4 out of 100,000 people.

Causes
Hepatic encephalopathy follows increasing blood ammonia levels. Normally, the ammonia produced by protein breakdown in the bowel is metabolized to urea in the liver. When portal blood shunts past the liver, ammonia directly enters the systemic circulation and is carried to the brain. Such shunting may result from the collateral venous circulation that develops in portal hypertension or from surgically created portal-systemic shunts. Cirrhosis further compounds this problem because impaired hepatocellular function prevents conversion of ammonia that reaches the liver.

Other factors that predispose a patient to increasing ammonia levels include excessive protein intake, sepsis, excessive accumulation of nitrogenous body wastes (from constipation or GI hemorrhage), and bacterial action on protein and urea to form ammonia. Certain other factors heighten the brain's sensitivity to ammonia intoxication: hypoxia, azotemia, impaired glucose metabolism, infection, and administration of sedatives, narcotics, and general anesthetics. Depletion of the intravascular volume, from bleeding or diuresis, reduces hepatic and renal perfusion and leads to contraction alkalosis. In turn, hypokalemia and alkalosis increase ammonia production and impair its excretion.

Clinical presentation
Clinical manifestations of hepatic encephalopathy vary (depending on the

severity of neurologic involvement) and develop in four stages:

■ In the prodromal stage, early signs and symptoms are commonly overlooked because they're so subtle: slight personality changes (disorientation, forgetfulness, and slurred speech) and a slight tremor.
■ During the impending stage, tremor progresses into asterixis, the hallmark of hepatic encephalopathy. Lethargy, aberrant behavior, and apraxia also occur.
■ At the stuporous stage, hyperventilation occurs; the patient is typically stuporous but becomes noisy and abusive when aroused.
■ In the comatose stage, the patient has hyperactive reflexes, a positive Babinski's sign, fetor hepaticus (musty, sweet odor to the breath), and coma.

Differential diagnoses
■ Trauma
■ Alcohol withdrawal syndrome
■ Meningitis
■ Drug use
■ Metabolic encephalopathy

Diagnosis
Clinical features, a positive history of liver disease, and elevated serum ammonia levels in venous and arterial samples confirm hepatic encephalopathy.

Other supportive laboratory values include:
■ electroencephalogram (EEG) that slows as the disease progresses
■ increase in spinal fluid glutamine
■ elevated bilirubin
■ prolonged prothrombin time.

Evoked potential testing may be a more specific indicator of encephalopathy, but its benefit over EEGs isn't yet clear.

Management
General
Effective treatment stops progression of encephalopathy by reducing blood ammonia levels. Treatment includes eliminating ammonia-producing substances from the GI tract by administration of neomycin to suppress bacterial flora (preventing them from converting amino acids into ammonia), performing sorbitol-induced catharsis to produce osmotic diarrhea and continuous aspiration of blood from the stomach, and reducing dietary protein intake. Hemodialysis is sometimes used to clear toxic blood temporarily. Exchange transfusions may provide dramatic but temporary improvement; however, these require an exceptionally large amount of blood.

Medication
The following medications may be used to treat hepatic encephalopathy:
■ lactulose — 20 to 30 g P.O. t.i.d. to q.i.d., or 300 ml mixed with 700 ml of water for retention enema
■ neomycin — 1 to 3 g P.O. q.i.d. for 5 to 6 days for hepatic coma
■ potassium supplements — according to potassium levels.

Albumin may be used to maintain fluid and electrolyte balance, replace depleted albumin levels, and restore plasma.

Referral
■ Refer the patient to a hepatologist.
■ Refer the patient to a hepatic transplant service, if appropriate.
■ Refer the family for emotional support for the patient in the terminal stage of encephalopathy.

Follow-up
If the patient is stable, see him monthly. If the condition worsens, see him weekly.

Patient teaching
- Tell the patient to maintain a low-protein diet, with carbohydrates supplying most of the calories.
- Tell the patient and family members to promote rest, comfort, and a quiet atmosphere. Discourage stressful exercise.

Complications
- Impaired state
- Disseminated intravascular coagulopathy
- Bleeding
- Hepatorenal syndrome
- Shock

Special considerations
- Record detailed assessments of patient's level of consciousness. Keep a record of the patient's handwriting to monitor progression of neurologic involvement.

• • • • • • • • • • • •

HEPATITIS, NONVIRAL

A nonviral inflammation of the liver (toxic or drug-induced hepatitis) is a form of hepatitis that usually results from exposure to certain chemicals or drugs. Most patients recover from this illness, although a few develop fulminating hepatitis or cirrhosis. Nonviral hepatitis cases occur in 8 out of 10,000 people.

Causes
Various hepatotoxins — carbon tetrachloride, acetaminophen, trichloroethylene, poisonous mushrooms, and vinyl chloride — can cause the toxic form of this disease. Following exposure to these agents, liver damage usually occurs within 24 to 48 hours, depending on the size of the dose or degree of exposure. Alcohol, anoxia, and preexisting liver disease exacerbate the toxic effects of some of these agents.

Drug-induced (idiosyncratic) hepatitis may stem from a hypersensitivity reaction unique to the affected individual, unlike toxic hepatitis, which appears to affect all people indiscriminately. Among the drugs that may cause this type of hepatitis are niacin, halothane, sulfonamides, isoniazid, methyldopa, and phenothiazines (cholestasis-induced hepatitis). In hypersensitive people, symptoms of hepatic dysfunction may appear at any time during or after exposure to these drugs but usually emerge after 2 to 5 weeks of therapy. Not all adverse drug reactions are toxic. Oral contraceptives, for example, can impair liver function and produce jaundice without causing necrosis, fatty infiltration of liver cells, or hypersensitivity.

Clinical presentation
Clinical features of toxic and drug-induced hepatitis vary with the severity of liver damage and the causative agent. In most patients, signs and symptoms resemble those of viral hepatitis:
- anorexia
- nausea
- vomiting
- jaundice
- dark urine
- hepatomegaly
- possible abdominal pain (with acute onset and massive necrosis)
- clay-colored stools
- pruritus

Carbon tetrachloride poisoning also produces headache, dizziness, drowsiness, and vasomotor collapse; halothane-related hepatitis produces fever, moderate leukocytosis, and eosinophilia; chlorpromazine toxicity produces abrupt fever, rash, arthralgia, lymphadenopathy, and epigastric or right upper quadrant pain.

Differential diagnoses
- Viral hepatitis
- Appendicitis
- Mononucleosis

Diagnosis
Diagnostic findings include:
- elevated serum aspartate aminotransferase
- elevated alanine aminotransferase
- elevated total and direct bilirubin (with cholestasis)
- elevated alkaline phosphatase
- elevated white blood cell (WBC) count, and eosinophil count (possible in drug-induced type).

Liver biopsy may help to identify the underlying pathology, especially infiltration with eosinophils and other WBCs. Liver function tests have limited value in distinguishing between nonviral and viral hepatitis.

Management
General
Effective treatment must remove the causative agent by lavage, catharsis, or hyperventilation, depending on the route of exposure.

Medication
The following medications may be used to treat nonviral hepatitis:
- Acetylcysteine (initially 140 mg/kg P.O., then 70 mg/kg every 4 hours for 17 doses) may serve as an antidote for toxic hepatitis caused by acetaminophen poisoning but doesn't prevent drug-induced hepatitis caused by other substances.
- Corticosteroids may be ordered for patients with drug-induced hepatitis.

Referral
- If the patient is unstable, refer him to the hospital for treatment.

Follow-up
The patient should be seen routinely to evaluate resolution of illness and assess for any other sequelae.

Patient teaching
- Preventive measures include instructing the patient about the proper use of drugs and proper handling of cleaning agents and solvents.

Complications
- Cirrhosis
- Dehydration

•••••••••••

HEPATITIS, VIRAL

Viral hepatitis is a fairly common systemic disease, marked by hepatic cell destruction, necrosis, and autolysis, leading to anorexia, jaundice, and hepatomegaly. In most patients, hepatic cells eventually regenerate with little or no residual damage. However, old age and serious underlying disorders make complications more likely. The prognosis is poor if edema and hepatic encephalopathy develop. More than 70,000 cases are reported annually in the United States.

There are six forms of hepatitis:
- Type A (infectious or short-incubation hepatitis) is rising among homosexuals and in people with immunosuppression related to human immunodeficiency virus (HIV) infection.
- Type B (serum or long-incubation hepatitis) also is increasing among HIV-positive individuals. Routine screening of donor blood for the hepatitis B surface antigen (HBsAg) has decreased the incidence of posttransfusion cases, but transmission by needles shared by drug abusers remains a major problem.

■ Type C accounts for about 20% of all viral hepatitis cases and for most posttransfusion cases.

■ Type D (delta hepatitis) is responsible for about 50% of all cases of fulminant hepatitis, which has a high mortality. Developing in 1% of patients, fulminant hepatitis causes unremitting liver failure with encephalopathy. It progresses to coma and commonly leads to death within 2 weeks. In the United States, type D is confined to people who are frequently exposed to blood and blood products, such as I.V. drug users and hemophiliacs.

■ Type E (formerly grouped with type C under the name non-A, non-B hepatitis) occurs primarily among patients who have recently returned from an endemic area (such as India, Africa, Asia, or Central America); it's more common in young adults and more severe in pregnant women.

■ Type G accounts for 0.3% of acute viral hepatitis. It's typically asymptomatic. Chronic infection develops in 90% to 100% of infected people; however, it doesn't cause clinically significant chronic disease.

Causes

The six major forms of viral hepatitis result from infection with the causative viruses: A, B, C, D, E, or G.

Type A hepatitis is highly contagious and usually transmitted by the fecal-oral route, but may also be transmitted parenterally. Hepatitis A usually results from ingestion of contaminated food, milk, or water. Many outbreaks of this type are traced to ingestion of seafood from polluted water.

Type B hepatitis, once thought to be transmitted only by the direct exchange of contaminated blood, is now known to be transmitted also by contact with human secretions and feces. As a result, nurses, doctors, laboratory technicians, and dentists are frequently exposed to type B hepatitis, in many cases as a result of wearing defective gloves. Transmission also occurs during intimate sexual contact as well as through perinatal transmission.

Although specific type C hepatitis viruses have been isolated, only a small percentage of patients test positive for them, perhaps reflecting the test's poor specificity. Usually, this type of hepatitis is transmitted through transfused blood from asymptomatic donors.

Type D hepatitis is found only in patients with an acute or chronic episode of hepatitis B and requires the presence of HBsAg. The type D virus depends on the double-shelled type B virus to replicate. For this reason, type D infection can't outlast a type B infection.

Type E hepatitis is transmitted enterically, much like type A. Because this virus is inconsistently shed in feces, detection is difficult.

Type G hepatitis is a newly identified virus. It's thought to be blood-borne, with transmission similar to hepatitis C.

Clinical presentation

Assessment findings are similar for the different types of hepatitis. Typically, signs and symptoms progress in several stages:

■ In the prodromal (preicteric) stage, the patient typically complains of easy fatigue and anorexia (possibly with mild weight loss), generalized malaise, depression, headache, weakness, arthralgia, myalgia, photophobia, and nausea with vomiting. He also may describe changes in his senses of taste and smell. Assessment of vital signs may reveal a fever of 100° to 102° F (37.8° to 38.9° C). As the prodromal stage draws to a close, usually 1 to 5 days before the onset of the clinical jaundice stage, inspection of urine

and stool specimens may reveal dark-colored urine and clay-colored stools.
- If the patient has progressed to the clinical jaundice stage, he may report pruritus, abdominal pain or tenderness, and indigestion. Early in this stage, he may complain of anorexia; later, his appetite may return. Inspection of the sclerae, mucous membranes, and skin may reveal jaundice, which can last for 1 to 2 weeks. Jaundice indicates that the damaged liver is unable to remove bilirubin from the blood but doesn't indicate the severity of the disease. Occasionally, hepatitis occurs without jaundice. During the clinical jaundice stage, inspection of the skin may disclose rashes, erythematous patches, or urticaria, especially if the patient has hepatitis B or C. Palpation may disclose abdominal tenderness in the right upper quadrant, an enlarged and tender liver and, in some cases, splenomegaly and cervical adenopathy.
- During the recovery (posticteric) stage, most of the patient's symptoms decrease or subside. On palpation, a decrease in liver enlargement may be noted. The recovery phase commonly lasts from 2 to 12 weeks; this phase sometimes lasts longer in patients with hepatitis B, C, or E.

Differential diagnoses
- Infectious mononucleosis
- Malignancy
- Drug- or alcohol-induced hepatitis

Diagnosis
A hepatitis profile, which identifies antibodies specific to the causative virus and establishes the type of hepatitis, is routine in suspected viral hepatitis:
- Type A — Detection of an antibody to hepatitis A confirms the diagnosis.
- Type B — The presence of HBsAg and hepatitis B antibodies confirms the diagnosis.

- Type C — Diagnosis depends on serologic testing for the specific antibody 1 month or more after the onset of acute hepatitis. Until then, the diagnosis is established primarily by obtaining negative test results for hepatitis A, B, and D.
- Type D — Detection of intrahepatic delta antigens or immunoglobulin (Ig) antidelta antigens in acute disease (or IgM and IgG in chronic disease) establishes the diagnosis.
- Type E — Detection of hepatitis E antigens supports the diagnosis; the diagnosis may also be determined by ruling out hepatitis C.
- Type G — Polymerase chain reaction assay is the only specific test for hepatitis G.

Additional findings from liver function studies support the diagnosis:
- Serum aspartate aminotransferase and serum alanine aminotransferase levels are increased in the prodromal stage of acute viral hepatitis.
- Serum alkaline phosphatase levels are slightly increased.
- Serum bilirubin levels are elevated. Levels may continue to be high late in the disease, especially in severe cases.
- Prothrombin time is prolonged (more than 3 seconds longer than normal indicates severe liver damage).
- White blood cell counts commonly reveal transient neutropenia and lymphopenia followed by lymphocytosis.
- Liver biopsy is performed if chronic hepatitis is suspected; it's performed for acute hepatitis only if the diagnosis is questionable.

Management
General
The patient is advised to rest in the early stages of the illness and combat anorexia by eating small, high-calorie, high-protein meals. (Protein intake should be reduced if signs or symptoms of pre-

coma—lethargy, confusion, and mental changes—develop.) Large meals are usually better tolerated in the morning because many patients experience nausea late in the day.

In acute viral hepatitis, hospitalization usually is required only for patients with severe symptoms or complications. Parenteral nutrition may be required if the patient experiences persistent vomiting and is unable to maintain oral intake.

Medication
No specific drug therapy has been developed for patients with hepatitis, with the exception of hepatitis C, which has been treated somewhat successfully with interferon alpha. The following medications may be used to relieve symptoms:
- trimethobenzamide—250 mg P.O. t.i.d. to q.i.d. or 200 mg I.M. or P.R. t.i.d. to q.i.d.
- cholestyramine—4 g P.O. a.c. and h.s.

Referral
- If the patient's condition is unstable, refer him to the hospital for treatment.

Follow-up
The patient should be monitored regularly for the first year after diagnosis by undergoing liver function tests every 2 to 4 weeks.

Patient teaching
- Encourage the patient to drink fluids (at least 4 L/day). Encourage the anorectic patient to drink fruit juices. Suggest chipped ice and effervescent soft drinks to maintain hydration without inducing vomiting.
- Advise the patient to take supplemental vitamins and commercial feedings, if necessary.
- Tell the patient to keep a record of weight changes.

- Warn the patient against using any alcohol or over-the-counter drugs.

Complications
- Cirrhosis
- Liver failure
- Carcinoma
- Death
- Necrosis

• • • • • • • • • • • •
HIATAL HERNIA

Hiatal hernia, also called hiatus hernia, is a defect in the diaphragm that permits a portion of the stomach to pass through the diaphragmatic opening into the chest. Hiatal hernia is the most common problem of the diaphragm affecting the alimentary canal. It occurs in most people over age 50.

Three types of hiatal hernia can occur: sliding hernia, paraesophageal (rolling) hernia, or mixed hernia, which includes features of both. In a sliding hernia, both the stomach and the gastroesophageal junction slip up into the chest, so the gastroesophageal junction is above the diaphragmatic hiatus. In paraesophageal hernia, a part of the greater curvature of the stomach rolls through the diaphragmatic defect. (See *Types of hiatal hernia.*)

Treatment can prevent complications, such as strangulation of the herniated intrathoracic portion of the stomach.

Causes
Hiatal hernia typically results from muscle weakening that's common with aging and may be secondary to esophageal carcinoma, kyphoscoliosis, trauma, or certain surgical procedures. It may also result from certain diaphragmatic malformations that cause congenital weakness.

In hiatal hernia, the muscular collar around the esophageal and diaphragmatic junction loosens, permitting the lower portion of the esophagus and the stomach to rise into the chest when intra-abdominal pressure increases (possibly causing gastroesophageal reflux). Such increased intra-abdominal pressure may result from ascites, pregnancy, obesity, constrictive clothing, bending, straining, coughing, Valsalva's maneuver, or extreme physical exertion.

Sliding hernias are three to ten times more common than paraesophageal and mixed hernias combined. The incidence of hiatal hernia increases with age, and prevalence is higher in women than in men (especially the paraesophageal type). Contributing factors include obesity, smoking, and trauma.

Clinical presentation

Typically, a paraesophageal hernia produces no symptoms; it's usually an incidental finding during a barium swallow or when testing for occult blood. Because this type of hernia leaves the closing mechanism of the cardiac sphincter unchanged, it rarely causes acid reflux or reflux esophagitis. Symptoms result from displacement or stretching of the stomach and may include a feeling of fullness in the chest or pain resembling angina pectoris. Even if it produces no symptoms, this type of hernia necessitates surgical treatment because of the high risk of strangulation that can occur when a large portion of stomach becomes caught above the diaphragm.

A sliding hernia without an incompetent sphincter produces no reflux or symptoms and, consequently, doesn't necessitate treatment. When a sliding hernia causes symptoms, they're typical of gastric reflux, resulting from the incompetent lower esophageal sphincter, and may include:

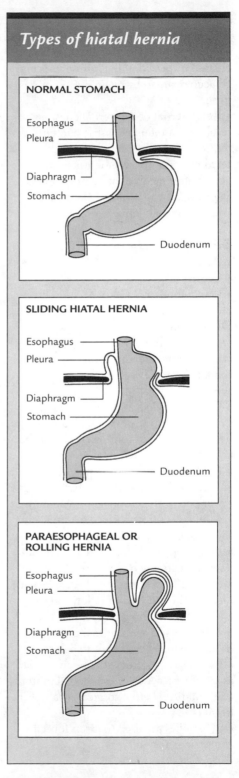

Types of hiatal hernia

NORMAL STOMACH

Esophagus
Pleura
Diaphragm
Stomach
Duodenum

SLIDING HIATAL HERNIA

Esophagus
Pleura
Diaphragm
Stomach
Duodenum

PARAESOPHAGEAL OR ROLLING HERNIA

Esophagus
Pleura
Diaphragm
Stomach
Duodenum

- Pyrosis (heartburn) occurs 1 to 4 hours after eating (especially overeating) and is aggravated by reclining, belching, and increased intra-abdominal pressure. It may be accompanied by regurgitation or vomiting.
- Retrosternal or substernal chest pain results from reflux of gastric contents, distention of the stomach, and spasm or altered motor activity. Chest pain usually occurs after meals or at bedtime and is aggravated by reclining, belching, and increased intra-abdominal pressure.

Differential diagnoses
- Angina
- Gastritis
- Gastrointestinal reflux disease

Diagnosis
Diagnosis of hiatal hernia is based on typical clinical features and the results of the following laboratory studies and procedures:
- Chest X-ray occasionally shows an air shadow behind the heart with a large hernia or infiltrates in lower lobes if the patient has aspirated.
- In barium study, hernia may appear as an outpouching containing barium at the lower end of the esophagus; small hernias are difficult to recognize. This study also shows diaphragmatic abnormalities.
- Endoscopy and biopsy are used to differentiate among hiatal hernia, varices, and other small gastroesophageal lesions; identify the mucosal junction and the edge of the diaphragm indenting the esophagus; and rule out malignancy that otherwise may be difficult to detect.
- Esophageal motility studies are used to assess the presence of esophageal motor abnormalities before surgical repair of the hernia.
- pH studies are used to assess for reflux of gastric contents.

- Acid perfusion (Bernstein) test indicates that heartburn results from esophageal reflux when perfusion of hydrochloric acid through the NG tube provokes this symptom.

The following laboratory test results may indicate GI bleeding as a complication of hiatal hernia:
- Complete blood count may show hypochromic microcytic anemia when bleeding from esophageal ulceration occurs.
- Stool guaiac test results may be positive.
- Analysis of gastric contents may reveal blood.

Management
General
The primary goals of treatment are to relieve symptoms by minimizing or correcting the incompetent cardia, and managing and preventing complications. Medical therapy is used first because symptoms usually respond to it and because hiatal hernia tends to recur after surgery. The goal of such therapy is to modify or reduce reflux by changing the quantity or quality of refluxed gastric contents, strengthening the lower esophageal sphincter muscle pharmacologically, or decreasing the amount of reflux through gravity. These measures include restricting any activity that increases intra-abdominal pressure, giving antiemetics and cough suppressants, avoiding constrictive clothing, modifying diet, giving stool softeners or laxatives to prevent straining during bowel movements, and discouraging smoking because it stimulates gastric acid production.

Modifying the diet by eating small, frequent, bland meals at least 2 hours before lying down (no bedtime snack), eating slowly, and avoiding spicy foods, fruit juices, alcoholic beverages, and coffee. To reduce the amount of reflux, the overweight patient should lose weight to decrease intra-abdominal pressure.

Medication
Medications used to treat a patient with hiatal hernia may include:
- calcium carbonate — 350 mg to 1.5 g P.O. 1 hour p.c. and h.s.
- cimetidine — 200 to 300 mg P.O. with meals and h.s.
- metoclopramide — 10 to 15 mg P.O. 30 minutes a.c. and h.s.

Surgical intervention
Surgical repair is necessary when symptoms can't be controlled medically or with the onset of complications such as stricture, bleeding, pulmonary aspiration, strangulation, or incarceration. Surgery typically involves creating an artificial closing mechanism at the gastroesophageal junction to strengthen the lower esophageal sphincter's barrier function. The surgeon may use an abdominal or a thoracic approach or he may repair the hernia by laparoscopic surgery, which allows for less dependence on an NG tube and a shorter hospital stay.

Referral
- The patient may need referral to a surgeon if treatment isn't successful.

Follow-up
The patient should be seen within 1 to 2 weeks after treatment is initiated.

Patient teaching
- Teach the patient what foods he can eat, and recommend eating small, frequent meals. Warn against activities that increase intra-abdominal pressure.
- To enhance compliance with treatment, teach the patient about this disorder. Explain treatments, diagnostic tests, and significant symptoms.

Complications
- Esophagitis
- Esophageal ulcer or stricture
- Incarceration
- Perforation of gastric ulcer
- Strangulation
- Gangrene (with strangulation)

• • • • • • • • • • • •

HIRSCHSPRUNG'S DISEASE

Hirschsprung's disease, also called congenital megacolon and congenital aganglionic megacolon, is a disorder of the large intestine. It's characterized by absence or marked reduction of parasympathetic ganglion cells in the colorectal wall. This congenital disorder impairs intestinal motility and causes severe, intractable constipation. Without prompt treatment, an infant with colonic obstruction may die within 24 hours from enterocolitis that leads to severe diarrhea and hypovolemic shock. With prompt treatment, the prognosis is good.

Causes and pathophysiology
In Hirschsprung's disease, the aganglionic bowel segment contracts without the reciprocal relaxation needed to propel feces forward. In 90% of patients, this aganglionic segment is in the rectosigmoid area, but it occasionally extends to the entire colon and parts of the small intestine.

Hirschsprung's disease is believed to be a familial, congenital defect, occurring in 1 out of 2,000 to 1 out of 5,000 live births. It's up to seven times more common in males than in females (although the aganglionic segment is usually shorter in males) and is more prevalent in whites. Total aganglionosis affects both sexes equally. Females with Hirschsprung's disease are at higher risk for having affected children. The disease commonly coexists with other congenital anomalies, especially Down syndrome and anomalies of the urinary tract such as megaloureter.

Clinical presentation

Clinical effects usually appear shortly after birth, but mild symptoms may not be recognized until later in childhood or during adolescence (usually) or adulthood (rarely). A neonate with Hirschsprung's disease may exhibit the following signs and symptoms:

- failure to pass meconium within 24 to 48 hours
- signs of obstruction
- irritability
- feeding difficulties
- failure to thrive
- dehydration
- overflow diarrhea
- abdominal distention.

Rectal examination, which may temporarily relieve GI symptoms, reveals a rectum empty of stool and, when the examining finger is withdrawn, an explosive gush of malodorous gas and liquid stool. In infants, the main cause of death is enterocolitis, caused by fecal stagnation that leads to bacterial overgrowth, production of bacterial toxins, intestinal irritation, profuse diarrhea, hypovolemic shock, and perforation.

A older child has intractable constipation (usually requiring laxatives and enemas), abdominal distention, and easily palpated fecal masses. In severe cases, failure to grow is characterized by wasted extremities and loss of subcutaneous tissue, with a large protuberant abdomen.

Adult megacolon, although rare, usually affects men. The patient has abdominal distention, rectal bleeding (rare), and a history of chronic intermittent constipation. He's generally in poor physical condition.

Differential diagnoses

- Bowel obstruction
- Intussusception

Diagnosis

Rectal biopsy provides a definitive diagnosis by showing the absence of ganglion cells. Suction aspiration using a small tube inserted into the rectum may be performed initially. If this test yields inconclusive findings, diagnosis requires full-thickness surgical biopsy under general anesthesia. In older infants, barium enema showing a narrowed segment of distal colon with a sawtooth appearance and a funnel-shaped segment above it confirms the diagnosis and is used to assess the extent of intestinal involvement.

Significantly, infants with Hirschsprung's disease retain barium longer than the usual 12 to 24 hours, so delayed films are usually helpful when other characteristic signs are absent. Other tests include rectal manometry, which detects failure of the internal anal sphincter to relax and contract, and upright plain films of the abdomen, which show marked colonic distention.

Management

General

Management of an infant until the time of surgery consists of daily colonic lavage to empty the bowel. Physiologic saline solution should be used rather than tap water. The patient can absorb large amounts of tap water, resulting in water intoxication. If total obstruction is present in the neonate, a temporary colostomy or ileostomy is necessary to decompress the colon.

Surgical intervention

Surgical treatment involves pulling the normal ganglionic segment through to the anus. However, corrective surgery is usually delayed until the infant is at least 10 months old and better able to withstand it. A preliminary bowel prep with an antibiotic, such as neomycin or nystatin, is necessary before surgery. The surgical technique used is based on the three main corrective procedures: the Duhamel, Soave, or Swenson's pullthrough operation.

Referral
- Refer the patient to a surgeon for treatment.

Follow-up
The patient should be seen within 1 to 2 weeks posthospitalization.

Patient teaching
- Teach parents to recognize the signs of fluid loss and dehydration and of enterocolitis.
- Before corrective surgery, instruct the parents to perform colonic lavage with normal saline solution to evacuate the colon at least once a day; ordinary enemas and laxatives won't clean it adequately.
- After corrective surgery, instruct parents to withhold foods that have previously increased the number of stools. Reassure them that their child will probably gain sphincter control and be able to eat a normal diet, but warn that complete continence may take several years to develop and constipation might recur at times.
- Because an infant with Hirschsprung's disease needs surgery and hospitalization so early in life, parents have difficulty establishing an emotional bond with their child. To promote bonding, encourage them to participate in their child's care as much as possible.

Complications
- Bowel obstruction
- Dehydration
- Death
- Enterocolitis

INGUINAL HERNIA

A hernia occurs when part of an internal organ protrudes through an abnormal opening in the containing wall of its cavity. Most hernias occur in the abdominal cavity. Although many kinds of abdominal hernias are possible, inguinal hernias (also called ruptures) are most common. In an inguinal hernia, the large or small intestine, omentum, or bladder protrudes into the inguinal canal. (See *Common sites of hernia*, page 424.)

Hernias may be reduced (if the hernia can be manipulated back into place with relative ease), incarcerated (if the hernia can't be reduced because adhesions have formed, obstructing the intestinal flow), or strangulated (if part of the herniated intestine becomes twisted or edematous, seriously interfering with normal blood flow and peristalsis and possibly leading to intestinal obstruction and necrosis). Yearly, 1 in 20 men in the United States will have a hernia that will require surgery. Men are 10 times more likely to have a hernia than women.

Causes
An inguinal hernia may be indirect or direct. An indirect inguinal hernia, the more common form, results from weakness in the fascial margin of the internal inguinal ring. In an indirect hernia, abdominal viscera leave the abdomen through the inguinal ring and follow the spermatic cord (in males) or round ligament (in females); they emerge at the ex-

Common sites of hernia

Umbilical hernia results from abnormal muscular structures around the umbilical cord. This hernia is quite common in neonates but also occurs in women who are obese or who have had several pregnancies. Because most umbilical hernias in infants close spontaneously, surgery is warranted only if the hernia persists for more than 4 or 5 years. Taping or binding the affected area or supporting it with a truss may relieve symptoms until the hernia closes. Severe congenital umbilical hernia allows the abdominal viscera to protrude outside the body. This condition necessitates immediate repair.

Incisional (ventral) hernia develops at the site of previous surgery, usually along vertical incisions. This hernia may result from a weakness in the abdominal wall, perhaps as a result of an infection or impaired wound healing. Inadequate nutrition, extreme abdominal distention, or obesity also predisposes a patient to incisional hernia. Palpation of an incisional hernia may reveal several defects in the surgical scar. Effective repair requires pulling the layers of the abdominal wall together without creating tension. If this isn't possible, surgical reconstruction uses Teflon or tantalum mesh to close the opening.

Inguinal hernia can be direct or indirect. Indirect inguinal hernia causes the

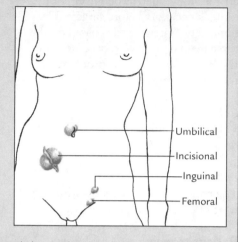

abdominal viscera to protrude through the inguinal ring and to follow the spermatic cord (in males) or round ligament (in females). Direct inguinal hernia results from a weakness in the fascial floor of the inguinal canal.

Femoral hernia occurs where the femoral artery passes into the femoral canal. Typically, a fatty deposit in the femoral canal enlarges and eventually creates a hole big enough to accommodate part of the peritoneum and bladder. A femoral hernia appears as a swelling or bulge at the pulse point of the large femoral artery. It's usually a soft, pliable, reducible, nontender mass but commonly becomes incarcerated or strangulated.

ternal ring and extend down the inguinal canal, commonly into the scrotum or labia. An indirect inguinal hernia may develop at any age, is three times more common in males, and is especially prevalent in infants younger than age 1.

A direct inguinal hernia results from a weakness in the fascial floor of the in-

guinal canal. Instead of entering the canal through the internal ring, the hernia passes through the posterior inguinal wall, protrudes directly through the transverse fascia of the canal (in an area known as Hesselbach's triangle), and comes out at the external ring.

In males, during the 7th month of gestation, the testicle normally descends into the scrotum, preceded by the peritoneal sac. If the sac closes improperly, it leaves an opening through which the intestine can slip. In either sex, a hernia can result from weak abdominal muscles (caused by congenital malformation, trauma, or aging) or increased intra-abdominal pressure (due to heavy lifting, pregnancy, obesity, or straining).

Clinical presentation

Inguinal hernia usually causes a lump to appear over the herniated area when the patient stands or strains. The lump disappears when the patient is supine. Tension on the herniated contents may cause a sharp, steady pain in the groin, which fades when the hernia is reduced. Strangulation produces severe pain and may lead to partial or complete bowel obstruction and even intestinal necrosis. Partial bowel obstruction may cause anorexia, vomiting, pain and tenderness in the groin, an irreducible mass, and diminished bowel sounds. Complete obstruction may cause shock, high fever, absent bowel sounds, and bloody stools. In an infant, an inguinal hernia commonly coexists with an undescended testicle or a hydrocele.

Differential diagnoses

- Hydrocele
- Varicocele
- Epididymitis
- Testicular tumor

Diagnosis

In a patient with a large hernia, physical examination reveals an obvious swelling or lump in the inguinal area. In the patient with a small hernia, the affected area may simply appear full. Palpation of the inguinal area while the patient is performing Valsalva's maneuver confirms the diagnosis.

A patient history of sharp or "catching" pain when lifting or straining may help to confirm the diagnosis. Suspected bowel obstruction requires X-rays and a white blood cell count (which may be elevated).

Management
General

If the hernia is reducible, pushing the hernia back into place may temporarily relieve the pain. A truss may keep the abdominal contents from protruding into the hernial sac, but this doesn't cure the hernia. This device is especially beneficial for an elderly or debilitated patient for whom surgery might be hazardous.

Surgical intervention

For infants, adults, and otherwise healthy elderly patients, herniorrhaphy is the treatment of choice. Herniorrhaphy replaces the contents of the hernial sac into the abdominal cavity and closes the opening. In many cases, this procedure is performed under local anesthesia in a short-term unit or as a single-day admission. Another effective surgical procedure for repairing hernia is hernioplasty, which reinforces the weakened area with steel mesh, fascia, or wire.

A strangulated or necrotic hernia necessitates bowel resection. Rarely, an extensive resection may require temporary colostomy. In either case, bowel resection lengthens postoperative recovery and necessitates administration of antibiotics, parenteral fluids, and electrolyte replacements.

Referral

- The patient may need referral to a surgeon.

Follow-up

The patient should be seen within 2 weeks after surgery.

Patient teaching

- If the patient has a truss, tell him to bathe daily and apply liberal amounts of cornstarch or baby powder to prevent skin irritation. Warn against applying the truss over clothing.
- After surgery (outpatient) teach the patient to check the incision and dressing for drainage, inflammation, or swelling and to watch for fever, and to report if any of these occur.
- To reduce scrotal swelling, have the patient support the scrotum with a rolled towel and apply an ice bag.
- Instruct the patient to drink plenty of fluids to maintain hydration and prevent constipation.
- Warn the patient against lifting heavy objects or straining during bowel movements.

Complications

- Strangulation
- Intestinal obstruction
- Infection (after surgery)

• • • • • • • • • • • •

INTUSSUSCEPTION

Intussusception is a telescoping (invagination) of a portion of the bowel into an adjacent distal portion. It's most common in infants and occurs in three times more males than females. Intussusception may be fatal, especially if treatment is delayed for more than 24 hours.

AGE ALERT Eighty-seven percent of children with intussusception are younger than age 2; 70% of these children are between ages 4 months and 11 months.

Causes

Studies suggest that intussusception may be linked to viral infections because seasonal peaks are noted in the spring and summer, coinciding with peak incidence of enteritis, and in the midwinter, coinciding with peak incidence of respiratory tract infections.

The cause of most cases of intussusception in infants is unknown. In older children, polyps, alterations in intestinal motility, hemangioma, lymphosarcoma, lymphoid hyperplasia, or Meckel's diverticulum may trigger the process. In adults, intussusception usually results from benign or malignant tumors (65% of patients). It may also result from polyps, Meckel's diverticulum, gastroenterostomy with herniation, or an appendiceal stump.

When a bowel segment (the intussusceptum) invaginates, peristalsis propels it along the bowel, pulling more bowel along with it; the receiving segment is the intussuscipiens. This invagination produces edema, hemorrhage from venous engorgement, incarceration, and obstruction. If treatment is delayed for longer than 24 hours, strangulation of the intestine usually occurs, with gangrene, shock, and perforation.

Clinical presentation

In an infant or child, intussusception produces four cardinal clinical effects:

- Intermittent attacks of colicky pain cause the child to scream, draw his legs up to his abdomen, turn pale and diaphoretic and, possibly, display grunting respirations.
- Vomiting of stomach contents may occur initially, followed by further vomiting of bile-stained or fecal material.
- "Currant jelly" stools, containing a mixture of blood and mucus, may be observed.

■ The patient will have a tender, distended abdomen, with a palpable, sausage-shaped abdominal mass; the viscera are usually absent from the right lower quadrant.

In adults, intussusception produces nonspecific, chronic, and intermittent symptoms, including colicky abdominal pain and tenderness, vomiting, diarrhea (occasionally constipation), bloody stools, and weight loss. Abdominal pain usually localizes in the right lower quadrant, radiates to the back, and increases with eating. Adults with severe intussusception may develop strangulation with excruciating pain, abdominal distention, and tachycardia.

Differential diagnoses
■ Appendicitis
■ Gastroenteritis
■ Adhesive band small bowel obstruction

Diagnosis
Barium enema confirms colonic intussusception when it shows the characteristic coiled spring sign; it also delineates the extent of intussusception.

Upright abdominal X-rays may show a soft-tissue mass and signs of complete or partial obstruction, with dilated loops of bowel. White blood cell count up to 15,000/µl indicates obstruction; more than 15,000/µl, strangulation; more than 20,000/µl, possible bowel infarction.

Management
General
During hydrostatic reduction, the radiologist drips a barium solution into the rectum from a height of no more than 3′ (0.9 m); fluoroscopy traces the progress of the barium. If the procedure is successful, the barium backwashes into the ileum and the mass disappears. If not, the procedure is stopped, and the patient is prepared for surgery.

Surgical intervention
In children, therapy may include hydrostatic reduction or surgery. Surgery is indicated for children with recurrent intussusception, for those who show signs of shock or peritonitis, and for those in whom symptoms have been present longer than 24 hours. In adults, surgery is always the treatment of choice.

During surgery, manual reduction is attempted first. After compressing the bowel above the intussusception, the surgeon attempts to milk the intussusception back through the bowel. However, if manual reduction fails, or if the bowel is gangrenous or strangulated, a resection of the affected bowel segment and most likely, a prophylactic appendectomy will be performed.

Referral
■ Refer the patient to a surgeon for treatment.

Follow-up
The patient should be seen 1 week after discharge from the hospital.

Patient teaching
■ If appropriate, encourage the patient to deep-breathe and cough productively. Teach him to splint the incision when he coughs.
■ To minimize the stress of hospitalization, encourage parents to participate in their child's care as much as possible.

Complications
■ Strangulation
■ Perforation
■ Ischemic bowel
■ Sepsis
■ Intestinal obstruction

Special considerations
■ Offer special reassurance and emotional support to the child and parents. This condition is a pediatric emergency, and parents are generally unprepared for their child's hospitalization and possible surgery; they may feel guilty for not seeking medical aid sooner. Similarly, the child is unprepared for a separation from his parents and home.

• • • • • • • • • • • •

IRRITABLE BOWEL SYNDROME

Irritable bowel syndrome, also called spastic colon and spastic colitis, is a common condition marked by chronic or periodic diarrhea, alternating with constipation, and accompanied by straining and abdominal cramps. Irritable bowel syndrome affects men and women alike and age isn't a factor. Fourteen percent to 24% of women and 5% to 19% of men are afflicted with irritable bowel syndrome. The prognosis is good. Supportive treatment or avoidance of a known irritant often relieves symptoms.

Causes
This functional disorder is generally associated with psychological stress; however, it may result from physical factors, such as diverticular disease, ingestion of irritants (coffee and raw fruits or vegetables), lactose intolerance, abuse of laxatives, food poisoning, or colon cancer.

Clinical presentation
Irritable bowel syndrome characteristically produces:
■ lower abdominal pain (usually relieved by defecation or passage of gas)
■ diarrhea that may alternate with constipation or normal bowel function

■ small stools that contain visible mucus
■ dyspepsia
■ abdominal distention.

Differential diagnoses
■ Amebiasis
■ Diverticulitis
■ Colon cancer
■ Lactose intolerance

Diagnosis
Diagnosis of irritable bowel syndrome requires a careful history to determine contributing psychological factors such as a recent stressful life change. Appropriate diagnostic procedures include sigmoidoscopy, colonoscopy, barium enema, rectal biopsy, and stool examination for blood, parasites, and bacteria.

Management
General
The goal of therapy is to relieve symptoms and includes counseling to help the patient understand the relationship between stress and illness. Strict dietary restrictions aren't beneficial, but food irritants should be investigated and the patient should be instructed to avoid them. Rest and heat applied to the abdomen are helpful. If the cause of irritable bowel syndrome is chronic laxative abuse, bowel training may help to correct the condition.

Medication
Medications used in the treatment of a patient with irritable bowel syndrome may include:
■ phenobarbital—30 to 120 mg/day P.O. in 2 to 3 divided doses
■ propantheline—15 mg P.O. t.i.d. a.c. and 30 mg P.O. h.s.
■ diphenoxylate with atropine sulfate—5 mg P.O. q.i.d. p.r.n.

With chronic use, the patient may become dependent on these drugs.

Referral
■ The patient may need to be referred for psychological counseling.

Follow-up
The patient should be seen every 2 to 3 weeks initially, then every 6 months.

Patient teaching
■ Tell the patient to avoid irritating foods, and encourage him to develop regular bowel habits.
■ Help the patient deal with stress, and warn against dependence on sedatives or antispasmodics.
■ Encourage regular checkups because irritable bowel syndrome is associated with a higher-than-normal incidence of diverticulitis and colon cancer. For patients over age 40, emphasize the need for an annual sigmoidoscopy and rectal examination.

Complications
■ Dependency on medication or laxatives

• • • • • • • • • • • •

PANCREATITIS

Pancreatitis, an inflammation of the pancreas, occurs in acute and chronic forms and may be due to edema, necrosis, or hemorrhage. In men, this disease is commonly associated with alcoholism, trauma, or peptic ulcer; in women, it's linked to biliary tract disease. The prognosis is good when pancreatitis follows biliary tract disease but poor when it follows alcoholism. Mortality increases to as high as 60% when pancreatitis is associated with necrosis and hemorrhage. (See

Chronic pancreatitis, page 430.) Acute pancreatitis affects 4 out of 10,000 people and chronic pancreatitis affects 2 out of 10,000 people. Men are affected more than women.

Causes
The most common causes of pancreatitis are biliary tract disease and alcoholism, but it can also result from pancreatic cancer, trauma, or use of certain drugs, such as glucocorticoids, sulfonamides, chlorothiazide, and azathioprine. This disease also may develop as a complication of peptic ulcer, mumps, or hypothermia. Rarer causes are stenosis or obstruction of the sphincter of Oddi, hyperlipidemia, metabolic endocrine disorders (hyperparathyroidism and hemochromatosis), vasculitis or vascular disease, viral infections, mycoplasmal pneumonia, pregnancy, trauma, and pancreatic tumor.

Diabetes, pancreatic insufficiency, and calcification occur in young people, probably from malnutrition and alcoholism, and lead to pancreatic atrophy. Regardless of the cause, pancreatitis involves autodigestion: The enzymes normally excreted by the pancreas digest pancreatic tissue. (See *Anatomy of the pancreas,* page 431.)

Clinical presentation
In many patients, the first and only symptom of mild pancreatitis is steady epigastric pain centered close to the umbilicus, radiating between the tenth thoracic and sixth lumbar vertebrae, and unrelieved by vomiting. However, a severe attack causes these signs and symptoms:
■ extreme pain
■ persistent vomiting
■ abdominal rigidity
■ diminished bowel activity (suggesting peritonitis)
■ crackles at lung bases

Chronic pancreatitis

Chronic pancreatitis is usually associated with alcoholism (in over half of all patients) but can also follow hyperparathyroidism (causing hypercalcemia), hyperlipidemia or, infrequently, gallstones, trauma, or peptic ulcer. Inflammation and fibrosis cause progressive pancreatic insufficiency and eventually destroy the pancreas. Symptoms of chronic pancreatitis include constant dull pain with occasional exacerbations, malabsorption, severe weight loss, and hyperglycemia (leading to diabetic symptoms). Diagnosis is based on the patient history, X-rays showing pancreatic calcification, elevated erythrocyte sedimentation rate, and examination of stool for steatorrhea.

Treatment also includes administration of analgesics; a low-fat diet; and oral administration of pancreatic enzymes, such as pancreatin or pancrelipase to control steatorrhea; insulin or oral hypoglycemics to curb hyperglycemia and, occasionally, surgical repair of biliary or pancreatic ducts or the sphincter of Oddi to reduce pressure and promote the flow of pancreatic juice. Prognosis is good if the patient can avoid alcohol; poor if he can't.

- left pleural effusion
- extreme malaise and restlessness
- mottled skin
- tachycardia
- low-grade fever (100° to 102° F [37.8° to 38.9° C])
- cold and sweaty extremities.

Fulminant pancreatitis causes massive hemorrhage and total destruction of the pancreas, resulting in diabetic acidosis, shock, or coma.

Differential diagnoses
- Perforated ulcer disease
- Acute cholecystitis
- Appendicitis
- Bowel infarction
- Bowel obstruction

Diagnosis
A thorough patient history (especially for alcoholism) and physical examination are the first steps in diagnosis, but the retroperitoneal position of the pancreas makes physical assessment difficult.

Dramatically elevated serum amylase levels — in many cases over 500 U/L — confirm pancreatitis. Similarly dramatic elevations of amylase also occur in urine, ascites, or pleural fluid. Characteristically, amylase levels return to normal 48 hours after the onset of pancreatitis, despite continuing symptoms.

Supportive laboratory values include:
- increased serum lipase levels, which increase more slowly than serum amylase
- low serum calcium levels (hypocalcemia) from fat necrosis and formation of calcium soaps
- white blood cell counts ranging from 8,000 to 20,000/µl, with increased polymorphonuclear leukocytes
- elevated glucose levels, as high as 500 to 900 mg/dl, indicating hyperglycemia.

Other tests used to diagnose pancreatitis may include:
- An electrocardiogram shows changes (prolonged QT segment but normal T wave) that help to diagnose hypocalcemia.
- Abdominal X-rays show dilation of the small or large bowel or calcification of the pancreas.

Anatomy of the pancreas

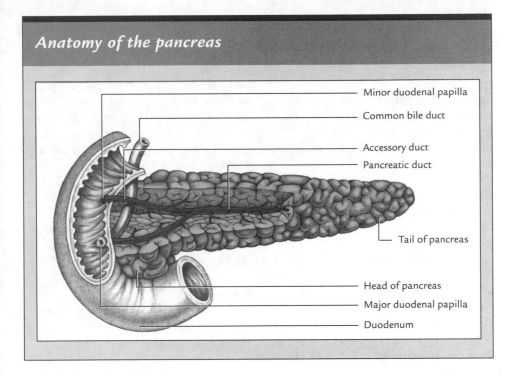

Minor duodenal papilla

Common bile duct

Accessory duct

Pancreatic duct

Tail of pancreas

Head of pancreas

Major duodenal papilla

Duodenum

■ A GI series indicates extrinsic pressure on the duodenum or stomach due to edema of the pancreas head.

■ Chest X-rays show left-sided pleural effusion.

■ An ultrasound or computed tomography scan reveals an increased pancreatic diameter and helps to distinguish acute cholecystitis from acute pancreatitis.

Management
General

The goal of therapy is to maintain circulation and fluid volume. Treatment measures must also relieve pain and decrease pancreatic secretions.

Emergency treatment of shock (which is the most common cause of death in early-stage pancreatitis) consists of vigorous I.V. replacement of electrolytes and proteins. Metabolic acidosis that develops secondary to hypovolemia

and impaired cellular perfusion requires vigorous fluid volume replacement.

After the emergency phase, continuing I.V. therapy for 5 to 7 days should provide adequate electrolytes and protein solutions that don't stimulate the pancreas. If the patient isn't ready to resume oral feedings by then, total parenteral nutrition may be necessary. Nonstimulating elemental gavage feedings may be safer because of the decreased risk of infection and overinfusion.

Medication

Medications used in the treatment of a patient with pancreatitis may include:

■ meperidine — 50 to 100 mg I.M. every 3 to 4 hours for acute pancreatitis

■ diazepam — 2 to 10 mg P.O. b.i.d. to t.i.d.

■ antibiotics — appropriate to cause

■ calcium gluconate — for low calcium levels

- insulin therapy—for elevated glucose levels.
- octreotide—50 to 200 mg S.C. every 8 hours

Surgical intervention
In extreme cases, laparotomy to debride the pancreatic bed, partial pancreatectomy, or a combination of both and feeding jejunostomy may be necessary.

Referral
- The patient may need referral to a surgeon.
- If the patient develops diabetes as a result of this illness, a referral to a diabetes educator may be appropriate.
- If the cause of pancreatitis is alcohol related, refer the patient to Alcoholics Anonymous.

Patient teaching
- Educate the patient and family members about pancreatitis, specifying the suspected cause and the outcomes.
- Encourage the patient to stop ingesting alcohol, if this is the cause of illness.

Complications
- Pseudocyst
- Diabetes mellitus
- Adult respiratory distress syndrome
- Sepsis
- Death

• • • • • • • • • • • •

PEPTIC ULCERS

Peptic ulcers—circumscribed lesions in the mucosal membrane—can develop in the lower esophagus, stomach, pylorus, duodenum, or jejunum. About 80% of all peptic ulcers are duodenal ulcers, which affect the proximal part of the small intestine.

Gastric ulcers, which affect the stomach mucosa, are most common in middle-aged and elderly men, especially in chronic users of nonsteroidal anti-inflammatory drugs (NSAIDs), alcohol, or tobacco. Gastric ulcers occur in 8 out of 10,000 people. They affect both men and women and occur more frequently in people over age 50. Duodenal ulcers occur in 7 out of 1,000 people. They occur more frequently in men over age 30.

Duodenal ulcers usually follow a chronic course, with remissions and exacerbations; 5% to 10% of patients develop complications that necessitate surgery.

Causes
Researchers recognize three major causes of peptic ulcer disease: infection with *Helicobacter pylori* (formerly known as *Campylobacter pylori*), use of NSAIDs, and pathologic hypersecretory disorders such as Zollinger-Ellison syndrome. (See *How peptic ulcers develop.*)

How *H. pylori* produce an ulcer isn't clear. Gastric acid, which was considered a primary cause, now appears mainly to contribute to the consequences of infection. Ongoing studies may soon unveil the full mechanism of ulcer formation.

Salicylates and other NSAIDs encourage ulcer formation by inhibiting the secretion of prostaglandins (the substances that suppress ulceration). Certain illnesses, such as pancreatitis, hepatic disease, Crohn's disease, preexisting gastritis, and Zollinger-Ellison syndrome, are also known causes.

Predisposing factors include:
- blood type (gastric ulcers tend to strike people with type A blood; duodenal ulcers tend to afflict people with type O blood) and other genetic factors
- exposure to irritants, such as alcohol, coffee, and tobacco; may contribute by

How peptic ulcers develop

Peptic ulcers can result from factors that increase gastric acid production or impair mucosal barrier protection.

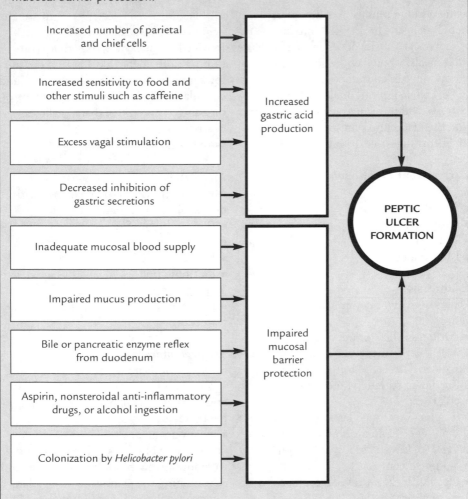

accelerating gastric acid emptying and promoting mucosal breakdown. Ulceration occurs when the acid secretion exceeds the buffering factors.

Physical trauma, emotional stress, and normal aging are additional predisposing conditions.

Clinical presentation

Heartburn and indigestion usually signal the beginning of a gastric ulcer attack. Eating stretches the gastric wall and may cause or, in some cases, relieve pain and feelings of fullness and distention. Other typical effects include weight loss and repeated episodes of massive GI bleeding.

Duodenal ulcers produce:
- pyrosis
- well-localized midepigastric pain (relieved by food)
- weight gain (because the patient eats to relieve discomfort)
- the peculiar sensation of hot water bubbling in the back of the throat.

Attacks usually occur about 2 hours after meals, whenever the stomach is empty, or after consumption of orange juice, coffee, aspirin, or alcohol. Exacerbations tend to recur several times a year and then fade into remission. Vomiting and other digestive disturbances are rare.

Differential diagnoses
- Gastritis
- *H. pylori* infection
- Crohn's disease
- Pancreatitis
- Malignancy

Diagnosis
Diagnosis may be confirmed by these tests:
- Barium swallow or upper GI and small-bowel series may reveal the presence of the ulcer. This is the initial test performed on a patient whose symptoms aren't severe.
- Esophagogastroduodenoscopy confirms the presence of an ulcer and permits cytologic studies and biopsy to rule out *H. pylori* or cancer.
- Upper GI tract X-rays reveal mucosal abnormalities.
- Laboratory analysis may disclose occult blood in stools.
- Serologic testing may disclose clinical signs of infection such as elevated white blood cell count.
- Gastric secretory studies show hyperchlorhydria.
- Carbon 13 urea breath test results reflect activity of *H. pylori*.

Management
General
Experts recommend treating every ulcer patient at least once to eradicate *H. pylori* because the infection can occur even with other causes, such as NSAID use. If GI bleeding occurs, emergency treatment begins with passage of an NG tube to allow iced saline lavage, sometimes containing norepinephrine. Gastroscopy allows visualization of the bleeding site and coagulation by laser or cautery to control bleeding. This type of therapy allows postponement of surgery until the patient's condition stabilizes.

Medication
Medications used to treat patients with peptic ulcers may include:
- tetracycline — 500 mg P.O. q.i.d. for 14 days
- bismuth — 525 mg P.O. q.i.d.
- metronidazole — 500 mg P.O. q.i.d. for 14 days
- famotidine — 40 mg P.O. h.s. for 4 to 8 weeks.

Surgical intervention
Surgery is indicated for perforation, unresponsiveness to conservative treatment, and suspected malignancy. Surgery for peptic ulcers may include:
- vagotomy and pyloroplasty — severing one or more branches of the vagus nerve to reduce hydrochloric acid secretion and refashioning the pylorus to create a larger lumen and facilitate gastric emptying
- distal subtotal gastrectomy (with or without vagotomy) — excising the antrum of the stomach, thereby removing the hormonal stimulus of the parietal cells, followed by anastomosis of the rest of the stomach to the duodenum or the jejunum
- pyloroplasty — surgical enlargement of the pylorus to provide drainage of gastric secretions.

Referral

- If symptoms persist, refer the patient to a gastroenterologist.
- The patient may need referral to a surgeon.
- If bleeding is suspected, refer the patient to the hospital for immediate treatment.

Follow-up

The patient should be seen 2 to 3 days after treatment is initiated and again in 2 weeks.

Patient teaching

- Advise any patient who uses antacids, has a history of cardiac disease, or follows a sodium-restricted diet to take only those antacids that contain small amounts of sodium.
- Warn the patient to avoid taking aspirin, steroids, and NSAIDs, because they irritate the gastric mucosa. For the same reason, advise the patient to stop smoking and avoid stressful situations, excessive intake of coffee, and ingestion of alcoholic beverages during exacerbations of peptic ulcer disease.
- Tell the patient taking bismuth subsalicylate that this drug may cause constipation.
- To avoid dumping syndrome, advise the patient to lie down after meals, drink fluids between meals rather than with meals, avoid eating large amounts of carbohydrates, and eat four to six small, high-protein, low-carbohydrate meals during the day.

Complications

- Hemorrhage
- Perforation
- Gastric outlet obstruction
- Pernicious anemia
- Dumping syndrome
- Iron or folate deficiency

• • • • • • • • • • • •
PERITONITIS

Peritonitis is an acute or a chronic inflammation of the peritoneum, the membrane that lines the abdominal cavity and covers the visceral organs. Inflammation may extend throughout the peritoneum or may be localized as an abscess. Peritonitis commonly decreases intestinal motility and causes intestinal distention with gas. Mortality is 10%, with death usually a result of bowel obstruction; the mortality rate was much higher before the introduction of antibiotics. There are two cases per 1 million people per year.

Causes

Although the GI tract normally contains bacteria, the peritoneum is sterile. When bacteria invade the peritoneum because of an inflammation and a perforation of the GI tract, peritonitis results. Bacterial invasion of the peritoneum typically results from appendicitis, diverticulitis, peptic ulcer, ulcerative colitis, volvulus, strangulated obstruction, abdominal neoplasm, or a stab wound. Peritonitis can also occur following chemical inflammation, as in the rupture of a fallopian or ovarian tube or the bladder, perforation of a gastric ulcer, or released pancreatic enzymes.

In chemical and bacterial inflammations, accumulated fluids containing protein and electrolytes make the transparent peritoneum opaque, red, inflamed, and edematous. Because the peritoneal cavity is so resistant to contamination, infection is commonly localized as an abscess instead of disseminated as a generalized infection.

Clinical presentation

The key symptom of peritonitis is sudden, severe, and diffuse abdominal pain that tends to intensify and localize in the area of the underlying disorder. For instance, if appendicitis causes the rupture, pain eventually localizes in the right lower quadrant. Many patients display weakness, pallor, excessive sweating, and cold skin as a result of excessive loss of fluid, electrolytes, and protein into the abdominal cavity. Decreased intestinal motility and paralytic ileus result from the effect of bacterial toxins on the intestinal muscles. Intestinal obstruction causes nausea, vomiting, and abdominal rigidity.

Other clinical characteristics include:
- hypotension
- tachycardia
- dehydration
- acutely tender abdomen associated with rebound tenderness
- temperature of 103° F (39.4° C) or higher
- hypokalemia.

An inflammation of the diaphragmatic peritoneum may cause shoulder pain and hiccups. Abdominal distention and resulting upward displacement of the diaphragm can decrease respiratory capacity. Typically, the patient with peritonitis tends to breathe shallowly and move as little as possible to minimize pain. He may lie on his back, with knees flexed, to relax abdominal muscles.

Differential diagnoses
- Appendicitis
- Pancreatitis
- Abscess
- Ileus

Diagnosis
Abdominal X-rays showing edematous and gaseous distention of the small and large bowel support the diagnosis. In the case of perforation of a visceral organ, the X-ray shows air lying under the diaphragm in the abdominal cavity. Other appropriate tests include:

- Chest X-ray may show elevation of the diaphragm.
- Blood studies show leukocytosis (greater than 20,000/µl).
- Paracentesis reveals bacteria, exudate, blood, pus, or urine.

Laparotomy may be necessary to identify the underlying cause.

Management
General
Early treatment of GI inflammatory conditions and preoperative and postoperative antibiotic therapy help to prevent peritonitis. After peritonitis develops, emergency treatment must combat infection, restore intestinal motility, and replace fluids and electrolytes. To decrease peristalsis and prevent perforation, the patient should receive nothing by mouth; he should receive supportive fluids and electrolytes parenterally. An NG tube may be inserted to decompress the bowel and, possibly, a rectal tube may be inserted to facilitate passage of flatus.

Medication
Antibiotic therapy may be used; examples include:
- cefotaxime — 2 to 12 g/day I.V. in divided doses
- ampicillin — 1 to 2 g I.V. every 6 hours; plus gentamicin — 1.5 mg/kg/dose; plus clindamycin — 600 to 900 mg I.V. every 8 hours.

An analgesia, such as morphine (2 to 4 mg I.V. or I.M. every 2 to 4 hours p.r.n.), may be given.

Surgical intervention
When peritonitis results from perforation, surgery is necessary as soon as possible. The goal of surgery is to eliminate the source of infection by evacuating the spilled contents and inserting drains.

Referral
- Refer the patient to the hospital for treatment.
- Refer the patient to a surgeon.

Follow-up
The patient should be seen posthospitalization within 1 to 2 weeks.

Patient teaching
- Encourage ambulation and coughing and deep breathing.
- Teach the patient about the signs of infection and instruct him to report them immediately.

Complications
- Sepsis
- Acute renal failure
- Abscess
- Hypovolemia

• • • • • • • • • • • •
PILONIDAL DISEASE

In pilonidal disease, a coccygeal cyst forms in the intergluteal cleft on the posterior surface of the lower sacrum. It usually contains hair and becomes infected, producing an abscess, a draining sinus, or a fistula. Incidence is 2.2 times higher in men than in women, occurring between puberty and age 40. It's more common in obese people as well as those with thick body hair. There are 26 cases per 100,000 people in the United States.

Causes
Pilonidal disease may develop congenitally from a tendency to hirsutism, or be acquired from stretching or irritation of the sacrococcygeal area (intergluteal fold) from prolonged rough exercise (such as horseback riding), heat, excessive perspiration, or constricting clothing.

Clinical presentation
Generally, a pilonidal cyst produces no symptoms until it becomes infected, causing local pain, tenderness, swelling, or heat. Other clinical features include continuous or intermittent purulent drainage, followed by development of an abscess, chills, fever, headache, and malaise.

Differential diagnoses
- Malignancy
- Anorectal fistula

Diagnosis
Physical examination confirms the diagnosis and may reveal a series of openings along the midline, with thin, brown, foul-smelling drainage or a protruding tuft of hair. Pressure on the sinus tract may produce a purulent drainage. Passing a probe back through the sinus tract toward the sacrum shouldn't reveal a perforation between the anterior sinus and anal canal. Cultures of discharge from the infected sinus may show staphylococci or skin bacteria but don't usually contain bowel bacteria.

Management
General
Conservative treatment of pilonidal disease consists of incision and drainage of abscesses, regular extraction of protruding hairs, and sitz baths (four to six times daily).

Medication
Ibuprofen (300 to 800 mg P.O. q.i.d.) may be given.

Surgical intervention
Persistent infections may necessitate surgical excision of the entire affected area.

Follow-up

After excision of a pilonidal abscess, the patient requires regular follow-up care to monitor wound healing. The surgeon may periodically palpate the wound during healing with a cotton-tipped applicator, curette excess granulation tissue, and extract loose hairs to promote wound healing from the inside out and to prevent dead cells from collecting in the wound. Complete healing may take several months.

Patient teaching

■ After surgery, tell the patient to report excessive bleeding.
■ Encourage the patient to walk as soon as possible after the procedure.
■ Tell the patient to place a gauze pad over the wound site after the dressing is removed to allow ventilation and prevent friction from clothing. Advise him to continue the use of sitz baths and to let the area air-dry instead of rubbing or patting it dry with a towel.
■ After healing, the patient should briskly wash the area daily with a washcloth to remove loose hairs.
■ Encourage obese patients to lose weight.

Complications

■ Anorectal fistula
■ Sepsis

• • • • • • • • • • • •

PROCTITIS

Proctitis is an acute or a chronic inflammation of the rectal mucosa. The prognosis is good unless massive bleeding occurs.

Causes

Contributing factors include chronic constipation, habitual laxative use, emotional upset, radiation (especially for cancer of the cervix and of the uterus), endocrine dysfunction, rectal injury, rectal medications, bacterial infections, allergies (especially to milk), vasomotor disturbance that interferes with normal muscle control, and food poisoning. This condition occurs with high frequency among homosexual men and women who engage in anal intercourse. Sexually transmitted diseases, such as gonorrhea and chlamydia, are also related to proctitis.

Clinical presentation

Key symptoms include:
■ tenesmus
■ constipation
■ feeling of rectal fullness
■ abdominal cramps on the left side
■ intense urge to defecate, which produces a small amount of stool that may contain blood and mucus.

Differential diagnoses

■ Ulcerative colitis
■ Crohn's disease
■ Infection
■ Malignancy

Diagnosis

A detailed patient history is essential. In acute proctitis, sigmoidoscopy shows edematous, bright red or pink rectal mucosa that is thick, shiny, friable and, possibly, ulcerated. In chronic proctitis, sigmoidoscopy shows thickened mucosa, loss of vascular pattern, and stricture of the rectal lumen. Other supportive tests include biopsy to rule out cancer and a bacteriologic examination.

Management
General
Primary treatment eliminates the underlying cause (fecal impaction, laxatives, or other medications). Soothing enemas or steroid (hydrocortisone) suppositories or enemas may be helpful if proctitis is due to radiation.

Medication
Depending on the cause, medication may include:
- mesalamine — topically, 4 g enema daily, or 800 mg P.O. t.i.d. for ulcerative proctitis
- ceftriaxone — 250 mg I.M. once; plus doxycycline — 100 mg P.O. b.i.d. for gonorrheal proctitis
- acyclovir — 200 mg P.O. five times per day for 10 days for herpetic proctitis
- tetracycline — 500 mg P.O. q.i.d. for chlamydial proctitis.

Referral
- Refer the patient to a gastroenterologist if treatment is unsuccessful.

Follow-up
The patient should be seen after 1 and 2 weeks, and then monthly for 6 months.

Patient teaching
- Tell the patient to watch for and report bleeding and other persistent symptoms.
- Fully explain proctitis and the treatment to help the patient understand the disorder and prevent its recurrence.

Complications
- Fistula
- Abscess
- Ulcerative colitis
- Perforation

PRURITUS ANI

Pruritus ani is perianal itching, irritation, or superficial burning. This disorder is more common in men than in women and is rare in children. Prognosis is good with use of medication or removal of the source.

Causes
Factors that contribute to pruritus ani include overcleaning of the perianal area (harsh soap, vigorous rubbing with washcloth or toilet paper); minor trauma caused by straining to defecate; poor hygiene; sensitivity to spicy foods, coffee, alcohol, food preservatives, perfumed or colored toilet paper, detergents, or certain fabrics; specific medications (antibiotics, antihypertensives, or antacids that cause diarrhea); excessive sweating (in occupations associated with physical labor or high stress levels); anal skin tags; systemic disease, especially diabetes; certain skin lesions, such as those associated with squamous cell carcinoma, basal cell carcinoma, Bowen's disease, Paget's disease, melanoma, syphilis, and tuberculosis; fungal or parasitic infection; and local anorectal disease (fissure, hemorrhoids, and fistula).

Clinical presentation
The key symptom of pruritus ani is perianal itching or burning after a bowel movement, during stress, or at night. In acute pruritus ani, scratching produces reddened skin, with weeping excoriations; in chronic pruritus ani, skin becomes thick and leathery, with excessive pigmentation.

Differential diagnoses
- Anorectal fissure or fistula
- Infection

- Allergies
- Dermatitis
- Diabetes mellitus
- Neoplasia

Diagnosis

A detailed patient history is essential. Allergy testing or biopsy may also be helpful.

Management

General

After elimination of the underlying cause, treatment is symptomatic.

Medication

Medication may include:
- clotrimazole with hydrocortisone 1% cream — apply to anal area b.i.d.
- vaseline — apply to anal area p.r.n.

Referral

- The patient may need referral to a gastroenterologist, if treatment fails.

Follow-up

The patient should be seen within 2 weeks following initiation of treatment, and then as needed.

Patient teaching

- Advise the patient to avoid self-prescribed creams or powders, perfumed soaps, and colored toilet paper because they may be irritating.
- Teach him to keep the perianal area clean and dry. Suggest witch hazel pads for wiping and cotton balls tucked between buttocks to absorb moisture.

Complications

- Excoriation
- Infection

• • • • • • • • • • • •

PSEUDOMEMBRANOUS ENTEROCOLITIS

Pseudomembranous enterocolitis is an acute inflammation and necrosis of the small and large intestines. It usually affects the mucosa but may extend into submucosa and, rarely, other layers. The incidence is 1 out of 1,000 people.

Causes

Pseudomembranous enterocolitis is thought to be caused by a change in the flora of the colon and an overgrowth of a toxin-producing strain of *Clostridium difficile*.

Pseudomembranous enterocolitis has occurred postoperatively in debilitated patients who undergo abdominal surgery or patients who have been treated with broad-spectrum antibiotics. Ampicillin, clindamycin, and cephalosporins are suspected causative factors. Immunocompromised patients (such as individuals with cystic fibrosis, neurologic disease, liver and renal disease, diabetes mellitus, malnutrition, and hematologic disorders) are at increased risk for this disease. Whatever the cause, necrosed mucosa is replaced by a pseudomembrane filled with staphylococci, leucocytes, mucus, fibrin, and inflammatory cells.

Clinical presentation

Pseudomembranous enterocolitis begins suddenly with copious watery diarrhea, abdominal pain, and fever. Diarrhea, with or without blood, and abdominal pain may occur within 48 hours after administration of a causative drug. Signs and symptoms may begin with mild to moderate watery diarrhea with lower abdominal cramping. As the disease progresses, the patient may have profuse watery diarrhea, with up to 30 stools per day, and abdominal pain. Low-grade fever, along with abdominal tenderness and leukocytosis, occurs. In a small number of patients, colitis develops with bradycardia, fever, abdominal pain, and distention.

Differential diagnoses
- Inflammatory bowel disease
- Enteric infection

Diagnosis
In this disorder, diagnosis is often difficult because of the abrupt onset of enterocolitis and the emergency situation it creates, so consideration of patient history is essential. A rectal biopsy through sigmoidoscopy confirms pseudomembranous enterocolitis. Stool cultures can identify C. *difficile*.

Management
General
A patient receiving broad-spectrum antibiotic therapy requires immediate discontinuation of the antibiotics. If possible, medications that slow peristalsis should be avoided. Supportive treatment must maintain fluid and electrolyte balance and combat hypotension.

Medication
Metronidazole (250 mg P.O. every 6 hours) may be given.

Referral
- Refer the patient to a physician for severe cases.

Follow-up
The patient should be seen every week until symptoms resolve.

Patient teaching
- Tell the patient to continue to drink fluids; encourage the use of commercial electrolyte solutions.
- Encourage good hygiene to prevent excoriation.

Complications
- Dehydration
- Hypovolemia
- Shock
- Bowel perforation
- Hypoalbuminemia
- Death

Special considerations
- Make sure to monitor the patient for signs of shock, especially if he's elderly.

• • • • • • • • • • • •

RECTAL PROLAPSE

Rectal prolapse is the circumferential protrusion of one or more layers of the mucous membrane through the anus. Prolapse may be complete (with displacement of the anal sphincter or bowel herniation) or partial (mucosal layer). (See *Types of rectal prolapse*, page 442.)

Rectal prolapse usually occurs in men under age 40, in women around age 45 (three times more often than in men), and in children ages 1 to 3 (especially those with cystic fibrosis). Prognosis is good with treatment.

Causes
Predisposing factors for rectal prolapse include:
- increased intra-abdominal pressure, especially from straining during defecation
- conditions that affect the pelvic floor or rectum, such as weak sphincters
- weak longitudinal, rectal, or levator ani muscles caused by neurologic disorders, injury, tumors, aging, and chronic wasting diseases, such as tuberculosis, cystic fibrosis, or whooping cough
- nutritional disorders.

Types of rectal prolapse

Partial rectal prolapse involves only the rectal mucosa and a small mass of radial mucosal folds. In complete rectal prolapse (also known as procidentia), the full rectal wall, sphincter muscle, and a large mass of concentric mucosal folds protrude. Ulceration is possible after complete prolapse.

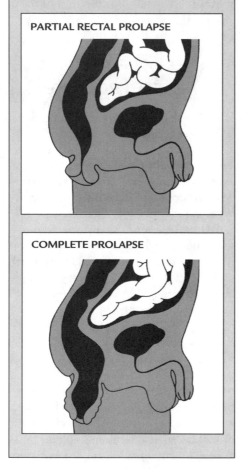

PARTIAL RECTAL PROLAPSE

COMPLETE PROLAPSE

Clinical presentation

In rectal prolapse, protrusion of tissue from the rectum may occur during defecation or walking. Hemorrhoids or rectal polyps may coexist with a prolapse. Other signs and symptoms include:

- persistent sensation of rectal fullness
- bloody diarrhea
- pain in the lower abdomen.

Differential diagnoses

- Rectal polyps
- Hemorrhoids
- Intussusception
- Tumor

Diagnosis

Typical clinical features and visual examination confirm the diagnosis. In complete prolapse, examination reveals the full thickness of the bowel wall and, possibly, the sphincter muscle protruding and mucosa falling into bulky, concentric folds. In partial prolapse, examination reveals only partially protruding mucosa and a smaller mass of radial mucosal folds. Straining during examination may disclose the full extent of the prolapse.

Management

General

In some cases, eliminating the underlying cause (straining, coughing, and nutritional disorders) is the only treatment necessary. In a child, prolapsed tissue usually diminishes as the child grows. In an older patient, injection of a sclerosing agent to cause a fibrotic reaction fixes the rectum in place.

Surgical intervention

Severe or chronic prolapse requires surgical repair by strengthening or tightening the sphincters with wire or by anterior or rectal resection of prolapsed tissue.

Referral

- The patient may need referral to a surgeon.

Follow-up

The patient should be seen monthly unless surgery has been done or the prolapse is resolved.

Patient teaching

■ Educate the patient about underlying causes and preoperative and postoperative support.
■ Help the patient to prevent constipation by teaching him the correct diet and stool-softening regimen. Advise the patient with severe prolapse and incontinence to wear a perineal pad.
■ Teach perineal strengthening exercises: Have the patient lie down, with his back flat on the mattress; then ask him to pull in his abdomen and squeeze while taking a deep breath; or have the patient repeatedly squeeze and relax his buttocks while sitting on a chair.

Complications

■ Necrosis
■ Stricture
■ Mucosal ulceration
■ Intestinal obstruction
■ Fecal impaction
■ Hemorrhage
■ Pelvic abscess
■ Rectal stenosis

• • • • • • • • • • • •

STOMATITIS AND OTHER ORAL INFECTIONS

Stomatitis is an inflammation of the oral mucosa that may extend to the buccal mucosa, lips, and palate. It's a common infection that may occur alone or as part of a systemic disease. There are two main types: acute herpetic stomatitis and aphthous stomatitis. Acute herpetic stomatitis is usually self-limiting; however, it may be severe and, in neonates, may be generalized and potentially fatal. Aphthous stomatitis usually heals spontaneously, without a scar, in 10 to 14 days. Other oral infections include gingivitis, periodontitis, and Vincent's angina. (See *Types of oral infections*, page 444.)

Causes

Acute herpetic stomatitis results from the herpes simplex virus. It's common in children ages 1 to 3. The cause of aphthous stomatitis is unknown, but predisposing factors include stress, fatigue, anxiety, febrile states, trauma, and solar overexposure. This type is common in girls and female adolescents.

Clinical presentation

Acute herpetic stomatitis begins suddenly with these signs and symptoms:
■ mouth pain
■ malaise
■ lethargy
■ anorexia
■ irritability
■ fever
■ swollen gums that bleed easily
■ extremely tender oral mucous membrane.

Papulovesicular ulcers appear in the mouth and throat and eventually become punched-out lesions with reddened areolae. Submaxillary lymphadenitis is common. Pain usually disappears from 2 to 4 days before healing of ulcers is complete. If the child with stomatitis sucks his thumb, these lesions spread to the hand.

A patient with aphthous stomatitis typically reports burning, tingling, and slight swelling of the mucous membrane. Single or multiple shallow ulcers with whitish centers and red borders appear and heal at one site and then reappear at another. (See *Examining aphthous stomatitis*, page 445.)

Types of oral infections

DISEASE AND CAUSES	SIGNS AND SYMPTOMS	TREATMENT
Gingivitis (inflammation of the gingiva) ■ Early sign of hypovitaminosis, diabetes, and blood dyscrasias ■ Occasionally related to use of oral contraceptives	■ Inflammation with painless swelling, redness, change of normal contours, bleeding, and periodontal pocket (gum detachment from teeth)	■ Removal of irritating factors (calculus and faulty dentures) ■ Good oral hygiene; regular dental checkups; and vigorous chewing ■ Oral or topical corticosteroids
Periodontitis (progression of gingivitis; inflammation of the oral mucosa) ■ Early sign of hypovitaminosis, diabetes, and blood dyscrasias ■ Occasionally related to use of oral contraceptives ■ Dental factors: calculus, poor oral hygiene, malocclusion; major cause of tooth loss after middle age	■ Acute onset of bright red gum inflammation, painless swelling of interdental papillae, easy bleeding ■ Loosening of teeth, typically without inflammatory symptoms, progressing to loss of teeth and alveolar bone ■ Acute systemic infection (fever and chills)	■ Scaling, root planing, and curettage for infection control ■ Periodontal surgery to prevent recurrence ■ Good oral hygiene, regular dental checkups, vigorous chewing
Vincent's angina (trench mouth and necrotizing ulcerative gingivitis) ■ Fusiform bacillus or spirochete infection ■ Predisposing factors: stress, poor oral hygiene, insufficient rest, nutritional deficiency, and smoking	■ Sudden onset: painful, superficial bleeding gingival ulcers (rarely, on buccal mucosa) covered with a graywhite membrane ■ Ulcers become punchedout lesions after slight pressure or irritation ■ Malaise, mild fever, excessive salivation, bad breath, pain on swallowing or talking, enlarged submaxillary lymph nodes	■ Removal of devitalized tissue with ultrasonic cavitron ■ Antibiotics for infection ■ Analgesics as needed ■ Hourly mouth rinses (with equal amounts of hydrogen peroxide and warm water) ■ Soft, nonirritating diet; rest; and no smoking ■ With treatment, improvement common within 24 hours
Glossitis (inflammation of the tongue) ■ Streptococcal infection ■ Irritation or injury; jagged teeth; ill-fitting dentures; biting during convulsions; alcohol; spicy foods; smoking ■ Vitamin B deficiency and anemia ■ Skin conditions: lichen planus, erythema multiforme, and pemphigus vulgaris	■ Reddened ulcerated or swollen tongue (may obstruct airway) ■ Painful chewing and swallowing ■ Speech difficulty ■ Painful tongue without inflammation	■ Treatment of underlying cause ■ Topical anesthetic mouthwash or systemic analgesics (aspirin and acetaminophen) for painful lesions ■ Good oral hygiene; regular dental checkups; and vigorous chewing ■ Avoidance of hot, cold, or spicy foods and alcohol

Differential diagnoses
- Squamous cell carcinoma
- Hand-foot-and-mouth disease
- Stevens-Johnson syndrome

Diagnosis
Diagnosis is based on the physical examination. In Vincent's angina, a smear of ulcer exudate allows identification of the causative organism. If herpes stomatitis is suspected, a Tzanck test should be done.

Management
General
For acute herpetic stomatitis, treatment is conservative. For local symptoms, supportive measures include warm water mouth rinses (antiseptic mouthwashes are contraindicated because they're irritating) and a topical anesthetic to relieve mouth ulcer pain. Supplementary treatment includes bland or liquid diet and, in severe cases, I.V. fluids and bed rest.

For aphthous stomatitis, primary treatment is application of a topical anesthetic. Effective long-term treatment requires alleviation or prevention of precipitating factors.

Medication
The following medications may be used to treat stomatitis:
- lidocaine viscous 2% — applied to affected area
- sucralfate suspension — 1 tsp swished in the mouth q.i.d.

Referral
- If treatment is unsuccessful, refer the patient to a physician.

Follow-up
The patient should be seen within 2 to 3 weeks after treatment is initiated.

Examining aphthous stomatitis

In aphthous stomatitis, numerous small, round vesicles appear. They soon break and leave shallow ulcers with red areolae.

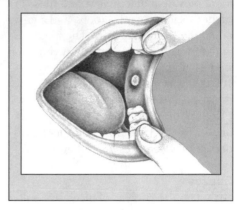

Patient teaching
- Review the causes for stomatitis and the treatment options.
- Recommend that the patient stop smoking, if appropriate.

Complications
- Intraoral scarring
- Oral stricture
- Death (gangrenous stomatitis)
- Ocular or central nervous system involvement (herpetic stomatitis)

• • • • • • • • • • • •

ULCERATIVE COLITIS

Ulcerative colitis is an inflammatory disease that affects the mucosa of the colon. It's chronic in many cases. It invariably begins in the rectum and sigmoid colon and commonly extends upward into the entire colon; it rarely affects the small intestine, except for the terminal ileum. Ulcerative colitis produces edema (leading to mucosal friability) and ulcerations. Severity ranges from a mild, localized disorder to a fulminant disease that may cause a perforated colon, progressing to potentially fatal peritonitis and toxemia.

Ulcerative colitis occurs mainly in young adults, especially women. It's also more prevalent among Jews and those in higher socioeconomic groups, and a familial tendency may exist. The incidence of the disease is unknown; however, some studies indicate as many as 100 out of 100,000 persons have the disease.

AGE ALERT Onset of symptoms of ulcerative colitis seems to peak between ages 15 and 20; another peak occurs between ages 55 and 60.

Causes

Although the etiology of ulcerative colitis is unknown, it's thought to be related to abnormal immune response in the GI tract, possibly associated with food or bacteria such as *Escherichia coli*. Stress was once thought to be a cause of ulcerative colitis, but studies show that, although it isn't a cause, it does increase the severity of the attack.

Clinical presentation

The hallmark of ulcerative colitis is recurrent attacks of bloody diarrhea, in many cases containing pus and mucus, interspersed with asymptomatic remissions. The intensity of these attacks varies with the extent of inflammation. A patient with ulcerative colitis is likely to have as many as 15 to 20 liquid, bloody stools daily. Other symptoms include spastic rectum and anus, abdominal pain, irritability, weight loss, weakness, anorexia, nausea, and vomiting.

Ulcerative colitis may lead to complications affecting many body systems, although it isn't known for certain why these complications outside the bowel

are linked to ulcerative colitis: Scientists think it may occur when the immune system triggers inflammation in other parts of the body. These disorders are usually mild and disappear when the colitis is treated.

Other clinical findings may include:
- blood — anemia from iron deficiency and coagulation defects due to vitamin K deficiency
- skin — erythema nodosum on the face and arms; pyoderma gangrenosum on the legs and ankles
- eye — uveitis
- liver — pericholangitis, sclerosing cholangitis, cirrhosis, and possible cholangiocarcinoma
- musculoskeletal — arthritis, ankylosing spondylitis, and loss of muscle mass
- GI — strictures, pseudopolyps, stenosis, and perforated colon, leading to peritonitis and toxemia.

Patients with ulcerative colitis have an increased risk of developing colorectal cancer, especially if onset of the disease occurs before age 15 or if it has persisted for longer than 10 years.

Differential diagnoses
- Hemorrhoids
- Neoplasm
- Crohn's disease
- Colonic diverticula
- Infection
- "Gay bowel" syndrome causes (herpes simplex, chlamydia trachomatis, cryptosporidium, and cytomegalovirus)

Diagnosis

Sigmoidoscopy showing increased mucosal friability, decreased mucosal detail, and thick inflammatory exudate suggests the diagnosis. Biopsy can help to confirm it.

Colonoscopy may be required to determine the extent of the disease and to evaluate areas of stricture and pseudopolyps. (Biopsy would be done during colonoscopy.) Barium enema can be used to assess the extent of the disease and detect complications, such as strictures and carcinoma.

A stool specimen should be cultured and analyzed for leukocytes, ova, and parasites. Other supportive laboratory values include decreased serum levels of potassium, magnesium, hemoglobin, and albumin as well as leukocytosis and an increased prothrombin time. Elevated erythrocyte sedimentation rate correlates with the severity of the attack.

Management
General
The goals of treatment are to control inflammation, replace nutritional losses and blood volume, and prevent complications. Supportive treatment includes bed rest, I.V. fluid replacement, and a clear-liquid diet. For patients awaiting surgery or showing signs of dehydration and debilitation from excessive diarrhea, parenteral alimentation rests the intestinal tract, decreases stool volume, and restores positive nitrogen balance. Blood transfusions or iron supplements may be needed to correct anemia.

Medication
Medications used to treat a patient with ulcerative colitis may include:
- sulfasalazine — 1 g P.O. every 6 to 8 hours
- prednisone — 40 to 60 mg/day P.O., gradually tapered over 2 months
- diphenoxylate — 5 mg P.O. q.i.d. initially, then p.r.n.; used only for patients with frequent, troublesome diarrheal stools whose ulcerative colitis is under control. This drug may precipitate massive dilation of the colon (toxic megacolon) and is generally contraindicated.

Surgical intervention
Surgery is the last resort and performed if the patient has toxic megacolon, fails to respond to drugs and supportive measures, or finds symptoms unbearable. A common surgical technique is proctocolectomy with ileostomy. Another procedure such as the ileoanal pull-through is becoming more common. This procedure entails performing a total proctocolectomy and mucosal stripping, creating a pouch from the terminal ileum, and anastomosing the pouch to the anal canal. A temporary ileostomy is created to divert stools and allow the rectal anastomosis to heal. The ileostomy is closed in 2 to 3 months, and the patient can then evacuate stools rectally. In this procedure, all potentially malignant epithelia of the rectum and colon are removed. Total colectomy and ileorectal anastomosis isn't common, because of its mortality rate (2% to 5%). This procedure is used to remove the entire colon and to anastomose the terminal ileum to the rectum; it requires observation of the remaining rectal stump for any signs of cancer or colitis.

Pouch ileostomy (Kock pouch or continent ileostomy), in which the surgeon creates a pouch from a small loop of the terminal ileum and a nipple valve from the distal ileum, may be an option. The resulting stoma opens just above the pubic hairline and the pouch is emptied periodically through a catheter inserted in the stoma. In ulcerative colitis, a colectomy may be performed after 10 years of active disease (because of the increased incidence of colon cancer in these patients). Performing a partial colectomy to prevent colon cancer is controversial.

Referral
- Refer the patient to a gastroenterologist for treatment.
- The patient may need to be referred to an enterostomal nurse for management after surgery.
- Refer the family to a local organization for education and support, such as the Crohn's & Colitis Foundation of America.

Follow-up
The patient should be seen according to the gastroenterologist's recommendation.

Patient teaching
- Teach the patient and family members about the disease process and possible outcomes of treatment.
- Tell the patient to follow a nutritionally balanced diet with an emphasis on fluid intake.
- Teach the patient about all medications and potential adverse effects.

Complications
- Perforation
- Colon cancer
- Toxic megacolon
- Liver disease
- Stricture

• • • • • • • • • • • •

SELECTED REFERENCES

Bickley, L.S., and Hoekelman, R.A. *Bate's Guide to Physical Examination and History Taking,* 7th ed. Philadelphia: Lippincott Williams & Wilkins, 1999.

Elkin, M.K., et al. *Nursing Interventions and Clinical Skills,* 2nd ed. St. Louis: Mosby–Year Book, Inc., 2000.

Fauci, A.S., et al., eds. *Harrison's Principles of Internal Medicine,* 15th ed. New York: McGraw-Hill Book Co., 2001.

Friedman, L.S., and Keeffe, E.B. *Handbook of Liver Disease.* Philadelphia: W.B. Saunders Co., 1998.

Handbook of Pathophysiology. Springhouse, Pa.: Springhouse Corp., 2001.

Ignatavicius, D., et al. *Medical-Surgical Nursing across the Health Care Continuum,* 3rd ed. Philadelphia: W.B. Saunders Co., 1999.

Kirsner, J.B., ed. *Inflammatory Bowel Disease,* 5th ed. Philadelphia: W.B. Saunders Co., 2000.

Lewis, A.M. "Gastrointestinal Emergency!" *Nursing99* 29(4):52-54, April 1999.

Nursing Procedures, 3rd ed. Springhouse, Pa.: Springhouse Corp., 2000.

Metabolic, endocrine, and nutritional disorders

M etabolic, endocrine, and nutritional disorders may affect a patient's growth and development, reproductive system, energy level, metabolic rate, or ability to adapt to stress. Many of these disorders, such as Cushing's syndrome or goiter, can cause disfigurement. Others, such as diabetes mellitus or obesity, may require extensive lifestyle changes.

• • • • • • • • • • • •

ASSESSMENT

To thoroughly assess the metabolic, endocrine, and nutritional status of your patient, you must take an accurate health history — including family history — and conduct a physical examination.

Physical examination
A physical examination should include a total body evaluation and a complete neurologic assessment. Begin by measuring the patient's vital signs, height, and weight. Then, to obtain the most objective findings, inspect, palpate, and auscultate the patient.

Inspection
Continue your physical assessment by systematically inspecting the patient's overall appearance and examining all areas of his body.

General appearance
Assess the patient's physical appearance and mental and emotional status. Note such factors as overall affect, speech, level of consciousness and orientation, appropriateness and neatness of dress and grooming, and activity level. Evaluate general body development, including posture, body build, body proportion, and distribution of body fat.

Skin, hair, and nails
Assess the patient's overall skin color, and inspect the skin and mucous membranes for lesions or areas of increased, decreased, or absent pigmentation. Con-

sider racial and ethnic variations. In a dark-skinned patient, color variations are best assessed in the sclera, conjunctiva, mouth, nail beds, and palms. Next, assess skin texture and hydration.

Inspect the patient's hair for amount, distribution, condition, and texture. Assess scalp and body hair, looking for abnormal patterns of growth or loss. Again, consider normal racial, ethnic, and sexual differences in hair growth and texture. Check the patient's fingernails for cracking, peeling, separation from the nail bed (onycholysis), and clubbing, and check the toenails for fungal infection, ingrown nails, discoloration, length, and thickness.

Head and neck

Assess the patient's face for overall color and presence of erythematous areas, especially in the cheeks. Note facial expression. Note the shape and symmetry of the eyes, and look for eyeball protrusion, incomplete eyelid closure, or periorbital edema. Have the patient extend his tongue, and inspect it for color, size, lesions, positioning, and tremors or unusual movements.

Standing in front of the patient, examine the neck — first with it held straight, then slightly extended, and finally while the patient swallows water. Check for neck symmetry and midline positioning and for symmetry of the trachea.

Chest

Evaluate the overall size, shape, and symmetry of the chest, noting any deformities. In females, assess the breasts for size, shape, symmetry, pigmentation (especially on the nipples and in skin creases), and nipple discharge (galactorrhea). In males, observe for bilateral or unilateral breast enlargement (gynecomastia) and nipple discharge.

Genitalia

Inspect the patient's external genitalia — particularly the testes and clitoris — for normal development.

Extremities

Inspect the patient's arms and hands for tremors. To do so, have him hold both arms outstretched in front with the palms down and fingers separated. Then place a sheet of paper on the outstretched fingers and watch for any trembling. Note any muscle wasting, especially in the upper arms, and have him grasp your hands to assess his grip.

Next, inspect the legs for muscle development, symmetry, color, and hair distribution. Then assess muscle strength by having the patient sit on the edge of the examination table and extend the legs horizontally. A patient who can maintain this position for 2 minutes usually exhibits normal strength. Examine the feet for size, and note any lesions, corns, calluses, or marks made from socks or shoes. Inspect the toes and the spaces between them for maceration and fissures.

Palpation

In many patients, you may not be able to palpate the thyroid gland. If you can, it should be smooth, finely lobulated, nontender, and either soft or firm. If palpable, you should be able to feel the gland's sections.

Use tangential lighting to aid visualization. An enlarged thyroid may be diffuse and asymmetrical. A thyroid nodule feels like a knot, a protuberance, or a swelling; a firm, fixed nodule may be a tumor. Be careful not to confuse thick neck musculature with an enlarged thyroid or a goiter. (See *Palpating the thyroid*.)

Palpating the thyroid

To palpate the thyroid from the front, stand in front of the patient and place your index and middle fingers below the cricoid cartilage on both sides of the trachea. Palpate for the thyroid isthmus as he swallows. Then ask the patient to flex his neck to the side being examined as you gently palpate each lobe. In most cases, you'll feel only the isthmus connecting the two lobes. However, if the patient has a thin neck, you may feel the whole gland. If he has a short, stocky neck, you may have trouble palpating even an enlarged thyroid.

To locate the right lobe, use your right hand to displace the thyroid cartilage slightly to your left. Hook your left index and middle fingers around the sternocleidomastoid muscle to palpate for thyroid enlargement. Then examine the left lobe, using your left hand to displace the thyroid cartilage and your right hand to palpate the lobe.

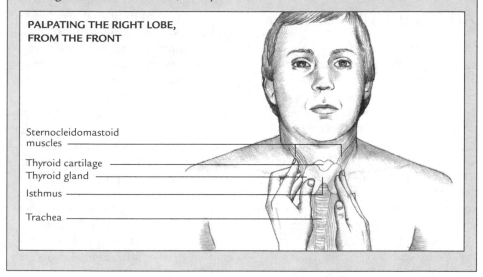

PALPATING THE RIGHT LOBE, FROM THE FRONT

Sternocleidomastoid muscles

Thyroid cartilage
Thyroid gland
Isthmus
Trachea

If you suspect that a patient has hypocalcemia (low serum calcium levels) related to deficient or ineffective parathyroid hormone secretion from hypoparathyroidism or surgical removal of the parathyroid glands, attempt to elicit Chvostek's sign and Trousseau's sign. To elicit Chvostek's sign, tap the facial nerve in front of the ear with a finger; if the facial muscles contract toward the ear, the test is positive for hypocalcemia. To elicit Trousseau's sign, place a blood pressure cuff on the arm and inflate it above the patient's systolic pressure. If the patient has a positive reaction, he'll exhibit carpal spasm (ventral contraction of the thumb and digits) within 3 minutes.

Milk the testes to the bottom of the scrotal sac for palpation. The testes should feel firm and smooth. The normal testis is about 2″ (5 cm) long.

Auscultation
If you palpate an enlarged thyroid, auscultate the gland for systolic bruits. Such bruits may indicate hyperthyroidism. To

auscultate for bruits, place the stethoscope's bell over one of the thyroid's lateral lobes; then listen for a low, soft, rushing sound. Have the patient hold his breath while you auscultate.

To distinguish a bruit from a venous hum, listen for the rushing sound; then gently occlude the jugular vein with your fingers on the side you're auscultating and listen again. A venous hum disappears during venous compression; a bruit doesn't.

• • • • • • • • • • •

ADRENAL HYPOFUNCTION

Primary adrenal hypofunction (also called adrenal insufficiency or Addison's disease) originates within the adrenal gland itself and is characterized by decreased mineralocorticoid, glucocorticoid, and androgen secretion. Adrenal hypofunction also can occur secondary to a disorder outside the gland (such as pituitary tumor, with corticotropin deficiency), but aldosterone secretion frequently continues intact. A relatively uncommon disorder, adrenal hypofunction can occur at any age and in both sexes. Secondary adrenal hypofunction occurs when a patient abruptly stops taking long-term exogenous steroid therapy. With early diagnosis and adequate replacement therapy, the prognosis for adrenal hypofunction is good.

CLINICAL CAUTION Adrenal crisis (addisonian crisis), a critical deficiency of mineralocorticoids and glucocorticoids, generally follows acute stress, sepsis, trauma, surgery, or omission of steroid therapy in patients who have chronic adrenal insufficiency. A medical emergency, adrenal crisis necessitates immediate, vigorous treatment.

Causes
Adrenal hypofunction occurs when more than 90% of both adrenal glands is destroyed, an occurrence that typically results from an autoimmune process in which circulating antibodies react specifically against the adrenal tissue. Other causes include tuberculosis (once the chief cause; now responsible for less than 10% of adult cases), bilateral adrenalectomy, hemorrhage into the adrenal gland, neoplasms, and infections (acquired immunodeficiency syndrome, histoplasmosis, cytomegalovirus). Rarely, a familial tendency to autoimmune disease predisposes the patient to adrenal hypofunction and other endocrinopathies.

Secondary adrenal hypofunction that results in glucocorticoid deficiency can stem from hypopituitarism (causing decreased corticotropin secretion), abrupt withdrawal of long-term corticosteroid therapy (long-term exogenous corticosteroid stimulation suppresses pituitary corticotropin secretion and results in adrenal gland atrophy), or removal of a nonendocrine, corticotropin-secreting tumor. Adrenal crisis follows when trauma, surgery, or other physiologic stress exhausts the body's stores of glucocorticoids in a person with adrenal hypofunction.

Clinical presentation
Adrenal hypofunction typically produces such effects as:
- weakness
- fatigue
- weight loss
- various GI disturbances.

When primary, the disorder usually causes a conspicuous bronze coloration of the skin. The patient appears to be deeply suntanned, especially in the creases of the hands and over the metacarpophalangeal joints, the elbows, and the knees. He also may exhibit a darkening of scars, areas of vitiligo, and increased pigmentation of the mucous membranes, especially the buccal mucosa. Abnormal skin and mucous membrane coloration results from decreased secretion of cortisol, which causes the pituitary gland to simultaneously secrete excessive amounts of corticotropin and melanocyte-stimulating hormone (MSH).

Associated cardiovascular abnormalities in adrenal hypofunction include orthostatic hypotension, decreased cardiac size and output, and a weak, irregular pulse. Other clinical effects include decreased tolerance for even minor stress, poor coordination, fasting hypoglycemia (due to decreased gluconeogenesis), and a craving for salty food. Adrenal hypofunction may also retard axillary and pubic hair growth in females, decrease the libido (from decreased androgen production) and, in severe cases, cause amenorrhea.

Secondary adrenal hypofunction produces similar clinical effects but without hyperpigmentation because corticotropin and MSH levels are low. Because aldosterone secretion may continue at fairly normal levels in secondary adrenal hypofunction, this condition doesn't necessarily cause accompanying hypotension and electrolyte abnormalities.

Adrenal crisis produces:
- profound weakness
- fatigue
- nausea
- vomiting
- hypotension
- dehydration
- high fever followed by hypothermia.

If untreated, adrenal crisis can ultimately lead to vascular collapse, renal shutdown, coma, and death.

Differential diagnoses
- Syndrome of inappropriate antidiuretic hormone
- Salt-losing nephritis
- Anorexia nervosa
- Hyperparathyroidism
- Heavy metal ingestion
- Secondary adrenocortical insufficiency: withdrawal of long-term corticosteroid use, surgical incision of pituitary gland, pituitary adenomas
- Tertiary adrenocortical insufficiency: trauma, hypothalamic tumor

Diagnosis
Diagnosis requires demonstration of decreased corticosteroid concentrations in plasma and an accurate classification of adrenal hypofunction as primary or secondary. If secondary adrenal hypofunction is suspected, the metyrapone test is indicated. This test requires oral or I.V. administration of metyrapone, which blocks cortisol production and should stimulate the release of corticotropin from the hypothalamic-pituitary system. In adrenal hypofunction, the hypothalamic-pituitary system responds normally, and plasma reveals high corticotropin levels; however, plasma levels of cortisol precursor and urinary concentrations of 17-hydroxycorticosteroids don't rise.

If either primary or secondary adrenal hypofunction is suspected, a short corticotropin stimulation test may be done. If adrenocorticotropic hormone and cortisol are low, the long corticotropin test may be done. This test involves I.V. corticotropin administration over 6 to 8 hours, after samples have been obtained to determine baseline plasma cortisol and 24-hour urine cortisol levels. In adrenal hypofunction, plasma and urine cortisol levels fail to rise normally in response to corticotropin; in secondary hypofunction, repeated doses of corticotropin over successive days produce a gradual increase in cortisol levels until normal values are reached.

In a patient with typical addisonian symptoms, these laboratory findings strongly suggest acute adrenal hypofunction:

- decreased cortisol levels in the plasma (less than 10 µg/dl in the morning, with lower levels in the evening) (However, this test is time-consuming, and emergency therapy shouldn't be postponed for test results.)
- decreased serum sodium and fasting blood glucose levels
- increased serum potassium and blood urea nitrogen levels
- elevated hematocrit and lymphocyte and eosinophil counts.

X-rays show a small heart and adrenal calcification.

Management
General
In adrenal crisis, monitor vital signs carefully, especially for hypotension, volume depletion, and other signs of shock (decreased level of consciousness and urine output). Watch for hyperkalemia before treatment and for hypokalemia after treatment (from excessive mineralocorticoid effect).

With proper treatment, adrenal crisis usually subsides quickly; the patient's blood pressure should stabilize, and water and sodium levels should return to normal. After the crisis, maintenance doses of hydrocortisone preserve physiologic stability.

Medication
Corticosteroid replacement therapy with one of these agents is the primary treatment for primary and secondary adrenal hypofunction and must continue throughout life:

- cortisone — 25 to 300 mg P.O. daily
- hydrocortisone — 5 to 30 mg P.O. b.i.d. to q.i.d.

Therapy for adrenal crisis is prompt administration of 100 mg hydrocortisone-sodium succinate given as an I.V. bolus. Later, 50- to 100-mg doses are given I.M. or are diluted with dextrose in saline solution and given I.V. until the patient's condition stabilizes.

Referral
- Refer the patient to an endocrinologist.
- Refer the patient to the National Addison's Disease Foundation for information and support.

Follow-up
Initially, the patient should be seen every week; thereafter, he should be seen every 2 to 4 weeks, depending on response to treatment.

Patient teaching
- Tell the patient to keep a weight record to help monitor volume depletion. Until onset of mineralocorticoid effect, tell him to force fluids to replace excessive fluid loss.
- Tell the patient to follow a high-protein, high-carbohydrate diet that maintains sodium and potassium balances.
- If the patient is anorectic, suggest six small meals per day to increase calorie intake. Tell him to keep a late-morning snack available in case he becomes hypoglycemic.
- Teach the patient the symptoms of under- or over-medicating. Tell the patient that the dosage may need to be increased during times of stress.
- Warn the patient that infection, injury, or profuse sweating in hot weather may precipitate adrenal crisis.
- Instruct the patient to always carry a medical identification card that states he

takes a steroid and that gives the name of the drug and the dosage.
- Teach the patient how to give himself an injection of hydrocortisone. Tell the patient to keep an emergency kit available containing hydrocortisone in a prepared syringe for use in times of stress.

Complications
- Addisonian crisis
- Hyperpyrexia
- Adverse effects from steroid treatment

Special considerations
- If the patient also has diabetes, periodically check blood glucose levels because steroid replacement therapy may require adjustment of the insulin dosage.
- If the patient is receiving only glucocorticoids, observe for orthostatic hypotension or electrolyte abnormalities, which may indicate a need for mineralocorticoid therapy.
- Be sure to explain that lifelong steroid therapy is necessary.

••••••••••••

ADRENOGENITAL SYNDROME

Adrenogenital syndrome results from disorders of adrenocortical steroid biosynthesis. This syndrome may be inherited (congenital adrenal hyperplasia [CAH]) or acquired, usually as a result of an adrenal tumor (adrenal virilism). CAH is the most prevalent adrenal disorder in infants and children; simple virilizing CAH and salt-losing CAH are the most common forms. Acquired adrenal virilism is rare and affects twice as many females as males.

AGE ALERT Salt-losing CAH may cause fatal adrenal crisis in neonates.

Causes and pathophysiology
CAH is transmitted as an autosomal recessive trait that causes deficiencies in the enzymes needed for adrenocortical secretion of cortisol and, possibly, aldosterone. Compensatory secretion of corticotropin produces varying degrees of adrenal hyperplasia. In simple virilizing CAH, deficiency of the enzyme 21-hydroxylase results in underproduction of cortisol. In turn, this cortisol deficiency stimulates increased secretion of corticotropin, producing large amounts of cortisol precursors and androgens that don't require 21-hydroxylase for synthesis.

In salt-losing CAH, 21-hydroxylase is almost completely absent. Corticotropin secretion increases, causing excessive production of cortisol precursors, including salt-wasting compounds. However, plasma cortisol and aldosterone levels — both dependent on 21-hydroxylase — fall precipitously and, in combination with the excessive production of salt-wasting compounds, precipitate acute adrenal crisis. Corticotropin hypersecretion stimulates adrenal androgens, possibly even more than in simple virilizing CAH, and produces masculinization. Other rare CAH enzyme deficiencies exist and lead to increased or decreased production of affected hormones.

Clinical presentation
The female neonate with simple virilizing CAH has ambiguous genitalia (enlarged clitoris, with urethral opening at the base; some labioscrotal fusion) but a normal genital tract and gonads. As she grows older, signs of progressive virilization develop: early appearance of pubic and axillary hair, deep voice, acne, and facial hair. The male neonate with this condition has no obvious abnormality; however, at prepuberty he shows accentuated masculine characteristics, such as

Acquired adrenal virilism

Acquired adrenal virilism results from virilizing adrenal tumors, carcinomas, or adenomas. This rare disorder is twice as common in females than in males. Although acquired adrenal virilism can develop at any age, its clinical effects vary with age at onset:

- Prepubescent girls — pubic hair, clitoral enlargement; at puberty, delayed breast development, delayed or absent menses
- Prepubescent boys — hirsutism, macrogenitosomia praecox (excessive body development, with marked enlargement of genitalia); occasionally, the penis and prostate equal those of an adult male in size; however, testicular maturation fails to occur
- Women (especially middle-aged) — dark hair on legs, arms, chest, back, and face; pubic hair extending toward navel; oily skin, sometimes with acne; menstrual irregularities; muscular hypertrophy (masculine resemblance); male pattern baldness; and atrophy of breasts and uterus
- Men — no overt signs; discovery of tumor usually accidental

- All patients — good muscular development; taller than average during childhood and adolescence; short stature as adults due to early closure of epiphyses.

DIAGNOSIS AND TREATMENT

Diagnostic tests for this disorder include:

- urinary total 17-ketosteroids (17-KS) level — greatly elevated, but vary daily; oral dexamethasone doesn't suppress 17-KS
- dehydroepiandrosterone — plasma levels greatly elevated
- serum electrolyte levels — normal
- kidney X-ray — may show downward displacement of kidneys by tumor.

Treatment requires surgical excision of tumor and metastases (if present), when possible, or radiation therapy and chemotherapy. Preoperative treatment may include glucocorticoids. With treatment, the prognosis is very good in patients with slow-growing and nonrecurring tumors. Periodic follow-up urine testing (for increased 17-KS levels) to check for tumor recurrence is essential.

deepened voice and an enlarged phallus, with frequent erections. At puberty, females fail to begin menstruation and males have small testes. Males and females with this condition may be taller than other children their age as a result of rapid bone and muscle growth, but because excessive androgen levels hasten epiphyseal closure, abnormally short adult stature results. (See *Acquired adrenal virilism.*)

Salt-losing CAH in females causes more complete virilization than the simple form and results in development of male external genitalia without testes.

Because males with this condition have no external genital abnormalities, immediate neonatal diagnosis is difficult and is commonly delayed until the neonate develops severe systemic symptoms. Characteristically, the neonate is apathetic, fails to eat, and has diarrhea; he develops symptoms of adrenal crisis in the 1st week of life (vomiting, dehydration from hyponatremia, hyperkalemia).

CLINICAL CAUTION Unless this condition is treated promptly, dehydration and hyperkalemia may lead to cardiovascular collapse and cardiac arrest.

Hermaphroditism

True hermaphroditism (hermaphrodism, intersexuality) is a rare condition characterized by ovarian and testicular tissues. External genitalia are usually ambiguous but may be completely male or female, which can mask hermaphroditism until puberty. The hermaphrodite almost always has a uterus (fertility is rare) and ambiguous gonads distributed as follows:

- bilaterally — testis and ovary on both sides, ovotestes
- unilaterally — ovary or testis on one side, an ovotestis on the other
- asymmetrically or laterally — an ovary and a testis on opposite sides.

CAUSES AND DIAGNOSIS

Because the Y chromosome is needed to develop testicular tissue, hermaphroditism in infants with XY karyotypes is particularly perplexing but may result from mosaicism (XX/XY, XX/XXY), hidden mosaicism, or hidden gene alterations. In patients with XX karyotype, ovaries are usually better developed than in those with XY karyotype. Fifty percent of hermaphrodites have a 46 XX karyotype, 20% have XY, and 30% are mosaics.

Although ambiguous external genitalia suggest hermaphroditism, chromosomal studies (particularly a buccal smear for Barr bodies, indicating an XX karyotype), a 24-hour urine specimen for 17-ketosteroids to rule out congenital adrenal hyperplasia, and gonadal biopsy are necessary to confirm it.

CRUCIAL EARLY TREATMENT

Sexual assignment, based on the anatomy of the external genitalia, and surgical reconstruction should be done as early as possible to prevent physical and psychological consequences of delayed reassignment. During surgery, inappropriate reproductive organs are removed to prevent incongruous secondary sex characteristics at puberty. Hormonal replacement may be necessary.

Differential diagnoses

- Androgen insensitivity syndrome
- Failure to thrive
- Sprue syndrome

Diagnosis

Physical examination revealing pseudohermaphroditism in females or precocious puberty in both sexes strongly suggests CAH. (See *Hermaphroditism*.) These laboratory findings confirm the diagnosis: elevated plasma 17-ketosteroids (17-KS), which can be suppressed by administering oral dexamethasone; elevated urinary levels of hormone metabolites, particularly pregnanetriol; elevated plasma 17-hydroxyprogesterone; and normal or decreased urinary levels of 17-hydroxycorticosteroids.

Adrenal hypofunction or adrenal crisis in the 1st week of life suggests salt-losing CAH. Hyperkalemia, hyponatremia, and hypochloremia with excessive urinary 17-KS and pregnanetriol and decreased urinary aldosterone levels confirm it.

Management
General

The neonate with salt-losing CAH in adrenal crisis requires immediate I.V. sodium chloride and glucose infusion to maintain fluid and electrolyte balance and to stabilize vital signs. If I.V. fluids don't control symptoms while the diagnosis is being established, then medication is necessary. Sex chromatin and karyotype studies determine the genetic sex of patients with ambiguous external genitalia.

Medication

Simple virilizing CAH requires correction of the cortisol deficiency and inhibition of excessive pituitary corticotropin production by daily administration of cortisone or hydrocortisone. Treatment returns androgen production to normal levels. Measurement of urinary 17-KS levels determines the initial dose of cortisone or hydrocortisone; this dose is usually large and is given I.M. Later dosage is modified according to decreasing urinary 17-KS levels. Infants must continue to receive cortisone or hydrocortisone I.M. until age 18 months; after that, they may take it orally.

Later, maintenance includes mineralocorticoid (desoxycorticosterone, fludrocortisone, or both) and glucocorticoid (cortisone or hydrocortisone) replacement.

Surgical intervention

Females with masculine external genitalia require reconstructive surgery, such as correction of the labial fusion and of the urogenital sinus. Surgery is usually scheduled between ages 1 and 3, after the effect of cortisone therapy has been assessed.

Referral

■ Refer the patient to an endocrinologist. If surgery is necessary, the patient may need to be referred to a surgeon.
■ Refer the family to the Ambiguous Genitalia Support Network for information and support.

Patient teaching

■ Teach the parents about the possible adverse effects (cushingoid symptoms) of long-term therapy. Explain that maintenance therapy with hydrocortisone, cortisone, or the mineralocorticoid fludrocortisone is essential for life. Warn them not to withdraw these drugs suddenly because potentially fatal adrenal hypofunction will result.
■ Instruct the parents to report stress and infection, which require increased steroid dosages.
■ Instruct the parents that the patient should wear a medical identification bracelet indicating that he's on prolonged steroid therapy and providing information about dosage.

Complications

■ Adrenal crisis
■ Death
■ Depression

Special considerations

■ Suspect CAH in infants hospitalized for failure to thrive, dehydration, or diarrhea, as well as in tall, sturdy-looking children with a record of numerous episodic illnesses.
■ Help the parents of a female infant with male genitalia to understand that she's physiologically a female and that this abnormality can be surgically corrected. Arrange for counseling, if necessary.

• • • • • • • • • • • •

CALCIUM IMBALANCE

Calcium plays an indispensable role in cell permeability, formation of bones and teeth, blood coagulation, transmission of nerve impulses, and normal muscle contraction. Nearly all (99%) of the body's calcium is found in the bones. The remaining 1% exists in ionized form in serum; the maintenance of this 1% of ionized calcium in the serum is critical to healthy neurologic function. The parathyroid glands regulate ionized calcium and determine its resorption into bone, absorption from the GI mucosa, and excretion in urine and feces. Severe calcium imbalance requires emergency treatment because hypocalcemia can lead to tetany and seizures; hypercalcemia can lead to cardiac arrhythmias and coma. (See *Clinical effects of calcium imbalance*, page 460.)

Causes

Common causes of hypocalcemia include:

- inadequate intake of calcium and vitamin D, in which inadequate levels of vitamin D inhibit intestinal absorption of calcium
- hypoparathyroidism resulting from injury, disease, or surgery that decreases or eliminates secretion of parathyroid hormone (PTH), which is necessary for calcium absorption and normal serum calcium levels
- malabsorption or loss of calcium from the GI tract caused by increased intestinal motility from severe diarrhea or laxative abuse; it can also result from inadequate levels of vitamin D or PTH or a reduction in gastric acidity, which decreases the solubility of calcium salts
- severe infections or burns in which diseased and burned tissue traps calcium from the extracellular fluid
- overcorrection of acidosis, resulting in alkalosis, which causes decreased ionized calcium and induces symptoms of hypocalcemia
- pancreatic insufficiency, which may cause malabsorption of calcium and subsequent calcium loss in feces; in pancre-

atitis, participation of calcium ions in saponification contributes to calcium loss
- renal failure, resulting in excessive excretion of calcium secondary to increased retention of phosphate
- hypomagnesemia, which causes decreased PTH secretion and blocks the peripheral action of that hormone.

Causes of hypercalcemia include:

- hyperparathyroidism, which increases serum calcium levels by promoting calcium absorption from the intestine, resorption from bone, and reabsorption from the kidneys
- hypervitaminosis D, which can promote increased absorption of calcium from the intestine
- tumors, which raise serum calcium levels by destroying bone or by releasing PTH or a PTH-like substance, osteoclast-activating factor, prostaglandins and, perhaps, a vitamin D–like sterol
- multiple fractures and prolonged immobilization, which release bone calcium and raise the serum calcium level
- multiple myeloma, which promotes loss of calcium from bone.

Other causes include milk-alkali syndrome, sarcoidosis, hyperthyroidism, adrenal insufficiency, thiazide diuretics, and loss of serum albumin secondary to renal disease.

Clinical presentation

Calcium deficit causes nerve fiber irritability and repetitive muscle spasms. Consequently, characteristic symptoms of hypocalcemia include:

- perioral paresthesia
- twitching
- carpopedal spasm
- tetany
- seizures
- cardiac arrhythmias
- Chvostek's sign

Clinical effects of calcium imbalance

DYSFUNCTION	HYPOCALCEMIA	HYPERCALCEMIA
Neurologic	▪ Anxiety, irritability, twitching around mouth, laryngospasm, seizures, Chvostek's sign, Trousseau's sign	▪ Drowsiness, lethargy, headaches, depression or apathy, irritability, confusion
Musculoskeletal	▪ Paresthesia (tingling and numbness of the fingers), tetany or painful tonic muscle spasms, facial spasms, abdominal cramps, muscle cramps, spasmodic contractions	▪ Weakness, muscle flaccidity, bone pain, pathologic fractures
Cardiovascular	▪ Arrhythmias, hypotension	▪ Signs of heart block, cardiac arrest, hypertension
GI	▪ Increased GI motility, diarrhea	▪ Anorexia, nausea, vomiting, constipation, dehydration, polydipsia
Other	▪ Blood-clotting abnormalities	▪ Renal polyuria, flank pain and, eventually, azotemia

▪ Trousseau's sign. (See *Trousseau's sign*, page 461, and *Chvostek's sign*, page 462.)

Clinical effects of hypercalcemia include:
▪ muscle weakness
▪ decreased muscle tone
▪ lethargy
▪ anorexia
▪ constipation
▪ nausea
▪ vomiting
▪ dehydration
▪ polydipsia
▪ polyuria.

CLINICAL CAUTION Severe hypercalcemia (serum levels that exceed 15 mg/dl) may produce cardiac arrhythmias and, eventually, coma.

Differential diagnoses
▪ Seizure disorder
▪ Myocardial infarction
▪ Specific cause of calcium imbalance would need to be diagnosed

Diagnosis
A serum calcium level less than 8.5 mg/dl confirms hypocalcemia; a level above 10.5 mg/dl confirms hypercalcemia. (However, because approximately one-half of serum calcium is bound to albumin, changes in serum protein must be considered when interpreting serum calcium levels.)

Urine analysis shows increased calcium precipitation in hypercalcemia. In hypocalcemia, an electrocardiogram (ECG) reveals lengthened QT interval, prolonged ST segment, and arrhythmias;

in hypercalcemia, an ECG indicates shortened QT interval and heart block.

Management
General
Treatment varies and requires correction of the acute imbalance, followed by maintenance therapy and correction of the underlying cause. Mild hypocalcemia may require nothing more than an adjustment in diet to allow adequate intake of calcium, vitamin D, and protein, possibly with oral calcium supplements. Treatment of hypercalcemia primarily eliminates excess serum calcium through hydration with normal saline solution, which promotes calcium excretion in the urine.

Medication
Acute hypocalcemia is an emergency that needs immediate correction by I.V. administration of calcium gluconate or calcium chloride. Chronic hypocalcemia also requires vitamin D supplements to facilitate GI absorption of calcium. To correct mild deficiency states, the amount of vitamin D in most multivitamin preparations is adequate. For severe deficiency, vitamin D is used in four forms: ergocalciferol (vitamin D_2), cholecalciferol (vitamin D_3), calcitriol, and dihydrotachysterol, a synthetic form of vitamin D_2.

These loop diuretics are administered to promote calcium excretion:
- ethacrynic acid — 50 to 200 mg/day P.O.
- furosemide — 20 to 80 mg/day P.O.

Thiazide diuretics are contraindicated in hypercalcemia because they inhibit calcium excretion.

These corticosteroids are helpful in treating sarcoidosis, hypervitaminosis D, and certain tumors:
- prednisone — 5 to 60 mg/day P.O. or every other day

Trousseau's sign

To check for Trousseau's sign, apply a blood pressure cuff to the patient's arm. A carpopedal spasm that causes thumb adduction and phalangeal extension, as shown, confirms tetany.

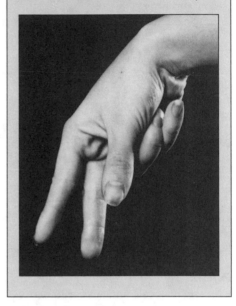

- hydrocortisone — 5 to 30 mg P.O. b.i.d., t.i.d., or q.i.d.

Plicamycin can also lower serum calcium levels and is especially effective against hypercalcemia secondary to certain tumors; it's given 15 to 25 mcg/kg/day I.V. over 4 to 6 hours for 3 to 4 days and may be repeated weekly.

Other medications that may be administered include:
- sodium phosphate solution — 20 to 30 ml solution mixed with 120 ml cold water or 135 ml P.R.
- calcitonin (salmon) — 4 IU/kg I.M. every 12 hours; may be increased to up to 8 IU/kg every 6 hours.

Chvostek's sign

To check for Chvostek's sign, tap the facial nerve above the mandibular angle, adjacent to the earlobe. A facial muscle spasm that causes the patient's upper lip to twitch, as shown, confirms tetany.

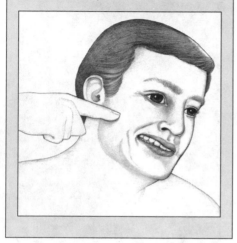

Referral
- Severe hypocalcemia may require hospitalization for immediate treatment.
- The patient may need to be referred to an endocrinologist to determine the cause of calcium imbalance.

Follow-up
Initially, the patient should be seen weekly and serum calcium levels should be measured weekly until they normalize. The cause of the calcium imbalance may also determine the follow-up schedule.

Patient teaching
- Tell the patient to take oral calcium supplements 1 to 1½ hours after meals or with milk.
- To prevent hypocalcemia, advise all patients — especially elderly ones — to eat foods rich in calcium, vitamin D, and protein, such as fortified milk and cheese. Explain how calcium is important for normal bone formation and blood coagulation.
- Discourage chronic use of laxatives. Also, warn patients with hypocalcemia not to overuse antacids because these may aggravate the condition.
- Tell patients with hypercalcemia to follow a low-calcium diet, with increased fluid intake, and to drink acid-ash fluids, such as cranberry or prune juice, because calcium salts are more soluble in acid than in alkali.

Complications
For hypocalcemia
- Cardiac arrhythmias
- Seizure
- Death

For hypercalcemia
- Renal damage
- Cardiac arrhythmias
- Renal calculi
- Pathologic fractures
- Ileus

Special considerations
- Watch for hypocalcemia in patients receiving massive transfusions of citrated blood; in those with chronic diarrhea, severe infections, and insufficient dietary intake of calcium and protein (especially elderly patients); and in those who are hyperventilating.
- Monitor the patient closely for a possible drug interaction if he's receiving cardiac glycosides and large doses of oral calcium supplements; watch for signs of digoxin toxicity.

• • • • • • • • • • • •
CHLORIDE IMBALANCE

Hypochloremia and hyperchloremia are, respectively, conditions of deficient or excessive serum levels of the chloride anion. A predominantly extracellular anion, chloride accounts for two-thirds of all serum anions. Secreted by stomach mucosa as hydrochloric acid, it provides an acid medium that aids digestion and activation of enzymes. Chloride also participates in maintaining acid-base and body-water balances, influences the osmolality or tonicity of extracellular fluid, plays a role in the exchange of oxygen and carbon dioxide (CO_2) in red blood cells, and helps activate salivary amylase (which, in turn, activates the digestive process).

Causes

Hypochloremia may result from:
- decreased chloride intake or absorption, as in low dietary-sodium intake, sodium deficiency, potassium deficiency, metabolic alkalosis; prolonged use of mercurial diuretics; or administration of dextrose I.V. without electrolytes
- excessive chloride loss resulting from prolonged diarrhea or diaphoresis; loss of hydrochloric acid in gastric secretions due to vomiting, gastric suctioning, or gastric surgery.

Hyperchloremia may result from:
- excessive chloride intake or absorption — as in hyperingestion of ammonium chloride or ureterointestinal anastomosis — allowing reabsorption of chloride by the bowel
- hemoconcentration due to dehydration
- compensatory mechanisms for other metabolic abnormalities, as in metabolic acidosis, brain stem injury causing neurogenic hyperventilation, and hyperparathyroidism.

Clinical presentation

Hypochloremia is usually associated with hyponatremia and its characteristic muscle weakness and twitching because renal chloride loss always accompanies sodium loss and sodium reabsorption isn't possible without chloride. However, if chloride depletion results from metabolic alkalosis secondary to loss of gastric secretions, chloride is lost independently from sodium; typical symptoms are:
- muscle hypertonicity
- tetany
- shallow, depressed breathing.

Because of the natural affinity of sodium and chloride ions, hyperchloremia usually produces clinical effects associated with hypernatremia and resulting extracellular fluid volume excess. Hyperchloremia associated with metabolic acidosis is due to excretion of base bicarbonate by the kidneys and induces deep, rapid breathing; weakness; diminished cognitive ability; and, ultimately, coma.

Differential diagnoses
- Respiratory failure
- Heart failure
- Sepsis

Diagnosis

Serum chloride level below 98 mEq/L confirms hypochloremia. (Supportive values in metabolic alkalosis include serum pH above 7.45 and serum CO_2 level above 32 mEq/L.) Serum chloride level above 108 mEq/L confirms hyperchloremia; with metabolic acidosis, serum pH is below 7.35 and serum CO_2 level is below 22 mEq/L.

Management
General

The aim of therapy for hypochloremia is to correct the condition that causes the chloride imbalance and to give oral replacement such as salty broth. When oral therapy isn't possible or when emergency measures are necessary, treatment may include normal saline solution I.V. (if hypovolemia is present) or chloride-containing drugs. Lactated Ringer's solution is administered for mild hyperchloremia; it converts to bicarbonate in the liver, thus increasing base bicarbonate to correct acidosis.

Medication

These medications may be used to treat a chloride imbalance (dosage depends on chloride level):
- ammonium chloride — to increase serum chloride levels
- potassium chloride — for metabolic alkalosis
- sodium bicarbonate — for severe hyperchloremic acidosis to raise the serum bicarbonate level and permit renal excretion of the chloride anion, because bicarbonate and chloride compete for combination with sodium (2 to 5 mEq/kg I.V. over 4- to 8-hour period).

Referral

- If the patient is acidotic, refer him to a hospital for treatment.

Follow-up

The underlying cause of the chloride imbalance will direct follow-up needs.

Patient teaching

- Teach the patient about any underlying condition and its effect on chloride levels.
- Teach the patient about any medications he is taking to correct chloride imbalance.

Complications

- Respiratory distress

Special considerations

- If the patient is receiving high doses of sodium bicarbonate, watch for signs of overcorrection (metabolic alkalosis, respiratory depression) or lingering signs of hyperchloremia, which indicate inadequate treatment.

• • • • • • • • • • • •

CUSHING'S SYNDROME

Cushing's syndrome is a cluster of clinical abnormalities caused by excessive levels of adrenocortical hormones (particularly cortisol) or related corticosteroids and, to a lesser extent, androgens and aldosterone. Its unmistakable signs include rapidly developing adiposity of the face (moon face), neck, and trunk, and purple striae on the skin. Cushing's syndrome is most common in females. The prognosis depends on the underlying cause; it's poor in untreated people and in those with untreatable ectopic corticotropin-producing carcinoma.

Causes

In approximately 70% of patients, Cushing's syndrome results from excessive production of corticotropin and consequent hyperplasia of the adrenal cortex. Overproduction of corticotropin may stem from pituitary hypersecretion (Cushing's disease), a corticotropin-producing tumor in another organ (particularly bronchogenic or pancreatic cancer), or excessive administration of exogenous glucocorticoids.

In the remaining 30% of patients, Cushing's syndrome results from a cortisol-secreting adrenal tumor, which is usually benign. In infants, the usual cause of Cushing's syndrome is adrenal carcinoma.

Clinical presentation

Like other endocrine disorders, Cushing's syndrome induces changes in multiple body systems, depending on the adrenocortical hormone involved. Clinical effects may include:

- endocrine and metabolic systems — diabetes mellitus, with decreased glucose tolerance, fasting hyperglycemia, and glycosuria
- musculoskeletal system — muscle weakness due to hypokalemia or loss of muscle mass from increased catabolism, pathologic fractures due to decreased bone mineral, and skeletal growth retardation in children
- skin — purplish striae; fat pads above the clavicles, over the upper back (buffalo hump), on the face (moon face), and throughout the trunk, with slender arms and legs; little or no scar formation; poor wound healing; acne and hirsutism in women. (See *Symptoms of cushingoid syndrome*, page 466.)
- GI system — peptic ulcer, resulting from increased gastric secretions and pepsin production, and decreased gastric mucus
- central nervous system — irritability and emotional lability, ranging from euphoric behavior to depression or psychosis; insomnia
- cardiovascular system — hypertension due to sodium and water retention; left ventricular hypertrophy; capillary weakness due to protein loss, which leads to bleeding, petechiae, and ecchymosis
- immune system — increased susceptibility to infection due to decreased lymphocyte production and suppressed antibody formation; decreased resistance to stress; suppressed inflammatory response, which may mask infection
- renal and urologic systems — sodium and secondary fluid retention, increased potassium excretion, inhibited antidiuretic hormone secretion, ureteral calculi from increased bone demineralization with hypercalciuria
- reproductive system — increased androgen production with clitoral hypertrophy, mild virilism, and amenorrhea or oligomenorrhea in females; sexual dysfunction also occurs.

Differential diagnoses

- Obesity related to diabetes mellitus
- Hypercortisolism secondary to alcoholism
- Adrenogenital syndrome

Diagnosis

Initially, diagnosis of Cushing's syndrome requires determination of plasma steroid levels. In people with normal hormone balance, plasma cortisol levels are higher in the morning and decrease gradually throughout the day (diurnal variation). In patients with Cushing's syndrome, cortisol levels don't fluctuate and typically remain consistently elevated; 24-hour urine specimen demonstrates elevated free cortisol levels. A low-dose dexamethasone suppression test confirms the diagnosis of Cushing's syndrome.

A high-dose dexamethasone suppression test can determine if Cushing's syndrome results from pituitary dysfunction (Cushing's disease). In this test, dexamethasone suppresses plasma cortisol levels, and urinary 17-hydroxycorticosteroid (17-OHCS) and 17-ketogenic steroid levels fall to 50% or less of basal levels. Failure to suppress these levels indicates that the syndrome results from an adrenal tumor or a nonendocrine, corticotropin-secreting tumor. This test can produce false-positive results.

In a stimulation test, administration of metyrapone, which blocks cortisol production by the adrenal glands, tests the ability of the pituitary gland and the hypothalamus to detect and correct low levels of plasma cortisol by increasing

Symptoms of cushingoid syndrome

Long-term treatment with corticosteroids may produce an adverse effect called cushingoid syndrome — a condition marked by obvious fat deposits between the shoulders and around the waist, and widespread systemic abnormalities.

In addition to the symptoms shown in the illustration, observe for signs of hypertension, renal disorders, hyperglycemia, tissue wasting, muscle weakness, and labile emotional state. The patient may also have amenorrhea and glycosuria.

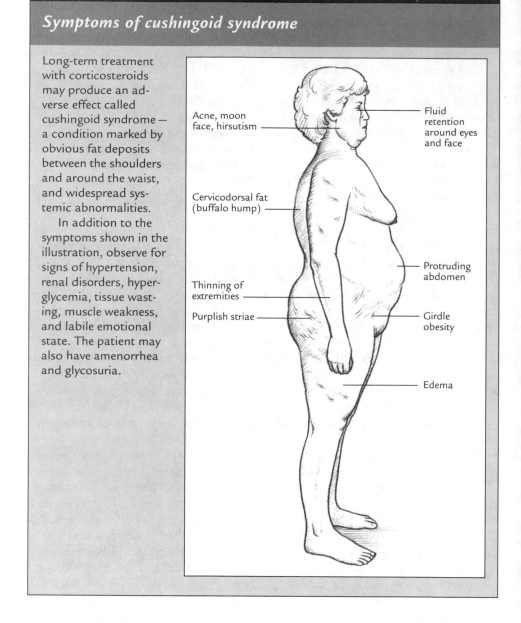

corticotropin production. The patient with Cushing's disease reacts to this stimulus by secreting an excess of plasma corticotropin as measured by levels of urinary 17-OHCS. If the patient has an adrenal or a nonendocrine corticotropin-secreting tumor, the pituitary gland — which is suppressed by the high cortisol levels — can't respond normally, so steroid levels remain stable or fall.

Ultrasound, computed tomography (CT) scan, or angiography localizes adrenal tumors; CT scan and magnetic resonance imaging of the head identify pituitary tumors.

Management
General
The goal of treatment is to restore hormone balance and reverse Cushing's syndrome.

Medication
To decrease cortisol levels, these medications have been beneficial for many cushingoid patients:
▪ aminoglutethimide—250 mg P.O. q.i.d. at 6-hour intervals
▪ ketoconazole—200 to 400 mg daily P.O.
    Aminoglutethimide alone, or in combination with metyrapone, may also be useful in metastatic adrenal carcinoma.
    Cortisol therapy (individualized dosage) is essential during and after surgery to help the patient tolerate the physiologic stress imposed by removal of the pituitary or adrenal gland. If normal cortisol production resumes, steroid therapy may be gradually tapered and eventually discontinued. However, bilateral adrenalectomy or total hypophysectomy mandates life-long steroid replacement therapy to correct hormonal deficiencies.
    The adrenal cytotoxic agent mitotane may be given (2 to 6 g/day in divided doses; may increase to 16 g/day).

Surgical intervention
Before surgery, the patient with cushingoid symptoms should have special management to control hypertension, edema, diabetes, and cardiovascular manifestations and to prevent infection. Glucocorticoid administration on the morning of surgery can help prevent acute adrenal hypofunction during surgery.
    Pituitary-dependent Cushing's syndrome with adrenal hyperplasia and severe cushingoid symptoms (such as psychosis, poorly controlled diabetes mellitus, osteoporosis, and severe pathologic fractures) may require partial or complete hypophysectomy or pituitary irradiation.

If the patient fails to respond, bilateral adrenalectomy may be performed. Nonendocrine corticotropin-producing tumors require excision of the tumor, followed by drug therapy to decrease cortisol levels if symptoms persist.

Referral
▪ The patient should be referred to an endocrinologist.
▪ The patient may need referral to a surgeon.

Follow-up
The patient's follow-up will depend on the type of therapy and the specialist.

Patient teaching
▪ Tell the patient to check for edema and to monitor daily weight and intake and output carefully.
▪ To minimize weight gain, edema, and hypertension, tell the patient to follow a diet that is high in protein and potassium but low in calories, carbohydrates, and sodium.

After surgery
▪ Advise the patient to take replacement steroids with antacids or meals to minimize gastric irritation. (Usually it's helpful to take two-thirds of the dose in the morning and the remaining third in the early afternoon to mimic diurnal adrenal secretion.)
▪ Tell the patient to carry a medical identification card and to immediately report physiologically stressful situations, which necessitate increased dosage.
▪ Instruct the patient to watch closely for signs of inadequate steroid dosage (fatigue, weakness, dizziness) and overdosage (severe edema, weight gain).

CLINICAL CAUTION Emphatically warn against abrupt discontinuation of steroid therapy because this may produce a fatal adrenal crisis.

Complications
- Osteoporosis
- Diabetes insipidus
- Hirsutism
- Increased susceptibility to infection
- Metastases of malignant tumors

Special considerations
- Watch for infection, a particular problem in Cushing's syndrome.

After bilateral adrenalectomy and pituitary surgery
- Monitor glucose levels for hypoglycemia due to removal of the source of cortisol.
- Check regularly for signs of adrenal hypofunction.

••••••••••••

DIABETES INSIPIDUS

Diabetes insipidus (also called pituitary diabetes insipidus) is a disorder of water metabolism resulting from a deficiency of circulating vasopressin (also called antidiuretic hormone [ADH]). It's characterized by excessive fluid intake and hypotonic polyuria. The disorder is more common in men than in women. Incidence is slightly higher today than in the past. In uncomplicated diabetes insipidus, the prognosis is good with adequate water replacement and replacement of ADH by tablet or nasal spray; patients usually lead normal lives.

AGE ALERT Diabetes insipidus may start in childhood or early adulthood (median age of onset is 21).

Causes
Diabetes insipidus results from intracranial neoplastic or metastatic lesions, hypophysectomy or other neurosurgery, a skull fracture, or head trauma that damages the neurohypophyseal structures. It can also result from infection, granulomatous disease, and vascular lesions; it may be idiopathic and, rarely, familial.

Note: Pituitary diabetes insipidus shouldn't be confused with nephrogenic diabetes insipidus, a rare congenital disturbance of water metabolism that results from renal tubular resistance to vasopressin.

Normally, the hypothalamus synthesizes vasopressin. The posterior pituitary gland (or neurohypophysis) stores vasopressin and releases it into general circulation, where it causes the kidneys to reabsorb water by making the distal tubules and collecting duct cells water-permeable. The absence of vasopressin in diabetes insipidus allows the filtered water to be excreted in the urine instead of being reabsorbed.

Clinical presentation
The patient's history typically shows an abrupt onset of extreme polyuria (usually 4 to 16 L/day of dilute urine, but sometimes as much as 30 L/day). As a result, the patient is extremely thirsty and drinks great quantities of water to compensate for the body's water loss. This disorder may also result in nocturia. In severe cases, it may lead to extreme fatigue from inadequate rest caused by frequent voiding and excessive thirst.

Other characteristic features of diabetes insipidus include signs and symptoms of dehydration. These symptoms usually begin abruptly, commonly appearing within 1 to 2 days after a basal skull fracture, a cerebrovascular accident, or surgery. Relieving cerebral edema or increased intracranial pressure may cause these symptoms to subside as rapidly as they began.

Differential diagnoses
- Increased fluid intake
- Diabetes mellitus

- Psychogenic polydipsia
- Nephrogenic diabetes insipidus

Diagnosis

Urinalysis reveals almost colorless urine of low osmolality (50 to 200 mOsm/kg, less than that of plasma) and low specific gravity (less than 1.005). Diagnosis requires evidence of vasopressin deficiency, resulting in the kidneys' inability to concentrate urine during a water deprivation test.

In this test, after baseline vital signs, weight, and urine and plasma osmolalities are obtained, the patient is deprived of fluids and observed to make sure he doesn't drink anything surreptitiously. Hourly measurements then record the total volume of urine output, body weight, urine osmolality or specific gravity, and plasma osmolality. Throughout the test, blood pressure and pulse rate must be monitored for signs of orthostatic hypotension. Fluid deprivation continues until the patient loses 3% of his body weight (indicating severe dehydration). When urine osmolality stops increasing in three consecutive hourly specimens, patients receive 5 units of aqueous vasopressin subcutaneously (S.C.).

Hourly measurements of urine volume and specific gravity continue after S.C. injection of aqueous vasopressin. Patients with pituitary diabetes insipidus respond to exogenous vasopressin with decreased urine output and increased specific gravity. Patients with nephrogenic diabetes insipidus show no response to vasopressin.

Management
General

Mild cases require no treatment other than fluid intake to replace fluid lost. Patient care includes monitoring symptoms to ensure that fluid balance is restored and maintained.

Medication

Until the cause of more severe cases of diabetes insipidus can be identified and eliminated, various forms of vasopressin or of a vasopressin stimulant can be given:
- vasopressin—5 to 10 U I.M. or S.C., b.i.d. to t.i.d., p.r.n.; intranasally in individualized doses
- desmopressin acetate—0.1 to 0.4 ml intranasally, one to three times/day; 0.5 to 1 ml/day I.V. or S.C. in two divided doses
- hydrochlorothiazide—25 to 100 mg/day P.O.; can be used in central and nephrogenic diabetes insipidus.

Referral

- The patient may need to be referred to an endocrinologist.
- Refer the patient to a mental health professional for additional counseling if necessary.

Follow-up

The patient will need to be monitored according to underlying cause and specialist.

Patient teaching

- If constipation develops, tell the patient to add more high-fiber foods and fruit juices to his diet and, if necessary, to take a mild laxative such as milk of magnesia.
- Instruct the patient to administer desmopressin by nasal spray only after the onset of polyuria—not before—to prevent excess fluid retention and water intoxication.
- Tell the patient to report weight gain, which may indicate that his medication dosage is too high. Recurrence of polyuria, as reflected on the intake and output sheet, indicates that the dosage is too low.
- Teach the parents of a child with diabetes insipidus about normal growth and

development. Discuss how their child may differ from others at his developmental stage.

■ Encourage the parents to help identify the child's strengths and to use them in developing coping strategies.

■ Advise the patient with diabetes insipidus to wear a medical identification bracelet and to carry his medication with him at all times.

Complications
■ Dehydration
■ Dilation of the urinary tract
■ Shock and renal failure

•••••••••••••

DIABETES MELLITUS

Diabetes mellitus is a chronic disease of absolute or relative insulin deficiency or resistance characterized by disturbances in carbohydrate, protein, and fat metabolism. A leading cause of death by disease in the United States, this syndrome is a contributing factor in about 50% of myocardial infarctions and about 75% of strokes as well as in renal failure and peripheral vascular disease. It's also the leading cause of new blindness.

Diabetes mellitus occurs in four forms classified by etiology: type 1, type 2, other specific types, and gestational diabetes mellitus (GDM). Type 1 is further subdivided into immune-mediated diabetes and idiopathic diabetes. Those who were previously in the type I diabetes group fall into this group. Children and adolescents with type 1 immune-mediated diabetes rapidly develop ketoacidosis, but most adults with this type experience only modest fasting hyperglycemia unless they develop an infection or experience another stressor. Patients with type 1 idiopathic diabetes are prone to ketoacidosis.

Most patients with type 2 diabetes are obese. Those who were previously in the type II diabetes group fall into this category. The "other specific types" category includes people who have diabetes as a result of a genetic defect, endocrinopathies, or exposure to certain drugs or chemicals. GDM occurs during pregnancy. In this type of diabetes, glucose tolerance levels usually return to normal after delivery.

Diabetes mellitus affects an estimated 5% of the population of the United States (16 million people), about half of whom are undiagnosed. Incidence is equal in males and females and rises with age.

Causes
In type 1 diabetes, pancreatic beta-cell destruction or a primary defect in beta-cell function results in failure to release insulin and ineffective glucose transport. Type 1 immune-mediated diabetes is caused by cell-mediated destruction of pancreatic beta cells. The rate of beta-cell destruction is usually higher in children than in adults. The idiopathic form of type 1 diabetes has no known cause. Patients with this form have no evidence of autoimmunity and don't produce insulin.

In type 2 diabetes, beta cells release insulin, but receptors are insulin-resistant and glucose transport is variable and ineffective. Risk factors for type 2 diabetes include:

■ obesity (even just an increased percentage of body fat primarily in the abdominal region); risk decreases with weight and drug therapy
■ lack of physical activity
■ history of GDM
■ hypertension or dyslipidemia
■ Black, Hispanic, or Native American origin

- strong family history of diabetes
- increasing age.

As the body ages, the cells become more resistant to insulin, thus reducing the older adult's ability to metabolize glucose. In addition, the release of insulin from the pancreatic beta cells is reduced and delayed. These combined processes result in hyperglycemia. In the older patient, sudden concentrations of glucose cause increased and more prolonged hyperglycemia.

The other specific types of diabetes mellitus result from various conditions (such as a genetic defect of the beta cells or endocrinopathies) or from use of or exposure to certain drugs or chemicals. GDM is considered present whenever a patient has any degree of abnormal glucose during pregnancy. This form may result from weight gain and increased levels of estrogen and placental hormones, which antagonize insulin.

Insulin transports glucose into the cell for use as energy and storage as glycogen. It also stimulates protein synthesis and free fatty acid storage in the fat deposits. Insulin deficiency compromises the body tissues' access to essential nutrients for fuel and storage.

Clinical presentation

Diabetes may begin dramatically with ketoacidosis or insidiously. Its most common symptom is fatigue from energy deficiency and a catabolic state. Insulin deficiency causes hyperglycemia, which pulls fluid from body tissues, causing:

- osmotic diuresis
- polyuria
- dehydration
- polydipsia
- dry mucous membranes
- poor skin turgor
- unexplained weight loss.

Because older adults' thirst mechanism functions less effectively, they may not report polydipsia, a hallmark of diabetes in younger adults.

In ketoacidosis and hyperosmolar hyperglycemic nonketotic syndrome (HHNS), dehydration may cause hypovolemia and shock. Wasting of glucose in the urine usually produces weight loss and hunger in type 1 diabetes, even if the patient eats voraciously.

Differential diagnoses

- Non-insulin-dependent diabetes versus insulin-dependent diabetes
- Glucose intolerance
- GDM
- Benign renal glycosuria
- Secondary diabetes: pancreatic disease, hormonal disorders, genetic disorders, drug-induced

Diagnosis

According to the American Diabetes Association's (ADA's) latest guidelines, diabetes mellitus can be diagnosed if any of these conditions exist:

- symptoms of diabetes (polyuria, polydipsia, unexplained weight loss) plus a casual plasma glucose value (obtained without regard to the time of the patient's last food intake) greater than or equal to 200 mg/dl
- a fasting plasma glucose level (no caloric intake for at least 8 hours) greater than or equal to 126 mg/dl
- a plasma glucose value in the 2-hour sample of the oral glucose tolerance test greater than or equal to 200 mg/dl. This test should be performed after a glucose load dose of 75 g of anhydrous glucose.

If results are questionable, the diagnosis should be confirmed by a repeat test on a different day. The ADA also recommends these testing guidelines:

Classifying blood glucose levels

The American Diabetes Association classifies blood glucose levels as follows:
- provisional diabetes — 126 mg/dl or more, confirmed by repeat test done on another day (previous guidelines — 140 mg/dl or more)
- impaired — 110 to 125 mg/dl
- normal — less than 110 mg/dl.

- people age 45 or older without symptoms — test every 3 years
- people with the classic symptoms — test immediately.

Certain high-risk groups should be tested frequently:
- Blacks, Hispanics, and Native Americans
- those who are obese (more than 20% over ideal body weight)
- those who have a close relative with diabetes
- those with high blood pressure (140/90 mm Hg or higher)
- those with high levels of high-density lipoprotein cholesterol (35 mg/dl or higher) or triglycerides (250 mg/dl or higher)
- women who have delivered a baby weighing more than 9 lb or who have a history of GDM
- those previously diagnosed with impaired glucose tolerance (IGT) or impaired fasting glucose (IFG).

Note: Individuals with IGT usually have normal blood levels unless challenged by a glucose load, such as a piece of pie or a glass of orange juice. Two hours after a glucose load, the glucose level ranges from 140 to 199 mg/dl. Individuals with IFG have an abnormal fasting glucose level between 110 and 125 mg/dl. Because the fasting plasma glucose test is sufficient to make the diagnosis of diabetes, it replaces the oral glucose tolerance test. (See *Classifying blood glucose levels.*)

An ophthalmologic examination may show diabetic retinopathy. Other diagnostic and monitoring tests include urinalysis for acetone level and blood testing for glycosylated hemoglobin (hemoglobin A) level, which reflects recent glucose cortisol.

Management
General
Effective treatment normalizes blood glucose level and decreases complications. In type 1 diabetes, this is achieved with insulin replacement, diet, and exercise. Treatment of all types of diabetes also requires a strict diet planned to meet nutritional needs, to control blood glucose levels, and to reach and maintain appropriate body weight. For the obese patient with type 2 diabetes, weight reduction is a goal. In type 1 diabetes, the calorie allotment may be high, depending on growth stage and activity level. For success, the diet must be followed consistently and meals must be eaten at regular times.

Any patient with a wound that has lasted longer than 8 weeks and who has tried standard wound care and revascularization without improvement should consider hyperbaric oxygen therapy. This treatment may speed healing by allowing more oxygen to get to the wound and may therefore result in fewer amputations.

The Diabetes Control and Complications Trial has shown that in type 1 diabetes, intensive drug therapy that focuses on keeping glucose at near-normal levels for 5 years or more reduces both the onset and progression of retinopathy (up to 63%), nephropathy (up to 54%), and neuropathy (up to 60%). The United Kingdom Diabetes Study Group demonstrated that in type 2 diabetes, blood pressure control as well as smoking cessation reduced the onset and progression of complications, including cardiovascular disease.

Medication
Current forms of insulin replacement include single-dose, mixed-dose, split-mixed dose, and multiple-dose regimens. The multiple-dose regimens may use an insulin pump. Insulin may be rapid-acting (Regular), intermediate-acting (NPH), long-acting (Ultralente), or a combination of rapid-acting and intermediate-acting (Mixtard); it may be standard or purified, and it may be derived from beef, pork, or human sources. Purified human insulin is commonly used today. Pancreas transplantation is experimental and requires chronic immunosuppression.

Type 2 diabetes may require oral antidiabetic drugs to stimulate endogenous insulin production, increase insulin sensitivity at the cellular level, and suppress hepatic gluconeogenesis. Five types of drugs have been used to treat diabetes:
- sulfonylureas, such as tolbutamide — 500 to 3,000 mg/day P.O.
- a stimulator for insulin release such as repaglinide — 0.5 to 4 mg P.O. with meals b.i.d., t.i.d., or q.i.d.
- biguanides such as metformin — 500 mg P.O. b.i.d. or 850 mg/day with a maximum dose of 2,550 mg in divided doses
- alpha-glucosidase inhibitors such as acarbose — 25 to 100 mg P.O. t.i.d. with meals.
- thiazolidinediones such as troglitazone — 200 to 600 mg/day P.O. with a meal.

Surgical intervention
Treatment of long-term diabetic complications may include transplantation or dialysis for renal failure, photocoagulation for retinopathy, and vascular surgery for large-vessel disease. Meticulous blood glucose control is essential.

Referral
- The patient may need to be referred to an endocrinologist.
- The patient may need to be referred to a diabetic educator.
- For further information and support, refer the patient to the Juvenile Diabetes Foundation, the ADA, and the American Association of Diabetes Educators.

Follow-up
The patient will need to be seen based on individual response to treatment and underlying medical conditions this disorder may affect.

Patient teaching
- Stress the importance of complying with the prescribed treatment program. Tailor your teaching to the patient's needs, abilities, and developmental stage. Include diet; purpose, administration, and possible adverse effects of medication; exercise; monitoring; hygiene; and the prevention and recognition of hypoglycemia and hyperglycemia.
- Stress the effect of blood glucose control on long-term health.
- Teach the patient to care for his feet by washing them daily, drying carefully between toes, and inspecting for corns, calluses, redness, swelling, bruises, and breaks in the skin. Urge him to report changes. Advise him to wear nonconstricting shoes and to avoid walking barefoot. Instruct him to use over-the-counter athlete's foot remedies and seek professional care if athlete's foot doesn't improve.
- Teach the patient how to manage his diabetes when he has a minor illness, such as a cold, flu, or upset stomach.
- To delay the clinical onset of diabetes, teach people at high risk to avoid risk

factors. Advise genetic counseling for young adult diabetics who are planning families.

Complications
- Microvascular: retinopathy, nephropathy, and neuropathy
- Macrovascular: coronary, peripheral, and cerebral artery disease
- Dyslipidemia
- Hypoglycemia
- Diabetic ketoacidosis
- HHNS
- Excessive weight gain
- Skin ulcerations
- Chronic renal failure

Special considerations
- Watch for diabetic effects on the cardiovascular system, such as cerebrovascular, coronary artery, and peripheral vascular impairment, and on the peripheral and autonomic nervous systems. Treat all injuries, cuts, and blisters (particularly on the legs or feet) meticulously. Be alert for signs of urinary tract infection and renal disease.
- Urge regular ophthalmologic examinations to detect diabetic retinopathy.
- Assess for signs of diabetic neuropathy. Stress the need for personal safety precautions because decreased sensation can mask injuries. Minimize complications by maintaining strict blood glucose control.

• • • • • • • • • • • •
HIRSUTISM

A distressing disorder usually found in women and children, hirsutism is the excessive growth of body hair, typically in an adult male distribution pattern. This condition commonly occurs spontaneously but may also develop as a secondary disorder of various underlying diseases. It must always be distinguished from hypertrichosis. The prognosis varies with the cause and the effectiveness of treatment.

Causes
Idiopathic hirsutism probably stems from a hereditary trait because the patient usually has a family history of the disorder. Causes of secondary hirsutism include endocrine abnormalities related to pituitary dysfunction (acromegaly, precocious puberty), adrenal dysfunction (Cushing's disease, congenital adrenal hyperplasia, or Cushing's syndrome), ovarian lesions (such as polycystic ovary syndrome), and iatrogenic factors (such as use of minoxidil, androgenic steroids, testosterone, diazoxide, glucocorticoids, and oral contraceptives). Other kinds of hirsutism have been reported. (See *Hypertrichosis.*)

Clinical presentation
Hirsutism typically produces enlarged hair follicles as well as enlargement and hyperpigmentation of the hairs themselves. Excessive facial hair growth is the complaint for which most patients seek medical help. Generally, hirsutism involves appearance of thick, pigmented hair in the beard area, upper back, shoulders, sternum, axillae, and pubic area. Frontotemporal scalp hair recession is often a coexisting condition. Patterns of hirsutism vary widely, depending on the patient's race and age. Elderly women commonly show increased hair growth on the chin and upper lip. In secondary hirsutism, signs of masculinization may appear, such as:
- deepening of the voice
- increased muscle mass
- increased size of genitalia
- menstrual irregularity
- decreased breast size.

Differential diagnoses

- Excessive ovarian or adrenal androgen production
- Ovarian or adrenal tumor
- Hypothyroidism
- Hyperprolactinemia
- Idiopathic cause

Diagnosis

A family history of hirsutism, absence of menstrual abnormalities or signs of masculinization, and a normal pelvic examination strongly suggest idiopathic hirsutism. Tests for secondary hirsutism depend on associated symptoms that suggest an underlying disorder. About 90% of women with hirsutism have an elevated free testosterone level.

Management
General

At the patient's request, treatment of idiopathic hirsutism consists of eliminating excess hair by scissors, shaving, depilatory creams, or removal of the entire hair shaft with tweezers or wax. Bleaching with hydrogen peroxide may also be satisfactory. Electrolysis can destroy hair bulbs permanently, but it works best when only a few hairs need to be removed. (A history of keloid formation contraindicates this procedure.) Treatment of secondary hirsutism varies, depending on the nature of the underlying disorder.

Medication

Hirsutism due to elevated androgen levels may require:
- low-dose dexamethasone—0.25 to 0.5 mg P.O. h.s.
- oral contraceptives (any brand).

An androgen receptor-competitive inhibitor such as spironolactone (100 to 200 mg/day P.O.) may also be used, but the drug varies in its effectiveness.

Hypertrichosis

Hypertrichosis is a localized or generalized condition in males and females that is marked by excessive hair growth. Localized hypertrichosis usually results from local trauma, chemical irritation, or hormonal stimulation; pigmented nevi (Becker's nevus, for example) may also contain hairs. Generalized hypertrichosis results from neurologic or psychiatric disorders, such as encephalitis, multiple sclerosis, concussion, anorexia nervosa, or schizophrenia; contributing factors include juvenile hypothyroidism, porphyria cutanea tarda, and the use of drugs such as phenytoin.

Hypertrichosis lanuginosa is a generalized proliferation of fine, lanugotype hair (sometimes called down, or woolly hair). Such hair may be present at birth but generally disappears shortly thereafter. This condition may become chronic, with persistent lanugo-type hair growing over the entire body, or may develop suddenly later in life. It's very rare and usually results from malignancy.

Referral

- Suggest consulting a cosmetologist about makeup or bleaching agents.

Follow-up

The patient should be seen after 6 months to evaluate treatment and assess for adverse medication effects.

Patient teaching

- Teach the patient about medications and explain that she may have to take them throughout her life.

• Tell the patient that the treatment may prevent further hair growth but won't reverse present hair growth.

Complications
▪ Dysfunctional uterine bleeding
▪ Poor self-image
▪ Increased cardiac risk
▪ Alteration in bone density

Special considerations
▪ Care for patients with idiopathic hirsutism focuses on emotional support and patient teaching; care for patients with secondary hirsutism depends on the treatment for the underlying disease.
▪ Watch for signs of contact dermatitis in patients being treated with depilatory creams, especially the elderly. Also watch for infection of hair follicles after hair removal with tweezers or wax.

• • • • • • • • • • •

HYPERTHYROIDISM

Hyperthyroidism (also known as Graves' disease, Basedow's disease, or thyrotoxicosis) is a metabolic imbalance that results from thyroid hormone overproduction. The most common form of hyperthyroidism is Graves' disease, which increases thyroxine (T_4) production, enlarges the thyroid gland (goiter), and causes multiple system changes.

With treatment, most patients can lead normal lives. However, thyroid storm — an acute exacerbation of hyperthyroidism — is a medical emergency that may lead to life-threatening cardiac, hepatic, or renal failure.

AGE ALERT Incidence of Graves' disease is highest between ages 30 and 40, especially in people with family histories of thyroid abnormalities; only 5% of hyperthyroid patients are younger than age 15.

Causes
Hyperthyroidism may result from genetic and immunologic factors. An increased incidence of this disorder in monozygotic twins, for example, points to an inherited factor, probably an autosomal recessive gene. This disease occasionally coexists with abnormal iodine metabolism and other endocrine abnormalities, such as diabetes mellitus, thyroiditis, and hyperparathyroidism. Hyperthyroidism is also associated with the production of autoantibodies (thyroid-stimulating immunoglobulin and thyroid-stimulating hormone [TSH]-binding inhibitory immunoglobulin), possibly due to a defect in suppressor-T-lymphocyte function that allows formation of autoantibodies.

In latent hyperthyroidism, excessive dietary intake of iodine and, possibly, stress can precipitate clinical hyperthyroidism. (See *Other forms of hyperthyroidism.*)

CLINICAL CAUTION In a person with inadequately treated hyperthyroidism, stress — including surgery, infection, toxemia of pregnancy, and diabetic ketoacidosis — can precipitate thyroid storm.

Clinical presentation
The classic features of hyperthyroidism are an enlarged thyroid (goiter), nervousness, heat intolerance, weight loss despite increased appetite, sweating, diarrhea, tremor, and palpitations. Exophthalmos is considered most characteristic but is absent in many patients with hyperthyroidism. Many other symptoms are common because hyperthyroidism profoundly affects virtually every body system:
▪ central nervous system — difficulty concentrating because increased T_4 se-

cretion accelerates cerebral function; excitability or nervousness due to increased basal metabolic rate; fine tremor, shaky handwriting, and clumsiness from increased activity in the spinal cord area that controls muscle tone; emotional instability and mood swings, ranging from occasional outbursts to overt psychosis
- skin, hair, and nails — smooth, warm, flushed skin (patient sleeps with minimal covers and little clothing); fine, soft hair; premature graying and increased hair loss in both sexes; friable nails and onycholysis (distal nail separated from the bed); pretibial myxedema (dermopathy), producing thickened skin, accentuated hair follicles, raised red patches of skin that are itchy and sometimes painful, with occasional nodule formation; microscopic examination shows increased mucin deposits
- cardiovascular system — tachycardia; full, bounding pulse; wide pulse pressure; cardiomegaly; increased cardiac output and blood volume; visible point of maximal impulse; paroxysmal supraventricular tachycardia and atrial fibrillation (especially in the elderly); and, occasionally, systolic murmur at the left sternal border
- respiratory system — dyspnea on exertion and at rest, possibly from cardiac decompensation and increased cellular oxygen utilization
- GI system — possible anorexia; nausea and vomiting due to increased GI mobility and peristalsis; increased defecation; soft stools or, with severe disease, diarrhea; and liver enlargement
- musculoskeletal system — weakness, fatigue, and muscle atrophy; rare coexistence with myasthenia gravis; possible generalized or localized paralysis associated with hypokalemia; and occasional acropachy (soft-tissue swelling, accompanied by underlying bone changes where new bone formation occurs)

Other forms of hyperthyroidism

- *Toxic adenoma* is a small, benign nodule in the thyroid gland that secretes thyroid hormone and is the second most common cause of hyperthyroidism. The cause of toxic adenoma is unknown; incidence is highest in the elderly. Clinical effects are essentially similar to those of Graves' disease, except that toxic adenoma doesn't induce ophthalmopathy, pretibial myxedema, or acropachy. Presence of adenoma is confirmed by radioactive iodine (^{131}I) uptake and thyroid scan, which shows a single hyperfunctioning nodule suppressing the rest of the gland. Treatment includes ^{131}I therapy or surgery to remove adenoma after antithyroid drugs achieve a euthyroid state.
- *Thyrotoxicosis factitia* results from chronic ingestion of thyroid hormone for thyrotropin suppression in patients with thyroid carcinoma or from thyroid hormone abuse by people who are trying to lose weight.
- *Functioning metastatic thyroid carcinoma* is a rare disease that causes excess production of thyroid hormone.
- *Thyroid-stimulating hormone–secreting pituitary tumor* causes overproduction of thyroid hormone.
- *Subacute thyroiditis* is a virus-induced granulomatous inflammation of the thyroid, producing transient hyperthyroidism associated with fever, pain, pharyngitis, and tenderness in the thyroid gland.
- *Silent thyroiditis* is a self-limiting, transient form of hyperthyroidism, with histologic thyroiditis but no inflammatory symptoms.

■ reproductive system — in females, oligomenorrhea or amenorrhea, decreased fertility, higher incidence of spontaneous abortions; in males, gynecomastia due to increased estrogen levels; in both sexes, diminished libido

■ eyes — exophthalmos (from the combined effects of accumulation of mucopolysaccharides and fluids in the retro-orbital tissues that force the eyeball outward and of lid retraction that produces the characteristic staring gaze); occasional inflammation of conjunctivae, corneas, or eye muscles; diplopia; and increased tearing.

When hyperthyroidism escalates to thyroid storm, these symptoms can be accompanied by extreme irritability, hypertension, tachycardia, vomiting, temperature up to 106° F (41.1° C), delirium, and coma.

Differential diagnoses

■ Malignancy
■ Anxiety
■ Diabetes
■ Pregnancy
■ Pheochromocytoma
■ Menopause

Diagnosis

The diagnosis of hyperthyroidism usually is straightforward and depends on a careful clinical history and physical examination, a high index of suspicion, and routine hormone determinations. These tests confirm the disorder:

■ Radioimmunoassay shows increased serum T_4 and triiodothyronine (T_3) concentrations.

■ Thyroid scan reveals increased uptake of radioactive iodine (^{131}I). This test is contraindicated if the patient is pregnant.

■ TSH levels are decreased.

■ Thyroid-releasing hormone (TRH) stimulation test indicates hyperthyroidism if the TSH level fails to rise within 30 minutes after the administration of TRH.

■ Ultrasonography confirms subclinical ophthalmopathy.

Management
General

A number of approaches are used to treat hyperthyroidism, primarily administration of antithyroid drugs, treatment with ^{131}I, and surgery. Appropriate treatment depends on the goiter's size, the causes, the patient's age and parity, and how long surgery will be delayed (if the patient is an appropriate candidate for surgery).

Medication

Antithyroid drug therapy is used for children, young adults, pregnant women, and patients who refuse surgery or ^{131}I treatment. Thyroid hormone antagonists include:

■ propylthiouracil — adults, 300 to 900 mg P.O. daily; children older than age 10, 150 to 300 mg/day P.O. in three divided doses

■ methimazole — adults, 15 to 60 mg P.O. daily; children, 0.4 mg/kg P.O. daily; although hypermetabolic symptoms subside within 4 to 8 weeks after such therapy begins, the patient must continue the medication for 6 months to 2 years, depending on the clinical circumstances

■ propranolol — adults, 4 to 240 mg/day P.O.; children, 1mg/kg/day P.O.

During pregnancy, antithyroid medication should be kept at the minimum dosage required to keep maternal thyroid function within the high-normal range until delivery and to minimize the risk of fetal hypothyroidism — even though most infants of hyperthyroid mothers are born with mild and transient hyperthyroidism. (Neonatal hyperthyroidism may even necessitate treatment with antithyroid medications and propranolol for 2 to 3 months.) Because hyperthyroidism is sometimes exacerbated in the puerperal period, continuous control of maternal thyroid function is essential. Approximately 3 to 6 months postpartum, antithyroid drug administration can be gradually tapered and thyroid function reassessed. The mother receiving low-dose antithyroid treatment may breast-feed as long as the infant's thyroid function is checked periodically. Small amounts of the drug can be found in breast milk.

A single oral dose of ^{131}I is the treatment of choice for patients not planning to have children. However, some patients may require a second dose.

Therapy for hyperthyroid ophthalmopathy includes local applications of topical medications but may require high doses of corticosteroids.

Surgical intervention
Subtotal (partial) thyroidectomy, which decreases the thyroid gland's capacity for hormone production, is indicated for patients with a large goiter whose hyperthyroidism has repeatedly relapsed after drug therapy or patients who refuse or aren't candidates for ^{131}I treatment. Preoperatively, the patient may receive iodides (Lugol's solution or saturated solution of potassium iodide), antithyroid drugs, or high doses of propranolol to help prevent thyroid storm. If euthyroidism isn't achieved, surgery should be delayed and propranolol administered to decrease the systemic effects (cardiac arrhythmias) caused by hyperthyroidism. After ablative treatment with ^{131}I or surgery, patients require regular medical supervision for the rest of their lives because they usually develop hypothyroidism, sometimes as long as several years after treatment.

A patient with severe exophthalmos that causes pressure on the optic nerve may require external beam radiation therapy or surgical decompression to lessen pressure on the orbital contents.

Referral
- Refer the patient to an endocrinologist.

Follow-up
The patient should be seen according to treatment plan. Thyroid function tests should be done after 6 weeks and then every 6 months. Stress the importance of regular medical follow-up after surgery because hypothyroidism may develop from 2 to 4 weeks postoperatively.

Patient teaching
- Promote weight gain by telling the patient to follow a balanced diet, with six meals a day. If the patient has edema, suggest a low-sodium diet.
- If iodide is part of the treatment, tell the patient to mix it with milk, juice, or water to prevent GI distress and to administer it through a straw to prevent tooth discoloration.
- Teach the patient to watch for signs of thyroid storm (tachycardia, hyperkinesis, fever, vomiting, hypertension).
- If the patient has exophthalmos or other ophthalmopathy, suggest sunglasses or eye patches to protect his eyes from light. Tell the patient to moisten the conjunctivae often with isotonic eye drops. Warn the patient with severe lid retraction to avoid sudden physical movements that might cause the lid to slip behind the eyeball.
- After ^{131}I therapy, tell the patient not to expectorate or cough freely because his saliva will be radioactive for 24 hours.

- Stress the need for repeated measurement of serum T_4 levels.
- Tell him to report fever, enlarged cervical lymph nodes, sore throat, mouth sores, and other signs of blood dyscrasias and rash or skin eruptions — these are signs of hypersensitivity.
- Watch the patient taking propranolol for signs of hypotension. Tell him to rise slowly after sitting or lying down to prevent orthostatic syncope.
- Instruct the patient receiving antithyroid drugs or ^{131}I therapy to report any symptoms of hypothyroidism.

Complications
- Thyroid storm
- Hypothyroidism
- Vision loss
- Muscle wasting
- Hypoparathyroidism (after surgery)
- Cardiac failure

Special considerations
- Patients with hyperthyroidism require vigilant care to prevent acute exacerbations and complications.
- If the patient is pregnant, tell her to watch closely during the first trimester for signs of spontaneous abortion and to report such signs immediately.
- Avoid excessive palpation of the thyroid to avoid precipitating thyroid storm.

• • • • • • • • • • • •

HYPOPITUITARISM

Hypopituitarism, which includes panhypopituitarism or dwarfism, is a complex syndrome marked by metabolic dysfunction, sexual immaturity, and growth retardation (when it occurs in childhood). It results from a deficiency of the hormones secreted by the anterior pituitary gland. Panhypopituitarism refers to a generalized condition caused by partial or total failure of the anterior pituitary's vital hormones — corticotropin, thyroid-stimulating hormone (TSH), luteinizing hormone (LH), follicle-stimulating hormone (FSH), human growth hormone (hGH), and prolactin — plus the posterior pituitary hormone, antidiuretic hormone. Partial hypopituitarism and complete hypopituitarism occur in adults and children; in children, these diseases may cause dwarfism and delayed puberty. The prognosis may be good with adequate replacement therapy and correction of the underlying causes.

Causes
The most common cause of primary hypopituitarism in adults is a tumor. Other causes include congenital defects (hypoplasia or aplasia of the pituitary gland); pituitary infarction (most often from postpartum hemorrhage); or partial or total hypophysectomy by surgery, irradiation, or chemical agents; and, rarely, granulomatous disease (tuberculosis, for example). Occasionally, hypopituitarism may have no identifiable cause, or it may be related to autoimmune destruction of the gland. Secondary hypopituitarism stems from a deficiency of releasing hormones produced by the hypothalamus — either idiopathic or possibly resulting from infection, trauma, or a tumor.

Primary hypopituitarism usually develops in a predictable pattern of hormonal failures. It generally starts with hypogonadism from gonadotropin failure (decreased FSH and LH levels). In adults, it causes cessation of menses in women and impotence in men. Deficient hGH levels follow; in children, this causes short stature, delayed growth, and delayed puberty. In adults, it causes osteoporosis, decreased lean-to-fat body mass index, adverse lipid changes, and subtle emotional dysphoria and lethargy. Subsequent failure of thyrotropin (decreased TSH levels) causes hypothyroidism; finally, adrenocorticotropic failure (decreased corticotropin levels) results in adrenal insufficiency. However, when hypopituitarism follows surgical ablation or trauma, the pattern of hormonal events may not necessarily follow this sequence. Sometimes, damage to the hypothalamus or neurohypophysis from surgical ablation or trauma leads to diabetes insipidus.

Clinical presentation

Clinical features of hypopituitarism develop slowly and vary with the severity of the disorder and the number of deficient hormones. Signs and symptoms of hypopituitarism in adults may include:

- gonadal failure
- diabetes insipidus
- hypothyroidism
- adrenocortical insufficiency.

Postpartum necrosis of the pituitary (Sheehan's syndrome) characteristically causes failure of lactation, menstruation, growth of pubic and axillary hair, and symptoms of thyroid and adrenocortical failure.

In children, hypopituitarism causes retarded growth or delayed puberty. Dwarfism usually isn't apparent at birth, but early signs begin to appear during the first few months of life; by age 6 months, growth retardation is obvious. Although these children generally enjoy good health, pituitary dwarfism may cause chubbiness due to fat deposits in the lower trunk, delayed secondary tooth eruption and, possibly, hypoglycemia. Growth continues at less than half the normal rate — sometimes extending into the patient's 20s or 30s — to an average height of 4' (122 cm), with normal proportions.

When hypopituitarism strikes before puberty, it prevents development of secondary sex characteristics (including facial and body hair). In males, it produces undersized testes, penis, and prostate gland; absent or minimal libido; and inability to initiate and maintain an erection. In females, it usually causes immature development of the breasts, sparse or absent pubic and axillary hair, and primary amenorrhea.

Panhypopituitarism may induce a host of mental and physiologic abnormalities, including:

- lethargy
- psychosis
- orthostatic hypotension
- bradycardia
- anemia
- anorexia.

Clinical manifestations of hormonal deficiencies resulting from pituitary destruction don't become apparent until 75% of the gland is destroyed. Total loss of all hormones released by the anterior pituitary is fatal unless treated.

Neurologic signs associated with hypopituitarism and produced by pituitary tumors include headache, bilateral temporal hemianopia, loss of visual acuity and, possibly, blindness. Acute hypopituitarism resulting from surgery or infection is often associated with fever, hypotension, vomiting, and hypoglycemia — all characteristic of adrenal insufficiency.

Differential diagnoses

- Primary hypothyroidism
- Anorexia nervosa
- Addison's disease
- Primary hypogonadism

Diagnosis

In suspected hypopituitarism, evaluation must confirm hormonal deficiency due to impairment or destruction of the anterior pituitary gland and rule out disease of the target organs (adrenals, gonads, and thyroid) or the hypothalamus. Low serum levels of thyroxine, for example, indicate diminished thyroid gland function, but further tests are necessary to identify the source of this dysfunction as the thyroid, pituitary, or hypothalamus.

Radioimmunoassay showing decreased plasma levels of some or all pituitary hormones, accompanied by end-organ hypofunction, suggests pituitary failure and eliminates target gland disease. Failure of thyrotropin-releasing hormone administration to increase TSH or prolactin concentrations rules out hypothalamic dysfunction as the cause of hormonal deficiency.

Provocative tests are helpful in pinpointing the source of low cortisol levels. Oral metyrapone blocks cortisol synthesis, which should stimulate pituitary secretion of corticotropin and the adrenal precursors of cortisol, measured in urine as hydroxycorticosteroids. Insulin-induced hypoglycemia also stimulates corticotropin secretion. Persistently low levels of corticotropin indicate pituitary or hypothalamic failure. These tests require careful medical supervision because they may precipitate an adrenal crisis.

Diagnosis of hypopituitarism requires measurement of hGH levels in the blood after administration of regular insulin (inducing hypoglycemia) or levodopa (causing hypotension). These drugs should provoke increased secretion of hGH. Persistently low hGH levels, despite provocative testing, confirm hGH deficiency. Computed tomography scanning, magnetic resonance imaging, or cerebral angiography confirms the presence of intrasellar or extrasellar tumors.

Management
Medication
Replacement of hormones secreted by the target glands is the most effective treatment for hypopituitarism. Hormone replacement therapy (dosage according to age and sex) includes cortisol, thyroxine, and androgen or cyclic estrogen.

Prolactin doesn't need to be replaced. The patient of reproductive age may benefit from administration of FSH and human chorionic gonadotropin to boost fertility. Replacement of hGH is recommended for adults as well as children. Replacement is done by administering daily subcutaneous injections of one of two recombinant deoxyribonucleic acid (DNA) growth hormones, accompanied by follow-up of serum insulin-like growth factor–1 levels. Lean body mass increases, whereas adipose tissue — particularly in the abdomen — decreases. Risk of cardiovascular disease and osteoporosis also decrease with treatment. Many patients also notice an improved sense of well-being.

Somatrem, which is identical to hGH but is the product of recombinant DNA technology, has replaced hGH derived from human sources. It's effective for treating dwarfism and stimulates growth increases of as much as 4″ to 6″ (10 to 15 cm) in the first year of treatment. The growth rate tapers off in subsequent years. After pubertal changes have occurred, the effects of somatrem therapy are limited. Occasionally, a child becomes unresponsive to somatrem therapy, even with larger doses, perhaps because antibodies have formed against it. In such refractory patients, small doses of androgen may again stimulate growth, but extreme caution is necessary to prevent premature closure of the epiphyses. Children with hypopituitarism may also need replacement of adrenal and thyroid hormones and, as they approach puberty, sex hormones.

Referral
▪ Refer the patient to an endocrinologist.
▪ Refer the family of a child with dwarfism to appropriate community resources for psychological counseling because the emotional stress caused by this disorder increases as the child becomes more aware of his condition.

Follow-up
The patient receiving hormonal therapy should be seen after 3 and 6 months to monitor treatment.

Patient teaching
▪ Instruct the patient to wear a medical identification bracelet. Teach him and family members how to administer steroids parenterally in case of an emergency.
▪ Teach the patient and family about any medication he'll be taking and the adverse effects to watch for and report.

Complications
▪ Blindness
▪ Adrenal crisis

Special considerations
▪ Caring for patients with hypopituitarism requires an understanding of hormonal effects and skilled physical and psychological support.

• • • • • • • • • • • • •

HYPOTHYROIDISM, ADULT

Hypothyroidism, a state of low serum thyroid hormone, results from hypothalamic, pituitary, or thyroid insufficiency. The disorder can progress to life-threatening myxedema coma. Hypothyroidism is eight times more prevalent in women.

AGE ALERT In the United States, the incidence of hypothyroidism is rising significantly in people ages 40 to 50.

Causes
Hypothyroidism results from inadequate production of thyroid hormone—usually because of dysfunction of the thyroid gland due to surgery (thyroidectomy), irradiation therapy (particularly with radioactive iodine), inflammation, chronic autoimmune thyroiditis (Hashimoto's disease) or, rarely, such conditions as amyloidosis and sarcoidosis. It may also result from pituitary failure to produce thyroid-stimulating hormone (TSH), hypothalamic failure to produce thyrotropin-releasing hormone, inborn errors of thyroid hormone synthesis, inability to synthesize thyroid hormone because of iodine deficiency (usually dietary), or the use of antithyroid medications such as propylthiouracil. In patients with hypothyroidism, infection, exposure to cold, and sedatives may precipitate myxedema coma.

Clinical presentation
Typically, the early clinical features of hypothyroidism are vague: fatigue, menstrual changes, hypercholesterolemia, forgetfulness, sensitivity to cold, unexplained weight gain, and constipation. As the disorder progresses, characteristic myxedematous signs and symptoms appear:
▪ decreasing mental stability
▪ dry, flaky, inelastic skin
▪ puffy face, hands, and feet
▪ hoarseness
▪ periorbital edema
▪ upper eyelid droop
▪ dry, sparse hair

Facial signs of myxedema

Characteristic myxedematous signs in adults include dry, flaky, inelastic skin; puffy face; and upper eyelid droop.

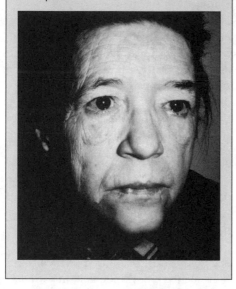

- thick, brittle nails. (See *Facial signs of myxedema.*)

Cardiovascular involvement leads to decreased cardiac output, slow pulse rate, signs of poor peripheral circulation and, occasionally, an enlarged heart. Other common effects include anorexia, abdominal distention, menorrhagia, decreased libido, infertility, ataxia, intention tremor, and nystagmus. Reflexes show delayed relaxation time (especially in the Achilles tendon).

Progression to myxedema coma is usually gradual, but when stress (such as hip fracture, infection, or myocardial infarction) aggravates severe or prolonged hypothyroidism, coma may develop abruptly. Clinical effects include progressive stupor, hypoventilation, hypoglycemia, hyponatremia, hypotension, and hypothermia.

Differential diagnoses
- Nephrotic syndrome
- Chronic autoimmune thyroiditis
- Radiation-induced thyroid damage
- Depression
- Medication-induced hypothyroidism
- Chronic nephritis
- Pituitary tumor

Diagnosis
Radioimmunoassay confirms hypothyroidism with low triiodothyronine (T_3) and thyroxine (T_4) levels.

Supportive laboratory findings include:
- increased TSH level when hypothyroidism is due to thyroid insufficiency; decreased TSH level when hypothyroidism is due to hypothalamic or pituitary insufficiency
- elevated levels of serum cholesterol, alkaline phosphatase, and triglycerides
- normocytic normochromic anemia.

In myxedema coma, laboratory tests may also show low serum sodium levels as well as decreased pH and increased partial pressure of carbon dioxide, indicating respiratory acidosis.

Management
General
During myxedema coma, effective treatment supports vital functions while restoring euthyroidism. To support blood pressure and pulse rate, treatment includes I.V. administration of levothyroxine and hydrocortisone to correct possible pituitary or adrenal insufficiency. Hypoventilation requires oxygenation and respiratory support. Other supportive measures include fluid replacement and antibiotics for infection.

Medication
Therapy for hypothyroidism consists of gradual thyroid replacement:

- levothyroxine (T_4) — 25 to 200 mcg/day P.O., increased by 25 mcg/day every 4 to 6 weeks until TSH is normal
- liothyronine (T_3) — 25 mcg/day P.O., increased by 12.5 to 25 mcg every 1 to 2 weeks until response is satisfactory.

Surgical intervention
Surgical excision, chemotherapy, or radiation may be necessary for tumors.

Referral
- The patient may need to be referred to an endocrinologist.

Follow-up
The patient should be seen every 6 weeks until his condition is stable, then every 3 to 6 months as needed.

Patient teaching
- Tell the patient to follow a high-bulk, low-calorie diet, and encourage activity to combat constipation and promote weight loss.
- After thyroid replacement therapy begins, tell the patient to watch for symptoms of hyperthyroidism, such as restlessness, sweating, and excessive weight loss.
- Tell the patient to report signs of aggravated cardiovascular disease, such as chest pain and tachycardia.
- To prevent myxedema coma, tell the patient to continue his course of thyroid medication even if his symptoms subside.
- Warn the patient to report infection immediately.

Complications
- Myxedema coma
- Adrenal crisis
- Megacolon

In patients with coronary disease
- Angina
- Cardiac arrhythmias
- Heart failure

HYPOTHYROIDISM, CONGENITAL

Deficiency of thyroid hormone secretion during fetal development or early infancy results in congenital hypothyroidism (infantile cretinism). Untreated hypothyroidism is characterized in infants by respiratory difficulties, persistent jaundice, and hoarse crying; in older children, it's characterized by stunted growth (dwarfism), bone and muscle dystrophy, and mental deficiency.

Congenital hypothyroidism is three times more common in girls than in boys. Early diagnosis and treatment allow the best prognosis; neonates treated before age 3 months usually grow and develop normally. However, athyroid children who remain untreated beyond age 3 months and children with acquired hypothyroidism who remain untreated beyond age 2 suffer irreversible mental retardation; their skeletal abnormalities are reversible with treatment.

Causes
In infants, congenital hypothyroidism usually results from defective embryonic development that causes congenital absence or underdevelopment of the thyroid gland. The next most common cause can be traced to an inherited enzymatic defect in the synthesis of thyroxine (T_4) caused by an autosomal recessive gene. Less commonly, antithyroid drugs taken during pregnancy produce congenital hypothyroidism in infants. In children older than age 2, congenital hypothyroidism usually results from chronic autoimmune thyroiditis.

Clinical presentation
The weight and length of an infant with congenital hypothyroidism appear normal at birth, but characteristic signs of

hypothyroidism develop by the time he's 3 to 6 months old. In a breast-fed infant, onset of most symptoms may be delayed until weaning because breast milk contains small amounts of thyroid hormone.

Typically, an infant with congenital hypothyroidism sleeps excessively, seldom cries (except for occasional hoarse crying), and is inactive. Because of this, his parents may describe him as a "good baby—no trouble at all." However, such behavior actually results from lowered metabolism and progressive mental impairment. The infant with congenital hypothyroidism also exhibits these signs and symptoms:

- abnormal deep tendon reflexes
- hypotonic abdominal muscles
- a protruding abdomen
- slow, awkward movements
- feeding difficulties
- constipation
- jaundice.

The infant's large, protruding tongue obstructs respiration, making breathing loud and noisy and forcing him to open his mouth to breathe. He may have dyspnea on exertion, anemia, abnormal facial features (such as a short forehead; puffy, wide-set eyes; wrinkled eyelids; a broad, short, upturned nose) and a dull expression resulting from mental retardation. His skin is cold and mottled because of poor circulation, and his hair is dry, brittle, and dull. Teeth erupt late and tend to decay early, body temperature is below normal, and pulse rate is slow.

In the child who acquires hypothyroidism after age 2, appropriate treatment can prevent mental retardation. However, growth retardation becomes apparent in short stature (due to delayed epiphyseal maturation, particularly in the legs), obesity, and a head that appears abnormally large because the arms and legs are stunted. An older child may show delayed or accelerated sexual development.

Differential diagnoses

- Chronic autoimmune thyroiditis
- Prenatal thyroid deficiency
- Congenital absence of thyroid gland
- Underdeveloped thyroid gland

Diagnosis

A high serum level of thyroid-stimulating hormone (TSH), associated with low triiodothyronine and T_4 levels, points to congenital hypothyroidism. Because early detection and treatment can minimize the effects of congenital hypothyroidism, many states require measurement of infant thyroid hormone levels at birth.

Thyroid scan and radioactive iodine (^{131}I) uptake tests show decreased uptake levels and confirm the absence of thyroid tissue in athyroid children. Increased gonadotropin levels are compatible with sexual precocity in older children and may coexist with hypothyroidism. Electrocardiography shows bradycardia and flat or inverted T waves in untreated infants. Hip, knee, and thigh X-rays reveal absence of the femoral or tibial epiphyseal line and delayed skeletal development that is markedly inappropriate for the child's chronological age. A low T_4 level associated with abnormal TSH level suggests hypothyroidism secondary to hypothalamic or pituitary disease, a rare condition.

Management
General

Early detection is mandatory to prevent irreversible mental retardation and permit normal physical development.

Medication

Treatment of infants younger than age 1 consists of replacement therapy with oral levothyroxine (25 to 50 mcg P.O. daily; children age 1 and older, 3 to 5 mcg/kg P.O. daily) doses.

Referral
- Refer the patient to an endocrinologist.
- Refer the patient and his family to appropriate community resources for support.

Patient teaching
- Inform the parents that the child will require lifelong treatment with thyroid supplements.
- Teach them to recognize signs of overdose: rapid pulse rate, irritability, insomnia, fever, sweating, and weight loss.
- Stress the need to comply with the treatment regimen to prevent further mental impairment.

Complications
- Irreversible mental retardation
- Learning disabilities
- Short stature
- Accelerated or delayed sexual maturation

Special considerations
- Provide support to help parents deal with a child with mental retardation. Help them adopt a positive but realistic attitude and focus on their child's strengths rather than his weaknesses.
- Encourage them to provide stimulating activities to help the child reach his maximum potential.

HEALTHY LIVING To prevent congenital hypothyroidism, emphasize the importance of adequate nutrition during pregnancy, including iodine-rich foods and the use of iodized salt or, in the case of sodium restriction, an iodine supplement.

•••••••••••

MAGNESIUM IMBALANCE

Magnesium is the second most common cation in intracellular fluid. Although its major function is to enhance neuromuscular integration, it also stimulates parathyroid hormone (PTH) secretion, thus regulating intracellular fluid calcium levels. Therefore, hypomagnesemia may result in transient hypoparathyroidism or interference with the peripheral action of PTH. Magnesium may also regulate skeletal muscles through its influence on calcium utilization by depressing acetylcholine release at synaptic junctions. In addition, magnesium activates many enzymes for proper carbohydrate and protein metabolism, aids in cell metabolism and the transport of sodium and potassium across cell membranes, and influences sodium, potassium, calcium, and protein levels.

Approximately one-third of magnesium taken into the body is absorbed through the small intestine and is eventually excreted in the urine; the remaining unabsorbed magnesium is excreted in the stool.

Because many common foods contain magnesium, a dietary deficiency is rare. Hypomagnesemia generally follows impaired absorption, too-rapid excretion, or inadequate intake during total parenteral nutrition. It frequently coexists with other electrolyte imbalances, especially low calcium and potassium levels. Hypermagnesemia is common in patients with renal failure and excessive intake of magnesium-containing antacids.

Causes
Hypomagnesemia usually results from impaired absorption of magnesium in the intestines or excessive excretion in urine or stool. Possible causes include:

Signs and symptoms of magnesium imbalance

DYSFUNCTION	HYPOMAGNESEMIA	HYPERMAGNESEMIA
Neuromuscular	■ Hyperirritability, tetany, leg and foot cramps, Chvostek's sign (facial muscle spasms induced by tapping the branches of the facial nerve)	■ Diminished reflexes, muscle weakness, flaccid paralysis, respiratory muscle paralysis that may cause respiratory embarrassment
Neurologic	■ Confusion, delusions, hallucinations, seizures	■ Drowsiness, flushing, lethargy, confusion, diminished sensorium
Cardiovascular	■ Arrhythmias, vasomotor changes (vasodilation and hypotension) and, occasionally, hypertension	■ Bradycardia, weak pulse, hypotension, heart block, cardiac arrest (common with serum levels of 25 mEq/L)

■ decreased magnesium intake or absorption, as in malabsorption syndrome, chronic diarrhea, or postoperative complications after bowel resection; chronic alcoholism; prolonged diuretic therapy, nasogastric suctioning, or administration of parenteral fluids without magnesium salts; and starvation or malnutrition

■ excessive loss of magnesium, as in severe dehydration and diabetic acidosis; hyperaldosteronism and hypoparathyroidism, which result in hypokalemia and hypocalcemia; hyperparathyroidism and hypercalcemia; excessive release of adrenocortical hormones; and diuretic therapy.

Hypermagnesemia results from the kidneys' inability to excrete magnesium that was either absorbed from the intestines or infused. Common causes of hypermagnesemia include:

■ chronic renal insufficiency

■ use of laxatives (magnesium sulfate, milk of magnesia, and magnesium citrate solutions), especially with renal insufficiency

■ overuse of magnesium-containing antacids

■ severe dehydration (resulting oliguria can cause magnesium retention)

■ overcorrection of hypomagnesemia.

Clinical presentation

Hypomagnesemia causes neuromuscular irritability and cardiac arrhythmias. Hypermagnesemia causes central nervous system and respiratory depression, in addition to neuromuscular and cardiac effects. (See *Signs and symptoms of magnesium imbalance.*)

Differential diagnoses

■ Respiratory failure
■ Stroke
■ Seizure disorder
■ Myocardial infarction
■ Imbalance of other electrolytes

Diagnosis

Serum magnesium levels less than 1.5 mEq/L confirm hypomagnesemia; levels greater than 2.5 mEq/L confirm hypermagnesemia.

Low levels of other serum electrolytes (especially potassium and calcium) often coexist with hypomagnesemia. In fact, unresponsiveness to correct treatment for hypokalemia strongly suggests hypomagnesemia. Similarly, elevated levels of other serum electrolytes are associated with hypermagnesemia.

Management
General
Therapy for magnesium imbalance aims to identify and correct the underlying cause. Therapy for hypermagnesemia includes increased fluid intake and loop diuretics, such as furosemide, with impaired renal function; calcium gluconate (10%), a magnesium antagonist, for temporary relief of symptoms in an emergency; and peritoneal dialysis or hemodialysis if renal function fails or if excess magnesium can't be eliminated.

Medication
■ For treatment of mild hypomagnesemia, magnesium supplements are given I.M. or P.O. depending on magnesium levels.
■ For treatment of severe hypomagnesemia, magnesium sulfate is given 1 g I.M. every 6 hours for 4 doses.
■ For treatment of magnesium intoxication, calcium gluconate is given I.V. depending on calcium levels.

Referral
■ The patient may require a referral to a specialist depending on the underlying cause of the magnesium imbalance.
■ The patient with severe magnesium imbalance should be referred to a hospital for treatment.

Follow-up
The underlying cause of the magnesium imbalance will direct follow-up care.

Patient teaching
■ Advise patients with hypomagnesemia to eat foods high in magnesium, such as fish and green vegetables.
■ Advise patients not to abuse laxatives and antacids containing magnesium, particularly the elderly or those patients with compromised renal function.

Complications
For hypomagnesemia
■ Bradycardia
■ Cardiac arrest
■ Heart block

For hypermagnesemia
■ Cardiac arrhythmias
■ Confusion
■ Seizure

Special considerations
■ The kidneys excrete excess magnesium; therefore, hypermagnesemia could occur with renal insufficiency.
■ Watch for signs of hypermagnesemia in predisposed patients. Observe closely for respiratory distress if magnesium serum levels rise above 10 mEq/L.

• • • • • • • • • • • •

MALNUTRITION, PROTEIN-CALORIE

One of the most prevalent and serious depletion disorders, protein-calorie malnutrition (PCM) occurs as marasmus (protein-calorie deficiency), which is characterized by growth failure and wasting, and as kwashiorkor (protein deficiency), which is characterized by tissue edema and damage. Both forms vary from mild to severe and may be fatal, depending on accompanying stress (particularly sepsis or injury) and duration of deprivation. PCM increases the risk of death from pneumonia, chickenpox, or measles.

Kwashiorkor (edematous PCM) and marasmus (nonedematous PCM) are common in underdeveloped countries and in areas where dietary amino acid content is insufficient to satisfy growth requirements. Kwashiorkor typically occurs at about age 1, after infants are weaned from breast milk to a protein-deficient diet of starchy gruels or sugar water, but it can develop at any time during the formative years. Marasmus affects infants ages 6 to 18 months as a result of breast-feeding failure or a debilitating condition such as chronic diarrhea.

Causes

In industrialized countries, PCM may occur secondary to chronic metabolic disease that decreases protein and calorie intake or absorption or trauma that increases protein and calorie requirements. In the United States, PCM is estimated to occur to some extent in 50% of surgical and 48% of medical patients. Those who aren't allowed anything by mouth for an extended period are at high risk for developing PCM. Conditions that increase protein-calorie requirements include severe burns and injuries, systemic infections, and cancer, which accounts for the largest group of hospitalized patients with PCM. Conditions that cause defective utilization of nutrients include malabsorption syndrome, short-bowel syndrome, and Crohn's disease.

Clinical presentation

Children with chronic PCM exhibit these signs and symptoms:
- small for chronological age
- tendency to be physically inactive
- mental apathy
- susceptibility to frequent infections
- anorexia
- diarrhea.

In acute PCM, children are small, gaunt, and emaciated, with no adipose tissue. Skin is dry and "baggy," and hair is sparse and dull brown or reddish yellow. Temperature is low; pulse rate and respirations are slowed. Such children are weak, irritable, and usually hungry, although they may have anorexia, with nausea and vomiting.

Unlike marasmus, chronic kwashiorkor allows the patient to grow in height, but adipose tissue diminishes as fat metabolizes to meet energy demands. Edema often masks severe muscle wasting; dry, peeling skin and hepatomegaly are common. Patients with secondary PCM show signs similar to marasmus, primarily loss of adipose tissue and lean body mass, lethargy, and edema. Severe secondary PCM may cause loss of immunocompetence.

Differential diagnoses

- Secondary growth failure due to malabsorption or congenital defects
- Cardiac failure
- Child abuse or neglect
- Anorexia nervosa
- Disorders of glycogen metabolism
- Cystic fibrosis
- Nephritis

Diagnosis

Clinical appearance, dietary history, and anthropometry confirm PCM. If the patient doesn't suffer from fluid retention, weight change over time is the best index of nutritional status.

These factors support the diagnosis:
- height and weight less than 80% of standard for the patient's age and sex; below-normal arm circumference and triceps skinfold
- moderate anemia
- serum albumin level less than 2.8 g/dl (normal: 3.3 to 4.3 g/dl)
- urinary creatinine (24-hour) level is used to show lean body mass status by relating creatinine excretion to height and

ideal body weight to yield creatinine-height index

■ skin tests with standard antigens to indicate degree of immunocompromise by determining reactivity expressed as a percentage of normal reaction.

Management
General
The aim of treatment is to provide sufficient proteins, calories, and other nutrients for nutritional rehabilitation and maintenance. When treating severe PCM, restoring fluid and electrolyte balance parenterally is the initial concern. A patient who shows normal absorption may receive enteral nutrition after anorexia has subsided. When possible, the preferred treatment is oral feeding of high-quality protein foods, especially milk, and protein-calorie supplements. A patient who is unwilling or unable to eat may require supplementary feedings through a nasogastric tube or total parenteral nutrition (TPN) through a central venous catheter. Cautious realimentation is essential to prevent complications from overloading the compromised metabolic system.

Medication
Medications used include antibiotics that don't inhibit protein synthesis if an infection is present and multivitamins and multiminerals for protein-calorie malnutrition.

Referral
■ Refer the patient to a nutritionist.
■ The patient may need a referral based on the underlying cause of this disorder.
■ The patient may need referral for psychological counseling.
■ The patient may need to be referred to a hospital for treatment.

Follow-up
The patient would need to be seen according to his nutritional state. If the patient is in a severely depleted nutritional state, more frequent visits would be warranted.

Patient teaching
■ Encourage the patient with PCM to consume as much nutritious food and beverage as possible. Have the family assist the patient to eat if necessary. Tell them to monitor intake.
■ If the patient is receiving parenteral nutrition at home, teach him and the family safe management techniques of the TPN and the infusion site.

Complications
■ Death
■ Electrolyte imbalance
■ Hypothermia
■ Circulatory failure

• • • • • • • • • • • •

OBESITY

Obesity is characterized by an excess of body fat, generally 20% above ideal body weight. The National Institute of Health estimates that approximately 97 million adults in the United States are overweight or obese. Approximately 22.5% are obese. The prognosis for correction of obesity is poor: Fewer than 30% of patients succeed in losing 20 lb (9 kg), and only half of these maintain the loss over a prolonged period.

Causes
Obesity results from excessive calorie intake and inadequate expenditure of energy. Theories to explain this condition include hypothalamic dysfunction of hunger and satiety centers, genetic predisposition, abnormal absorption of nu-

trients, and impaired action of GI and growth hormones and of hormonal regulators, such as insulin. An inverse relationship between socioeconomic status and the prevalence of obesity has been documented, especially in women. Obesity in parents increases the probability of obesity in children, from genetic or environmental factors, such as activity levels and learned eating patterns. Psychological factors may also contribute to obesity.

Clinical presentation

Observation and comparison of height and weight to a standard table indicate obesity. Weight alone may not be an accurate measure of obesity because muscle tissue weighs more than fat.

Differential diagnoses

- Hypothyroidism
- Eating disorder

Diagnosis

Measurement of the thickness of subcutaneous fat folds with calipers provides an approximation of total body fat (body mass index [BMI]. Although this measurement is reliable and isn't subject to daily fluctuations, it has little meaning for the patient in monitoring subsequent weight loss. A BMI of 30 or greater indicates obesity.

Management

General

Successful management of obesity must decrease the patient's daily calorie intake, while increasing his activity level. Effective treatment must be based on a balanced, low-calorie diet that eliminates foods high in fat or sugar. To achieve long-term benefits, lifelong maintenance of these improved eating and exercise patterns is necessary.

The popular low-carbohydrate diets offer no long-term advantage; rapid early weight reduction is due to loss of water, not fat. These and other crash or fad diets have the overwhelming drawback that they don't teach the patient long-term modification of eating patterns and often lead to the "yo-yo syndrome"— episodes of repeated weight loss followed by weight gain.

Total fasting is an effective method of rapid weight reduction but requires close monitoring and supervision to minimize risks of ketonemia, electrolyte imbalance, hypotension, and loss of lean body mass. Prolonged fasting and very-low-calorie diets have been associated with sudden death, possibly resulting from cardiac arrhythmias caused by electrolyte abnormalities. These methods also neglect patient reeducation, which is necessary for long-term weight maintenance.

Treatment may also include hypnosis and behavior modification techniques, which promote fundamental changes in eating habits and activity patterns. In addition, psychotherapy may be beneficial for some patients, because weight reduction may lead to depression or even psychosis.

Medication

Amphetamines and amphetamine congeners have been used to enhance compliance with a prescribed diet by temporarily suppressing the appetite and creating a feeling of well-being. However, because their value in long-term weight control is questionable and they have a significant potential for dependence and abuse, their use is generally avoided. If these drugs are used at all, they should be prescribed only for short-term therapy and should be monitored carefully.

Recently, drugs such as sibutramine hydrochloride monohydrate (Meridia) have been approved by the Food and Drug Administration for weight loss.

However, Meridia can increase blood pressure in some patients and is contraindicated in those with a history of coronary artery disease, arrhythmias, heart failure, and stroke.

Surgical intervention
As a last resort, morbid obesity (body weight 200% or greater than standard) may be treated surgically with various restrictive procedures. The two most popular procedures are vertical banded gastroplasty and gastric bypass. These procedures decrease the volume of food that the stomach can hold or bypass the stomach and thus produce satiety with small intake. The latter also induces diarrhea when concentrated sweets are ingested. These techniques cause fewer complications than jejunoileal bypass, which induces a permanent malabsorption syndrome.

Referral
- Refer the patient to a nutritionist.
- The patient may need to be referred to an endocrinologist.
- The patient may need to be referred to a weight-reduction program, such as Weight Watchers, for counseling and support.

Follow-up
The patient should be followed every 2 weeks initially, and then monthly, unless enrolled in a weight-reduction program, then follow-up would depend on the amount of weight loss needed.

Patient teaching
- Ask the patient to keep a careful record of what, where, and when he eats to help identify situations that normally provoke overeating.
- Explain the prescribed diet carefully, and encourage compliance to improve health status.

- To increase calorie expenditure, promote increased physical activity, including an exercise program. Recommend varying activity levels according to the patient's general condition and cardiovascular status.
- Teach the grossly obese patient the importance of good skin care to prevent breakdown in moist skin folds. Recommend regular use of powder to keep skin dry.
- To help prevent obesity in children, teach parents to avoid overfeeding their infants and to familiarize themselves with actual nutritional needs and optimum growth rates. Discourage parents from using food to reward or console their children, from emphasizing the importance of "cleaning plates," and from allowing eating to prevent hunger rather than to satisfy it.

Complications
- Diabetes mellitus
- Cardiovascular disease
- Hypertension
- Hyperlipidemia
- Gallbladder disease
- Sleep apnea
- Depression
- Poor self-image

Special considerations
- Obtain an accurate diet history to identify the patient's eating patterns and the importance of food to his lifestyle.

• • • • • • • • • • • •

PHEOCHROMOCYTOMA

A pheochromocytoma is a chromaffin-cell tumor of the adrenal medulla that secretes an excess of the catecholamines epinephrine and norepinephrine, which results in severe hypertension, increased metabolism, and hyperglycemia. This disorder is potentially fatal, but the prognosis is generally good with treatment. However, pheochromocytoma-induced kidney damage is irreversible.

AGE ALERT Pheochromocytoma occurs primarily between ages 30 and 40.

Causes

A pheochromocytoma may result from an inherited autosomal dominant trait. According to some estimates, about 0.5% of newly diagnosed patients with hypertension have pheochromocytoma. Although this tumor is usually benign, it may be malignant in as many as 10% of these patients. It affects all races and both sexes.

Clinical presentation

The cardinal sign of pheochromocytoma is persistent or paroxysmal hypertension. Common clinical effects include:

- palpitations
- tachycardia
- headache
- diaphoresis
- pallor
- warmth or flushing
- paresthesia
- tremor
- excitation
- fright
- nervousness
- feelings of impending doom
- abdominal pain
- tachypnea
- nausea and vomiting.

Orthostatic hypotension and paradoxical response to antihypertensive drugs are common, as are associated glycosuria, hyperglycemia, and hypermetabolism. Patients with hypermetabolism may show marked weight loss, but some patients with pheochromocytomas are obese. Symptomatic episodes may recur as seldom as once every 2 months or as

often as 25 times per day. They may occur spontaneously or may follow certain precipitating events, such as postural change, exercise, laughing, smoking, induction of anesthesia, urination, or a change in environmental or body temperature.

Pheochromocytoma is commonly diagnosed during pregnancy, when uterine pressure on the tumor induces more frequent attacks; such attacks can prove fatal for both mother and fetus as a result of cerebrovascular accident, acute pulmonary edema, cardiac arrhythmias, or hypoxia. In such patients, the risk of spontaneous abortion is high, but most fetal deaths occur during labor or immediately after birth.

Differential diagnoses

- Anxiety and panic attacks
- Labile essential hypertension
- Paroxysmal cardiac arrhythmias
- Withdrawal of adrenergic-inhibiting medications
- Hyperventilation
- Thyrotoxicosis
- Amphetamine or cocaine use
- Angina
- Sympathomimetic ingestion
- Menopausal syndrome
- Hypoglycemia
- Migraine headache

Diagnosis

The most common presentation for pheochromocytoma is continuous hypertension with or without orthostatic hypotension. A history of acute episodes of hypertension, headache, sweating, and tachycardia — particularly in a patient with hyperglycemia, glycosuria, and hypermetabolism — strongly suggests pheochromocytoma. A patient who has intermittent attacks may have no symptoms during a latent phase. The tumor is rarely palpable; when it is, palpation of the surrounding area may induce an acute attack and help confirm the diagnosis. Generally, diagnosis depends on laboratory findings. Increased urinary excretion of total free catecholamines and their metabolites, vanillylmandelic acid (VMA) and metanephrine, as measured by analysis of a 24-hour urine specimen, confirms pheochromocytoma.

Labile blood pressure necessitates urine collection during a hypertensive episode and comparison of this specimen with a baseline specimen. Direct assay of total plasma catecholamines shows levels 10 to 50 times higher than normal.

Provocative tests with glucagon and phentolamine suggest the diagnosis; however, because they may precipitate a hypertensive crisis or induce a false-positive or false-negative result, they're seldom used. The clonidine suppression test will cause decreased plasma catecholamine levels in normal patients but no change in those with pheochromocytoma. After demonstrating biochemical evidence of pheochromocytoma, computed tomography scanning or magnetic resonance imaging of the abdomen (where 95% of pheochromocytomas are located) is warranted. If a tumor isn't located—or if there is more than one—an ^{131}I-metaiodobenzylguanidine nuclear scan usually confirms the diagnosis in unclear cases. Angiography and excretory urography are no longer used; adrenal venography is used, but rarely.

Management
Medication
- If surgery isn't feasible, alpha-adrenergic blockers such as phenoxybenzamine are used; 10 mg/day P.O., increased every 2 days until blood pressure is controlled.
- Beta-adrenergic blockers such as propranolol are also used (10 mg P.O. t.i.d. to q.i.d.).

- These agents are used for hypertensive crisis:
  - phentolamine—2.5 to 5 mg by I.V. push
  - nitroprusside—0.25 to 0.3 mcg/kg/minute I.V. titrated to a maximum of 10 mcg/kg/minute.

Surgical intervention
Surgical removal of the tumor is the treatment of choice. To decrease blood pressure, alpha-adrenergic blockers are given from 1 to 2 weeks before surgery. A beta-adrenergic blocker may also be used after achieving alpha blockade. Postoperatively, I.V. fluids, plasma volume expanders, vasopressors and, possibly, transfusions may be required for hypotension. Persistent hypertension in the immediate postoperative period can occur.

Referral
- Refer the patient to a surgeon for treatment.
- If autosomal dominant transmission of pheochromocytoma is suspected, the patient's family should also be referred for genetic counseling.

Follow-up
Prior to surgery, the patient should be seen daily for blood pressure monitoring. After surgery, the patient should have 24-hour urine analysis for catecholamine and metanephrine levels for 2 consecutive weeks, then yearly if values are normal.

Patient teaching
- Tell the patient to report headaches, palpitations, nervousness, or other symptoms of an acute attack.

Complications
- Hypertensive crisis
- Pulmonary edema (with beta-adrenergic blockade)

■ Postural hypotension (with alpha-adrenergic blockade)

Special considerations

■ To ensure the reliability of urine catecholamine measurements, make sure the patient avoids foods high in vanillin (such as coffee, nuts, chocolate, and bananas) for 2 days before urine collection of VMA. Also, be aware of possible drug therapy that may interfere with the accurate determination of VMA (such as guaifenesin and salicylates).

• • • • • • • • • • • •

PHOSPHORUS IMBALANCE

Phosphorus exists primarily in inorganic combination with calcium in teeth and bones. In extracellular fluid, the phosphate ion supports several metabolic functions: utilization of B vitamins, acid-base homeostasis, bone formation, nerve and muscle activity, cell division, transmission of hereditary traits, and metabolism of carbohydrates, proteins, and fats. Renal tubular reabsorption of phosphate is inversely regulated by calcium levels — an increase in phosphorus causes a decrease in calcium. An imbalance causes hypophosphatemia or hyperphosphatemia. Incidence of hypophosphatemia varies with the underlying cause; hyperphosphatemia occurs most commonly in children, who tend to consume more phosphorus-rich foods and beverages than adults, and in children and adults with renal insufficiency. The prognosis for both conditions depends on the underlying cause.

Causes

Hypophosphatemia is usually the result of inadequate dietary intake; it's often related to malnutrition resulting from a prolonged catabolic state or chronic alcoholism. It may also stem from intestinal malabsorption, chronic diarrhea, hyperparathyroidism with resultant hypercalcemia, hypomagnesemia, or deficiency of vitamin D, which is necessary for intestinal phosphorus absorption. Other causes include chronic use of antacids containing aluminum hydroxide, use of parenteral nutrition solution with inadequate phosphate content, renal tubular defects, tissue damage in which phosphorus is released by injured cells, and diabetic acidosis.

Hyperphosphatemia is generally secondary to hypocalcemia, hypervitaminosis D, hypoparathyroidism, or renal failure (commonly due to stress or injury). It may also result from overuse of laxatives with phosphates or phosphate enemas.

Clinical presentation

Hypophosphatemia produces these signs and symptoms:
■ anorexia
■ muscle weakness
■ tremor
■ paresthesia
■ osteomalacia.

Impaired red blood cell functions may occur in hypophosphatemia due to alterations in oxyhemoglobin dissociation, which may result in peripheral hypoxia. Hyperphosphatemia usually remains asymptomatic unless it results in hypocalcemia, with tetany and seizures.

Differential diagnoses

■ Neoplasm
■ Hypocalcemia
■ Hypoparathyroidism
■ Renal failure
■ Laxative abuse
■ Alcoholism

Diagnosis

Serum phosphorus levels less than 1.7 mEq/L or 2.5 mg/dl confirm hypophos-

Foods high in phosphorus

FOOD	PORTION	AMOUNT (MG)
Almonds	⅔ cup	475
Beef liver (fried)	3½ oz	476
Broccoli (cooked)	⅔ cup	62
Carbonated beverages	12 oz	Up to 500
Milk (whole)	8 oz	93
Turkey (roasted)	3½ oz	251

phatemia. Urine phosphorus levels above 1.3 g/24 hours support this diagnosis.

Serum phosphorus levels over 2.6 mEq/L or 4.5 mg/dl confirm hyperphosphatemia. Supportive values include decreased levels of serum calcium (less than 9 mg/dl) and urine phosphorus (less than 0.9 g/24 hours).

Management
General
The treatment goal is to correct the underlying cause of phosphorus imbalance. Hypophosphatemia should be managed with a high-phosphorous diet and supplements. (See *Foods high in phosphorus*.) Severe hyperphosphatemia may require peritoneal dialysis or hemodialysis to lower the serum phosphorus level.

Medication
These supplements are given for hypophosphatemia (dosage based on phosphorous levels):
- phosphate salt tablets or capsules
- potassium phosphate infusion.

Referral
- The patient with a severe phosphorous imbalance may need to be referred to a hospital.
- Refer the patient to a dietitian if the condition results from chronic renal insufficiency.

Follow-up
The patient will need to be seen depending on the underlying cause and the severity of the phosphorous imbalance.

Patient teaching
- For hypophosphatemia, advise the patient to follow a high-phosphorus diet containing milk and milk products, kidney, liver, turkey, and dried fruits.
- For hyperphosphatemia, advise the patient to follow a low-phosphorus diet containing fruit juices, grains, and noncola soft drinks, and to avoid high-phosphorous foods.

Complications
- Respiratory failure
- Myalgia

- Malaise
- Cardiac irregularities

Special considerations
- Assess renal function, and be alert for hypocalcemia when giving phosphate supplements. If phosphate salt tablets cause nausea, use capsules instead.
- Watch for signs of hypocalcemia, such as muscle twitching and tetany, which often accompany hyperphosphatemia.

• • • • • • • • • • • •

POTASSIUM IMBALANCE

Potassium, a cation that is the dominant cellular electrolyte, facilitates contraction of both skeletal and smooth muscles—including myocardial contraction—and figures prominently in nerve impulse conduction, acid-base balance, enzyme action, and cell membrane function. Because serum potassium level has such a narrow range (3.5 to 5 mEq/L), a slight deviation in either direction can produce profound clinical consequences. Paradoxically, both hypokalemia and hyperkalemia can lead to muscle weakness and flaccid paralysis, because both create an ionic imbalance in neuromuscular tissue excitability. Both conditions also diminish excitability and conduction rate of the heart muscle, which may lead to cardiac arrest. (See *Clinical effects of potassium imbalance*.)

Causes
Because many foods contain potassium, hypokalemia seldom results from a dietary deficiency. Instead, potassium loss may result from:
- excessive GI or urinary losses, such as vomiting, gastric suction, diarrhea, dehydration, anorexia, or chronic laxative abuse

- trauma (injury, burns, or surgery), in which damaged cells release potassium, which enters serum or extracellular fluid, to be excreted in the urine
- chronic renal disease, with tubular potassium wasting
- certain drugs, especially potassium-wasting diuretics, steroids, and certain sodium-containing antibiotics (carbenicillin)
- acid-base imbalances, which cause potassium shifting into cells without true depletion in alkalosis
- prolonged potassium-free I.V. therapy
- hyperglycemia, causing osmotic diuresis and glycosuria
- Cushing's syndrome, primary hyperaldosteronism, excessive ingestion of licorice, and severe serum magnesium deficiency.

Hyperkalemia results from the kidneys' inability to excrete excessive amounts of potassium infused I.V. or administered orally; from decreased urine output, renal dysfunction or failure; or the use of potassium-sparing diuretics, such as triamterene, by patients with renal disease. It may also result from injuries or conditions that release cellular potassium or favor its retention, such as burns, crushing injuries, failing renal function, adrenal gland insufficiency, dehydration, or diabetic acidosis.

Clinical presentation
Hypokalemia may produce these clinical effects:
- acne
- constipation
- vomiting
- abdominal distention
- frequent urination with large volumes
- constant fatigue
- cardiac arrhythmias.

Hyperkalemia may cause these signs and symptoms:
- weakness

Clinical effects of potassium imbalance

DYSFUNCTION	HYPOKALEMIA	HYPERKALEMIA
Cardiovascular	▪ Dizziness, hypotension, arrhythmias, electrocardiogram (ECG) changes (flattened T waves, elevated U waves, depressed ST segment), cardiac arrest (with serum potassium levels < 2.5 mEq/L)	▪ Tachycardia and later bradycardia, ECG changes (tented and elevated T waves, widened QRS complex, prolonged PR interval, flattened or absent P waves, depressed ST segment), cardiac arrest (with levels > 7 mEq/L)
GI	▪ Nausea, vomiting, anorexia, diarrhea, abdominal distention, paralytic ileus, or decreased peristalsis	▪ Nausea, diarrhea, abdominal cramps
Musculoskeletal	▪ Muscle weakness and fatigue, leg cramps	▪ Muscle weakness, flaccid paralysis
Genitourinary	▪ Polyuria	▪ Oliguria, anuria
Neurologic	▪ Malaise, irritability, confusion, mental depression, speech changes, decreased reflexes, respiratory paralysis	▪ Hyperreflexia progressing to weakness, numbness, tingling, flaccid paralysis
Acid-base balance	▪ Metabolic alkalosis	▪ Metabolic acidosis

- tingling
- depressed reflexes
- cardiac arrhythmias.

Differential diagnoses
- Cardiac arrhythmias
- Hypocalcemia
- Secondary hypokalemia: inadequate dietary intake, laxative or diuretic use, diarrhea, vomiting, renal or adrenal disease

Diagnosis
Serum potassium levels less than 3.5 mEq/L confirm hypokalemia; serum levels greater than 5 mEq/L confirm hyperkalemia.

Additional tests may be necessary to determine the underlying cause of the imbalance.

Management
General
Hemodialysis or peritoneal dialysis aids in the removal of excess potassium. Low potassium levels may be corrected through the use of a high-potassium diet or supplements.

Medication
Dosage depends on the extent of the potassium imbalance and any medical conditions present.

For hypokalemia
- Potassium chloride I.V. or P.O.

For hyperkalemia
- 10% calcium gluconate I.V. decreases myocardial irritability and temporarily prevents cardiac arrest but doesn't correct serum potassium excess; it's also contraindicated in patients receiving cardiac glycosides.
- Sodium bicarbonate I.V. (as an emergency measure) increases pH and causes potassium to shift back into the cells.
- Insulin and 10% to 50% glucose I.V. cause potassium to move back into cells. Infusions should be followed by dextrose 5% in water because infusion of 10% to 15% glucose will stimulate secretion of endogenous insulin.
- Sodium polystyrene sulfonate 15 g P.O. or P.R. daily to q.i.d. with 70% sorbitol produces exchange of sodium ions for potassium ions in the intestine.

Referral
- The patient may need to be referred to a dietitian.
- For severe imbalances, refer the patient to a hospital for immediate treatment.

Follow-up
The patient will need to be seen according to the severity of the potassium imbalance and any medical conditions present.

Patient teaching
- To prevent hypokalemia, instruct patients (especially those predisposed to hypokalemia due to long-term diuretic therapy) to include potassium-rich foods in their diet—oranges, bananas, tomatoes, dark green leafy vegetables, milk, dried fruits, apricots, and peanuts.
- Tell patients with renal disorders to follow a low-potassium diet.

Complications
For hypokalemia
- Cardiac conduction defects or arrhythmias
- Ileus
- Muscle weakness
- Hypertension
- Renal injury
- Overcorrection of imbalance

For hyperkalemia
- Cardiac conduction defects or arrhythmias
- Death
- Hypocalcemia
- Overcorrection of imbalance

Special considerations
- Carefully monitor patients receiving cardiac glycosides because hypokalemia enhances the action of these drugs and may produce signs of digoxin toxicity (anorexia, nausea, vomiting, blurred vision, and arrhythmias).
- Watch for signs of hyperkalemia in predisposed patients, especially those with poor urine output or those receiving potassium supplements orally or I.V.

• • • • • • • • • • • •

SODIUM IMBALANCE

Sodium is the major cation (90%) in extracellular fluid; potassium is the major cation in intracellular fluid. During repolarization, the sodium-potassium pump continually shifts sodium into the cells and potassium out of the cells; during depolarization, it does the reverse. Sodium cation functions include maintaining tonicity and concentration of extracellular fluid, acid-base balance (reabsorption of sodium ion and excretion of hydrogen ion), nerve conduction and neuromuscular function, glandular secretion, and water balance. Although the body requires only 2 to 4 g of sodium daily, most Americans consume 6 to 10 g daily (mostly sodium chloride, as table salt), excreting excess sodium through the kidneys and skin.

A low-sodium diet or excessive use of diuretics may induce hyponatremia; dehydration may induce hypernatremia.

Causes
Hyponatremia can result from:
- excessive GI loss of water and electrolytes due to vomiting, suctioning, or diarrhea; excessive perspiration or fever; use of potent diuretics; or tap-water enemas. When such losses decrease circulating fluid volume, increased secretion of antidiuretic hormone (ADH) promotes maximum water reabsorption, which further dilutes serum sodium. These factors are especially likely to cause hyponatremia when combined with excessive intake of free water
- excessive drinking of water, infusion of I.V. dextrose in water without other solutes, malnutrition or starvation, and a low-sodium diet, usually in combination with one of the other causes
- trauma, surgery (wound drainage), or burns, which cause sodium to shift into damaged cells
- adrenal gland insufficiency (Addison's disease) or hypoaldosteronism
- cirrhosis of the liver with ascites
- syndrome of inappropriate antidiuretic hormone (SIADH) secretion, resulting from brain tumor, cerebrovascular accident, pulmonary disease, or neoplasm with ectopic ADH production. Certain drugs, such as chlorpropamide and clofibrate, may produce an SIADH-like syndrome.

Causes of hypernatremia include:
- decreased water intake (when severe vomiting and diarrhea cause water loss that exceeds sodium loss, serum sodium levels rise, but overall extracellular fluid volume decreases)
- excess adrenocortical hormones, as in Cushing's syndrome
- ADH deficiency (diabetes insipidus)
- salt intoxication (less common), which may be produced by excessive ingestion of table salt.

Clinical presentation
Sodium imbalance has profound physiologic effects and can induce severe central nervous system, cardiovascular, and GI abnormalities. For example, hyponatremia may cause renal dysfunction or, if serum sodium loss is abrupt or severe, seizures; hypernatremia may produce pulmonary edema, circulatory disorders, and decreased level of consciousness. (See *Clinical effects of sodium imbalance*, page 502.)

Differential diagnoses
- Diabetes insipidus
- Hyperosmotic coma
- Salt ingestion
- Hypertonic dehydration
- Secondary hyponatremia: vomiting, diarrhea, third spacing, skin loss, diuretic use
- Renal loss
- Mineralocorticoid deficiency
- Hypothyroidism

Diagnosis
Hyponatremia is defined as serum sodium level less than 135 mEq/L; hypernatremia, as serum sodium level greater than 145 mEq/L. However, additional laboratory studies are necessary to determine etiology and to differentiate between a true deficit and an apparent deficit due to sodium shift or to hypervolemia or hypovolemia. In true hyponatremia, supportive values include urine sodium greater than 100 mEq/24 hours, with low serum osmolality; in true hypernatremia, urine sodi-

Clinical effects of sodium imbalance

DYSFUNCTION	HYPONATREMIA	HYPERNATREMIA
Neurologic	▪ Anxiety, headaches, muscle twitching and weakness, seizures	▪ Fever, agitation, restlessness, seizures
Cardiovascular	▪ Hypotension; tachycardia; with severe deficit, vasomotor collapse, thready pulse	▪ Hypertension, tachycardia, pitting edema, excessive weight gain
GI	▪ Nausea, vomiting, abdominal cramps	▪ Rough, dry tongue; intense thirst
Genitourinary	▪ Oliguria or anuria	▪ Oliguria
Respiratory	▪ Cyanosis with severe deficiency	▪ Dyspnea, respiratory arrest, and death (from dramatic rise in osmotic pressure)
Cutaneous	▪ Cold, clammy skin; decreased skin turgor	▪ Flushed skin; dry, sticky mucous membranes

um level is less than 40 mEq/24 hours, with high serum osmolality.

Management
General
Therapy for mild hyponatremia usually consists of restricted free-water intake when it's due to hemodilution, SIADH, or such conditions as heart failure, cirrhosis of the liver, and renal failure. The aim of treatment of secondary hyponatremia is to correct the underlying disorder. For hypernatremia, treatment would include a sodium-restricted diet and discontinuation of drugs that promote sodium retention.

Medication
For hyponatremia
▪ Demeclocycline or lithium, which blocks ADH action in the renal tubules, can be used to promote water excretion.

▪ 3% or 5% saline solution infusion for rare instances of severe symptomatic hyponatremia, when serum sodium levels fall below 110 mEq/L

For hypernatremia
▪ Salt-free solutions (such as dextrose in water) to return serum sodium levels to normal, followed by infusion of half-normal saline solution to prevent hyponatremia.

Referral
▪ Refer the patient on maintenance dosage of diuretics to a dietitian for instruction about dietary sodium intake.
▪ If severe hyponatremia is present, refer the patient to a facility for treatment.

Follow-up
The patient will need to be seen according to the severity of the sodium imbalance and any medical conditions present.

Patient teaching
- Explain the importance of sodium restriction, and teach the patient how to plan a low-sodium diet. Closely monitor the serum sodium levels of high-risk patients.

Complications
For hyponatremia
- Hypervolemia
- Brain damage
- Death

For hypernatremia
- Seizures
- Mental retardation
- Central nervous system thrombosis or hemorrhage
- Shock

Special considerations
- Obtain a drug history to check for drugs that promote sodium retention.

• • • • • • • • • • • •

SELECTED REFERENCES

Aronson, B.S. "Update on Acute Pancreatitis," *Medsurg Nursing* 8(1):9-16, February 1999.

Bunevicius, R., et al. "Effects of Thyroxine as Compared with Thyroxine Plus Triiodothyronine in Patients with Hypothyroidism," *New England Journal of Medicine* 340(6):424-29, February 11, 1999.

Diseases, 3rd ed. Springhouse, Pa.: Springhouse Corp., 2001.

Dudek, S.G. *Nutrition Handbook for Nursing Practice*, 4th ed. Philadelphia: Lippincott Williams & Wilkins, 2001.

Fauci, A.S., et al., eds. *Harrison's Principles of Internal Medicine*, 15th ed. New York: McGraw-Hill Book Co., 2001.

Fluids & Electrolytes Made Incredibly Easy, 2nd ed. Springhouse, Pa.: Springhouse Corp., 2001.

Handbook of Geriatric Nursing Care. Springhouse, Pa.: Springhouse Corp., 1999.

Heitz, U.E., et al. *Pocket Guide to Fluid, Electrolyte, and Acid-Base Balance*, 4th ed. St. Louis: Mosby–Year Book Inc., 2000.

Katz, D.L. *Nutrition in Clinical Practice*. Philadelphia: Lippincott Williams & Wilkins, 2001.

Mahan, L.K., and Escott-Stump, S. *Krause's Food, Nutrition, and Diet Therapy*, 10th ed. Philadelphia: W.B. Saunders Co., 2000.

Rakel, R.E., ed. *Conn's Current Therapy, 2001*. Philadelphia: W.B. Saunders Co., 2001.

Smeltzer, S., and Bare, B. *Brunner & Suddarth's Textbook of Medical-Surgical Nursing*, 9th ed. Philadelphia: Lippincott Williams & Wilkins, 2000.

Reproductive disorders

Because misinformation and cultural taboos surround the reproductive system, reproductive disorders present a formidable challenge. Patients with such disorders as impotence, abnormal uterine bleeding, and infertility require sensitive counseling and straightforward teaching. You'll have to help many of these patients overcome feelings of vulnerability, guilt, and embarrassment.

• • • • • • • • • • • • •

ASSESSMENT

Assessing the reproductive system is an essential — but potentially uncomfortable — part of a health assessment. Performed with sensitivity and tact, your assessment may uncover important information and concerns that the patient was previously unwilling to share.

Physical examination

For the male patient, physical assessment involves inspecting and palpating the groin, penis, and scrotum. If the patient is over age 40 or has a high likelihood of having prostate problems, you'll also palpate the prostate gland. For the female patient, assessment may involve the external genitalia or a complete gynecologic examination.

Examining the male patient

Instruct the patient to urinate before the examination and to undress and put on a gown.

Explain each step before performing it, and expose only the necessary areas.

Inspection

To begin physical assessment of the male reproductive system, inspect the patient's genitals and inguinal area.

Penis

Evaluate the color and integrity of the penile skin. This should appear loose and wrinkled over the shaft, and taut and smooth over the glans penis. The skin should be pink to light brown in whites and light to dark brown in blacks and free from scars, lesions, ulcers, or breaks.

Ask an uncircumcised patient to retract his prepuce to expose the glans penis. The urethral meatus, a slitlike opening, should be located at the tip of the glans. The urethral meatus should have no discharge.

Scrotum
Evaluate the amount, distribution, color, and texture of pubic hair. Inspect the scrotal skin for obvious lesions, ulcerations, induration, or reddened areas, and evaluate the scrotal sac for symmetry and size. It should be coarse and more deeply pigmented than the body skin. The left testis usually hangs slightly lower than the right.

Inguinal area
Check this area for obvious bulges — a sign of hernias. Then ask the patient to bear down as you inspect again. Also check for enlarged lymph nodes, a sign of infection.

Palpation
After inspection, palpate the penis and scrotum for structural abnormalities; then palpate the inguinal area for hernias.

Penis
To palpate this organ, gently grasp the shaft between the thumb and first two fingers and palpate along its entire length, noting any indurated, tender, or lumpy areas. The flaccid penis should feel soft and have no nodules.

Scrotum
Palpate the scrotum, also using the thumb and first two fingers. Begin by feeling the scrotal skin for nodules, lesions, or ulcers.

Next, palpate the scrotal sac. Normally, the right and left halves of the sac have identical contents and feel the same. Their surface should feel smooth and even in contour. Slight compression of the testes should elicit a dull, aching

sensation that radiates to the patient's lower abdomen. This pressure-pain sensation shouldn't occur when the other structures are compressed. No other pain or tenderness should be present.

The absence of a testis may result from temporary migration. This contraction is normal and may occur at any time during the assessment.

Palpate the epididymis on the posterolateral surface by grasping each testis between the thumb and forefinger and feeling from the epididymis to the spermatic cord or vas deferens up to the inguinal ring. The epididymis should feel like a ridge of tissue lying vertically on the testicular surface. The vas deferens should feel like a smooth cord and be freely movable. The arteries, veins, lymph vessels, and nerves may feel like indefinite threads.

Transilluminate any swellings, lumps, or nodular areas. If the swollen area contains serous fluid, it will glow orange-red; if it contains blood or tissue, it won't. Describe a lump or mass anywhere in the scrotal sac according to its placement, size, shape, consistency, tenderness, and response to transillumination.

Inguinal area
Palpate this area for hernias. (See *Palpating the inguinal area*, page 506.)

Examining the female patient
Preparing for the assessment
Before beginning the assessment, gather the necessary equipment and supplies.

If this is the patient's first gynecologic assessment, explain the procedure so she knows what to expect. Tell her to empty her bladder before the examination begins.

Palpating the inguinal area

Palpate the inguinal area to assess for inguinal and femoral hernias.

INGUINAL HERNIAS

To palpate for an inguinal hernia, first place the index and middle finger of each hand over each external inguinal ring and ask the patient to bear down or cough to increase intra-abdominal pressure momentarily. Then, with the patient relaxed, gently insert the middle or index finger (if the patient is an adult) or the little finger (if the patient is a young child) into the scrotal sac and follow the spermatic cord upward to the external inguinal ring, to an opening just above and lateral to the pubic tubercle known as Hesselbach's triangle. Holding the finger at this spot, ask the patient to bear down or cough again. A hernia will feel like a mass or bulge.

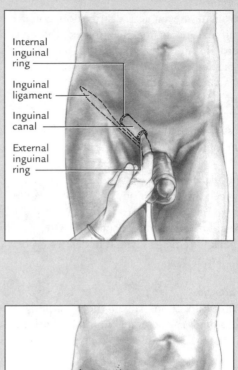

Internal inguinal ring

Inguinal ligament

Inguinal canal

External inguinal ring

FEMORAL HERNIAS

To palpate for a femoral hernia, place your right hand on the patient's thigh, with the index finger over the femoral artery. The femoral canal is then under the ring finger in an adult patient and between the index and ring finger in a child. A hernia here will feel like a soft bulge or mass.

Femoral vein

Femoral artery

Positioning

The patient usually must assume the lithotomy position for the assessment. Her heels should be secure in the stirrups and her knees comfortably placed in the knee supports if they are used. Adjust the foot or knee supports so that the legs are comfortably separated and balanced.

The patient's buttocks must extend about ½" (1.3 cm) over the table end.

The hips and knees will be flexed and the thighs abducted. A pillow placed beneath her head may help her to relax the abdominal muscles. Raising the head of the examination table helps maintain eye contact and doesn't hinder the examination.

Beginning the assessment

Describe what the patient will feel. Show her how to relax by inhaling slowly and deeply through the nose, exhaling through the mouth, and concentrating on breathing regularly to relax the muscles. If the patient begins to tense up, remind her to breathe and relax. Assure the patient that the assessment takes little time and that she'll be told what to expect before each new step. (See *Avoiding embarrassment*.)

If the examiner is male, a female assistant should attend the examination for the patient's comfort and the examiner's legal protection.

Inspection

Sometimes only the patient's external genitalia need be inspected to determine the origin of sores or itching.

Place the patient in a supine position with the pubic area uncovered, and begin the assessment by determining sexual maturity. Inspect pubic hair for amount and pattern. It's usually thick and appears on the mons pubis as well as the inner aspects of the upper thighs. Using a gloved index finger and thumb, gently spread the labia majora and look for the labia minora. The labia should be pink and moist with no lesions. Normal cervical discharge varies in color and consistency; it's clear and stretchy before ovulation, white and opaque after ovulation, and usually odorless and nonirritating to the mucosa. No other discharge should be present. Specimens of all dis-

> ## Avoiding embarrassment
>
> Occasionally, a male patient may be uncomfortable being examined by a female, and a female patient may feel the same way about a male. If the male patient objects to being examined by a female, a male nurse practitioner should perform the examination. Likewise, if a female patient objects to being examined by a male, a female nurse practitioner should perform the examination.
>
> Remember, if the examiner is male, a female assistant should attend the examination for the patient's emotional comfort and the examiner's legal protection.

charges should be cultured or examined microscopically in the laboratory.

Gynecologic assessment

In some facilities, you may perform complete gynecologic assessments. As part of this assessment, obtain a Papanicolaou test after inspecting the cervix. (Obtain the test before touching the cervix in any manner.) Also obtain other specimens if an abnormal cervical or vaginal discharge indicates infection.

• • • • • • • • • • • •

ABNORMAL PREMENOPAUSAL BLEEDING

Abnormal premenopausal bleeding refers to bleeding that deviates from the normal menstrual cycle before menopause. These deviations include menstrual bleeding that is abnormally infrequent (oligomenorrhea), abnormally frequent (polymenorrhea), excessive (menorrhagia or hypermenorrhea), deficient (hypomenorrhea), or irregular (metrorrhagia [uterine bleeding between menses]). Rarely, menstrual symptoms aren't accompanied by external bleeding (cryptomenorrhea). Premenopausal bleeding may merely be troublesome or can result in severe hemorrhage; the prognosis depends on the underlying cause. In many instances, abnormal bleeding patterns often respond to hormonal or other therapy.

Causes
Causes of abnormal premenopausal bleeding vary with the type of bleeding:
- Oligomenorrhea and polymenorrhea usually result from anovulation due to an endocrine or systemic disorder.
- Menorrhagia usually results from local lesions, such as uterine leiomyomas, endometrial polyps, and endometrial hyperplasia. It may also result from endometritis, salpingitis, and anovulation.
- Hypomenorrhea results from local, endocrine, or systemic disorders or from blockage due to partial obstruction by the hymen or to cervical obstruction.
- Cryptomenorrhea may result from an imperforate hymen or cervical stenosis.
- Metrorrhagia usually results from slight physiologic bleeding from the endometrium during ovulation but may also result from local disorders, such as uterine malignancy, cervical erosions, polyps (which tend to bleed after intercourse), or inappropriate estrogen therapy. Complications of pregnancy can also cause premenopausal bleeding. Such bleeding may be as mild as spotting or as severe as menorrhagia. (See *Causes of abnormal premenopausal bleeding.*)

Clinical presentation
Bleeding not associated with abnormal pregnancy is usually painless, but it may be severely painful. When bleeding is associated with abnormal pregnancy, other symptoms include:
- nausea
- breast tenderness
- bloating
- fluid retention.

Severe or prolonged bleeding causes anemia, especially in patients with underlying disease (such as blood dyscrasia) and in patients receiving anticoagulants.

Differential diagnoses
- Ectopic pregnancy
- Leiomyoma
- Adenomyosis
- Endometrial polyps, carcinoma
- Endometriosis
- Coagulation defects
- Ovarian abnormalities
- Thyroid dysfunction
- Stress
- Drug use
- Morbid obesity

Diagnosis
The typical clinical picture confirms abnormal premenopausal bleeding. Special tests identify the underlying cause:
- Serum hormone levels reflect adrenal, pituitary, or thyroid dysfunction.
- Urinary 17-ketosteroids reveal adrenal hyperplasia, hypopituitarism, or polycystic ovarian disease.
- Endometrial sampling rules out malignant tumors and should be performed in all patients with premenopausal bleeding.
- Pelvic examination, Papanicolaou (Pap) test, and patient history rule out local or malignant causes.
- Complete blood count rules out anemia.

If testing rules out pelvic and hormonal causes of abnormal bleeding, a complete hematologic survey (including platelet count and bleeding time) is appropriate to determine clotting abnormalities.

Causes of abnormal premenopausal bleeding

	HYPOMENORRHEA	OLIGOMENORRHEA	METRORRHAGIA	POLYMENORRHEA	MENORRHAGIA
Malnutrition	●	●			
Hyperthyroidism	●	●			
Hypothyroidism				●	●
Severe psychological trauma	●	●			●
Blood dyscrasias			●	●	●
Severe infections	●	●			
Endometritis			●		
Drugs (such as cardiac glycosides, corticosteroids, anticoagulants)				●	
Uterine tumors			●		●

Management
General
Treatment depends on the type of bleeding abnormality and its cause. Menstrual irregularity alone may not require therapy unless it interferes with the patient's attempt to achieve or avoid conception or leads to anemia.

Medication
These medications may be given for abnormal premenopausal bleeding:
- oral contraceptives (low dose)
- clomiphene — 50 mg/day P.O. for 5 days starting on day 5 of the menstrual cycle induces ovulation
- progesterone — 5 to 10 mg/day I.M. for six days
- ferrous sulfate — 300 mg P.O. b.i.d.

Surgical intervention
Electrocautery, chemical cautery, or cryosurgery can remove cervical polyps; dilatation and curettage can remove uterine polyps. Organic disorders (such as cervical or uterine malignancy) may necessitate hysterectomy, radium or X-ray therapy, or both of these treatments, depending on the site and extent of the disease. Of course, anemia and infections require appropriate treatment.

Referral
■ Refer the patient to a gynecologist if abnormal bleeding continues.

Follow-up
The patient should have regular yearly check-ups unless anemia is present; then the patient should be monitored every 3 to 6 months to evaluate treatment.

Patient teaching
■ If a patient complains of abnormal bleeding, tell her to record the dates of the bleeding and the number of tampons or pads she uses per day. This helps to assess the cyclic pattern and the amount of bleeding.
■ Instruct the patient to report abnormal bleeding immediately to help rule out major hemorrhagic disorders such as those that occur in abnormal pregnancy.
■ Explain how to take medications (such as oral contraceptives) in order for them to be effective.

Complications
■ Anemia
■ Adverse effects of medication

HEALTHY LIVING To prevent abnormal bleeding due to organic causes, and for early detection of malignancy, encourage the patient to have a Pap test and a pelvic examination annually.

• • • • • • • • • • • •

AMENORRHEA

Amenorrhea is the abnormal absence or suppression of menstruation. Primary amenorrhea is the absence of menarche in an adolescent (by age 18). Secondary amenorrhea is the failure of menstruation for at least 3 months after normal onset of menarche.

Causes and pathophysiology
Amenorrhea is normal before puberty, after menopause, or during pregnancy and breast-feeding; it's pathologic at any other time. It usually results from anovulation due to hormonal abnormalities, such as decreased secretion of estrogen, gonadotropins, luteinizing hormone, and follicle-stimulating hormone; lack of ovarian response to gonadotropins; or constant presence of progesterone or other endocrine abnormalities.

Amenorrhea may also result from the absence of a uterus, endometrial damage, or from ovarian, adrenal, or pituitary tumors. It's also linked to emotional disorders and is common in patients with such severe disorders as depression and anorexia nervosa. Mild emotional disturbances tend merely to distort the ovulatory cycle, while severe psychic trauma may abruptly change the bleeding pattern or may completely suppress one or more full ovulatory cycles. Amenorrhea may also result from malnutrition, intense exercise, and prolonged use of oral contraceptives.

Clinical presentation
Clinical features of amenorrhea include:
■ failure to menstruate
■ change in menstrual pattern.

Differential diagnoses
■ Pregnancy
■ Imperforate hymen
■ Cervical stenosis
■ Menopause
■ Premature ovarian failure
■ Hyperprolactinemia
■ Gonadal dysgenesis
■ Missed abortion
■ Inhibited gonadotropin-releasing hormone

Diagnosis

A history of failure to menstruate in a female over age 18 confirms primary amenorrhea.

Secondary amenorrhea can be diagnosed when a change is noted in a previously established menstrual pattern (absence of menstruation for 3 months). A thorough physical and pelvic examination rules out pregnancy, as well as anatomic abnormalities (such as cervical stenosis) that may cause false amenorrhea (cryptomenorrhea), in which menstruation occurs without external bleeding.

Onset of menstruation within 1 week after administration of pure progestational agents, such as medroxyprogesterone and progesterone, indicates a functioning uterus. If menstruation doesn't occur, special diagnostic studies are appropriate.

Blood and urine studies may reveal hormonal imbalances, such as lack of ovarian response to gonadotropins (elevated pituitary gonadotropins), failure of gonadotropin secretion (low pituitary gonadotropin levels), and abnormal thyroid levels. Tests for identification of dominant or missing hormones include examination for cervical mucus ferning, vaginal cytologic examinations, basal body temperature, endometrial biopsy (during dilatation and curettage), urinary 17-ketosteroid levels, and plasma progesterone, testosterone, and androgen levels. A complete medical workup, including appropriate X-rays, laparoscopy, and biopsy, may detect ovarian, adrenal, and pituitary tumors.

Management
General

Treatment of amenorrhea not related to hormone deficiency depends on the cause.

Medication

These medications may be given for amenorrhea:
- medroxyprogesterone — 5 mg/day P.O. b.i.d. for 5 days
- conjugated estrogens — 25 mg I.V. or I.M. repeated in 6 to 12 hours p.r.n.
- calcium supplement — 1,500 mg/day P.O. if the cause is hypoestrogenism.

Surgical intervention

Amenorrhea that results from a tumor usually requires surgery. A hymenectomy would need to be done if the cause of amenorrhea is imperforate hymen.

Referral

- The patient may need a referral to a gynecologist once pregnancy or menopause has been ruled out as the cause of amenorrhea.
- Psychiatric counseling may be necessary if amenorrhea results from emotional disturbances.

Follow-up

After the workup is complete, the patient should be seen yearly.

Patient teaching

- After treatment, teach the patient how to keep an accurate record of her menstrual cycles to aid early detection of recurrent amenorrhea.
- Instruct the patient how to take all medication appropriately and tell her about any adverse effects that may occur.

Complications

- Estrogen deficiency syndrome
- Osteoporosis

Chancroidal lesion

Chancroid produces a soft, painful chancre, similar to that of syphilis. Without treatment, it may progress to inguinal adenitis and formation of buboes (enlarged, inflamed lymph nodes).

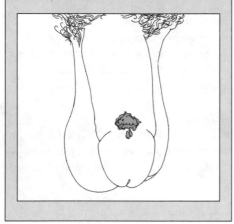

• • • • • • • • • • • •

CHANCROID

Chancroid (also known as soft chancre) is a sexually transmitted disease (STD) characterized by painful genital ulcers and inguinal adenitis. This infection occurs worldwide but is particularly common in tropical countries; it affects more males than females. Chancroidal lesions may heal spontaneously and usually respond well to treatment in the absence of secondary infections. A high rate of human immunodeficiency virus (HIV) infection has been reported among patients with chancroid.

Causes

Chancroid results from *Haemophilus ducreyi*, a gram-negative streptobacillus, and is transmitted through sexual contact. Poor hygiene may predispose males—especially those who are uncircumcised—to this disease.

Clinical presentation

After a 3- to 5-day incubation period, a small papule appears at the entry site, usually the groin or inner thigh; in the male, it may appear on the penis; in the female, on the vulva, vagina, or cervix. (See *Chancroidal lesion.*) Occasionally, this papule may erupt on the tongue, lip, breast, or navel. The papule rapidly ulcerates, becoming painful, soft, and malodorous; it bleeds easily and produces pus. It's gray and shallow, with irregular edges, and measures up to 1″ (2.5 cm) in diameter. Within 2 to 3 weeks, inguinal adenitis develops, creating suppurated, inflamed nodes that may rupture into large ulcers or buboes. Headache and malaise occur in 50% of patients. During the healing stage, phimosis may develop.

Differential diagnoses

- Syphilis
- Genital herpes
- Granuloma inguinale

Diagnosis

Gram stain smears of ulcer exudate or bubo aspirate are 50% reliable; blood agar cultures are 75% reliable. Biopsy confirms the diagnosis but is reserved for resistant cases or cases in which cancer is suspected. Dark-field examination and serologic testing rule out other STDs that cause similar ulcers. Testing for HIV infection should be done at the time of diagnosis.

Management
Medication

These medications may be given in the treatment of chancroid:

- azithromycin—1 g P.O. in a single dose

- erythromycin — 500 mg P.O. q.i.d. for 7 to 14 days
- ceftriaxone — 250 mg I.M. in a single dose.

Surgical intervention
Aspiration of fluid-filled nodes helps prevent spread of the infection.

Referral
- If the patient isn't responding to treatment, refer him to an infectious disease specialist.

Follow-up
The patient should be seen 1 week following initiation of treatment, and then in 3 months for HIV testing.

Patient teaching
- Instruct the patient not to apply lotions, creams, or oils on or near the genitalia or on other lesion sites.
- Tell the patient to abstain from sexual contact until healing is complete (usually about 2 weeks after treatment begins) and to wash the genitalia daily with soap and water. Instruct uncircumcised males to retract the foreskin for thorough cleaning.
- To prevent chancroid, advise patients to avoid sexual contact with infected people, to use condoms during sexual activity, and to wash the genitalia with soap and water after sexual activity.

Complications
- Phimosis
- Balanoposthitis
- Rupture of buboes
- Increased risk of HIV

•••••••••••••

CHLAMYDIAL INFECTIONS

Chlamydial infections — including urethritis in men and urethritis and cervicitis in women — are a group of infections that are linked to one organism: *Chlamydia trachomatis*. These infections are the most common sexually transmitted diseases in the United States, affecting an estimated 4 million Americans each year.

Trachoma inclusion conjunctivitis, a chlamydial infection that seldom occurs in the United States, is a leading cause of blindness in Third World countries. Lymphogranuloma venereum, a rare disease in the United States, is also caused by *C. trachomatis*. (See *Lymphogranuloma venereum*, page 514.)

Causes
Transmission of *C. trachomatis* primarily follows vaginal or rectal intercourse or orogenital contact with an infected person. Because symptoms of chlamydial infections commonly appear late in the course of the disease, sexual transmission of the organism typically occurs unknowingly.

Children born of mothers who have chlamydial infections may contract associated conjunctivitis, otitis media, and pneumonia during passage through the birth canal.

Clinical presentation
Men and women with chlamydial infections may be asymptomatic or may show signs of infection on physical examination. Individual signs and symptoms vary with the specific type of chlamydial infection and are determined by the organism's transmission route to susceptible tissue:
- Women who have cervicitis may develop cervical erosion, mucopurulent discharge, pelvic pain, and dyspareunia.

Lymphogranuloma venereum

A rare disease in the United States, lymphogranuloma venereum (LGV) is caused by serovars L_1, L_2, or L_3 of *Chlamydia trachomatis*. The most common clinical manifestation of LGV among heterosexuals, especially male patients, is enlarged inguinal lymph nodes (usually unilateral). These nodes may become fluctuant, tender masses. Regional nodes draining the initial lesion may enlarge and appear as a series of bilateral buboes. Untreated buboes may rupture and form sinus tracts that discharge a thick, yellow, granular secretion.

Women and homosexually active men may have proctocolitis or inflammatory involvement of perirectal or perianal lymphatic tissues, resulting in fistulas and strictures.

DIAGNOSIS

By the time most patients seek treatment, the self-limited genital ulcer that sometimes occurs at the site of inoculation is no longer present. The diagnosis usually is made serologically and by excluding other causes of inguinal lymphadenopathy or genital ulcers.

TREATMENT

The treatment of choice is doxycycline. Treatment cures infection and prevents ongoing tissue damage, although the patient may develop a scar or an indurated inguinal mass. Buboes may require aspiration or incision and drainage through intact skin.

■ Women who have endometritis or salpingitis may experience signs of pelvic inflammatory disease (PID), such as pain and tenderness of the abdomen, cervix, uterus, and lymph nodes; chills; fever; breakthrough bleeding; bleeding after intercourse; and vaginal discharge. They may also have dysuria.
■ Women with urethral syndrome may experience dysuria, pyuria, and urinary frequency.
■ Men who have urethritis may experience dysuria, erythema, tenderness of the urethral meatus, urinary frequency, pruritus, and urethral discharge. In urethritis, such discharge may be copious and purulent or scant and clear or mucoid.
■ Men with epididymitis may experience painful scrotal swelling and urethral discharge.
■ Men who have prostatitis may have low back pain, urinary frequency, dysuria, nocturia, and painful ejaculation.
■ In proctitis, patients may have diarrhea, tenesmus, pruritus, bloody or mucopurulent discharge, and diffuse or discrete ulceration in the rectosigmoid colon.

Differential diagnoses

■ Gonorrhea
■ Macropurulent cervicitis
■ Salpingitis
■ PID

Diagnosis

A swab from the infection site (urethra, cervix, or rectum) establishes a diagnosis of urethritis, cervicitis, salpingitis, endometritis, or proctitis. A culture of aspirated material establishes a diagnosis of epididymitis.

Antigen detection methods, including the enzyme-linked immunosorbent assay and the direct fluorescent antibody test, have long been used for identifying chlamydial infection. Tissue cell cultures, however, are more sensitive and specific. Newer nucleic acid probes using polymerase chain reactions are also commercially available and have become the diagnostic tests of choice.

Management
Medication
These medications may be given for chlamydial infection:
- doxycycline — 100 mg/day P.O. for 7 days
- azithromycin — 1 g P.O. in a single dose
- erythromycin — 500 mg P.O. q.i.d. for 7 days.

Referral
- Refer the patient to a gynecologist or an infectious disease specialist if not responding to treatment.
- If the problem is recurrent, refer the patient for risk-reduction counseling.

Follow-up
The patient may be retested after treatment, but it isn't routine.

Patient teaching
- Make sure the patient fully understands the dosage requirements of any prescribed medication for this infection.
- Stress the importance of completing the entire course of drug therapy, even after the symptoms subside.
- Teach the patient to follow meticulous personal hygiene measures as recommended.
- To prevent eye contamination, instruct the patient to avoid touching any discharge and to wash and dry his hands thoroughly before touching his eyes.
- To prevent reinfection during treatment, urge the patient to abstain from intercourse until he and his partner are cured.

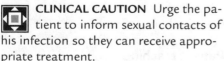 **CLINICAL CAUTION** Urge the patient to inform sexual contacts of his infection so they can receive appropriate treatment.

Complications
- Increased risk of human immunodeficiency virus (HIV)

Male
- Transient oligospermia
- Acute epididymitis

Female
- Tubal infertility
- Tubal pregnancy
- Chronic pelvic pain
- PID
- Sterility
- Salpingitis

Special considerations
- If required in your state, report all cases of chlamydial infection to the appropriate local public health authorities, who will then conduct follow-up notification of the patient's sexual contacts.
- Suggest that the patient and his sexual partners receive HIV testing.
- Check neonates of infected mothers for signs of chlamydial infection. Obtain appropriate specimens for diagnostic testing.

• • • • • • • • • • • •

DYSFUNCTIONAL UTERINE BLEEDING

Dysfunctional uterine bleeding (DUB) refers to abnormal endometrial bleeding without recognizable organic lesions. The prognosis varies with the cause. DUB is the indication for almost 25% of gynecologic surgical procedures.

Causes
DUB usually results from an imbalance in the hormonal-endometrial relationship, where persistent and unopposed stimulation of the endometrium by estrogen occurs. Disorders that cause sustained high estrogen levels are polycystic

ovary syndrome, obesity, immaturity of the hypothalamic-pituitary-ovarian mechanism (in postpubertal teenagers), and anovulation (in women in their late 30s or early 40s).

In most cases of DUB, the endometrium shows no pathologic changes. However, in chronic unopposed estrogen stimulation (as from a hormone-producing ovarian tumor), the endometrium may show hyperplastic or malignant changes.

Clinical presentation

DUB usually occurs as one or more of the following:
■ metrorrhagia (episodes of vaginal bleeding between menses)
■ hypermenorrhea (heavy or prolonged menses, longer than 8 days)
■ chronic polymenorrhea (menstrual cycle of less than 18 days).

Differential diagnoses

■ Pregnancy
■ Ectopic pregnancy
■ Leiomyoma
■ Endometriosis
■ Thyroid dysfunction
■ Drugs
■ Morbid obesity
■ Ovarian abnormalities
■ Endometrial polyps, carcinoma
■ Coagulation defects
■ Stress

Diagnosis

Diagnostic studies must rule out other causes of excessive vaginal bleeding. Dilatation and curettage (D&C) and biopsy results confirm the diagnosis by revealing endometrial hyperplasia. Hysteroscopy is a visualization of the endometrium through a scope to identify polyps, fibroids, or structural abnormalities.

Hemoglobin levels and hematocrit determine the need for blood or iron replacement.

Management

General

Regardless of the primary treatment, the patient may need iron replacement or transfusions of packed cells or whole blood, as indicated, because of anemia caused by recurrent bleeding.

Medication

These medications are given in the treatment of DUB:
■ oral contraceptives — a high dose q.i.d. for 5 to 7 days, then continue in usual fashion
■ medroxyprogesterone — 10 mg/day P.O. on cycle days 16 to 25 of each month
■ conjugated estrogens —25 mg I.V. or I.M. repeated in 6 to 12 hours p.r.n.
■ ferrous sulfate — 300 mg P.O. b.i.d.

Surgical intervention

In patients over age 35, endometrial biopsy is necessary before the start of estrogen therapy to rule out endometrial adenocarcinoma.

If drug therapy is ineffective, a D&C serves as a supplementary treatment, through removal of a large portion of the bleeding endometrium. Also, a D&C can help determine the original cause of hormonal imbalance and can aid in planning further therapy.

Referral

■ The patient may need to be referred to a gynecologist if treatment is ineffective.

Follow-up

The patient may need to be reevaluated if bleeding continues; otherwise, an annual check-up is appropriate.

Patient teaching

■ Explain the importance of adhering to the prescribed hormonal therapy. If a

D&C is ordered, explain this procedure and its purpose.
- Stress the need for regular checkups to assess the treatment's effectiveness.

Complications
- Anemia
- Adenocarcinoma
- Adverse effects of prescribed medication

• • • • • • • • • • • •

DYSMENORRHEA

Dysmenorrhea— painful menstruation—is the most common gynecologic complaint and a leading cause of absenteeism from school (affecting 10% of high school girls each month) and work (causing about 140 million lost work hours annually). Dysmenorrhea can occur as a primary disorder or secondary to an underlying disease. Because primary dysmenorrhea is self-limiting, the prognosis is generally good. The prognosis for secondary dysmenorrhea depends on the underlying disorder.

Causes
Although primary dysmenorrhea has no known single cause, possible contributing factors include hormonal imbalances and psychogenic factors. The pain of dysmenorrhea probably results from increased prostaglandin secretion, which intensifies normal uterine contractions. (See *Causes of pelvic pain.*) Dysmenorrhea may also be secondary to such gynecologic disorders as endometriosis, cervical stenosis, uterine leiomyomas, uterine malposition, pelvic inflammatory disease, pelvic tumors, or adenomyosis.

Because dysmenorrhea almost always follows an ovulatory cycle, both the primary and secondary forms are rare during

Causes of pelvic pain

The characteristic pelvic pain of dysmenorrhea must be distinguished from the acute pain caused by many other disorders, such as:
- GI disorders — appendicitis, acute diverticulitis, acute or chronic cholecystitis, chronic cholelithiasis, acute pancreatitis, peptic ulcer perforation, intestinal obstruction
- urinary tract disorders — cystitis, renal calculi
- reproductive disorders — acute salpingitis, chronic inflammation, degenerating fibroid, ovarian cyst torsion
- pregnancy disorders — impending abortion (pain and bleeding early in pregnancy), ectopic pregnancy, abruptio placentae, uterine rupture, leiomyoma degeneration, toxemia
- emotional conflicts — psychogenic (functional) pain.

Other conditions that may mimic dysmenorrhea include ovulation and normal uterine contractions experienced in pregnancy.

the anovulatory cycles of menses. After age 20, dysmenorrhea is generally secondary.

Clinical presentation
Dysmenorrhea produces sharp, intermittent, cramping, lower abdominal pain, which usually radiates to the back, thighs, groin, and vulva. Such pain— sometimes compared to labor pains— typically starts with or immediately before menstrual flow and peaks within 24 hours. Dysmenorrhea may also be associated with the characteristic signs and symptoms of premenstrual syndrome.

Differential diagnoses
- Endometriosis
- Obstructive defects
- Adenomyosis
- Leiomyoma
- Pelvic inflammatory disease
- Pelvic tumors
- Urinary tract infection
- Endometrial polyps, carcinoma

Diagnosis
Pelvic examination and a detailed patient history may help suggest the cause of dysmenorrhea.

Primary dysmenorrhea is diagnosed when secondary causes are ruled out. Appropriate tests (such as laparoscopy, dilatation and curettage, and pelvic ultrasound) are used to diagnose underlying disorders in secondary dysmenorrhea.

Management
General
Initial treatment aims to relieve pain. Pain-relief measures may include heat applied locally to the lower abdomen (may relieve discomfort in mature women but isn't recommended in young adolescents because appendicitis may mimic dysmenorrhea) and medication. Because persistently severe dysmenorrhea may have a psychogenic cause, psychological evaluation and appropriate counseling may be helpful.

Medication
These medications may be used to treat dysmenorrhea:
- aspirin — 325 to 650 mg P.O. every 4 hours p.r.n. for mild to moderate pain (most effective when taken 24 to 48 hours before onset of menses; is especially effective for treating dysmenorrhea because it also inhibits prostaglandin synthesis)
- naproxen sodium — 550 mg initially, then 275 mg P.O. every 6 to 8 hours
- ibuprofen — 400 mg P.O. q.i.d.

For primary dysmenorrhea, administration of sex steroids is an effective alternative to treatment with antiprostaglandins or analgesics, to relieve pain by suppressing ovulation. However, patients who are attempting pregnancy should rely on antiprostaglandin therapy instead of oral contraceptives to relieve symptoms of primary dysmenorrhea.

Surgical intervention
In secondary dysmenorrhea, treatment is designed to identify and correct the underlying cause. This may include surgical treatment of underlying disorders, such as endometriosis or uterine leiomyomas. However, surgical treatment is recommended only after conservative therapy fails.

Referral
- The patient may need to be referred to a gynecologist if treatment is unsuccessful.
- Refer the patient to a psychologist for counseling if a psychogenic cause is suspected.

Follow-up
The patient should be seen for 3 consecutive months to evaluate treatment.

Patient teaching
- Explain normal female anatomy and physiology to the patient as well as the nature of dysmenorrhea. This may be a good opportunity, depending on circumstances, to provide the adolescent patient with information on pregnancy and contraception.
- Encourage the patient to keep a detailed record of her menstrual symptoms.
- Stress the importance of exercise, nutrition, and relaxation techniques.

Complications
- Anxiety
- Depression
- Infertility

Special considerations
- Obtain a complete history, focusing on the patient's gynecologic complaints, including detailed information on any symptoms of pelvic disease, such as excessive bleeding, changes in bleeding pattern, vaginal discharge, and dyspareunia.

• • • • • • • • • • • •

DYSPAREUNIA

Dyspareunia is genital pain associated with intercourse. It may be mild, or it may be severe enough to affect enjoyment of intercourse. Dyspareunia is commonly associated with physical problems; less commonly it's associated with a psychological disorder. The prognosis is good if the underlying disorder can be treated successfully.

Causes
Physical causes of dyspareunia include an intact hymen; deformities or lesions of the introitus or vagina; marked retroversion of the uterus; genital, rectal, or pelvic scar tissue; acute or chronic infections of the genitourinary tract; and disorders of the surrounding viscera (including residual effects of pelvic inflammatory disease or disease of the adnexal and broad ligaments).

Among the many other possible physical causes are:
- endometriosis
- benign and malignant growths and tumors
- insufficient lubrication
- radiation to the area

- allergic reactions to diaphragms, condoms, or other contraceptives.

Psychological causes include fear of pain or of injury during intercourse, recollection of a previous painful experience, guilt feelings about sex, fear of pregnancy or injury to the fetus during pregnancy, anxiety caused by a new sexual partner or technique, and mental or physical fatigue.

Clinical presentation
Dyspareunia produces discomfort ranging from mild aches to severe pain before, during, or after intercourse. It also may be associated with vaginal itching or burning.

Differential diagnoses
- Urethritis
- Pelvic inflammatory disease
- Vulvovaginitis
- Uterine prolapse
- Psychological factors
- Cystitis
- Urethral syndrome
- Muscle spasm
- Hymenal strands
- Scar tissue
- Cervicitis
- Episiotomy
- Lack of sexual foreplay

Diagnosis
Physical examination and laboratory tests help determine the underlying disorder. Diagnosis also depends on a detailed sexual history.

When the disorder causes marked distress or interpersonal difficulty, it may fulfill the diagnostic criteria for a diagnosis as defined in the American Psychiatric Association's *Diagnostic and Statistical Manual of Mental Disorders*, 4th ed.

Management
General
The patient may be advised to change her coital position to reduce pain on deep penetration. Methods of treating psychologically based dyspareunia vary with the particular patient. Sensate focus exercises deemphasize intercourse itself and teach appropriate foreplay techniques. Education about contraception methods can reduce fear of pregnancy; education about sexual activity during pregnancy can relieve fear of harming the fetus.

Medication
Treatment of physical causes may include:
- creams and water-soluble gels for inadequate lubrication
- appropriate antibiotic for infections.

Surgical intervention
Surgery may be indicated for excision of hymenal scars and gentle stretching of painful scars at the vaginal opening.

Referral
- The patient may need to be referred to a gynecologist.
- The patient may need to be referred to a surgeon.
- Refer the patient for psychosexual counseling if appropriate.

Follow-up
The patient's follow-up depends on the cause of the disorder.

Patient teaching
- Provide instruction concerning anatomy and physiology of the reproductive system, contraception, and the human sexual response cycle.
- When appropriate, provide advice and information on drugs that may affect the patient sexually and on lubricating gels and creams.

Complications
- Genital infections
- Psychosexual dysfunction

• • • • • • • • • • • •

ENDOMETRIOSIS

Endometriosis is the presence of endometrial tissue outside the lining of the uterine cavity. Such ectopic tissue is generally confined to the pelvic area, most commonly around the ovaries, uterovesical peritoneum, uterosacral ligaments, and cul-de-sac, but it can appear anywhere in the body. This ectopic endometrial tissue responds to normal stimulation the same way the endometrium does. During menstruation, the ectopic tissue bleeds, which causes inflammation of the surrounding tissues. This inflammation causes fibrosis, leading to adhesions that produce pain and infertility.

AGE ALERT Severe symptoms of endometriosis may have an abrupt onset or may develop over many years. This disorder usually becomes progressively severe during the menstrual years; after menopause, it tends to subside. Active endometriosis usually occurs between ages 30 and 40, especially in women who postpone childbearing; it's uncommon before age 20.

Causes
The mechanism by which endometriosis causes symptoms, including infertility, are unknown. The main theories to explain this disorder are:
- transtubal regurgitation of endometrial cells and implantation at ectopic sites
- coelomic metaplasia (repeated inflammation may induce metaplasia of meso-

thelial cells to the endometrial epithelium)
- lymphatic or hematogenous spread to explain extraperitoneal disease.

Clinical presentation

The classic symptom of endometriosis is acquired dysmenorrhea, which may produce constant pain in the lower abdomen and in the vagina, posterior pelvis, and back. This pain usually begins from 5 to 7 days before menses reaches its peak and lasts for 2 to 3 days. It differs from primary dysmenorrheal pain, which is more cramplike and concentrated in the abdominal midline. The severity of pain, however, doesn't necessarily indicate the extent of the disease.

Other clinical features depend on the location of the ectopic tissue:
- ovaries and oviducts — infertility and profuse menses
- ovaries or cul-de-sac — deep-thrust dyspareunia
- bladder — suprapubic pain, dysuria, hematuria
- small bowel and appendix — nausea and vomiting, which worsen before menses, and abdominal cramps
- cervix, vagina, and perineum — bleeding from endometrial deposits in these areas during menses.

The primary complication of endometriosis is infertility.

Differential diagnoses

- Chronic pelvic inflammatory disease
- Recurrent acute salpingitis
- Ovarian neoplasm (benign or malignant)
- Ectopic pregnancy
- Adenomyosis
- Hemorrhagic corpus luteum

Diagnosis

Pelvic examination suggests endometriosis. Palpation may detect multiple tender nodules on uterosacral ligaments or in the rectovaginal septum in one-third of patients. These nodules enlarge and become more tender during menses. Palpation may also uncover ovarian enlargement in the presence of endometrial cysts on the ovaries or thickened, nodular adnexa (as in pelvic inflammatory disease). Laparoscopy must confirm the diagnosis and determine the stage of the disease before treatment is initiated. The American Society for Reproductive Medicine has proposed that endometriosis be classified in stages: Stage I, mild; Stage II, moderate; Stage III, severe; and Stage IV, extensive.

Management

General

Treatment varies according to the stage of the disease and the patient's age and desire to have children.

Medication

Conservative therapy for young women who want to have children includes:
- danazol — 100 to 800 mg/day P.O. in two divided doses for 6 to 9 months; this androgen produces a temporary remission in Stages I and II
- progestins and oral contraceptives — (dosage and instruction varies) help relieve symptoms
- leuprolide — 3.75 mg I.M. once monthly for up to 6 months; this gonadotropin-releasing hormone (Gn-RH) agonist induces a pseudomenopause and, thus, a "medical oophorectomy." (Gn-RH agonists have shown a remission of disease and are commonly used.)

Surgical intervention

When ovarian masses are present, surgery must rule out cancer. Conservative surgery includes laparoscopic removal of endometrial implants with conventional or laser techniques and presacral neurectomy for severe dysmenorrhea. The treatment of choice for women who don't want to bear children or for extensive disease is a total abdominal hysterectomy with bilateral salpingo-oophorectomy.

Referral
■ Refer the patient to a gynecologist if treatment is unsuccessful.
■ The patient may need to be referred for psychological counseling to deal with any life-altering treatments (such as a hysterectomy).

Follow-up
The patient should be seen initially 2 weeks after treatment is initiated, and then every 3 to 4 months.

Patient teaching
■ Advise adolescents to use sanitary napkins instead of tampons; this can help prevent retrograde flow in girls with a narrow vagina or small introitus.
■ Because infertility is a possible complication, advise the patient who wants children not to postpone childbearing.

Complications
■ Infertility
■ Chronic pelvic pain
■ Hysterectomy

Special considerations
■ Minor gynecologic procedures are contraindicated immediately before and during menstruation.

• • • • • • • • • • • •

ERECTILE DISORDER

Erectile disorder, or impotence, refers to a male's inability to attain or maintain penile erection sufficient to complete intercourse. The patient with primary impotence has never achieved a sufficient erection; secondary impotence, which is more common and less serious than the primary form, implies that, despite present inability, the patient has succeeded in completing intercourse in the past.

Transient periods of impotence aren't considered dysfunction and probably occur in half of adult males. Erectile disorder affects all age-groups but increases in frequency with age. The prognosis depends on the severity and duration of impotence and the underlying cause.

Causes
Psychogenic factors are responsible for approximately 50% to 60% of cases of erectile disorder; organic factors account for the rest. In some patients, psychogenic and organic factors coexist, making isolation of the primary cause difficult.

Psychogenic causes may be intrapersonal, reflecting personal sexual anxieties, or interpersonal, reflecting a disturbed sexual relationship. Intrapersonal factors generally involve guilt, fear, depression, or feelings of inadequacy resulting from previous traumatic sexual experience, rejection by parents or peers, exaggerated religious orthodoxy, abnormal mother-son intimacy, or homosexual experiences. Interpersonal factors may stem from differences in sexual preferences between partners, lack of communication, insufficient knowledge of sexual function, or nonsexual personal conflicts. Situational impotence, a temporary condition, may develop in response to stress, as in performance anxiety.

Organic causes may include chronic diseases, such as cardiopulmonary disease, diabetes, multiple sclerosis, or renal failure; spinal cord trauma; complications of surgery; drug- or alcohol-induced dysfunction; and, rarely, genital anomalies or central nervous system defects.

Clinical presentation

Secondary erectile disorder is classified as:

■ partial — the patient is unable to achieve a full erection.

■ intermittent — the patient is sometimes potent with the same partner.

■ selective — the patient is potent only with certain partners.

Some men lose erectile function suddenly; others lose it gradually. If the cause isn't organic, erection may still be achieved through masturbation.

Patients with psychogenic impotence may appear anxious, with sweating and palpitations, or may lose interest in sexual activity. Patients with psychogenic or drug-induced impotence may suffer severe depression, which may cause the impotence or result from it.

Differential diagnoses

■ Psychosocial dysfunction
■ Diabetes
■ Cardiac disease
■ Multiple sclerosis
■ Drug- or alcohol-related neuropathy

Diagnosis

A detailed sexual history helps differentiate between organic and psychogenic factors and between primary and secondary impotence. Questions should include: Does the patient have intermittent, selective, nocturnal, or early-morning erections? Can he achieve erections through other sexual activity? When did his dysfunction begin, and what was his life situation at that time? Did erectile problems occur suddenly or gradually? Is he taking large quantities of prescription or nonprescription drugs?

Diagnosis must rule out chronic diseases, such as diabetes, and other vascular, neurologic, or urogenital problems.

When the disorder causes marked distress or interpersonal difficulty, it may fulfill the diagnostic criteria for a diagnosis as defined in the American Psychiatric Association's *Diagnostic and Statistical Manual of Mental Disorders*, 4th ed.

Management

General

Sex therapy, which should include both partners, may effectively cure psychogenic impotence. The course and content of such therapy depend on the specific cause of the dysfunction and the nature of the relationship. Usually, therapy includes sensate focus exercises, which restrict the couple's sexual activity and encourage them to become more attuned to the physical sensations of touching. Sex therapy also includes improving verbal communication skills, eliminating unreasonable guilt, and reevaluating attitudes toward sex and sexual roles.

Treatment of organic impotence focuses on reversing the cause, if possible. If not, psychological counseling may help the couple deal realistically with their situation and explore alternatives for sexual expression. Medication may also help improve erectile function.

Medication

Sildenafil citrate may be given for erectile disorder; the typical dosage is 50 mg P.O. p.r.n. about 1 hour before sexual activity for adults under age 65 and 25 mg P.O. p.r.n. about 1 hour before sexual activity for adults over age 65.

CLINICAL CAUTION Serious cardiovascular events, including cardiac arrest, have been reported in temporal association with drug use.

Surgical intervention

Certain patients suffering from organic impotence may benefit from surgically inserted inflatable or noninflatable penile implants.

Referral

■ The patient may need to be referred for psychosexual counseling.
■ The patient may need to be referred to a urologist if treatment isn't successful.

Follow-up

The patient should be seen 2 weeks after treatment is initiated, and then annually if treatment is effective.

Patient teaching

■ After penile implant surgery, instruct the patient to avoid intercourse until the incision heals, usually in 6 weeks.
■ Provide information about resuming sexual activity for any patient with a condition that requires modification of daily activities. Such patients include those with cardiac disease, diabetes, hypertension, and chronic obstructive pulmonary disease and all postoperative patients.

Complications

■ Depression
■ Dependent on therapy

Special considerations

■ To help prevent impotence, promote establishment of responsible health and sex education programs at primary, secondary, and college levels.

• • • • • • • • • • • •
GENITAL HERPES

Genital herpes is an acute inflammatory disease of the genitalia. The prognosis varies, depending on the patient's age, the status of the immune system, and the infection site. Primary genital herpes usually is self-limiting but may cause painful local or systemic disease. (See *Understanding the genital herpes cycle*.) In neonates and immunocompromised patients, such as those with acquired immunodeficiency syndrome, genital herpes is commonly severe, resulting in complications and a high mortality.

Causes

Genital herpes usually is caused by infection with herpes simplex virus type 2, but some studies report increasing incidence of infection with herpes simplex virus type 1. This disease typically is transmitted through sexual intercourse, orogenital sexual activity, kissing, and hand-to-body contact. Pregnant women may transmit the infection to neonates during vaginal delivery if an active infection is present. Such transmitted infection may be localized (for instance, in the eyes) or disseminated, and may be associated with central nervous system involvement.

Clinical presentation

After a 3- to 7-day incubation period, fluid-filled vesicles appear, usually on the cervix (the primary infection site) and possibly on the labia, perianal skin, vulva, or vagina of the female and on the glans penis, foreskin, or penile shaft of the male. Extragenital lesions may appear on the mouth or anus. In both males and females, the vesicles, usually painless at first, will rupture and develop into extensive, shallow, painful ulcers, with redness, marked edema, tender inguinal lymph nodes, and the characteristic yellow, oozing centers.

Other features of initial mucocutaneous infection include fever, malaise, dysuria and, in females, leukorrhea.

Differential diagnoses

■ Chancroid
■ Primary syphilis

Understanding the genital herpes cycle

After a patient is infected with genital herpes, a latency period follows. The virus takes up permanent residence in the nerve cells surrounding the lesions, and intermittent viral shedding may take place.

Repeated outbreaks may develop at any time, again followed by a latent stage during which the lesions heal completely. Outbreaks may recur as often as three to eight times yearly.

Although the cycle continues indefinitely, some people remain symptom-free for years.

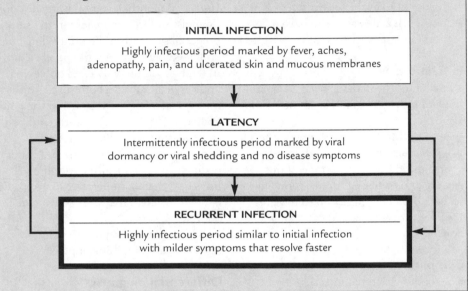

INITIAL INFECTION

Highly infectious period marked by fever, aches, adenopathy, pain, and ulcerated skin and mucous membranes

LATENCY

Intermittently infectious period marked by viral dormancy or viral shedding and no disease symptoms

RECURRENT INFECTION

Highly infectious period similar to initial infection with milder symptoms that resolve faster

---

- Lymphogranuloma venereum
- Mucocutaneous manifestations of Crohn's disease

Diagnosis

Diagnosis is based on the physical examination and patient history. Helpful (but nondiagnostic) measures include laboratory data showing increased antibody titers, smears of genital lesions showing atypical cells, and cytologic preparations (Tzanck test) that reveal giant cells. Diagnosis can be confirmed by demonstration of the herpes simplex virus in vesicular fluid, using tissue culture techniques, or by antigen tests that identify specific antigens.

Management
Medication

These medications may be given for genital herpes:

- acyclovir sodium—primary herpes, 200 mg P.O. five times/day for 7 to 10 days; recurrent herpes, 200 mg P.O. five times/day for 5 days; daily suppression, 200 mg P.O. three to five times/day
- famciclovir—125 mg P.O. b.i.d. for 5 days

- valacyclovir—initial episode of herpes, 1 g P.O. b.i.d. for 10 days; recurrent herpes, 500 mg P.O. b.i.d. for 5 days.

Referral
- Refer patients to the Herpes Resource Center, which has local chapters nationwide, for support.

Follow-up
The patient should be seen after 2 weeks of treatment to evaluate effectiveness. Advise the female patient to have a Papanicolaou test every 6 months.

Patient teaching
- Encourage the patient to get adequate rest and nutrition and to keep the lesions dry.

CLINICAL CAUTION Advise the patient to avoid sexual intercourse during the active stage of this disease and to use condoms during all sexual exposures. Urge him to have his sexual partners seek medical examination.

Complications
- Secondary bacterial infection
- Transmission to neonate
- Urine retention

• • • • • • • • • • • •
GENITAL WARTS

Genital warts (also known as venereal warts or condylomata acuminata) consist of papillomas with fibrous tissue overgrowth from the dermis and thickened epithelial coverings. They are uncommon before puberty and after menopause. Certain types of human papillomavirus (HPV) infections have been strongly associated with genital dysplasia and, over a period of years (depending on the viral strain), with cervical neoplasia.

Causes
Infection with one of the more than 60 known strains of HPV causes genital warts, which are transmitted through sexual contact. The warts grow rapidly in the presence of heavy perspiration, poor hygiene, or pregnancy, and commonly accompany other genital infections.

Clinical presentation
After a 1- to 6-month incubation period (usually 2 months), genital warts develop on moist surfaces: in males, on the subpreputial sac, within the urethral meatus and, less commonly, on the penile shaft; in females, on the vulva and on vaginal and cervical walls. In both sexes, papillomas spread to the perineum and the perianal area. These painless warts start as tiny red or pink swellings that grow (sometimes up to 4″ [10 cm]) and become pedunculated. Typically, multiple swellings give them a cauliflower-like appearance. If infected, the warts become malodorous.

Most patients report no symptoms; a few complain of itching or pain.

Differential diagnoses
- Condylomata lata
- Carcinoma
- Concomitant sexually transmitted diseases
- Molluscum contagiosum

Diagnosis
Dark-field examination of scrapings from wart cells shows marked vascularization of epidermal cells, which helps to differentiate genital warts from condylomata lata associated with second-stage syphilis. Applying 5% acetic acid (white vinegar) to the warts turns them white. Warts are usually diagnosed early by visual inspection; biopsy is indicated only when neoplasia is strongly suspected.

Management
General
Treatment is mostly for cosmetic reasons and should be guided by the patient's preference. Treatment aims to remove exophytic warts and to ameliorate signs and symptoms. No therapy has proved effective in eradicating HPV. Relapse is common.

Medication
Topical drug therapy used for genital warts includes:
- podophyllum 10% to 20% in tincture of benzoin — apply to wart, wash off after 1 to 4 hours; apply again weekly for 3 weeks; contraindicated in pregnancy
- trichloroacetic acid 80% to 90% — apply to warts and powder with talc to remove excess acid; use weekly up to 6 weeks
- podofilox 0.5% — apply to warts b.i.d. for 3 days, followed by no treatment for 4 days; repeat cycle four times if needed.

Surgical intervention
Warts larger than 1″ (2.5 cm) are generally removed by carbon dioxide laser treatment, cryosurgery, or electrocautery. Electrodiathermy is also performed as an office procedure when the lesion is confined to the cervix and there's no evidence of endocervical or invasive disease.

Referral
- Depending on the extent of the lesion, the patient may need to be referred to a gynecologist for treatment.

Follow-up
The patient receiving cryotherapy should initially be seen weekly and then every 2 weeks. Patients receiving topical treatment should be seen every 2 weeks. The female patient should have biannual Papanicolaou tests for 2 years following treatment and then annually if she has no reoccurrence.

Patient teaching
- Recommend the use of condoms.
- Teach the patient proper use of topical medication to avoid injury to healthy tissue.

Complications
Male
- Penile cancer
- Rectal cancer
- Urethral obstruction

Female
- Cervical cancer
- Cervical dysplasia
- Rectal cancer

Special considerations
- Encourage the patient's sexual partners to be examined for HPV, human immunodeficiency virus, and other sexually transmitted diseases.

•••••••••••

GONORRHEA

A common sexually transmitted disease, gonorrhea is an infection of the genitourinary tract (especially the urethra and cervix) and, occasionally, the rectum, pharynx, and eyes. Untreated gonorrhea can spread through the blood to the joints, tendons, meninges, and endocardium; in females, it can also lead to chronic pelvic inflammatory disease (PID) and sterility. After adequate treatment, the prognosis for males and females is excellent, although reinfection is common.

AGE ALERT Gonorrhea is especially prevalent among young people and people with multiple partners, particularly those between ages 19 and 25.

Causes

Transmission of *Neisseria gonorrhoeae*, the organism that causes gonorrhea, almost always follows sexual contact with an infected person. Children born of infected mothers can contract gonococcal ophthalmia neonatorum during passage through the birth canal. Children and adults with gonorrhea can contract gonococcal conjunctivitis by touching their eyes with contaminated hands.

Clinical presentation

Many infected males may be asymptomatic; however, after a 3- to 6-day incubation period, some develop symptoms of urethritis, including dysuria and purulent urethral discharge, with redness and swelling at the infection site. Most infected females remain asymptomatic but may develop inflammation and a greenish yellow discharge from the cervix — the most common gonorrheal symptoms in females. (See *What happens in gonorrhea.*)

Other clinical features vary according to the site involved:

- urethra — dysuria, urinary frequency and incontinence, purulent discharge, itching, and red and edematous meatus
- vulva — occasional itching, burning, and pain due to exudate from an adjacent infected area (symptoms tend to be more severe before puberty or after menopause)
- vagina (most common site in children over age 1) — engorgement, redness, swelling, and profuse purulent discharge
- liver — right upper quadrant pain in patients with perihepatitis
- pelvis — severe pelvic and lower abdominal pain, muscle rigidity, tenderness, and abdominal distention.

As the infection spreads, nausea, vomiting, fever, and tachycardia may develop in patients with salpingitis or PID.

Other possible symptoms include pharyngitis, tonsillitis, and rectal burning, itching, and bloody mucopurulent discharge.

Gonococcal septicemia is more common in females than in males. Its characteristic signs include tender papillary skin lesions on the hands and feet; these lesions may be pustular, hemorrhagic, or necrotic. Gonococcal septicemia may also produce migratory polyarthralgia and polyarthritis and tenosynovitis of the wrists, fingers, knees, or ankles. Untreated septic arthritis leads to progressive joint destruction.

Signs of gonococcal ophthalmia neonatorum include lid edema, bilateral conjunctival infection, and abundant purulent discharge 2 to 3 days after birth. Adult conjunctivitis, most common in men, causes unilateral conjunctival redness and swelling. Untreated gonococcal conjunctivitis can progress to corneal ulceration and blindness.

Differential diagnoses

- *Chlamydia trachomatis* infection
- Mucopurulent cervicitis

Diagnosis

A culture from the infection site (urethra, cervix, rectum, or pharynx) usually establishes the diagnosis by isolating *N. gonorrhoeae*. (See Neisseria gonorrhoeae, page 530.) A Gram stain showing gram-negative diplococci supports the diagnosis and may be sufficient to confirm gonorrhea in males.

Confirmation of gonococcal arthritis requires identification of gram-negative diplococci on smears made from joint fluid and skin lesions. Complement fixation and immunofluorescent assays of serum reveal antibody titers four times the nor-

What happens in gonorrhea

After exposure to *Neisseria gonorrhoeae*, the epithelial cells at the infection site become infected; then the disease begins to spread locally. The disease pattern depends on the individual infected and the infection site.

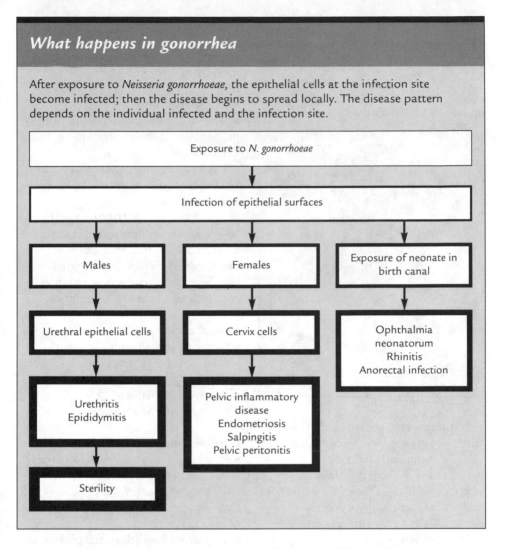

mal rate. Culture of conjunctival scrapings confirms gonococcal conjunctivitis.

Management
Medication
■ For uncomplicated gonorrhea caused by susceptible non–penicillinase-producing *N. gonorrhoeae,* a single 125-mg dose of ceftriaxone I.M is recommended; a single dose of ceftriaxone 125 mg I.M. with erythromycin (500 mg P.O. q.i.d. for 7 days) is recommended for pregnant patients and those allergic to penicillin.

■ The recommended initial regimen for disseminated gonococcal infection in adults and adolescents is:
– ceftriaxone — 1 to 2 g I.M. or I.V. every 24 hours
– spectinomycin — 2 g I.M. every 12 hours for 24 to 48 hours for patients allergic to beta-lactam drugs.
■ For presumptive treatment of concurrent *Chlamydia trachomatis* infection, 100 mg doxycycline is given P.O. b.i.d. for 7 days.
■ All regimens should be continued for 24 to 48 hours after improvement begins;

Neisseria gonorrhoeae

In gonorrhea, microscopic examination reveals gram-negative diplococcus — *N. gonorrhoeae*, the causative organism.

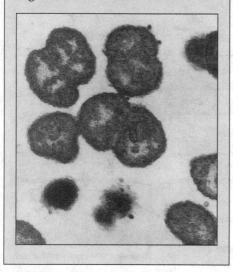

then therapy may be switched to one of the following regimens to complete a full week of antimicrobial therapy:
– cefixime — 400 mg P.O. daily
– ciprofloxacin — 500 mg P.O. b.i.d.; contraindicated for children, adolescents under age 18, and pregnant and breast-feeding women.
■ Treatment of gonococcal conjunctivitis requires a single dose of ceftriaxone (1 g I.M.) and lavage of the infected eye with saline solution once.
■ Routine instillation of 1% silver nitrate drops or erythromycin ointment into neonates' eyes soon after delivery has greatly reduced the incidence of gonococcal ophthalmia neonatorum.

Referral
■ The patient may need to be referred to a hospital for treatment.

Follow-up
Because treatment failure is rare, follow-up testing isn't necessary. Retest if symptoms recur.

Patient teaching
■ Warn the patient that, until cultures prove negative, he can transmit gonococcal infection.
■ If the patient has gonococcal arthritis, tell him to apply moist heat to ease pain in affected joints.

CLINICAL CAUTION Urge the patient to inform sexual contacts of his infection so that they can seek treatment, even if cultures are negative. Advise the patient to avoid sexual intercourse until treatment is complete.

Complications
■ Corneal scarring after eye infection
■ Cardiac valve destruction
■ Death
■ Infertility (female)
■ Urethral stricture (male)

Special considerations
■ Report gonorrhea cases to local public health authorities for follow-up with sexual contacts. Examine and test all people exposed to gonorrhea as well as children of infected mothers.
■ To prevent gonorrhea, tell patients to use condoms during intercourse, to wash genitals with soap and water before and after intercourse, and to avoid sharing washcloths or douche equipment.
■ Report gonorrhea cases in children to child abuse authorities.

• • • • • • • • • • • •
INFERTILITY, FEMALE

Infertility, the inability to conceive after regular intercourse for at least 1 year without contraception, affects approximately 10% to 15% of couples in the United States. About 30% to 40% of infertility is attributed to the female and 30% to 40% to the male; about 20% is due to a combination of male and female factors. Following extensive investigation and treatment, approximately 50% of these infertile couples achieve pregnancy. Of the 50% who don't, 10% have no pathologic basis for infertility; the prognosis for this group becomes extremely poor if pregnancy isn't achieved within 3 years.

Causes
Functional
Complex hormonal interactions determine the normal function of the female reproductive tract and require an intact hypothalamic-pituitary-ovarian axis—a system that stimulates and regulates the production of hormones necessary for normal sexual development and function. Any defect or malfunction of this axis can cause infertility due to insufficient gonadotropin secretions (luteinizing hormone [LH] and follicle-stimulating hormone). The ovary controls and is controlled by the hypothalamus through a system of negative and positive feedback mediated by estrogen production. Insufficient gonadotropin levels may result from infections, tumors, or neurologic disease of the hypothalamus or pituitary gland. Hypothyroidism also impairs fertility.

Anatomic
Ovarian factors are related to anovulation and oligo-ovulation (infrequent ovulation) and are a major cause of infertility. Pregnancy or direct visualization provides irrefutable evidence of ovulation. Presumptive signs of ovulation include regular menses, cyclic changes reflected in basal body temperature readings, postovulatory progesterone levels, and endometrial changes due to the presence of progesterone. Absence of presumptive signs suggests anovulation. Ovarian failure, in which no ova are produced by the ovaries, may result from ovarian dysgenesis or premature menopause. Amenorrhea is often associated with ovarian failure. Oligo-ovulation may be due to a mild hormonal imbalance in gonadotropin production and regulation and may be caused by polycystic disease of the ovary or abnormalities in the adrenal or thyroid gland that adversely affect hypothalamic-pituitary functioning.

Uterine fibroids or uterine abnormalities rarely cause infertility; however, such abnormalities may include congenitally absent uterus, bicornuate or double uterus, leiomyomas, or Asherman's syndrome, in which the anterior and posterior uterine walls adhere because of scar tissue formation.

Tubal and peritoneal factors are due to faulty tubal transport mechanisms and unfavorable environmental influences affecting the sperm, ova, or recently fertilized ovum. Tubal loss or impairment may occur secondary to ectopic pregnancy. In many cases, tubal and peritoneal factors result from anatomic abnormalities: bilateral occlusion of the tubes due to salpingitis (resulting from gonorrhea, tuberculosis, or puerperal sepsis), peritubal adhesions (resulting from endometriosis, pelvic inflammatory disease [PID], diverticulosis, or childhood rupture of the appendix), and uterotubal obstruction due to tubal spasm.

Cervical factors may include a malfunctioning cervix that produces deficient or excessively viscous mucus and is impervious to sperm, preventing entry into the uterus. In cervical infection, viscous mucus may contain spermicidal macrophages. The possible existence of cervical antibodies that immobilize sperm is also under investigation.

Psychosocial

Psychosocial problems probably account for relatively few cases of infertility. Occasionally, ovulation may stop under stress due to failure of LH release. The frequency of intercourse may be related. More commonly, however, psychosocial problems result from, rather than cause, infertility.

Clinical presentation

The obvious indication of female infertility is the inability to conceive after regular intercourse for at least 1 year without contraception. Other clinical features are based on the underlying cause.

In addition, female infertility may cause emotional frustration in a couple, including feelings of anger, guilt, and low self-esteem.

Differential diagnoses
■ Any of the many causes

Diagnosis

Inability to achieve pregnancy after having regular intercourse without contraception for at least 1 year suggests infertility. (In women over age 35, many clinicians use 6 months rather than 1 year as a cutoff point.)

Diagnosis requires a complete physical examination and health history, including specific questions on the patient's reproductive and sexual function, past diseases, mental state, previous surgery, types of contraception used in the past, and family history. Irregular, painless menses may indicate anovulation. A history of PID may suggest fallopian tube blockage. Sometimes PID is silent and no history may be known.

These tests assess ovulation:
■ Basal body temperature graph shows a sustained elevation in body temperature postovulation until just before onset of menses, indicating the approximate time of ovulation.
■ Endometrial biopsy, done on or about day 5 after the basal body temperature elevates, provides histologic evidence that ovulation has occurred.
■ Progesterone blood levels, measured when they should be highest, can show a luteal phase deficiency or presumptive evidence of ovulation.

These procedures assess structural integrity of the fallopian tubes, the ovaries, and the uterus:
■ Urinary LH kits, available without a prescription, can sensitively detect the LH surge about 24 hours preovulation, allowing couples to time coitus.
■ Hysterosalpingography provides radiologic evidence of tubal obstruction and abnormalities of the uterine cavity by injecting radiopaque contrast fluid through the cervix.
■ Endoscopy confirms the results of hysterosalpingography and visualizes the endometrial cavity by hysteroscopy or explores the posterior surface of the uterus, fallopian tubes, and ovaries by culdoscopy. Laparoscopy allows visualization of the abdominal and pelvic areas.

Male-female interaction studies include:
■ Postcoital test examines the cervical mucus for motile sperm cells following intercourse that takes place at midcycle (as close to ovulation as possible).
■ Immunologic or antibody testing detects spermicidal antibodies in the fe-

male's sera. Further research is being conducted in this area.

Management
General
Treatment depends on identifying the underlying abnormality or dysfunction within the hypothalamic-pituitary-ovarian complex. Some options are controversial and involve emotional and financial cost, such as surrogate mothering, frozen embryos, or in vitro fertilization (IVF). In view of its good success rate (about 20%), IVF may be used instead of surgery in many cases.

Medication
These medications may be used in treatment of female infertility:
- hormone therapy for hyperactivity or hypoactivity of the adrenal or thyroid gland
- progesterone replacement for deficiency
- clomiphene — 50 mg/day P.O. for 5 days starting on day 5 of the menstrual cycle (may increase dose to 100 mg if bleeding doesn't occur) for anovulation; if mucus production decreases (an adverse effect), small doses of estrogen may be given concomitantly to improve the quality of cervical mucus (however, such intervention remains unproven)
- danazol — 100 to 200 mg P.O. b.i.d. for 3 to 6 months, depending on the severity, or noncyclic administration of oral contraceptives for endometriosis continued for 9 months.

Surgical intervention
Surgical restoration may correct certain anatomic causes of infertility such as fallopian tube obstruction. Surgery may also be necessary to remove tumors located within or near the hypothalamus or pituitary gland. Surgical removal of areas of endometriosis may be necessary, along with drug therapy.

Referral
- Refer the patient to a fertility specialist for a workup.
- The couple may need psychological counseling to cope with this problem.
- Refer the patient to organizations such as the American Infertility Organization for information and support.

Follow-up
Follow-up will depend on the cause of infertility and the treatment.

Patient teaching
- An infertile couple may suffer loss of self-esteem; they may feel angry, guilty, or inadequate, and the diagnostic procedures for this disorder may intensify their fear and anxiety. You can help by explaining these procedures thoroughly. Above all, encourage the patient and her partner to talk about their feelings, and listen to what they say with a nonjudgmental attitude.
- If the patient requires surgery, tell her what to expect postoperatively; this, of course, depends on which procedure is to be performed.

Complications
- Depression
- Multiple births
- Disruption of regular lifestyle
- Marital difficulties

••••••••••••

INFERTILITY, MALE

Male infertility may be suspected whenever a couple fails to achieve pregnancy after about 1 year of regular, unprotected intercourse. Approximately 40% to 50% of infertility problems in the United States are totally or partially attributed to the male.

Causes

Some of the factors associated with male infertility include:

- varicocele, a mass of dilated and tortuous varicose veins in the spermatic cord
- semen disorders, such as volume or motility disturbances and inadequate sperm density
- proliferation of abnormal or immature sperm, with variations in the size and shape of the head
- systemic disease, such as diabetes mellitus, neoplasms, hepatic and renal diseases, and viral disturbances, especially mumps-related orchitis
- genital infections, such as gonorrhea, tuberculosis, and herpes
- disorders of the testes, such as cryptorchidism, Sertoli-cell–only syndrome, and ductal obstruction (caused by absence or ligation of vas deferens or infection)
- genetic defects, such as Klinefelter's and Reifenstein's syndromes
- immunologic disorders, such as autoimmune infertility and allergic orchitis
- endocrine imbalances that disrupt pituitary gonadotropins, inhibiting spermatogenesis, testosterone production, or both (as in Kallmann's syndrome, panhypopituitarism, hypothyroidism, and congenital adrenal hyperplasia)
- chemicals and drugs that can inhibit gonadotropins or interfere with spermatogenesis, such as arsenic, methotrexate, medroxyprogesterone acetate, nitrofurantoin, monoamine oxidase inhibitors, and some antihypertensives
- sexual problems, such as erectile disorder, ejaculatory incompetence, and low libido.

Age, occupation, and traumatic injury to the testes can also contribute to male infertility.

Clinical presentation

The obvious indication of male infertility is, of course, failure to impregnate a fertile woman. In addition, male infertility may induce troublesome negative emotions in a couple — anger, hurt, disgust, guilt, and loss of self-esteem. Clinical features may include:

- atrophied testes
- empty scrotum
- scrotal edema
- varicocele or anteversion of the epididymis
- inflamed seminal vesicles
- beading or abnormal nodes on the spermatic cord and vas deferens
- penile nodes
- warts
- plaques
- hypospadias
- prostatic enlargement
- nodules
- swelling
- tenderness.

Differential diagnoses

- Any of the many causes

Diagnosis

A detailed patient history may reveal abnormal sexual development, delayed puberty, infertility in previous relationships, and a medical history of prolonged fever, mumps, impaired nutritional status, previous surgery, or trauma to genitalia. After a thorough patient history and physical examination, the most conclusive test for male infertility is semen analysis.

Other laboratory tests include gonadotropin assay to determine the integrity of the pituitary gonadal axis, serum testosterone levels to determine end organ response to luteinizing hormone (LH), urine 17-ketosteroid levels to measure testicular function, and testicular biopsy to help clarify unexplained oligospermia and azoospermia. Vasography and seminal vesiculography may be necessary.

Management
General

When anatomic dysfunction or infection causes infertility, treatment consists of correcting the underlying problem. For patients with sexual dysfunction, treatment includes education, counseling or therapy (on sexual techniques, coital frequency, and reproductive physiology), and proper nutrition with vitamin supplements

Patients with oligospermia who have a normal history and physical examination, normal hormonal assays, and no signs of systemic disease require emotional support and counseling, adequate nutrition, multivitamins, and selective therapeutic agents. Alternatives to such treatment are adoption and artificial insemination.

Medication

These medications may be given to treat male infertility:
- vitamin B therapy for decreased follicle-stimulating hormone levels
- human chorionic gonadotropin therapy for decreased LH levels, decreased testosterone levels, decreased semen motility, and volume disturbances
- testosterone (low dosages) for normal or elevated LH level.

Surgical intervention

A varicocele requires surgical repair or removal.

Referral

- Refer the patient to a fertility specialist for evaluation.
- The couple may need psychological counseling to cope with this problem.
- Refer the patient to organizations such as the American Infertility Organization for information and support.

Follow-up

Follow-up would depend on the cause of infertility and the treatment.

Patient teaching

- Educate the couple as necessary regarding reproductive and sexual function and about factors that may interfere with fertility, such as the use of lubricants and douches.
- Urge men with oligospermia to avoid habits that may interfere with normal spermatogenesis by elevating scrotal temperature, such as wearing tight underwear and athletic supporters, taking hot tub baths, or habitually riding a bicycle. Explain that cool scrotal temperature is essential for normal spermatogenesis.

Complications

- Depression
- Marital difficulties

HEALTHY LIVING Help prevent male infertility by encouraging patients to have regular physical examinations, protect gonads during athletic activity, receive early treatment for sexually transmitted diseases, and undergo surgical correction for anatomic defects.

• • • • • • • • • • • •

MENOPAUSE

Menopause is the cessation of menstruation. It results from a complex syndrome of physiologic changes — the climacteric — caused by declining ovarian function. The climacteric produces various body changes, the most dramatic being menopause.

Causes

Menopause occurs in three forms:
- Physiologic menopause, the normal decline in ovarian function due to aging, begins in most women between ages 40

and 50 and results in infrequent ovulation, decreased menstrual function and, eventually, cessation of menstruation (usually between ages 45 and 55).

■ Pathologic (premature) menopause, the gradual or abrupt cessation of menstruation before age 40, occurs idiopathically in about 5% of women in the United States. However, certain diseases, especially severe infections and reproductive tract tumors, may cause pathologic menopause by seriously impairing ovarian function. Other factors that may precipitate pathologic menopause include malnutrition, debilitation, extreme emotional stress, excessive radiation exposure, and surgical procedures that impair ovarian blood supply.

■ Artificial menopause may follow radiation therapy or surgical procedures such as oophorectomy.

Clinical presentation

Many menopausal women are asymptomatic, but some have severe symptoms. The decline in ovarian function and consequent decreased estrogen level produce menstrual irregularities: a decrease in the amount and duration of menstrual flow, spotting, and episodes of amenorrhea and polymenorrhea (possibly with hypermenorrhea). Irregularities may last a few months or persist for several years before menstruation ceases permanently.

These body system changes may occur (usually after the permanent cessation of menstruation):

■ reproductive system — menopause may cause shrinkage of vulval structures and loss of subcutaneous fat, possibly leading to atrophic vulvitis; atrophy of vaginal mucosa and flattening of vaginal rugae, possibly causing bleeding after coitus or douching; vaginal itching and discharge from bacterial invasion; and loss of capillaries in the atrophying vaginal wall, causing the pink, rugal lining to become

smooth and white. Menopause may also produce excessive vaginal dryness and dyspareunia due to decreased lubrication from the vaginal walls and decreased secretion from Bartholin's glands; smaller ovaries and oviducts; and progressive pelvic relaxation as the supporting structures lose their tone because of the absence of estrogen. As a woman ages, atrophy causes the vagina to shorten and the mucous lining to become thin, dry, less elastic, and pale as a result of decreased vascularity. In addition, the pH of vaginal secretions increases, making the vaginal environment more alkaline. The type of flora also changes, increasing the older woman's chance of vaginal infections.

■ urinary system — atrophic cystitis due to the effects of decreased estrogen levels on bladder mucosa and related structures may cause pyuria; dysuria; and urinary frequency, urgency, and incontinence. Urethral carbuncles from loss of urethral tone and mucosal thinning may cause dysuria, meatal tenderness, and hematuria.

■ mammary system — breast size decreases.

■ integumentary system — the patient may experience loss of skin elasticity and turgor due to estrogen deprivation, loss of pubic and axillary hair and, occasionally, slight alopecia.

■ autonomic nervous system — the patient may exhibit hot flashes and night sweats (in 60% of women), vertigo, syncope, tachycardia, dyspnea, tinnitus, emotional disturbances (irritability, nervousness, crying spells, fits of anger), and exacerbation of preexisting depression, anxiety, and compulsive, manic, or schizoid behavior.

Menopause may also induce atherosclerosis, and a decrease in estrogen level contributes to osteoporosis.

Ovarian activity in younger women is believed to provide a protective effect on the cardiovascular system, and the loss of this function at menopause may partly explain the increased death rate from myocardial infarction in older women. Also, estrogen has been found to increase levels of high-density lipoprotein cholesterol.

Artificial menopause produces symptoms within 2 to 5 years in 95% of women. In many cases, cessation of menstruation in pathologic and artificial menopause is abrupt and may cause severe vasomotor and emotional disturbances. Menstrual bleeding after 1 year of amenorrhea may indicate organic disease.

Differential diagnoses
- Hypothalamic, pituitary tumor
- Infection (viral)
- Thyroid disease
- Tuberculosis
- Alcoholism

Diagnosis
The patient history and typical clinical features suggest menopause. A Papanicolaou (Pap) test may show the influence of estrogen deficiency on vaginal mucosa. Radioimmunoassay shows these blood hormone levels:
- estrogen — 0 to 14 ng/dl
- plasma estradiol — 15 to 40 pg/ml
- estrone — 25 to 50 pg/ml.

Radioimmunoassay also shows these urine values:
- estrogen — 6 to 28 μg/24 hours
- pregnanediol (urinary secretion of progesterone) — 0.3 to 0.9 mg/24 hours.

Follicle-stimulating hormone production may increase as much as 15 times its normal level; luteinizing hormone production, as much as 5 times.

Pelvic examination, endometrial biopsy, and dilatation and curettage may rule out organic disease in patients with abnormal menstrual bleeding.

Management
Medication
Estrogen is the treatment of choice in relieving vasomotor symptoms and symptoms caused by vaginal and urethral mucosal atrophy.

CLINICAL CAUTION Because of the controversy over the effect of estrogen replacement therapy (ERT) on breast cancer, the patient should first have a screening mammogram.

ERT may be administered cyclically or continuously. Patients usually receive the lowest dosage that effectively treats symptoms and prevents osteoporosis. Severe hot flashes may require a higher dosage for a limited period, followed by a gradual reduction to the standard dosage.

In women who haven't had a hysterectomy, the addition of a progestin (such as medroxyprogesterone acetate) during the last 12 days of estrogen administration lowers the incidence of hyperplasia and endometrial cancer. In women who don't have a uterus, progestin's relationship to breast cancer is unknown.

The oral route is preferred for estrogen-progestin therapy; the transdermal route reduces GI adverse effects such as nausea, and topical estrogen relieves symptoms of vaginal atrophy. Regardless of the route, patients need to know about the risk of endometrial hyperplasia and have regular checkups to detect it early. (See *Estrogen-progestin guidelines*, page 538.)

Referral
- The patient may need to be referred for psychotherapy to help relieve psychological disturbances.

Follow-up
The patient should be seen approximately 1 month after treatment is initiated

Estrogen-progestin guidelines

If the patient is receiving sequential estrogen-progestin therapy, alert her to the possibility of monthly withdrawal bleeding after the cessation of progestin therapy, and tell her that such bleeding is benign. (If breakthrough bleeding occurs before day 6 of progestin therapy, an endometrial biopsy is needed to rule out hyperplasia.) Other adverse effects of progestins include breast tenderness, fluid retention, weight gain, dysmenorrhea, and depression.

Without a progestin, however, long-term estrogen replacement therapy carries an increased risk of endometrial hyperplasia and, eventually, endometrial cancer. With this in mind, consider these guidelines:

■ Symptoms associated with the progestin component may resolve when the daily dose of medroxyprogesterone is reduced from 10 mg to 5 mg. The lower dose, however, doesn't offer as much protection as the higher one.
■ Withdrawal bleeding often can be eliminated by reducing the conjugated estrogens dose from 0.625 mg to 0.3 mg or by adding 2.5 mg of medroxyprogesterone daily. This lower dose of estrogen may be ineffective in relieving climacteric symptoms and in protecting against osteoporosis.
■ If estrogen-only therapy is given, an endometrial biopsy should be performed before therapy begins and annually thereafter. If endometrial hyperplasia develops, the patient must either stop estrogen therapy or add a progestin. In either case, a repeat biopsy is essential to ensure that the hyperplasia has resolved. Transvaginal ultrasonography can detect excessive endometrial proliferation.

and then every 3 to 6 months depending on success of treatment.

Patient teaching

■ Provide the patient with all the facts about ERT. Make sure she realizes the need for regular monitoring.
■ Before ERT begins, have the patient undergo a baseline physical examination, Pap test, and mammogram.
■ Advise the patient not to discontinue contraceptive measures until cessation of menstruation has been confirmed.
■ Tell the patient to immediately report vaginal bleeding or spotting after menstruation has ceased.

Complications

■ Osteoporosis
■ Coronary heart disease
■ Psychological symptoms
■ Vaginal atrophy
■ Arteriosclerosis

• • • • • • • • • • •

OVARIAN CYST

An ovarian cyst is usually a nonneoplastic sac on an ovary that contains fluid or semisolid material. Although these cysts are usually small and produce no symptoms, they require thorough investigation as possible sites of malignant change. Common ovarian cysts include follicular cysts, lutein cysts (granulosa-lutein [corpus luteum] and theca-lutein cysts), and polycystic ovarian disease. Ovarian cysts can develop any time between puberty and menopause, including during pregnancy. Granulosa-lutein cysts are uncommon and usually occur during early pregnancy. The prognosis for nonneoplastic ovarian cysts is excellent.

Causes

Follicular cysts are generally very small and arise from follicles that overdistend. When such cysts persist into menopause, they secrete excessive amounts of estrogen in response to the hypersecretion of follicle-stimulating hormone and luteinizing hormone that normally occurs during menopause. (See *Follicular cyst.*)

Granulosa-lutein cysts, which occur within the corpus luteum, are functional, nonneoplastic enlargements of the ovaries caused by excessive accumulation of blood during the hemorrhagic phase of the menstrual cycle. Theca-lutein cysts are commonly bilateral and filled with clear, straw-colored fluid; they are often associated with hydatidiform mole, choriocarcinoma, or hormone therapy (with human chorionic gonadotropin [hCG] or clomiphene citrate).

Polycystic ovarian disease is part of the Stein-Leventhal syndrome and stems from endocrine abnormalities.

Clinical presentation

Small ovarian cysts (such as follicular cysts) usually don't produce symptoms unless torsion or rupture causes signs of an acute abdomen. Ovarian cysts with torsion induce acute abdominal pain similar to that of appendicitis. Large or multiple cysts may induce these signs and symptoms:
- mild pelvic discomfort
- low back pain
- dyspareunia
- abnormal uterine bleeding secondary to a disturbed ovulatory pattern.

Granulosa-lutein cysts that appear early in pregnancy may grow as large as 2″ to 2½″ (5 to 6 cm) in diameter and produce unilateral pelvic discomfort and, if rupture occurs, massive intraperitoneal hemorrhage. In nonpregnant women, these cysts may cause delayed menses, followed by prolonged or irregular bleed-

Follicular cyst

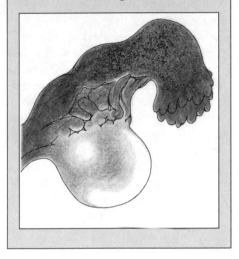

A common type of ovarian cyst, a follicular cyst is usually semitransparent and overdistended with watery fluid that is visible through its thin walls.

ing. Polycystic ovarian disease may also produce secondary amenorrhea, oligomenorrhea, or infertility.

Differential diagnoses
- Pelvic inflammatory disease
- Endometriosis
- Uterine leiomyomas
- Pelvic kidney
- Pregnancy

Diagnosis

Generally, characteristic clinical features suggest ovarian cysts. Visualization of the ovary through ultrasound, laparoscopy, or surgery (commonly for another condition) confirms ovarian cysts.

Extremely elevated hCG titers strongly suggest theca-lutein cysts.

In polycystic ovarian disease, physical examination demonstrates bilaterally enlarged polycystic ovaries. Tests reveal slight elevation of urinary 17-ketosteroids and anovulation (shown by basal body temperature graphs and endometrial biopsy). Direct visualization must rule out paraovarian cysts of the broad ligament, salpingitis, endometriosis, and neoplastic cysts.

Management
General
Follicular cysts generally don't require treatment because they tend to disappear spontaneously within 60 days. Treatment for granulosa-lutein cysts that occur during pregnancy is aimed at relieving symptoms because these cysts diminish during the third trimester and rarely require surgery. Theca-lutein cysts disappear spontaneously after elimination of the hydatidiform mole, destruction of choriocarcinoma, or discontinuation of hCG or clomiphene citrate therapy.

Medication
These medications may be given for follicular cysts:
- clomiphene citrate — 50 to 100 mg/day P.O. for 5 days
- progesterone — 5 to 10 mg/day I.M. for 6 days.

In functional cysts, oral contraceptives may also accelerate involution.

These medications may be given for polycystic ovarian disease:
- clomiphene citrate — 50 mg/day P.O. for 5 days starting on day 5 of the menstrual cycle (may increase to 100 mg/day P.O. if bleeding doesn't occur) to induce ovulation
- medroxyprogesterone acetate — 10 mg/ day P.O. for 10 days beginning on day 16 of menstrual cycle for the patient who doesn't want to become pregnant
- oral contraceptives (low-dose) for the patient who needs reliable contraception.

Surgical intervention
Surgery, in the form of laparoscopy or exploratory laparotomy with possible ovarian cystectomy or oophorectomy, may become necessary if an ovarian cyst is persistent or suspicious.

Referral
- If the patient is premenarcheal or postmenopausal and a palpable adnexal mass is detected, immediately refer her to a gynecologist for treatment.

Follow-up
The patient should be seen 1 month after treatment is initiated and then in 3 to 6 months depending on the treatment's effectiveness.

Patient teaching
- Carefully explain the nature of the cyst, the type of discomfort — if any — the patient is apt to experience, and how long the condition is expected to last.
- Tell the patient to watch for signs of cyst rupture, such as increasing abdominal pain, distention, and rigidity.

Complications
- Rupture
- Torsion
- Peritonitis

• • • • • • • • • • • •

PELVIC INFLAMMATORY DISEASE

Pelvic inflammatory disease (PID) is any acute, subacute, recurrent, or chronic infection of the oviducts and ovaries, with adjacent tissue involvement. It includes inflammation of the fallopian tubes (salpingitis) and ovaries (oophoritis), which can extend to the connective tissue lying between the broad ligaments (parametritis). Early diagnosis and treatment prevent damage to the reproductive system. Untreated PID may cause infertility and may lead to potentially fatal septicemia and shock.

Causes

PID can result from infection with aerobic or anaerobic organisms. The organisms *Neisseria gonorrhoeae* and *Chlamydia trachomatis* are the most common causes because they most readily penetrate the bacteriostatic barrier of cervical mucus.

Normally, cervical secretions have a protective and defensive function. Therefore, conditions or procedures that alter or destroy cervical mucus impair this bacteriostatic mechanism and allow bacteria present in the cervix or vagina to ascend into the uterine cavity; such procedures include conization or cauterization of the cervix.

Uterine infection can also follow the transfer of contaminated cervical mucus into the endometrial cavity by instrumentation. Consequently, PID can follow insertion of an intrauterine device (IUD), use of a biopsy curet or an irrigation catheter, or tubal insufflation. Other predisposing factors include abortion, pelvic surgery, and infection during or after pregnancy.

Bacteria may also enter the uterine cavity through the bloodstream or from drainage from a chronically infected fallopian tube, a pelvic abscess, a ruptured appendix, diverticulitis of the sigmoid colon, or other infectious foci.

Common bacteria found in cervical mucus are staphylococci, streptococci, diphtheroids, chlamydiae, and coliforms, including *Pseudomonas* and *Escherichia coli*. Uterine infection can result from any one or several of these organisms or may follow the multiplication of normally nonpathogenic bacteria in an altered endometrial environment. Bacterial multiplication is most common during parturition because the endometrium is atrophic, quiescent, and not stimulated by estrogen.

Clinical presentation

Clinical features of PID vary with the affected area but generally include a profuse, purulent vaginal discharge, sometimes accompanied by low-grade fever and malaise (particularly if gonorrhea is the cause). The patient experiences lower abdomen pain; movement of the cervix or palpation of the adnexa may be extremely painful. (See *Forms of pelvic inflammatory disease*, page 542.)

Differential diagnoses

- Ectopic pregnancy
- Ruptured corpus luteum cyst
- Septic abortion
- Appendicitis
- Pyelonephritis
- Endometriosis
- Endometritis
- Ulcerative colitis
- Torsion of an adnexal mass
- Degeneration of a leiomyoma

Diagnosis

Diagnostic tests generally include:

- gram stain of secretions from the endocervix or cul-de-sac; culture and sensitivity (aids selection of the appropriate antibiotic); cultures of urethral and rectal secretions
- C-reactive protein levels (highly specific for PID)
- complete blood count (white blood cell count is elevated [greater than 10,000 µl] and the erythrocyte sedimentation rate is elevated)
- ultrasonography (identifies an adnexal or uterine mass).

In addition, patient history is significant. In general, PID is associated with recent sexual intercourse, insertion of an

Forms of pelvic inflammatory disease

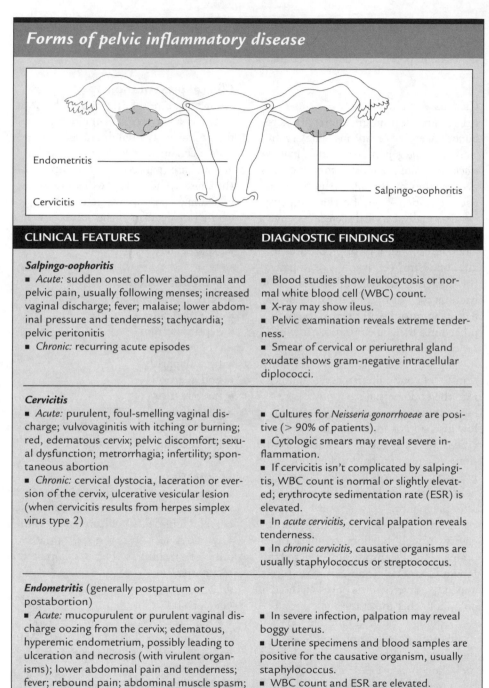

Endometritis

Cervicitis

Salpingo-oophoritis

CLINICAL FEATURES

DIAGNOSTIC FINDINGS

Salpingo-oophoritis
- *Acute:* sudden onset of lower abdominal and pelvic pain, usually following menses; increased vaginal discharge; fever; malaise; lower abdominal pressure and tenderness; tachycardia; pelvic peritonitis
- *Chronic:* recurring acute episodes

- Blood studies show leukocytosis or normal white blood cell (WBC) count.
- X-ray may show ileus.
- Pelvic examination reveals extreme tenderness.
- Smear of cervical or periurethral gland exudate shows gram-negative intracellular diplococci.

Cervicitis
- *Acute:* purulent, foul-smelling vaginal discharge; vulvovaginitis with itching or burning; red, edematous cervix; pelvic discomfort; sexual dysfunction; metrorrhagia; infertility; spontaneous abortion
- *Chronic:* cervical dystocia, laceration or eversion of the cervix, ulcerative vesicular lesion (when cervicitis results from herpes simplex virus type 2)

- Cultures for *Neisseria gonorrhoeae* are positive (> 90% of patients).
- Cytologic smears may reveal severe inflammation.
- If cervicitis isn't complicated by salpingitis, WBC count is normal or slightly elevated; erythrocyte sedimentation rate (ESR) is elevated.
- In *acute cervicitis,* cervical palpation reveals tenderness.
- In *chronic cervicitis,* causative organisms are usually staphylococcus or streptococcus.

Endometritis (generally postpartum or postabortion)
- *Acute:* mucopurulent or purulent vaginal discharge oozing from the cervix; edematous, hyperemic endometrium, possibly leading to ulceration and necrosis (with virulent organisms); lower abdominal pain and tenderness; fever; rebound pain; abdominal muscle spasm; thrombophlebitis of uterine and pelvic vessels (in severe forms)
- *Chronic:* recurring acute episodes (increasingly common because of widespread use of intrauterine devices)

- In severe infection, palpation may reveal boggy uterus.
- Uterine specimens and blood samples are positive for the causative organism, usually staphylococcus.
- WBC count and ESR are elevated.

IUD, childbirth, abortion, or a sexually transmitted disease.

Management
Medication
To prevent progression of PID, antibiotic therapy begins immediately after culture specimens are obtained. Such therapy can be reevaluated as soon as laboratory results are available (usually after 24 to 48 hours). Infection may become chronic if treated inadequately.

The guidelines of the Centers for Disease Control and Prevention (CDC) for outpatient treatment include:
- ofloxacin (400 mg P.O. b.i.d.) with metronidazole (500 mg P.O. b.i.d.) for 14 days
- ceftriaxone (250 mg I.M.) with doxycycline (100 mg P.O. b.i.d.) for 14 days.

The CDC guidelines for inpatient treatment include doxycycline (100 mg P.O. b.i.d.) with cefoxitin (2 g I.V. every 6 hours) for 48 hours after clinical improvement.

Surgical intervention
Development of a pelvic abscess necessitates adequate drainage. A ruptured abscess is life-threatening. If this complication develops, the patient may need a total abdominal hysterectomy with bilateral salpingo-oophorectomy. Alternatively, laparoscopic drainage with preservation of the ovaries and uterus appears to hold promise.

Referral
- The patient may need to be referred to a hospital for treatment.

Follow-up
For outpatient treatment, see the patient 72 hours after treatment is initiated and then in 2 weeks and as needed.

Patient teaching
- To prevent a recurrence, explain the nature and seriousness of PID, and encourage the patient to comply with the treatment regimen.
- Stress the need for the patient's sexual partner to be examined and, if necessary, treated for infection.
- To prevent infection after minor gynecologic procedures, such as dilatation and curettage, tell the patient to immediately report any fever, increased vaginal discharge, or pain. After such procedures, instruct her to avoid douching and intercourse for at least 7 days.

Complications
- Pelvic abscess
- Recurrent infection
- Ruptured pelvic abscess
- Infertility
- Chronic pain

• • • • • • • • • • • •

POSTMENOPAUSAL BLEEDING

Postmenopausal bleeding is defined as bleeding from the reproductive tract that occurs 1 year or more after cessation of menses. Sites of bleeding include the vulva, vagina, cervix, and endometrium. The prognosis varies with the cause.

Causes
Postmenopausal bleeding may result from:
- exogenous estrogen, when administration is excessive or prolonged or when small amounts are given in the presence of a hypersensitive endometrium
- endogenous estrogen production, especially when levels are high, as in persons with estrogen-producing ovarian tumor. (However, in some persons, even slight

fluctuation in estrogen levels may cause bleeding.)
- atrophic endometrium due to low estrogen levels
- atrophic vaginitis, usually triggered by trauma during coitus in the absence of estrogen production
- aging, which increases vascular vulnerability by thinning epithelial surfaces, increasing vascular fragility, producing degenerative tissue changes, and decreasing resistance to infections
- cervical or endometrial cancer (more common after age 60)
- adenomatous hyperplasia or atypical adenomatous hyperplasia (usually considered a premalignant lesion).

Clinical presentation
Vaginal bleeding, the primary symptom, ranges from spotting to outright hemorrhage; its duration also varies. Other symptoms depend on the cause. Excessive estrogen stimulation, for example, may also produce copious cervical mucus; estrogen deficiency may cause vaginal mucosa to atrophy.

Differential diagnoses
- Endometrial carcinoma
- Cervical carcinoma
- Adenomatous hyperplasia
- Atrophic vaginitis
- Atrophic endometrium

Diagnosis
Diagnostic evaluation of the patient with postmenopausal bleeding should include physical examination (especially pelvic examination), a detailed history, standard laboratory tests (such as complete blood count), and cytologic examination of smears from the cervix and the endocervical canal. An endometrial biopsy or dilatation and curettage (D&C) reveals pathologic findings in the endometrium.

Diagnosis must rule out underlying degenerative or systemic disease. Before testing for estrogen levels, the patient must stop all sources of exogenous estrogen intake — including face and body creams that contain estrogen — to rule out excessive exogenous estrogen as a cause.

Management
General
Therapy varies according to the underlying cause. Emergency treatment to control massive hemorrhage is rarely necessary, except in advanced cancer.

Medication
Estrogen creams and suppositories are usually effective in correcting estrogen deficiency because they are rapidly absorbed.

Surgical intervention
Treatment may include D&C to relieve bleeding. Hysterectomy is indicated for repeated episodes of postmenopausal bleeding from the endometrial cavity. Such bleeding may indicate endometrial cancer.

Referral
- The patient may need a referral to a gynecologist for treatment.

Follow-up
Follow-up will depend on the underlying cause and treatment plan.

Patient teaching
- To prevent disorders that cause postmenopausal bleeding, stress the fact that periodic gynecologic examinations are as important after menopause as they were before.

Complications

- Iron deficiency anemia
- Endometrial adenocarcinoma

Special considerations

- Obtain a detailed patient history to rule out excessive exogenous estrogen as a cause of bleeding.
- Ask the patient about use of cosmetics (especially face and body creams), drugs, and other products that may contain estrogen.
- Discuss the risks and benefits of estrogen replacement therapy with the patient.

• • • • • • • • • • • •

PREMENSTRUAL SYNDROME

Also designated "late luteal phase dysphoric disorder" in the American Psychiatric Association's *Diagnostic and Statistical Manual of Mental Disorders*, 4th ed., premenstrual syndrome (PMS) is characterized by varying symptoms that appear 7 to 14 days before menses and usually subside with its onset. The effects of PMS range from minimal discomfort to severe, disruptive symptoms and can include nervousness, irritability, depression, and multiple somatic complaints.

AGE ALERT Researchers believe that 70% to 90% of women experience PMS at some time during their childbearing years, usually between ages 25 and 45.

Causes

The list of biological theories offered to explain the cause of PMS is impressive. It includes such conditions as a progesterone deficiency in the luteal phase of the menstrual cycle and vitamin deficiencies. Although there is no evidence that PMS is hormonally mediated, failure to identify a specific disorder with a specific mechanism suggests that PMS represents various manifestations triggered by normal physiologic hormonal changes.

Clinical presentation

Clinical effects vary widely among patients and may include any combination of the following:

- behavioral — mild to severe personality changes, nervousness, hostility, irritability, agitation, sleep disturbances, fatigue, lethargy, and depression
- somatic — breast tenderness or swelling, abdominal tenderness or bloating, joint pain, headache, edema, diarrhea or constipation, and exacerbations of skin problems (such as acne or rashes), respiratory problems (such as asthma), or neurologic problems (such as seizures).

Differential diagnoses

- Depression
- Perimenopause
- Hypothyroidism
- Nutritional deficiency
- Diabetes mellitus
- Dysfunctional marriage
- Stress
- Hypoglycemia
- Hyperlactinemia
- Cyclothymic disorder
- Alcoholism
- Drug addiction

Diagnosis

The patient history shows typical symptoms related to the menstrual cycle. To help ensure an accurate history, the patient may be asked to record menstrual symptoms and body temperature on a calendar for 2 to 3 months prior to diagnosis. Estrogen and progesterone blood levels may be evaluated to help rule out hormonal imbalance. A psychological evaluation is also recommended to rule out or detect an underlying psychiatric disorder.

Management
General
Educating and reassuring patients that PMS is a real physiologic syndrome are important parts of treatment. Because treatment is predominantly symptomatic, each patient must learn to cope with her own individual set of symptoms. For treatment to be effective, the patient may have to maintain a diet that is low in simple sugars, caffeine, and salt.

Medication
Treatment may include:
- alprazolam — 0.25 to 0.5 mg P.O., b.i.d. to t.i.d., during the luteal phase
- vitamin and mineral supplement — 1 multivitamin tablet/day P.O.
- fluoxetine — 20 mg/day P.O.
- ibuprofen — 400 mg P.O. every 6 hours
- spironolactone — 25 to 200 mg P.O. q.i.d. during the luteal phase, only when absolutely necessary
- mefenamic acid — 500 mg P.O. t.i.d. for 3 days.

Referral
- The patient may need to be referred for psychological counseling.
- Refer the patient to self-help groups for women with PMS.

Follow-up
The patient should be seen after 2 months of treatment for evaluation and modification.

Patient teaching
- Discuss ways in which the patient can modify her lifestyle, such as making changes in her diet and avoiding stimulants and alcohol.

Complications
- Lifestyle disruption
- Depression

Special considerations
- Obtain a complete patient history to help identify emotional problems that may contribute to PMS.

• • • • • • • • • • •

SYPHILIS

A chronic, infectious, sexually transmitted disease, syphilis begins in the mucous membranes and quickly becomes systemic, spreading to nearby lymph nodes and the bloodstream. This disease, when untreated, is characterized by progressive stages: primary, secondary, latent, and late (formerly called tertiary). About 34,000 cases of syphilis, in primary and secondary stages, are reported annually in the United States. Untreated syphilis leads to crippling or death, but the prognosis is excellent with early treatment.

AGE ALERT Incidence of syphilis is highest among urban populations, especially in people between ages 15 and 39, drug users, and those infected with the human immunodeficiency virus (HIV).

Causes
Infection from the spirochete *Treponema pallidum* causes syphilis. Transmission occurs primarily through sexual contact during the primary, secondary, and early latent stages of infection. Prenatal transmission from an infected mother to her fetus is also possible. (See *Prenatal syphilis.*)

Clinical presentation
Signs and symptoms of syphilis vary according to the stage of development:

Prenatal syphilis

A woman can transmit syphilis transplacentally to her unborn child throughout pregnancy. This type of syphilis is often called congenital, but prenatal is a more accurate term. Approximately 50% of infected fetuses die before or shortly after birth. The prognosis is better for infants who develop overt infection after age 2.

SIGNS AND SYMPTOMS
The infant with prenatal syphilis may appear healthy at birth but usually develops characteristic lesions — vesicular, bullous eruptions, commonly on the palms and soles — 3 weeks later. Shortly afterward, a maculopapular rash similar to that in secondary syphilis may erupt on the face, mouth, genitalia, palms, or soles. Condylomata lata commonly occur around the anus. Lesions may erupt on the mucous membranes of the mouth, pharynx, and nose. When the infant's larynx is affected, his cry becomes weak and forced. If nasal mucous membranes are involved, he may also develop nasal discharge, which can be slight and mucopurulent or copious with blood-tinged pus. Visceral and bone lesions, liver or spleen enlargement with ascites, and nephrotic syndrome may also occur.

Late prenatal syphilis becomes apparent after age 2; it may be identifiable only through blood studies or may cause unmistakable syphilitic changes: screwdriver-shaped central incisors, deformed molars or cusps, thick clavicles, saber shins, bowed tibias, nasal septum perforation, eighth nerve deafness, and neurosyphilis.

DIAGNOSIS AND TREATMENT
In the infant with prenatal syphilis, the Venereal Disease Research Laboratory titer, if reactive at birth, stays the same or rises, indicating active disease. The infant's titer drops in 3 months if the mother has received effective prenatal treatment. Absolute diagnosis necessitates dark-field examination of umbilical vein blood or lesion drainage.

An infant with abnormal cerebrospinal fluid (CSF) may be treated with aqueous crystalline penicillin G, I.M. or I.V. (50,000 U/kg of body weight/day divided in two doses for at least 10 days), or aqueous penicillin G procaine I.M. (50,000 U/kg of body weight/day for at least 10 days). An infant with normal CSF may be treated with a single injection of penicillin G benzathine (50,000 U/kg of body weight).

When caring for a child with prenatal syphilis, record the extent of the rash, and watch for signs of systemic involvement, especially laryngeal swelling, jaundice, and decreasing urine output.

■ Primary syphilis develops after an incubation period that generally lasts about 3 weeks. Initially, one or more chancres erupt on the genitalia; others may erupt on the anus, fingers, lips, tongue, nipples, tonsils, or eyelids. These chancres, which are usually painless, start as papules and then erode; they have indurated, raised edges and clear bases. Chancres typically disappear after 3 to 6 weeks, even when untreated. They're usually associated with regional lymphadenopathy (unilateral or bilateral). In females, chancres are commonly overlooked because they usually develop on internal structures — the cervix or the vaginal wall.

■ The development of symmetrical mucocutaneous lesions and general lymphadenopathy signals the onset of secondary syphilis, which may develop within a few days or up to 8 weeks after onset of initial chancres. The rash of secondary syphilis can be macular, papular, pustular, or nodular. Lesions are well defined, generalized, and of uniform size. Macules commonly erupt between rolls of fat on the trunk and, proximally, on the arms, palms, soles, face, and scalp. In warm, moist areas (perineum, scrotum, vulva, and between rolls of fat), the lesions enlarge and erode, producing highly contagious, pink or grayish white lesions (condylomata lata).

Mild constitutional symptoms of syphilis appear in the second stage and may include headache, malaise, anorexia, weight loss, nausea, vomiting, sore throat and, possibly, slight fever. Alopecia may occur, with or without treatment, and is usually temporary. Nails become brittle and pitted.

▪ Latent syphilis is characterized by an absence of clinical symptoms but a reactive serologic test for syphilis. Because infectious mucocutaneous lesions may reappear when infection is of less than 4 years' duration, early latent syphilis is considered contagious. Approximately two-thirds of patients remain asymptomatic in the late latent stage, until death. The rest develop characteristic late-stage symptoms.

▪ Late syphilis is the final, destructive but noninfectious stage of the disease. It has three subtypes, any or all of which may affect the patient: late benign syphilis, cardiovascular syphilis, and neurosyphilis. The lesions of late benign syphilis, which develop between 1 and 10 years after becoming infected, appear on the skin, bones, mucous membranes, upper respiratory tract, liver, or stomach. The typical lesion is a gumma—a chronic, superficial nodule or deep, granulomatous lesion that is solitary, asymmetrical, painless, and indurated. Gummas can be found on any bone—particularly the long bones of the legs—and in any organ. If late syphilis involves the liver, it can cause epigastric pain, tenderness, enlarged spleen, and anemia; if it involves the upper respiratory tract, it may cause perforation of the nasal septum or the palate. In severe cases, late benign syphilis results in destruction of bones or organs, which eventually causes death.

▪ Cardiovascular syphilis develops about 10 years after the initial infection in approximately 10% of patients with late, untreated syphilis. It causes fibrosis of elastic tissue of the aorta and leads to aortitis, most often in the ascending and transverse sections of the aortic arch. Cardiovascular syphilis may be asymptomatic or may cause aortic insufficiency or aneurysm.

▪ Symptoms of neurosyphilis develop in about 8% of patients with late, untreated syphilis and appear from 5 to 35 years after infection. These clinical effects consist of meningitis and widespread central nervous system damage that may include general paresis, personality changes, and arm and leg weakness.

Differential diagnoses
For primary syphilis
▪ Chancroid
▪ Granuloma inguinale
▪ Lymphogranuloma venereum
▪ Herpes genitalis
▪ Carcinoma
▪ Scabies
▪ Trauma
▪ Psoriasis
▪ Lichen planus

For secondary syphilis
▪ Pityriasis rosea
▪ Psoriasis
▪ Tinea versicolor
▪ Parasitic infection

- Infectious mononucleosis
- Alopecia
- Drug eruption
- Lichen planus

Diagnosis

Identifying *T. pallidum* from a lesion on dark-field examination confirms the diagnosis of syphilis. This method is most effective when moist lesions are present, as in primary, secondary, and prenatal syphilis. (See *Treponema pallidum*.)

The fluorescent treponemal antibody-absorption test identifies antigens of *T. pallidum* in tissue, ocular fluid, cerebrospinal fluid (CSF), tracheobronchial secretions, and exudates from lesions. This is the most sensitive test available for detecting syphilis in all stages. Once reactive, it remains so permanently.

Other appropriate procedures include:
- Venereal Disease Research Laboratory (VDRL) slide test and rapid plasma reagin test detect nonspecific antibodies. Both tests, if positive, become reactive within 1 to 2 weeks after the primary lesion appears or 4 to 5 weeks after the infection begins.
- CSF examination identifies neurosyphilis when the total protein level is above 40 mg/dl, the VDRL slide test is reactive, and the cell count exceeds five mononuclear cells/µl.

Management
Medication

These medications may be used to treat syphilis:
- penicillin G benzathine — 2.4 million U I.M. as a single dose for early syphilis; 2.4 million U I.M. weekly for 3 weeks for syphilis of more than 1 year's duration
- doxycycline — 100 mg P.O. b.i.d. for 14 days for early syphilis or 28 days for la-

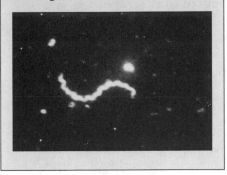

Treponema pallidum

In syphilis, a dark-field examination that shows spiral-shaped bacterial organisms — *T. pallidum* — confirms the diagnosis.

tent or late syphilis for nonpregnant patients who are allergic to penicillin.

Nonpenicillin therapy for latent or late syphilis should be used only after neurosyphilis has been excluded.

Referral

- Refer the patient to an infectious disease specialist if treatment fails.
- Refer the patient and his sexual partners for HIV testing.

Follow-up

The patient should have VDRL testing after 3, 6, 12, and 24 months to detect possible relapse. Patients treated for latent or late syphilis should receive blood tests at 6-month intervals for 2 years.

Patient teaching

- Stress the importance of completing the full course of antibiotic therapy even after symptoms subside.

CLINICAL CAUTION Urge the patient to inform sexual partners of his infection so they can also receive treatment.

Complications
- Cardiovascular disease
- Irreversible neurologic disease
- Irreversible organ damage
- Membranous glomerulonephritis
- Death

Special considerations
- Be sure to report all cases of syphilis to local public health authorities.

• • • • • • • • • • • •

TRICHOMONIASIS

A protozoal infection of the lower genitourinary tract, trichomoniasis affects about 15% of sexually active females and 10% of sexually active males. This infection, which occurs worldwide, may be acute or chronic in females. The risk of recurrence is minimized when sexual partners are treated concurrently.

Causes
Trichomonas vaginalis — a tetraflagellated, motile protozoan — causes trichomoniasis in females by infecting the vagina, the urethra and, possibly, the endocervix, bladder, Bartholin's glands, or Skene's glands. In males, it infects the lower urethra and, possibly, the prostate gland, seminal vesicles, or epididymis.

T. *vaginalis* grows best when the vaginal mucosa is more alkaline than normal (pH about 5.5 to 5.8). Therefore, factors that raise the vaginal pH — use of oral contraceptives, pregnancy, bacterial overgrowth, exudative cervical or vaginal lesions, or frequent douching, which disturbs lactobacilli that normally live in the vagina and maintain acidity — may predispose a woman to trichomoniasis.

Trichomoniasis is usually transmitted by intercourse; less often, by contaminated douche equipment or moist washcloths.

Clinical presentation
Approximately 70% of females — including those with chronic infections — and most males with trichomoniasis are asymptomatic. In females, acute infection may produce variable signs, such as:
- gray or greenish yellow and possibly profuse and frothy, malodorous vaginal discharge
- severe itching
- redness
- swelling
- tenderness
- dyspareunia
- dysuria
- urinary frequency
- postcoital spotting
- menorrhagia
- dysmenorrhea.

Such symptoms may persist for a week to several months and may be more pronounced just after menstruation or during pregnancy. If trichomoniasis is untreated, symptoms may subside, although T. *vaginalis* infection persists, possibly associated with an abnormal cytologic smear of the cervix.

In males, trichomoniasis may produce mild to severe transient urethritis, possibly with dysuria and frequency.

Differential diagnoses
- Bacterial vaginosis
- Candidiasis
- Cytolytic vaginosis
- Foreign body vaginitis

Diagnosis
Direct microscopic examination of vaginal or seminal discharge is decisive when it reveals T. *vaginalis,* a motile, pear-shaped organism. Examination of clear urine specimens may also reveal T. *vaginalis*.

Physical examination of symptomatic females shows vaginal erythema; edema; frank excoriation; a frothy, malodorous, greenish yellow vaginal discharge; and, rarely, a thin, gray pseudomembrane over the vagina. Cervical examination demonstrates punctate cervical hemorrhages, giving the cervix a strawberry appearance that is almost pathognomonic for this disorder.

Management
General
Sitz baths may be used to help relieve symptoms.

Medication
These medications are used to treat trichomoniasis:
■ metronidazole—2 g P.O. as a single dose or 250 mg P.O. t.i.d. for 7 days given to both sexual partners; oral metronidazole hasn't been proven safe during the first trimester of pregnancy but can be considered for use if symptoms are severe
■ clotrimazole—100 mg vaginal tablets h.s. for 14 days; only has a 20% to 25% cure rate.

Follow-up
The patient won't need follow-up if treatment is effective.

Patient teaching
■ Instruct the patient to refrain from douching before being examined for trichomoniasis.
■ Urge abstinence from intercourse until the patient is cured. Refer partners for treatment.
■ Tell the patient to avoid using tampons.
■ Warn the patient to abstain from alcoholic beverages while taking metronidazole because alcohol consumption may provoke a disulfiram-type reaction (confusion, headache, cramps, vomiting, and seizures). Also, tell the patient that this drug may turn urine dark brown.

■ Caution the patient to avoid over-the-counter douches and vaginal sprays because chronic use can alter vaginal pH.
■ Advise the patient to scrub the bathtub with a disinfecting cleaner before and after sitz baths.

Complications
■ Recurrent infections

HEALTHY LIVING Tell patients that they can reduce the risk of genitourinary bacterial growth by wearing loose-fitting, cotton underwear, which allows ventilation; bacteria flourish in a warm, dark, moist environment.

VAGINISMUS

Vaginismus is involuntary spastic constriction of the lower vaginal muscles, usually from fear of vaginal penetration. This disorder may coexist with dyspareunia and, if severe, may prevent intercourse (a common cause of unconsummated marriages). Vaginismus affects females of all ages and backgrounds. The prognosis is excellent for a motivated patient who doesn't have untreatable organic abnormalities.

Causes
Vaginismus may be physical or psychological in origin. It may occur spontaneously as a protective reflex to pain or result from organic causes, such as hymenal abnormalities, genital herpes, obstetric trauma, and atrophic vaginitis.

Psychological causes may include:
■ childhood and adolescent exposure to rigid, punitive, and guilt-ridden attitudes toward sex
■ fears resulting from painful or traumatic sexual experiences, such as incest or rape

- early traumatic experience with pelvic examinations
- fear of pregnancy, sexually transmitted disease, or cancer.

Clinical presentation

The female with vaginismus typically experiences muscle spasm with constriction and pain on insertion of any object into the vagina, such as a tampon, diaphragm, or speculum. She may profess a lack of sexual interest or a normal level of sexual desire.

Differential diagnoses

- Psychological cause
- Dyspareunia

Diagnosis

Diagnosis depends on the sexual history and pelvic examination to rule out physical disorders. The sexual history must include early childhood experiences and family attitudes toward sex, previous and current sexual responses, contraceptive practices and reproductive goals, feelings about her sexual partner, and specific details about pain on insertion of any object into the vagina. A carefully performed pelvic examination confirms the diagnosis by showing involuntary constriction of the musculature surrounding the outer portion of the vagina.

When the disorder causes marked distress or interpersonal difficulty, it may fulfill the diagnostic criteria for a diagnosis as defined in the American Psychiatric Association's *Diagnostic and Statistical Manual of Mental Disorders*, 4th ed.

Management

General

Treatment is designed to eliminate maladaptive muscle constriction and underlying psychological problems. In Masters and Johnson therapy, the patient uses a graduated series of dilators, which she inserts into her vagina while tensing and relaxing her pelvic muscles. The patient controls the amount of time that the dilator is left in place and the movement of the dilator. Together with her sexual partner, she begins sensate focus and counseling therapy to increase sexual responsiveness, improve communication skills, and resolve any underlying conflicts.

Kaplan therapy also uses progressive insertion of dilators or fingers (in vivo/desensitization therapy), with behavior therapy (imagining vaginal penetration until it can be tolerated) and, if necessary, psychoanalysis and hypnosis. Practitioners of both Masters and Johnson and Kaplan therapies claim a 100% cure rate.

Referral

- The patient may need a referral to a sex therapist.

Follow-up

The patient will need to be seen based on the treatment modality.

Patient teaching

- Teach the patient about the anatomy and physiology of the reproductive system, contraception, and human sexual response. This can be done quite naturally during the pelvic examination.
- Teach the patient about any medication that may affect her sexual response, such as antihypertensives, tranquilizers, or steroids. If she has insufficient lubrication for intercourse, tell her about lubricating gels and creams.

Complications

- Difficulty with intimate relationships
- Psychiatric illness

• • • • • • • • • • • •
VULVOVAGINITIS

Vulvovaginitis is inflammation of the vulva (vulvitis) and vagina (vaginitis). Because of the proximity of these two structures, inflammation of one occasionally causes inflammation of the other. Vulvovaginitis may occur at any age and affects most females at some time. The prognosis is excellent with treatment.

Causes
Common causes of vaginitis (with or without consequent vulvitis) include:
- infection with *Trichomonas vaginalis*, a protozoan flagellate, usually transmitted through sexual intercourse
- infection with *Candida albicans*, a fungus that requires glucose for growth; incidence rises during the secretory phase of the menstrual cycle (Such infection is twice as common in pregnant females as in nonpregnant females. It also commonly affects users of oral contraceptives, diabetics, and patients receiving systemic therapy with broad-spectrum antibiotics [incidence may reach 75%].)
- infection with *Gardnerella vaginalis*, a gram-negative bacillus.
    Common causes of vulvitis include:
- parasitic infection (*Phthirus pubis* [crab louse])
- trauma (Skin breakdown may lead to secondary infection.)
- poor personal hygiene
- chemical irritations, or allergic reactions to hygiene sprays, douches, detergents, clothing, or toilet paper
- vulval atrophy in menopausal women due to decreasing estrogen levels
- retention of a foreign body, such as a tampon or diaphragm.

Clinical presentation
- In trichomonas vaginitis, vaginal discharge is thin, bubbly, green-tinged, and malodorous. This infection causes marked irritation and itching and urinary symptoms, such as burning and frequency.
- Candidal vaginitis produces a thick, white, cottage cheese–like discharge and red, edematous mucous membranes, with white flecks adhering to the vaginal wall, and is often accompanied by intense itching.
- Bacterial vaginosis produces a gray, foul, "fishy"-smelling discharge.
- Acute vulvitis causes a mild to severe inflammatory reaction, including edema, erythema, burning, and pruritus. Severe pain during urination and dyspareunia may necessitate immediate treatment. Herpes infection may cause painful ulceration or vesicle formation during the active phase.
- Chronic vulvitis generally causes relatively mild inflammation, possibly associated with severe edema that may involve the entire perineum.

Differential diagnoses
- Trichomonas vaginitis
- Candidiasis
- Bacterial vaginosis
- Allergic contact dermatitis
- Foreign body vaginitis

Diagnosis
Diagnosis of vaginitis requires identification of the infectious organism during microscopic examination of vaginal exudate on a wet slide preparation (a drop of vaginal exudate placed in normal saline solution).
- In trichomonal infections, the presence of motile, flagellated trichomonads confirms the diagnosis.
- In candidal vaginitis, 10% potassium hydroxide is added to the slide; diagnosis requires identification of *C. albicans* fungi.

■ In bacterial vaginosis, wet mount shows the presence of clue cells (epithelial cells with obscured borders).

Diagnosis of vulvitis or suspected sexually transmitted disease may require complete blood count, urinalysis, cytology screening, biopsy of chronic lesions to rule out malignancy, culture of exudate from acute lesions, and possible human immunodeficiency virus testing.

Management
General
Cold compresses or cool sitz baths may provide relief from pruritus in acute vulvitis; severe inflammation may require warm compresses. Other therapy includes avoiding drying soaps and wearing loose clothing to promote air circulation.

Medication
These medications may be used to treat vulvovaginitis:
■ hydrocortisone cream — applied q.i.d. to reduce inflammation
■ diflorasone cream 0.05% — applied b.i.d to q.i.d.
■ estrogen — 0.625 mg/day P.O. to treat atrophic vulvovaginitis
■ acyclovir ointment — apply six times per day; this doesn't cure herpesvirus infections, but the duration and symptoms of active lesions may be reduced.

These medications may be used to treat bacterial vaginosis:
■ metronidazole — 500 mg P.O. b.i.d. for 7 days or 0.75% vaginal gel intravaginally h.s. for 5 days
■ clindamycin vaginal cream 2% — intravaginally h.s. for 7 days.

These medications may be used to treat candidiasis:
■ miconazole vaginal cream 2% — intravaginally h.s. for 7 days
■ clotrimazole vaginal creme 1% — intravaginally h.s. for 7 to 14 days

■ fluconazole — 150 mg P.O. as a single dose.

Trichomoniasis is treated with metronidazole — 2 g P.O. as a single dose, 250 mg P.O. t.i.d. for 7 days, or 500 mg P.O. b.i.d. for 7 days for the patient and her sexual partner.

Referral
■ Refer the patient to a gynecologist if infections are recurrent.

Follow-up
The patient should be seen again if treatment isn't successful.

Patient teaching
■ Teach the patient how to insert vaginal ointments and suppositories. Tell her to remain prone for at least 30 minutes after insertion to promote absorption (insertion at bedtime is ideal). Suggest she wear a pad to prevent staining her underclothing.
■ Encourage good hygiene. Advise the patient with a history of recurrent vulvovaginitis to wear all-cotton underpants. Advise her to avoid wearing tight-fitting pants and panty hose, which encourage the growth of the infecting organisms.

Complications
■ Secondary infection
■ Pelvic abscess
■ Pelvic inflammatory disease
■ Intrauterine infection
■ Preterm labor
■ Fetal loss

Special considerations
■ Report notifiable cases of sexually transmitted diseases to local public health authorities.
■ Persistent, recurring candidiasis may suggest diabetes or undiagnosed pregnancy.

••••••••••••

SELECTED REFERENCES

Association of Women's Health, Obstetric, and Neonatal Nurses, Mandeville, L.K., and Troiano, N.H., eds. *AWHONN's High Risk and Critical Care Intrapartum Nursing,* 2nd ed. Philadelphia: Lippincott Williams & Wilkins, 1999.

Burroughs, A., and Leifer, G. *Maternity Nursing: An Introductory Text,* 8th ed. Philadelphia: W.B. Saunders Co., 2001.

Diagnostic and Statistical Manual of Mental Disorders, 4th ed. Washington, D.C.: American Psychiatric Association, 1994.

Gilbert, E.S., and Harmon, J.S. *Manual of High Risk Pregnancy and Delivery,* 2nd ed. St. Louis: Mosby–Year Book, Inc., 1998.

Leifer, G. *Thompson's Introduction to Maternity and Pediatric Nursing,* 3rd ed. Philadelphia: W.B. Saunders Co., 1999.

Lowdermilk, D.L., et al. *Maternity Nursing,* 5th ed. St. Louis: Mosby–Year Book, Inc., 1999.

Maas, M., et al. *Nursing Care of Older Adults: Diagnoses, Outcomes, and Interventions.* St. Louis: Mosby–Year Book, Inc., 2000.

Melson, K.A., et al. *Maternal-Infant Care Planning,* 3rd ed. Springhouse, Pa.: Springhouse Corp., 1999.

Novak, J.C., and Broom, B.L. *Ingalls and Salerno's Maternal and Child Health Nursing,* 9th ed. St. Louis: Mosby–Year Book, Inc., 1999.

Nursing Procedures, 3rd ed. Springhouse, Pa.: Springhouse Corp., 2000.

Pillitteri, A. *Maternal and Child Health Nursing: Care of the Childbearing and Childrearing Family,* 3rd ed. Philadelphia: Lippincott Williams & Wilkins, 1999.

Thiedke, C., and Rosenfeld, J.A. *Women's Health (American Academy of Family Physicians).* Philadelphia: Lippincott Williams & Wilkins, 2000.

Zerbe, K.J. *Women's Mental Health in Primary Care.* Philadelphia: W.B. Saunders Co., 1999.

Eye, ear, nose, and throat disorders

Disorders that affect the eye generally lead to vision loss or impairment; routine ophthalmic examinations and early treatment can help prevent vision loss through early detection. Ear, nose, and throat disorders require careful nursing assessment and, in many cases, recommendations for follow-up treatment. Untreated hearing loss or deafness may impair a person's ability to interact with society. Ear disorders also have the ability to impair equilibrium. Nasal disorders can cause changes in facial features and interfere with breathing and tasting. Diseases arising in the throat may threaten airway patency and interfere with speech. In addition, these disorders can cause considerable discomfort and pain for the patient and require thorough assessment and prompt treatment.

ASSESSMENT

Assessment of the eye includes testing the patient's vision and extraocular muscle function, inspecting the external ocular structures, and inspecting internal structures with an ophthalmoscope.

Use inspection and palpation to assess the patient's ears, nose, and throat.

Assessing the eyes

For a basic eye assessment, obtain a Snellen eye chart, a piece of newsprint, an eye occluder or an opaque 3″ × 5″ card, a penlight, a wisp of cotton, a pencil or other narrow cylindrical article, and an ophthalmoscope. A patient who normally wears corrective lenses should wear them for the distance- and near-vision tests.

Distance vision

To test the distance vision of a patient who can read English, use the Snellen alphabet chart, which is printed with lines of various letters in decreasing sizes from top to bottom. For patients who are illiterate or unable to speak English, use the Snellen E chart, which displays the letter E in varying sizes and positions. The patient indicates the position of the E by duplicating the position with his fingers. Picture charts can be used for children.

Each line of the chart is labeled with a number, such as 20/20 or 20/100. The denominator, which ranges from 10 to 200, indicates the distance from which a person with normal vision can read the chart. For example, if the patient can only read a line identified by the numbers 20/100, this means that he can read from 20′ (6.1 m) what a person with normal vision can read from 100′ (31 m). If he reads the 20/20 line correctly, this is considered "normal" visual acuity.

Be certain to position the patient 20′ from the chart. Test each eye separately by first covering the left eye, and then the right, with an opaque 3″ × 5″ card or an eye occluder. Afterward, test binocular vision by having the patient read the chart with both eyes uncovered. Start with the line marked 20/40. Continue down the chart until the patient can read a line correctly with no more than two errors. That line indicates the patient's distance visual acuity.

Near vision
Test the patient's near vision by holding either a Snellen chart or a card with newsprint 12″ to 14″ (30.5 to 35.5 cm) in front of the patient's eyes. As with distance vision, test each eye separately and then together. Any patient who complains of blurring with the card at 12″ to 14″ or who is unable to read it accurately needs retesting and then referral to an ophthalmologist, if necessary. Keep in mind that a patient who is illiterate may be too embarrassed to say so. If a patient seems to be struggling to read the type or stares at it without attempting to read, change to the Snellen E chart.

Color perception
People with color blindness can't distinguish among red, green, and blue. The most common test to detect color blindness involves asking a patient to identify patterns of colored dots on colored plates. A patient who can't discern colors is unable to discern the patterns.

Extraocular muscle function
To assess extraocular muscle function, first inspect the eyes for position and alignment, making sure they're parallel. Next, perform the following tests: the six cardinal positions of gaze test, the cover-uncover test, and the corneal light reflex test.

To perform the six cardinal positions of gaze test, sit directly in front of the patient, and ask him to remain still while you hold a cylindrical object, such as a penlight, directly in front of, and about 18″ (46 cm) away from, the patient's nose. Ask him to hold his head still and to watch the object as you move it from straight ahead to up and to the right, to the right side, down and to the right, straight down, down and to the left, to the left side, and up and to the left. Throughout the test, the patient's eyes should remain parallel as they move.

The cover-uncover test is used to assess the fusion reflex, which makes binocular vision possible. To perform this test, have the patient stare at an object on a distant wall that's straight ahead. Cover the patient's left eye with an opaque card and observe the uncovered right eye for movement or wandering. Next, remove the card from the left eye. The left eye should remain steady, without moving or wandering. Repeat the procedure on the right eye.

To perform the corneal light reflex test, ask the patient to stare straight ahead while you shine a penlight on the bridge of his nose from a distance of 12″ to 15″ (30.5 to 38 cm). Check to make sure that the cornea reflects the light in exactly the same place in both eyes.

Peripheral vision

Assessment of peripheral vision is done to test the optic nerve (cranial nerve II) and measure the retina's ability to receive stimuli from the periphery of its field. You can grossly evaluate the patient's visual fields by comparing the patient's peripheral vision with your own. However, because this assumes you have normal vision, the test can be subjective and inaccurate. (See *Testing peripheral vision*.)

Inspection

Next inspect the eyelids, eyelashes, and lacrimal apparatus. Then inspect the eyeball, the conjunctiva, sclera, cornea, anterior chamber, iris, and pupil. Using an ophthalmoscope, inspect the vitreous humor and retina.

Eyelids, eyelashes, eyeball, and lacrimal apparatus

Inspect these structures for general appearance. The eyes are normally bright and clear. The eyelids should close completely over the sclera and, when opened, the margins of the upper eyelids should fall between the superior pupil margin and the superior limbus, covering a small portion of the iris. The eyelids should be free from edema, scaling, or lesions, and the eyelashes should curve outward and be equally distributed along the upper and lower eyelid margins. Inspect the palpebral folds for symmetry and the eyes for nystagmus and lid lag. Further inspect the eyes for excessive tearing or dryness and the puncta for inflammation and swelling.

Conjunctiva and sclera

View the white sclera through the bulbar portion of the conjunctiva. The conjunctiva should be free from engorged blood vessels and mucus.

Inspect the color of the sclera, which is normally white. However, it isn't unusual for patients with dark complexions, such as blacks and those from the Middle East, to have small, darkly pigmented spots on the sclera.

Cornea, anterior chamber, and iris

To inspect the cornea and anterior chamber, shine a penlight into the patient's eye from several side angles (tangentially). Normally, the cornea and anterior chamber are clear and transparent. Calculate the depth of the anterior chamber from the side by figuring the distance between the cornea and the iris. The iris should illuminate with the side lighting.

The surface of the cornea normally appears shiny and bright without any scars or irregularities. The lids of both eyes should close when you touch either cornea.

Inspect the iris for shape and color. The iris should have a rather flat appearance when it's viewed from the side.

Pupil

Examine the pupil of each eye for equality of size, shape, reaction to light, and accommodation. To test for accommodation, ask the patient to stare at an object across the room. Normally, the pupils should dilate. Then ask him to stare at your index finger or at a pencil held about 14″ (35.5 cm) away. The pupils should constrict and converge equally on the object. (See *Documenting with PERRLA*, page 560.)

Palpation

After inspection, palpate the eye and related structures. Begin by gently palpat-

Testing peripheral vision

To test peripheral visual fields, follow this procedure. Sit facing the patient, about 2' (61 cm) away, with your eyes at the same level as the patient's. Ask the patient to stare straight ahead. Cover one of your eyes with an opaque cover or your hand and ask the patient to cover the eye directly opposite your covered eye. Next, bring an object such as a penlight from the periphery of the superior field toward the center of the field of vision, as shown in the illustration below. The object should be equidistant between you and the patient. Ask the patient to tell you the moment the object appears. If your peripheral vision is intact, you and the patient should see the object at the same time.

inferior, nasal, and temporal visual fields, as shown in the diagram below. When testing the temporal field, it's difficult to move the penlight far enough out so that neither person can see it. So, test the temporal field by placing the penlight somewhat behind the patient and out of the patient's visual field; slowly bring the penlight around until the patient can see it.

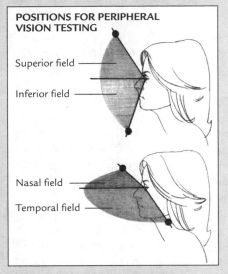

POSITIONS FOR PERIPHERAL VISION TESTING

Superior field

Inferior field

Nasal field

Temporal field

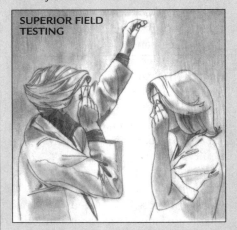

SUPERIOR FIELD TESTING

Repeat the procedure clockwise at 45-degree angles, checking the superior,

The normal field of vision is about 50 degrees upward, 60 degrees medially, 70 degrees downward, and 110 degrees laterally. Remember that this test discovers only large peripheral vision defects such as blindness in one-quarter to one-half of the visual field.

ing the eyelids for swelling and tenderness. Next, palpate the eyeballs by placing the tips of both index fingers on the eyelids over the sclerae while the patient looks down. The eyeballs should feel equally firm. However, never do this when you suspect traumatic eye injury.

Next, palpate the lacrimal sac by pressing the index finger against the patient's lower orbital rim on the side closest to his nose. While pressing, observe the punctum for any abnormal regurgitation of purulent material or excessive

Documenting with PERRLA

To document a normal pupil assessment, use the abbreviation PERRLA. By using this common acronym, which stands for **p**upils **e**qual, **r**ound, **r**eactive to **l**ight, and **a**ccommodation, you can speed up your documentation. Also, remember to use the terms direct and consensual when documenting a normal pupil response to light.

tears, which could indicate blockage of the nasolacrimal duct.

Ophthalmoscopic examination

Before beginning, practice holding and using the ophthalmoscope until you feel comfortable with it. The "0" lens is glass without any refraction. Set the lens at 0 and then slowly move toward a positive number, such as 6 or 8, or until the patient's optic disk becomes sharply focused.

An ophthalmoscopic examination can be used to detect many disorders of the optic disk and retina, but mastering the technique and interpreting abnormalities require skill, experience, and knowledge. (See *Performing an ophthalmoscopic examination*.)

Assessing the ears, nose, and throat

Use inspection and palpation to assess the ears, nose, and throat. If appropriate, also use a head mirror, postnasal mirrors, an otoscope, and a nasal speculum.

Inspecting and palpating the ears

Examine ear color and size. The ears should be similarly shaped, colored the

same as the face, and sized in proportion to the head. Look for drainage, nodules, or lesions. Some ears normally drain large amounts of cerumen. Check behind the ear for inflammation, masses, or lesions.

Palpate the external ear and the mastoid process to discover any areas of tenderness, swelling, nodules, or lesions, and then gently pull the helix of the ear backward to detect pain or tenderness.

Otoscopic examination

Before examining the auditory canal and the tympanic membrane, become familiar with the function of the otoscope. (See *Performing an otoscopic examination*, page 563.)

Assessing the temporomandibular joints

Inspect and palpate the temporomandibular joints, which are located anterior to and slightly below the auricle. To palpate these joints, place the middle three fingers of each hand bilaterally over each joint. Then gently press on the joints as the patient opens and closes his mouth. Evaluate the joints for movability, approximation (drawing of bones together), and discomfort. Normally, this process should be smooth and painless for the patient.

Assessing the nose

Inspect the nose for symmetry and contour, noting any foreign bodies, unusual or foul odors, and areas of deformity, swelling, or discoloration. To assess nasal symmetry, ask the patient to tilt his head back and observe the position of the nasal septum. The septum should be aligned with the bridge of the nose. With the head in the same position, evaluate flaring of the nostrils. Some flaring during quiet breathing is normal, but marked flaring may indicate respiratory distress. The nose should be intact and symmetri-

Performing an ophthalmoscopic examination

Use an ophthalmoscope to identify inner eye abnormalities. Place the patient in a darkened or semidarkened room, with neither you nor the patient wearing glasses unless you're very myopic or astigmatic. You or the patient may wear contact lenses.

1. Sit or stand in front of the patient with your head about 1½' (46 cm) in front of and about 15 degrees to the right of the patient's line of vision in the right eye. Hold the ophthalmoscope in your right hand with the viewing aperture as close to your right eye as possible. Place your left thumb on the patient's right eyebrow to prevent hitting the patient with the ophthalmoscope as you move in close. Keep your right index finger on the lens selector to adjust the lens as necessary, as shown here. To examine the left eye, perform these steps on the patient's left side.

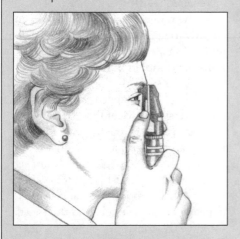

2. Instruct the patient to look straight ahead at a fixed point on the wall at eye level. Next, approaching from an oblique angle about 15″ (38 cm) out and with the diopter at 0, focus a small circle of light on the pupil as shown at the top of the next column. Look for the orange-red glow of the red reflex, which should be sharp and distinct through the pupil. The red reflex indicates that the lens is free from opacity and clouding.

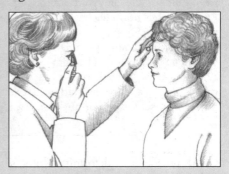

3. Move closer to the patient, changing the lens with your forefinger to keep the retinal structures in focus, as shown below.

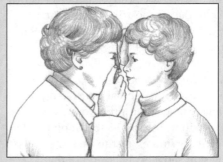

4. Change to a positive diopter to view the vitreous humor, observing for any opacity.
5. Next, view the retina, using a strong negative lens. Look for a retinal blood vessel, and follow that vessel toward the patient's nose, rotating the lens selector to keep the vessel in focus. Examine all the retinal structures, including the retinal vessels, the optic disc, the retinal background, the macula, and the fovea.

(continued)

Performing an ophthalmoscopic examination (continued)

6. Examine the vessels for their color, the size ratio of arterioles to veins, the arteriole light reflex, and the arteriovenous (AV) crossing. The crossing points should be smooth, without nicks or narrowing, and the vessels should be free from exudate, bleeding, and narrowing. Retinal vessels normally have an AV ratio of 2:3 or 4:5.

7. Evaluate the color of the retinal structures. The retina should be light yellow to orange and the background free from hemorrhages, aneurysms, and exudates. The optic disc, located on the nasal side

of the retina, should be orange-red with distinct margins. The physiologic cup is about one-third the size of the optic disc and is normally yellow-white and readily visible.

8. Examine the macula last and as briefly as possible because it's very light-sensitive. The macula, which is darker than the rest of the retinal background, is free from vessels and located temporally to the optic disc. The fovea centralis is a slight depression in the center of the macula.

---

cal, with no edema or deformity. Note the character and amount of any drainage from the nostrils.

Next, palpate the nose, checking for painful or tender areas, swelling, or deformities. Evaluate nostril patency by gently occluding one nostril with your finger and having the patient exhale through the other.

Assessing the sinuses

To assess the paranasal sinuses, inspect, palpate, and percuss the frontal and maxillary sinuses. To assess the frontal and maxillary sinuses, first inspect the external skin surfaces above and to the side of the nose for inflammation or edema. Then palpate and percuss the sinuses.

Assessing the mouth and oropharynx

Put on gloves, and ask the patient to remove any partial or complete dentures.

When examining the oral mucosa, observe the gingivae and teeth. Gingival surfaces should appear pink, moist, and slightly irregular, with no spongy or edematous areas. The edges of the teeth should be clearly defined, with a shallow

crevice visible between the gingivae and teeth. Note any missing, broken, loose, or repaired teeth.

The tongue should appear pink and slightly rough, with a midline depression and a V-shaped division (sulcus terminalis), and should move freely.

Also inspect the hard and soft palates. They should appear pink to light red, with symmetrical lines. Normally, the hard palate is rougher and a lighter pink than the soft palate.

Examine the oropharynx, using a tongue blade and flashlight, if necessary. Observe the position, size, and overall appearance of the uvula and the tonsils. Observe the tonsils for enlargement. Then place the tongue blade firmly on the midpoint of the tongue, almost far enough back to elicit the gag reflex, and ask the patient to say "ah." The soft palate and uvula should rise symmetrically.

Performing an otoscopic examination

Have the patient sit in a comfortable position or lie down on the side opposite the ear you wish to examine. Hold the otoscope's handle in the space between your thumb and index finger. Assist the patient to tilt her head toward the shoulder opposite the ear you're examining. While envisioning how the ear canal curves in an adult, gently grasp the auricle and pull it up and back to straighten the ear canal before inserting the speculum as shown below.

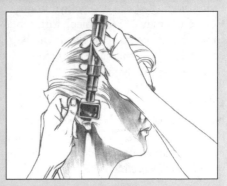

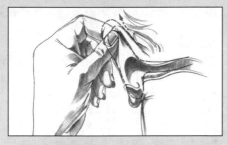

Keep in mind the sensitivity of the skin in the ear canal. Using an improper technique at this time can cause the patient considerable discomfort or even pain.

If you're examining a child's ear, pull the auricle gently downward to straighten the ear canal before inserting the speculum.

Grasp the otoscope in your dominant hand with the handle parallel to the patient's head and the speculum at the patient's ear, as shown at the top of the next column. Holding the otoscope

with the handle facing up allows you to brace your hand against the patient's head to stabilize the instrument. This helps to prevent injury if the patient moves her head quickly.

Inspect the auditory canal for cerumen, redness, or swelling. You'll see hairs and cerumen in the distal two-thirds of the ear canal. Note if excessive cerumen obstructs your view; you may need to remove it to complete your inspection.

Inspect the tympanic membrane. Typically, middle ear problems are evident from the appearance of the tympanic membrane. Focus on the membrane's color and contour; it should be pearly gray and appear concave at the umbo. Then move the otoscope to identify landmarks on the tympanic membrane, including the umbo, handle of malleus, and cone of light. Be alert for perforations, bulging, missing landmarks, or a distorted cone of light.

•••••••••••

BLEPHARITIS

Blepharitis is a common inflammation that produces a red-rimmed appearance of the margins of the eyelids. It's commonly chronic and bilateral and can affect both upper and lower lids. Seborrhe-

ic blepharitis is characterized by formation of waxy scales and symptoms of burning and foreign-body sensation and is common in elderly patients and in patients with red hair. Staphylococcal (ulcerative) blepharitis is characterized by formation of dry scales along the inflamed lid margins, which also have ulcerated areas. It's more common in females and may be associated with keratoconjunctivitis sicca (KES), a dry-eye syndrome. Both types may coexist. Blepharitis tends to recur and become chronic. It can be controlled if treatment begins before onset of ocular involvement.

Causes
Seborrheic blepharitis may be seen in conjunction with seborrhea of the scalp, eyebrows, and ears; ulcerative blepharitis, with *Staphylococcus aureus* infection.

Clinical presentation
Clinical features of blepharitis include:
- itching
- burning
- foreign-body sensation
- sticky, crusted eyelids on waking.

Constant irritation results in unconscious rubbing of the eyes (causing reddened rims) or continual blinking. Other signs include waxy scales in seborrheic blepharitis; flaky scales on lashes, loss of lashes, and ulcerated areas on lid margins in ulcerative blepharitis. In association with KES, dry eyes may also be a problem.

Differential diagnoses
- Anaphylaxis
- Insect bites
- Chalazion
- Orbital infections
- Hordeolum or stye
- Cavernous sinus thrombosis
- Dacryocystitis

Diagnosis
Diagnosis depends on the patient's history and characteristic symptoms. In ulcerative blepharitis, culture of the ulcerated lid margin shows *S. aureus*.

Management
General
The goals of therapy are to control the disease, maintain vision, and avoid secondary complications. Treatment depends on the type of blepharitis:
- Seborrheic blepharitis — Perform daily lid hygiene (using a mild shampoo on a damp applicator stick or a washcloth) and use hot compresses to remove scales from the lid margins; also, frequently shampoo the scalp and eyebrows.
- Ulcerative blepharitis — Warm compresses and an antibiotic may be applied.
- Blepharitis resulting from pediculosis — Remove nits (with forceps or ointment).

Medication
The following medications may be used to treat blepharitis:
- bacitracin ophthalmic ointment — apply to lid margin b.i.d. to q.i.d. for 2 weeks
- erythromycin ophthalmic ointment — apply to lid margin b.i.d. to q.i.d. for 2 weeks
- tetracycline — 250 mg P.O. q.i.d. for 2 weeks
- physostigmine ophthalmic ointment — insecticide used to treat the patient with blepharitis resulting from pediculosis.

Referral
- If there's no improvement in signs and symptoms in 24 to 48 hours, refer the patient to an ophthalmologist.

Follow-up
The patient should be seen after 2 weeks of treatment and then every month until the condition is completely controlled.

Patient teaching
- Instruct the patient to gently remove scales from the lid margins daily, using an applicator stick or a clean washcloth.

- Teach the patient the following method for applying warm compresses:
  – Run warm water into a clean bowl.
  – Immerse a clean cloth in the water and wring it out.
  – Place the warm cloth against the closed eyelid (be careful not to burn the skin). Hold the compress in place until it cools.
  – Continue this procedure for 15 minutes.
  – Antibiotic ophthalmic ointment should be applied after warm compresses.
- Tell the patient that blepharitis is a chronic condition that requires long-term eyelid hygiene.

Complications
- Scarring of the eyelid margin
- Corneal infection
- Hordeolum

Special considerations
- Treatment of seborrheic blepharitis also necessitates attention to the face and scalp.

• • • • • • • • • • • •
CATARACT

A cataract is a gradually developing opacity of the lens or lens capsule of the eye. It's the most common cause of correctable vision loss. Cataracts commonly occur bilaterally, with each progressing independently. Exceptions are traumatic cataracts, which are usually unilateral, and congenital cataracts, which may not progress. The prognosis is generally good; surgery improves vision in 95% of affected people.

AGE ALERT More than one-half of people older than age 65 have a cataract.

Causes
Cataracts have various causes:
- Senile cataracts develop in elderly patients, probably because of degenerative changes in the chemical state of lens proteins.
- Congenital cataracts occur in neonates as genetic defects or as sequelae of maternal rubella during the first trimester.
- Traumatic cataracts develop after a foreign object injures the lens with sufficient force to allow aqueous or vitreous humor to enter the lens capsule. Trauma may also dislocate the lens.
- Complicated cataracts develop as secondary effects in patients with uveitis, glaucoma, or retinitis pigmentosa or in the course of a systemic disease, such as diabetes, hypoparathyroidism, or atopic dermatitis. They can also result from exposure to ionizing radiation or infrared rays.
- Toxic cataracts result from drug or chemical toxicity from prednisone, ergot alkaloids, dinitrophenol, naphthalene, phenothiazines, or pilocarpine. They can also result from extended exposure to ultraviolet rays.

Clinical presentation
Characteristically, a patient with a cataract experiences painless, gradual blurring and loss of vision. As the cataract progresses, the normally black pupil appears hazy, and when a mature cataract develops, the white lens may be seen through the pupil. Some patients complain of:
- blinding glare from headlights when they drive at night
- poor reading vision
- unpleasant glare and poor vision in bright sunlight.

Patients with central opacities report better vision in dim light than in bright light because the cataract is nuclear and, as the pupils dilate, patients can see around the lens opacity.

Differential diagnoses
- Trauma
- Myopia
- Diabetic retinopathy
- Retinitis pigmentosa

Diagnosis
On examination, visual acuity is decreased, and the lens remains unnoticeable until the cataract is advanced. Ophthalmoscopy or slit-lamp examination confirms the diagnosis by revealing a dark area in the normally homogeneous red reflex.

Management
General
The best treatment for cataracts is surgical removal. Without surgery, a patient's eyesight deteriorates to blindness.

Surgical intervention
Treatment consists of surgical extraction of the cataractous lens and intraoperative correction of visual deficits, generally as a same-day procedure. Surgical procedures include:
- In extracapsular cataract extraction (ECCE), the anterior lens capsule and cortex are removed, leaving the posterior capsule intact. A posterior chamber intraocular lens (IOL) is implanted where the patient's own lens used to be. (A posterior chamber IOL is the most common type used in the United States.) This procedure is appropriate for use in patients of all ages.
- In phacoemulsification, ultrasonic vibrations are used to fragment and then emulsify the lens, which is then aspirated through a small incision.
- In intracapsular cataract extraction, the entire lens is removed from the intact capsule. This procedure is seldom performed;

ECCE with phacoemulsification has replaced it as the most common procedure.
- Discission and aspiration can still be used for children with soft cataracts, but this procedure has largely been replaced by phacoemulsification.

A patient with an IOL implant may have improved vision shortly after surgery if there's no corneal or retinal pathology. Most IOLs correct for distance vision, but a new generation of IOLs are multifocal. Most patients still need either corrective reading glasses or a corrective contact lens, which is fitted sometime between 4 and 6 weeks after surgery.

When no IOL is implanted, the patient may receive temporary aphakic cataract glasses; in about 4 to 8 weeks, the patient is refracted for his own glasses.

In some cases, a patient who has an ECCE develops a secondary membrane in the posterior lens capsule (which has been left intact) that causes decreased visual acuity. However this membrane can be removed by laser surgery, which cuts an area out of the center of the membrane, thereby restoring vision. Laser therapy isn't used to remove a cataract.

Posterior capsular opacification occurs in approximately 15% to 20% of all patients within 2 years after cataract surgery.

Referral
- Refer the patient to an ophthalmologist for treatment.

Follow-up
The patient should be seen 1 to 2 days after discharge from surgery.

Patient teaching
- Tell the patient to avoid activities that increase intraocular pressure such as straining.
- Urge the patient to protect the eye from accidental injury at night by wear-

ing a plastic or metal shield with perforations; a shield or glasses should be worn for protection during the day.

• Teach the patient to administer antibiotic ointment or drops to prevent infection and steroids to reduce inflammation; combination steroid and antibiotic eyedrops may be used.

• Advise the patient to watch for and immediately report complications such as a sharp pain in the eye that's uncontrolled by analgesics; this can be caused by hyphema (clouding in the anterior chamber) and may herald an infection.

• Advise the patient about activity restrictions, and caution him that it will take several weeks for him to receive his corrective reading glasses or lenses.

Complications
• Blindness
• Postoperative infection
• Hyphema
• Pupillary block glaucoma
• Retinal detachment

• • • • • • • • • • • •

CHALAZION

A chalazion is a chronic granulomatous inflammation of a meibomian (sebaceous) gland or gland of Zeis in the upper or lower eyelid. This common eye disorder is characterized by localized swelling within the tarsal plate, or it may break through the conjunctival or skin side; mild irritation and blurred vision usually develop slowly over several weeks. (See *Recognizing chalazion.*)

A chalazion may become large enough to press on the eyeball, producing astigmatism; a large chalazion seldom subsides spontaneously. It's generally benign and chronic and can occur at any age; in some patients, recurrence is likely.

> ### Recognizing chalazion
>
> The chalazion depicted below is a nontender granulomatous inflammation of a meibomian gland on the upper eyelid.
>
>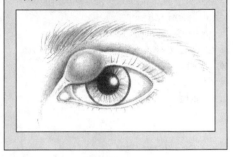

Causes
Obstruction of the meibomian gland duct causes a chalazion.

Clinical presentation
A chalazion usually occurs as a painless, hard lump that usually points *toward* the conjunctival side of the eyelid. Eversion of the lid reveals a red or red-yellow raised area on the conjunctival surface. In some cases, a chalazion is an indurated bump under the skin of the upper eyelid.

Differential diagnoses
• Hordeolum
• Stye
• Blepharitis
• Meibomianitis
• Meibomian cell carcinoma

Diagnosis
Diagnosis requires visual examination and palpation of the eyelid, revealing a small bump or nodule. Persistently recurrent chalazion, especially in an adult, necessitates biopsy to rule out meibomian cancer.

Management

General

The initial treatment for chalazion is to apply warm compresses to open the lumen of the gland.

Medication

Medication used to treat a patient with chalazion include:

- gentamicin ophthalmic eyedrops — 1 to 2 drops every 4 hours into the affected eye
- erythromycin ophthalmic ointment — applied to the affected eye b.i.d. for 2 to 8 days.

Surgical intervention

If the above therapy fails, or if the chalazion presses on the eyeball or causes a severe cosmetic problem, steroid injection or incision and curettage under local anesthetic may be necessary.

Referral

- The patient may need referral to an ophthalmologist if he doesn't respond to treatment.

Follow-up

The patient should be seen after 1 to 2 weeks of treatment to evaluate improvement.

Patient teaching

- Instruct the patient how to properly apply warm compresses: Tell him to take special care to avoid burning the skin, to always use a clean cloth, and to discard used compresses. Also tell him to start applying warm compresses at the first sign of lid irritation to increase the blood supply and to keep the lumen open.
- Teach the patient about eyelid hygiene to prevent reoccurrence.

Complications

- Cellulitis of the eyelid or orbit
- Astigmatism

• • • • • • • • • • •

CONJUNCTIVITIS

Conjunctivitis is characterized by hyperemia of the conjunctiva due to infection, allergy, or chemical reactions. (See *Recognizing conjunctivitis*.) This disorder usually occurs as benign, self-limiting pinkeye; it may also be chronic, possibly indicating degenerative changes or damage from repeated acute attacks. In the Western Hemisphere, conjunctivitis is probably the most common eye disorder.

Causes

The most common causative organisms are:

- bacterial — *Staphylococcus aureus, Streptococcus pneumoniae, Neisseria gonorrhoeae, N. meningitides*
- chlamydial — *Chlamydia trachomatis* (inclusion conjunctivitis)
- viral — adenovirus types 3, 7, and 8; herpes simplex virus, type 1.

Other causes include allergic reactions to pollen, grass, topical medication, air pollutants, smoke, or unknown seasonal allergens (vernal conjunctivitis); environmental (wind, dust, smoke) and occupational irritants (acids and alkalies); and a hypersensitivity to contact lenses or solutions.

Vernal conjunctivitis (so-called because symptoms tend to be worse in the spring) is a severe form of immunoglobulin E-mediated mast cell hypersensitivity reaction. This form of conjunctivitis is bilateral. It usually begins between ages 3 and 5 and persists for about 10 years. It's sometimes associated with other signs of allergy commonly related to pollens, asthma, and allergic rhinitis.

Epidemic keratoconjunctivitis is an acute, highly contagious viral conjunctivitis. Health care providers must be careful to wash their hands and sterilize equipment to prevent the spread of this disease.

Clinical presentation

Conjunctivitis commonly produces the following signs and symptoms:

- hyperemia of the conjunctiva, sometimes accompanied by discharge
- tearing
- pain and photophobia.

It generally doesn't affect vision. Conjunctivitis usually begins in one eye and rapidly spreads to the other by contamination of towels, washcloths, or the patient's own hand.

Acute bacterial conjunctivitis (pinkeye) usually lasts only 2 weeks. The patient typically complains of:

- itching
- burning
- sensation of a foreign object in the eye.

The eyelids show a crust of sticky, mucopurulent discharge; if the disorder is due to *N. gonorrhoeae*, the patient exhibits a profuse, purulent discharge.

Viral conjunctivitis produces copious tearing with minimal exudate and enlargement of the preauricular lymph node. Some viruses follow a chronic course and produce severe disabling disease; others last 2 to 3 weeks and are self-limiting.

Differential diagnoses

- Corneal abrasion
- Acute angle closure glaucoma
- Herpes zoster
- Otic herpes zoster
- Iritis
- Uveitis
- Scleritis
- Reiter's syndrome

Recognizing conjunctivitis

Itching is the hallmark of allergy. Giant papillae resembling cobblestones may be seen on the palpebral conjunctiva, as shown here.

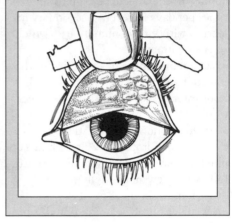

Diagnosis

Physical examination reveals peripheral injection of the bulbar conjunctival vessels. In children, possible systemic symptoms include sore throat or fever, if the conjunctivitis is suspected of being of adenoviral origin.

Lymphocytes are predominant in stained smears of conjunctival scrapings if a virus causes conjunctivitis. Polymorphonuclear cells (neutrophils) predominate if conjunctivitis is due to bacteria; eosinophils predominate if it's allergy-related. Culture and sensitivity tests are used to identify the causative bacterial organism and to select the appropriate antibiotic therapy.

Management
General

Patients may be contagious for several weeks after onset. The most important aspect of treatment is preventing transmission. Cold compresses are applied to relieve itching.

Medication

Treatment of conjunctivitis varies with the cause:

- bacitracin ophthalmic ointment—applied to affected eye q.d. or more for bacterial conjunctivitis.
- erythromycin ophthalmic ointment—applied to the infected eye up to six times per day to prevent a secondary infection with viral conjunctivitis (which resists treatment).
- vidarabine ointment—applied to the infected eyelid five times per day at 3-hour intervals for herpes simplex infection.
- prednisolone acetate ophthalmic solution—1 to 2 drops every 3 to 4 hours applied for vernal (allergic) conjunctivitis, followed by cromolyn sodium, 1 to 2 drops four to six times per day.
- 1% silver nitrate solution (Credé's procedure)—one time dose administered to prevent gonococcal conjunctivitis in neonates.

Referral

- Refer the patient to an ophthalmologist if treatment is unsuccessful.

Follow-up

The patient should be checked in 48 hours for improvement and then in 2 weeks.

Patient teaching

- Teach proper hand-washing technique because bacterial and viral conjunctivitis are highly contagious. Stress the risk of spreading infection to family members by sharing washcloths, towels, and pillows. Warn against rubbing the infected eye, which can spread the infection to the other eye and to other people.
- Teach the patient to instill eyedrops and ointments correctly, without touching the bottle tip to his eye or lashes.

Complications

With bacterial conjunctivitis

- Chronic marginal blepharitis
- Corneal ulcer or perforation
- Conjunctival scar if membrane disrupted

With viral conjunctivitis

- Bacterial superinfection
- Corneal scars with herpes simplex
- Corneal scars, lid scars, entropion

With allergic conjunctivitis

- Bacterial superinfection

Special considerations

- Caution a patient who wears contact lenses to remove them while the eyes are infected.
- Stress the importance of safety glasses for the patient who works near chemical irritants.
- Notify public health authorities if cultures show *N. gonorrhoeae*.

• • • • • • • • • • • •

CORNEAL ABRASION

A corneal abrasion is a scratch on the surface epithelium of the cornea. An abrasion, or foreign object in the eye, is the most common eye injury. With treatment, the prognosis is usually good.

Causes

A corneal abrasion usually results from a foreign object—such as a cinder or piece of dust, dirt, or grit—that becomes embedded under the eyelid. Even if tears wash out the foreign substance, it can still injure the cornea. In some cases, a small piece of metal that gets in the eye of a worker who doesn't wear protective glasses quickly forms a rust ring on the cornea and causes corneal abrasion.

Corneal abrasions also commonly occur in the eyes of people who fall asleep wearing hard contact lenses or whose lenses aren't fitted properly.

A corneal scratch produced by a fingernail, a piece of paper, or another organic substance can cause a persistent lesion. The epithelium doesn't always heal properly, and recurrent corneal erosion may develop, with delayed effects more severe than the original injury.

Clinical presentation

A corneal abrasion typically produces the following signs and symptoms:
- redness
- increased tearing
- discomfort with blinking
- sensation of "something in the eye"
- pain disproportionate to the size of the injury.

It may also affect visual acuity, depending on the size and location of the injury.

Differential diagnoses

- Herpetic keratitis
- Recurrent corneal erosion syndrome
- Corneal ulcer
- Corneal laceration
- Corneal dystrophy
- Hyphema
- Iris prolapse
- Foreign object

Diagnosis

History of eye trauma or prolonged wearing of contact lenses and typical symptoms suggest corneal abrasion. Staining the cornea with fluorescein stain confirms the diagnosis: The injured area appears green when examined with a flashlight. Slit-lamp examination discloses the depth and allows measurement of the abrasion.

Examining the eye with a flashlight may reveal a foreign object on the cornea; the eyelid must be everted to check for a foreign object embedded under the lid.

Before beginning treatment, a test to determine visual acuity provides a medical baseline and a legal safeguard.

Management
General

Application of a pressure patch prevents further corneal irritation when the patient blinks. If the patient wears contact lenses, he may need to abstain from wearing the lenses until the corneal abrasion heals.

Medication

Medications used to treat a patient with corneal abrasion include:
- ciprofloxacin 0.3% ophthalmic drops — 2 drops every 15 minutes for the first 6 hours, then 2 drops every 30 minutes for the remainder of the first day, 2 drops every hour on day 2, then every 4 hours on days 3 to 14
- erythromycin 0.5% ointment — apply to the eye every 4 hours
- sulfacetamide 10% solution — 1 to 2 drops every 2 to 3 hours.

Surgical intervention

Topical anesthetic eyedrops are instilled in the affected eye before a foreign body spud is used to remove a superficial foreign object. A rust ring on the cornea must be removed with an ophthalmic burr. When only partial removal is possible, reepithelialization lifts the ring again to the surface and allows complete removal the next day.

Referral

- Refer the patient to an ophthalmologist for treatment.

Follow-up

The patient should be seen according to the ophthalmologist's recommendation.

Patient teaching

- Tell the patient with an eye patch to leave it in place for 6 to 12 hours. Warn that a patch alters depth perception, so advise caution in daily activities, such as climbing stairs or stepping off a curb.
- Reassure the patient that the corneal epithelium usually heals in 24 to 48 hours.
- Stress the importance of instilling antibiotic eyedrops, as ordered, because an untreated corneal abrasion can become infected, which can lead to a corneal ulcer and permanent vision loss. Teach the patient the proper way to instill eye medication.

Complications

- Blindness
- Vision loss
- Infection

Special considerations

- If a foreign object is visible, carefully irrigate with normal saline solution.
- Emphasize the importance of safety glasses to protect workers' eyes from flying fragments.
- To prevent further trauma, review instructions for wearing and caring for contact lenses.

• • • • • • • • • • • • •

CORNEAL ULCERS

Corneal ulcers produce corneal scarring or perforation. They occur in the central or marginal areas of the cornea, vary in shape and size, and may be singular or multiple; marginal ulcers are most common. Corneal ulcers are a major cause of blindness worldwide. Prompt treatment (within hours of onset) can prevent visual impairment.

Causes

Corneal ulcers generally result from protozoan, bacterial, viral, or fungal infections. Common bacterial sources include *Staphylococcus aureus, Pseudomonas aeruginosa, Streptococcus viridans, Streptococcus (Diplococcus) pneumoniae*, and *Moraxella liquefaciens*. Viral sources include herpes simplex type 1, variola, vaccinia, and varicella-zoster viruses. Common fungal sources include *Candida, Fusarium*, and *Cephalosporium*.

Other causes include trauma, exposure, reactions to bacterial infections, toxins, allergens, and wearing contact lenses. (See *What happens in corneal ulceration.*) Tuberculoprotein causes a classic phlyctenular keratoconjunctivitis; vitamin A deficiency results in xerophthalmia; and fifth cranial nerve lesions cause neurotropic ulcers.

Clinical presentation

Typically, corneal ulceration begins with pain (aggravated by blinking) and photophobia, followed by increased tearing. Eventually, central corneal ulceration produces pronounced visual blurring. The eye may look as if it's infected. If a bacterial ulcer is present, purulent discharge is possible.

Differential diagnoses

- Conjunctivitis
- Corneal abrasion
- Glaucoma
- Iritis
- Uveitis
- Foreign object
- Blepharitis

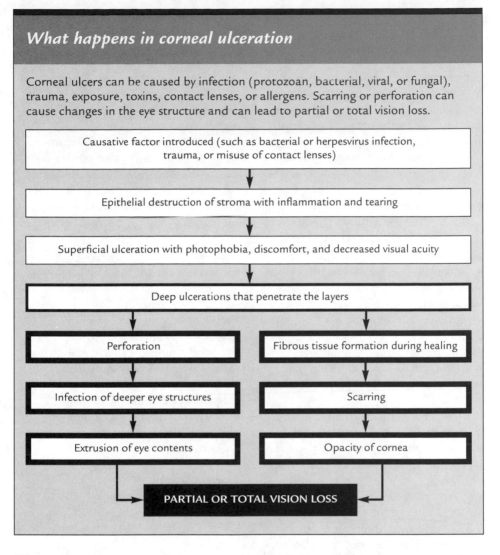

What happens in corneal ulceration

Corneal ulcers can be caused by infection (protozoan, bacterial, viral, or fungal), trauma, exposure, toxins, contact lenses, or allergens. Scarring or perforation can cause changes in the eye structure and can lead to partial or total vision loss.

Causative factor introduced (such as bacterial or herpesvirus infection, trauma, or misuse of contact lenses)

↓

Epithelial destruction of stroma with inflammation and tearing

↓

Superficial ulceration with photophobia, discomfort, and decreased visual acuity

↓

Deep ulcerations that penetrate the layers

↓ ↓

Perforation | Fibrous tissue formation during healing

↓ ↓

Infection of deeper eye structures | Scarring

↓ ↓

Extrusion of eye contents | Opacity of cornea

→ **PARTIAL OR TOTAL VISION LOSS** ←

Diagnosis

A history of trauma or use of contact lenses and flashlight examination that reveals an irregular corneal surface suggests corneal ulcer. Exudate may be present on the cornea, and a hypopyon (accumulation of white cells in the anterior chamber) may appear as a white crescent moon that moves when the head is tilted. Fluorescein dye, instilled in the conjunctival sac, stains the outline of the ulcer and confirms the diagnosis.

Culture and sensitivity testing of corneal scrapings may be used to identify the causative bacteria or fungus and determine an appropriate antibiotic or antifungal therapy.

Management
General

Prompt treatment is essential for all forms of corneal ulcer, to prevent complications and permanent visual impairment. The goals of treatment are to eliminate the underlying cause of the ulcer and to relieve pain.

Medication

Treatment usually consists of systemic and topical broad-spectrum antibiotics until culture results identify the causative organism. After the organism is identified, various treatments must be followed.

A patient with infection by *P. aeruginosa* must be treated immediately and isolated. This type of corneal ulcer spreads rapidly and can cause corneal perforation and loss of the eye within 48 hours. Medications used to treat this type of corneal ulcer include:

- polymyxin B — 1 to 3 drops of 0.1% to 0.25% hourly or up to 10,000 U injected subconjunctivally daily
- gentamicin ophthalmic solution — 1 to 2 drops every 4 hours up to a maximum of 2 drops every hour
- tobramycin — 1 to 2 drops every 4 hours or 1 cm ointment every 8 to 12 hours.

For a patient with an infection by herpes simplex type 1 virus, treat with vidarabine ointment (apply to the infected eyelid five times daily at 3-hour intervals).

For a patient with an infection by varicella zoster, treat with sulfacetamide 10% (1 drop q.i.d. to prevent secondary infection). These lesions are unilateral, following the pathway of the fifth cranial nerve, and are typically quite painful. Or, treat a patient with scopolamine (1 to 2 drops of 0.25% up to q.i.d.) for associated anterior uveitis. Watch for signs of secondary glaucoma (transient vision loss and halos around lights).

For a patient with an infection by fungi, treat with natamycin (1 drop every 1 to 6 hours) for infection by *Fusarium*, *Cephalosporium*, and *Candida*.

For a patient with hypovitaminosis A, treat by correcting dietary deficiency or GI malabsorption of vitamin A.

For a patient with neurotropic ulcers or exposure keratitis, treat with frequent instillation of artificial tears or lubricating ointments and use a plastic bubble eye shield for protection.

CLINICAL CAUTION Treatment for a patient with a corneal ulcer due to bacterial infection should *never* include an eye patch because patching creates a dark, warm, moist environment that's ideal for bacterial growth.

Referral

- Refer the patient to an ophthalmologist.

Follow-up

The patient should be seen according to the ophthalmologist's recommendation, usually after 1 week of treatment.

Patient teaching

- Teach the patient how to properly clean and wear contact lenses to prevent a recurrence.

Complications

- Vision loss
- Corneal scarring

• • • • • • • • • • • •

DACRYOCYSTITIS

Dacryocystitis is an infection of the lacrimal sac. In infants, it results from congenital atresia of the nasolacrimal duct; in adults, it results from an obstruction (dacryostenosis) of the nasolacrimal duct (most often in women over age 40). Dacryocystitis can be acute or chronic.

Causes

Atresia of the nasolacrimal ducts results from failure of canalization or, in the first few months of life, from blockage when the membrane that separates the lower part of the nasolacrimal duct and the inferior nasal meatus fails to open spontaneously before tear secretion. Bony obstruction of the duct may also occur.

In acute dacryocystitis, *Staphylococcus aureus* and, occasionally, beta-hemolytic streptococci are the cause. In chronic dacryocystitis, *Streptococcus pneumoniae* or, sometimes, a fungus — such as *Actinomyces* or *Candida albicans* — is the causative organism. Primary lumps and secondary tumors from the sinuses, nose, and orbits have also been reported as causes.

Clinical presentation

Dacryocystitis is extremely painful for the patient. The hallmark of both the acute and chronic forms of dacryocystitis is constant tearing. Other symptoms of dacryocystitis include inflammation and tenderness over the nasolacrimal sac; pressure over this area may fail to produce purulent discharge from the punctum.

Differential diagnoses

- Anaphylaxis
- Insect bites
- Chalazion
- Orbital infections
- Hordeolum (stye)
- Cavernous sinus thrombosis
- Blepharitis

Diagnosis

Clinical features and findings of a physical examination suggest dacryocystitis. Culture of the discharged material reveals *S. aureus* and, occasionally, beta-hemolytic streptococci in acute dacryocystitis and *S. pneumoniae* or *C. albicans*

in the chronic form. The patient's white blood cell count may be elevated in the acute form; in the chronic form, it's generally normal. An X-ray after injection of a radiopaque medium (dacryocystography) locates the atresia in infants.

Management

General

Treatment for a patient with acute dacryocystitis consists of warm compresses, along with topical and systemic antibiotics. Therapy for nasolacrimal duct obstruction in an infant consists of careful massage of the area over the lacrimal sac four times a day for 6 to 9 months. If this fails to open the duct, dilation of the punctum and probing of the duct are necessary.

Medication

Medications used to treat a patient with dacryocystitis include:
- polymyxin B — 1 to 3 drops every hour
- ofloxacin 0.3% solution — 1 to 2 drops every 2 to 4 hours while awake for 2 days, then q.i.d. for 5 more days
- cephalexin — 500 mg P.O. every 12 hours
- erythromycin — 500 mg P.O. every 12 hours.

Surgical intervention

Chronic dacryocystitis may eventually require dacryocystorhinostomy.

Referral

- Refer the patient to an ophthalmologist if an obstruction is present.

Follow-up

The patient should be seen as per the ophthalmologist's recommendation.

Patient teaching

- Teach the patient about the prescribed medication and how to apply warm compresses. Make sure you tell him that this treatment doesn't relieve any obstruction and that surgery may be required.
- Tell the adult patient what to expect after surgery: He'll have ice compresses over the surgical site and will have bruising and swelling. Tell him to place a small adhesive bandage over the suture line to protect it from damage.

Complications

- Abscess formation
- Periorbital cellulitis

• • • • • • • • • • • •

EARDRUM PERFORATION

Perforation of the eardrum is a rupture of the tympanic membrane. Such injury can cause otitis media and hearing loss.

Causes

The usual cause of a perforated eardrum is trauma, such as the deliberate or accidental insertion of foreign objects (cotton swabs or bobby pins) or sudden excessive changes in pressure (due to an explosion, a blow to the head, flying, or diving). A perforated eardrum may result from untreated otitis media and, in children, from acute otitis media.

Clinical presentation

Sudden onset of a severe earache and bleeding from the ear are the first signs of a perforated eardrum. Other symptoms include:

- hearing loss
- tinnitus
- vertigo.

Purulent otorrhea within 24 to 48 hours of injury signals infection.

Differential diagnoses

- Barotrauma
- Foreign object in ear
- Temporal bone fracture
- Otitis media
- Otitis externa
- Child abuse
- Trauma

Diagnosis

A severe earache and bleeding from the ear with a history of trauma strongly suggest a perforated eardrum; direct visualization of the perforated tympanic membrane with an otoscope confirms it.

Additional diagnostic measures include audiometric testing and a check of voluntary facial movements to rule out facial nerve damage.

Management

General

A sterile dressing may be applied over the outer ear if there's evidence of bleeding.

Medication

Medications used to treat a patient with a perforated eardrum include:

- acetaminophen — 325 to 650 mg P.O. every 4 to 6 hours: follow the package directions for pediatric dosage.
- amoxicillin-clavulanate — for a patient who weighs more than 88 lb (40 kg), 250 mg P.O. every 8 hours, or 500 mg every 12 hours; less than 88 lb (40 kg), 20 to 45 mg/kg/day P.O. divided every 8 to 12 hours.

Surgical intervention

A large perforation with uncontrolled bleeding may necessitate immediate surgery to approximate the ruptured edges.

Referral
- Refer the patient to an otolaryngologist if the perforation isn't healing.

Follow-up
The patient should be seen within 1 week to assess healing. After the perforation has healed, the patient should have an audiogram to determine whether hearing loss has occurred.

Patient teaching
- Tell the patient or parent not to irrigate the ear for any reason.
- Tell the patient or parent not to blow the nose or get water in the ear canal until the perforation heals.

Complications
- Middle ear infection
- Cholesteatoma
- Hearing loss

Special considerations
- Find out the cause of the injury and report suspected child abuse.

• • • • • • • • • • • •

EPISTAXIS

Epistaxis, commonly known as a nosebleed, may either be a primary disorder or occur secondary to another condition. Epistaxis is twice as common in children as in adults. Such bleeding in children generally originates in the anterior nasal septum and tends to be mild. In adults, such bleeding is most likely to originate in the posterior septum and can be severe. Exsanguination from epistaxis is rare.

Causes
Epistaxis usually follows trauma from an external or internal cause: a blow to the nose, nose picking, or insertion of a foreign object. Less commonly, it follows polyps; such acute or chronic infections as sinusitis and rhinitis, which cause congestion and eventual bleeding of the capillary blood vessels; or inhalation of chemicals that irritate the nasal mucosa.

Predisposing factors include anticoagulant therapy, hypertension, long-term use of aspirin, living at high altitude or in a dry climate, sclerotic vessel disease, Hodgkin's disease, neoplastic disorders (such as juvenile nasopharyngeal angiofibromas), scurvy, vitamin K deficiency, rheumatic fever, and blood dyscrasias (hemophilia, purpura, leukemia, and anemias).

Clinical presentation
Blood oozing from the nostrils usually originates in the anterior nose and is bright red. Blood from the back of the throat originates in the posterior area and may be dark or bright red (commonly mistaken for hemoptysis due to expectoration). Epistaxis is generally unilateral, except when it's due to dyscrasia or severe trauma. In severe epistaxis, blood may seep behind the nasal septum; it may also appear in the middle ear or corners of the eyes.

Associated clinical effects depend on the severity of bleeding. Moderate blood loss may produce:
- light-headedness
- dizziness
- slight respiratory difficulty.
Severe hemorrhage causes:
- hypotension
- rapid and bounding pulse
- dyspnea
- pallor.

Bleeding is considered severe if it persists longer than 10 minutes after pressure is applied and causes blood loss as great as 1 L/hour in adults.

Inserting an anterior-posterior nasal pack

The first step in the insertion of an anterior-posterior nasal pack is the insertion of catheters into the nostrils. After the catheters are drawn through the mouth, a suture from the pack is tied to each (as shown below).

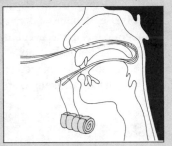

This positions the pack in place as the catheters are drawn back through the nostrils. While the sutures are held tightly, packing is inserted into the anterior nose (as shown below).

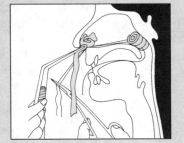

The sutures are then secured around a dental roll; the middle suture extends from the mouth (as shown below) and is taped to the cheek.

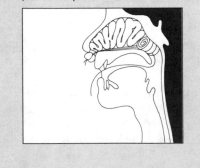

Differential diagnoses
- Barotrauma
- Disseminated intravascular coagulation
- Nasal foreign body
- Hemophilia A and B
- Sinusitis
- Drug toxicity (cocaine, coumarin, nonsteroidal anti-inflammatory drugs [NSAIDs], salicylate)
- Plant poisoning, glycosides
- Trauma

Diagnosis
Simple observation confirms epistaxis. Inspection with a bright light and a nasal speculum is necessary to locate the site of bleeding.

Relevant laboratory values include:
- gradual reduction in hemoglobin levels and hematocrit (HCT), which is commonly inaccurate immediately after epistaxis because of hemoconcentration)
- decreased platelet count in a patient with blood dyscrasia
- prothrombin time and partial thromboplastin time showing a coagulation time twice the control because of a bleeding disorder or anticoagulant therapy.

Bleeding tests are indicated if any of the following is present:
- family history of a bleeding disorder
- medical history of easy bleeding
- spontaneous bleeding at other sites
- bleeding that won't clot with direct pressure
- bleeding that lasts longer than 30 minutes
- onset before age 2 or decreased HCT due to epistaxis.

Management
General
For anterior bleeding, treatment consists of application of a cotton ball saturated with vasoconstrictor solution and external pressure to the bleeding site, followed

by cauterization with electrocautery or a silver nitrate stick. If these measures don't control the bleeding, petroleum gauze nasal packing may be needed.

For posterior bleeding, therapy includes gauze packing inserted through the nose, or postnasal packing inserted through the mouth, depending on the bleeding site. (Gauze packing generally remains in place for 24 to 48 hours; postnasal packing remains in place for 3 to 5 days.) (See *Inserting an anterior-posterior nasal pack.*) An alternate method, using a nasal balloon catheter, also controls bleeding effectively.

If local measures fail to control bleeding, additional treatment may include supplemental vitamin K and, for severe bleeding, blood transfusions.

Medication
Medications may include:
- phenylephrine 0.125% to 1% solution — 1 or 2 sprays into nostril
- cocaine 4% solution — applied to cotton ball before application to nasal cavity
- cephalexin — 250 mg P.O. every 6 hours if packing must remain in place for longer than 24 hours.

Surgical intervention
Surgical ligation or embolization of a bleeding artery may be necessary.

Referral
- Refer the patient to the emergency department if you're unable to control the bleeding.
- The patient should be seen by a ear, nose, and throat specialist within 24 to 48 hours if packing is needed.

Follow-up
The patient should be seen within 48 hours if bleeding recurs. Further follow-up depends on the cause of bleeding.

Patient teaching
- Tell the patient to keep his head at a 45-degree angle and to apply cold compresses or an ice collar to the nose.
- Instruct the patient to breathe through his mouth and not to swallow blood, talk, or blow his nose.
- To prevent recurrence of epistaxis, instruct the patient not to pick his nose or insert foreign objects into it and to avoid bending or lifting. Advise prompt treatment of any nasal infection or irritation.
- Suggest humidifiers for a patient who lives in a dry climate or at a high elevation or one whose home is heated with circulating hot air.
- Tell the patient to avoid aspirin or aspirin products and NSAIDs.

Complications
- Hypovolemia
- Shock
- Sinusitis
- Septal hematoma
- Septal abscess
- Septal perforation

• • • • • • • • • • • •

GLAUCOMA

Glaucoma is a group of disorders characterized by an abnormally high intraocular pressure (IOP), which can damage the optic nerve. Untreated glaucoma can lead to gradual peripheral vision loss and, ultimately, blindness. Glaucoma occurs in several forms: chronic open-angle (primary), acute angle-closure, congenital (inherited as an autosomal recessive trait), and secondary to other causes.

About 80,000 Americans are blind from glaucoma; 1.5 to 2 million people over age 40 have been diagnosed with the disease; another 5 to 10 million have elevated IOP. Glaucoma accounts for

Blindness

Blindness affects 28 million people worldwide. In the United States, blindness is legally defined as optimal visual acuity of 20/200 or less in the better eye after best correction, or a visual field of 20 degrees or less in the better eye.

According to the World Health Organization, the most common causes of preventable blindness worldwide are trachoma, cataracts, onchocerciasis (microfilarial infection transmitted by a blackfly and other species of Simulium), and xerophthalmia (dryness of the conjunctiva and cornea from vitamin A deficiency).

In the United States, the most common causes of acquired blindness are glaucoma, age-related macular degeneration, and diabetic retinopathy. (The incidence of blindness from glaucoma is decreasing thanks to early detection and treatment.) Rarer causes of acquired blindness include herpes simplex keratitis, cataracts, and retinal detachment.

12% of all new cases of blindness in the United States. (See *Blindness.*) Incidence is highest among blacks. The prognosis for maintaining vision is good with early treatment.

Causes

Chronic open-angle glaucoma results from overproduction of aqueous humor or obstruction to its outflow through the trabecular meshwork or the canal of Schlemm. (See *Normal flow of aqueous humor.*) This form of glaucoma is commonly familial in origin and affects 90% of all patients with glaucoma. Diabetes

and systemic hypertension have also been associated with this form of glaucoma.

Acute angle-closure (narrow-angle) glaucoma results from obstruction to the outflow of aqueous humor due to anatomically narrow angles between the anterior iris and the posterior corneal surface, shallow anterior chambers, a thickened iris that causes angle closure on pupil dilation, or a bulging iris that presses on the trabeculae and closes the angle (peripheral anterior synechiae).

Congenital glaucoma occurs when there's an abnormal fluid drainage angle of the eye. It may be caused by congenital infections such as TORCH (toxoplasmosis, other [varicella, mumps, parvovirus, human immunodeficiency virus], rubella, cytomegalovirus, and herpes), Sturge-Weber syndrome, and retinopathy of prematurity.

Secondary glaucoma can result from uveitis, trauma, or drugs (such as steroids). Neovascularization in the angle can result from vein occlusion or diabetes.

Clinical presentation

Chronic open-angle glaucoma is usually bilateral, with insidious onset and a slowly progressive course. Symptoms appear late in the disease and include:
- mild aching in the eyes
- loss of peripheral vision
- seeing halos around lights
- reduced visual acuity (especially at night; not correctable with glasses).

Acute angle-closure glaucoma typically has a rapid onset and is an ophthalmic emergency. Symptoms include:
- acute pain in a unilaterally inflamed eye, with pressure over the eye
- moderate pupil dilation that is nonreactive to light
- cloudy cornea
- blurring and decreased visual acuity

Normal flow of aqueous humor

Aqueous humor, a plasmalike fluid produced by the ciliary epithelium of the ciliary body, flows from the posterior chamber to the anterior chamber through the pupil. Here it flows peripherally and filters through the trabecular meshwork to the canal of Schlemm, through which the fluid ultimately enters venous circulation.

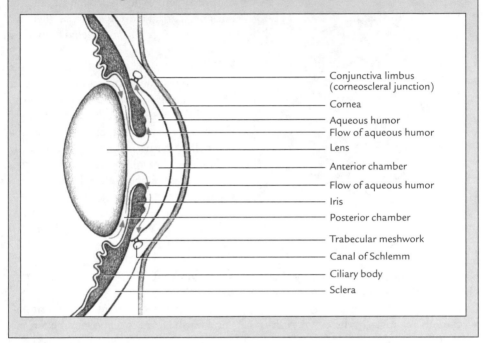

- Conjunctiva limbus (corneoscleral junction)
- Cornea
- Aqueous humor
- Flow of aqueous humor
- Lens
- Anterior chamber
- Flow of aqueous humor
- Iris
- Posterior chamber
- Trabecular meshwork
- Canal of Schlemm
- Ciliary body
- Sclera

- photophobia
- seeing halos around lights.

  Increased IOP may induce nausea and vomiting, which can cause misinterpretation of glaucoma as GI distress.

 CLINICAL CAUTION Unless treated promptly, acute angle-closure glaucoma produces blindness in 3 to 5 days.

Differential diagnoses
- Conjunctivitis
- Corneal abrasion or laceration
- Keratitis
- Retinal artery occlusion
- Temporal arteritis

- Acute angle closure glaucoma
- Globe rupture
- Herpes zoster
- Cavernous sinus thrombosis
- Scleritis
- Iritis
- Uveitis
- Periorbital infection
- Anisocoria
- Headache, migraine tension

Diagnosis
Loss of peripheral vision and disk changes confirms that glaucoma is present.

Optic disk changes

Ophthalmoscopy and slit-lamp examination show cupping of the optic disk, as depicted below, which is characteristic of chronic glaucoma.

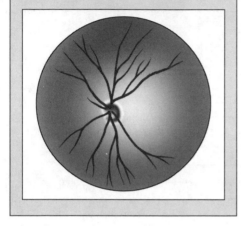

Diagnosis is made by:
- testing IOP
- measuring the visual field and noting changes such as an enlarged blind spot and loss of peripheral vision field
- observing changes in the cup to disk ratio of the optic nerve head.

Relevant diagnostic tests include:
- Tonometry (using an applanation tonopen or air puff tonometer) measures the IOP and provides a baseline for reference. Normal IOP ranges from 8 to 21 mm Hg. However, patients whose IOP are within this normal range can develop signs and symptoms of glaucoma, and patients who have abnormally high pressure may have no clinical effects. Fingertip tension is another way to measure IOP. On gentle palpation of closed eyelids, one eye feels harder than does the other in acute angle-closure glaucoma.
- Slit-lamp examination facilitates examination of the anterior structures of the eye, including the cornea, iris, and lens with a slit lamp.
- Gonioscopy determines the angle of the anterior chamber of the eye and enables differentiation between chronic open-angle glaucoma and acute angle-closure glaucoma. The angle is normal in chronic open-angle glaucoma. In older patients, partial closure of the angle can occur, so that two forms of glaucoma may coexist.
- Ophthalmoscopy enables the examiner to look at the fundus to establish if there are any changes such as cupping of the optic disk. (See *Optic disk changes*.) These changes appear later in chronic glaucoma if the disease isn't brought under control.
- Fundus photography takes pictures of the optic nerve head to track changes.
- Perimetry or visual field tests reveal the extent of damage to the optic neurons, signaled by an enlarged blind spot and loss of peripheral vision.

Management
Medication
Medications used to treat the patient depend on the form of glaucoma. Severe pain may necessitate administration of narcotic analgesics.

For chronic open-angle glaucoma
- timolol 0.25 to 0.50% — 1 drop into the affected eye q.d. to b.i.d.
- betaxolol 0.5% — 1 to 2 drops into the affected eye b.i.d.
- dorzolamide 2% — 1 drop into the affected eye t.i.d.
- pilocarpine 2% — 1 to 2 drops q.i.d. into the affected eye

For acute open-angle glaucoma
- acetazolamide — 500 mg I.V., then 125 to 250 mg P.O. every 4 hours
- glycerin — 1 to 2 g/kg P.O. 60 to 90 minutes preoperatively

- mannitol 20% — 1 to 2 g/kg I.V. over 45 minutes, administered 60 to 90 minutes preoperatively
- pilocarpine hydrochloride 2% — 1 drop into the affected eye every 5 minutes for 3 to 6 doses followed by 1 drop every 1 to 3 hours until pressure is controlled
- timolol 0.25 to 0.50% — 1 drop into the affected eye b.i.d.
- prednisolone acetate 1% — 1 to 2 drops into the affected eye may be used hourly, then taper to every 4 to 6 hours

Surgical intervention

Patients who are unresponsive to drug therapy may be candidates for argon laser trabeculoplasty (ALT) or a surgical filtering procedure called trabeculectomy, which creates an opening for aqueous outflow. In ALT, an argon laser beam is focused on the trabecular meshwork of an open angle. This produces a thermal burn that changes the surface of the meshwork and increases the outflow of aqueous humor. In trabeculectomy, a flap of sclera is dissected free to expose the trabecular meshwork. Then this discrete tissue block is removed and a peripheral iridectomy is performed. This produces an opening for aqueous outflow under the conjunctiva, creating a filtering bleb. In chronic refractory glaucoma, a tuboplast or tube shunt, such as a Moltino or a Braerveldt valve, is used to keep IOP within normal limits.

Acute angle-closure glaucoma is an ocular emergency requiring immediate treatment to decrease IOP. Preoperative drug therapy decreases IOP and is used first. If pressure doesn't decrease with drug therapy, laser iridotomy or surgical peripheral iridectomy must be performed promptly to save the patient's vision. Iridectomy relieves pressure by excising part of the iris to reestablish aqueous humor outflow. A prophylactic iridectomy is performed a few days later on the other eye to prevent an acute episode of glaucoma in the normal eye.

Referral
- Refer the patient to an ophthalmologist for treatment.

Follow-up
The patient should be seen according to the ophthalmologist's recommendation.

Patient teaching
- Stress the importance of meticulous compliance with prescribed drug therapy to prevent an increase in IOP and resulting disk changes and vision loss.

Complications
- Blindness
- Chronic corneal edema
- Corneal fibrosis and vascularization
- Optic atrophy

Special considerations
- Cycloplegics used postoperatively must be used only in the affected eye. The use of these drops in the normal eye may precipitate an attack of acute angle-closure glaucoma in this eye, threatening the patient's residual vision.

HEALTHY LIVING Glaucoma screening is important for early detection and prevention. Anyone over age 35, especially one with a family history of glaucoma, should have an annual tonometric examination.

• • • • • • • • • • • •

HEARING LOSS

Hearing loss (partial or total) results from a mechanical or nervous impediment to the transmission of sound waves. The major forms of hearing loss are classified as conductive loss (interrupted passage of sound from the external ear to the junction of the stapes and oval window); sensorineural loss (impaired cochlea or acoustic [eighth cranial] nerve dysfunction, causing failure of transmission of sound impulses in the inner ear or brain); or mixed loss (combined dysfunction of conduction and sensorineural transmission). Minor hearing loss is normal and affects one in five people by age 55.

Causes

Congenital hearing loss may be transmitted as a dominant, autosomal dominant, autosomal recessive, or sex-linked recessive trait. Hearing loss in neonates may also result from trauma, toxicity, or infection during pregnancy or delivery. Predisposing factors include a family history of hearing loss or known hereditary disorders (otosclerosis, for example), maternal exposure to rubella or syphilis during pregnancy, use of ototoxic drugs during pregnancy, prolonged fetal anoxia during delivery, and congenital abnormalities of the ears, nose, or throat. Premature or low-birth-weight infants are most likely to have structural or functional hearing impairment; those with serum bilirubin levels above 20 mg/dl also risk hearing impairment from the toxic effect of high serum bilirubin levels on the brain. Trauma during delivery can cause intracranial hemorrhage and may damage the cochlea or the acoustic nerve.

Sudden deafness refers to sudden hearing loss in a person with no prior hearing impairment. This condition is a medical emergency; prompt treatment may restore full hearing. Causes and predisposing factors may include:
■ acute infections, especially mumps (most common cause of unilateral sensorineural hearing loss in children), other bacterial and viral infections (such

as rubella, rubeola, influenza, herpes zoster, and infectious mononucleosis) and mycoplasma infections
■ metabolic disorders (diabetes mellitus, hypothyroidism, hyperlipoproteinemia)
■ vascular disorders (hypertension, arteriosclerosis)
■ head trauma or brain tumors
■ ototoxic drugs (tobramycin, streptomycin, quinine, gentamicin, furosemide, ethacrynic acid)
■ neurologic disorders (multiple sclerosis, neurosyphilis)
■ blood dyscrasias (leukemia, hypercoagulation).

Noise-induced hearing loss, which may be transient or permanent, may follow prolonged exposure to loud noise (85 to 90 dB) or brief exposure to extremely loud noise (greater than 90 dB). Such hearing loss is common in workers subjected to constant industrial noise and in military personnel, hunters, and rock musicians.

Presbycusis, an otologic effect of aging, results from a loss of hair cells in the organ of Corti. This disorder causes progressive, symmetrical, bilateral sensorineural hearing loss, usually of high-frequency tones.

Clinical presentation

A congenital hearing loss may produce no obvious signs of hearing impairment at birth, but a deficient response to auditory stimuli generally becomes apparent within 2 to 3 days. As the child grows older, hearing loss impairs speech development.

Sudden deafness may be conductive, sensorineural, or mixed, depending on etiology. Associated clinical features depend on the underlying cause.

Noise-induced hearing loss causes sensorineural damage, the extent of which depends on the duration and intensity of the noise. Initially, the patient loses perception of certain frequencies (around 4,000 Hz) but, with continued exposure, eventually loses perception of all frequencies.

Presbycusis usually produces tinnitus and inability to understand spoken words. A deaf infant's behavior can appear normal and mislead parents as well as health care professionals, especially if the infant has autosomal recessive deafness and is the first child of parents who are carriers.

Differential diagnoses
Conductive loss
- Foreign object in ear
- Chronic otitis media
- Otitis externa
- Cerumen impaction
- Tympanic membrane perforation
- Otosclerosis
- Developmental defects
- Glomus tumors
- Exostoses

Sensorineural loss
- Barotrauma
- Ménière's disease
- Drug toxicity
- Acoustic neuroma
- Cholestea
- Presbycusis
- Noise-induced loss
- Multiple sclerosis
- Congenital syphilis

Diagnosis
Patient, family, and occupational histories and a complete audiologic examination usually provide ample evidence of hearing loss and suggest possible causes or predisposing factors.

Partial or total hearing loss is calculated from this American Medical Association formula: Hearing is 1.5% im-

paired for every decibel that the pure tone average exceeds 25 dB. The Weber, the Rinne, and specialized audiologic tests are conducted to differentiate between conductive and sensorineural hearing loss.

Management
General
After the underlying cause is identified, therapy for congenital hearing loss refractory to surgery includes teaching the patient to communicate through sign language, speech reading, or other effective means. Measures to prevent congenital hearing loss include aggressively immunizing children against rubella to reduce the risk of maternal exposure during pregnancy; educating pregnant women about the dangers of exposure to drugs, chemicals, or infection; and careful monitoring during labor and delivery to prevent fetal anoxia.

Treatment of sudden deafness requires prompt identification of the underlying cause. Preventive measures include educating patients and health care professionals about the many causes of sudden deafness and ways to recognize and treat them.

Hyperbilirubinemia can be controlled by phototherapy and exchange transfusions. Children need the appropriate immunizations. Medication that may be ototoxic should be used judiciously in children and monitored closely. Avoiding exposure to loud noises generally prevents high-frequency hearing loss.

In people with noise-induced hearing loss, overnight rest usually restores normal hearing in those exposed to noise levels greater than 90 dB for several hours, unless they have been exposed to such noise repeatedly. As hearing deteriorates, treatment must include speech and hearing rehabilitation because hearing aids are seldom helpful. Preventing noise-induced hearing loss requires public education on the dangers of noise exposure and the use — as mandated by law — of protective devices such as earplugs during occupational exposure to noise.

Amplifying sound, as with a hearing aid, helps some patients with presbycusis, but many patients have an intolerance to loud noise and wouldn't be helped by a hearing aid.

Medication
Medications used to treat a patient with hearing loss are listed here.

For cerumen impaction
- triethanolamine polypeptide oleate-condensate — fill the ear canal with solution and insert a cotton plug; remove after 15 to 30 minutes and flush with warm water

For otitis media
- erythromycin — adults, 250 mg P.O. q.i.d. for 10 days; children, 30 to 50 mg/kg/day P.O. in divided doses for 10 days

For otitis externa
- hydrocortisone, neomycin sulfate, polymyxin B otic solution — adults, 4 drops into the affected ear q.i.d.; children, 3 drops q.i.d.

Referral
- Refer a child with suspected hearing loss to an audiologist or otolaryngologist for further evaluation.
- If any child fails a language screening examination, refer him to a speech pathologist for language evaluation. The child with a mild language delay may benefit from a home language enrichment program.

- Refer the patient and family members to programs for the deaf for education and support.

Follow-up
Follow-up is based on the cause of the hearing loss.

Patient teaching
- When the patient needs a hearing aid, teach how the aid works and how to maintain it.
- Teach the patient or family members about prescribed medication; emphasize the importance of following instructions for their use.

Complications
- Increased hearing loss
- Total deafness
- Chronic ear problems
- Chronic tinnitus

Special considerations
- When speaking to a patient with a hearing loss who can read lips, stand directly in front of him, with the light on your face, and speak slowly and distinctly. If possible, speak to him at eye level. Approach the patient within his visual range and get his attention by raising your arm or waving; touching him may be unnecessarily startling.
- When addressing an older patient, speak slowly and distinctly, in a low tone; avoid shouting.

HEALTHY LIVING To help prevent hearing loss, watch for signs of hearing impairment in patients receiving ototoxic drugs. Emphasize the danger of excessive exposure to noise; stress the danger to pregnant women of exposure to drugs, chemicals, and infection (especially rubella); and encourage the use of protective devices in a noisy environment.

• • • • • • • • • • •
INCLUSION CONJUNCTIVITIS

Inclusion conjunctivitis (also called inclusion blennorrhea) is an acute ocular inflammation resulting from infection by *Chlamydia trachomatis*. Although inclusion conjunctivitis occasionally becomes chronic, the prognosis is usually good.

Causes
C. trachomatis is an obligate intracellular organism of the lymphogranuloma venereum serotype group. Serotypes D through K are sexually transmitted, and secondary eye involvement in adults occurs in about 1 in 300 genital cases. Because contaminated cervical secretions infect the eyes of the neonate during birth, inclusion conjunctivitis is an important cause of ophthalmia neonatorum.

AGE ALERT Ocular chlamydial disease occurs most frequently in adults between ages 18 and 30.

Clinical presentation
Inclusion conjunctivitis develops 5 to 12 days after contamination (it takes longer to develop than gonococcal ophthalmia). In a neonate, reddened eyelids and tearing with moderate mucoid discharge are presenting symptoms. In a neonate, pseudomembranes may form, which can lead to conjunctival scarring. In adults, follicles appear inside the lower eyelids; such follicles don't form in infants because the lymphoid tissue isn't yet well developed. Children and adults also develop preauricular lymphadenopathy. Inclusion conjunctivitis may persist for weeks or months, possibly with superficial corneal involvement.

Differential diagnoses
- Conjunctivitis
- Uveitides

- Trachoma
- Toxic reactions
- Gonorrhea infection
- Adenoviral infection
- Molluscum infection
- Pneumonitis (in infants)

Diagnosis
Clinical features and a history of sexual contact with an infected individual suggest inclusion conjunctivitis. Examination of Giemsa-stained conjunctival scraping reveals cytoplasmic inclusion bodies in conjunctival epithelial cells and is effective in detecting chlamydial infection in infants. The direct fluorescent monoclonal antibody and enzyme immunosorbent assay tests are most effective in adults.

Management
General
Treatment is primarily through antibiotic therapy.

Medication
Medications used in treatment for inclusion conjunctivitis include:
- erythromycin stearate — infants, 30 to 50 mg/kg/day P.O. divided q.i.d. for 2 weeks; adults, 250 mg q.i.d. for 2 weeks
- tetracycline — adults, 250 to 500 mg P.O. q.i.d. for 2 to 3 weeks; children younger than age 8, 25 to 50 mg/kg/day divided q.i.d. P.O.
- doxycycline — 100 mg P.O. b.i.d. on 1st day, then 100 mg q.d. to b.i.d.
- prophylactic tetracycline or erythromycin ointment — applied once, 1 hour after delivery (not significantly more effective than Credé's method [1% silver nitrate]).

Referral
- Refer the patient to an ophthalmologist if he doesn't respond to treatment.

An infant should be referred to an ophthalmologist.

Follow-up

The patient should be seen within 1 week after treatment is initiated and again after treatment is complete.

Patient teaching

- Teach the patient to keep his eyes as clean as possible. Tell him to clean the eyes from the inner to the outer canthus and to apply warm soaks as needed.
- Remind the patient not to rub his eyes, which can irritate them.
- If the patient's eyes are sensitive to light, tell him to keep the room dark or suggest wearing dark glasses.

Complications

- Corneal scarring or laceration
- Intraocular infection
- Vision loss
- Otitis media (in children)

Special considerations

- Genital examination of the mother of an infected neonate or of any adult with inclusion conjunctivitis is suggested.
- Urge the patient to inform all sexual contacts so that they may be examined for chlamydial infection.

• • • • • • • • • • • •

KERATITIS

Keratitis — an inflammation of the cornea — may result from bacterial, fungal, or viral infection. If untreated, the infection can lead to blindness.

Causes

The most common cause of keratitis is infection by herpes simplex virus type 1 (known as dendritic corneal ulcer be-

cause of a characteristic branched lesion of the cornea resembling the veins of a leaf). Bacterial corneal ulcers commonly occur as a result of an infected corneal abrasion or a contaminated contact lens. Fungal keratitis is more frequently encountered in tropical climates. Poor lid closure can result in exposure keratitis; chemicals accidentally splashed into the eye can also produce keratitis.

Clinical presentation

Keratitis is usually unilateral. The patient may present with:

- decreased vision
- discomfort ranging from mild irritation to acute pain
- tearing
- photophobia.

On examination with a penlight, the corneal light reflex may appear distorted. When keratitis results from exposure, it usually affects the lower portion of the cornea.

Differential diagnoses

- Infection
- Allergy
- Foreign body
- Subconjunctival hemorrhage
- Scleritis
- Corneal abrasion, laceration, or ulceration
- Herpes simplex or zoster
- Blepharitis
- Iritis or uveitis
- Dacryocystitis
- Glaucoma
- Cellulitis

Diagnosis

Visual acuity may be decreased if the lesion is central. Slit-lamp examination confirms keratitis. Staining the eye with a sterile fluorescein strip enables the examiner to discern the extent and depth of the corneal lesion.

Patient history may reveal a recent infection of the upper respiratory tract accompanied by cold sores or eye irritation from wearing contact lenses.

Management
General
Treatment depends on the cause of keratitis.

Medication
Depending on the cause of keratitis, the following medications may be used.

For herpes simplex-related keratitis
- trifluridine solution — 1 drop every 2 hours, up to 9 times per day until reepithelialization occurs, then 1 drop every 4 hours for 7 more days
- vidarabine 3% ointment — 1 cm to lower conjunctival sac five times daily at 3-hour intervals

For bacterial corneal ulcers
- ciprofloxacin solution — 2 drops every 15 minutes for 6 hours, then every 30 minutes for the rest of the 1st day, then 2 drops every hour for 24 hours, then every 4 hours until reepithelialization occurs
- erythromycin ointment — thin strip of ointment to lower conjunctival sac up to 6 times per day

For fungal keratitis
- natamycin — 1 drop every 1 to 6 hours

Surgical intervention
Vision may be restored by penetrating keratoplasty (corneal transplant) in blindness resulting from corneal scarring.

Referral
- Refer the patient to an ophthalmologist for slit-lamp examination as soon as possible for intensive treatment.

Follow-up
Follow-up is based on the type and severity of keratitis.

Patient teaching
- Teach the patient the proper method of applying eyedrops and ointment.
- Stress to the patient the importance of following the medication schedule.

Complications
- Vision loss
- Squamous cell carcinoma

Special considerations
- Be aware that the patient with a red eye may have keratitis. Check for a history of contact lens wear, cold sores, or recent sensation of having something in the eye.

• • • • • • • • • • •
LARYNGITIS

Laryngitis, a common disorder, is an acute or chronic inflammation of the vocal cords. Acute laryngitis may occur as an isolated infection or as part of a generalized bacterial or viral upper respiratory tract infection. Repeated attacks of acute laryngitis produce inflammatory changes associated with chronic laryngitis.

Causes
Acute laryngitis usually results from infection (primarily viral) or excessive use of the voice, which is an occupational hazard in vocations such as teaching, public speaking, and singing, for example. It may also result from leisure activi-

ties (such as cheering at a sports event), inhalation of smoke or fumes, or aspiration of caustic chemicals. Chronic laryngitis may be caused by chronic upper respiratory tract disorders (sinusitis, bronchitis, nasal polyps, or allergy), breathing through the mouth, smoking, constant exposure to dust or other irritants, and alcohol abuse.

Clinical presentation

Acute laryngitis typically begins with hoarseness, ranging from mild to complete loss of voice. Associated clinical features include:
- pain (especially when swallowing or speaking)
- persistent dry cough
- fever
- laryngeal edema
- malaise.

In chronic laryngitis, persistent hoarseness is usually the only symptom.

Differential diagnoses
- Foreign object in the throat
- Diphtheria
- Esophagitis
- Aspiration
- Upper respiratory infection
- GI reflux
- Tumor
- Excessive use of voice
- Epiglottiditis
- Vocal cord paralysis
- Excessive smoking
- Inhalation of irritant gases
- Vocal cord nodules
- Seasonal allergies

Diagnosis

Indirect laryngoscopy is used to confirm the diagnosis by revealing red, inflamed and, occasionally, hemorrhagic vocal cords, with rounded rather than sharp

edges and exudate. Bilateral swelling may be present.

In severe cases or if toxicity is a concern, obtain a culture of the exudate. Consider 24-hour pH probe testing in chronic laryngitis and gastroesophageal reflux disease (GERD). Also consider biopsy in chronic laryngitis in an adult with a history of smoking or alcohol abuse.

Management
General

The primary treatment is resting the voice. Steam inhalation may be beneficial, as are smoking cessation, reducing alcohol intake, and changing or modifying the patient's job. Severe, acute laryngitis may necessitate hospitalization. In chronic laryngitis, effective treatment must eliminate the underlying cause.

Medication

Medications used to treat a patient with laryngitis depend on the cause.

For viral infection
- acetaminophen — 325 to 650 mg P.O. every 4 hours p.r.n.
- throat lozenges

For bacterial infection
- amoxicillin — 250 to 500 mg P.O. every 8 hours for 10 days
- erythromycin — adults, 250 mg P.O. q.i.d. for 10 days; children, 30 to 50 mg/kg daily P.O. in divided doses for 10 days

For GERD
- calcium carbonate — 350 mg to 1.5 g P.O. 1 hour after meals
- famotidine — 10 mg P.O. a.c. (or histamine-2 blockers may be used)

Surgical intervention

When laryngeal edema causes airway obstruction, a tracheostomy may be necessary.

Referral

■ Refer the patient to an appropriate program for assistance with smoking cessation and changing other predisposing habits or occupational hazards.

Follow-up

The patient should be reevaluated in 2 weeks and then as needed.

Patient teaching

■ Explain to the patient and family members why the patient shouldn't talk.
■ For the patient with a bacterial infection, stress the importance of completing the full course of antibiotic therapy.
■ Suggest that the patient maintain adequate humidification by using a vaporizer or humidifier during the winter, avoiding air conditioning during the summer (because it dehumidifies), using medicated throat lozenges, and refraining from smoking.

Complications

■ Hoarseness

Special considerations

■ Obtain a detailed patient history to help determine the cause of chronic laryngitis. Encourage the patient to change predisposing habits, especially to stop smoking.

• • • • • • • • • • • •

MACULAR DEGENERATION, AGE-RELATED

Macular degeneration — atrophy or degeneration of the macular region of the retina — is the most common cause of legal blindness in adults. It accounts for about 12% of blindness cases in the United States and for about 17% of new blindness cases. It's also one cause of severe, irreversible loss of central vision in elderly patients. Most patients are of white European descent.

Two types of age-related macular degeneration (ARMD) occur. The dry or atrophic form is characterized by atrophic pigment epithelial changes and is most often associated with a slow, progressive, and mild vision loss. The wet, exudative form causes progressive visual distortion leading to vision loss. It's characterized by subretinal neovascularization that causes leakage, hemorrhage, and fibrovascular scar formation, which produce significant loss of central vision.

Causes

ARMD results from underlying pathologic changes that occur primarily at the level of the retinal pigment epithelium, Bruch's membrane, and the choriocapillaris in the macular region. Drusen (bumps), which are common in elderly patients, appear as yellow deposits beneath the pigment epithelium and may be prominent in the macula. No predisposing conditions have been identified; however, some forms of the disorder are hereditary.

Clinical presentation

The patient notices a change in central vision. Initially, straight lines (for example, of buildings) become distorted; later, a blank area appears in the center of a printed page (central scotoma).

Differential diagnoses
- Diabetic retinopathy
- Hypertensive retinopathy
- Idiopathic subretinal neovascularization

Diagnosis
The following procedures help diagnose ARMD:
- Indirect ophthalmoscopy — fundus examination through a dilated pupil may reveal gross macular changes.
- I.V. fluorescein angiography — sequential photographs may show leaking vessels as fluorescein dye flows into the tissues from the subretinal neovascular net.
- Amsler's chart — used to monitor visual field loss.

Management
General
Laser photocoagulation reduces the incidence of severe vision loss in patients with subretinal neovascularization, turning serous ARMD to the dry form.

Medication
Medication may include:
- supplements — vitamins A, E, and C
- zinc sulfate (ophthalmic) — 1 to 2 drops b.i.d. to q.i.d.

Referral
- Refer the patient to an ophthalmologist.
- Refer a patient with bilateral central vision loss to visual rehabilitation services.

Follow-up
Schedule follow-up monitoring and treatment according to the ophthalmologist's recommendation.

Patient teaching
- Teach the patient about special devices, such as low-vision optical aids, that are available to improve the quality of life in patients with good peripheral vision.
- Tell the patient to follow a diet high in vitamins A, E, and C; beta-carotene; and zinc to help prevent cellular damage and to retard vision loss.

Complications
- Blindness

• • • • • • • • • • • •
MÉNIÈRE'S DISEASE

Ménière's disease, a labyrinthine dysfunction also known as endolymphatic hydrops, produces severe vertigo, sensorineural hearing loss, and tinnitus. After multiple attacks over several years, this disorder leads to residual tinnitus and hearing loss. Usually only one ear is involved. This disease affects approximately 200 out of 100,000 people.

AGE ALERT Ménière's disease usually affects adults between ages 30 and 60; it affects men slightly more frequently than women.

Causes
Ménière's disease may result from overproduction or decreased absorption of endolymph, which causes endolymphatic hydrops or endolymphatic hypertension, with consequent degeneration of the vestibular and cochlear hair cells. This condition also may stem from autonomic nervous system dysfunction that produces a temporary constriction of blood vessels supplying the inner ear. In some women, premenstrual edema may precipitate attacks of Ménière's disease.

Clinical presentation

Ménière's disease produces three characteristic effects:
- severe episodic vertigo
- tinnitus
- sensorineural hearing loss.

A feeling of fullness or blockage in the ear is also common. Violent paroxysmal attacks last from 10 minutes to several hours. During an acute attack, other symptoms may include:
- severe nausea
- vomiting
- sweating
- giddiness
- nystagmus.

Vertigo may cause loss of balance and falling to the affected side. Symptoms tend to wax and wane as the endolymphatic pressure increases and decreases. To reduce these symptoms, the patient may assume a characteristic posture: lying on the side of the unaffected ear and looking in the direction of the affected ear.

Initially, the patient may be asymptomatic between attacks, except for residual tinnitus that worsens during an attack. Such attacks may occur several times a year, or remissions may last as long as several years. These attacks become less frequent as hearing loss progresses (usually unilaterally); they may cease when hearing loss is total. All symptoms are aggravated by motion.

Differential diagnoses

Otologic disorders
- Chronic otitis media
- Benign positional vertigo
- Labyrinthitis
- Acoustic neuroma
- Otosclerosis

Systemic disorders
- Vertebrobasilar disorders
- Cerebrovascular accident
- Basilar migraine
- Epilepsy
- Multiple sclerosis
- Paget's disease
- Thyroid disease
- Autoimmune disease
- Syphilis

Diagnosis

Presence of all three typical symptoms suggests Ménière's disease. Audiometric studies indicate a loss of hearing after an attack and then hearing gets better. Electronystagmography, electrocochleography, computed tomography scan, magnetic resonance imaging, and X-rays of the internal meatus may be necessary for a differential diagnosis.

Laboratory studies, including thyroid and lipid studies, may be performed to rule out other conditions such as *Treponema pallidum*.

Caloric testing may reveal loss or impairment of thermally induced nystagmus on the involved side.

CLINICAL CAUTION During diagnosis, don't overlook an acoustic tumor, which produces an identical clinical picture.

Management

General
Treatment for Ménière's disease varies as the condition progresses.

Medication
For an acute attack
- atropine — 0.1 to 0.4 mg I.V.
- lorazepam — 0.5 mg P.O. every 12 hours
- dimenhydrinate — 50 mg I.M.
- transdermal scopolamine patch — 1 patch applied to the skin and left on for a minimum of 3 days

For long-term management
- hydrochlorothiazide — 25 to 100 mg P.O. q.d.
- meclizine — 25 to 100 mg P.O. q.d. in divided doses
- diazepam — 2 mg or less P.O. t.i.d.
- dimenhydrinate — 25 to 50 mg P.O. t.i.d.

Surgical intervention
If Ménière's disease persists after 2 years of treatment, produces incapacitating vertigo, or resists medical management, surgery may be necessary. Destruction of the affected labyrinth permanently relieves symptoms but results in irreversible hearing loss. If medical therapy fails and the patient is disabled by vertigo, surgical decompression of the endolymphatic sac may bring relief.

Referral
- The patient may need referral to an otolaryngologist for a definitive diagnosis and hearing evaluation.

Follow-up
Follow-up should be arranged according to the otolaryngologist's recommendation.

Patient teaching
- During an attack of Ménière's disease, advise the patient to avoid reading and exposure to glaring lights to reduce dizziness.
- Instruct the patient to avoid sudden position changes and any tasks that vertigo makes hazardous because an attack can begin rapidly.

Complications
- Hearing loss
- Injury secondary to loss of balance
- Change in lifestyle

• • • • • • • • • • • •
MOTION SICKNESS

Motion sickness is characterized by transient loss of equilibrium and associated nausea and vomiting that result from irregular or rhythmic movements or from the sensation of motion. Motion sickness can also be induced when a person's pattern of motion changes such as riding backward.

Motion sickness from cars, elevators, trains, and swings is most common in children; from boats and airplanes, in adults.

Causes
Motion sickness may result from excessive stimulation of the labyrinthine receptors of the inner ear by certain motions, such as those experienced in a car, boat, plane, or swing. The disorder may also be caused by confusion in the cerebellum from conflicting sensory input; the visual stimulus (a moving horizon) conflicts with labyrinthine perception. Predisposing factors include tension or fear, offensive odors, or sights and sounds associated with a previous attack. People who suffer from one kind of motion sickness aren't necessarily susceptible to other types.

Clinical presentation
Typically, motion sickness induces:
- nausea
- vomiting
- headache
- dizziness
- fatigue
- diaphoresis
- difficulty breathing (occasionally, leading to a sensation of suffocation).

These symptoms usually subside when the precipitating stimulus is removed, but they may persist for several hours or days.

Differential diagnoses

- Migraine headache
- Benign positional vertigo
- Vestibular neuronitis
- Decompression sickness
- Labyrinthitis
- Ménière's disease
- Tumor
- Intracranial hemorrhage
- Autonomic dysfunction

Management

General

The best way to treat motion sickness is to stop the action that's causing it. If this isn't possible, the patient will benefit from lying down, closing his eyes, and trying to sleep.

Medication

Medications may include:
- scopolamine transdermal patch — apply 6 hours before travel
- dimenhydrinate — adults, 50 to 100 mg P.O. every 4 hours; children age 6 to 12, 25 to 50 mg P.O. every 6 to 8 hours; age 2 to 6, 12 to 25 mg P.O. every 6 to 8 hours
- meclizine — 25 to 50 mg/day P.O. 1 hour before travel.

Referral

- Referral isn't necessary.

Follow-up

Treatment should be evaluated after travel.

Patient teaching

- Tell the patient to avoid exposure to precipitating motion whenever possible. A traveler can minimize motion sickness by sitting where motion is least apparent (near the wing section in an aircraft, in the center of a boat, or in the front seat of an automobile). Instruct him to keep his head still and his eyes closed or focused on a distant and stationary object. An elevated car seat may prevent motion sickness in a child, because it allows him to see out the front window.
- Instruct the patient to avoid eating or drinking for at least 4 hours before traveling and to take an antiemetic 30 to 60 minutes before traveling or apply a transdermal scopolamine patch at least 4 hours before traveling.

Complications

- Hypotension
- Dehydration
- Depression
- Panic

• • • • • • • • • • • •

NOSE, FRACTURED

The most common facial fracture, a fractured nose usually results from blunt injury and may be associated with other facial fractures. The severity of the fracture depends on the direction, force, and type of blow the patient receives. A severe, comminuted fracture may cause extreme swelling or bleeding that may partially obstruct the airway. Inadequate or delayed treatment can cause permanent nasal displacement, septal deviation, and obstruction.

Clinical presentation

Immediately after injury, a nosebleed may occur. Soft-tissue swelling may quickly obscure the break. After several hours, pain, periorbital ecchymoses, and nasal displacement and deformity are prominent.

Differential diagnoses

- Mandible dislocation or fracture
- Nasoethmoid fracture
- Avulsed teeth (dentate)
- Fractured teeth (dentate)

- Le Fort fractures
- Orbital fractures
- Globe rupture
- Neck trauma
- Child abuse
- Domestic violence
- Elder abuse
- Sexual assault
- Intracranial hemorrhage
- Retinal detachment
- Corneal injuries

Diagnosis

Palpation, X-rays, and clinical findings, such as a deviated septum, confirm a nasal fracture.

Diagnosis also requires a complete patient history, including the cause of the injury and the amount of nasal bleeding. Watch for clear fluid drainage, which may suggest cerebrospinal fluid (CSF) leakage and a basilar skull fracture. If the patient is pregnant, a computed tomography (CT) scan is necessary.

Management

General

Treatment restores normal facial appearance and reestablishes bilateral nasal passage after swelling subsides. Severe swelling can delay treatment. CSF leakage calls for close observation, a CT scan of the basilar skull, and antibiotic therapy; septal hematoma requires incision and drainage to prevent necrosis. Start treatment immediately. While waiting for X-rays, apply ice packs to the nose to minimize swelling. Wrap the ice packs in a light towel to prevent ice from directly contacting the skin. To control anterior bleeding, gently apply local pressure. Posterior bleeding is rare and requires an internal tamponade applied in the emergency department.

Medication

The following medications may be administered:
- acetaminophen — 325 to 650 mg P.O. for analgesia
- ibuprofen — 300 to 800 mg P.O. t.i.d. to q.i.d.

Surgical intervention

Reduction of the fracture corrects alignment; immobilization (intranasal packing and an external splint shaped to the nose and taped) maintains it. Reduction is best accomplished in the operating room under local anesthesia for adults and general anesthesia for children.

Referral

- Refer the patient to an ear, nose, and throat specialist or orthopedic surgeon for treatment.

Follow-up

Follow-up care should be scheduled according to the specialist's recommendation.

Patient teaching

- Because the patient will find breathing more difficult as swelling increases, instruct him to breathe slowly through his mouth. To warm the inhaled air during cold weather, tell the patient to cover his mouth with a handkerchief or scarf. To prevent subcutaneous emphysema or intracranial air penetration (and potential meningitis), warn him not to blow his nose.

Complications

- Sinusitis
- Obstructed air flow
- Meningitis
- Septal hematoma
- Abscess
- Avascular septal necrosis
- Saddle nose deformity

OTITIS EXTERNA

Otitis externa, inflammation of the skin of the external ear canal and auricle, may be acute or chronic. Also known as external otitis and swimmer's ear, it's most common in the summer. With treatment, acute otitis externa usually subsides within 7 days — although it may become chronic — and tends to recur.

Causes and incidence
Otitis externa usually results from bacteria, such as *Pseudomonas*, *Proteus vulgaris*, *Staphylococcus aureus*, and streptococci and, sometimes, from such fungi as *Aspergillus niger* and *Candida albicans*. Fungal otitis externa is most common in tropical regions. Occasionally, chronic otitis externa results from dermatologic conditions, such as seborrhea and psoriasis. Allergic reactions due to nickel or chromium earrings, chemicals in hair spray, cosmetics, hearing aids, and medication (such as sulfonamide and neomycin) that's commonly used to treat otitis externa can also cause otitis externa.

Predisposing factors include:
- swimming in contaminated water (cerumen creates a culture medium for the waterborne organism)
- cleaning the ear canal with a cotton swab, bobby pin, finger, or other foreign object (this irritates the ear canal and may introduce the infecting microorganism)
- exposure to dust, perfumes, hair care products, or other irritants that cause the patient to scratch the ear, excoriating the auricle and canal
- regular use of earphones, earplugs, or earmuffs, which trap moisture in the ear canal, creating a culture medium for infection (especially if earplugs don't fit properly)
- chronic drainage from a perforated tympanic membrane
- self-administered eardrops.

Clinical presentation
Acute otitis externa characteristically produces moderate to severe pain that's exacerbated by manipulating the auricle or tragus, clenching the teeth, opening the mouth, or chewing. Other clinical effects may include:
- fever
- foul-smelling discharge
- crusting in the external ear
- regional cellulitis
- partial hearing loss
- itching.

It may be difficult to view the tympanic membrane due to pain in the external canal. Hearing acuity is normal unless complete occlusion occurs.

Fungal otitis externa may be asymptomatic, although A. *niger* produces a black or gray, blotting, paperlike growth in the ear canal. In chronic otitis externa, pruritus replaces pain, and scratching may lead to scaling and skin thickening. Aural discharge may also occur.

Differential diagnoses
- Malignant otitis externa
- Otitis media
- Folliculitis from obstructed sebaceous glands
- Otic foreign body
- Herpes zoster
- Parotitis
- Periauricular adenitis
- Mastoiditis
- Dental abscess
- Sinusitis
- Tonsillitis
- Pharyngitis
- Temporomandibular pain

Differentiating acute otitis externa from acute otitis media

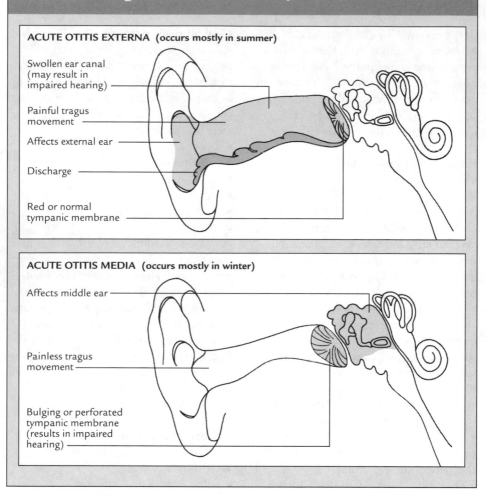

ACUTE OTITIS EXTERNA (occurs mostly in summer)

Swollen ear canal (may result in impaired hearing)

Painful tragus movement

Affects external ear

Discharge

Red or normal tympanic membrane

ACUTE OTITIS MEDIA (occurs mostly in winter)

Affects middle ear

Painless tragus movement

Bulging or perforated tympanic membrane (results in impaired hearing)

Diagnosis

Physical examination findings confirm otitis externa. In acute otitis externa, otoscopy reveals a swollen external ear canal (sometimes to the point of complete closure), periauricular lymphadenopathy and, occasionally, regional cellulitis.

In fungal otitis externa, removal of the growth reveals thick, red epithelium. Microscopic examination or culture and sensitivity tests can be used to identify the causative organism and determine antibiotic treatment. Pain on palpation of the tragus or auricle distinguishes acute otitis externa from otitis media. (See *Differentiating acute otitis externa from acute otitis media.*)

In chronic otitis externa, physical examination discloses thick, red epithelium in the ear canal. Severe chronic otitis externa may reflect underlying diabetes mellitus, hypothyroidism, or nephritis. Microscopic examination or culture and sensitivity tests can be used to identify the causative organism and determine antibiotic treatment.

Management
General
To help relieve the pain of acute otitis externa, apply heat therapy to the periauricular region (heat lamp; hot, damp compresses; heating pad). If the ear canal is too edematous to instill eardrops, an ear wick may be used for the first few days. In chronic otitis externa, primary treatment consists of cleaning the ear and removing debris. For mild chronic otitis externa, treatment may include instilling antibiotic eardrops once or twice weekly and wearing specially fitted earplugs while showering, shampooing, or swimming.

Medication
Medications used to treat a patient with otitis externa may include:
- aspirin — 325 to 650 mg P.O. every 4 hours
- ibuprofen — adults, 300 to 800 mg P.O. t.i.d. to q.i.d.; children, 30 to 50 mg/kg in 3 to 4 divided doses per day
- hydrocortisone cream — apply to affected ear q.d. to q.i.d.
- acetic acid solution — 1 to 2 drops every 4 to 6 hours
- systemic antibiotic — specific for infection
- aluminum acetate — apply to ear canal on cotton to clean area.

To help treat otitis externa resulting from candidal organisms, 2% salicylic acid in cream containing nystatin may be used. Instillation of slightly acidic eardrops creates an unfavorable environment in the ear canal for most fungi and for *Pseudomonas*.

No specific treatment exists for otitis externa caused by A. *niger*, except re-

peated cleaning of the ear canal with baby oil.

Referral
- Referral to a specialist generally isn't necessary.

Follow-up
The patient should be seen in 1 week to evaluate the tympanic membrane and to make sure it's intact.

Patient teaching
- If the patient has acute otitis externa, tell him to not participate in any swimming activity during the acute phase.
- To prevent otitis externa, suggest using lamb's wool earplugs coated with petroleum jelly to keep water out of the ears when showering or shampooing.
- Tell the patient to wear earplugs or to keep his head above water when swimming and to instill 2 or 3 drops of 3% boric acid solution in 70% alcohol before and after swimming to toughen the skin of the external ear canal.
- Warn against cleaning the ears with cotton swabs or other objects.
- Children who have an intact tympanic membrane but are predisposed to otitis externa from swimming should instill 2 to 3 drops of a 1:1 solution of white vinegar and 70% ethyl alcohol into their ears before and after swimming.

Complications
- Malignant otitis externa
- Chondritis

Special considerations
- If the patient is diabetic, evaluate him for malignant otitis externa.

• • • • • • • • • • • •
OTITIS MEDIA

Otitis media, inflammation of the middle ear, may be suppurative or secretory, acute, persistent, unresponsive, or chronic. Acute otitis media is common in children; its incidence increases during the winter months, paralleling the seasonal increase in nonbacterial respiratory tract infections. With prompt treatment, the prognosis for a patient with acute otitis media is excellent; however, prolonged accumulation of fluid in the middle ear cavity causes chronic otitis media and, sometimes, perforation of the tympanic membrane. (See *Site of otitis media.*)

Chronic suppurative otitis media can lead to scarring, adhesions, and severe structural or functional ear damage. Chronic secretory otitis media, with its persistent inflammation and pressure, can cause conductive hearing loss. It most commonly occurs in children with tympanostomy tubes or a perforated tympanic membrane.

Recurrent otitis media is defined as three near-acute otitis media episodes within 6 months or four episodes of acute otitis media within 1 year.

Otitis media with complications can damage middle ear structures by causing adhesions, retraction, pockets, cholesteatoma, and intratemporal and intracranial complications.

Causes
Otitis media results from disruption of eustachian tube patency. In the suppurative form, respiratory tract infection, allergic reaction, nasotracheal intubation, or positional changes allow nasopharyngeal flora to reflux through the eustachian tube and colonize the middle ear. Suppurative otitis media usually results from bacterial infection with pneumococcus, *Haemophilus influenzae* (the most common cause in children under age 6), *Moraxella catarrhalis*, beta-hemolytic streptococci, staphylococci (the most common cause in children age 6 or older), or gram-negative bacteria.

Predisposing factors include the normally wider, shorter, more horizontal eustachian tubes and increased lymphoid tissue in children, as well as anatomic anomalies. Chronic suppurative otitis media results from inadequate treatment of acute otitis episodes, infection by resistant strains of bacteria or, rarely, tuberculosis.

Secretory otitis media results from obstruction of the eustachian tube. This causes a buildup of negative pressure in the middle ear that promotes transudation of sterile serous fluid from blood vessels in the membrane of the middle ear. Such effusion may be secondary to eustachian tube dysfunction from viral infection or allergy. It may also follow barotrauma (pressure injury caused by inability to equalize pressures between the environment and the middle ear), as occurs during rapid aircraft descent in a person with an upper respiratory tract infection or during rapid underwater ascent in scuba diving (barotitis media).

Chronic secretory otitis media follows persistent eustachian tube dysfunction from mechanical obstruction (adenoidal tissue overgrowth, tumors), edema (allergic rhinitis, chronic sinus infection), or inadequate treatment of acute suppurative otitis media.

Clinical presentation
Many patients are asymptomatic. Clinical features of acute suppurative otitis media include:
■ severe, deep, throbbing pain (from pressure behind the tympanic membrane)
■ signs of upper respiratory tract infection (sneezing, coughing)

Site of otitis media

Otitis media can affect any part of the shaded area in the drawing below.

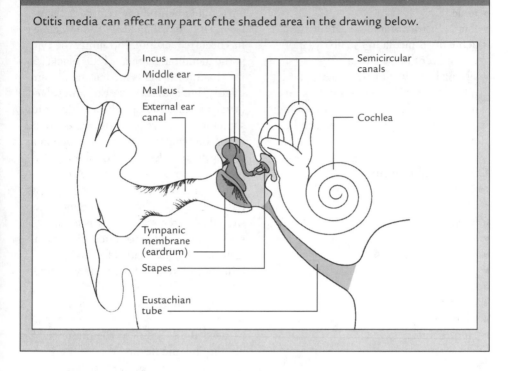

mild to very high fever
hearing loss (usually mild and conductive)
tinnitus
dizziness
nausea
vomiting
bulging of the tympanic membrane, with concomitant erythema
purulent drainage in the ear canal from tympanic membrane rupture. However, many patients are asymptomatic.

Acute secretory otitis media produces a severe conductive hearing loss — which varies from 15 to 35 dB, depending on the thickness and amount of fluid in the middle ear cavity — and, possibly, a sensation of fullness in the ear and popping, crackling, or clicking sounds on swallowing or with jaw movement. Accumulation of fluid can also cause the pa-

tient to hear an echo when he speaks and to experience a vague feeling of top heaviness.

The cumulative effects of chronic otitis media include:
thickening and scarring of the tympanic membrane
decreased or absent tympanic membrane mobility
cholesteatoma (a cystlike mass in the middle ear)
painless, purulent discharge, in chronic suppurative otitis media.

The extent of associated conductive hearing loss varies with the size and type of tympanic membrane perforation and ossicular destruction. If the tympanic membrane has ruptured, the patient may report that the pain suddenly stopped.

The following factors increase a child's risk for otitis media:

- day care
- formula feeding
- smoking in the household
- male sex
- family history of middle ear disease
- acute otitis media in the first year of life (recurrent otitis media)
- sibling history of otitis media.

Acute otitis media may not cause symptoms in the first few months of life; irritability is sometimes the only indication of earache.

Differential diagnoses
Infection
- Otitis externa
- Mastoiditis
- Dental abscess
- Peritonsillar abscess
- Sinusitis
- Lymphadenitis
- Parotitis
- Meningitis
- Herpes zoster

Trauma
- Perforated tympanic membrane
- Foreign body
- Barotrauma
- Instrumentation

Diagnosis
In acute suppurative otitis media, otoscopy reveals obscured or distorted bony landmarks of the tympanic membrane. Pneumatoscopy can show decreased tympanic membrane mobility, but this procedure is painful with an obviously bulging, erythematous tympanic membrane. The pain pattern is diagnostically significant; for example, in acute suppurative otitis media, pulling the auricle *does not* exacerbate the pain. A culture of the ear drainage identifies the causative organism.

In acute secretory otitis media, otoscopic examination reveals tympanic membrane retraction, which causes the bony landmarks to appear more prominent.

Examination also discloses clear or amber fluid behind the tympanic membrane. If hemorrhage into the middle ear has occurred, as in barotrauma, the tympanic membrane appears blue-black.

In chronic otitis media, the patient history discloses recurrent or unresolved otitis media. Otoscopy shows thickening, sometimes scarring, and decreased mobility of the tympanic membrane; pneumatoscopy shows decreased or absent tympanic membrane movement. A history of recent air travel or scuba diving suggests barotitis media. The following measures should be taken to treat otitis media:
- Tympanocentesis for microbiologic diagnosis is recommended for treatment failures and may be followed by myringotomy.
- Tympanometry, acoustic reflex measurement, or acoustic reflectometry may be needed to document the presence of fluid in the middle ear.
- Blood tests may be used to determine higher white blood cell counts, which indicate bacterial otitis media.

Management
General
Concomitant treatment of the underlying cause (such as eliminating allergens or adenoidectomy for hypertrophied adenoids) may be helpful in correcting this disorder. In acute secretory otitis media, inflation of the eustachian tube using Valsalva's maneuver several times per day may be the only treatment required.

Medication
For patients with acute otitis media
- amoxicillin — adults, 250 to 500 mg P.O. t.i.d. for 10 days; children, 20 to 40 mg/kg/day in three divided doses for 10 days

■ amoxicillin/clavulanate—patients weighing more than 88 lb (40 kg), 250 to 500 mg P.O. every 8 to 12 hours in areas with a high incidence of beta-lactamase-producing *H. influenzae* and in patients who aren't responding to amoxicillin; patients weighing less than 88 lb (40 kg), 20 to 45 mg/kg/day P.O. in divided doses
■ cefaclor—children, 20 to 40 mg/kg/day P.O. in 2 to 3 doses
■ cefixime—children, 8 mg/kg/day P.O. in a single or divided dose
■ ceftriaxone—children, 50 to 75 mg/kg/day I.M. or I.V. in divided doses.

For patients with chronic otitis media
■ amoxicillin—20 to 40 mg/kg/day P.O. for 3 to 6 months
■ oxymetazoline nasal solution—2 to 3 sprays in each nostril b.i.d. for 3 to 5 days.

Surgical intervention
Severe, painful bulging of the tympanic membrane usually necessitates myringotomy.

If decongestant therapy fails, myringotomy and aspiration of middle ear fluid are necessary, followed by insertion of a polyethylene tube into the tympanic membrane, for immediate and prolonged pressure equalization. The tube falls out spontaneously after 9 to 12 months.

Referral
■ If treatment isn't successful or if the condition becomes chronic, refer the patient to an otolaryngologist.

Follow-up
The patient should be reevaluated after 48 hours of treatment.

Patient teaching
■ After myringotomy, tell the patient or his parents to not place cotton or plugs deep in the ear canal; they may place sterile cotton loosely in the external ear to absorb drainage. Instruct then to change the cotton whenever it gets damp and to wash the hands before and after giving ear care to prevent infection. Advise them to watch for and report headache, fever, severe pain, or disorientation.
■ After tympanoplasty, tell the patient or his parents to watch for and report excessive bleeding from the ear canal. Advise against blowing the nose or getting the ear wet when bathing.
■ Encourage the patient to complete the prescribed course of antibiotic treatment. If nasopharyngeal decongestants are ordered, teach him how to instill them correctly.
■ Suggest applying heat to the ear to relieve pain.
■ Advise the patient with acute secretory otitis media to watch for and immediately report pain and fever, which are signs of secondary infection.
■ To promote eustachian tube patency, instruct the patient to perform Valsalva's maneuver several times daily.

HEALTHY LIVING To prevent otitis media, instruct the parents not to feed their infant in a supine position or put him to bed with a bottle. This prevents reflux of nasopharyngeal flora.

Complications
■ Perforated eardrum
■ Hearing loss
■ Acute mastoiditis
■ Meningitis
■ Atrophy and scarring of the eardrum
■ Chronic perforation and otorrhea
■ Abscess
■ Sigmoid sinus or jugular vein thrombosis
■ Septicemia
■ Facial paralysis
■ Otitis externa

• • • • • • • • • • • •
PHARYNGITIS

Pharyngitis is an acute or chronic inflammation of the pharynx. It's the most common throat disorder and is widespread among adults who live or work in dusty or very dry environments, use their voices excessively, habitually use tobacco or alcohol, or suffer from chronic sinusitis, persistent coughs, or allergies. It frequently accompanies the common cold.

Causes
Pharyngitis is usually caused by a virus. The most common bacterial cause is group A beta-hemolytic streptococci. Other common causes include *Mycoplasma* and *Chlamydia*.

Clinical presentation
Pharyngitis produces a sore throat and slight difficulty in swallowing. Swallowing saliva is usually more painful than swallowing food. Pharyngitis can also cause the sensation of a lump in the throat as well as a constant, aggravating urge to swallow. Associated features can include:
- mild fever
- headache
- muscle and joint pain
- coryza
- rhinorrhea.

Over 90% of cases of sore throat and fever in children are of viral origin. Associated symptoms usually include a runny nose and nonproductive cough. Uncomplicated pharyngitis usually subsides in 3 to 10 days.

Differential diagnoses
- Candidiasis
- Diphtheria
- Epiglottiditis, adult
- Gonorrhea
- Herpes simplex
- Mononucleosis
- Peritonsillar abscess
- Pneumonia, mycoplasma
- Retropharyngeal abscess
- Rheumatic fever
- Gastrointestinal reflux disease

Diagnosis
Physical examination of the pharynx reveals generalized redness and inflammation of the posterior wall and red, edematous mucous membranes studded with white or yellow follicles. Exudate is usually confined to the lymphoid areas of the throat, sparing the tonsillar pillars. Bacterial pharyngitis usually produces a large amount of exudate.

A throat culture may be performed to identify bacterial organisms that may be the cause of the inflammation.

Management
General
Treatment for a patient with acute viral pharyngitis is usually symptomatic and consists mainly of rest, warm saline gargles, throat lozenges containing a mild anesthetic, and plenty of fluids. If the patient can't swallow fluids, I.V. hydration may be required. Chronic pharyngitis necessitates the same supportive measures as acute pharyngitis but with greater emphasis on eliminating the underlying cause, such as an allergen. Preventive measures include adequate humidification and avoiding excessive exposure to air conditioning. In addition, the patient should be urged to stop smoking.

Medication
For acute and chronic pharyngitis
- acetaminophen—adults, 325 to 650 mg P.O. every 4 hours p.r.n.; children, dosage per package directions

For bacterial pharyngitis
- penicillin V — adults, 125 to 250 mg P.O. every 6 hours for 10 days; for children, 500 mg/day P.O. in divided doses
- erythromycin ethylsuccinate — 400 to 800 mg P.O. every 6 hours for 10 days

Referral
- If treatment isn't successful, refer the patient to an otolaryngologist.
- Refer the patient to a self-help group to stop smoking, if appropriate.

Follow-up
The patient should be reevaluated after 48 hours of treatment.

Patient teaching
- Encourage the patient to drink plenty of fluids.
- If the patient has acute bacterial pharyngitis, emphasize the importance of completing the full course of antibiotic therapy.
- Teach the patient with chronic pharyngitis how to minimize sources of throat irritation in the environment such as using a bedside humidifier.

Complications
- Rheumatic fever
- Post-streptococcal glomerulonephritis
- Systemic infection
- Otitis media
- Peritonsillar abscess
- Sinusitis

Special considerations
- Children attending school should receive at least 24 hours of therapy before returning to school.
- If a patient has exhibited three or more documented infections within 6 months, consider daily penicillin prophylaxis during the winter months. Also, consider treatment for carriers who live in closed or semiclosed communities.

••••••••••••

RETINAL DETACHMENT

Retinal detachment occurs when the outer retinal pigment epithelium splits from the neural retina, creating subretinal space. This space then fills with fluid, called subretinal fluid. Retinal detachment is twice as common in males (perhaps due to increased incidence of trauma among males). Retinal detachment usually involves only one eye but may later involve the other eye. Surgical reattachment is often successful; the prognosis for good vision depends on which area of the retina is affected.

Causes
Any retinal tear or hole allows the liquid vitreous to seep between the retinal layers, separating the retina from its choroidal blood supply. Predisposing factors include myopia, intraocular surgery, and trauma. In adults, retinal detachment usually results from degenerative changes of aging, which cause a spontaneous retinal hole.

Retinal detachment may also result from seepage of fluid into the subretinal space (because of inflammation, tumors, or systemic diseases) or from traction that's placed on the retina by vitreous bands or membranes (due to proliferative diabetic retinopathy, posterior uveitis, or a traumatic intraocular foreign body).

Retinal detachment is rare in children, but occasionally develops as a result of retinopathy of prematurity, tumors (retinoblastomas), trauma, or myopia (which tends to run in families).

Clinical presentation
Initially, the patient may complain of floating spots and recurrent flashes of light (photopsia). However, as detachment progresses, gradual, painless vision loss may be described as a veil, curtain, or

cobweb that eliminates a portion of the visual field.

Differential diagnoses
- Senile retinoschisis
- Juvenile retinoschisis
- Choroidal detachment
- Inflammation of retina
- Trauma
- Child abuse
- Domestic violence

Diagnosis
Diagnosis depends on ophthalmoscopy after full pupil dilation. Examination shows the usually transparent retina as gray and opaque; in severe detachment, it reveals folds in the retina and ballooning out of the area. Indirect ophthalmoscopy is used to search for retinal tears. Ultrasound is performed if the lens is opaque.

Management
General
Treatment depends on the location and severity of the detachment. It may include restriction of eye movements and complete bed rest until surgical reattachment is done. A hole in the peripheral retina can be treated with cryothermy (freeze-bonding) in the posterior portion and laser therapy.

Surgical intervention
Retinal detachment usually requires a scleral buckling procedure, pneumatic retinoplexy or, for more complicated and severe detachments, a vitrectomy to reattach the retina.

Referral
- Refer the patient to an ophthalmologist for treatment.

Follow-up
The patient should be seen as per the ophthalmologist's recommendation.

Patient teaching
- Postoperatively, tell the patient to lie facedown on his right or left side and with the head of the bed raised. Discourage straining when defecating, bending down, hard coughing, sneezing, or vomiting, which can raise intraocular pressure. Antiemetics may be indicated.
- Tell the patient to protect the eye with a shield or glasses.
- To reduce edema and discomfort, tell the patient to apply ice packs.
- Teach the patient how to properly instill eyedrops and emphasize compliance and follow-up care. Suggest dark glasses to compensate for light sensitivity caused by cycloplegia.

Complications
- Posterior vitreous detachment
- Vision loss
- Infection

• • • • • • • • • • • •
SINUSITIS

Sinusitis — inflammation of the paranasal sinuses — may be acute, subacute, chronic, allergic, or hyperplastic.
- Acute sinusitis usually results from the common cold and lingers in subacute form in only about 10% of patients.
- Chronic sinusitis follows persistent bacterial infection.
- Allergic sinusitis accompanies allergic rhinitis.
- Hyperplastic sinusitis is a combination of purulent acute sinusitis and allergic sinusitis or rhinitis. The prognosis is good for all types.

Causes

Sinusitis usually results from viral or bacterial infection. The bacteria responsible for acute sinusitis are usually pneumococci, other streptococci, *Haemophilus influenzae*, and *Moraxella catarrhalis*. Staphylococci and gram-negative bacteria are more likely to cause sinusitis in chronic cases or in intensive care patients.

Predisposing factors include any condition that interferes with drainage and ventilation of the sinuses, such as chronic nasal edema, deviated septum, viscous mucus, nasal polyps, allergic rhinitis, nasal intubation, or debilitation due to chemotherapy, malnutrition, diabetes, blood dyscrasia, chronic use of steroids, or immunodeficiency. Bacterial invasion commonly results from the previously mentioned predisposing factors or from a viral infection or swimming in contaminated water.

The incidence of both acute and chronic sinusitis increases in later childhood. Sinusitis may be more prevalent in children who have had tonsils and adenoids removed.

Clinical presentation

The primary indication of acute sinusitis is nasal congestion, followed by a gradual buildup of pressure in the affected sinus. For 24 to 48 hours after onset, nasal discharge may be present and later may become purulent. Associated symptoms include malaise, sore throat, headache, and low-grade fever of 99° to 99.5° F [37.2° to 37.5° C]).

Characteristic pain depends on the affected sinus:
- maxillary sinusitis — pain over the cheeks and upper teeth
- ethmoid sinusitis — pain over the eyes
- frontal sinusitis — pain over the eyebrows
- sphenoid sinusitis (rare) — pain behind the eyes.

Purulent nasal drainage that continues for longer than 3 weeks after an acute infection subsides suggests subacute sinusitis. Other clinical features of the subacute form include:
- stuffy nose
- vague facial discomfort
- fatigue
- nonproductive cough.

The effects of chronic sinusitis are similar to those of acute sinusitis, but the chronic form causes continuous mucopurulent discharge.

The effects of allergic sinusitis are the same as those of allergic rhinitis. In both conditions, the prominent signs and symptoms include:
- sneezing
- frontal headache
- watery nasal discharge
- stuffy, burning, itchy nose.

In hyperplastic sinusitis, bacterial growth on the diseased tissue causes pronounced tissue edema; thickening of the mucosal lining and the development of mucosal polyps combine to produce chronic stuffiness of the nose as well as headaches.

Differential diagnoses

- Chronic sinusitis
- Allergic rhinitis
- Polyps
- Tumor or cyst
- Nasal foreign body
- Vasculitides
- Otitis media
- Dental infection
- Upper respiratory infection
- Headache, migraine cluster, or tension

Diagnosis

The following diagnostic measures are useful:
- Nasal examination reveals inflammation and pus.

- Sinus X-rays reveal cloudiness in the affected sinus, air and fluid, and any thickening of the mucosal lining.
- Antral puncture promotes drainage of purulent material. It may also be used to provide a specimen for culture and sensitivity testing of the infecting organism, but it's seldom performed.
- Ultrasound and computed tomography (CT) scan aid in diagnosing suspected complications. CT scanning is more sensitive than routine X-rays in detecting sinusitis.
- Transillumination is a simple diagnostic tool that involves shining a light into the patient's mouth with his lips closed around it. Infected sinuses look dark, and normal sinuses transilluminate.

Management
General
Steam inhalation along with decongestants may be helpful. Local applications of heat may help to relieve pain and congestion.

Medication
Medications for treatment of sinusitis may include:
- oxymetazoline — 2 to 3 drops/nostril b.i.d. for 3 days
- phenylephrine — 1 to 2 sprays/nostril every 3 to 4 hours for 3 days
- pseudoephedrine hydrochloride — adults, 60 mg P.O. every 4 to 6 hours or sustained release 120 mg every 12 hours; children older than age 5, 30 mg P.O. every 4 to 6 hours; children ages 2 to 5, 15 mg P.O. every 4 to 6 hours
- amoxicillin — adults, 250 to 875 mg P.O. every 12 hours; children, 20 to 40 mg/kg/day P.O. in 3 divided doses
- amoxicillin/clavulanate — adults, 250 to 500 mg P.O. every 12 hours; children, weighing less than 88 lb (40 kg), 20 to 45 mg/kg P.O. in 3 divided doses

- clarithromycin — 500 mg P.O. every 12 hours for 10 to 14 days
- azithromycin — 500 mg initial dose, then 250 mg/day P.O. for 4 days.

In subacute sinusitis, antibiotics and decongestants may be helpful.

Treatment for allergic sinusitis must include treatment for allergic rhinitis: administering antihistamines, identifying allergens through skin testing, and desensitization through immunotherapy.

Surgical intervention
If subacute infection persists, the sinuses may be irrigated. If irrigation fails to relieve symptoms, endoscopic sinus surgery may be required to obtain a histologic diagnosis, remove polyps, and provide adequate ventilation of the infected sinuses. Partial or total resection of the middle turbinate as well as more radical procedures, such as total sphenoethmoidectomy, may be performed.

Referral
- Refer the patient to an ear, nose, and throat specialist if treatment is unsuccessful.

Follow-up
The patient should be seen after 48 to 72 hours of treatment and then in 2 weeks.

Patient teaching
- Encourage bed rest and tell the patient to drink plenty of fluids to promote drainage.
- To relieve pain and promote drainage, tell the patient to apply warm compresses continuously or four times daily for 2-hour intervals.
- Tell the patient to finish the prescribed antibiotics, even if his symptoms disappear.
- If surgery is necessary, tell the patient what to expect postoperatively: nasal packing will be in place for 12 to 24 hours

after surgery; he'll have to breathe through his mouth and won't be able to blow his nose. Tell the patient that even after the packing is removed, nose blowing can cause bleeding and swelling. If the patient is a smoker, instruct him not to smoke for at least 2 or 3 days after surgery.

Complications
- Meningitis
- Abscess
- Orbital infection
- Osteomyelitis
- Septic cavernous thrombosis

• • • • • • • • • • •

STYE

A stye (or hordeolum) is a localized, purulent staphylococcal infection that can occur externally (in the lumen of the smaller glands of Zeis or in Moll's glands) or internally (in the larger meibomian gland). A stye can occur at any age. Generally, styes are self-limiting and respond well to hot moist compresses. If untreated, a stye can eventually lead to cellulitis of the eyelid.

Clinical presentation
Typically, a stye produces redness, swelling, and pain. An abscess commonly forms at the lid margin, with an eyelash pointing outward from its center. (See *Recognizing a stye.*)

Differential diagnoses
- Chalazion
- Conjunctivitis
- Corneal abrasion

Diagnosis
Visual examination generally confirms this infection. Culture of purulent material from the abscess usually reveals a staphylococcal organism.

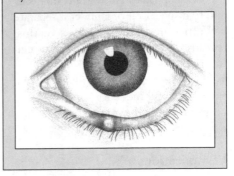

Recognizing a stye

A stye is a localized red, swollen, and tender abscess of the glands in an eyelid.

Management
General
Treatment consists of warm compresses applied for 10 to 15 minutes, four times per day for 3 to 4 days, to facilitate drainage of the abscess, relieve pain and inflammation, and promote suppuration.

Medication
The following medications may be prescribed to treat a stye:
- sulfacetamide sodium ophthalmic ointment 10% — ½" to 1" (1 to 2.5 cm) into the conjunctival sac q.i.d. and h.s. for 7 to 14 days; 10% solution — 2 drops in the affected eye every 3 hours for 7 to 14 days
- bacitracin or polymyxin B ointment — ½" to 1" into the conjunctival sac every 4 hours for 7 to 14 days.

Surgical intervention
If conservative treatment fails, incision and drainage may be necessary.

Referral
- Refer the patient to an ophthalmologist if treatment isn't successful.

Follow-up

The patient should be seen in 2 weeks to be reevaluated.

Patient teaching

- Instruct the patient to use a clean cloth for each application of warm compresses and to dispose of it or launder it separately.
- Warn against squeezing the stye; this spreads the infection and can cause cellulitis.
- Teach the patient or family members the proper technique for instilling eyedrops or ointments into the cul-de-sac of the lower eyelid.

Complications

- Cellulitis of the eyelid

• • • • • • • • • • •

TONSILLITIS

Tonsillitis — inflammation of the tonsils — can be acute or chronic. The uncomplicated acute form usually lasts 4 to 6 days and commonly affects children between ages 5 and 10. The presence of proven chronic tonsillitis justifies tonsillectomy, the only effective treatment. Tonsils tend to hypertrophy during childhood and atrophy after puberty.

Causes

Tonsillitis generally results from infection with group A beta-hemolytic streptococci but can result from other bacteria or viruses or from oral anaerobes.

Clinical presentation

Acute tonsillitis commonly begins with a mild to severe sore throat. A very young child, unable to describe a sore throat, may stop eating. Tonsillitis may also produce:

- dysphagia
- fever

- swelling and tender lymph glands in the submandibular area
- muscle and joint pain
- chills
- malaise
- headache
- pain (frequently referred to the ears).

Excess secretions can cause a constant urge to swallow, and the back of the throat may feel constricted. Such discomfort usually subsides after 72 hours.

Chronic tonsillitis produces a recurrent sore throat and purulent drainage in the tonsillar crypts. Frequent attacks of acute tonsillitis may also occur.

Differential diagnoses

- Coxsackie virus
- Scarlet fever
- Peritonsillar abscess
- Mononucleosis
- Diphtheria
- Mediastinitis
- Retropharyngeal abscess
- Malignancy

Diagnosis

Diagnostic confirmation requires a thorough throat examination that reveals:

- generalized inflammation of the pharyngeal wall
- swollen tonsils that project from between the pillars of the fauces and exude white or yellow follicles
- purulent drainage when pressure is applied to the tonsillar pillars
- a possible edematous and inflamed uvula.

Culture may be used to determine the infecting organism and appropriate antibiotic therapy. Leukocytosis is also usually present.

Management

General

Treatment for acute tonsillitis requires rest, adequate fluid intake, and administration of analgesics and antibiotics.

Medication

The following medications may be used to treat tonsillitis:

- acetaminophen—adults, 325 to 650 mg P.O. every 4 hours p.r.n.; children, dosage per package directions
- ibuprofen—adults, 200 to 400 mg P.O. every 4 to 6 hours p.r.n.; children, dosage per package directions
- penicillin V—adults, 250 to 500 mg P.O. every 6 hours for 10 days; children, 500 mg/day P.O. in divided doses
- erythromycin—adults, 250 to 500 mg P.O. q.i.d. for 10 days; children, 30 to 50 mg/kg/day P.O. in divided doses.

Surgical intervention

Chronic tonsillitis or complications (obstructions from tonsillar hypertrophy, peritonsillar abscess) may necessitate a tonsillectomy but only after the patient has been free from tonsillar or respiratory tract infections for 3 to 4 weeks.

Referral

- Refer the patient to an ear, nose, and throat specialist if treatment is unsuccessful or if the condition is chronic.

Follow-up

The patient should be reevaluated after 2 weeks.

Patient teaching

- Urge the patient to drink plenty of fluids, especially if he has a fever. Parents may offer a child ice cream and flavored drinks and ices. Suggest gargling to soothe the throat, unless it exacerbates pain.
- Make sure that the patient and his parents understand the importance of completing the prescribed course of antibiotic therapy.
- After surgery, tell the patient and parents to expect a white scab to form in the throat between 5 and 10 days postoperatively and to report bleeding, ear discomfort, or a fever that lasts longer than 3 days.

Complications

- Systemic infection
- Peritonsillar abscess or cellulitis
- Scarlet fever
- Poststreptococcal glomerulonephritis

• • • • • • • • • • • •

UVEITIS

Uveitis is inflammation of the uveal tract. It occurs as anterior uveitis, which affects the iris (iritis), or the iris and the ciliary body (iridocyclitis); as posterior uveitis, which affects the choroid (choroiditis), or the choroid and the retina (chorioretinitis); or as panuveitis, which affects the entire uveal tract.

Untreated anterior uveitis may result in elevated intraocular pressure (IOP) leading to vision loss. With immediate treatment, anterior uveitis usually subsides after a few days to several weeks; however, recurrence can occur. Posterior uveitis may lead to vision loss if the macula is involved.

Causes

Typically, uveitis is idiopathic; however, it can result from allergy, bacteria, viruses, fungi, chemicals, trauma, or surgery or it may be associated with systemic diseases, such as rheumatoid arthritis, ankylosing spondylitis, and toxoplasmosis.

Granulomatous and nongranulomatous uveitis

FACTOR	GRANULOMATOUS	NONGRANULOMATOUS
Location	Usually posterior part of uveal tract	Anterior part of the iris and ciliary body
Onset	Insidious	Acute
Pain	None or slight	Marked
Photophobia	Slight	Marked
Course	Chronic	Acute
Prognosis	Fair to poor	Good
Recurrence	Occasional	Common
Blurred vision	Marked	Moderate

Clinical presentation

Anterior uveitis produces:
- moderate to severe unilateral eye pain
- severe ciliary injection
- photophobia
- tearing
- small, nonreactive pupil
- blurred vision (due to the increased number of cells in the aqueous humor).

It sometimes produces deposits called keratic precipitates on the back of the cornea, which may be seen in the anterior chamber. The iris may adhere to the lens, causing posterior synechiae and pupillary distortion; pain and photophobia may occur. Onset may be acute or insidious.

Although clinical distinction isn't always possible, anterior uveitis occurs in two forms — granulomatous and nongranulomatous. Granulomatous uveitis was once thought to be caused by tuberculosis bacilli; nongranulomatous uveitis, by streptococci. Although this isn't true, the terms are still used. (See *Granulomatous and nongranulomatous uveitis*.)

Posterior uveitis begins insidiously, with complaints of slightly decreased or blurred vision or floating spots. Posterior uveitis may be acute or chronic and affect one or both eyes. Retinal damage caused by lesions from toxoplasmosis and retinal detachments can occur.

Differential diagnoses
- Retinal detachment
- Conjunctivitis
- Corneal abrasion or laceration
- Ulcerative keratitis
- Acute angle glaucoma
- Scleritis
- Foreign body
- Sarcoidosis

Diagnosis

In anterior and posterior uveitis, a slit-lamp examination shows a "flare and cell" pattern, which looks like particles dancing in a sunbeam. With a special lens, slit-lamp and ophthalmoscopic examination can also identify active inflammatory fundus lesions involving the retina and choroid, although a hazy vitreous may obscure the view.

In posterior uveitis, serologic tests may be used to rule out toxoplasmosis.

Management
General
Uveitis requires vigorous and prompt management, which includes treatment of any known underlying cause and application of a topical cycloplegic.

Medication
Medications may include:
- 1% atropine sulfate — 1 to 2 drops up to q.i.d.
- prednisolone acetate 1% ophthalmic solution — 2 drops into the affected eye every hour initially, tapering to q.i.d. with improvement.

Referral
- Refer the patient to an ophthalmologist to receive a dilated fundus examination and for treatment, including treatment for local systemic diseases.

Follow-up
The patient should be seen according to the ophthalmologist's recommendation.

Patient teaching
- Encourage the patient to rest during the acute phase.
- Teach the patient the proper method of instilling eyedrops.
- Suggest the use of dark glasses to ease the discomfort of photophobia.
- Instruct the patient to watch for and report adverse effects of systemic corticosteroid therapy.
- Stress the importance of follow-up care to check high IOP while the patient is taking steroids. Tell the patient to seek treatment immediately at the first sign of iritis.

Complications
- Vision loss
- Increased IOP
- Cataract formation
- Macular edema
- Optic nerve damage
- Retinal damage
- Retinal detachment

• • • • • • • • • • • •

VASCULAR RETINOPATHIES

Vascular retinopathies are noninflammatory retinal disorders that result from interference with the blood supply to the eyes. The five distinct types of vascular retinopathy are central retinal artery occlusion, central retinal vein occlusion, diabetic retinopathy, hypertensive retinopathy, and sickle cell retinopathy.

Causes
When one of the arteries maintaining blood circulation in the retina becomes obstructed, the diminished blood flow causes visual deficits. (See *A close look at vascular retinopathy,* page 614.)

Central retinal artery occlusion may be idiopathic or may result from embolism, atherosclerosis, infection, or conditions that retard blood flow, such as temporal arteritis, carotid occlusion, and heart failure. Central retinal artery occlusion is rare, occurs unilaterally, and usually affects elderly patients. However, if it occurs in a younger person, the obstruction may have originated in the heart (such as embolization from plaque material from valve vegetations) and should be investigated accordingly.

Causes of central retinal vein occlusion include atherosclerosis, hypertension, optic disk edema, hypercoagulable states (polycythemia, leukemia, sickle cell disease), glaucoma, retrobulbar compression (such as an orbital tumor), and

A close look at vascular retinopathy

The figure here depicts several possible findings found during an ophthalmic examination.

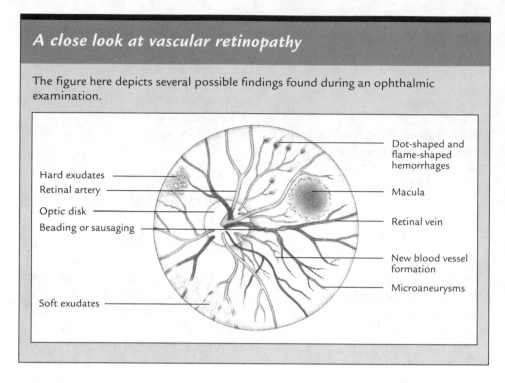

- Hard exudates
- Retinal artery
- Optic disk
- Beading or sausaging
- Soft exudates
- Dot-shaped and flame-shaped hemorrhages
- Macula
- Retinal vein
- New blood vessel formation
- Microaneurysms

drugs such as oral contraceptives. This form of vascular retinopathy is most prevalent in elderly patients and is characterized by impaired venous outflow.

Diabetic retinopathy results from juvenile or adult diabetes. Microcirculatory changes occur more rapidly when diabetes is poorly controlled. About 90% of patients with juvenile diabetes develop retinopathy within 20 years of onset of diabetes. In adults with diabetes, incidence increases with the duration of diabetes; 80% of patients who have had diabetes for 20 to 25 years develop retinopathy. This condition is a leading cause of acquired adult blindness.

Hypertensive retinopathy results from prolonged hypertensive disease, producing retinal vasospasm, and consequent damage and arteriolar narrowing.

Sickle cell retinopathy results from impaired ability of the sickled cell to pass through microvasculature, producing vaso-occlusion. This leads to microaneurysms, chorioretinal infarction, and retinal detachment.

Clinical presentation

Clinical effects depend on the type of retinopathy present:

- Central retinal artery occlusion produces sudden, painless, unilateral loss of vision (partial or complete). It may follow amaurosis fugax or transient episodes of unilateral loss of vision lasting from a few seconds to minutes, probably due to vasospasm. This condition typically causes permanent blindness. However, some patients experience spontaneous resolution within hours and regain partial vision.

- Central retinal vein occlusion causes reduced visual acuity, allowing perception of only hand movement and light. This condition is painless, except when it results in secondary neovascular glaucoma (uncontrolled proliferation of weak blood vessels). The prognosis is poor;

some patients with this condition develop secondary glaucoma within 3 to 4 months after occlusion.

■ Nonproliferative diabetic retinopathy produces changes in the lining of the retinal blood vessels that cause the vessels to leak plasma or fatty substances, which decrease or block blood flow (nonperfusion) in the retina. This disorder may also produce microaneurysms and small hemorrhages. Nonproliferative retinopathy causes no symptoms in some patients; in others, leakage of fluid into the macular region causes significant loss of central visual acuity (necessary for reading and driving) and diminished night vision.

■ Proliferative diabetic retinopathy produces fragile new blood vessels on the disk (neovascularization) and elsewhere in the fundus. These vessels can grow into the vitreous and then rupture, causing vitreous hemorrhage with corresponding sudden vision loss. Scar tissue that may form along the new blood vessels can pull on the retina, causing it to tear or even detach.

■ Hypertensive retinopathy is characterized by blurred vision, commonly accompanied by headache. Ophthalmoscopic examination may reveal diffuse binocular narrowing, venular tortuosity, silver wire reflexes, macular scars, and swelling of the head of the optic nerve (disk edema). Severe, prolonged disease eventually produces blindness; mild, prolonged disease, visual defects.

■ Sickle cell retinopathy include peripheral arteriolar occlusions, peripheral arteriovenous anastomoses, sea fan neurovascular fronds, vitreous hemorrhage as tractional forces and vitreous collapse tear fragile neovascular membranes and, with advanced disease, severe vitreous traction and retinal detachment.

Differential diagnoses
■ Giant cell or temporal arteritis
■ Anterior ischemic optic neuropathy
■ Central retinal artery occlusion
■ Optic neuritis
■ Tumor
■ Edema
■ Hyphema
■ Trauma
■ Psychogenic causes

Diagnosis
Check the patient's visual acuity and then vital signs, including blood pressure. Diagnosis is made on fundal examination with an ophthalmoscope. Determine if female patients are pregnant; hypertensive retinopathy may be an early sign of preeclampsia. (See *Diagnostic tests for vascular retinopathies*, page 616.)

Management
General
There's no treatment to control central retinal artery occlusion. However, an attempt is made to release the occlusion into the peripheral circulation. Treatment of nonproliferative diabetic retinopathy is prophylactic. Careful control of blood glucose levels may reduce the severity of the retinopathy or delay its onset. Patients with early symptoms of microaneurysms should have frequent eye examinations (three to four times a year); children with diabetes should have an annual eye examination.

Treatment of hypertensive retinopathy includes controlling blood pressure with appropriate drugs, diet, and exercise. Treating the systemic hypertension should improve the condition of the eyes. If left untreated, hypertensive retinopathy results in severe vision loss.

Treatment of sickle cell retinopathy is to reduce the risk of or prevent or eliminate the retinal neovascularization. Patients with symptoms should have ocular

Diagnostic tests for vascular retinopathies

CENTRAL RETINAL ARTERY OCCLUSION

■ *Ophthalmoscopy (direct or indirect)* shows blockage of retinal arterioles during transient attack.

■ *Retinal examination* within 2 hours of onset shows clumps or segmentation in artery; later, milky white retina around disk due to swelling and necrosis of ganglion cells caused by reduced blood supply; also shows cherry-red spot in macula that subsides after several weeks.

■ *Color Doppler tests* evaluate carotid occlusion with no need for arteriography.

■ *Physical examination* reveals underlying cause of vascular retinopathy, for example, diabetes or hypertension.

CENTRAL RETINAL VEIN OCCLUSION

■ *Ophthalmoscopy (direct or indirect)* shows flame-shaped hemorrhages, retinal vein engorgement, white patches among hemorrhages, edema around the disk.

■ *Color Doppler tests* confirm or rule out occlusion of blood vessels.

■ *Physical examination* reveals underlying cause.

DIABETIC RETINOPATHY

■ *Indirect ophthalmoscopic examination* shows retinal changes, such as microaneurysms (earliest change), retinal hemorrhages and edema, venous dilation and beading, lipid exudates, fibrous bands in the vitreous, and growth of new blood vessels. Infarcts of the nerve fiber layer are observed.

■ *Fluorescein angiography* shows leakage of fluorescein from weak-walled vessels and "lights up" microaneurysms, differentiating them from true hemorrhages.

■ *History* reveals diabetes.

HYPERTENSIVE RETINOPATHY

■ *Ophthalmoscopy (direct or indirect)* in early stages, shows hard, shiny deposits; flame-shaped hemorrhages; silver wire appearance of narrowed arterioles; and nicking of veins where arteries cross them (atrioventricular nicking). In late stages, shows cotton wool patches, lipid exudates, retinal edema, papilledema due to ischemia and capillary insufficiency, hemorrhages, and microaneurysms in both eyes.

■ *Physical examination* reveals elevated blood pressure.

■ *History* reveals decreased vision, headache, nausea, and acute or malignant hypertension.

---

examinations and dilated retinal evaluation twice a year. Proliferative disease should be treated with fluorescein angiography and panretinal photocoagulation. Cryotherapy hasn't been proven to be effective and has a high complication rate.

Medication

Aspirin (325 to 650 mg P.O. every 4 to 6 hours p.r.n.) may be given.

Surgical intervention

Anterior chamber paracentesis may be needed to try to move the arterial obstruction into the peripheral field. Laser photocoagulation can reduce the risk of neovascular glaucoma for some patients whose eyes have widespread capillary nonperfusion.

Treatment for proliferative diabetic retinopathy or severe macular edema is also laser photocoagulation, which cauterizes the leaking blood vessels. Laser treatment may be focal (aimed at new blood vessels) or panretinal (placing burns throughout the peripheral retina). Despite treatment, neovascularization continues to proliferate, and vitreous hemorrhage, with or without retinal detachment, may follow. If the blood isn't absorbed in 6 weeks to 3 months, vitrectomy may restore partial vision.

Referral
■ Refer the patient to an ophthalmologist for treatment.

Follow-up
The patient should be seen according to the ophthalmologist's recommendation.

Patient teaching
■ Encourage a diabetic patient to comply with the prescribed regimen.
■ For a patient with hypertensive retinopathy, stress the importance of complying with antihypertensive therapy.

Complications
■ Vision loss
■ Progressive myopia
■ Cataracts

• • • • • • • • • • • •

SELECTED REFERENCES

Bickley, L.S., and Hoekelman, R.A. *Bates Guide to Physical Examination and History Taking*, 7th ed. Philadelphia: Lippincott Williams & Wilkins, 1999.

Chernecky, C.C., and Berger, B.J. *Laboratory Tests and Diagnostic Procedures*, 3rd ed. Philadelphia: W.B. Saunders Co., 2001.

Christensen, B.L., and Kockrow, E.O. *Foundations of Nursing*, 3rd ed. St. Louis: Mosby–Year Book, Inc., 1999.

Diseases, 3rd ed. Springhouse, Pa.: Springhouse Corp., 2001.

Fraunfelder, F.T., and Roy, F.H. *Current Ocular Therapy*, 5th ed. Philadelphia: W.B. Saunders Co., 2000.

Fauci, A.S., et al., eds. *Harrison's Principles of Internal Medicine*, 15th ed. New York: McGraw-Hill Book Co., 2001.

Lamkin, J.C. *Massachusetts Eye & Ear Infirmary Review Manual for Ophthalmology*, 2nd ed. Philadelphia: Lippincott Williams & Wilkins, 1999.

Lee, K.J. *Essential Otolaryngology: Head and Neck Surgery*, 7th ed. Stamford, Conn.: Appleton & Lange, 1999.

Lewis, S.M., et al., ed. *Medical-Surgical Nursing: Assessment and Management of Clinical Problems*, 5th ed. St. Louis: Mosby–Year Book, Inc., 2000.

Rakel, R.E., and Edward T. Bope, E.T., eds. *Conn's Current Therapy 2001*. Philadelphia: W.B. Saunders Co., 2001.

Rhee, D.J., and Pyfer, M.F. *The Wills Eye Manual: Office and Emergency Room Diagnosis and Treatment of Eye Disease*, 3rd ed. Philadelphia: Lippincott Williams & Wilkins, 1999.

Smeltzer, S.C., and Bare, B.G., eds. *Brunner and Suddarth's Textbook of Medical-Surgical Nursing*, 9th ed. Philadelphia: Lippincott Williams & Wilkins, 2000.

Vaughan, D., et al. *General Ophthalmology*, 15th ed. Stamford, Conn.: Appleton & Lange, 1999.

Infectious diseases

Despite improved methods of treating and preventing infection — potent antibiotics, complex immunizations, and modern sanitation — infectious diseases still account for much serious illness, even in highly industrialized countries. In developing countries, infectious diseases are some of the most critical health problems.

. . . .

UNDERSTANDING INFECTION

Infection is the invasion and proliferation of microorganisms in or on body tissue that produce signs and symptoms as well as an immune response. Reproduction of such microorganisms injures the host by causing cellular damage from microorganism-produced toxins or intracellular multiplication or by competing with the host's metabolism. The host's own immune response sometimes compounds the tissue damage, which may be localized (as in infected pressure ulcers) or systemic. The severity of the infection varies with the pathogenicity and num-

ber of the invading microorganisms and the strength of host defenses. The young and the old are especially susceptible to infections.

Why are the microorganisms that cause infectious diseases so difficult to overcome? There are many complex reasons:

- Some bacteria develop a resistance to antibiotics.
- Some microorganisms, such as the human immunodeficiency virus, include so many different strains that a single vaccine can't provide protection against all of them.
- Most viruses resist antiviral drugs.
- Some microorganisms localize in areas that make treatment difficult, such as the central nervous system and bone.

Even some factors that contribute to improved health — such as the affluence that allows good nutrition and living conditions and advances in medical science — can indirectly lead to increased risk of infection. For example, travel can expose people to diseases for which they have little natural immunity. The expanded use of immunosuppressants, surgery, and other invasive procedures also increases the risk of infection.

Types of infection

A laboratory-verified infection that causes no signs or symptoms is called a *subclinical, silent,* or *asymptomatic infection.* A multiplication of microbes that produces no signs, symptoms, or immune response is called a *colonization.* A person with a subclinical infection or colonization may be a carrier and transmit infection to others. A latent infection occurs after a microorganism has been dormant in the host, sometimes for years. An *exogenous infection* results from environmental pathogens; an *endogenous infection* results from the host's normal flora (such as a urinary tract infection that results from *Escherichia coli* from the colon).

Microorganisms responsible for infectious diseases include bacteria, viruses, rickettsiae, chlamydiae, fungi (yeasts and molds), and protozoa. Some larger organisms, such as helminths (parasitic worms) and other roundworms or flatworms, also cause infectious diseases.

Bacteria

Bacteria are single-cell microorganisms with well-defined cell walls that can grow independently on artificial media without the need for other cells. Bacteria inhabit the intestines of humans and other animals as normal flora used in the digestion of food. Other bacteria are vital to soil fertility. These microorganisms break down dead tissue, which allows it to be used by other organisms.

Despite the many types of known bacteria, only a small percentage are harmful to humans. In developing countries, where poor sanitation increases the risk of infection, bacterial diseases commonly result in death and disability. In industrialized countries, bacterial infections are the most common fatal infec-

tious diseases. (See *How bacteria damage tissue,* page 620.)

Bacteria can be classified according to shape. Spherical bacterial cells are called *cocci;* rod-shaped bacteria, *bacilli;* and spiral-shaped bacteria, *spirilla.* Bacteria can also be classified according to their response to staining (gram-positive, gram-negative, or acid-fast bacteria), their motility (motile or nonmotile bacteria), their tendency toward encapsulation (encapsulated or nonencapsulated bacteria), and their capacity to form spores (sporulating or nonsporulating bacteria).

Spirochetes are bacteria with flexible, slender, undulating spiral rods that have cell walls. Most are anaerobic. The three pathogenic forms in humans include *Treponema, Leptospira,* and *Borrelia.*

Viruses

Viruses are subcellular organisms made up only of a ribonucleic acid or a deoxyribonucleic acid nucleus covered with proteins. They're the smallest known organisms (so tiny that they're visible only through an electron microscope). Independent of host cells, viruses can't replicate. Rather, they invade a host cell and stimulate it to participate in the formation of additional virus particles. The estimated 400 viruses that infect humans are classified according to their size, shape (spherical, rod shaped, or cubic), or mode of transmission (respiratory, fecal, oral, or sexual).

Rickettsiae

Rickettsiae are relatively uncommon in the United States. These small, gram-negative organisms are classified as bacteria that commonly induce life-threatening infections. Like viruses, they require a host cell for replication. Three genera of rickettsiae include *Rickettsia, Coxiella,* and *Rochalimaea.*

How bacteria damage tissue

The human body is constantly infected by bacteria and other infectious organisms. Some are beneficial, such as the intestinal bacteria that produce vitamins. Others are harmful, causing illnesses ranging from the common cold to life-threatening septic shock.

To infect a host, bacteria must first enter it. They do this either by adhering to the mucosal surface and directly invading the host cell or by attaching to epithelial cells and producing toxins, which invade host cells. To survive and multiply in a host, bacteria or their toxins adversely affect biochemical reactions in cells. The result is a disruption of normal cell function or cell death (see illustration below). For example, the diphtheria toxin damages heart muscle by inhibiting protein synthesis. In addition, as some organisms multiply, they extend into deeper tissue and eventually gain access to the bloodstream.

Some toxins cause blood to clot in small blood vessels. The tissues supplied by these vessels may be deprived of blood and damaged (see illustration below).

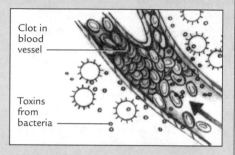

Clot in blood vessel

Toxins from bacteria

Other toxins can damage the cell walls of small blood vessels, causing leakage. This fluid loss results in decreased blood pressure, which in turn impairs the heart's ability to pump enough blood to vital organs (see illustration below).

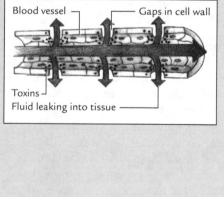

Blood vessel — Gaps in cell wall

Toxins —
Fluid leaking into tissue —

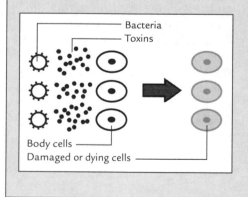

Bacteria
Toxins

Body cells —
Damaged or dying cells —

Chlamydiae

Chlamydiae are smaller than rickettsiae and bacteria but larger than viruses. They too depend on host cells for replication; however, unlike viruses, they're susceptible to antibiotics.

Fungi

Fungi are single-cell organisms, with nuclei enveloped by nuclear membranes. They have rigid cell walls like plant cells but lack chlorophyll, the green matter necessary for photosynthesis; they also show relatively little cellular specialization. Fungi occur as yeasts (single-cell oval-shaped organisms) or molds (organisms with hyphae, or branching filaments). Depending on the environment, some fungi may occur in both forms. Fungal diseases in humans are called mycoses.

Protozoa

Protozoa are the simplest single-cell organisms of the animal kingdom but show a high level of cellular specialization. Like other animal cells, they have cell membranes rather than cell walls, and their nuclei are surrounded by nuclear membranes.

Nosocomial infections

A nosocomial infection is one that develops after a patient is admitted to a hospital or other institution, such as a nursing home or long-term care facility. This type of infection is usually transmitted by direct contact. Less commonly, transmission occurs by inhalation or by contact with contaminated equipment and solutions.

Despite hospital infection control programs that include surveillance, prevention, and education, about 5% of patients who enter hospitals contract nosocomial infections. Since the 1960s, staphylococcal infections have been declining; however, gram-negative bacilli, resistant enterococci, and fungal infections have been steadily increasing.

Nosocomial infections continue to be a difficult problem because most hospital patients are older and more debilitated than in the past. Moreover, the increased use of invasive and surgical procedures, immunosuppressants, and antibiotics predisposes patients to infection and superinfection. At the same time, the growing number of personnel that come in contact with each patient makes the risk of exposure greater.

Here's how you can prevent nosocomial infections:
- Follow strict infection-control procedures. (See *Standard precautions*, pages 622 and 623, and *CDC isolation precautions*, pages 624 and 625.)
- Document hospital infections as they occur.
- Identify outbreaks early, and take steps to prevent their spread.
- Eliminate unnecessary procedures that contribute to infection.
- Strictly follow necessary isolation techniques.
- Observe *all* patients for signs of infection, especially those who are at high risk.
- Always follow proper hand-washing technique, and encourage other staff members to follow these guidelines.
- Keep staff members and visitors with obvious infection as well as known carriers away from susceptible, high-risk patients.
- Take special precautions with vulnerable patients, such as those with indwelling urinary catheters, mechanical ventilators, or I.V. lines, and those recuperating from surgery.

Modes of transmission

Most infectious diseases are transmitted in one of four ways:
- In *contact transmission*, the susceptible host comes into direct contact (as in sexually transmitted disease) or indirect contact (contaminated inanimate objects or the close-range spread of respiratory droplets) with the source. The most common mode of contact transmission is by contaminated hands.
- *Airborne transmission* results from inhaling contaminated aerosolized droplets (as in pulmonary tuberculosis).
- In *enteric (oral-fecal) transmission*, the infecting organisms are found in feces and are ingested by susceptible victims, in many cases through fecally contami-

Standard precautions

The Centers for Disease Control and Prevention recommends using the following standard blood and body fluid precautions for *all* patients. This is especially important in emergency care settings, where the risk of blood exposure is increased and the patient's infection status is usually unknown. Implementing standard precautions doesn't eliminate the need for other transmission-based precautions, such as airborne, droplet, and contact precautions.

SOURCES OF POTENTIAL EXPOSURE
Standard precautions apply to blood, semen, vaginal secretions, cerebrospinal fluid, synovial fluid, pleural fluid, peritoneal fluid, pericardial fluid, and amniotic fluid. These fluids are most likely to transmit human immunodeficiency virus (HIV). Standard precautions also apply to other body fluids, including feces, nasal secretions, saliva, sputum, tears, vomitus, and breast milk.

BARRIER PRECAUTIONS
- Wear gloves when touching blood, body fluids, mucous membranes, or the broken skin of all patients; when handling items or touching surfaces soiled with blood or body fluids; and when performing venipuncture and other vascular access procedures.
- Change gloves and wash your hands after contact with each patient.
- Wear a mask and protective eyewear or a face shield to protect mucous membranes of the mouth, nose, and eyes during procedures that may generate drops of blood or other body fluids.
- In addition to a mask and protective eyewear or a face shield, wear a gown or an apron during procedures that are likely to generate splashing of blood or other body fluids.
- After removing gloves, thoroughly wash your hands and other skin surfaces that may be contaminated with blood or other body fluids.

PRECAUTIONS FOR INVASIVE PROCEDURES
- During all invasive procedures, wear gloves and a surgical mask.
- During procedures that commonly generate droplets or splashes of blood or other body fluids or that generate bone chips, wear protective eyewear and a mask or a face shield.
- During invasive procedures that are likely to cause splashing or splattering of blood or other body fluids, wear a gown or an impervious apron.
- If you perform or assist in vaginal or cesarean deliveries, wear gloves and a gown when handling the placenta or the infant and during umbilical cord care.

WORK PRACTICE PRECAUTIONS
Prevent injuries caused by needles, scalpels, and other sharp instruments when disposing of used needles and when handling sharp instruments after procedures:
- To prevent needle-stick injuries, don't recap used needles, bend or break needles, remove them from disposable syringes, or manipulate them.
- Place disposable syringes and needles, scalpel blades, and other sharp items in puncture-resistant containers for disposal; make sure these containers are located near the area of use.
- Place large-bore reusable needles in a puncture-resistant container for transport to the reprocessing area.

Standard precautions *(continued)*

■ If a glove tears or a needle-stick or other injury occurs, remove the gloves, wash your hands, and wash the injury site thoroughly, then put on new gloves as quickly as patient safety permits. Remove the needle or instrument involved in the incident from the sterile field. Promptly report injuries and mucous membrane exposure to the appropriate infection-control officer.

ADDITIONAL PRECAUTIONS
■ Make sure mouthpieces, one-way valve masks, resuscitation bags, or other ventilation devices are available in areas where the need for resuscitation is likely. *Note:* Saliva hasn't been implicated in HIV transmission.
■ If you have exudative lesions or weeping dermatitis, refrain from direct patient care and handling patient care equipment until the condition resolves.

---

nated food or water (as in salmonella infections).
■ *Vectorborne transmission* occurs when an intermediate carrier (vector), such as a flea or a mosquito, transfers an organism.

Methods to prevent the transmission of infectious diseases include:
■ comprehensive immunization (including the required immunization of travelers to or emigrants from endemic areas)
■ drug prophylaxis
■ improved nutrition, living conditions, and sanitation
■ correction of environmental factors
■ widespread disease tracking. (See *Reportable infectious diseases,* page 626.)

Immunization can be used to control many diseases, including diphtheria, pertussis, measles, rubella, some forms of meningitis, poliovirus, hepatitis B, pneumococcal pneumonia, influenza, rabies, and tetanus. Smallpox (variola) — which killed and disfigured millions — has been virtually eradicated by a comprehensive World Health Organization program of surveillance and immunization.

Vaccines, which contain live but attenuated (weakened) or killed microorganisms, and toxoids, which contain modified bacterial exotoxins, induce active immunity against bacterial and viral diseases by stimulating antibody formation. Natural active immunity is produced as a patient who has the disease forms antibodies against it, thus preventing the recurrence of the disease. Immune globulins contain previously formed antibodies from hyperimmunized donors or pooled plasma and provide temporary passive immunity. Generally, passive immunization is used when active immunization is perilous or impossible or when complete protection requires both active and passive immunization. Maternal passive immunity crosses the placental barrier from mother to fetus and is also provided to the infant by antibodies present in breast milk.

Although prophylactic antibiotic therapy may prevent certain diseases, the risk of superinfection and the emergence of drug-resistant strains may outweigh the benefits; therefore, prophylactic antibiotics are usually reserved for patients at high risk for exposure to dangerous infections. Antibiotic-resistant bacteria are on the increase mainly because antibiotics are misused and overused. Some

CDC isolation precautions

The Centers for Disease Control and Prevention (CDC) and the Hospital Infection Control Practices Advisory Committee developed the CDC *Guideline for Isolation Precautions in Hospitals* to help hospitals maintain up-to-date isolation practices.

STANDARD PRECAUTIONS

The latest (1997) guidelines contain two tiers of precautions. The first — called standard precautions — are to be used when caring for all hospital patients, regardless of their diagnoses or presumed infections. Standard precautions are the primary strategy for preventing nosocomial infection and take the place of the earlier, universal precautions. Standard precautions refer to protection from:
- blood
- all body fluids, secretions, and excretions, except sweat, regardless of whether they contain visible blood
- skin that isn't intact
- mucous membranes.

TRANSMISSION-BASED PRECAUTIONS

The second tier is known as transmission-based precautions. These precautions are instituted when caring for patients with known or suspected highly transmissible infections that necessitate more stringent precautions than those described in the standard precautions. There are three types of transmission-based precautions: airborne precautions, droplet precautions, and contact precautions.

AIRBORNE PRECAUTIONS

Airborne precautions reduce the risk of airborne transmission of infectious agents. Microorganisms carried through the air can be dispersed widely by air currents, making them available for inhalation or deposit on a susceptible host in the same room or a longer distance away from the infected patient. Airborne precautions include special air-handling and ventilation procedures to prevent the spread of infection. They require the use of respiratory protection, such as a mask — in addition to standard precautions — when entering an infected patient's room.

DROPLET PRECAUTIONS

Droplet precautions reduce the risk of transmitting infectious agents in large-particle (exceeding 5 micrometers) droplets. Such transmission involves the contact of infectious agents to the conjunctivae or to the nasal or oral mucous membranes of a susceptible person. Large-particle droplets don't remain in the air and generally travel short distances of 3' (0.9 m) or less. They require the use of a mask — in addition to standard precautions — to protect the mucous membranes.

CONTACT PRECAUTIONS

Contact precautions reduce the risk of transmitting infectious agents by direct or indirect contact. Direct-contact transmission can occur through patient care activities that require physical contact. Indirect-contact transmission involves a susceptible host coming in contact with a contaminated object, usually inanimate, in the patient's environment. Contact precautions include the use of gloves, a mask, and a gown — in addition to standard precautions — to avoid contact with the infectious agent. Stringent hand washing is also necessary after removing the protective items.

Refer to the following table for examples of patients with whom specific precautions should be used.

CDC isolation precautions *(continued)*

PRECAUTIONS	INDICATIONS
Standard precautions	All patients regardless of diagnosis or presumed infection
Airborne precautions (used in addition to standard precautions)	Patients known to have or suspected of having a serious illness transmitted by airborne droplet nuclei, such as: ■ measles ■ varicella ■ tuberculosis
Droplet precautions (used in addition to standard precautions)	Patients known to have or suspected of having a serious illness transmitted by large-particle droplets, such as: ■ invasive *Haemophilus influenzae* type b disease, including meningitis, pneumonia, epiglottiditis, and sepsis ■ invasive *Neisseria meningitidis* disease, including meningitis, pneumonia, and sepsis ■ other serious bacterial respiratory infections spread by droplets, such as diphtheria; mycoplasma pneumonia; pertussis; pneumonic plague; streptococcal pharyngitis, pneumonia, or scarlet fever in infants and young children ■ other serious viral infections spread by droplets, including adenovirus, influenza, mumps, rubella, human parvovirus B19
Contact precautions (used in addition to standard precautions)	Patients known to have or suspected of having a serious illness easily transmitted by direct patient contact or by contact with items in the patient's environment, including: ■ GI, respiratory, skin, or wound infections or colonization with multidrug-resistant bacteria judged by the infection control program (based on current state, regional, or national recommendations) to be of special clinical and epidemiologic significance ■ enteric infections with a low infectious dose or prolonged environmental survival, including *Clostridium difficile;* for diapered or incontinent patients, enterohemorrhagic *Escherichia coli, Shigella,* hepatitis A, or rotavirus ■ respiratory syncytial virus, parainfluenza virus, or enteroviral infections in infants and young children ■ skin infections that are highly contagious or that may occur on dry skin, including diphtheria (cutaneous); herpes simplex (neonatal or mucocutaneous); impetigo; major (noncontained) abscesses, cellulitis, or decubiti; pediculosis; scabies; staphylococcal furunculosis in infants and young children; zoster (disseminated or in the immunocompromised host) ■ viral or hemorrhagic conjunctivitis ■ viral hemorrhagic infections (Ebola, Lassa, or Marburg)

bacteria, such as enterococci, have developed mutant strains that don't respond to antibiotic therapy.

ASSESSMENT

Accurate assessment can help to identify patients with infectious diseases and prevent complications. A complete assess-

Reportable infectious diseases

Disease reporting laws vary from state to state. Local agencies report certain diseases to state health departments, which determine which diseases are reported to the Centers for Disease Control and Prevention. Reportable infectious diseases include:

- acquired immunodeficiency syndrome
- amebiasis
- anthrax (cutaneous or pulmonary)
- arbovirus
- botulism
- brucellosis
- campylobacteriosis
- chancroid
- chlamydial infections
- cholera
- coccidioidomycosis
- *Coxiella* burnetti (Q fever)
- cryptosporidiosis
- cyclosporiasis
- diarrhea of the neonate (epidemic)
- diphtheria (cutaneous or pharyngeal)
- ehrlichiosis
- encephalitis (postinfectious or primary)
- enterohemorrhagic *Escherichia* coli
- food poisoning
- gastroenteritis (hospital outbreak)

- giardiasis
- gonococcal infections
- Guillain-Barré syndrome
- Hantavaris pulmonary syndrome
- hepatitis (all types)
- histoplasmosis
- human immunodeficiency virus
- influenza
- Kawasaki disease
- lead poisoning
- *Legionella* infections
- leprosy
- leptospirosis
- listeriosis
- Lyme disease
- lymphogranuloma venereum
- malaria
- measles
- meningococcal disease
- mumps
- neonatal hypothyroidism
- pertussis
- phenylketonuria
- plague

- poliomyelitis
- psittacosis
- rabies
- Reye's syndrome
- rheumatic fever
- rickettsial diseases (including Rocky Mountain spotted fever)
- rubella and congenital rubella syndrome
- salmonellosis
- shigellosis
- staphylococcal infections (neonatal)
- streptococcal infections (group A, invasive, toxic shock syndrome)
- syphilis (all types)
- tetanus
- toxic shock syndrome
- toxoplasmosis
- trichinosis
- tuberculosis
- tularemia
- typhoid, and paratyphoid fever
- typhus
- varicella (deaths only)
- yellow fever.

ment begins with a patient history, physical examination findings, and laboratory data.

The history should include the patient's sex, age, address, occupation, and place of work; known exposure to illness and recent medications, including antibiotics; and date of disease onset. Signs and symptoms — including their duration and whether they occurred suddenly or gradually, precipitating factors, relief measures, and weight loss or gain — should also be included in the history. Detail information about recent hospitalization, blood transfusions, blood donation denial by the Red Cross or other agencies, vaccination, travel or camping trips, and exposure to animals. (See *Immunization schedule*.)

Immunization schedule

Before an immunization, obtain the child's medication, illness, and allergy history. Instruct the parents to report a severe reaction to the vaccine. Childhood immunizations are usually given on a fixed schedule.

AGE	IMMUNIZATION
Birth to 2 months	First dose: hepatitis B vaccine
1 to 4 months	Second dose: hepatitis B vaccine[1]
2 months	First dose: diphtheria and tetanus toxoids and acellular pertussis vaccine (DTaP); inactivated poliovirus vaccine (IPV); *Haemophilus influenzae* type b conjugate vaccine (Hib); and consider rotovirus vaccine (Rv)
4 months	Second dose: DTaP, IPV, and Hib, 2nd dose of Rv
6 months	Third dose: DTaP and Hib and Rv[4]
6 to 18 months	Third dose: hepatitis B vaccine and IPV
12 to 15 months	First dose: Measles-mumps-rubella (MMR) vaccine Fourth dose: Hib
12 to 18 months	Fourth dose: DTaP[2] First dose: varicella-zoster virus vaccine
4 to 6 years	Fifth dose: DTaP Fourth dose: IPV Second dose: MMR vaccine
11 to 12 years	MMR vaccine (if not given at age 4 to 6); varicella-zoster virus vaccine (catch-up vaccination[3])
11 to 16 years	Tetanus vaccine (booster every 10 years) Hepatitis vaccine series (if not previously given)

[1] The second dose of hepatitis B vaccine is given at least 1 month after the first dose. The third dose is given at least 4 months after the first dose and at least 2 months after the 2nd dose. The infant should be at least 6 months of age for the third dose.
[2] A fourth dose of DTaP may be given as early as age 12 months through 18 months, provided that 6 months have elapsed since the third dose. The acellular form of the vaccine can now be used for all doses in the vaccination series, even for children who started the series with standard whole-cell D vaccine.
[3] Unvaccinated children with no history of chickenpox should be vaccinated at ages 11 to 12 with 2 doses at least 4 weeks apart.
[4] All doses of Rv vaccine series should be given by age 1.

If applicable, ask about possible exposure to sexually transmitted diseases or about drug abuse. Also, try to determine the patient's resistance to infectious disease. Ask about usual dietary patterns, (*Text continues on page 630.*)

How to collect specimens for culture

Identifying a causative organism begins with properly collecting specimens for culture. Label specimens to be used for culturing with the date, time, patient's name, suspected diagnosis, and specimen's source. Always try to obtain specimens before the first dose of antibiotics. If antibiotics are given before specimen collection, obtain the specimen as soon as possible. Don't withhold treatment of the patient to await specimen collection if a delay is anticipated.

CULTURE SITE	SPECIMEN SOURCE	SPECIAL CONSIDERATIONS
Infected wound	■ Aspiration of exudate with syringe (preferred technique) ■ Applicator swab	■ Use only a sterile syringe. A pungent odor suggests the presence of anaerobes. Use oxygen-free collection tubes, if available. ■ Firmly but gently insert the swab deep into the wound, and saturate it with exudate from the infected site. If the surface is dry, moisten the swab with sterile saline solution before taking the culture.
Skin lesions	■ Excision or puncture	■ Thoroughly clean the skin before excision or puncture, and follow the procedure for an infected wound.
Upper respiratory tract	■ Nasopharyngeal swab (generally used to detect carriers of *Staphylococcus aureus* and viral infections) ■ Throat swab	■ Gently pass the swab through the nose into the nasopharynx. Send the specimen to the laboratory for culture immediately. ■ Under adequate light, swab the area of inflammation or exudation.
Lower respiratory tract	■ Expectorated sputum ■ Induced sputum (used when patient can't expectorate sputum) ■ Nasotracheal suction ■ Pleural tap	■ Instruct the patient to cough deeply and to expectorate into a cup. Culture requires expectorated sputum, not just saliva. The best time to obtain a sputum specimen is first thing in the morning, before eating. ■ Use aerosol mist spray of saline solution or water to induce sputum production. Perform cupping and postural drainage, if needed. ■ Measure the approximate distance from the patient's nose to his ear. Note the distance, and then insert a sterile suction catheter this length, with a collection vial attached, into his nose. Maintain suction during catheter withdrawal. ■ Warn the patient that he may feel discomfort even though his skin will be anesthetized before this procedure. After the tap, check the site often for local swelling, and report dyspnea and other adverse reactions.

How to collect specimens for culture *(continued)*

CULTURE SITE	SPECIMEN SOURCE	SPECIAL CONSIDERATIONS
Lower intestinal tract	■ Rectal swab	■ A lesion on the colon or rectal wall may require a colonoscopy or sigmoidoscopy to obtain the specimen. If so, explain the procedure. Help the patient to assume a left lateral decubitus or knee-chest position.
	■ Stool specimen	■ The specimen should contain any pus or blood present in feces and a sampling of the first, middle, and last portion of stool. Urine with stool can invalidate results. Send the specimen to the laboratory at once in a clean, tightly covered container, especially stools being examined for ova and parasites.
Eye	■ Cotton swab	■ Carefully retract the lower lid, and gently swab the conjunctiva.
	■ Corneal scrapings	■ Use a swab loop to scrape the specimen from the site of corneal infection. Reassure the patient that the procedure is quick and discomfort is minimal.
Genital tract	■ Swab specimen	■ A specimen from a male should contain urethral discharge or prostatic fluid; from a female, urethral or cervical specimens. Always collect specimens on two swabs simultaneously.
Urinary tract	■ Midstream clean-catch urine specimen	■ A midstream clean-catch specimen in an infected person should contain fewer than 10,000 bacteria/ml. ■ Teach the patient how to collect the specimen or supervise collection. In males, retract the foreskin and clean the glans penis; in females, clean and separate the labia so the urinary meatus is clearly visible; then clean the meatus. Tell the patient to void 25 to 30 ml first, then, without stopping the urine stream, collect the specimen. ■ In infants, apply the collection bag carefully and check it frequently to avoid mechanical urethral obstruction. ■ Send the urine specimen to the laboratory immediately, or refrigerate it to retard growth.
	■ Indwelling urinary catheter specimen	■ Clean the specimen port of the catheter with povidone-iodine, and aspirate urine with a sterile needle, or from a latex catheter, at a point distal to the "Y" branch.

(continued)

	How to collect specimens for culture (continued)	
CULTURE SITE	**SPECIMEN SOURCE**	**SPECIAL CONSIDERATIONS**
Body fluids	■ Needle aspiration	■ Send peritoneal and synovial fluid and cerebrospinal fluid (CSF) to the laboratory at once. Don't retard the growth of CSF organisms by refrigerating the specimen.
Blood	■ Venous or arterial aspiration	■ Using a sterile syringe, collect 12 to 15 ml of blood, changing needles before injecting blood into the aerobic and anaerobic collection bottles. ■ If the patient is receiving antibiotics, note this on the laboratory slip because the laboratory may add enzymes or resins to the culture to inactivate the drug.

unusual fatigue, and conditions — such as neoplastic disease or alcoholism — that might predispose him to infection. Notice if the patient is listless or uneasy, lacks concentration, or has any obvious abnormality of mood or affect.

When infection is suspected, assess the skin, mucous membranes, liver, spleen, and lymph nodes. Check for and note the location of and type of drainage from skin lesions. Record skin color, temperature, and turgor; ask if the patient has pruritus. Take his temperature, using the same route consistently, and watch for a fever. Note and record the pattern of temperature change and the effect of antipyretics. Be aware that some analgesics contain antipyretics. With high fever, especially in children, watch for seizures.

Check the patient's pulse rate; infection commonly increases pulse rate, but some infections, notably typhoid fever and psittacosis, may decrease it. In severe infection or when complications are pos-sible, watch for hypotension, hematuria, oliguria, hepatomegaly, jaundice, bleeding from gums or into joints, and altered level of consciousness. Obtain laboratory studies and appropriate cultures. (See *How to collect specimens for culture*, pages 628 to 630.)

• • • • • • • • • • • •
ASCARIASIS

Ascariasis (roundworm infection) is caused by *Ascaris lumbricoides*, a large roundworm that resembles an earthworm. This disease occurs worldwide; it's most common in tropical areas with poor sanitation and in Asia, where farmers use human feces as fertilizer. In the United States, it's more prevalent in the South.

Approximately 1 billion people are affected worldwide, and the outcome is usually good even without treatment.

AGE ALERT Ascariasis is prevalent among children ages 4 to 12.

Causes

Ascariasis is transmitted to humans by ingestion of soil contaminated with human feces that harbor *A. lumbricoides* ova. Ingestion occurs directly (by eating contaminated soil) or indirectly (by eating poorly washed raw vegetables grown in contaminated soil).

Ascariasis never passes directly from person to person. After ingestion, *A. lumbricoides* ova hatch and release larvae, which penetrate the intestinal wall and reach the lungs through the bloodstream. After about 10 days in pulmonary capillaries and alveoli, the larvae migrate to the bronchioles, bronchi, trachea, and epiglottis. There they're swallowed and return to the intestine to mature into worms.

Clinical presentation

Ascariasis produces two phases of infection: early pulmonary and prolonged intestinal. Mild intestinal infection may cause only vague stomach discomfort. The first clue may be vomiting a worm or passing a worm in the stool. Severe infection causes stomach pain, vomiting, restlessness, disturbed sleep and, in extreme cases, intestinal obstruction. Larvae migrating by the lymphatic and the circulatory systems cause symptoms that vary; for instance, when they invade the lungs, pneumonitis may result.

Differential diagnoses

- Asthma
- Infection with other parasites
- Pneumonia
- Other causes of pancreatitis
- Anemia
- Malnutrition
- Appendicitis
- Duodenitis
- Esophagitis

Diagnosis

The key to diagnosis is identifying ova in the stool or adult worms, which may be passed rectally or by mouth.

When migrating larvae invade alveoli, X-rays may show characteristic bronchovascular markings: infiltrates, patchy areas of pneumonitis, and widening of hilar shadows. In a patient with ascariasis, these findings usually accompany a complete blood count that shows eosinophilia.

Management

General

In intestinal obstruction, nasogastric suctioning controls vomiting. When vomiting is controlled, medication can be administered.

Medication

Medications used in the treatment of patients with ascariasis include:

- pyrantel — 11 mg/kg P.O. as a single dose, not to exceed 1 g
- mebendazole — 100 mg P.O. b.i.d. for 3 days; repeat in 3 weeks if infection persists.

In multiple helminth infection, one of these drugs must be the first treatment; using some other anthelmintic first may stimulate *A. lumbricoides'* perforation into other organs. No specific treatment exists for migratory infection because anthelmintics affect only mature worms.

Referral

- Refer the patient to an infectious disease specialist if infection isn't responding to treatment.

Follow-up

Repeat stool studies 2 weeks after treatment is initiated.

Patient teaching

- Tell the patient and family members to properly dispose of feces and soiled linen and to use proper hand-washing technique.
- Teach the patient to prevent reinfection by washing his hands thoroughly, especially before eating and after defecation, and by bathing and changing underwear and bed linens daily.
- Inform the patient about possible adverse drug effects.

Complications

- Cholangitis
- Pancreatitis
- Appendicitis
- Diverticulitis
- Liver abscess
- Intestinal obstruction
- Anemia

• • • • • • • • • • • •

CANDIDIASIS

Candidiasis (also called candidosis or moniliasis) is usually a mild, superficial fungal infection caused by the genus *Candida*. It usually infects the nails (onychomycosis), skin (diaper rash), or mucous membranes, especially the oropharynx (thrush), vagina (moniliasis), esophagus, and GI tract. Rarely, these fungi enter the bloodstream and invade the kidneys, lungs, endocardium, brain, or other structures, causing serious infections. The prognosis varies, depending on the patient's resistance.

CLINICAL CAUTION Systemic infection is most prevalent among drug abusers and patients who are already hospitalized, especially diabetics, immunosuppressed patients, or patients receiving broad-spectrum antibiotics.

Causes

Most cases of *Candida* infection result from *C. albicans*. Other infective strains include *C. parapsilosis*, *C. tropicalis*, and *C. guilliermondii*. These fungi are part of the normal flora of the GI tract, mouth, vagina, and skin. They cause infection when some change in the body (increasing glucose levels from diabetes mellitus; decreased resistance from an immunosuppressive drug, radiation, aging, or a disease such as cancer or human immunodeficiency virus [HIV] infection) permits their sudden proliferation or when they're introduced systemically by I.V. or urinary catheters, drug abuse, hyperalimentation, or surgery. The incidence of candidiasis is increasing because of the widespread use of I.V. therapy and greater number of immunocompromised patients, especially those with HIV infection. Nonetheless, the most common predisposing factor is the use of broad-spectrum antibiotics, which decrease the number of normal flora and permit an increasing number of candidal organisms to proliferate.

The neonate of a mother with vaginal candidiasis can contract oral thrush while passing through the birth canal. Thrush also occurs in many neonates who are breast-fed.

Clinical presentation

Symptoms of superficial candidiasis vary with the site of infection:

- skin — scaly, erythematous, papular rash, sometimes covered with exudate, appearing below the breast, between fingers, and at the axillae, groin, and umbilicus; in diaper rash, papules at the edges of the rash

- nails—red, swollen, darkened nail bed; occasionally, purulent discharge and the separation of a pruritic nail from the nail bed
- oropharyngeal mucosa (thrush)—cream-colored or bluish white patches of exudate on the tongue, mouth, or pharynx that reveal bloody engorgement when scraped; they may swell, causing respiratory distress in infants; may be painful or cause a burning sensation in the throats and mouths of adults (see *Recognizing candidiasis.*)
- esophageal mucosa—dysphagia, retrosternal pain, regurgitation and, occasionally, scales in the mouth and throat
- vaginal mucosa—white or yellow discharge, with pruritus and local excoriation; white or gray raised patches on vaginal walls, with local inflammation; dyspareunia.

Systemic infection produces chills; high, spiking fever; hypotension; prostration; myalgias; arthralgias; and a rash. Specific signs and symptoms depend on the site of infection:

- pulmonary—hemoptysis, cough, fever
- renal—fever, flank pain, dysuria, hematuria, pyuria, cloudy urine
- brain—headache, nuchal rigidity, seizures, focal neurologic deficits
- endocardium—systolic or diastolic murmur, fever, chest pain, embolic phenomena
- eye—endophthalmitis, blurred vision, orbital or periorbital pain, scotoma, exudate.

Differential diagnoses
Oral cavity
- Aphthous stomatitis
- Leukoplakia

Female genitalia
- Bacterial vaginosis
- Pediculosis pubis

Recognizing candidiasis

Candidiasis of the oropharyngeal mucosa (thrush) causes cream-colored or bluish white pseudomembranous patches on the tongue, mouth, or pharynx. Fungal invasion may extend to circumoral tissues.

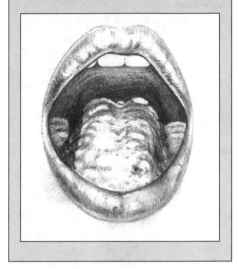

- *Trichomonas*
- Allergic contact dermatitis

Male genitalia
- Bacterial infection
- Tinea
- Psoriasis

Diagnosis
Diagnosis of superficial candidiasis depends on evidence of *Candida* on a Gram stain of skin, vaginal scrapings, pus, or sputum or on skin scrapings prepared in potassium hydroxide solution. Diagnosis of systemic infection requires blood or tissue culture.

Management

General

The goal of treatment is to first improve the underlying condition that predisposes the patient to candidiasis, such as controlling diabetes or discontinuing antibiotic therapy and catheterization, if possible.

Medication

Medications used in the treatment of a patient with candidiasis may include:

- nystatin — oral suspension, swish and swallow 5 to 10 ml over 20 minutes 4 to 5 times per day; cream, apply to affected area b.i.d. for 2 weeks; vaginal tab, 1 daily for 2 weeks
- clotrimazole — 10 mg troches, P.O., slowly dissolve in mouth 5 times per day for 14 days; 1% cream, 1 applicator full intravaginally h.s. for 7 days, or apply to affected area; suppository, 100 mg intravaginally h.s. for 7 days or 200 mg h.s. for 3 days
- fluconazole — 150 mg P.O. 1 time for vaginal candidiasis; 200 mg on day 1 then 100 mg/day P.O. for 2 weeks for oral and esophageal candidiasis; children 6 mg/kg P.O. on first day, then 3 mg/kg daily for 2 weeks
- miconazole — 2% cream, 1 applicator full intravaginally (Monistat 7) h.s. for 7 days or apply to affected area b.i.d.; suppository, 100 mg intravaginally h.s. for 7 days or 200 mg intravaginally h.s. for 3 days.

For systemic infection, medication may include:

- amphotericin B — 0.25 to 1.0 mg/kg/day I.V. for 4 to 10 weeks
- fluconazole — 400 mg/day P.O. or I.V. for 1st day, then 200 mg for 4 weeks.

Referral

- If candidiasis disseminates, refer the patient to an infectious disease specialist.

Follow-up

The patient should be seen in 2 weeks if treatment isn't successful. Otherwise, follow-up isn't necessary.

Patient teaching

- Instruct a patient using nystatin solution to swish it around in the mouth for several minutes before swallowing it.
- Tell parents to swab nystatin on the oral mucosa of an infant with thrush. Treat the infant after feeding because feeding washes the medication away. The infant's mother should also be treated to prevent the infection from being passed back and forth.

Complications

Disseminated candidiasis

- Pyelonephritis
- Endocarditis
- Myocarditis
- Pneumonitis
- Arthritis
- Central nervous system infection

Special considerations

- Assess the patient with candidiasis for underlying causes such as diabetes mellitus.

HEALTHY LIVING Encourage a woman in the third trimester of pregnancy to be examined for vaginal candidiasis to protect the neonate from infection at birth.

• • • • • • • • • • • •

CLOSTRIDIUM DIFFICILE INFECTION

Clostridium difficile infection is caused by a gram-positive anaerobic bacterium. It most often results in antibiotic-associated diarrhea. Symptoms range from asymptomatic carrier states to severe pseudomembranous colitis and are caused by the exo-toxins produced by the organism: Toxin A is an enterotoxin and toxin B is a cyto-toxin.

High-risk groups include individuals on great numbers of antibiotics, those having abdominal surgery, patients receiving antineoplastic agents that have an antibiotic activity, immunocompromised individuals, pediatric patients (commonly in day-care centers), and nursing home patients.

Prognosis is good; however, relapse does occur.

Causes
C. *difficile* colitis can be caused by almost any antibiotic that disrupts the bowel flora, but it's classically associated with clindamycin use. Other factors that alter normal intestinal flora include enemas and intestinal stimulants.

C. *difficile* is most commonly transmitted directly from patient to patient by contaminated hands of facility personnel; it also may be indirectly spread by contaminated equipment such as bedpans, urinals, call bells, rectal thermometers, nasogastric tubes, and contaminated surfaces such as bed rails, floors, and toilet seats.

Clinical presentation
Risk of C. *difficile* begins 1 to 2 days after antibiotic therapy is started and extends for as long as 2 to 3 months after the last dose. The patient may be asymptomatic or exhibit any of the following symptoms: soft, unformed, or watery diarrhea that may be foul smelling (more than 3 stools in a 24-hour period) or grossly bloody; abdominal pain, cramping, or tenderness; and fever. The patient's white blood cell count may be elevated to 20,000/µl. In severe cases, toxic megacolon, colonic perforation, and peritonitis can develop.

Differential diagnoses
- Parasitic infection
- Intestinal obstruction
- Viral infection
- Adverse drug reaction
- Food poisoning
- Bacterial infection
- Dietary intolerance
- Colitis

Diagnosis
Diagnosis is by identifying the toxin through one of these acceptable methods.
- Cell cytotoxin test — tests for toxins A and B; this takes 2 days to perform. It's highly sensitive and specific for C. *difficile*.
- Enzyme immunoassays — slightly less sensitive than the cell cytotoxin test but has a turnaround time of only a few hours. Specificity is excellent.
- Stool culture — the most sensitive test; has a turnaround time of 2 days to obtain results. Non-toxin-producing strains of C. *difficile* can be easily identified and must be further tested for presence of the toxin.
- Endoscopy (flexible sigmoidoscopy) — may be used in a patient who presents with an acute abdomen but no diarrhea, making it difficult to obtain a stool specimen. If pseudomembranes are visualized, treatment for C. *difficile* is usually initiated.

Management
General
After withdrawing the causative antibiotic (if possible), symptoms resolve in patients who are mildly symptomatic. This is usually the only treatment needed. In more severe cases, medication is needed.

Medication
Medications used to treat a patient with C. *difficile* infection may include:

■ metronidazole — 250 mg P.O. q.i.d. or
500 mg P.O. t.i.d.
■ vancomycin — 125 mg P.O. q.i.d. for
10 days.

Ten percent to 20% of patients may
have a recurrence with the same organism
within 14 to 30 days of treatment. Beyond
30 days, a recurrence may be a relapse or
reinfection of *C. difficile*. If the previous
treatment was by metronidazole, low-dose
vancomycin (125 mg q.i.d. for 21 days)
may be effective. An alternative treatment combines metronidazole (500 mg
P.O. t.i.d.) and rifampin (600 mg/day P.O.
b.i.d.) and is given for 10 days.

There's no evidence that eating yogurt or taking lactobacillus is effective.
Other experimental treatments involve
the administration of yeast, *Saccharomy-
ces boulardii*, with metronidazole or vancomycin and biologic vaccines to restore
normal GI flora.

Referral
■ A referral to an infectious disease specialist may be necessary if treatment is
unsuccessful.

Follow-up
The patient should be seen in 2 weeks,
and stools should be retested if there's no
improvement in condition.

Patient teaching
■ Teach good hand-washing technique to
prevent the spread of the infection.
■ Review proper disinfection of contaminated clothing or household items.

Complications
■ Electrolyte abnormalities
■ Hypovolemic shock
■ Anasarca (caused by hypoalbumine-
mia)
■ Toxic megacolon
■ Colonic perforation
■ Peritonitis

■ Sepsis
■ Hemorrhage
■ Death

• • • • • • • • • • • •

COCCIDIOIDOMYCOSIS

Coccidioidomycosis, also called valley
fever or San Joaquin Valley fever, is
caused by the fungus *Coccidioides immitis*
and is primarily a respiratory infection.
Secondary sites of infection include the
skin, bones, joints, and meninges. Generalized dissemination is also possible. The
primary pulmonary form is usually self-
limiting and seldom fatal. The rare secondary form (which is progressive and disseminated) produces abscesses throughout
the body and carries a mortality of up to
60%, even with treatment. Such dissemination is more common in dark-skinned
men, pregnant women, and patients receiving immunosuppressants.

Causes
Coccidioidomycosis is endemic to the
southwestern United States, especially
between the San Joaquin Valley in California and southwestern Texas; it's also
found in Mexico, Guatemala, Honduras,
Venezuela, Colombia, Argentina, and
Paraguay. It may result from inhalation of
C. immitis spores found in the soil in
these areas or from inhalation of spores
from dressings or plaster casts of infected
people. It's most prevalent during warm,
dry months.

Because of population distribution
and an occupational link (it's common in
migrant farm laborers), coccidioidomycosis generally strikes Philippine Americans, Mexican Americans, Native Americans, and African Americans. In primary
infection, the incubation period is from 1
to 4 weeks.

Clinical presentation

Primary coccidioidomycosis usually produces acute or subacute respiratory signs and symptoms (dry cough, pleuritic chest pain, and pleural effusion), fever, sore throat, dyspnea, chills, malaise, headache, and an itchy macular rash. Occasionally, the sole sign is a fever that persists for weeks. From 3 days to several weeks after onset, some patients, especially white women, develop tender red nodules (erythema nodosum) on their legs, especially the shins, with joint pain in the knees and ankles. Generally, primary disease heals spontaneously within a few weeks.

In rare cases, coccidioidomycosis disseminates to other organs several weeks or months after the primary infection. Disseminated coccidioidomycosis causes fever and abscesses throughout the body, especially in skeletal, central nervous system (CNS), splenic, hepatic, renal, and subcutaneous tissues. Depending on the location of these abscesses, disseminated coccidioidomycosis may cause bone pain and meningitis. Chronic pulmonary cavitation, which can occur in the primary and disseminated forms, causes hemoptysis with or without chest pain.

Differential diagnoses

- Pneumonia
- Tuberculosis
- Lung carcinoma
- Lymphoma
- Sarcoidosis
- Lung abscess
- Meningitis

Diagnosis

Typical clinical features and skin and serologic studies confirm this diagnosis. The primary form—and sometimes the disseminated form—produces a positive coccidioidin skin test.

In the first week of illness, complement fixation for immunoglobulin G antibodies or, in the first month, positive serum precipitins (immunoglobulins) also establish the diagnosis. Examination or, more recently, immunodiffusion testing of sputum, pus from lesions, and a tissue biopsy may show *C. immitis* spores. The presence of antibodies in pleural and joint fluid and an increasing serum or body fluid antibody titer indicate dissemination. Chest X-ray shows bilateral diffuse infiltrates.

Other abnormal laboratory results include:
- increased white blood cell (WBC) count
- eosinophilia
- increased erythrocyte sedimentation rate
- cerebrospinal fluid analysis showing an increased WBC count to more than 500/μl (primarily due to mononuclear leukocytes), increased protein levels, and decreased glucose levels in coccidioidal meningitis
- ventricular fluid obtained from the brain may contain complement fixation antibodies.

After diagnosis, order serial skin tests, blood cultures, and serologic tests to document the effectiveness of therapy.

Management

General

Usually, a patient with mild primary coccidioidomycosis requires only bed rest and symptom relief. Severe primary disease and dissemination also necessitate long-term I.V. infusion (or, in CNS dissemination, intrathecal administration) of medication.

Medication

Medications used to treat a patient with coccidioidomycosis may include:

- amphotericin B—.25 to 1.0 mg/kg/day I.V. for 8 weeks or more
- fluconazole—400 mg/day P.O. or I.V. for 1 week, then maintenance of 200 mg/day P.O. for 4 weeks.
- ibuprofen—200 to 400 mg P.O. every 4 hours p.r.n.

Surgical intervention
Excision or drainage of lesions may be necessary. Severe pulmonary lesions may necessitate lobectomy.

Referral
- The patient may need referral to an infectious disease specialist or pulmonologist if treatment is ineffective or if the disease is severe.

Follow-up
The patient should be seen every 2 weeks until serology titers decrease and the patient shows clinical improvement.

Patient teaching
- In mild primary disease, encourage bed rest and adequate fluid intake. Tell the patient to record the amount and color of sputum. Also tell him to report shortness of breath that may point to pleural effusion.
- If the patient has draining lesions, stress a "no touch" dressing technique and careful hand washing.
- Tell the patient to immediately report hearing loss, tinnitus, dizziness, and all signs of medication toxicity. To ease adverse effects of amphotericin B, tell the patient to take antiemetics and antipyretics.

Complications
- Lung tissue destruction
- Hemoptysis
- Death

• • • • • • • • • • • •
COMMON COLD

The common cold (also known as acute coryza) is an acute, usually afebrile viral infection that causes inflammation of the upper respiratory tract. It's the most common infectious disease, accounting for more time lost from school or work than any other cause. Although a cold is benign and self-limiting, it can lead to secondary bacterial infections.

The common cold is more prevalent in children than in adults, in adolescent boys than in girls, and in women than in men. In temperate zones, it's more common in the colder months; in the tropics, during the rainy season.

Causes
About 90% of colds result from a viral infection of the upper respiratory passages and consequent mucous membrane inflammation; occasionally, a cold results from a mycoplasmal infection. (See *What happens in the common cold.*) More than 100 different viruses can cause the common cold. Major culprits include rhinoviruses, coronaviruses, myxoviruses, adenoviruses, coxsackieviruses, and echoviruses.

Transmission occurs through airborne respiratory droplets, contact with contaminated objects, and hand-to-hand transmission. Children acquire new strains from their schoolmates and pass them on to family members. Fatigue or drafts don't increase susceptibility.

Clinical presentation
After a 1- to 4-day incubation period, the common cold produces pharyngitis, nasal congestion, coryza, headache, and burning, watery eyes. Additional effects may include fever (in children), chills, myalgia, arthralgia, malaise, lethargy, and a

What happens in the common cold

Virus-infected droplets enter the body and attack the cells lining the throat and nose. The virus particles then multiply rapidly.

The immune system responds by sending lymphocytes to the infected mucosa, causing blood vessels in the nasal mucosa to swell. This swelling causes secretion of excess fluid—the classic cold symptom of a runny nose.

Phagocytes engulf and destroy dead virus particles and damaged cells. Soon the cold symptoms disappear.

Some lymphocytes immobilize the virus particles with virus-specific proteins (antibodies); others kill infected cells with a chemical substance.

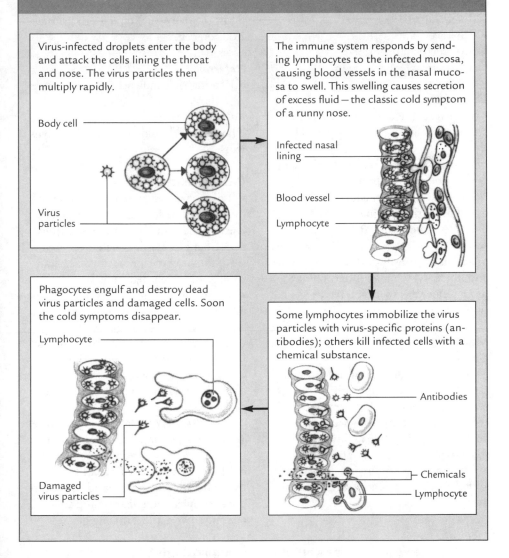

hacking, nonproductive, or nocturnal cough.

As the cold progresses, clinical features develop more fully. After a day, signs and symptoms include a feeling of fullness with a copious nasal discharge that commonly irritates the nose, adding to discomfort. About 3 days after onset,

major signs and symptoms diminish, but the "stuffed up" feeling generally persists for about a week. Reinfection (with productive cough) is common, but complications are rare. A cold is communicable for 2 to 3 days after the onset of symptoms.

Differential diagnoses

- Sinusitis
- Allergic rhinitis
- Otitis media
- Pneumonia
- Rubeola
- Streptococcal infection
- Influenza

Diagnosis

There's no explicit diagnostic test to isolate the specific organism responsible for the common cold. Diagnosis rests on the typically mild, localized, and afebrile upper respiratory symptoms. Despite infection, white blood cell counts and differential are within normal limits. A temperature higher than 100° F (37.8° C), severe malaise, anorexia, tachycardia, exudate on the tonsils or throat, petechiae, and tender lymph glands may point to more serious disorders and require additional diagnostic tests.

Management

General

The primary treatment measures — aspirin or acetaminophen, fluids, and rest — are symptomatic; the common cold has no cure. Steam encourages expectoration. There are no known measures to prevent the common cold. Vitamin therapy, interferon administration, and ultraviolet irradiation are under investigation.

Medication

Medications used to treat a patient with the common cold may include:

- aspirin — 325 to 650 mg P.O. every 4 hours p.r.n.
- acetaminophen — 325 to 650 mg P.O. every 4 to 6 hours p.r.n.
- ibuprofen — 200 to 400 mg P.O. every 6 hours p.r.n.
- oxymetazoline — 2 sprays each nostril b.i.d. for 3 to 5 days

- oral decongestant — over-the-counter (OTC); refer to instructions on package
- throat lozenges — OTC; refer to instructions on package
- antitussives — OTC; refer to instructions on package.

Referral

- Referral isn't indicated.

Follow-up

The patient should be seen if symptoms worsen.

Patient teaching

- Tell the patient to maintain bed rest during the first few days, to use a lubricant on the nostrils to decrease irritation, to use hard candy or cough drops to relieve throat irritation, to increase fluid intake, and to eat light meals.
- Warm baths or heating pads can reduce aches and pains but don't hasten a cure. Suggest hot- or cold-steam vaporizers. Commercial expectorants are available, but their effectiveness is questionable.
- Advise against overuse of nose drops or sprays because they may cause rebound congestion.

HEALTHY LIVING To help prevent colds, warn the patient to minimize contact with people who have colds. To avoid spreading colds, teach the patient to wash his hands often, to cover coughs and sneezes, and to avoid sharing towels and drinking glasses.

Complications

- Sinusitis
- Lower respiratory tract infection
- Otitis media
- Pneumonia

Special considerations

- Emphasize that antibiotics don't cure the common cold.

• • • • • • • • • • •
CYTOMEGALOVIRUS INFECTION

Cytomegalovirus (CMV) infection is caused by the cytomegalovirus, a deoxyribonucleic acid, ether-sensitive virus belonging to the herpes family. It's also known as generalized salivary gland disease or cytomegalic inclusion disease. CMV infection occurs worldwide and is transmitted by human contact. About four out of five people over age 35 have been infected with CMV, usually during childhood or early adulthood. In most of these people, the disease is so mild that it's overlooked. However, CMV infection during pregnancy can be hazardous to the fetus, possibly leading to stillbirth, brain damage, and other birth defects or to severe neonatal illness. About 1% of all neonates have CMV.

Causes
CMV has been found in saliva, urine, semen, breast milk, feces, blood, and vaginal and cervical secretions of infected people. The virus is usually transmitted through contact with these infected secretions, which harbor the virus for months or even years. It may be transmitted by sexual contact and can travel across the placenta, causing a congenital infection. Recipients of blood transfusions from donors with positive CMV antibodies are at some risk.

CLINICAL CAUTION Immunosuppressed patients, especially organ transplant recipients, have a 90% chance of contracting CMV infection.

Clinical presentation
CMV probably spreads through the body in lymphocytes or mononuclear cells to the lungs, liver, GI tract, eyes, and central nervous system, where it commonly produces inflammatory reactions. Most patients with CMV infection have mild, nonspecific complaints or none at all, even though antibody titers indicate infection. In these patients, the disease usually runs a self-limiting course.

Immunodeficient patients and those receiving immunosuppressants may develop pneumonia or other secondary infections. In patients with acquired immunodeficiency syndrome, disseminated CMV infection may cause chorioretinitis (resulting in blindness), colitis, encephalitis, abdominal pain, diarrhea, or weight loss. Infected infants ages 3 to 6 months usually appear asymptomatic but may develop hepatic dysfunction, hepatosplenomegaly, spider angiomas, pneumonitis, and lymphadenopathy.

Congenital CMV infection is seldom apparent at birth, although the neonate's urine contains the virus. CMV can cause brain damage that may not show up for months after birth. It can also produce a rapidly fatal neonatal illness characterized by jaundice, petechial rash, hepatosplenomegaly, thrombocytopenia, hemolytic anemia, microcephaly, psychomotor retardation, mental deficiency, and hearing loss. Occasionally, this form is rapidly fatal.

In some adults, CMV may cause CMV mononucleosis, with 3 weeks or more of irregular, high fever. Other findings may include a normal or elevated white blood cell (WBC) count, lymphocytosis, and increased atypical lymphocytes.

Differential diagnoses
- Toxoplasmosis
- Rubella
- Syphilis
- Viral hepatitis
- Infectious mononucleosis

Diagnosis

Isolation of the virus in urine is the most sensitive laboratory method; diagnosis can also rest on virus isolation from saliva, throat, cervix, WBC, and biopsy specimens.

Other laboratory tests support the diagnosis, including complement fixation studies, hemagglutination inhibition antibody tests and, for congenital infections, indirect immunofluorescent tests for CMV immunoglobulin M antibody.

Management

General

Treatment includes measures to relieve symptoms and prevent complications.

Medication

Medications used in the treatment of an immunosuppressed patient may include:
- acyclovir—adults, 5 mg/kg I.V. over 1 hour every 8 hours for 7 to 14 days; children younger than age 12, 250 mg/m² I.V. over 1 hour every 8 hours for 7 days
- ganciclovir—5 mg/kg I.V. every 12 hours for 14 to 21 days, then daily for 7 days or 1 g P.O. t.i.d.
- foscarnet—60 mg/kg I.V. every 8 hours for 2 to 3 weeks, then 90 to 120 mg/kg/day I.V.

Referral

- Refer the patient to a health care facility for treatment.
- For information and support, refer the patient and family members to a local chapter of the National Center for Infectious Diseases.

Follow-up

Follow-up depends on the severity of the illness.

Patient teaching

- Urge patients with CMV infection to wash their hands thoroughly to prevent spreading the virus. Stress this with young children.

Complications

- Colitis
- Death
- Brain damage
- Deafness
- Mental retardation
- Encephalitis

HEALTHY LIVING To help prevent spreading CMV infection, warn immunosuppressed patients and pregnant women to avoid exposure to confirmed or suspected CMV infection.

• • • • • • • • • • •

ENTEROBIASIS

Enterobiasis (also called pinworm, seatworm, or threadworm infection or oxyuriasis) is a benign intestinal disease caused by the nematode *Enterobius vermicularis*. Infection occurs worldwide, even in temperate regions with good sanitation. It's the most prevalent helminthic infection in the United States with an estimated 40 million persons infected.

Enterobiasis infection and reinfection occur most often in children between ages 5 and 14 and in certain institutionalized groups because of poor hygiene and frequent hand-to-mouth activity. Crowded living conditions increase the likelihood of it spreading to several members of a family. There's a 90% cure rate with proper treatment; however, reinfection is common.

Causes

Adult pinworms live in the intestine; female worms migrate to the perianal region to deposit their ova. Direct transmission occurs when the patient's hands transfer infective eggs from the anus to the mouth. Indirect transmission occurs when a person comes in contact with contaminated articles, such as linens and clothing.

Clinical presentation
Asymptomatic enterobiasis is commonly overlooked. However, intense perianal pruritus can occur, especially at night, when the female worm leaves the anus to deposit ova. Pruritus causes irritability, scratching, skin irritation and, sometimes, vaginitis. Rarely, complications include appendicitis, salpingitis, and pelvic granuloma.

Differential diagnoses
- Contact dermatitis
- Other intestinal parasites
- Atopic dermatitis
- Psoriasis
- Scabies
- Vaginitis
- Poor hygiene

Diagnosis
A history of anal pruritus suggests enterobiasis; identification of *Enterobius* ova recovered from the perianal area with a cellophane tape swab confirms it.

This test is done before the patient bathes and defecates in the morning. A stool sample is usually ova- and worm-free because the worms deposit ova outside the intestine and die after return to the anus.

Management
General
The goal of treatment is to eradicate the infective organism.

Medication
Medications used to treat a patient with enterobiasis may include:

- pyrantel — 11 mg/kg P.O. as a single dose, not to exceed 1 g; repeat in 2 weeks
- mebendazole — 100 mg P.O. as a single dose; repeat in 2 to 3 weeks if infection persists.

Referral
- Referral isn't indicated.

Follow-up
The patient needs to be seen if symptoms persist for more than 2 weeks or recur.

Patient teaching
- Tell the patient and family members that pyrantel colors the stool bright red and may cause vomiting (vomitus will also be red).
- To help prevent enterobiasis infection, tell parents to bathe children daily (showers are preferable to tub baths) and to change underwear and bed linens daily. Educate children in proper personal hygiene, and stress the need for hand washing after defecation and before handling food. Discourage nail biting; if the child can't stop, suggest that he wear gloves until the infection clears.

Complications
- Pancreatitis
- Cholangitis
- Endometritis
- Liver abscess
- Diverticulosis
- Impetigo
- Vulvovaginitis
- Urinary tract infection

Special considerations
- Effective eradication requires simultaneous treatment of family members and, in health care facilities, other patients.
- Report *all* outbreaks of enterobiasis to school authorities.

• • • • • • • • • • •

GIARDIASIS

Giardiasis (also called *Giardia* enteritis or lambliasis) is an infection of the small bowel caused by the symmetrical flagellate protozoan *Giardia lamblia*. Giardiasis occurs worldwide but is most common in developing countries and other areas where sanitation and hygiene are poor. In the United States, giardiasis is most common in travelers who have recently returned from endemic areas and in campers who drink nonpurified water from contaminated streams. In untreated giardiasis, symptoms wax and wane; with treatment, recovery is complete.

Causes

G. lamblia has two stages: the cystic stage and the trophozoite stage. Ingestion of *G. lamblia* cysts in fecally contaminated water or the fecal-oral transfer of cysts by an infected person results in giardiasis. Giardiasis may be transmitted through sexual contact (direct or indirect fecal-oral contact). When cysts enter the small bowel, they become trophozoites and attach themselves with their sucking disks to the bowel's epithelial surface. After this, the trophozoites encyst again, travel down the colon, and are excreted. Unformed feces that pass quickly through the intestine may contain trophozoites as well as cysts.

Probably because of frequent hand-to-mouth activity, children are more likely to become infected with G. *lamblia* than adults. Hypogammaglobulinemia also appears to predispose people to this disorder. Giardiasis doesn't confer immunity, so reinfections may occur.

Clinical presentation

Attachment of G. *lamblia* to the intestinal lumen causes superficial mucosal invasion and destruction, inflammation, and irritation. All of these destructive effects decrease food transit time through the small intestine and result in malabsorption. Such malabsorption produces chronic GI complaints—such as abdominal cramps—and pale, loose, greasy, malodorous, and frequent stools (from 2 to 10 per day) with concurrent nausea. Stools may contain mucus but not pus or blood. Chronic giardiasis may produce fatigue and weight loss in addition to these typical signs and symptoms. A mild infection may not produce intestinal symptoms.

Differential diagnoses

- Food allergy
- Irritable bowel syndrome (if not accompanied by weight loss)
- Crohn's disease
- Celiac sprue
- Infectious cause

Diagnosis

Suspect giardiasis when travelers to endemic areas or campers who may have drunk nonpurified water develop symptoms. Actual diagnosis requires laboratory examination of a fresh stool specimen for cysts or examination of duodenal aspirate for trophozoites. An antibody test of the stool for giardiasis is also very effective in diagnosis.

A barium X-ray of the small bowel may show mucosal edema and barium segmentation. Diagnosis must also rule out other causes of diarrhea and malabsorption.

HEALTHY LIVING To help prevent giardiasis, warn travelers to endemic areas not to drink water or eat uncooked and unpeeled fruits or vegetables (they may have been rinsed in contaminated water). Prophylactic drug therapy isn't recommended. Advise campers to purify all stream water before drinking it.

Management
General
A patient with severe diarrhea may require parenteral fluid replacement to prevent dehydration if oral fluid intake is inadequate.

Medication
Medications used to treat a patient with giardiasis may include:
- metronidazole — 750 mg P.O. t.i.d. for 5 to 10 days
- furazolidone — adults, 100 mg q.i.d. P.O.; children older than age 5, 25 to 50 mg q.i.d. P.O.

Referral
- Referral isn't necessary.

Follow-up
The patient should be seen 2 weeks after treatment is initiated, with a repeat stool culture 3 to 4 weeks after treatment is started.

Patient teaching
- Inform the patient receiving metronidazole of the possible adverse effects of this drug: commonly, headache, anorexia, and nausea and, less commonly, vomiting, diarrhea, and abdominal cramps. Warn against drinking alcoholic beverages, which may provoke a disulfiram-like reaction.
- Teach good personal hygiene, particularly proper hand-washing technique.

Complications
- Dehydration
- Weight loss
- Malnutrition
- Electrolyte imbalance

Special considerations
- If the patient is a woman, ask if she's pregnant because metronidazole is contraindicated during pregnancy.

- When talking to family members and other suspected contacts, emphasize the importance of stool examinations for G. *lamblia* cysts.
- Report epidemic situations to the public health authorities.

• • • • • • • • • • • •

HAEMOPHILUS INFLUENZAE INFECTION

Haemophilus influenzae is a bacterium that causes disease in many organ systems but most commonly attacks the respiratory system. It's a common cause of epiglottiditis, laryngotracheobronchitis, pneumonia, bronchiolitis, otitis media, and meningitis. Less commonly, it causes bacterial endocarditis, conjunctivitis, facial cellulitis, septic arthritis, and osteomyelitis. *H. influenzae* pneumonia is an increasingly common nosocomial infection. It tends to infect about half of all children before age 1 and virtually all children by age 3; a vaccine given at ages 2, 4, and 6 months has reduced this incidence.

Causes
H. influenzae, the cause of this infection, is a small, gram-negative, pleomorphic aerobic bacillus that appears predominantly in coccobacillary exudates. Transmission occurs by direct contact with secretions or by airborne droplets.

Clinical presentation
H. influenzae provokes a characteristic tissue response, acute suppurative inflammation. When *H. influenzae* infects the larynx, the trachea, and the bronchial tree, it leads to irritable cough, dyspnea, mucosal edema, and thick, purulent exudate. When it invades the lungs, it leads to bronchopneumonia. In the pharynx, *H. influenzae* usually produces no remarkable changes, except when it causes

epiglottiditis, which generally affects the laryngeal and pharyngeal surfaces. The pharyngeal mucosa may be reddened, rarely with soft yellow exudate. Usually, though, it appears normal or shows only slight diffuse redness, even though severe pain can make swallowing difficult or impossible. *H. influenzae* infections typically cause high fever and generalized malaise.

Differential diagnoses
- Other bacterial infections.

Diagnosis
Isolation of the organism, usually by blood culture, confirms the diagnosis of *H. influenzae* infection. Other laboratory findings include:
- polymorphonuclear leukocytosis (15,000 to 30,000 leukocytes/µl)
- leukopenia (2,000 to 3,000 leukocytes/µl) in young children with severe infection
- *H. influenzae* bacteremia (found in many patients with meningitis).

Management
General
Treatment consists of antibiotic therapy, along with comfort measures dependent on the patient's symptoms, such as oxygen administration, clear liquids for difficulty in swallowing, or measures to reduce fever.

Medication
Medications used to treat a patient with *H. influenzae* may include:
- ampicillin—250 to 500 mg P.O. every 6 hours or 1 to 12 g/day I.M. or I.V. in divided doses; children weighing less than 88 lb (40 kg), 25 to 100 mg/kg/day P.O. in divided doses or 25 to 50 mg/kg/day I.M. or I.V. in divided doses
- cefotaxime—4 to 12 g daily divided in doses every 6 to 8 hours; patients weighing less than 110 lb (50 kg) 50 to 180 mg/kg/day I.M. or I.V. in 4 to 6 divided doses
- ceftriaxone—adults, 1 to 2 g I.M. or I.V. daily divided in doses every 8 to 12 hours; children younger than age 12, 50 to 75 mg/kg I.V. every 6 to 8 hours.

Resistant strains are becoming more common; alternative treatment includes chloramphenicol (50 to 100 mg/kg/day I.V. in divided doses every 6 hours).

Referral
- The patient may need referral to an infectious disease specialist.
- Refer the patient to a health care facility for treatment, if appropriate.

Follow-up
The patient should be seen within 3 to 4 days to evaluate treatment, then in 2 to 3 weeks.

Patient teaching
- Teach the patient and parent the importance of completing all medication regimens.
- Tell the patient to report worsening respiratory symptoms immediately.
- Inform the parents of a child infected with *H. influenzae* about the high risk of acquiring this infection at day-care centers.
- Encourage parents to have their young children receive the *H. influenzae* vaccine to prevent these infections.

Complications
- Meningitis
- Pneumonia
- Septicemia
- Death

Special considerations
- Monitor complete blood count for signs of bone marrow depression when therapy includes ampicillin or chloramphenicol.

• • • • • • • • • • • •

HANTAVIRUS PULMONARY SYNDROME

Hantavirus pulmonary syndrome is a viral disease first reported in May 1993. It occurs mainly in the southwestern United States but isn't confined to that area. The syndrome, which rapidly progresses from flulike symptoms to respiratory failure and, possibly, death, is known for its high mortality. The hantavirus strain that causes disease (mainly hemorrhagic fever and renal disease) in Asia and Europe is distinctly different from the one currently described in North America.

Causes

The genus *Hantavirus* (a member of the Bunyaviridae family that was first isolated in 1977) is responsible for hantavirus pulmonary syndrome. Disease transmission is associated with exposure to infected rodents, the primary reservoir for this virus. Data suggest that the deer mouse is the main source, but piñon mice, brush mice, and western chipmunks in close proximity to humans in rural areas are also sources. Hantavirus infections have been documented in people whose activities are associated with rodent contact, such as farming, hiking or camping in rodent-infested areas, and occupying rodent-infested dwellings.

Infected rodents manifest no apparent illness but shed the virus in feces, urine, and saliva. Human infection may occur from inhalation, ingestion (of contaminated food or water, for example), contact with rodent excrement, or rodent bites. Transmission from person to person or by mosquitoes, fleas, or other arthropods hasn't been reported.

Clinical presentation

Noncardiogenic pulmonary edema distinguishes the syndrome. Common reasons for seeking care include:

- myalgia
- fever
- headache
- nausea
- vomiting
- cough.

Respiratory distress typically follows the onset of a cough. Hypoxia and, in some patients, serious hypotension may develop.

Other signs and symptoms include an increasing respiratory rate (28 breaths/minute or more) and an increased heart rate (120 beats/minute or more).

Differential diagnoses

- Pulmonary edema
- Respiratory failure
- Sepsis
- Pneumonia

Diagnosis

Diagnosis currently is based on clinical suspicion along with a process of elimination developed by the Centers for Disease Control and Prevention (CDC) with the Council of State and Territorial Epidemiologists. The CDC and state health departments can perform definitive testing for hantavirus exposure and antibody formation. Efforts are ongoing to identify clinical and laboratory features that distinguish hantavirus pulmonary syndrome from other infections with similar features. (See *Screening for hantavirus pulmonary syndrome*, page 648.)

Laboratory tests usually reveal an elevated white blood cell count with a predominance of neutrophils, myeloid precursors, and atypical lymphocytes; elevated hematocrit; decreased platelet count; elevated partial thromboplastin time; and

Screening for hantavirus pulmonary syndrome

The Centers for Disease Control and Prevention (CDC) has developed a screening procedure to track cases of hantavirus pulmonary syndrome. The screening criteria identify potential and actual cases.

POTENTIAL CASES

For a diagnosis of possible hantavirus pulmonary syndrome, a patient must have one of the following:

- febrile illness (temperature equal to or above 101° F [38.3° C]) occurring in a previously healthy person and characterized by unexplained adult respiratory distress syndrome
- bilateral interstitial pulmonary infiltrates that develop within 1 week of hospitalization with respiratory compromise that requires supplemental oxygen
- unexplained respiratory illness resulting in death and autopsy findings demonstrating noncardiogenic pulmonary edema without an identifiable specific cause of death.

Exclusions

Of the patients who meet the criteria for having potential hantavirus pulmonary syndrome, the CDC excludes those who have any of the following:

- predisposing underlying medical condition (for example, severe underlying pulmonary disease, solid tumors or hematologic cancers, congenital or ac-

quired immunodeficiency disorders) or medical conditions or treatments — such as rheumatoid arthritis or organ transplantation — requiring immunosuppressive drug therapy (for example, steroids or cytotoxic chemotherapy)

- acute illness that provides a likely explanation for the respiratory illness (for example, a recent major trauma, burn, or surgery; recent seizures or history of aspiration; bacterial sepsis; another respiratory disorder such as respiratory syncytial virus in young children; influenza; or legionella pneumonia).

CONFIRMED CASES

Cases of confirmed hantavirus pulmonary syndrome must include:

- at least one serum or tissue specimen available for laboratory testing for evidence of hantavirus infection
- in a patient with a compatible clinical illness, serologic evidence (presence of hantavirus-specific immunoglobulin M [IgM] or increasing titers of IgG), polymerase chain reaction for hantavirus ribonucleic acid, or positive immunohistochemistry for hantavirus antigen.

a normal fibrinogen level. Usually, laboratory findings demonstrate only minimal abnormalities in renal function, with serum creatinine levels no higher than 2.5 mg/dl.

Chest X-rays eventually show bilateral diffuse infiltrates in almost all patients, a finding consistent with adult respiratory distress syndrome.

Management
General

Treatment is primarily supportive and consists of maintaining adequate oxygenation and hemodynamic stability. Fluid volume replacement may be ordered (with precautions not to overhydrate the patient).

Medication

Medications used to treat a patient with hantavirus may include:

■ dopamine — 1 to 20 mcg/kg/minute by I.V. infusion, titrated for hypotension
■ ribavirin — solution in concentration of 20 mg/ml to deliver aerosol mist with a concentration of 190 mcg/L for 12 to 18 hours/day for 3 to 7 days has been used for children, but its efficacy for adults hasn't been proven.

Referral

■ If appropriate, refer the patient to a pulmonologist for treatment.
■ Refer the patient to a health care facility for emergency treatment, if needed.

Follow-up

The patient should be seen according to the severity of illness and complications that occur.

Patient teaching

■ Provide prevention guidelines to the patient and family members. Until more is known about hantavirus pulmonary syndrome, preventive measures currently focus on rodent control.
■ Tell the patient and family members to report any signs of respiratory distress.

Complications

■ Respiratory distress
■ Respiratory failure
■ Death

Special considerations

■ Report cases of hantavirus pulmonary syndrome to your state health department.

HERPES SIMPLEX

Herpes simplex is a recurrent viral infection caused by *Herpesvirus hominis* (HSV), a widespread infectious agent. Herpes type 1 affects the skin and mucous membranes, commonly producing cold sores and fever blisters. Herpes type 2 mainly affects the genital area.

Herpes simplex is equally common among males and females and is worldwide in distribution. It's most prevalent among children in lower socioeconomic groups who live in crowded environments. Herpes type 1 is the leading cause of childhood gingivostomatitis in children ages 1 to 3. It causes the most common form of nonepidemic encephalitis and is the second most common viral infection in pregnant women. It can pass to the fetus transplacentally and, in early pregnancy, can cause spontaneous abortion or premature birth.

Causes

Saliva, stool, skin lesions, purulent eye exudate, and urine are potential sources of herpes infection. Herpes type 1 is transmitted by oral and respiratory secretions. Herpes type 2 is transmitted by sexual contact. However, cross-infection may result from orogenital sex.

After first being infected by HSV, a patient becomes a carrier and is susceptible to recurrent infections, which may be provoked by fever, menses, stress, heat, and cold.

Clinical presentation

In neonates, symptoms of herpes usually appear 1 to 2 weeks after birth. They range from localized skin lesions to a disseminated infection of such organs as the liver, lungs, or brain. Up to 90% of infants with disseminated disease die.

Primary infection in childhood may be localized or generalized and occurs after an incubation period of 2 to 12 days. After brief prodromal tingling and itching, localized infection causes typical primary lesions. These erupt as vesicles on an erythematous base, eventually rupturing and leaving a painful ulcer, followed by a yellowish crust. Vesicles may form on any part of the oral mucosa, especially the tongue, gingiva, and cheeks. Healing begins 7 to 10 days after onset and is complete in 3 weeks.

Generalized infection begins with:
- fever
- pharyngitis
- erythema
- edema.

Vesicles occur with submaxillary lymphadenopathy, increased salivation, halitosis, anorexia, and a fever of up to 105° F (40.6° C). Herpetic stomatitis can lead to severe dehydration in children. A generalized infection usually runs its course in 4 to 10 days. In this form, virus reactivation causes cold sores (a single or group of vesicles in and around the mouth).

Genital herpes, type 2, usually affects adolescents and young adults. Typically painful, the initial attack produces fluid-filled vesicles that ulcerate and heal in 1 to 3 weeks. Other signs and symptoms include:
- fever
- regional lymphadenopathy
- dysuria.

Usually, herpetic keratoconjunctivitis is unilateral and causes only local signs and symptoms, including:
- conjunctivitis
- regional adenopathy
- blepharitis
- vesicles on the eyelid
- excessive lacrimation
- edema

- chemosis
- photophobia
- purulent exudate.

Both types of herpes can cause acute sporadic encephalitis with altered level of consciousness, personality changes, and seizures. Other effects may include smell and taste hallucinations and neurologic abnormalities such as aphasia.

CLINICAL CAUTION Herpetic whitlow, an HSV finger infection, affects many nurses. First the finger tingles and then it becomes red, swollen, and painful. Vesicles with a red halo erupt and may ulcerate or coalesce. Other effects may include satellite vesicles, fever, chills, malaise, and a red streak up the arm.

Differential diagnoses
- Impetigo
- Aphthous stomatitis
- Herpes zoster
- Syphilitic chancre
- Herpangina
- Stevens-Johnson syndrome

Diagnosis
Typical lesions may suggest infection by HSV. However, confirmation requires isolation of the virus from local lesions and histologic biopsy.

An increase in antibodies and moderate leukocytosis may support the diagnosis.

Management
General
There's no cure for herpes; however, recurrences tend to be milder and of shorter duration than the primary infection. Symptomatic and supportive therapy is essential. Generalized primary infection usually requires an analgesic-antipyretic to reduce fever and relieve pain. Anesthetic mouthwashes may reduce the pain

of gingivostomatitis, enabling the patient to eat and preventing dehydration. (Tell patients to avoid alcohol-based mouthwashes.) Drying agents, such as calamine lotion, ease the pain of labial or skin lesions. Avoid petroleum-based ointments, which promote viral spread and slow healing.

Medication

Medications used to treat a patient with herpes may include:

- acetaminophen — 325 to 650 mg P.O. every 4 to 6 hours p.r.n.
- ibuprofen — adults, 400 mg P.O. every 6 hours p.r.n.; children ages 6 months to 12 years, 5mg/kg P.O. every 6 to 8 hours
- lidocaine viscous — apply locally every 8 hours p.r.n.
- acyclovir — initial treatment, 200 mg P.O. 5 times/day for 10 days; for recurrent treatment, 200 mg P.O. 5 times/day for 5 days; for mild symptoms, topical ointment every 4 hours for 7 days
- valacyclovir — 1 g P.O. b.i.d. for 10 days; for recurrent treatment, 500 mg P.O. b.i.d. for 5 days
- foscarnet — 40 mg/kg I.V. over 1 hour every 8 to 12 hours for 2 to 3 weeks (used to treat patients with HSV resistant to acyclovir).

Referral

- Referral to an ophthalmologist may be necessary for a patient with an eye infection.

Follow-up

The patient should be seen 1 week after treatment is initiated and then every 2 weeks until lesions heal. For pregnant women with HSV infection, recommend weekly viral cultures of the cervix and external genitalia starting at 32 weeks' gestation.

Patient teaching

- Teach the patient with genital herpes to use warm compresses or take sitz baths several times a day, use a drying agent such as povidone-iodine solution, increase fluid intake, and avoid all sexual contact during the outbreaks of active infection.
- Instruct patients with herpetic whitlow not to share towels or eating utensils. Educate other susceptible people about the risk of contagion.
- Tell patients with cold sores not to kiss infants or people with eczema.

Complications

- Herpes encephalitis
- Herpes pneumonia
- Herpes septicemia
- Aseptic meningitis

• • • • • • • • • • • •

HERPES ZOSTER

Herpes zoster (also called shingles) is an acute unilateral and segmental inflammation of the dorsal root ganglia caused by infection with the herpesvirus varicella-zoster, which also causes chickenpox. This infection produces localized vesicular skin lesions confined to a dermatome and severe neuralgic pain in peripheral areas innervated by the nerves arising in the inflamed root ganglia.

Herpes zoster occurs mainly in adults, especially those past age 50. It seldom recurs. It's also seen in HIV-positive patients. The prognosis is good unless the infection spreads to the brain. Eventually, most patients recover completely, except for possible scarring and, with corneal damage, visual impairment. Occasionally, neuralgia persists for months or years.

Recognizing shingles

The characteristic skin lesions in herpes zoster (shingles) are fluid-filled vesicles that dry and form scabs after about 10 days.

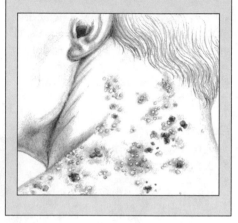

Causes and pathophysiology

Herpes zoster results from reactivation of varicella virus that has lain dormant in the cerebral ganglia (extramedullary ganglia of the cranial nerves) or the ganglia of posterior nerve roots since a previous episode of chickenpox. Exactly how or why this reactivation occurs isn't clear. Some believe that the virus multiplies as it's reactivated and that it's neutralized by antibodies remaining from the initial infection. However, if effective antibodies aren't present, the virus continues to multiply in the ganglia, destroy the host neuron, and spread down the sensory nerves to the skin.

Clinical presentation

Herpes zoster begins with fever and malaise. Within 2 to 4 days, severe deep pain, pruritus, and paresthesia or hyperesthesia develops, usually on the trunk and occasionally on the arms and legs in a dermatomal distribution. Pain may be continuous or intermittent and usually lasts from 1 to 4 weeks. Up to 2 weeks after the first symptoms, small red nodular skin lesions erupt on the painful areas. These lesions commonly spread unilaterally around the thorax or vertically over the arms or legs. Sometimes nodules don't appear at all, but when they do, they quickly become vesicles filled with clear fluid or pus. About 10 days after they appear, the vesicles dry and form scabs. (See *Recognizing shingles*.) When ruptured, such lesions often become infected and, in severe cases, may lead to enlargement of regional lymph nodes; they may even become gangrenous. Intense pain may occur before the rash appears and after the scabs form.

Occasionally, herpes zoster involves the cranial nerves, especially the trigeminal and geniculate ganglia or the oculomotor nerve. Geniculate zoster can cause vesicle formation in the external auditory canal, ipsilateral facial palsy, hearing loss, dizziness, and loss of taste. Trigeminal ganglion involvement causes eye pain and, possibly, corneal and scleral damage and impaired vision. Rarely, oculomotor involvement causes conjunctivitis, extraocular weakness, ptosis, and paralytic mydriasis.

In rare cases, herpes zoster leads to:
- generalized central nervous system infection
- muscle atrophy
- motor paralysis (usually transient)
- acute transverse myelitis
- ascending myelitis.

More commonly, generalized infection causes acute urine retention and unilateral diaphragm paralysis. In postherpetic neuralgia, a complication most common in elderly patients, intractable neurologic pain may persist for years. Scars may be permanent.

Differential diagnoses
- Herpes simplex
- Coxsackievirus
- Contact dermatitis
- Cholecystitis
- Pleuritis
- Myocardial infarction

Diagnosis
Diagnosis of herpes zoster usually isn't possible until the characteristic skin lesions develop. Before then, the pain might mimic that of appendicitis, pleurisy, or other conditions. Examination of vesicular fluid and infected tissue shows eosinophilic intranuclear inclusions and varicella virus. Also, a lumbar puncture shows increased pressure; examination of cerebrospinal fluid shows increased protein levels and, possibly, pleocytosis. To differentiate herpes zoster from localized herpes simplex, antibodies from vesicular fluid are stained for identification under fluorescent light.

Management
General
The primary goal of supportive treatment is to relieve itching and neuralgic pain. Use of transcutaneous electrical nerve stimulation may be helpful in treating a patient with postherpetic neuralgia. The treatment plan includes keeping the patient comfortable, maintaining meticulous hygiene, and preventing infection. During the acute phase, adequate rest and supportive care can promote proper healing of lesions.

Medication
Medications used to treat a patient with herpes zoster may include:
- acyclovir — 800 mg/day P.O. 5 times for 7 to 10 days; for immunocompromised patients
- amitriptyline — 50 to 100 mg P.O. h.s.
- calamine lotion — apply locally p.r.n.
- aspirin — 325 to 650 mg P.O. every 4 hours p.r.n.
- codeine — 15 to 60 mg P.O. every 4 to 6 hours p.r.n.
- capsaicin cream — apply to area t.i.d. to q.i.d.
- cortisone — 25 to 300 mg/day P.O. (dosage is highly individualized)
- interferon — for patients with cancer when the herpetic lesions are limited to the dermatome.

If bacteria have infected ruptured vesicles, the treatment plan usually includes an appropriate systemic antibiotic.

Referral
- If the patient experiences postherpetic neuralgia, refer him to a pain specialist to maximize pain relief without risking tolerance to the analgesic

Follow-up
The patient should be seen according to the severity of symptoms and complications.

Patient teaching
- Tell the patient who uses calamine lotion to apply it liberally to the lesions. If lesions are severe and widespread, tell him to apply a wet dressing.
- Instruct the patient to avoid scratching the lesions.
- If vesicles rupture, tell the patient to apply a cold compress.
- To decrease the pain of oral lesions, tell the patient to use a soft toothbrush, eat soft foods, and use a saline or bicarbonate mouthwash.

Complications
- Postherpetic neuralgia
- Meningoencephalitis
- Cutaneous dissemination
- Ocular involvement with facial zoster
- Hepatitis
- Pneumonitis

- Peripheral motor weakness
- Guillain-Barré syndrome
- Cranial nerve syndrome

Special considerations
- Repeatedly reassure the patient that herpetic pain will eventually subside. Encourage diversionary or relaxation activity.

• • • • • • • • • • • •

HOOKWORM DISEASE

Hookworm disease, also called uncinariasis or ground itch, is an infection of the upper intestine caused by *Ancylostoma duodenale* (found in the eastern hemisphere) or *Necator americanus* (in the western hemisphere). Sandy soil, high humidity, a warm climate, and failure to wear shoes all favor its transmission. In the United States, hookworm disease is rare. In lesser developed countries with moist tropical climates, prevalence of the disease is approximately 80%. Although this disease can cause cardiopulmonary complications, it's rarely fatal, except in debilitated individuals and infants under age 1. Prognosis is good with appropriate treatment.

Causes
Both forms of hookworm disease are transmitted to humans through direct skin penetration (usually in the foot) by hookworm larvae in soil contaminated with feces containing hookworm ova. These ova develop into infectious larvae in 1 to 3 days. Larvae travel through the lymphatics to the pulmonary capillaries, where they penetrate alveoli and move up the bronchial tree to the trachea and epiglottis. There they're swallowed and enter the GI tract. When they reach the small intestine, they mature, attach to the jejunal mucosa, and suck blood, oxygen, and glucose from the intestinal wall. The mature worms then deposit ova, which are excreted in the stool, starting a new cycle. Hookworm larvae mature in approximately 5 to 6 weeks.

Clinical presentation
Most cases of hookworm disease produce few symptoms and may be overlooked until worms are passed in the stool. The earliest signs and symptoms include irritation, pruritus, and edema at the site of entry, which are sometimes accompanied by secondary bacterial infection with pustule formation.

When the larvae reach the lungs, they might cause:
- pneumonitis
- hemorrhage with fever
- sore throat
- crackles
- cough.

Finally, intestinal infection can cause:
- fatigue
- nausea
- weight loss
- dizziness
- melena
- uncontrolled diarrhea.

In severe and chronic infection, anemia may also occur.

Differential diagnoses
- Pneumonitis
- Heart failure
- Cardiomegaly
- GI infection of another source
- Lung cancer
- Anemia
- Tinea

Diagnosis
Identification of hookworm ova in the stool confirms the diagnosis. Anemia suggests severe chronic infection.

In infected patients, blood studies show:

- hemoglobin level—5 to 9 g/dl (in severe cases)
- leukocyte count—as high as 47,000/µl
- eosinophil count—500 to 700/µl.

Management

General

Treatment generally involves administration of drugs to destroy the infecting organism. Anemia may need to be treated with blood transfusions, if severe.

Medication

Medications used to treat a patient with hookworms may include:

- mebendazole—100 mg P.O. b.i.d. for 3 days, repeat if infection persists 3 weeks later
- ferrous sulfate—100 to 200 mg P.O. t.i.d.

Referral

- Referral isn't necessary.

Follow-up

The stool culture should be repeated in 2 to 3 weeks.

Patient teaching

- To help prevent reinfection, educate the patient in proper hand-washing technique and sanitary disposal of feces. Tell him to wear shoes in endemic areas.
- To combat malnutrition, emphasize the importance of good nutrition, with particular attention to foods high in iron and protein. If the patient receives iron supplements, explain that they will darken stools.
- Tell the patient to take anthelmintic medication on an empty stomach but without a purgative.

Complications

- Anemia
- Respiratory failure
- Cardiomegaly
- Heart failure
- Secondary infection
- Dehydration
- Malnutrition

Special considerations

- Obtain a complete history, with special attention to travel or residency in endemic areas. Note the sequence and onset of symptoms. Interview family members and other close contacts to see if they too have any symptoms.

• • • • • • • • • • • •

INFLUENZA

Influenza (also called the grippe or the flu), an acute, highly contagious infection of the respiratory tract, results from three different types of *Myxovirus influenzae*. It occurs sporadically or in epidemics (usually during the colder months). Epidemics tend to peak within 2 to 3 weeks after initial cases and subside within a month.

Influenza affects people in all age groups; incidence is highest in school-age children, and its effects are most severe in young patients, elderly patients, and those with chronic diseases. In these groups, influenza can even lead to death. The catastrophic pandemic of 1918 caused an estimated 20 million deaths. The most recent pandemics (in 1957, 1968, and 1977) began in mainland China.

Causes

Transmission of influenza occurs through inhalation of a respiratory droplet from an infected person or by indirect contact with a contaminated object such as a drinking glass. The influenza virus then invades the epithelium of the respiratory tract, causing inflammation and desquamation.

One of the remarkable features of the influenza virus is its capacity for antigenic variation into numerous distinct strains, allowing it to infect new populations that have little or no immunologic resistance. Antigenic variation is characterized as antigenic drift (minor changes that occur yearly or every few years) and antigenic shift (major changes that lead to pandemics). Influenza viruses are classified into three groups:

- Type A, the most prevalent, strikes every year, with new serotypes causing epidemics every 3 years.
- Type B also strikes annually but causes epidemics only every 4 to 6 years.
- Type C is endemic and causes only sporadic cases.

Clinical presentation
After an incubation period of 24 to 48 hours, the following flu signs and symptoms begin to appear:
- sudden onset of chills
- temperature of 101° to 104° F (38.3° to 40° C)
- headache
- malaise
- myalgia (particularly in the back and limbs)
- nonproductive cough.

Occasionally, the following signs also occur:
- laryngitis
- hoarseness
- conjunctivitis
- rhinitis
- rhinorrhea.

These signs and symptoms usually subside in 3 to 5 days, but cough and weakness may persist. Fever is usually higher in children than in adults. Also, cervical adenopathy and croup are likely to be associated with influenza in children. In some patients (especially elderly patients), lack of energy and easy fatigability may persist for several weeks.

Fever that persists longer than 3 to 5 days signals the onset of complications. The most common complication is pneumonia, which occurs as primary influenza virus pneumonia or secondary to bacterial infection.

Differential diagnoses
- Respiratory viral infection
- Bronchitis
- Pneumonia
- Infectious mononucleosis
- Common cold
- Chlamydia

Diagnosis
At the beginning of an influenza epidemic, early cases are usually mistaken for other respiratory disorders. Because signs and symptoms aren't pathognomonic, isolation of M. *influenzae* through inoculation of chicken embryos (with nasal secretions from infected patients) is essential at the first sign of an epidemic. In addition, nose and throat cultures and increased serum antibody titers help to confirm this diagnosis.

After these measures confirm an influenza epidemic, diagnosis requires only observation of clinical signs and symptoms. Patients with uncomplicated disease show a decreased white blood cell count with an increase in lymphocytes.

Management
General
Treatment for a patient with uncomplicated influenza includes bed rest and adequate fluid intake, with medication (usually over the counter) to relieve fever, muscle pain, and nonproductive coughing. In influenza complicated by pneumonia, supportive care (fluid and electrolyte supplements, oxygen, and assisted venti-

lation) and appropriate antibiotic therapy for bacterial superinfection are necessary.

Medication

Medications used to treat a patient with influenza may include:

- aspirin—adults only, 325 to 650 mg P.O. every 4 hours p.r.n.
- acetaminophen—325 to 650 mg P.O. every 4 to 6 hours p.r.n.
- dextromethorphan—10 to 20 mg P.O. every 4 hours or 30 mg every 6 to 8 hours
- amantadine—adults, 200 mg P.O. once daily; children ages 1 to 9, 4.4 to 8.8 mg/kg/day divided into 1 or 2 doses; children ages 9 to 12, 100 mg P.O. b.i.d.
- oseltamivir phosphate—75 mg P.O. b.i.d. for 5 days (for patients who are symptomatic for 2 days or less)
- zanamivir—adults and children older than age 12, two oral inhalations every 12 hours for 5 days (for patients who are symptomatic for 2 days or less).

Referral

- Referral isn't necessary.

Follow-up

The patient should be seen weekly until the condition improves.

Patient teaching

- Advise the patient to use mouthwash and increase fluid intake. Warm baths or heating pads may relieve myalgia. Tell him to take nonnarcotic analgesic-antipyretics as needed.
- Teach the patient how to properly dispose of tissues and how to properly wash his hands to prevent the virus from spreading.

Complications

- Croup
- Pneumonia
- Otitis media
- Acute sinusitis
- Bronchitis
- Death
- Myositis
- Reye's syndrome
- Exacerbation of chronic obstructive pulmonary disease

Special considerations

- Inform people receiving the influenza vaccine of possible adverse effects. Although the vaccine hasn't been proven harmful to fetuses, it isn't recommended for pregnant women, except those who are highly susceptible to influenza, such as those with chronic diseases.

HEALTHY LIVING High-risk patients and health care personnel should receive the influenza vaccine annually. The vaccine administered is based on the previous year's virus and is usually about 75% effective.

• • • • • • • • • • •

LYME DISEASE

Lyme disease is a multisystemic disorder caused by the spirochete *Borrelia burgdorferi*, which is carried by the minute tick *Ixodes dammini* or another tick in the Ixodidae family. It commonly begins in the summer with a papule that becomes red and warm but isn't painful. This classic skin lesion is called erythema chronicum migrans. Weeks or months later, cardiac or neurologic abnormalities sometimes develop, possibly followed by arthritis of the large joints.

Lyme disease was first identified in a group of children in Lyme, Connecticut. Now it's known to occur primarily in three parts of the United States: in the Northeast, from Massachusetts down to Maryland; in the Midwest (Wisconsin and Minnesota); and in the West (California and Oregon).

In the United States, it's estimated that 6 out of 100,000 people are affected. However, epidemiologic data suggest that actual incidence may be as much as 10 times higher than that reported by the Centers for Disease Control and Prevention.

Causes

Lyme disease occurs when a tick injects spirochete-laden saliva into the bloodstream or deposits fecal matter on the skin. After incubating for 3 to 32 days, the spirochetes migrate out to the skin, causing erythema chronicum migrans. Then they disseminate to other skin sites or organs by the bloodstream or lymph system. The spirochetes' life cycle isn't completely clear. They may survive for years in the joints or they may trigger an inflammatory response in the host and then die.

Clinical presentation

Typically, Lyme disease has three stages. Erythema chronicum migrans heralds stage one with a red macule or papule, commonly at the site of a tick bite. This lesion typically feels hot and itchy and may grow to over 20″ (50.8 cm) in diameter; it resembles a bull's eye or target. Within a few days, more lesions may erupt, and a migratory, ringlike rash; conjunctivitis; or diffuse urticaria occurs. In 3 to 4 weeks, lesions are replaced by small red blotches, which persist for several more weeks. Malaise and fatigue are constant, but other findings are intermittent and include:

- headache
- neck stiffness
- fever
- chills
- achiness
- regional lymphadenopathy.
    Less common effects include:
- meningeal irritation
- mild encephalopathy

- migrating musculoskeletal pain
- hepatitis
- splenomegaly.
    A persistent sore throat and dry cough may appear several days before erythema chronicum migrans.

Weeks to months later, the second stage begins with neurologic abnormalities—fluctuating meningoencephalitis with peripheral and cranial neuropathy—that usually resolve after days or months. Facial palsy is especially noticeable. Cardiac abnormalities, such as a brief, fluctuating atrioventricular heart block, left ventricular dysfunction, or cardiomegaly may also develop. Cardiac involvement lasts only a few weeks but can be fatal.

Stage three begins weeks or years later and is characterized by arthritis. Migrating musculoskeletal pain leads to frank arthritis with marked swelling, especially in the large joints. Recurrent attacks may precede chronic arthritis with severe cartilage and bone erosion.

Differential diagnoses

- Juvenile rheumatoid arthritis
- Viral syndromes
- Influenza
- Later symptoms may mimic other diseases

Diagnosis

Because isolation of B. *burgdorferi* is unusual in humans and because indirect immunofluorescent antibody tests are marginally sensitive, diagnosis is usually based on the characteristic erythema chronicum migrans lesion and related clinical findings, especially in endemic areas. Mild anemia and an elevated erythrocyte sedimentation rate, leukocyte count, and serum immunoglobulin M and aspartate aminotransferase levels support the diagnosis.

Management
General
Treatment generally involves antibiotic therapy, along with symptomatic treatment, depending on which stage of Lyme disease is present.

Medication
Medications used to treat a patient with Lyme disease may include:
■ doxycycline—adults, 100 mg P.O. every 12 hours on 1st day, then 100 mg P.O. daily; children older than age 8 but weighing less than 99 lb (45 kg), 4.4 mg /kg P.O. or I.V. every 12 hours on 1st day, then 2.2 to 4.4 mg/kg daily.
■ amoxicillin—adults, 250 to 500 mg P.O. t.i.d. to q.i.d. for 10 to 30 days; children, 20 to 50 mg/kg/day P.O. every 8 hours at a maximum of 1 to 2 g/day for 10 to 30 days
■ ceftriaxone—adults, 1 to 2 g I.V. or I.M. daily; children younger than age 12, 50 to 75 mg/kg I.V. divided every 12 hours (for late stages) for 14 to 28 days.

Referral
■ If the patient is in the late stages of the disease, refer him to a dermatologist, neurologist, or an infectious disease specialist.

Follow-up
The patient should be seen every 1 to 2 weeks, depending on the severity of the disease.

Patient teaching
■ Teach the patient the importance of completing all medication regimens.

HEALTHY LIVING To prevent tick bites, instruct patients to wear light-colored clothing, tuck pant legs into socks, wear a hat and long sleeved shirt, avoid tall grass and brush, and spray exposed skin and clothing with a bug repellent containing diethyltoluamide.

Complications
■ Recurrent tendinitis
■ Recurrent bursitis
■ Recurrent synovitis
■ Chronic neurologic symptoms

• • • • • • • • • • •
MENINGOCOCCAL INFECTIONS

Two major meningococcal infections (meningitis and meningococcemia) are caused by the gram-negative bacteria *Neisseria meningitidis*, which also causes primary pneumonia, purulent conjunctivitis, endocarditis, sinusitis, and genital infection. Meningococcemia occurs as simple bacteremia, fulminating meningococcemia and, rarely, chronic meningococcemia. It commonly accompanies meningitis.

Meningococcal infections usually occur among children (ages 6 months to 1 year) and men, usually military recruits, because of overcrowding. Infections occur sporadically or in epidemics; virulent infections may be fatal within a matter of hours.

Causes
N. meningitidis includes seven serogroups (A, B, C, D, X, Y, and Z); group A causes most epidemics. The disease is transmitted by inhalation of an infected droplet from a carrier. The bacteria localize in the nasopharynx. After incubating for approximately 3 to 4 days, they spread through the bloodstream to joints, skin, adrenal glands, lungs, and the central nervous system. The tissue damage that results (possibly due to the effects of bacterial endotoxins) produces symptoms

and, in fulminating meningococcemia and meningococcal bacteremia, hemorrhage, thrombosis, and necrosis.

Clinical presentation
Features of meningococcal infections include:
- sudden spiking fever
- headache
- sore throat
- cough
- chills
- myalgia (in back and legs)
- arthralgia
- tachycardia
- tachypnea
- mild hypotension
- petechial, nodular, or maculopapular rash.

In about 10% to 20% of patients, these features progress to fulminating meningococcemia, with extreme prostration, enlargement of skin lesions, disseminated intravascular coagulation, and shock. Without prompt treatment, death from respiratory or heart failure occurs in 6 to 24 hours.

Characteristics of the rare chronic meningococcemia include intermittent fever, a rash, joint pain, and an enlarged spleen.

Differential diagnoses
- Septicemia from other organisms
- Influenza
- Meningitis from other bacteria
- Acute bacterial endocarditis
- Rocky Mountain spotted fever
- Vascular purpuras

Diagnosis
Isolation of N. *meningitidis* through a positive blood culture, cerebrospinal fluid (CSF) culture, or lesion scraping confirms the diagnosis, except in nasopharyngeal infections because N. *meningitidis*

is part of the normal nasopharyngeal flora.

Test results that support the diagnosis include counterimmunoelectrophoresis of CSF or blood, low white blood cell count and, in patients with skin or adrenal hemorrhages, decreased platelet and clotting levels.

Management
General
Supportive measures include fluid and electrolyte maintenance, ventilation (patent airway and oxygen, if necessary), insertion of an arterial or central venous pressure line to monitor cardiovascular status, and bed rest.

Medication
Medications used to treat a patient with meningococcal infections may include:
- penicillin G potassium (for meningitis) — adults, 1.2 to 24 million U/day I.M. or I.V. in divided doses esvery 4 to 6 hours; children, 25,000 to 400,000 U/kg/day I.M. or I.V. in divided doses every 4 to 6 hours; (for other infections, use half this dose)
- ampicillin — 150 to 200 mg/kg/day I.V. in divided doses every 3 to 4 hours
- cefoxitin — adults, 1 to 2 g I.V. or I.M. every 6 to 8 hours; children, 80 to 160 mg/kg/day I.V. or I.M. in 4 to 6 divided doses
- chloramphenicol (for meningitis) — adults, 1 g I.V. every 6 hours; children, 12.5 mg/kg I.V. every 6 hours
- rifampin (prophylaxis for people in close contact with the patient) — adults, 600 mg P.O. every 12 hours for 2 days; children younger than age 12, 10 mg/kg P.O. or I.V. every 12 hours for 2 days
- minocycline — 100 mg P.O. every 12 hours for 5 days to temporarily eradicate the infection in carriers.

Referral
- Refer the patient to the hospital for treatment.
- If neurologic deficits occur, refer the patient to a neurologist.

Follow-up
The patient should be seen 1 week after discharge from the hospital, then every 3 months.

Patient teaching
- Teach family members and the patient about the risk of contracting meningococcal infections.

Complications
- Disseminated intravascular coagulation
- Acute tubular necrosis
- Seizures
- Focal neurologic deficit
- Cranial nerve palsies
- Sensorineural hearing loss
- Arthritis
- Endocarditis
- Pneumonia

Special considerations
- Impose respiratory isolation until the patient has had antibiotic therapy for 24 hours.
- Report all meningococcal infections to public health department officials.

• • • • • • • • • • • •

METHICILLIN-RESISTANT *STAPHYLOCOCCUS AUREUS* INFECTION

Methicillin-resistant *Staphylococcus aureus* (MRSA) is a mutation of a common bacterium. In patients whose natural defense systems break down, such as after an invasive procedure, trauma, or chemo-therapy, the normally benign bacteria can invade tissues, proliferate, and cause infection. The bacteria are spread easily by direct person-to-person contact. Once limited to teaching hospitals and tertiary care centers, MRSA infection is now endemic in nursing homes, long-term care facilities, and community hospitals.

Although difficult to treat, MRSA still can be successfully cured.

Causes
MRSA enters health care facilities through an infected or colonized patient or a colonized health care worker. Although MRSA has been recovered from environmental surfaces, it's transmitted mainly by health care workers' hands. Many colonized individuals become silent carriers. The most frequent site of colonization is the anterior nares (40% of adults and most children become transient nasal carriers). Other sites include the groin, axilla, and the gut, although these sites aren't as common.

Persons most at risk for MRSA infection are immunosuppressed patients, burn patients, intubated patients, and those with central venous catheters, surgical wounds, or dermatitis. Others at risk include those with prosthetic devices, heart valves, and postoperative wound infections. Other risk factors include prolonged hospital stays, extended therapy with multiple or broad-spectrum antibiotics, and close proximity to those colonized or infected with MRSA. Also at risk are patients with acute endocarditis, bacteremia, cervicitis, meningitis, pericarditis, and pneumonia.

CLINICAL CAUTION MRSA infection has become prevalent with the overuse of antibiotics. Today, up to 90% of *S. aureus* isolates or strains are penicillin resistant, and about 27% of all *S. aureus* isolates are resistant to methicillin, a penicillin derivative. These strains may also resist cephalosporins, aminoglycosides, erythromycin, tetracycline, and clindamycin.

Clinical presentation

There are no specific signs or symptoms related to MRSA infection. However, the patient may display signs of infection affecting a specific body system, for example:

- pneumonia
- enterocotitis
- osteomyelitis
- skin infections.

These infections are resistant to methicillin treatment and won't show improvement if treated with medication that isn't susceptible to MRSA. The causative agent may be found incidentally when culture results show the organism.

Differential diagnoses

- Infection from another causative agent

Diagnosis

Typically, MRSA colonization is diagnosed by isolating bacteria from nasal secretions. MRSA can be cultured from the suspected site.

Management

General

Most facilities keep patients in isolation until surveillance cultures are negative.

Medication

Medications used to treat a patient with MRSA may include:

- mupirocin—single-use tube for each nostril (apply ½ tube per nostril b.i.d. for 5 days)
- linezolid—600 mg I.V. or P.O. every 12 hours for 10 to 14 days.

- vancomycin—adults, 1 to 1.5 g I.V. every 12 hours; children, 10 mg/kg I.V. every 6 hours
- quinupristin/dalfopristin—7.5 mg/kg I.V. every 12 hours for 7 days.

Referral

- Refer the patient to the hospital for treatment.

Follow-up

Cultures should be repeated after 5 to 7 days of treatment.

Patient teaching

- Teach family members proper handwashing technique to prevent the spread of MRSA.
- Instruct family members and friends to wear protective clothing when they visit the patient and show them how to dispose of it.
- Instruct the patient to take antibiotics for the full prescription period, even if he begins to feel better.

Complications

- Septicemia
- Spread of MRSA to others

• • • • • • • • • • •

MONONUCLEOSIS, INFECTIOUS

Infectious mononucleosis is an acute infectious disease caused by the Epstein-Barr virus (EBV), a member of the herpes group. It primarily affects young adults and children, although in children it's usually so mild that it's generally overlooked. This infection characteristically produces fever, sore throat, and cervical lymphadenopathy (the hallmarks of the disease) as well as hepatic dysfunction, increased lymphocyte and monocyte counts, and development and persistence of heterophil antibodies.

Infectious mononucleosis is fairly common in the United States, Canada, and Europe and affects both sexes equally. Incidence varies seasonally among college students but not among the general population. The prognosis is excellent, and major complications are uncommon.

Causes

Infectious mononucleosis probably spreads by the oral-pharyngeal route because about 80% of patients carry EBV in the throat during the acute infection and for an indefinite period afterward. It can also be transmitted by blood transfusions and has been reported after cardiac surgery as post-pump perfusion syndrome. Infectious mononucleosis is probably contagious from before symptoms develop until the fever subsides and oral-pharyngeal lesions disappear.

Clinical presentation

The symptoms of mononucleosis mimic those of many other infectious diseases, including hepatitis, rubella, and toxoplasmosis. Typically, after an incubation period of about 10 days in children and from 30 to 50 days in adults, infectious mononucleosis produces prodromal symptoms including headache, malaise, and fatigue. After 3 to 5 days, patients typically develop a triad of symptoms that include:

- sore throat
- cervical lymphadenopathy
- temperature fluctuations, with an evening peak of 101° to 102° F (38.3° to 38.9° C).

Other signs include:

- splenomegaly
- hepatomegaly
- stomatitis
- exudative tonsillitis
- pharyngitis may also develop.

Early in the illness, a maculopapular rash that resembles rubella sometimes develops; also, jaundice occurs in about 5% of patients. Symptoms usually subside about 6 to 10 days after onset of the disease but may persist for weeks.

Differential diagnoses

- Cytomegalovirus
- Streptococcal pharyngitis
- Viral tonsillitis
- Hepatitis
- Roseola
- Rubella
- Lymphocytic leukemia
- Adenovirus
- Toxoplasmosis
- Drug adverse effects

Diagnosis

Physical examination demonstrating the clinical triad suggests infectious mononucleosis. The following abnormal laboratory results confirm the diagnosis:

- Leukocyte count increases to 10,000 to 20,000/µl during the 2nd and 3rd weeks of illness. Lymphocytes and monocytes account for 50% to 70% of the total white blood cell count; 10% of the lymphocytes are atypical.
- Heterophil antibodies (agglutinins for sheep red blood cells) in serum drawn during the acute illness and at 3- to 4-week intervals increase to four times normal.
- Indirect immunofluorescence shows antibodies to EBV and cellular antigens. Such testing is usually more definitive than heterophil antibodies.
- Liver function study results are abnormal.

Management
General

Infectious mononucleosis resists prevention and antimicrobial treatment. Thus, therapy is essentially supportive: relief of symptoms, bed rest during the acute febrile period, and aspirin or another salicylate for headache and sore throat. If severe throat inflammation causes airway obstruction, steroids can be used to relieve swelling and, therefore, avoid tracheotomy. About 20% of patients with infectious mononucleosis also have streptococcal pharyngotonsillitis; these patients should receive antibiotic therapy for at least 10 days.

Medication
Medications used to treat a patient with mononucleosis may include:
- acetaminophen — 325 to 650 mg P.O. every 4 to 6 hours p.r.n.
- erythromycin — 250 to 500 mg P.O. q.i.d.
- prednisone — 5 to 60 mg/day P.O. (highly individualized)

Surgical intervention
Splenic rupture, marked by sudden abdominal pain, necessitates splenectomy.

Referral
- Refer the patient to an otolaryngologist if he has marked tonsillar swelling or a central nervous system complication.

Follow-up
The patient should be seen every 1 to 2 weeks until clinical signs improve.

Patient teaching
- During acute illness, stress the need for bed rest. If the patient is a student, tell him he may continue less demanding school assignments and see his friends but should avoid long, difficult projects until after recovery.
- To minimize throat discomfort, encourage the patient to drink milk shakes, fruit juices, and broths and to eat cool, bland foods. Advise gargling with saline mouthwash and taking aspirin or acetaminophen as needed.

Complications
- Splenic rupture
- Hemolytic anemia
- Thrombocytopenic purpura
- Coagulopathy
- Pleural effusion
- Pericarditis
- Myocarditis
- Pneumonitis
- Aplastic anemia
- Guillain-Barré syndrome
- Reye's syndrome
- Nephrotic syndrome
- Staphylococcal infection

• • • • • • • • • • • •

MUMPS

Mumps, also known as infectious or epidemic parotitis, is an acute viral disease caused by a paramyxovirus. Peak incidence occurs during late winter and early spring. The prognosis for complete recovery is good, although mumps sometimes causes complications. Approximately 1,500 cases a year are reported.

AGE ALERT Mumps is most prevalent in children between ages 6 and 8. Infants less than age 1 seldom get this disease because of passive immunity from maternal antibodies.

Causes
The mumps paramyxovirus is found in the saliva of an infected person and is transmitted by droplets or by direct contact. The virus is present in the saliva 6 days before to 9 days after onset of parotid gland swelling. The 48-hour period immediately before the onset of swelling is probably the time of highest communi-

cability. The incubation period ranges from 14 to 25 days (the average is 18). One attack of mumps (even if unilateral) almost always confers lifelong immunity.

Clinical presentation

The clinical features of mumps vary widely. An estimated 30% of susceptible people have subclinical illness.

Mumps usually begins with prodromal symptoms that last for 24 hours and include:

- myalgia
- anorexia
- malaise
- headache
- low-grade fever (followed by earache aggravated by chewing)
- parotid gland tenderness and swelling
- temperature of 101° to 104° F (38.3° to 40° C)
- pain (when chewing or drinking sour or acidic liquids).

Simultaneously with the swelling of the parotid gland or several days later, one or more of the other salivary glands may become swollen.

Differential diagnoses

- Parainfluenza parotitis
- Allergic parotitis
- Salivary gland tumors
- Lymphadenitis from any cause
- Mikulicz's syndrome

Diagnosis

Diagnosis is usually made after the characteristic signs and symptoms develop, especially parotid gland enlargement after exposure to mumps. Serologic antibody testing can verify the diagnosis when parotid or other salivary gland enlargement is absent. If comparison between a blood specimen obtained during the acute phase of illness and another specimen obtained 3 weeks later shows a fourfold increase in antibody titer, the patient most likely had mumps.

Management

General

Treatment includes analgesics for pain, antipyretics for fever, and adequate fluid intake to prevent dehydration from fever and anorexia. A soft diet may make it easier to eat. If the patient can't swallow, consider I.V. fluid replacement.

Medication

Medications used to treat a patient with mumps may include:

- acetaminophen — 325 to 650 mg P.O. every 4 to 6 hours p.r.n.
- Measles-mumps-rubella vaccine — 0.5 ml S.C. (1 dose for adults, 1 dose for children at age 12 to 15 months and again at either age 4 to 6 or age 11 to 12).

Referral

- Refer the patient to a hospital for treatment if he's experiencing a high fever and testicular pain.
- Refer the patient to a urologist if acute orchitis develops.

Follow-up

The patient should be rechecked in 48 hours to assess for improvement. Most cases are mild and may not require follow-up unless complications occur.

Patient teaching

- Stress the need for bed rest during the febrile period. Tell the patient to take analgesics and apply warm or cool compresses to the neck to relieve pain. Antipyretics and tepid sponge baths may help with fever.
- To prevent dehydration, encourage the patient to drink fluids; to minimize pain and anorexia, advise him to avoid spicy, irritating foods and those that require a

lot of chewing. Advise the patient to fol-low a soft, bland diet.
- Advise family members to follow respi-ratory isolation precautions until symp-toms subside.

Complications
- Epididymo-orchitis
- Pancreatitis
- Meningoencephalitis
- Deafness
- Nephritis
- Arthritis
- Meningitis

Special considerations
- Report all cases of mumps to local pub-lic health authorities.

HEALTHY LIVING Routine immu-nization with live attenuated mumps virus (paramyxovirus) at age 15 months and for susceptible patients (es-pecially males) who are approaching or are past puberty is strongly recommend-ed. Immunization within 24 hours of ex-posure may prevent or attenuate the dis-ease. Immunity against mumps lasts at least 12 years.

• • • • • • • • • • • •

NECROTIZING FASCIITIS

Necrotizing fasciitis is a progressive, rapidly spreading inflammatory infection arising in deep fascia. Group A beta-hemolytic *Streptococcus* (GAS) and *Staphylococcus aureus*, working alone or together, are commonly the primary in-fecting bacteria. Because it destroys fascia and fat, with secondary necrosis of subcu-taneous tissue, necrotizing fasciitis is most commonly called "flesh-eating bac-teria." It's also known as hemolytic strep-tococcal gangrene, acute dermal gan-grene, suppurative fasciitis, and synergis-tic necrotizing cellulitis.

High mortality rates (70% to 80%) associated with necrotizing fasciitis have been attributed to the emergence of more virulent strains of streptococci caused by changes in the bacteria's DNA. This would account for an increase in the fre-quency and severity of cases reported since 1985, following 50 to 60 years of insignificant clinical disease. In 1999, 9,400 cases of GAS were reported; 600 of them were found to be necrotizing fasci-itis.

Men are three times more likely than women to develop this rare condi-tion. Mortality decreases significantly and prognosis improves with early inter-vention and treatment. Cases treated ag-gressively with surgery, antibiotics, and hyperbaric oxygen therapy reduce mor-tality rates to as low as 9% to 20%.

AGE ALERT This disease rarely occurs in children except in coun-tries with poor hygiene practices. The mean age of the population contracting necrotizing fasciitis is 38 to 44.

Causes
Necrotizing fasciitis is most commonly caused by the pathogenic bacteria *Strepto-coccus pyogenes*. More than 80 types of *S. pyogenes* exist, making the epidemiology of GAS infections complex. Other aero-bic and anaerobic pathogens — including *Bacteroides, Clostridium, Peptostreptococ-cus,* Enterobacteriaceae, coliforms, *Pro-teus, Pseudomonas,* and *Klebsiella* — may be present, proliferating in an environ-ment of tissue hypoxia caused by trauma, recent surgery, or medical compromise.

Causative bacteria enter the host by local tissue injury or through a breach in the integrity of a mucous membrane bar-rier. Wounds as minor as pinpricks, nee-dle punctures, bruises, blisters, and abra-sions or as serious as a traumatic injury or surgical incision can provide an opportu-nity for bacteria to enter the body. The infection leads to necrosis of the surrounding tissue, accelerating the disease process by creating a favorable environment for invading organisms.

Risk factors for contracting necrotizing fasciitis include patients with advanced age, human immunodeficiency virus infection, alcohol abuse, and varicellar infection. Patients with chronic illnesses, such as cancer, diabetes, cardiac and pulmonary disease, and kidney disease requiring hemodialysis, and those using steroids are more susceptible to GAS infection due to debilitated immune responsiveness.

Clinical presentation

Infection may begin at the site of a small insignificant wound or a surgical incision and is characterized by invasive and progressive necrosis of the soft tissue and underlying blood supply. Pain, out of proportion to the size of the wound or an injury it's associated with, is usually the first symptom of necrotizing fasciitis and generally presents before other physical findings.

The infective process usually begins with a mild area of erythema at the site of insult, which quickly progresses within the first 24 hours. During the first 24- to 48-hour period, the erythema changes from red to purple in color and then blue, with the formation of fluid-filled blisters and bullae appearing, indicating rapid progression of the necrotizing process. By days 4 and 5, multiple patches of erythema form, producing large areas of gangrenous skin. By days 7 to 10, dead skin begins to separate at the margins of the erythema, revealing extensive necrosis of the subcutaneous tissue. At this stage, fascial necrosis is typically more advanced than appearance suggests.

Other clinical signs include:
- fever
- hypovolemia
- hypotension
- respiratory insufficiency
- sepsis.

In the most severe cases, necrosis advances rapidly until several large areas are involved, causing the patient to become mentally cloudy, delirious, or even unresponsive secondary to the intoxication.

Differential diagnoses
- Cellulitis
- GAS gangrene
- Fournier's gangrene
- Hernias
- Toxic shock syndrome

Diagnosis

Tissue biopsy is the best method for diagnosing necrotizing fasciitis. Cultures of microorganisms can be obtained locally from the periphery of the spreading infection or from deeper tissues during surgical debridement. Gram stain and culturing of biopsied tissue are useful in identifying the invasive organisms and effective treatment against them.

Radiographic studies can be used to locate subcutaneous gases. Computed tomography scans can be used to pinpoint the site of involvement by revealing necrosis. In combination with clinical assessment, magnetic resonance imaging is used to determine areas of necrosis and the need for surgical debridement.

Other supportive studies may include complete blood count with differential, urinalysis, and analysis of electrolytes, glucose, blood urea nitrogen, creatinine, and arterial blood gases.

Management
General

Reports suggest that using hyperbaric oxygen treatment (HBOT) decreases the mortality rate, significantly improves the tissues' defense against infection, and prevents necrosis from spreading by increasing the normal oxygen saturations of infected wounds a thousandfold, causing a bactericidal effect. HBOT should be started aggressively after the first surgical debridement and continued for 10 to 15 sessions.

Medication

Drug recommendations continue to change as new antibiotics are developed and new resistance emerges. Specific drugs are determined by the sensitivity of the organisms in culture. Medication in combination must be used when the infection is polymicrobial.

Medications that may be used to treat a patient with necrotizing fasciitis include:

- penicillin G sodium — adults, 1.2 to 24 million U/day I.M. or I.V. in divided doses every 4 to 6 hours; children younger than age 12, 25,000 to 400,000 U/kg/day I.M. or I.V. in divided doses every 4 to 6 hours
- clindamycin — 150 to 450 mg P.O. every 6 hours or 300 to 600 mg I.M. or I.V. every 6 to 12 hours
- metronidazole — initially 15 mg/kg I.V., then 7.5 mg/kg I.V. every 6 hours
- ceftriaxone — 1 to 2 g/day I.M. or I.V.
- gentamicin — adults, 3 mg/kg/day I.V. or I.M. in divided doses every 8 hours; children, 2.0 to 2.5 mg/kg I.M. or I.V. every 8 hours
- chloramphenicol — 50 to 100 mg/kg/day I.V. in divided doses every 6 hours
- ampicillin — adults, 250 to 500 mg P.O. every 6 hours or 1 to 12 g/day I.M. or I.V. in divided doses every 4 to 6 hours; children weighing less than 88 lb (40 kg), 25 to 100 mg/kg P.O. in divided doses every 6 hours or 25 to 50 mg/kg I.M. or I.V. in divided doses every 6 to 8 hours.

Surgical intervention

Prompt and aggressive exploration and debridement of suspected necrotizing fasciitis is necessary to provide an early and definitive diagnosis and to enhance the patient's prognosis. Ninety percent of patients presenting with clinical signs and symptoms need immediate surgical debridement, fasciotomy, or amputation.

Referral

- Refer the patient to an infectious disease specialist.
- Refer the patient to the hospital for treatment.
- For education and support, refer the patient and family members to organizations such as the National Necrotizing Fasciitis Foundation.

Follow-up

The patient should be seen after hospitalization according to the specialist's recommendation; follow-up measures depend on the severity of illness.

Patient teaching

- Teach family members about the illness and what outcomes to expect according to the area affected.

Complications

- Renal failure
- Septic shock
- Scarring with cosmetic deformities
- Myositis
- Myonecrosis
- Amputation

• • • • • • • • • • • •

RABIES

Rabies, also known as hydrophobia, is an acute central nervous system (CNS) infection caused by a virus that's transmitted by the saliva of an infected animal. If symptoms occur, rabies is almost always fatal; treatment soon after exposure may prevent fatal CNS invasion.

In the United States, dog vaccinations have reduced the incidence of rabies transmission to humans. Wild animals, such as skunks, foxes, raccoons, and bats, account for 70% of rabies cases. In 1998, there were 7,962 cases of rabies reported in animals, with 44% occurrence in raccoons. There was 1 case of rabies reported in humans. Hawaii has never reported a case of rabies.

Causes
The rabies virus is usually transmitted to a human through the bite of an infected animal, which introduces the virus through the skin or mucous membranes. The virus begins to replicate in the striated muscle cells at the bite site. Then it spreads up the nerve to the CNS and replicates in the brain. Finally, it moves through the nerves into other tissues, including the salivary glands. Occasionally, airborne droplets and infected tissue transplants transmit the virus.

Rabies symptoms appear earlier if the head or face is severely bitten. If the bite is on the face, the risk of developing rabies is about 60%; on the upper extremities, 15% to 40%; and on the lower extremities, about 10%.

Clinical presentation
After an incubation period of 1 to 3 months, rabies typically produces local or radiating pain or burning and a sensation of cold, pruritus, and tingling at the bite site. It also produces prodromal signs and symptoms, such as:
- slight fever (100° to 102° F [37.8° to 38.9° C])
- malaise
- headache
- anorexia
- nausea

- sore throat
- persistent loose cough
- nervousness
- anxiety
- irritability
- hyperesthesia
- photophobia
- sensitivity to loud noises
- pupillary dilation
- tachycardia
- shallow respirations
- pain and paresthesia in the bitten area
- excessive salivation, lacrimation, and perspiration.

About 2 to 10 days after the onset of prodromal symptoms, a phase of excitation begins. It's characterized by:
- agitation
- marked restlessness
- anxiety
- apprehension
- cranial nerve dysfunction (causes ocular palsies)
- strabismus
- asymmetrical pupillary dilation or constriction
- absence of corneal reflexes
- weakness of facial muscles
- hoarseness.

Severe systemic symptoms include tachycardia or bradycardia, cyclic respirations, urine retention, and a temperature of about 103° F (39.4° C).

About 50% of affected patients exhibit hydrophobia (fear of water), during which forceful, painful pharyngeal muscle spasms expel liquids from the mouth and cause dehydration and, possibly, apnea, cyanosis, and death. Difficulty swallowing causes frothy saliva to drool from the patient's mouth. Eventually, just the sight, mention, or thought of water causes uncontrollable pharyngeal muscle spasms and excessive salivation. Between episodes of excitation and hydrophobia, the patient commonly is cooperative and lucid. After about 3 days, excitation and hydrophobia subside and the progressively paralytic, terminal phase of the illness begins.

The patient experiences progressive, generalized, flaccid paralysis that ultimately leads to peripheral vascular collapse, coma, and death.

Differential diagnoses
- Encephalitis (from another cause)

Diagnosis
Because rabies is fatal unless treated promptly, always suspect rabies in any person who reports an unprovoked animal bite until you can prove otherwise. Isolation of the virus from the patient's saliva or throat and examination of his blood for direct fluorescent rabies antibody (dFA) are the most accurate diagnostic tests.

Other results typically include elevated white blood cell count, with increased polymorphonuclear and large mononuclear cells, and elevated urinary glucose, acetone, and protein levels.

Confinement of the suspected animal for 10 days of observation by a veterinarian aids diagnosis. If the animal appears rabid, it should be killed and its brain tissue tested for dFA and Negri bodies (oval or round masses that confirm rabies).

Management
General
Treatment consists of wound treatment and immunization as soon as possible after exposure. Thoroughly wash all bite wounds and scratches with soap and water to remove any infected saliva. (See *First aid in animal bites*.) Check the patient's immunization status, and administer tetanus-diphtheria prophylaxis, if needed.

Medication
Medications used to treat a patient with rabies may include:
- rabies immune globulin, human — 20 IU/kg I.M. given once
- rabies vaccine, human diploid cell — 1 ml I.M. given as soon as possible after exposure, then additional doses on day 3, 7, 14, and 28.

Surgical intervention
If the wound requires suturing, special treatment and suturing techniques must be used to allow proper wound drainage.

Referral
- Refer the patient to the hospital if the wound is serious or encephalitis has developed.

Follow-up
The patient should be seen for postexposure treatment according to the medication schedule.

Patient teaching

- Teach family members what to expect in the course of the illness.
- Teach the patient about careful wound cleansing.

HEALTHY LIVING To help prevent rabies, stress the need for vaccination of household pets that may be exposed to rabid wild animals. Advise against touching wild animals, especially if they appear ill or overly docile (a possible sign of rabies). Prophylactic rabies vaccine is available for high-risk people, such as farm workers, forest rangers, spelunkers (cave explorers), and veterinarians.

Complications

- Death

Special considerations

- Cooperate with public health authorities to determine the vaccination status of the animal. If the animal is proven rabid, help to identify others at risk.

• • • • • • • • • • • •

RESPIRATORY SYNCYTIAL VIRUS INFECTION

Respiratory syncytial virus (RSV) infection results from a subgroup of the myxoviruses that resemble paramyxovirus. Antibody titers seem to indicate that few children under age 4 escape contracting some form of RSV, even if it's mild. In fact, RSV is the only viral disease that has its maximum impact during the first few months of life (incidence of RSV bronchiolitis peaks at age 2 months). This virus occurs in annual epidemics during the late winter and early spring in temperate climates and during the rainy season in the tropics.

RSV causes death in infants but, in older children and adults, the disease may only be mild.

AGE ALERT RSV is the leading cause of lower respiratory tract infections in infants and young children. It's the major cause of pneumonia, tracheobronchitis, and bronchiolitis in this age-group and a suspected cause of the fatal respiratory diseases of infancy.

Causes

The organism that causes RSV is transmitted from person to person by respiratory secretions and has an incubation period of 4 to 5 days. School-age children, adolescents, and young adults with mild reinfections are probably the source of infection for infants and young children.

Clinical presentation

Clinical features of RSV infection vary in severity from mild, coldlike symptoms to bronchiolitis or bronchopneumonia and, in a few patients, severe, life-threatening lower respiratory tract infections. Symptoms usually include the following:

- coughing
- wheezing
- malaise
- pharyngitis
- dyspnea
- inflamed mucous membranes (nose and throat).

Reinfection is common, producing milder symptoms than the primary infection.

RSV has been identified in patients with a variety of central nervous system disorders, such as meningitis and myelitis.

Differential diagnoses

- Cold (non-RSV)
- Sinusitis

- Croup
- Allergic rhinitis
- Pneumonia
- Bronchitis

Diagnosis
Diagnosis is usually based on clinical findings and epidemiologic information.
- Cultures of nasal and pharyngeal secretions may show RSV; however, the virus is labile, so cultures aren't always reliable.
- Serum antibody titers may be elevated, but before age 6 months, maternal antibodies can impair test results.
- Two recently developed serologic techniques are the indirect immunofluorescent and the enzyme-linked immunosorbent assay methods.
- Chest X-rays help to detect pneumonia.

Management
General
Goals of treatment are to support respiratory function, maintain fluid balance, and relieve symptoms.

Medication
Medications used to treat a patient with RSV may include:
- ribavirin — 20 mg/ml mist 12 to 18 hours/day for 3 to 7 days (may be administered to severely ill patients or those at high risk for complications)
- albuterol nebulizer — dose appropriate for age, every 4 hours
- RSV immune globulin — maximum dose is 750 mg/kg I.V. infusion given monthly (for high-risk infants).

Referral
- Refer the patient to the hospital if complications occur.

Follow-up
The patient should be seen if the condition worsens, otherwise recovery should be uneventful.

Patient teaching
- Tell family members to continue to hold and cuddle infants and talk to and play with toddlers. Tell them to offer diversionary activities that are appropriate for the child's condition and age.
- Teach good hand-washing technique to family members to prevent spreading the illness.

Complications
- Pneumonia
- Sudden infant death syndrome
- Otitis media
- Bronchiolitis
- Croup
- Residual lung damage

• • • • • • • • • • • •

ROCKY MOUNTAIN SPOTTED FEVER

Rocky Mountain spotted fever (RMSF) is a febrile, rash-producing illness caused by *Rickettsia rickettsii*. The disease is transmitted to humans by a tick bite. It's endemic throughout the continental United States and is most prevalent in the southeast and southwest. Because RMSF is associated with outdoor activities, such as camping and backpacking, incidence is usually greater in the spring and summer. Epidemiologic surveillance reports for RMSF indicate that the incidence is 8 out of 100,000 people. It affects white men and boys more than women. RMSF is fatal in about 5% of patients. Mortality increases when treatment is delayed and in older patients.

AGE ALERT Two-thirds of reported cases of RMSF have been in children ages 5 to 9.

Causes

R. rickettsii is transmitted to a human or small animal by a prolonged bite (4 to 6 hours) of an adult tick (the wood tick [*Dermacentor andersoni*] in the West and the dog tick [*D. variabilis*] in the East). (See *Close-up of a tick.*) Occasionally, RMSF is acquired through inhalation of or contact of abraded skin with tick excreta or tissue juices; that's why people shouldn't crush ticks between their fingers when removing them from other people and animals. In most tick-infested areas, 1% to 5% of the ticks harbor *R. rickettsii*.

Clinical presentation

The incubation period of RMSF is usually about 7 days but can range from 2 to 14 days. Generally, the shorter the incubation time, the more severe the infection. Signs and symptoms, which usually begin abruptly, includes:

- persistent temperature of 102° to 104° F (38.9° to 40° C)
- generalized, excruciating headache
- nausea and vomiting
- aching in the bones, muscles, joints, and back.

In addition, the tongue is covered with a thick white coating that gradually turns brown as the patient's fever persists and temperature rises.

Initially, the skin may simply appear flushed. Between days 2 and 5, eruptions begin around the wrists, ankles, or forehead; within 2 days, they cover the entire body, including the scalp, palms, and soles. The rash consists of erythematous macules 0.04″ to 0.20″ (1 to 5 mm) in diameter that blanch on pressure; if untreated, the rash may become petechial

Close-up of a tick

Rocky Mountain spotted fever is transmitted by the bite of an adult tick like the one depicted below.

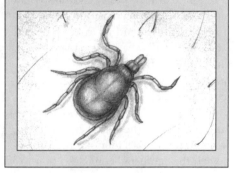

and maculopapular. By the third week, the skin peels off and may become gangrenous over the elbows, fingers, and toes.

The patient's pulse is strong initially, but gradually becomes rapid (possibly reaching 150 beats/minute) and thready. A rapid pulse rate and hypotension herald imminent death from complete vascular collapse.

Other signs and symptoms include:

- bronchial cough
- rapid respiratory rate (as many as 60 breaths/minute)
- anorexia
- constipation
- abdominal pain
- hepatomegaly
- splenomegaly
- insomnia
- restlessness
- delirium (in extreme cases).

Urine output decreases to half the normal level or less; the urine is dark and contains albumin.

Differential diagnoses

- Measles
- Meningoencephalitis

- Lyme disease
- Infectious mononucleosis
- Typhoid

Diagnosis

Diagnosis is usually based on a history of a tick bite or travel to a tick-infested area and a positive complement fixation test (which shows a fourfold increase in convalescent antibody titer compared with acute titers). Blood cultures should be performed to isolate the organism and confirm the diagnosis.

Another common but less reliable antibody test is the Weil-Felix reaction, which also shows a fourfold increase between the acute and convalescent sera titer levels. Increased titers usually develop after 10 to 14 days and persist for several months.

Additional recommended laboratory tests consist of a platelet count showing thrombocytopenia (12,000 to 150,000/µl) and a white blood cell count elevated to 11,000 to 33,000/µl during the 2nd week of illness.

Management

General

Treatment initially requires carefully removing the tick. Treatment also includes symptomatic measures.

Medication

Medications that may be used to treat a patient with RMSF include:
- chloramphenicol—50 to 100 mg/kg/day P.O. in 4 divided doses
- doxycycline—adults, 100 mg P.O. b.i.d. on 1st day, then 100 mg/day P.O.; children older than age 8 and weighing less than 99 lb (45 kg), 2.2 to 4.4 mg/kg P.O. in divided doses for 7 days
- acetaminophen—325 to 650 mg every 4 to 6 hours p.r.n.

Referral

- Refer the patient to an infectious disease specialist if complications occur.

Follow-up

The patient should be seen 2 days after treatment is initiated and when it's completed.

Patient teaching

- Instruct the patient to report any recurrent symptoms at once so that treatment measures may resume immediately.
- Advise the patient to avoid tick-infested areas (woods, meadows, streams, and canyons), if possible. If not possible, tell him to apply insect repellant to exposed skin and to clothing.
- Offer printed and illustrated instructions, if available, that teach the patient and family members or other caregivers how to correctly and safely remove a tick. Or show them how to use tweezers or forceps and how to apply steady traction to release the whole tick without leaving its mouth parts in the skin.

Complications

- Lobar pneumonia
- Otitis media
- Parotitis
- Disseminated intravascular coagulation
- Renal failure
- Death

• • • • • • • • • • • •

ROSEOLA INFANTUM

Roseola infantum (exanthema subitum), is an acute, benign, presumably viral infection. Characteristically, it first causes a high fever and then a rash that accompanies an abrupt drop to normal temperature.

Roseola affects boys and girls alike. It occurs year-round but is most prevalent in the spring and fall. Overt roseola, the most common exanthem in infants under age 2, affects 30% of all children; inapparent roseola (febrile illness without a rash) may affect the rest.

 AGE ALERT Roseola usually affects infants and young children ages 6 months to 3 years.

Causes

Human herpesvirus 6 is thought to cause roseola, although this is unconfirmed. The mode of transmission isn't known. Only rarely does an infected child transmit roseola to a sibling.

Clinical presentation

After a 10- to 15-day incubation period, the infant with roseola develops the following:
- abrupt increasing fever (peaks at 103° to 105° F [39.4° to 40.6° C] for 3 to 5 days then suddenly decreases)
- seizures
- anorexia
- irritability
- listlessness.

Simultaneously with an abrupt drop in temperature, the child develops a maculopapular, nonpruritic rash that blanches on pressure. The rash is profuse on the trunk, arms, and neck and mild on the face and legs. fading within 24 hours. Complications are extremely rare.

Differential diagnoses
- Measles
- Otitis media
- Meningitis
- Sepsis
- Rubella
- Drug eruption

Diagnosis

Diagnosis requires observation of the typical rash that appears about 48 hours after fever subsides.

Management
General

Because roseola is self-limiting, treatment is supportive and symptomatic.

Medication

Medications used to treat a patient with roseola may include:
- acetaminophen — follow package directions for dosage
- ibuprofen — follow package directions for dosage
- phenobarbital — 3 to 6 mg/kg/day P.O. in 2 divided doses (if seizures occur).

Referral
- If febrile seizures occur, refer the patient to the hospital.

Follow-up

The patient shouldn't need to be seen after the rash appears.

Patient teaching
- Teach parents how to reduce their infant's fever by giving tepid baths, keeping him in lightweight clothes, and maintaining normal room temperature.
- Stress the need for adequate fluid intake. Strict bed rest and isolation aren't necessary.

Complications
- Febrile seizures
- Encephalitis

• • • • • • • • • • • •

RUBELLA

Rubella, commonly called German measles, is an acute, mildly contagious viral disease that produces a distinctive 3-day rash and lymphadenopathy. Rubella flourishes worldwide during the spring (especially in big cities), and epidemics occur sporadically. This disease is self-limiting, with an excellent prognosis.

AGE ALERT Rubella usually occurs among children ages 5 to 9, adolescents, and young adults.

Causes
The rubella virus is transmitted through contact with the blood, urine, stool, or nasopharyngeal secretions of an infected person and, possibly, by contact with contaminated articles of clothing. Humans are the only known hosts for the rubella virus. The disease is contagious from about 10 days before the rash appears until 5 days after. Transplacental transmission, especially in the first trimester of pregnancy, can cause serious birth defects, such as microcephaly, mental retardation, patent ductus arteriosus, glaucoma, and bone defects. (See *Congenital rubella syndrome*.)

Clinical presentation
In children, after an incubation period of 14 to 21 days, an exanthematous, maculopapular rash erupts abruptly. (See *Incubation and duration of common rash-producing infections,* page 678.) In adolescents and adults, prodromal signs and symptoms appear first, including:
- headache
- malaise
- anorexia
- low-grade fever
- coryza
- lymphadenopathy
- conjunctivitis.

Suboccipital, postauricular, and postcervical lymph node enlargement is characteristic of this disease.

Typically, the rubella rash begins on the face and spreads rapidly, in many cases covering the trunk and extremities within hours. Small, red, petechial macules on the soft palate (Forschheimer spots) may precede or accompany the rash. By the end of the 2nd day, the facial rash begins to fade, but the rash on the trunk may be confluent and may be mistaken for scarlet fever. The rash continues to fade in the downward order in which it appeared. It generally disappears on the 3rd day, but may persist for 4 or 5 days, and is sometimes accompanied by mild coryza and conjunctivitis. The rapid appearance and disappearance of the rubella rash distinguishes it from rubeola. In rare cases, rubella can occur without a rash. Low-grade fever may accompany the rash (99° to 101° F [37.2° to 38.3° C]), but it usually doesn't persist after the 1st day of the rash; rarely, the patient's temperature reaches 104° F (40° C).

Differential diagnoses
- Rubeola
- Scarlet fever
- Drug eruptions
- Toxoplasmosis
- Infectious mononucleosis

With congenital rubella
- Cytomegalovirus
- Herpes simplex
- Varicella-zoster virus
- Poliovirus
- Congenital syphilis
- Hepatitis B

Diagnosis
The rubella rash, lymphadenopathy, other characteristic signs, and a history of exposure to an infected person usually permit clinical diagnosis without laboratory tests. However, cell cultures of the throat, blood, urine, and cerebrospinal fluid can confirm the virus' presence. Convalescent serum that shows a four-fold increase in antibody titers confirms the diagnosis.

Management

General

Because the rubella rash is self-limiting and only mildly pruritic, the patient doesn't require topical or systemic medication. Bed rest isn't necessary, but the patient should be isolated until the rash disappears.

Medication

A patient with rubella may be treated with the administration of acetaminophen. Follow package directions for dosage.

Referral

- Refer the patient to an infectious disease specialist if congenital rubella is confirmed.

Follow-up

The patient should be checked for improvement 3 days after the diagnosis is made.

HEALTHY LIVING Immunization with live virus vaccine RA27/3, the only rubella vaccine available in the United States, is necessary for prevention and appears to be more immunogenic than previous vaccines. The rubella vaccine should be given with measles and mumps vaccines at age 15 months to decrease the cost and number of injections.

Patient teaching

- Teach parents how to reduce their infant's fever by giving tepid baths, keeping him in lightweight clothes, and maintaining normal room temperature.

Complications

- Thrombocytopenic purpura
- Postinfectious encephalitis
- Congenital rubella
- Transient arthritis

Congenital rubella syndrome

Congenital rubella is by far the most serious form of rubella. Intrauterine rubella infection, especially during the first trimester, can lead to spontaneous abortion or stillbirth as well as single or multiple birth defects. (As a rule, the earlier the infection occurs during pregnancy, the greater the damage to the fetus.)

The combination of cataracts, deafness, and cardiac disease characterizes congenital rubella syndrome. Low birth weight, microcephaly, and mental retardation are other common manifestations. However, researchers now believe that congenital rubella can cause other disorders, many of which don't appear until later in life. These include dental abnormalities, thrombocytopenic purpura, hemolytic and hypoplastic anemia, encephalitis, giant-cell hepatitis, seborrheic dermatitis, and diabetes mellitus. Congenital rubella may be considered a lifelong disease; this theory is supported by the fact that the rubella virus has been isolated from urine 15 years after its acquisition in the uterus.

Infants born with congenital rubella should be isolated immediately because they excrete the virus for several months to a year after birth. Cataracts and cardiac defects may necessitate surgery. The prognosis depends on the particular malformations that occur. The overall mortality for infants with rubella is 6%, but this rate is higher for infants born with thrombocytopenic purpura, congenital cardiac disease, or encephalitis. Parents of affected children need emotional support and guidance in finding help from community resources and organizations.

Incubation and duration of common rash-producing infections

INFECTION	INCUBATION (DAYS)	DURATION (DAYS)
Herpes simplex	2 to 12	7 to 21
Roseola infantum	10 to 15	3 to 6
Rubella	14 to 21	3
Rubeola	8 to 14	5
Varicella	14 to 17	7 to 14

Special considerations

■ Report confirmed cases of rubella to local public health officials.
■ Give the vaccine at least 3 months after any administration of immune globulin or blood, which could have antibodies that neutralize the vaccine.

CLINICAL CAUTION Don't vaccinate any immunocompromised patients, patients with immunodeficiency diseases, or those receiving immunosuppressive, radiation, or corticosteroid therapy. Instead, administer immune serum globulin to prevent or reduce infection in susceptible patients.

• • • • • • • • • • • •

RUBEOLA

Rubeola, also known as measles or morbilli, is an acute, highly contagious paramyxovirus infection that may be one of the most common and most serious of all communicable childhood diseases. Use of the vaccine has reduced the occurrence of measles during childhood; as a result, measles is becoming more prevalent in adolescents and adults. (See *Administering the measles vaccine*.)

In temperate zones, incidence is highest in late winter and early spring. Before the availability of the measles vaccine, epidemics occurred every 2 to 5 years in large urban areas. In the United States, the prognosis is usually excellent; however, measles is a major cause of death in children in underdeveloped countries.

Causes

Measles is spread by direct contact or by contaminated airborne respiratory droplets. The portal of entry is the upper respiratory tract.

Clinical presentation

Incubation is from 8 to 14 days. Initial symptoms begin and greatest communicability occurs during the prodromal phase, about 11 days after exposure to the virus. This phase lasts from 4 to 5 days; signs and symptoms include:
■ fever
■ photophobia
■ malaise
■ anorexia
■ conjunctivitis
■ coryza
■ hoarseness
■ hacking cough.

Administering the measles vaccine

Generally, one bout of measles provides immunity (a second infection is extremely rare and may indicate a misdiagnosis); infants younger than age 4 months may be immune because of circulating maternal antibodies. Under normal conditions, measles vaccine isn't administered to children younger than age 15 months. However, during an epidemic, infants as young as 6 months may receive the vaccine and then be reimmunized at age 15 months. An alternative approach calls for administering gamma globulin to infants between ages 6 and 15 months who are likely to be exposed to measles.

The following are other guidelines for administering the measles vaccine:

■ Ask the patient about known allergies, especially to neomycin (each dose contains a small amount). *Note:* A patient who is allergic to eggs may receive the vaccine even though it contains minimal amounts of albumin and yolk components.

■ Avoid giving the vaccine to a pregnant woman (ask every woman for the date of her last menstrual period). Warn female patients to avoid pregnancy for at least 3 months after receiving the vaccine.

■ Don't vaccinate children with untreated tuberculosis, immunodeficiencies, leukemia, or lymphoma or those receiving immunosuppressants. If such children are exposed to the virus, recommend that they receive gamma globulin (gamma globulin won't prevent measles but will lessen its severity). Older unimmunized children who have been exposed to measles for more than 5 days may also require gamma globulin. Be sure to immunize them 3 months later.

■ Delay vaccination for 8 to 12 weeks after administration of whole blood, plasma, or gamma globulin because measles antibodies in these components may neutralize the vaccine.

■ Watch for signs of anaphylaxis for 30 minutes after vaccination. Have epinephrine 1:1,000 available.

■ Warn the patient or his parents that possible adverse effects are anorexia, malaise, rash, mild thrombocytopenia or leukopenia, and fever. Advise them that mild reactions may occur, usually within 7 to 10 days. If swelling occurs within 24 hours after vaccination, tell the patient to apply cold compresses to the injection site to promote vasoconstriction and to prevent antigenic cyst formation.

At the end of the prodromal phase, Koplik's spots, the hallmark of the disease, appear. These spots look like tiny, bluish white specks surrounded by a red halo. They appear on the oral mucosa opposite the molars and occasionally bleed. About 5 days after Koplik's spots appear, the patient's temperature rises sharply, spots slough off, and a slightly pruritic rash appears. This characteristic rash starts as faint macules behind the ears and on the neck and cheeks. The macules become papular and erythematous, rapidly spreading over the entire face, neck, eyelids, arms, chest, back, abdomen, and thighs. When the rash reaches the feet (2 to 3 days later), it begins to fade in the same sequence that it appeared, leaving a brownish discoloration that disappears in 7 to 10 days.

The disease climax occurs 2 to 3 days after the rash appears and is marked by a fever of 103° to 105° F (39.4° to 40.6° C), severe cough, puffy red eyes, and rhinorrhea. About 5 days after the rash appears, other symptoms disappear and communicability ends. Symptoms are usually mild in patients with partial immunity (conferred by administration of gamma globulin) or infants with transplacental antibodies. More severe symptoms and complications are more likely to develop in young infants, adolescents, adults, and immunocompromised patients than in young children.

Atypical measles may appear in patients who received the killed measles vaccine. These patients are acutely ill with a fever and maculopapular rash that's most obvious in the arms and legs or with pulmonary involvement and no skin lesions.

Differential diagnoses
- Drug eruption
- Rubella
- Roseola
- Erythema infectiosum
- Infectious mononucleosis

Diagnosis
Diagnosis rests on distinctive clinical features, especially Koplik's spots. Mild measles may resemble rubella, roseola infantum, enterovirus infection, toxoplasmosis, and drug eruptions; laboratory tests are required for a differential diagnosis. If necessary, measles virus may be isolated from the blood, nasopharyngeal secretions, and urine during the febrile period. Serum antibodies appear within 3 days after onset of the rash and reach peak titers 2 to 4 weeks later.

Management
General
Treatment for measles requires bed rest, relief of symptoms, and respiratory isolation throughout the communicable period. Vaporizers and a warm environment help reduce respiratory irritation, and an-

tipyretics can reduce fever. Therapy must also combat complications.

Medication
Medications that may be given in the treatment of rubeola include:
- acetaminophen — 325 to 650 mg P.O. every 4 to 6 hours p.r.n.
- immune globulin — 0.25 ml/kg I.M. within 6 days after exposure; for immunocompromised patients, 0.5 ml/kg I.M. within 6 days after exposure (maximum dose is 15 ml).

Referral
- Referral usually isn't needed.

Follow-up
The patient will need to be seen if complications occur.

Patient teaching
- Teach parents supportive measures, and stress the need for isolation, plenty of rest, and increased fluid intake. Advise them to cope with photophobia by darkening the room or providing sunglasses and to reduce fever by giving antipyretics and tepid sponge baths.
- Warn parents to watch for and report the early signs and symptoms of complications, such as encephalitis, otitis media, and pneumonia.

Complications
- Otitis media
- Bronchitis
- Pneumonia
- Encephalitis

• • • • • • • • • • • •

SALMONELLOSIS

Salmonellosis is caused by gram-negative bacilli of the genus *Salmonella,* a member of the Enterobacteriaceae family. It's a common infection in the United States, occurring as enterocolitis, bacteremia, localized infection, typhoid, or paratyphoid fever. Nontyphoidal forms usually produce mild to moderate illness with low mortality. (See *Types of salmonellosis,* page 682.)

Typhoid, the most severe form of salmonellosis, usually lasts from 1 to 4 weeks. Mortality is about 3% in patients who are treated. In those who are untreated, 10% of infections result in fatality, usually as a result of intestinal perforation or hemorrhage, cerebral thrombosis, toxemia, pneumonia, or acute circulatory failure. Salmonellosis is 20 times more common in patients with acquired immunodeficiency syndrome. Features are increased incidence of bacteremia, inability to identify the infection source, and tendency of infection recurring after therapy is stopped.

Causes

Of an estimated 1,700 serotypes of *Salmonella,* 10 cause the diseases most common in the United States; all 10 can survive for weeks in water, ice, sewage, or food. Nontyphoidal salmonellosis generally follows the ingestion of contaminated or inadequately processed foods, especially eggs, chicken, turkey, and duck. Proper cooking reduces the risk of contracting salmonellosis. Other causes include contact with infected people or animals or ingestion of contaminated dry milk, chocolate bars, or drugs of animal origin. Salmonellosis may occur in children under age 5 from fecal-oral spread. Enterocolitis and bacteremia are common (and more virulent) among infants, elderly people, and people already weakened by other infections; paratyphoid fever is rare in the United States.

Typhoid usually results from drinking water contaminated by excretions of a carrier or from ingesting contaminated

shellfish. (Contamination of shellfish occurs by leakage of sewage from offshore disposal systems.) Most typhoid patients are under age 30; most carriers are women over age 50. Incidence of typhoid in the United States is increasing as a result of travel to endemic areas.

Clinical presentation

Clinical manifestations of salmonellosis vary but usually include:
- fever
- abdominal pain
- severe diarrhea with enterocolitis.

Headache, increasing fever, and constipation are more common in typhoidal infection.

Differential diagnoses
- Viral gastroenteritis
- Bacterial infection from another source
- Pseudomembranous colitis
- Perforated viscous

Diagnosis

Generally, diagnosis depends on isolation of the organism in a culture, particularly blood (in typhoid, paratyphoid, and bacteremia) or feces (in enterocolitis, paratyphoid, and typhoid). Other appropriate culture specimens include urine, bone marrow, pus, and vomitus. In endemic areas, clinical symptoms of enterocolitis allow a working diagnosis before the cultures are positive. The presence of S. *typhi* in stool 1 or more years after treatment indicates that the patient is a carrier, which is true of 3% of patients.

Widal's test, an agglutination reaction against somatic and flagellar antigens, may suggest typhoid with a fourfold increase in titer. However, drug use or hepatic disease can also increase these titers and invalidate test results. Other supportive laboratory values that may be found include transient leukocytosis during the first week of typhoidal salmonel-

Types of salmonellosis

TYPE	CAUSE	CLINICAL FEATURES
Bacteremia	Any *Salmonella* species, but most commonly *S. choleraesuis;* incubation period varies	Fever, chills, anorexia, weight loss (without GI symptoms), and joint pain
Enterocolitis	Any species of nontyphoidal *Salmonella*, but usually *S. enteritidis;* incubation period, 6 to 48 hours	Mild to severe abdominal pain, diarrhea, sudden fever of up to 102° F (38.9° C), nausea, and vomiting; usually self-limiting, but may progress to enteric fever (resembling typhoid), local abscesses (usually abdominal), dehydration, and septicemia
Localized infections	Usually follows bacteremia caused by *Salmonella* species	Site of localization determines symptoms; localized abscesses may cause osteomyelitis, endocarditis, bronchopneumonia, pyelonephritis, and arthritis
Paratyphoid	*S. paratyphi* and *S. schottmuelleri* (formerly *S. paratyphi B*); incubation period, 3 weeks or more	Fever and transient diarrhea; generally resembles typhoid but less severe
Typhoid fever	*S. typhi* entering GI tract and invading the bloodstream via the lymphatics, setting up intracellular sites; during this phase, infection of biliary tract leading to intestinal seeding with millions of bacilli; involved lymphoid tissues (especially Peyer's patches in ilium) enlarging, ulcerating, and necrosing, resulting in hemorrhage; incubation period, usually 1 to 2 weeks	Symptoms of enterocolitis may develop within hours of ingestion of *S. typhi*; they usually subside before onset of typhoid fever symptoms *First week:* gradually increasing fever, anorexia, myalgia, malaise, headache, and slow pulse *Second week:* remittent fever up to 104° F (40° C) usually in the evening, chills, diaphoresis, weakness, delirium, increasing abdominal pain and distention, diarrhea or constipation, cough, moist crackles, tender abdomen with enlarged spleen, and maculopapular rash (especially on abdomen) *Third week:* persistent fever, increasing fatigue and weakness; usually subsides end of third week, although relapses may occur *Complications:* intestinal perforation or hemorrhage, abscesses, thrombophlebitis, cerebral thrombosis, pneumonia, osteomyelitis, myocarditis, acute circulatory failure, and chronic carrier state

losis, leukopenia during the third week, and leukocytosis in local infection.

Management

General

Treatment of the patient with salmonellosis includes bed rest and fluid and electrolyte replacement.

Medication

Antimicrobial therapy for typhoid, paratyphoid, and bacteremia depends on organism sensitivity but may not be necessary unless the infection spreads from the intestines. It may include:
- ampicillin — adults, 500 mg P.O. every 6 hours for 10 to 14 days; children weighing less than 88 lb (40 kg), 100 mg/kg/day in 4 divided doses
- ciprofloxacin — 500 mg P.O. every 12 hours for 3 to 7 days
- co-trimoxazole — adults, 1 double strength tablet P.O. every 12 hours for 10 to 14 days; children, 8 mg/kg/day trimethoprim and 50 mg/kg/day sulfamethoxazole in 2 divided doses for 10 to 14 days.

   Additional medication may include:
- diphenoxylate hydrochloride and atropine sulfate — adults, 5 mg P.O. p.r.n.; children, 0.3 to 0.4 mg/kg/day liquid form P.O. in 4 divided doses p.r.n.
- codeine — adults, 15 to 60 mg P.O., S.C., I.M., or I.V. every 4 to 6 hours p.r.n.; children, 0.5 mg/kg P.O., S.C., or I.M. every 4 hours p.r.n.

Surgical intervention

Localized abscesses may need surgical drainage. A patient with enterocolitis requires a short course of antibiotics only if it causes septicemia or prolonged fever.

Referral
- If the patient is severely dehydrated or septic, refer him to the hospital.

Follow-up

The patient should be seen 2 weeks after medication is initiated. Stool cultures should be repeated after 6 months and again after 1 year.

Patient teaching
- Teach the patient and family members the importance of proper hand washing.
- Tell the patient to use a different bathroom than other family members, if possible (while on antibiotics); to wash his hands afterward; and to avoid preparing uncooked foods, such as salads, for family members.

HEALTHY LIVING To prevent salmonellosis, advise patients to refrigerate meat and cooked foods promptly and to avoid consuming raw eggs or beverages made with raw eggs.

Complications
- Dehydration
- Hypovolemic shock
- Abscess formation
- Sepsis
- Toxic megacolon

Special considerations
- Report all infections caused by *Salmonella* to the state health department.
- An attack of typhoid confers lifelong immunity, although the patient may become a carrier.

• • • • • • • • • • • •

SHIGELLOSIS

Shigellosis, also known as bacillary dysentery, is an acute intestinal infection caused by the bacteria *Shigella*, a short, nonmotile, gram-negative rod. *Shigella* can be classified into four groups, all of which may cause shigellosis: group A (*S. dysenteriae*), which is most common in Central America and causes particularly severe infection and septicemia; group B (*S. flexneri*); group C (*S. boydii*); and group D (*S. sonnei*). Typically, shigellosis causes a high fever (especially in children), acute self-limiting diarrhea with tenesmus (ineffectual straining at stool) and, possibly, electrolyte imbalance and dehydration.

Shigellosis is endemic in North America, Europe, and the tropics. In the United States, about 18,000 cases appear annually, usually in children or in elderly, debilitated, or malnourished people. Shigellosis commonly occurs among confined populations such as those in mental institutions; it's also common in hospitals.

AGE ALERT Shigellosis is most common in children ages 1 to 4; however, many adults acquire the illness from children.

The prognosis is good. Mild infections usually subside within 10 days; severe infections may persist for 2 to 6 weeks. With prompt treatment, shigellosis is fatal in only 1% of cases; however, in severe *S. dysenteriae* epidemics, mortality may reach 8%.

Causes

Transmission occurs through the fecal-oral route, by direct contact with contaminated objects, or through ingestion of contaminated food or water. Occasionally, the housefly is a vector.

Clinical presentation

After an incubation period of 1 to 4 days, *Shigella* organisms invade the intestinal mucosa and cause inflammation. In children, shigellosis usually produces :
- high fever
- diarrhea with tenesmus
- nausea
- vomiting
- irritability
- drowsiness

- abdominal pain and distention.

Within a few days, the child's stool may contain pus, mucus, and—from the superficial intestinal ulceration typical of this infection—blood. Without treatment, dehydration and weight loss are rapid and overwhelming.

In adults, shigellosis produces sporadic, intense abdominal pain, which may be relieved at first by passing formed stools. Eventually, however, it causes rectal irritability, tenesmus and, in severe infection, headache and prostration. Stools may contain pus, mucus, and blood. In adults, shigellosis doesn't usually cause fever.

Differential diagnoses
- Ulcerative colitis
- Drug reaction
- Pseudomembranous colitis
- Diverticulitis
- Other bacterial source
- Viral enterocolitis

Diagnosis

Fever (in children) and diarrhea with stools containing blood, pus, and mucus point to this diagnosis; microscopic bacteriologic studies and culture help to confirm it.

Microscopic examination of a fresh stool may reveal mucus, red blood cells, and polymorphonuclear leukocytes; direct immunofluorescence with specific antisera, *Shigella*. Severe infection increases hemagglutinating antibodies. Sigmoidoscopy or proctoscopy may reveal typical superficial ulcerations.

Management
General

Treatment for a patient with shigellosis includes enteric precautions, low-residue diet and, most important, replacement of fluids and electrolytes with I.V. infusions of normal saline solution (with electrolytes) in sufficient quantities to maintain a urine output of 40 to 50 ml/hour.

Medication

The value of antibiotics is questionable, but they may be used in an attempt to eliminate the pathogen and thereby prevent further spread. They may include:
- ampicillin — adults, 500 mg P.O. every 6 hours for 10 to 14 days; children, 50 to 100 mg/kg/day in 4 divided doses
- ciprofloxacin — 500 mg P.O. every 12 hours
- co-trimoxazole — adults, 1 double strength tablet P.O. b.i.d. for 5 days; children, 8 mg/kg/day trimethoprim and 40 mg/kg/day sulfamethoxazole in 2 divided doses for 5 days.

Antidiarrheals that slow intestinal motility are contraindicated in shigellosis because they delay fecal excretion of *Shigella* and prolong fever and diarrhea. An investigational vaccine containing attenuated strains of *Shigella* appears to be promising in preventing shigellosis.

Referral

- Refer the patient to the hospital if he's severely dehydrated or producing bloody stools.

Follow-up

The patient should be seen in 5 days if diarrhea isn't resolved.

Patient teaching

- Encourage fluid intake to prevent dehydration.
- Teach the patient and family members the importance of proper hand washing.
- Tell the patient to use a different bathroom than other family members, if possible.

Complications

- Electrolyte imbalance
- Metabolic acidosis
- Shock
- Reiter's syndrome
- Conjunctivitis
- Iritis
- Arthritis
- Rectal prolapse
- Secondary bacterial infection
- Acute blood loss from mucosal ulcers
- Toxic neuritis

• • • • • • • • • • •

TETANUS

Tetanus, also known as lockjaw, is an acute exotoxin-mediated infection caused by the anaerobic, spore-forming, gram-positive bacillus *Clostridium tetani*. This infection is usually systemic; less often, localized. Tetanus is fatal in up to 60% of unimmunized people, usually within 10 days of onset. When symptoms develop within 3 days after exposure, the prognosis is poor.

Tetanus occurs worldwide, but it's more prevalent in agricultural regions and developing countries that lack mass immunization programs. It's one of the most common causes of neonatal deaths in developing countries, where neonates of unimmunized mothers are delivered under unsterile conditions. In such neonates, the unhealed umbilical cord is the portal of entry.

In the United States, approximately 110 cases occur each year, all in patients who aren't immunized or whose immunization has expired. About 75% of all cases occur between April and September.

HEALTHY LIVING Stress the importance of maintaining active tetanus immunization with a booster dose of tetanus toxoid every 10 years.

Causes

Normally, transmission occurs through a puncture wound that's contaminated by soil, dust, or animal excreta containing *C. tetani* or by way of burns and minor wounds. After *C. tetani* enters the body, it causes local infection and tissue necrosis. It also produces toxins that then enter the bloodstream and lymphatics and eventually spread to central nervous system tissue.

Clinical presentation

The incubation period varies from 3 to 4 weeks in mild tetanus to less than 2 days in severe tetanus. When symptoms occur within 3 days after injury, death is more likely. If tetanus remains localized, signs of onset are spasm and increased muscle tone near the wound.

If tetanus is generalized (systemic), indications include marked muscle hypertonicity, hyperactive deep tendon reflexes, tachycardia, profuse sweating, low-grade fever, and the following forms of painful, involuntary muscle contractions:
- neck and facial muscles, especially cheek muscles — locked jaw (trismus), painful spasms of masticatory muscles, difficulty opening the mouth, and *risus sardonicus*, a grotesque, grinning expression produced by spasm of facial muscles
- somatic muscles — arched-back rigidity (opisthotonos); boardlike abdominal rigidity
- intermittent tonic seizures lasting several minutes, which may result in cyanosis and sudden death by asphyxiation.

Despite such pronounced neuromuscular symptoms, cerebral and sensory functions remain normal. Complications include atelectasis, pneumonia, pulmonary emboli, acute gastric ulcers, flexion contractures, and cardiac arrhythmias.

Neonatal tetanus is always generalized. The first clinical sign is difficulty in sucking, which usually appears 3 to 10 days after birth. It progresses to total inability to suck with excessive crying, irritability, and nuchal rigidity.

Differential diagnoses

- Dental abscess
- Adverse effect of phenothiazines
- Strychnine poisoning
- Hypocalcemic tetany
- Meningitis
- Rabies

Diagnosis

In many cases, diagnosis must rest on clinical features, a history of trauma, and no previous tetanus immunization. Blood cultures and tetanus antibody tests may be negative; only one-third of patients have a positive wound culture. Cerebrospinal fluid pressure is sometimes greater than normal.

Management
General

The patient with tetany needs close airway maintenance, intravenous hydration, and quiet observation.

Medication

The patient with tetanus may require these medications:
- tetanus immune globulin — 3,000 to 6,000 U I.M.; infiltrate half around the wound and give the remainder I.M. in a different syringe
- tetanus toxoid — 0.5 ml I.M. (if not previously immunized); repeat in 1 month and in 6 to 12 months
- diazepam — adults, 5 to 10 mg I.M. or I.V. every 3 to 4 hours p.r.n.; children ages 30 days to 5 years, 1 to 2 mg I.M. or I.V. every 3 to 4 hours p.r.n.

Referral

- Refer the patient to the hospital for observation and treatment.

Follow-up
The patient should be seen after hospitalization, within 5 days.

Patient teaching
- Because even minimal external stimulation evokes muscle spasms, tell family members to keep the patient's room dark and quiet. Warn them not to upset or overstimulate the patient.
- Teach family members and the patient about the potential outcomes of this illness.

Complications
- Airway obstruction
- Respiratory arrest
- Heart failure
- Pneumonia
- Fractures
- Rhabdomyolysis
- Death

• • • • • • • • • • •

TOXOPLASMOSIS

Toxoplasmosis, one of the most common infectious diseases, is caused by the protozoa *Toxoplasma gondii*. It's found worldwide but is less common in cold or hot, arid climates and at high elevations. It usually causes localized infection but may produce significant generalized infection, especially in immunodeficient patients or neonates. Congenital toxoplasmosis, characterized by lesions in the central nervous system (CNS), may result in stillbirth or serious birth defects.

 CLINICAL CAUTION Pregnant women should avoid cleaning cat litter boxes to decrease the risk of contracting toxoplasmosis.

Causes
T. gondii exists in trophozoite forms in the acute stages of infection and in cystic forms (tissue cysts and oocysts) in the latent stages. Ingestion of tissue cysts in raw or uncooked meat (heating, drying, or freezing destroys these cysts) or fecal-oral contamination from infected cats transmits toxoplasmosis. However, toxoplasmosis also occurs in vegetarians who aren't exposed to cats, so other means of transmission may exist. Congenital toxoplasmosis follows transplacental transmission from a chronically infected mother or one who acquired toxoplasmosis shortly before or during pregnancy.

AGE ALERT Toxoplasmosis in the United States is most prevalent among women between ages 15 and 45.

Clinical presentation
Toxoplasmosis acquired in the first trimester of pregnancy commonly results in stillbirth. About one-third of neonates who survive have congenital toxoplasmosis. The later in pregnancy that maternal infection occurs, the greater the risk of congenital infection in the neonate. Obvious signs of congenital toxoplasmosis include:
- retinochoroiditis
- hydrocephalus or microcephalus
- cerebral calcification
- seizures
- lymphadenopathy
- fever
- hepatosplenomegaly
- jaundice
- rash.

Other defects, which may become apparent months or years later, include strabismus, blindness, epilepsy, and mental retardation. (See *Ocular toxoplasmosis*, page 688.)

Acquired toxoplasmosis can cause localized (mild lymphatic) or generalized (fulminating, disseminated) infection. Localized infection produces fever and a mononucleosis-like syndrome and lymphadenopathy. Generalized infection

Ocular toxoplasmosis

Ocular toxoplasmosis (active retino-choroiditis), characterized by focal necrotizing retinitis, accounts for about 25% of all cases of granulomatous uveitis. It's usually the result of congenital infection but may not appear until adolescence or young adulthood, when infection is reactivated. Symptoms include blurred vision, scotoma, pain, photophobia, and impairment or loss of central vision. Vision improves as inflammation subsides but usually without recovery of lost visual acuity. Ocular toxoplasmosis may subside after treatment with prednisone.

produces encephalitis, fever, headache, vomiting, delirium, seizures, and a diffuse maculopapular rash (except on the palms, soles, and scalp).

Differential diagnoses
- Lymphoma
- Infectious mononucleosis
- Cytomegalovirus
- Cat scratch disease
- Sarcoidosis
- Tuberculosis
- Carcinoma
- Leukemia

With congenital toxoplasmosis
- Rubella
- Cytomegalovirus
- Herpes simplex
- Syphilis
- Listeria
- Other infectious encephalopathies

Diagnosis
Identification of *T. gondii* in an appropriate tissue specimen confirms the diagnosis of toxoplasmosis. Serologic tests may be useful and, in patients with toxoplasmosis encephalitis, computed tomography scans and magnetic resonance imaging disclose lesions.

Management
General
Treatment for patients with toxoplasmosis is generally determined according to presenting symptoms. Comfort measures for fever, malaise, headache, and sore throat should be instituted.

Medication
Medications that may be used in combination to treat a patient with toxoplasmosis include:
- sulfadiazine — adults, 2 to 8 g P.O. in divided doses every 6 hours; children, 100 mg/kg/day up to 6 g/day
- pyrimethamine — adults, 50 to 75 mg P.O. (with sulfadiazine) for 1 to 3 weeks then reduce this dosage by half and continue for 4 to 5 weeks; children, 1 mg/kg/day P.O. initially in two equal doses for 2 to 4 days, then 0.5 mg/kg/day for 4 weeks.

Referral
- Refer the patient to the hospital if immunocompromised or having CNS effects.

Follow-up
The patient should be seen every 2 weeks until the condition improves, then monthly until treatment is concluded.

Patient teaching
- Teach all patients to wash their hands after working with soil (because it may be contaminated with cat oocysts), cook meat thoroughly and freeze it promptly if it isn't for immediate use, change cat litter daily (cat oocysts don't become infective until 1 to 4 days after excretion),

cover children's sandboxes, and keep flies away from food (flies transport oocysts).
■ Advise all pregnant women to avoid cleaning and handling cat litter boxes. If this can't be avoided, advise them to wear gloves.

Complications
■ Seizure disorder
■ Vision loss
■ Mental retardation
■ Deafness
■ Generalized infection
■ Stillbirth

Special considerations
■ Report all cases of toxoplasmosis to your local public health department.
■ Patients who are receiving immunosuppressants are susceptible to toxoplasmosis. Warn them of the risks and suggest having all cats that go outdoors tested for toxoplasmosis.

• • • • • • • • • • • •

VANCOMYCIN-RESISTANT ENTEROCOCCUS INFECTION

Vancomycin-resistant enterococcus (VRE) is a mutation of a very common bacterium that's spread easily by direct person-to-person contact. Facilities in more than 40 states have reported VRE infection, with rates as high as 14% in oncology units of large teaching facilities. Although difficult to treat, VRE is curable.

Causes
VRE enters health care facilities through an infected or colonized patient or a colonized health care worker. VRE spreads through direct contact between the patient and caregiver or between patients.

It can also be spread through patient contact with contaminated surfaces such as an overbed table. It's capable of living for weeks on surfaces. It has also been detected on patient gowns, bed linens, and handrails.

Patients most at risk for VRE infection include:
■ immunosuppressed patients or those with severe underlying disease
■ patients with a history of taking vancomycin, third-generation cephalosporins, or antibiotics targeted at anaerobic bacteria (such as *Clostridium difficile*)
■ patients with indwelling urinary or central venous catheters
■ elderly patients, especially those with prolonged or repeated hospital admissions
■ patients with cancer or chronic renal failure
■ patients undergoing cardiothoracic or intra-abdominal surgery or organ transplants
■ patients with wounds with an opening to the pelvic or intra-abdominal area, including surgical wounds, burns, and pressure ulcers
■ patients with enterococcal bacteremia, often associated with endocarditis
■ patients exposed to contaminated equipment or to a VRE-positive patient.

Clinical presentation
There are no specific signs or symptoms related to VRE infection. The causative agent may be found incidentally when culture results show the organism.

Differential diagnoses
■ Infection (by another source)

Diagnosis
Someone with no signs or symptoms of infection is considered colonized if VRE can be isolated from stool or a rectal swab.

When colonized, a patient is more than 10 times as likely to become infected with VRE, for example, through a breach in the immune system.

Management

General

There's no specific treatment at this time for eradicating VRE. Recently, the Centers for Disease Control and Prevention and the Hospital Infection Control Practices Advisory Committee proposed a two-level system of precautions to simplify isolation. The first level calls for standard precautions, which incorporate features of universal blood and body fluid precautions and body substance isolation precautions, to be used for all patient care. The second level calls for transmission-based precautions, which are implemented when a particular infection is suspected.

To prevent the spread of VRE, some facilities perform weekly surveillance cultures on at-risk patients in intensive care units or oncology units and on patients who were transferred from a long-term care facility. Any colonized patient is then placed in contact isolation until culture-negative or until discharged. Colonization can last indefinitely, and no protocol has been established for the length of time a patient should remain in isolation.

Medication

Medications used in the treatment of patients with VRE may include:
■ quinupristin/dalfopristin — 7.5 mg/kg I.V. infusion every 8 hours
■ linezolid — 600 mg P.O. every 12 hours for 14 to 28 days.

Referral

■ Refer the patient to the hospital for treatment, if appropriate.
■ The patient may need referral to an infectious disease specialist.

Follow-up

Follow-up depends on the type of VRE infection.

Patient teaching

■ Instruct family members and friends to wear protective garb around the patient, and teach them good hand-washing technique.
■ Instruct patients to take antibiotics for the full prescription period, even if they begin to feel better.

Complications

■ Sepsis

CLINICAL CAUTION Good hand washing is the most effective way to prevent VRE from spreading.

• • • • • • • • • • •

VARICELLA

Varicella, commonly known as chickenpox, is a common, acute, and highly contagious infection caused by the herpesvirus varicella-zoster, the same virus that, in its latent stage, causes herpes zoster (shingles).

There are approximately 3 million cases of varicella in the United States every year, with most cases occurring in late winter and spring. Chickenpox occurs worldwide and is endemic in large cities. Outbreaks occur sporadically, usually in areas with large groups of susceptible children. It affects all races and both sexes equally.

AGE ALERT Chickenpox can occur at any age, but 90% of cases occur in children younger than age 12.

Congenital varicella may affect neonates whose mothers had acute infections in their first or early second trimester. Neonatal infection is rare, probably because of transient maternal immunity. Second attacks are also rare.

Most children recover completely. Potentially fatal complications may affect children receiving corticosteroids, antimetabolites, or other immunosuppressants, and in those with leukemia, other neoplasms, or immunodeficiency disorders. Congenital and adult varicella may also have severe effects.

Causes
Varicella is transmitted by direct contact (primarily with respiratory secretions; less often, with skin lesions) and indirect contact (airwaves). The incubation period usually lasts 14 to 17 days. Chickenpox is probably communicable from 1 day before lesions erupt to 6 days after vesicles form (it's most contagious in the early stages of eruption of skin lesions).

Clinical presentation
Chickenpox produces distinctive signs and symptoms, notably a pruritic rash. During the prodromal phase, the patient has slight fever, malaise, and anorexia. Within 24 hours, the rash typically begins as crops of small, erythematous macules on the trunk or scalp that progress to papules and then clear vesicles on an erythematous base (the so-called dewdrop on a rose petal). The vesicles become cloudy and break easily; then scabs form.

The rash spreads to the face and over the trunk of the body, then to the limbs, buccal mucosa, axillae, upper respiratory tract, conjunctivae and, occasionally, the genitalia. New vesicles continue to appear for 3 or 4 days, so the rash contains a combination of red papules, vesicles, and scabs in various stages.

Congenital varicella causes hypoplastic deformity and scarring of a limb, retarded growth, and central nervous system and eye manifestations. In progressive varicella, an immunocompromised patient has lesions and a high fever for longer than 7 days.

Differential diagnoses
- Herpes simplex
- Herpes zoster
- Impetigo
- Coxsackievirus
- Scabies
- Drug rash

Diagnosis
Diagnosis rests on the characteristic clinical signs and usually doesn't require laboratory tests. However, the virus can be isolated from vesicular fluid within the 1st 3 or 4 days of the rash; Giemsa stain distinguishes varicella-zoster from vaccinia and variola viruses. Serum contains antibodies 7 days after onset.

Management
General
Chickenpox calls for strict isolation until all the vesicles and most of the scabs disappear (usually for 1 week after the onset of the rash). Children with only a few remaining scabs are no longer contagious and can return to school. Congenital chickenpox requires no isolation.

HEALTHY LIVING A vaccine for chickenpox has been available in the United States since 1995. It's effective 70% to 90% of the time. It should be administered between ages 12 months and 13 years. Adults receiving the vaccination need 2 doses for it to be optimally effective.

Medication
Medications used to treat a patient with chickenpox may include:
- acetaminophen—adults, 325 to 650 mg P.O. every 4 to 6 hours p.r.n.; children, follow instructions on package
- diphenhydramine—adults, 25 to 50 mg P.O. t.i.d. to q.i.d.; children weighing

greater than 20 lb (9 kg), 12.5 to 25 mg P.O. t.i.d. to q.i.d.

■ acyclovir — adults, 800 mg P.O. q.i.d. for 5 days; children weighing less than 88 lb (40 kg), 20 mg/kg/dose P.O. every 6 hours for 5 days

■ varicella-zoster immune globulin — adults and children, 625 U I.M. for 1 dose; children weighing less than 88 lb (40 kg), 125 U/10 kg I.M. for 1 dose

■ varicella vaccine — adults, 0.5 ml S.C. for 2 doses 4 to 8 weeks apart; children ages 12 months to 12 years, 0.5 ml S.C. for 1 dose.

Referral
■ The patient shouldn't need a referral unless complications occur.

Follow-up
There's no follow-up necessary unless complications occur.

Patient teaching
■ Teach the child and family members how to apply topical antipruritic medication correctly. Stress the importance of good hygiene.
■ Tell the patient not to scratch the lesions. However, because the need to scratch may be overwhelming, parents should trim the child's fingernails or tie mittens on his hands.
■ Warn parents to watch for and immediately report signs of complications. Severe skin pain and burning may indicate a serious secondary infection and require prompt medical attention.

Complications
■ Infection secondary to severe scratching
■ Scarring
■ Impetigo
■ Furuncles
■ Cellulitis
■ Pneumonia

■ Myocarditis
■ Fulminating encephalitis (Reye's syndrome)
■ Bleeding disorders
■ Arthritis
■ Nephritis
■ Hepatitis
■ Acute myositis

• • • • • • • • • • • •
VARIOLA

Variola, or smallpox, was an acute, highly contagious infectious disease caused by the poxvirus variola. After a global eradication program, the World Health Organization pronounced smallpox eradicated on October 26, 1979, 2 years after the last naturally occurring case was reported in Somalia. Vaccination is no longer recommended, except for certain laboratory workers. The last known case in the United States was reported in 1949. Although naturally occurring smallpox has been eradicated, variola virus preserved in laboratories remains an unlikely source of infection.

Smallpox developed in three major forms: *variola major* (classic smallpox), which carried a high mortality; *variola minor*, a mild form that occurred in nonvaccinated people and resulted from a less virulent strain; and *varioloid*, a mild variant of smallpox that occurred in previously vaccinated people who had only partial immunity.

Causes
Smallpox affected people of all ages. In temperate zones, incidence was highest during the winter; in the tropics, during the hot, dry months. Smallpox was transmitted directly by respiratory droplets or dried scales of virus-containing lesions or indirectly through contact with contaminated linens or other objects. Variola ma-

jor was contagious from onset until after the last scab was shed.

Clinical presentation

Characteristically, after an incubation period of 10 to 14 days, smallpox caused an abrupt onset of chills (and possible seizures in children), high fever (above 104° F [40° C]), headache, backache, severe malaise, vomiting (especially in children), marked prostration and, occasionally, violent delirium, stupor, or coma.

Two days after onset, symptoms became more severe, but by the 3rd day the patient began to feel better. However, the patient soon developed a sore throat and cough as well as lesions on the mucous membranes of the mouth, throat, and respiratory tract. Within days, skin lesions also appeared, progressing from macular to papular, vesicular, and pustular (pustules were as large as ⅓″ [8.5 mm] in diameter). During the pustular stage, the patient's temperature again rose, and early symptoms returned. By day 10, the pustules began to rupture and eventually dried and formed scabs. Symptoms finally subsided about 14 days after onset. Desquamation of the scabs took another 1 to 2 weeks, caused intense pruritus, and commonly left permanently disfiguring scars.

In fatal cases, a diffuse dusky appearance came over the patient's face and upper chest. Death resulted from encephalitic manifestations, extensive bleeding from any or all orifices, or secondary bacterial infections.

Differential diagnoses

- Measles
- Influenza

Diagnosis

Smallpox was readily recognizable, especially during an epidemic or after known contact. The most conclusive laboratory test was a culture of variola virus isolated from an aspirate of vesicles and pustules. Other laboratory tests included microscopic examination of smears from lesion scrapings and complement fixation to detect virus or antibodies to the virus in the patient's blood.

Management

General

The patient with smallpox would need immediate strict isolation. There's no cure for smallpox. Supportive measures to prevent dehydration and spread of infection would be required.

Medication

Medications used to treat a patient with smallpox may include:

- acetaminophen — 325 to 650 mg P.O. every 4 to 6 hours p.r.n.
- antibiotics — specific for isolated organism of secondary infection
- morphine — 2 to 10 mg every hour I.V. p.r.n.

Referral

- Refer the patient to the hospital for isolation and treatment, if appropriate.

Follow-up

Follow-up treatment depends on the extent and complications of the illness.

Patient teaching

- Teach family members the potential course of the illness.
- Stress to family members the importance of isolating the patient.

Complications

- Deafness
- Secondary infection
- Death
- Scarring
- Blindness

•••••••••••••

WEST NILE ENCEPHALITIS

West Nile encephalitis, like other encephalitic diseases, primarily causes an inflammation of the brain. The etiology stems from the West Nile virus, a flavivirus commonly found in humans, birds, and other vertebrates in Africa, West Asia, and the Middle East. This disease is part of a family of vectorborne diseases that also include malaria, yellow fever, and Lyme disease.

The virus was first documented in the Western Hemisphere late in August 1999. A virus found in numerous dead birds in New York, New Jersey, and Connecticut was identified by genetic sequencing as the West Nile virus. Scientists in the United States discovered the rare strain initially in and around the Bronx Zoo and believe birds may have carried the disease that spread as mosquitoes fed on the infected birds.

In temperate areas of the world, West Nile encephalitis cases occur mostly in late summer or early fall. In southern climates where temperatures are milder, West Nile encephalitis can occur year-round.

Health officials at the Centers for Disease Control and Prevention (CDC) have reported that, as of November 17, 1999, 56 cases (31 confirmed and 25 probable) of West Nile virus infection have been identified, including 7 deaths.

The risk of contracting West Nile encephalitis is greater for all residents of areas where active cases have been identified, but persons older than age 50 or those with compromised immune systems are at the greatest risk. At present, there's no documented evidence that a pregnant woman's fetus is at risk due to an infection with West Nile virus. The mortality rate of West Nile encephalitis is measured by case-fatality rates, which range from 3% to 15% (higher in the elderly population).

Causes

West Nile virus is transmitted to humans by the bite of a mosquito (primarily a *Culex* species) that's carrying the virus. They're considered the primary vector for West Nile virus and the source of the August 1999 outbreak in New York, New Jersey, and Connecticut. Mosquitoes become infected by feeding on birds contaminated with the West Nile virus and then transmitting the virus to humans and animals when taking a blood meal.

Ticks have been found infected with West Nile virus in Africa and Asia only. The role of ticks in the transmission and maintenance of the virus remains uncertain, and to date they aren't considered vectors for West Nile virus in the United States.

The CDC has reported that there's no evidence that a person can contract the virus from handling live or dead infected birds. However, avoid bare-handed contact when handling dead animals, including dead birds, and use gloves or double plastic bags to place the carcass in a garbage can. Report the finding to the nearest Emergency Management Office.

Clinical presentation

Mild infections by the virus are more common and include:
- fever
- headache
- body aches
- skin rash
- swollen lymph glands.

   Severe infections can be manifested by:
- headache
- high fever
- neck stiffness
- stupor
- disorientation

- coma
- tremors
- occasional convulsions
- paralysis
- death (rarely).

The incubation period for West Nile encephalitis is anywhere from 5 to 15 days after exposure.

Most patients bitten by an infected mosquito develop no symptoms at all. It's estimated that only 1 in 300 people bitten by infected mosquitoes actually get sick.

Differential diagnoses
- Encephalitis (from another source)
- Meningitis
- Seizure disorder
- Influenza
- Rocky Mountain spotted fever

Diagnosis
Obtain an extensive history of the patient's recent whereabouts within the last 2 to 3 weeks (especially around bodies of water, such as lakes and ponds), presence of dead birds, and recent mosquito bites.

The enzyme-linked immunosorbent assay (ELISA) is the test of choice for rapid definitive diagnosis. The major advantage of ELISA laboratory analysis is the high probability of accurate diagnosis of West Nile virus infection when performed only with acute serum or cerebrospinal fluid specimens obtained while the patient is hospitalized.

Encephalitis can be caused by numerous viral and bacterial infections, so all data must be examined to determine a definitive diagnosis.

Management
General
There's no specific therapy for treating patients with West Nile encephalitis and no known cure. Treatment is generally aimed at controlling specific symptoms.

Supportive care, such as I.V. fluid administration, fever control, and respiratory support is provided when necessary.

Medication
There's no vaccine to prevent West Nile encephalitis. The patient may be treated with acetaminophen (325 to 650 mg P.O. every 4 to 6 hours p.r.n.).

Referral
- Refer the patient to an infectious disease specialist.

Follow-up
Follow-up measures depend on the course of illness and complications that occur.

Patient teaching
- Teach family members and the patient about the expected course and outcomes of the illness.
- Encourage the patient to drink fluids to avoid dehydration.

HEALTHY LIVING To reduce the risk of infection with West Nile encephalitis, instruct persons at risk to:
– stay indoors at dawn and dusk and in the early evening
– wear long-sleeved shirts and long pants whenever outdoors
– apply insect repellent with diethyltoluamide sparingly to exposed skin. Spray clothing with repellents.

Complications
- Neurologic impairment
- Seizures
- Death

Special considerations
- Report any suspected cases of West Nile encephalitis to the appropriate state department of health.

• • • • • • • • • • • •

SELECTED REFERENCES

Bartlett, J.G. 2000 *Pocket Book of Infectious Disease Therapy*. Philadelphia: Lippincott Williams & Wilkins, 2000.

Fauci, A.S., et al., eds. *Harrison's Principles of Internal Medicine*, 15th ed. New York: McGraw-Hill Book Co., 2001.

Humes, H.D., et al. *Kelley's Textbook of Internal Medicine*, 4th ed. Philadelphia: Lippincott Williams & Wilkins, 2000.

Stone, D.R., and Gorbach, L.S. *Atlas of Infectious Disease*. Philadelphia: W.B. Saunders Co., 2000.

Dermatologic disorders

The skin and its appendages (the hair, the nails, and certain glands) protect the inner organs, bones, muscles, and blood vessels. They help to regulate body temperature and provide sensory information. What's more, they prevent body fluids from escaping and eliminate body wastes through more than 2 million pores.

• • • • • • • • • • •

ASSESSMENT

Assessment begins with a complete patient history. Remember that skin disorders may involve or stem from other disorders in other body systems. Don't discount minor symptoms or systemic complaints.

Physical examination
Physical assessment of the skin, hair, and nails requires inspection and palpation.

Preparing for skin assessment
Wash your hands and gather the necessary equipment: bright, even light source;

penlight; tongue blade; centimeter ruler; glass slide; flashlight with transilluminator; Wood's lamp (ultraviolet light); and gloves for palpating moist lesions or mucous membranes. (See *Keeping your patient comfortable*, page 698.) Sequentially expose areas for inspection and palpation.

Assessing appearance
Systematically assess all of the skin, hair, nails, and mucous membranes, even if the patient reports only a local lesion. Failure to assess the entire skin surface can lead to incorrect diagnosis.

Be alert for variations in lesion color, vascular supply, and pattern compared with other lesions. Also check for lesion distribution over the whole body.

Inspection
Begin by observing the patient's overall appearance from a distance of 3' to 5' (1 to 1.5 m), noting complexion, general color, color variations, and general appearance.

Note disturbances in pigmentation (light or dark areas compared with the rest of the skin), freckles, moles (nevi), and tanning (usually considered normal variations). Though usually benign, nevi that occur in large numbers (more than 40) and are irregular in size, shape, and color may be precursors to melanoma.

Next, note the color of healthy skin as well as problem areas. Rashes or lesions may range from red to brown to hypopigmented (as in vitiligo).

Alterations in skin vasculature usually appear as red or purple pigmented lesions. Some vascular lesions occur in people in good health. For example, blood vessel hypertrophy (enlargement) may result in hemangiomas, which vary from bright red to purple. Press on the lesion with a lucite rule or glass slide; observe and note the color change. Ecchymotic areas remain unchanged when pressure is applied, but areas of dilated blood vessels blanch (lose color or fade) when compressed. Permanently dilated superficial blood vessels (telangiectasia or spider veins) can indicate disease, but are normal in many cases.

Skin lesions
Carefully observe and document lesion morphology, distribution, and configuration.

MORPHOLOGY Note the lesion's size (measure and record its dimensions), shape or configuration, color, elevation or depression, pedunculation (connection to the skin by a stem or stalk), and texture. Note odor, color, consistency, and amount of exudate. Use a flashlight to assess the color of the lesion and elevation of its borders. Use a transilluminator to assess fluid in a lesion by darkening the room and placing the tip of the transilluminator against the side of the lesion: A fluid-filled lesion glows red, whereas a solid lesion does not. Use a Wood's lamp to assess pigmented or depigmented lesions.

Primary skin lesions appear on previously healthy skin in response to disease or external irritation. Modified lesions are described as secondary lesions. (See *Recognizing skin lesions*, pages 699 and 700.)

DISTRIBUTION. Assessment of distribution includes the extent and pattern of involvement. Is the pattern of lesions local (in one small area), regional (in one large area), or general (over the entire body)? Note characteristic locations, such as dermatomes (along cutaneous nerve endings), flexor or extensor surfaces, intertriginous areas, clothing or jewelry lines, or palms or soles. Also note if the lesions appear randomly.

CONFIGURATION. Is the pattern of lesions discrete (separate), grouped, linear, annular (circular), or arciform (arranged in a curve or arc)? Also note polycyclic (two or more circles of lesions) and dermatonal (along the course of cutaneous nerves) configurations.

Palpation
Assess skin texture, consistency, temperature, moisture, and turgor. Also use palpation to evaluate changes in or tenderness of particular lesions.

Recognizing skin lesions

The illustrations below depict the most common primary and secondary lesions.

PRIMARY LESIONS

Bulla
Fluid-filled lesion greater than ⅜″ (1 cm) in diameter (also called a blister) — for example, severe poison oak or ivy dermatitis, bullous pemphigoid, second-degree burn

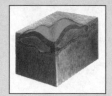

Macule
Flat, pigmented, circumscribed area less than ⅜″ (in diameter — for example, a freckle, rubella

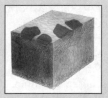

Nodule
Firm, raised lesion; deeper than a papule, extending into dermal layer more than ⅜″ in diameter — for example, intradermal nevus

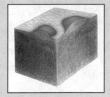

Papule
Firm, inflammatory, raised lesion less than ⅜″ in diameter; may be same color as skin or pigmented — for example, acne papule, lichen planus

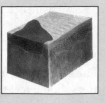

Patch
Flat, pigmented, circumscribed area greater than ⅜″ in diameter — for example, herald patch

Plaque
Circumscribed, solid, elevated lesion greater than ⅜″ in diameter; elevation above skin surface occupies larger surface area in comparison with height — for example, psoriasis

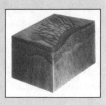

Pustule
Raised, circumscribed lesion usually less than ⅜″ in diameter; contains purulent material, making it a yellow-white color — for example, acne pustule, impetigo, furuncle

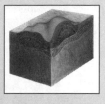

Tumor
Elevated solid lesion larger than ¾″ (1.9 cm) in diameter, extending into dermal and subcutaneous layers — for example, dermatofibroma

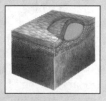

Vesicle
Raised, circumscribed, fluid-filled lesion less than ⅜″ in diameter — for example, herpes simplex

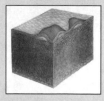

(continued)

Recognizing skin lesions (continued)

SECONDARY LESIONS

Crust
Dried sebum, serous, sanguineous, or purulent exudate, overlying an erosion or weeping vesicle, bullae, or pustule — for example, impetigo

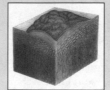

Erosion
Circumscribed lesion involving loss of superficial epidermis — for example, rug burn, abrasion

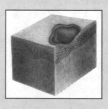

Excoriation
Linear scratched or abraded areas, may be self-induced — for example, abraded acne lesions, eczema

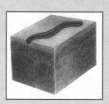

Fissure
Linear cracking of the skin extending into the dermal layer — for example, hand dermatitis (chapped skin)

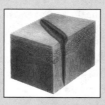

Lichenification
Thickened, prominent skin markings caused by constant rubbing — for example, chronic atopic dermatitis

Scale
Thin, dry flakes of shedding skin — for example, psoriasis, dry skin, newborn desquamation

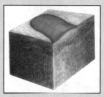

Scar
Fibrous tissue caused by trauma, deep inflammation, or surgical incision; red and raised (recent), pink and flat (6 weeks), or pale and depressed (old) — for example, a healed surgical incision

Ulcer
Epidermal and dermal destruction, may extend into subcutaneous tissue; usually heals with scarring — for example, pressure ulcer or stasis ulcer

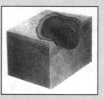

Texture and consistency
Skin texture refers to smoothness or coarseness; consistency refers to changes in skin thickness or firmness and relates more to changes associated with lesions.

While assessing texture and consistency, lightly rub the patient's skin. If it sloughs, leaving a moist base, this is a positive Nikolsky's sign, which characterizes staphylococcal scalded skin syndrome and other blistering conditions.

Temperature
The skin should feel warm to cool, and areas should feel the same bilaterally. A

localized area of warmth may indicate a bacterial infection such as cellulitis.

Turgor
Assess turgor by gently grasping and pulling up a fold of skin, releasing it, and observing how quickly it returns to normal shape. Normal skin usually resumes its flat shape immediately. Poor turgor may indicate dehydration and connective tissue disorders.

Lesions
Palpate skin lesions to obtain details about their morphology, distribution, location, and configuration.

Hair and scalp
Note the quantity, texture, color, and distribution of hair. Hair distribution varies greatly. Rub a few strands of hair between your index finger and thumb. Feel for dryness, brittleness, oiliness, and thickness.

Nails
Inspect the nails for color, consistency, smoothness, symmetry, and freedom from ridges and cracks as well as for length, jagged or bitten edges, and cleanliness.

Assess the nail base for firmness and the nail for firm adherence to the nail bed; sponginess and swelling accompany infection.

• • • • • • • • • • • •
ACNE VULGARIS

Acne vulgaris is an inflammatory disease of the sebaceous follicles that primarily affects adolescents. Although acne strikes boys more commonly and more severely, it usually occurs in girls at an earlier age and tends to last longer, sometimes into adulthood. The prognosis is good with treatment.

AGE ALERT Acne vulgaris usually occurs between ages 15 and 18, although lesions can appear as early as age 8.

Causes
The cause of acne is multifactorial, but theories regarding dietary influences appear to be groundless. Research now centers on follicular occlusion, androgen-stimulated sebum production, and *Propionibacterium acnes* as possible primary causes.

Predisposing factors include heredity; oral contraceptives (many females experience an acne flare-up during their first few menstrual cycles after starting or discontinuing oral contraceptives); androgen stimulation; certain drugs, including corticosteroids, corticotropin, androgens, iodides, bromides, trimethadione, phenytoin, isoniazid, lithium, and halothane; cobalt irradiation; and hyperalimentation. Other possible factors are trauma or rubbing from tight clothing, cosmetics, emotional stress, unfavorable climate, and exposure to heavy oils, greases, or tars.

More is known about the pathogenesis of acne. (See *What happens in acne*, page 702.) Androgens stimulate sebaceous gland growth and production of sebum, which is secreted into dilated hair follicles that contain bacteria. The bacteria, usually *P. acnes* and *Staphylococcus epidermidis* (which are normal skin flora), secrete lipase. This enzyme interacts with sebum to produce free fatty acids, which provoke inflammation. Also, the hair follicles produce more keratin, which joins with the sebum to form a plug in the dilated follicle.

Clinical presentation
The acne plug may appear as a closed comedo, or whitehead (if it doesn't protrude from the follicle and is covered by the epidermis), or as an open comedo, or

What happens in acne

In acne vulgaris, hormonal, bacterial, and inflammatory responses in the skin interact to produce the disorder.

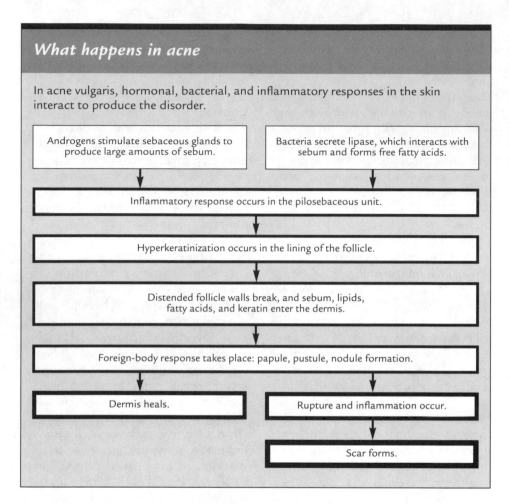

blackhead (if it does protrude and isn't covered by the epidermis). The black coloration is caused by the melanin or pigment of the follicle. Rupture or leakage of an enlarged plug into the dermis produces:
- inflammation and characteristic acne pustules
- papules
- acne cysts or abscesses (severe).

Chronic, recurring lesions produce acne scars.

Differential diagnoses
- Adult acne rosacea
- Folliculitis
- Tinea infections

Diagnosis
The appearance of characteristic acne lesions, especially in an adolescent patient, confirms the presence of acne vulgaris.

Management
General
Exposure to ultraviolet light (but never when a photosensitizing agent such as tretinoin is being used) and cryotherapy may be used to treat acne vulgaris.

Medication
Current therapy for acne includes topical and oral agents. The treatment for non-inflammatory acne consisting of open and closed comedones is:

- tretinoin gel—apply to affected area nightly initially, then every other night
- benzoyl peroxide—initially 5% applied to skin b.i.d.; increased strength as needed
- tetracycline—initially 250 mg P.O. every 6 hours, then 125 to 500 mg/day P.O. or every other day or 0.22% solution applied to skin b.i.d.
- erythromycin—500 mg P.O. b.i.d. for 3 to 6 weeks or 2% solution or gel applied to skin b.i.d.
- clindamycin 1% solution, gel, or lotion—thin film b.i.d., topical and systemic
- doxycycline—50 to 200 mg/day P.O.
- minocycline—50 to 200 mg/day P.O.
- isotretinoin—0.5 to 2mg/kg/day P.O. in two divided doses.

Because of its severe adverse effects, the 16- to 20-week course of isotretinoin is limited to people with severe papulopustular or cystic acne that doesn't respond to conventional therapy. Because this drug is known to cause birth defects, the manufacturer, with the Food and Drug Administration's approval, recommends these precautions:
- testing for pregnancy before dispensing
- dispensing only a 30-day supply
- repeating pregnancy testing throughout the treatment period
- providing effective contraception during treatment
- obtaining informed consent of the patient or parents regarding the drug's adverse effects.

Exacerbation of pustules or abscesses during antibiotic therapy requires a culture to identify a possible secondary bacterial infection.

Referral
- Refer a patient with moderate acne that resists conventional therapy to a dermatologist.
- If appropriate, refer the patient for counseling.

Follow-up
The patient should initially be seen monthly to evaluate treatment. A serum triglyceride level and liver enzymes should be measured before isotretinoin therapy begins and at 2-week intervals throughout its course.

Patient teaching
- Explain the causes of acne to the patient and family. Make sure they understand that the prescribed treatment is more likely to improve acne than a strict diet and fanatical scrubbing with soap and water. Provide written instructions regarding treatment.
- Tell the patient taking isotretinoin to avoid vitamin A supplements, which can worsen adverse effects. Also, teach him how to deal with the dry skin and mucous membranes that usually occur during treatment. Tell the female patient about the severe risk of teratogenicity. Monitor liver function and lipid levels.
- Inform the patient that acne takes a long time to clear—possibly even years for complete resolution. Encourage continued local skin care even after acne clears. Explain the adverse effects of all drugs.

Complications
- Scarring
- Secondary bacterial infection
- Acne conglobata
- Psychological scarring

Special considerations
- Pay special attention to the patient's perception of his physical appearance; he may need emotional support.

• • • • • • • • • • • •

ALOPECIA

Alopecia, or hair loss, usually occurs on the scalp but can also occur on bearded areas, eyebrows, and eyelashes. Hair loss elsewhere on the body is less common and less conspicuous. In the nonscarring form of this disorder (noncicatricial alopecia), hair loss may occur in association with many systemic diseases and the hair follicle can generally regrow hair. Scarring alopecia usually destroys the hair follicle, making hair loss irreversible. The most common form of nonscarring alopecia is male pattern alopecia, which appears to be related to androgen levels and aging. Genetic predisposition commonly influences time of onset, degree of baldness, speed with which it spreads, and pattern of hair loss. Women may experience diffuse thinning over the top of the scalp.

Other forms of nonscarring alopecia include:

- physiologic alopecia (usually temporary) — sudden hair loss in infants, loss of straight hairline in adolescents, and diffuse hair loss after childbirth
- alopecia areata (idiopathic form) — generally reversible and self-limiting; occurs most commonly in young and middle-age adults of both sexes (see *Alopecia areata*)
- trichotillomania — compulsive pulling out of one's own hair; most common in children.

Causes

Predisposing factors of nonscarring alopecia include radiation, many types of drug therapies and drug reactions, bacterial and fungal infections, psoriasis, seborrhea, and endocrine disorders, such as thyroid, parathyroid, and pituitary dysfunctions.

Scarring alopecia causes irreversible hair loss. It may result from physical or chemical trauma or chronic tension on a hair shaft, as occurs in braiding. Diseases that produce alopecia include destructive skin tumors, granulomas, lupus erythematosus, scleroderma, follicular lichen planus, and severe fungal, bacterial, or vi-

ral infections, such as kerion, folliculitis, or herpes simplex.

Clinical presentation

In male pattern alopecia, hair loss is gradual and usually affects the thinner, shorter, and less pigmented hairs of the frontal and parietal portions of the scalp. In women, hair loss is generally more diffuse; completely bald areas are uncommon but may occur.

Alopecia areata affects small patches of the scalp but may also occur as alopecia totalis, which involves the entire scalp, or as alopecia universalis, which involves the entire body. Although mild erythema may occur initially, affected areas of scalp or skin appear normal. "Exclamation point" hairs (loose hairs with dark, rough, brushlike tips on narrow, less pigmented shafts) occur at the periphery of new patches. Regrowth initially appears as fine, white, dry hair, which is replaced by normal hair.

In trichotillomania, patchy, incomplete areas of hair loss with many broken hairs appear on the scalp but may occur on other areas such as the eyebrows.

Differential diagnoses

- Bacterial infection
- Fungal infection
- Systemic disorders
- Secondary syphilis
- Thyroid disease
- Iron deficiency anemia
- Pituitary insufficiency

Diagnosis

Physical examination is usually sufficient to confirm alopecia. In trichotillomania, an occlusive dressing can establish the diagnosis by allowing new hair to grow, revealing that the hair is being pulled out. Diagnosis must also identify an underlying disorder.

Management
General
Hair loss that persists for longer than 1 year has a poor prognosis for regrowth. In trichotillomania, an occlusive dressing encourages normal hair growth simply by identifying the cause of hair loss.

Medication
The following medications are used for androgenic alopecia:
- minoxidil — 1 ml to total affected areas of the scalp b.i.d.
- finasteride — 1 mg/day P.O.
- estradiol — 0.5 to 2 mg P.O. in cycles of 21 days on and 7 days off (most effective in postmenopausal women).

The following medications are used for alopecia areata:
- hydrocortisone cream or gel — apply small amount to area q.d. to q.i.d. (beneficial for small patches and may produce regrowth in 4 to 6 weeks)
- cortisone — local injection to affected area monthly
- minoxidil — 1 ml to affected areas b.i.d.
- anthralin cream — apply to area once daily; remove after 1 hour.

Surgical intervention
An alternative treatment is surgical redistribution of hair follicles by autografting.

Referral
- Refer the patient to a dermatologist.
- Refer the patient to a local chapter of the National Alopecia Areata Foundation for further information and support.
- Refer the patient for counseling, if appropriate.

Follow-up
The patient should be seen every 4 months or as required by the dermatologist.

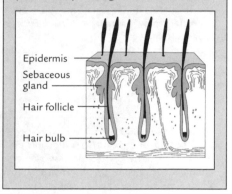

Alopecia areata

"Exclamation point" hairs commonly border new patches of alopecia areata. Not seen in any other type of alopecia, these hairs indicate that the patch is expanding.

Epidermis
Sebaceous gland
Hair follicle
Hair bulb

Patient teaching
- If the patient has alopecia areata, explain the disorder and give reassurance that complete regrowth is possible.
- Teach the patient about medications and their adverse effects.
- Tell the patient the reason for hair loss and if regrowth is possible.

Complications
- Psychological problems

Special considerations
- Reassure a woman with female pattern alopecia that it doesn't lead to total baldness. Suggest that she wear a wig.

• • • • • • • • • • • •

ATOPIC DERMATITIS

Atopic dermatitis, or eczema, is a chronic skin disorder that's characterized by superficial skin inflammation and intense itching. (See *Types of dermatitis*, pages 706 to 709.) Although this disorder may (*Text continues on page 708.*)

Types of dermatitis

TYPE	CAUSES	SIGNS AND SYMPTOMS
Seborrheic dermatitis An acute or subacute skin disease that affects the scalp, face, and occasionally other areas and is characterized by lesions covered with yellow or brownish gray scales	■ Unknown; stress and neurologic conditions may be predisposing factors; may be related to the yeast *Malassezia ovalis*	■ Eruptions in areas with many sebaceous glands (usually scalp, face, and trunk) and in skin folds ■ Itching, redness, and inflammation of affected areas; lesions may appear greasy; fissures may occur ■ Indistinct, occasionally yellowish, scaly patches from excess stratum corneum (dandruff may be a mild seborrheic dermatitis) ■ Generally worse in winter
Nummular dermatitis Chronic form of dermatitis that's characterized by inflammation of coin-shaped, vesicular, crusted scales and, possibly, pruritic lesions	■ Possibly precipitated by stress, skin dryness, irritants, scratching, or bathing with hot water	■ Round, nummular (coin-shaped) lesions, usually on arms and legs, with distinct borders of crusts and scales ■ Possible oozing and severe itching ■ Summertime remissions common, with wintertime recurrence
Contact dermatitis Often sharply demarcated inflammation and irritation of the skin due to contact with concentrated substances to which the skin is sensitive, such as perfumes, soaps, or chemicals	■ Mild irritants: chronic exposure to detergents or solvents ■ Strong irritants: damage on contact with acids or alkalis ■ Allergens: sensitization after repeated exposure	■ Mild irritants and allergens: erythema and small vesicles that ooze, scale, and itch ■ Strong irritants: blisters and ulcerations ■ Classic allergic response: clearly defined lesions, with straight lines following points of contact ■ Severe allergic reaction: marked edema of affected areas
Chronic dermatitis Characterized by inflammatory eruptions of the hands and feet	■ Usually unknown but may result from progressive contact dermatitis ■ Secondary (possibly perpetuating) factors: trauma, infections, redistribution of normal flora, photosensitivity, and food sensitivity	■ Thick, lichenified, single or multiple lesions on any part of the body (commonly on the hands) ■ Inflammation and scaling ■ Recurrence following long remissions

DIAGNOSIS	TREATMENT AND INTERVENTION
■ Patient history and physical findings, especially distribution of lesions in sebaceous gland areas, confirm seborrheic dermatitis. ■ Diagnosis must rule out psoriasis.	■ Removal of scales with frequent washing and shampooing with selenium sulfide suspension (most effective), zinc pyrithione, or tar and salicylic acid shampoo ■ Application of fluorinated corticosteroids to nonhairy areas
■ Physical findings and patient history confirm nummular dermatitis; a middle-age or older patient may have a history of atopic dermatitis. ■ Diagnosis must rule out fungal infections, atopic or contact dermatitis, and psoriasis.	■ Elimination of known irritants ■ Measures to relieve dry skin: increased humidification, limited frequency of baths and use of bland soap and bath oils, and application of emollients ■ Application of wet dressings in acute phase ■ Topical corticosteroids (occlusive dressings or intralesional injections) for persistent lesions ■ Tar preparations and antihistamines to control itching ■ Antibiotics for secondary infection ■ Other interventions as for atopic dermatitis
■ Patient history, patch testing to identify allergens, and shape and distribution of lesions suggest contact dermatitis.	■ Elimination of known allergens and decreased exposure to irritants; wearing protective clothing such as gloves; and washing immediately after contact with irritants or allergens ■ Topical anti-inflammatory agents (including corticosteroids), systemic corticosteroids for edema and bullae, antihistamines, and local applications of Burow's solution (for blisters) ■ Montoring for sensitization to topical medications ■ Other interventions as for atopic dermatitis
■ No characteristic pattern or course; diagnosis of chronic dermatitis relies on detailed patient history and physical findings.	■ Antibiotics for secondary infection ■ Avoidance of excessive washing and drying of hands and of accumulation of soaps and detergents under rings ■ Use of emollients with topical steroids ■ Other interventions as for contact dermatitis

(continued)

Types of dermatitis (continued)

TYPE	CAUSES	SIGNS AND SYMPTOMS
Localized neurodermatitis (lichen simplex chronicus, essential pruritus)		
Superficial inflammation of the skin characterized by itching and papular eruptions that appear on thickened, hyperpigmented skin	• Chronic scratching or rubbing of a primary lesion, insect bite, or other skin irritation	• Intense, sometimes continual scratching • Thick, sharp-bordered, possibly dry, scaly lesions with raised papules • Usually affects easily reached areas, such as ankles, lower legs, anogenital area, back of neck, and ears
Exfoliative dermatitis		
Severe, chronic skin inflammation characterized by redness and widespread erythema and scaling	• Usually, preexisting skin lesions progress to exfoliative stage, such as in contact dermatitis, drug reaction, lymphoma, or leukemia	• Generalized dermatitis, with acute loss of stratum corneum, and erythema and scaling • Sensation of tight skin • Hair loss • Possible fever, sensitivity to cold, shivering, gynecomastia, and lymphadenopathy
Stasis dermatitis		
Condition usually caused by impaired circulation and characterized by eczema of the legs with edema, hyperpigmentation, and persistent inflammation	• Secondary to peripheral vascular diseases affecting legs, such as recurrent thrombophlebitis and resultant chronic venous insufficiency	• Varicosities and edema common, but obvious vascular insufficiency not always present • Usually affects the lower leg, just above internal malleolus, or sites of trauma or irritation • Early signs: dusky red deposits of hemosiderin in skin, with itching and dimpling of subcutaneous tissue. Later signs: edema, redness, and scaling of large area of legs • Possible fissures, crusts, and ulcers

appear at any age, it typically begins during infancy or early childhood. It may then subside spontaneously, followed by exacerbations in late childhood, adolescence, or early adulthood. Atopic dermatitis affects approximately 3% of the U.S. population.

Causes

The cause of atopic dermatitis is unknown. However, several theories attempt to explain its pathogenesis. One theory suggests an underlying metabolically or biochemically induced skin disorder that's genetically linked to elevated serum immunoglobulin E (IgE) levels.

DIAGNOSIS	TREATMENT AND INTERVENTION
■ Physical findings confirm diagnosis of localized neurodermatitis.	■ Elimination of scratching so lesions will disappear (takes about 2 weeks) ■ Fixed dressing or Unna's boot to cover affected area ■ Topical corticosteroids under occlusion or by intralesional injection ■ Antihistamines and open wet dressings ■ Emollients ■ Discussion of underlying cause with patient
■ Diagnosis of exfoliative dermatitis requires identification of the underlying cause.	■ Hospitalization, with protective isolation and hygienic measures to prevent secondary bacterial infection ■ Open wet dressings, with colloidal baths ■ Bland lotions over topical corticosteroids ■ Maintenance of constant environmental temperature to prevent chilling or overheating ■ Careful monitoring of renal and cardiac status ■ Systemic antibiotics and steroids ■ Other interventions as for atopic dermatitis
■ Diagnosis of stasis dermatitis requires positive history of venous insufficiency and physical findings such as varicosities.	■ Measures to prevent venous stasis: avoidance of prolonged sitting or standing, use of support stockings, and weight reduction in obesity ■ Corrective surgery for underlying cause ■ After ulcer develops, encourage rest periods, with legs elevated; open, wet dressings; Unna's boot (zinc gelatin dressing provides continuous pressure to affected areas); and antibiotics for secondary infection after wound culture

Another theory suggests defective T-cell function.

Exacerbating factors of atopic dermatitis include irritants, infections (commonly caused by *Staphylococcus aureus*), and some allergens. Although no reliable link exists between atopic dermatitis and exposure to inhalant allergens (such as house dust and animal dander), exposure to food allergens (such as soybeans, fish, and nuts) may coincide with flare-ups of atopic dermatitis.

Clinical presentation

Scratching the skin causes vasoconstriction and intensifies pruritus, resulting in erythematous, weeping lesions. Eventually, the lesions become scaly and lichenified. Usually, they're located in areas of flexion and extension, such as the neck, antecubital fossa, popliteal folds, and behind the ears. A patient with atopic dermatitis is prone to unusually severe viral infections, bacterial and fungal skin infections, ocular complications, and allergic contact dermatitis.

Differential diagnoses
- Photosensitivity rash
- Contact dermatitis
- Seborrheic dermatitis
- Scabies
- Psoriasis
- Ichthyosis
- Lichen simplex chronicus

Diagnosis
Typically, the patient has a history of atopy, such as asthma, hay fever, or urticaria; his family may have a similar history. Laboratory tests reveal eosinophilia and elevated serum IgE levels. In addition, other types of dermatitis must have been ruled out.

Management
General
Measures to ease this chronic disorder include meticulous skin care, environmental control of offending allergens, and drug therapy. Because dry skin aggravates itching, frequent application of nonirritating topical lubricants is important, especially after bathing or showering. Minimizing exposure to allergens and irritants, such as wools and harsh detergents, also helps control symptoms.

Medication
The following medications may be used in the treatment of atopic dermatitis:
- hydrocortisone 1% cream—apply to area b.i.d to q.i.d.
- fluocinolone acetonide—apply to area b.i.d to q.i.d.
- flurandrenolide—apply to area b.i.d to t.i.d.
- hydroxyzine—25 mg P.O. q.i.d.; children ages 6 to 12 years, 50 to 100 mg P.O. in divided doses; children younger than age 6, 50 mg/day in divided doses.

If secondary infection develops, antibiotics are necessary.

Referral
- Because this disorder may frustrate the patient and strain family ties, counseling may play a role in treatment.
- Refer the patient to a dermatologist if he doesn't respond to conventional treatment.

Follow-up
The patient should be seen in 1 week and then 1 month or as required by the dermatologist.

Patient teaching
- Teach the patient when and how to apply topical corticosteroids.
- Emphasize the importance of regular personal hygiene using only water with minimal use of soap.
- Teach the patient how to recognize signs and symptoms of secondary infection
- If the patient's diet is modified to exclude food allergens, monitor his nutritional status.

Complications
- Secondary skin infection
- Adverse effects from cortisone treatment
- Psychological problems

Special considerations
- Discourage use of laundry additives.
- Dissuade the patient from scratching during urticaria to help prevent infection.

••••••••••••
BASAL CELL EPITHELIOMA

Basal cell epithelioma, also known as basal cell carcinoma, is a slow-growing, destructive skin tumor. This carcinoma typically occurs in people over age 40; it's more prevalent in blond, fair-skinned males and is the most common malignant tumor affecting whites. It affects approximately one million Americans each year and is the most common type of cancer.

Causes
Prolonged sun exposure is the most common cause of basal cell epithelioma, but arsenic ingestion, radiation exposure, burns, and immunosuppression are other possible causes.

Although the pathogenesis of basal cell epithelioma is uncertain, some experts now hypothesize that it originates when, under certain conditions, undifferentiated basal cells become carcinomatous instead of differentiating into sweat glands, sebum, and hair.

Clinical presentation
Three types of basal cell epithelioma occur:
- Noduloulcerative lesions usually occur on the face, particularly the forehead, eyelid margins, and nasolabial folds. In early stages, these lesions are small, smooth, pinkish, translucent papules. Telangiectatic vessels cross the surface, and the lesions are occasionally pigmented. As the lesions enlarge, their centers become depressed and their borders become firm and elevated. Ulceration and local invasion eventually occur. These ulcerated tumors, known as "rodent ulcers," rarely metastasize. However, if untreated, they can spread to vital areas and become infected or cause massive hemorrhage if they invade large blood vessels.
- Superficial basal cell epitheliomas are multiple in many cases and commonly occur on the chest and back. They're oval or irregularly shaped, lightly pigmented plaques with sharply defined, slightly elevated threadlike borders. Due to superficial erosion, these lesions appear scaly and have small, atrophic areas in the center that resemble psoriasis or eczema. They're usually chronic and tend not to invade other areas. Superficial basal cell epitheliomas are related to ingestion of or exposure to arsenic-containing compounds.
- Sclerosing basal cell epitheliomas (morphea-like epitheliomas) are waxy, sclerotic, yellow to white plaques without distinct borders. Occurring on the head and neck, sclerosing basal cell epitheliomas may look like small patches of scleroderma.

Differential diagnoses
- Actinic keratosis
- Leukoplakia
- Sebaceous hyperplasia
- Common nevus
- Seborrheic keratosis
- Molluscum contagiosum

Diagnosis
All types of basal cell epitheliomas are diagnosed by clinical appearance, incisional or excisional biopsy, and histologic study.

Management
General
Irradiation is used for tumor locations and for elderly or debilitated patients who might not withstand surgery. Cryotherapy with liquid nitrogen freezes and kills the cells.

Medication

For superficial lesions, apply 5-fluorouracil cream or solution to the affected area 1 to 2 times daily for 2 to 6 weeks.

Surgical intervention

Curettage and electrodesiccation offer good cosmetic results for small lesions. Microscopically controlled surgical excision carefully removes recurrent lesions until a tumor-free plane is achieved. After removal of large lesions, skin grafting may be required.

Chemosurgery is generally necessary for persistent or recurrent lesions. Chemosurgery consists of periodic applications of a fixative paste (such as zinc chloride) and subsequent removal of fixed pathologic tissue. Treatment continues until tumor removal is complete.

Referral

- The patient may need to be referred to a dermatologist for treatment.

Follow-up

The patient should be seen every month for 3 months and then every 6 months, or as required by the dermatologist.

Patient teaching

- Instruct the patient to eat frequent small meals that are high in protein. Suggest "blenderized" foods or liquid protein supplements if the lesion has invaded the oral cavity and causes eating problems.
- Advise the patient to relieve local inflammation from topical fluorouracil with cool compresses or corticosteroid ointment.
- Instruct the patient with noduloulcerative basal cell epithelioma to wash his face gently when ulcerations and crusting occur; scrubbing too vigorously may cause bleeding.

HEALTHY LIVING Tell the patient to avoid excessive sun exposure and to always use a strong sunscreen or sunshade to protect his skin from damage by ultraviolet rays in order to prevent basal cell epithelioma.

Complications

- Local recurrence
- Metastasis

• • • • • • • • • • • •

CORNS AND CALLUSES

Corns and calluses are acquired skin conditions marked by hyperkeratosis of the stratum corneum, usually on areas of repeated trauma (especially the feet). The prognosis is good with proper foot care.

Causes and incidence

A corn (also known as a clavus) is a hyperkeratotic area that usually results from external pressure, such as that from ill-fitting shoes or, less commonly, from internal pressure, such as that caused by a protruding underlying bone (due to arthritis, for example). A callus, generally found on the foot or hand, is an area of thickened skin produced by external pressure or friction. People whose activities produce repeated trauma (for example, manual laborers or guitarists) commonly develop calluses.

The severity of a corn or callus depends on the degree and duration of trauma.

Clinical presentation

Corns and calluses cause pain through pressure on underlying tissue by localized thickened skin. Corns contain a central keratinous core, are smaller and more clearly defined than calluses, and are usually more painful. The pain they cause may be dull and constant or sharp when pressure is applied. Soft corns have the following features:

- caused by the pressure of a bony prominence
- appear as whitish thickenings
- commonly found between toes, most often in the fourth interdigital web.

Hard corns have the following features:

- sharply delineated and conical
- appear most frequently over the dorsolateral aspect of the fifth toe.

Although calluses commonly appear over plantar warts, they're distinguished from these warts by normal skin markings.

Calluses have these characteristics:

- indefinite borders
- may be large
- usually produce dull pain on pressure, rather than constant pain.

Differential diagnoses

- Warts

Diagnosis

Diagnosis depends on careful physical examination of the affected area and on patient history revealing chronic trauma.

Management

General

The simplest and best treatment is essentially preventive—avoidance of trauma. Corns and calluses disappear after the source of trauma has been removed. Metatarsal pads may redistribute the weight-bearing areas of the foot; corn pads may prevent painful pressure. (See *Aids for relieving painful pressure*.)

Medication

The following medications may be used to treat corns and calluses:

- 40% salicylic acid plasters—apply to affected areas following the package directions

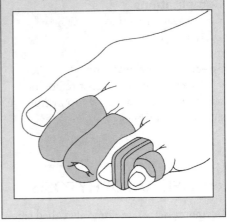

Aids for relieving painful pressure

Metatarsal and corn pads can help to relieve painful pressure. Commercial products available include, from left to right, foam toe cap, foam toe sleeve, soft corn shield, and hard corn (fifth toe) shield.

- corticosteroids—local injection.

Surgical intervention

Surgical debridement, usually under a local anesthetic after warm-water soaking, may be performed to remove the nucleus of a corn.

Referral

- A patient with persistent corns or calluses requires a referral to a podiatrist or dermatologist.
- A patient with corns or calluses caused by a bony malformation, as in arthritis, requires an orthopedic consultation.

Follow-up

The patient should be seen if there's a persistent problem or according to the specialist.

Patient teaching

- Teach the patient how to apply salicylic acid plasters. Make sure the plaster is large enough to cover the affected area.
- Advise the patient to wear properly fitted shoes. Suggest the use of metatarsal or corn pads to relieve pressure.
- Teach the patient about good foot care.

Complications

- Secondary infection
- Change in gait

Special considerations

- Warn the patient against removing corns or calluses with a sharp instrument such as a razor blade.

• • • • • • • • • • • •

DERMATOPHYTOSIS

Dermatophytosis, commonly called tinea, may affect the scalp (tinea capitis), body (tinea corporis), nails (tinea unguium), feet (tinea pedis), groin (tinea cruris), and bearded skin (tinea barbae). Tinea infections are quite prevalent in the United States and are usually more common in males than in females. One out of five people gets a fungal infection. With effective treatment, the cure rate is very high, although about 20% of infected people develop chronic conditions.

Causes

Tinea infections (except for tinea versicolor) result from dermatophytes (fungi) of the genera *Trichophyton*, *Microsporum*, and *Epidermophyton*.

Transmission can occur directly (through contact with infected lesions) or indirectly (through contact with contaminated articles, such as shoes, towels, and shower stalls).

Clinical presentation

Lesions vary in appearance and duration according to the types of dermatophytosis:

- Tinea capitis, which mainly affects children, is characterized by small, spreading papules on the scalp, causing patchy hair loss with scaling. The cardinal clue is broken-off hair, or stubs. The papules may progress to inflamed, pus-filled lesions (kerions).
- Tinea corporis (body ringworm) produces flat lesions on the skin at any site except the scalp, bearded skin, or feet. These lesions may be dry and scaly or moist and crusty; as they enlarge, their centers heal, causing the classic ring-shaped appearance. In tinea unguium (onychomycosis), infection typically starts at the tip of one or more toenails (fingernail infection is less common) and produces gradual thickening, discoloration, and crumbling of the nail, with accumulation of subungual debris. Eventually, the nail may be destroyed completely.
- Tinea pedis, or athlete's foot, causes scaling and blisters between the toes. Severe infection may result in inflammation, with severe itching and pain on walking. A dry, squamous inflammation may affect the entire sole. (See *Athlete's foot*.)
- Tinea cruris (jock itch) produces red, raised, sharply defined, itchy lesions in the groin that may extend to the buttocks, inner thighs, and the external genitalia. Warm weather and tight clothing encourage fungus growth.
- Tinea barbae is an uncommon infection that affects the bearded facial area of men.

Differential diagnoses

- Seborrheic dermatitis
- Atopic dermatitis
- Pityriasis

Diagnosis

Microscopic examination of lesion scrapings prepared in potassium hydroxide solution reveals branching fungal hyphae. Gently heating the slide helps separate epithelial cells and hyphae. Lowering the microscope condenser and dimming the light make hyphae easier to identify, as does adding a drop of ink to the potassium hydroxide.

Other diagnostic procedures include Wood's light examination (useful in only about 5% of cases of tinea capitis) and culture of the infecting organism, which is important for identifying hair and nail fungal infections.

There are other dermatological problems that can cause scaling. Making a firm diagnosis is important because use of an antifungal agent makes subsequent diagnosis by a dermatologist difficult.

Management

General

Supportive measures include open wet dressings, removal of scabs and scales, and application of keratolytics such as salicylic acid to soften and remove hyperkeratotic lesions of the heels or soles.

Medication

The following medications may be used to treat tinea infections:
- clotrimazole 1% cream—apply to lesions b.i.d. until 1 week after resolution
- griseofulvin—500 mg of microsize P.O. daily for 2 to 8 weeks
- itraconazole—200 mg/day P.O. for 12 weeks
- ketoconazole—200 to 400 mg/day P.O.; children older than age 2, 3.3 to 6.6 mg/kg/day for 6 to 8 weeks.

Referral

- Refer the patient to a dermatologist when diagnosis is unclear or treatment fails.

Athlete's foot

Dermatophytosis of the feet (tinea pedis) is commonly called athlete's foot. This infection causes macerated, scaling lesions, which may spread from the interdigital spaces to the sole. Diagnosis must rule out other possible causes of signs and symptoms, for example, eczema, psoriasis, contact dermatitis, and maceration by tight, ill-fitting shoes.

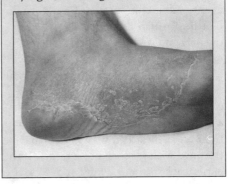

Follow-up

The patient should be seen in 2 weeks for evaluation and sooner if bacterial infection occurs. Liver function should be monitored before treatment and frequently during the course of therapy.

Patient teaching

- To prevent spread of infection to others, advise the patient to wash his towels, bedclothes, and combs frequently in hot water and to avoid sharing them. Suggest that family members be checked for tinea capitis.
- For tinea unguium, tell the patient to keep nails short and straight. Gently remove debris under the nails with an emery board. Prepare the patient for prolonged therapy and possible adverse effects of griseofulvin, such as headache, nausea, vomiting, and photosensitivity.

- For tinea pedis, encourage the patient to expose his feet to air whenever possible and to wear sandals or leather shoes and clean cotton socks. Instruct the patient to wash his feet twice daily and, after drying them thoroughly, to apply antifungal cream followed by antifungal powder to absorb perspiration and prevent excoriation.
- For tinea cruris, instruct the patient to dry the affected area thoroughly after bathing and to evenly apply antifungal powder after applying a topical antifungal agent. Advise him to wear loose-fitting clothing, which should be changed frequently and washed in hot water.
- For tinea corporis, tell the patient with excessive abdominal girth to use abdominal pads between skin folds and to change the pads frequently.
- For tinea barbae, suggest that the patient let his beard grow (whiskers may be trimmed with scissors, not a razor). If the patient insists that he must shave, advise him to use an electric razor instead of a blade.

Complications
- Secondary infection
- Permanent scarring
- Hair loss

• • • • • • • • • • • •

FOLLICULITIS, FURUNCULOSIS, AND CARBUNCULOSIS

Folliculitis is a bacterial infection of the hair follicle that causes the formation of a pustule. The infection can be superficial (follicular impetigo or Bockhart's impetigo) or deep (sycosis barbae). Folliculitis may also lead to the development of furuncles (furunculosis), deep-seated infections of the hair follicle and adjacent subcutaneous tissue, commonly known as boils. It may also cause carbuncles (carbunculosis), neglected or mishandled lesions of furunculosis. The prognosis depends on the infection's severity and on the patient's physical condition and ability to resist infection.

Causes
The most common cause of folliculitis, furunculosis, and carbunculosis is coagulase-positive *Staphylococcus aureus*. Predisposing factors include an infected wound, poor hygiene, debilitation, diabetes, alcoholism, occlusive cosmetics, tight clothes, friction, chafing, exposure to chemicals, and treatment of skin lesions with tar or with occlusive therapy, using steroids. "Hot tub folliculitis" is another type of folliculitis that occurs 1 to 4 days after bathing in a hot tub, whirlpool, or public swimming pool. The causative organism is *Pseudomonas aeruginosa*. Furunculosis often follows folliculitis exacerbated by irritation, pressure, friction, or perspiration. Carbunculosis follows persistent *S. aureus* infection and furunculosis.

Clinical presentation
Pustules of folliculitis usually appear in a hair follicle on the scalp, arms, and legs in children; on the face of bearded men (sycosis barbae); and on the eyelids (styes). Deep folliculitis may be painful.

Folliculitis may progress to the hard, painful nodules of furunculosis, which commonly develop on the neck, face, axillae, and buttocks. For several days these nodules enlarge, and then rupture, discharging pus and necrotic material. After the nodules rupture, pain subsides, but erythema and edema may persist for days or weeks.

Carbunculosis is marked by extremely painful, deep abscesses that drain through

Follicular skin infections

Degree of hair follicle involvement in bacterial skin infection ranges from superficial erythema and pustule of a single follicle to deep abscesses (carbuncles) involving several follicles.

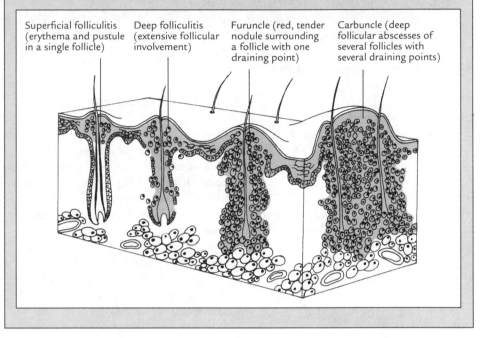

Superficial folliculitis (erythema and pustule in a single follicle)

Deep folliculitis (extensive follicular involvement)

Furuncle (red, tender nodule surrounding a follicle with one draining point)

Carbuncle (deep follicular abscesses of several follicles with several draining points)

multiple openings onto the skin surface, usually around several hair follicles. Fever and malaise may accompany these lesions. (See *Follicular skin infections*.)

Differential diagnoses
- Acne vulgaris
- Pustular miliaria
- Impetigo
- Fungal infections

Diagnosis
The obvious skin lesion confirms folliculitis, furunculosis, or carbunculosis. Wound culture shows S. *aureus*.

In carbunculosis, patient history reveals preexisting furunculosis. A complete blood count may reveal an elevated white blood cell count (leukocytosis).

Management
General
Treatment of folliculitis consists of cleaning the infected area thoroughly with soap and water; applying warm, wet compresses to promote vasodilation and drainage from the lesions; topical antibiotics; and, in extensive infection, systemic antibiotics. Daily repacking of gauze is necessary until the wound heals from the inside out.

Medication
The following medications may be used for treatment:

- mupirocin 2% ointment—apply to affected area t.i.d.
- dicloxacillin—adults, 125 to 250 mg P.O. q.i.d. for 5 to 7 days; children weighing less than 88 lb (40 kg), 12.5 to 25 mg/kg/day P.O. in divided doses
- cephalexin—250 to 500 mg P.O. q.i.d. for 5 to 7 days
- erythromycin—250 to 500 mg P.O. t.i.d. for 5 to 7 days
- ciprofloxacin—500 to 750 mg P.O. b.i.d. for 5 to 7 days.

Surgical intervention
Furunculosis and carbunculosis may require incision and drainage of ripe lesions after application of warm, wet compresses.

Referral
- The patient should be referred to a dermatologist if the condition hasn't improved after 5 days of treatment.
- The patient may need to be referred to a surgeon if a complex furnuncle or carbuncle requires incision and drainage.

Follow-up
The patient with folliculitis should be seen within 48 hours if he has a history of diabetes or if he's immunocompromised.

Patient teaching
- To avoid spreading bacteria to family members, urge the patient not to share towels and washcloths. Tell him that these items should be laundered in hot water before being reused. The patient should change his clothes and bed sheets daily, and they should also be washed in hot water. Encourage the patient to change dressings frequently and to discard them promptly in paper bags.

Complications
- Scarring
- Septecemia

Special considerations
- Caution the patient never to squeeze a boil because this may cause it to rupture into the surrounding area.
- The patient with recurrent furunculosis may have an underlying disease such as diabetes.
- Trauma resulting from hairstyles such as cornrowing can cause folliculitis.

• • • • • • • • • • • •

IMPETIGO

Impetigo is a contagious, superficial skin infection that occurs in nonbullous and bullous forms. It occurs when bacteria get beneath small cuts, scratches, or insect bites. This vesiculopustular eruptive disorder spreads most easily among infants, young children, and elderly patients.

AGE ALERT Impetigo most commonly affects children between ages 2 and 5. Predisposing factors, such as poor hygiene, anemia, malnutrition, and warm climate, favor outbreaks of this infection—most of which occur during the late summer and early fall. In the United States, impetigo occurs most commonly in southern states. Impetigo can complicate chickenpox, eczema, or other skin conditions marked by open lesions.

Causes
Coagulase-positive *Staphylococcus aureus* and, less commonly, group A beta-hemolytic streptococci usually produce nonbullous impetigo; *S. aureus* generally causes bullous impetigo.

Clinical presentation
Common nonbullous impetigo typically begins with a small red macule that turns into a vesicle, becoming pustular with a honey-colored crust within hours. When

the vesicle breaks, a thick yellow crust forms from the exudate. (See *Recognizing impetigo*.)

Autoinoculation may cause satellite lesions. Although it can occur anywhere, impetigo usually occurs on the face, around the mouth and nose. Other features include pruritus, burning, and regional lymphadenopathy.

In bullous impetigo, a thin-walled vesicle opens, and a thin, clear crust forms from the exudate. The lesion consists of a central clearing, circumscribed by an outer rim — much like a ringworm lesion — and commonly appears on the face or other exposed areas. Both forms usually produce painless itching; they may appear simultaneously and be clinically indistinguishable.

Ecthyma is a skin infection resembling impetigo. (See *Understanding ecthyma*, page 720.)

Differential diagnoses
- Allergic contact dermatitis
- Herpes simplex
- Fungal infection
- Ecthyma

Diagnosis
Culture and sensitivity testing of fluid or denuded skin may indicate the most appropriate antibiotic, but therapy shouldn't be delayed for laboratory results, which can take 3 days. White blood cell count may be elevated in the presence of infection.

Management
General
Topical therapy is most effective by removal of the exudate by washing the lesions two or three times per day with antibacterial soap and water or, for stubborn crusts, warm soaks or compresses of normal saline or a diluted soap solution.

Recognizing impetigo

In impetigo, when the vesicles break, crust forms from the exudate. This infection is especially contagious among young children.

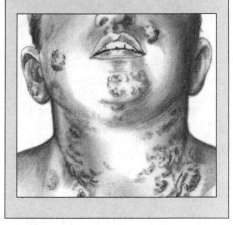

Medication
The following medications may be used in the treatment of impetigo:
- mupirocin 2 % ointment — apply to affected area t.i.d. for 10 days
- dicloxacillin — 125 to 250 mg P.O. q.i.d. for 5 to 7 days; children weighing less than 88 lb (40 kg), 12.5 to 25 mg/kg/day P.O. in divided doses
- cephalexin — 250 to 500 mg P.O. q.i.d. for 5 to 7 days
- erythromycin — 250 to 500 mg P.O. q.i.d. for 5 to 7 days.

Referral
- Refer the patient to a dermatologist if he isn't responding to conventional treatment.

Follow-up
The patient doesn't need follow-up unless treatment is unsuccessful or complications occur.

Understanding ecthyma

Ecthyma is a superficial skin infection that usually causes scarring. It generally results from infection by *Staphylococcus aureus* or group A beta-hemolytic streptococci. Ecthyma differs from impetigo in that its characteristic ulcer results from deeper penetration of the skin by the infecting organism (involving the lower epidermis and dermis), and the overlying crust tends to be piled high (¼″ to 1¼″ [1 to 3 cm]). These lesions are usually found on the legs after a scratch or bug bite. Autoinoculation can transmit ecthyma to other parts of the body, especially to sites that have been scratched open. Therapy is basically the same as for impetigo, beginning with removal of the crust, but response may be slower. Parenteral antibiotics (usually a penicillinase-resistant penicillin) are also used.

Patient teaching
■ Urge the patient not to scratch because this spreads impetigo. Advise parents to cut the child's fingernails.
■ Stress the need to continue prescribed medications for 7 to 10 days, even after lesions have healed.
■ Teach the patient or family how to care for impetiginous lesions. To prevent further spread of this highly contagious infection, encourage frequent bathing using a bactericidal soap. Tell the patient not to share towels, washcloths, or bed linens with family members. Emphasize the importance of following proper hand-washing technique.

Complications
■ Ecthyma
■ Bacteremia

■ Poststreptococcal acute glomerulonephritis
■ Deep cellulitis
■ Septic arthritis
■ Osteomyelitis
■ Erysipelas

Special considerations
■ Check family members for impetigo. If this infection is present in a school-age child, notify his school.
■ In black patients, impetigo often causes deeper dermal inflammation than in whites. This results in postinflammatory hyperpigmentation.

• • • • • • • • • • • •

LICHEN PLANUS

Lichen planus is a benign but pruritic skin eruption that usually produces scaling and purple papules marked by white lines or spots. Such eruptions occur most commonly in middle-age people and are uncommon in young or elderly people. Lichen planus, a relatively rare disorder, is found in all geographic areas, with equal distribution among races. In most patients, it resolves spontaneously in 6 to 18 months; in a few, chronic lichen planus may persist for several years.

Causes
The cause of lichen planus is unknown. Eruptions similar to lichen planus have been induced by arsenic, bismuth, gold, quinidine, propranolol, and naproxen. Exposure to developers used in color photography may likewise cause an eruption that is indistinguishable from lichen planus.

Clinical presentation
Lichen planus may develop suddenly or insidiously. Initial lesions commonly ap-

pear on the arms or legs (generally on the wrist and medial sides of the thighs) and evolve into the generalized eruption of flat, glistening, purple papules marked with white lines or spots (Wickham's striae). These lesions may be linear from scratching or may coalesce into plaques. Lesions often affect the mucous membranes (especially the buccal mucosa), male genitalia and, less often, the nails. Mild to severe pruritus is common.

Differential diagnoses
- Psoriasis
- Syphilis

Diagnosis
Although characteristic skin lesions usually establish the diagnosis of lichen planus, confirmation may require a skin biopsy.

Management
General
Treatment is essentially symptomatic.

Medication
The following medications may be used in the treatment of lichens planus:
- triamcinolone 1% — apply to affected area b.i.d. to t.i.d.
- hydroxyzine — 50 to 100 mg P.O. every 6 hours
- tretinoin 0.05% — apply to affected areas once daily and lightly cover
- methylprednisolone — 5 to 60 mg/day P.O. in divided doses; individualized
- isotretinoin — 0.5 to 2.0 mg/kg/day P.O. in 2 divided doses for 15 to 20 weeks.

Referral
- Refer the patient to a dermatologist if his case is severe or he doesn't respond to treatment.

Follow-up
The patient should be seen after 2 weeks to assess treatment.

Patient teaching
- Teach the patient about medication and potential adverse effects.
- Teach the patient stress reduction techniques, if appropriate.

Complications
- Alopecia
- Nail destruction
- Oral cancer

• • • • • • • • • • •

PEDICULOSIS

Pediculosis is caused by parasitic forms of lice: *Pediculus humanus capitis* causes pediculosis capitis, or head lice; *Pediculus humanus corporis* causes pediculosis corporis, or body lice; and *Phthirus pubis* causes pediculosis pubis, or crab lice. (See *Types of lice*, page 722.)

These lice feed on human blood and lay their eggs (nits) in body hairs or clothing fibers. After the nits hatch, the lice must feed within 24 hours or die; they mature in about 2 to 3 weeks. When a louse bites, it injects a toxin into the skin that produces mild irritation and a purpuric spot. Repeated bites cause sensitization to the toxin, leading to more serious inflammation. Treatment can effectively eliminate lice.

Causes
P. humanus capitis, which is the most common species, feeds on the scalp and, rarely, on the eyebrows, eyelashes, and beard. It's most commonly seen on the back of the head and neck and behind the ears. This form of pediculosis is caused by overcrowded conditions and

Types of lice

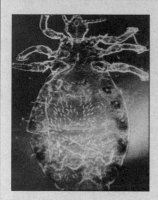 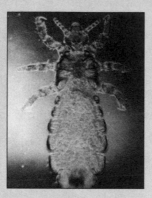 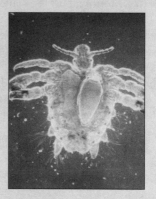

HEAD LOUSE
Pediculus humanus capitis
(head louse) is similar in
appearance to *Pediculus
humanus corporis* (see middle photograph).

BODY LOUSE
Pediculus humanus corporis
(body louse) has a long
abdomen, and all of its
legs are approximately
the same length.

PUBIC LOUSE
Phthirus pubis (pubic or
"crab lice") is slightly
translucent; its first set of
legs is shorter than its
second or third.

poor personal hygiene and commonly affects children, especially girls. It spreads through shared clothing, hats, combs, and hairbrushes. It's estimated that 6 to 10 million children a year are infested with lice.

P. humanus corporis lives in the seams of clothing, next to the skin, leaving only to feed on blood. Common causes include prolonged wearing of the same clothing (which might occur in cold climates), overcrowding, and poor personal hygiene. It spreads through shared clothing and bed sheets.

P. pubis is primarily found in pubic hairs, but this species may extend to the eyebrows, eyelashes, and axillary or body hair. Pediculosis pubis is transmitted through sexual intercourse or by contact with clothes, bed sheets, or towels harboring lice.

Clinical presentation

P. humanus capitis produces the following clinical features:
- itching
- excoriation (with severe itching)
- matted, foul-smelling, lusterless hair (in severe cases)
- occipital and cervical lymphadenopathy (posterior cervical lymphadenopathy without obvious disease)
- rash on the trunk (probably due to sensitization).

Adult lice migrate from the scalp and deposit oval, gray-white nits on hair shafts.

P. humanus corporis produces the following clinical features:
- Initially, small, red papules are produced, usually on the shoulders, trunk, or buttocks.
- Later, wheals may develop (probably a sensitivity reaction).

■ Untreated *P. humanus corporis* leads to vertical excoriations and ultimately to dry, discolored, thickly encrusted, scaly skin with bacterial infection and scarring.

In severe cases, headache, fever, and malaise may accompany cutaneous symptoms.

P. pubis causes:

■ skin irritation from scratching (more obvious than the bites)

■ small gray-blue spots (maculae ceruleae) on the thighs or upper body

■ small red spots in the patient's underclothing.

Differential diagnoses
■ Seborrheic dermatitis
■ Scabies
■ Anogenital pruritus
■ Eczema

Diagnosis
Pediculosis is visible on physical examination:

■ *P. humanus capitis* — oval, grayish nits that can't be shaken loose like dandruff (the closer the nits are to the end of the hair shaft, the longer the infection has been present, because the ova are laid close to the scalp)

■ *P. humanus corporis* — characteristic skin lesions; nits found on clothing

■ *P. pubis* — nits attached to pubic hairs, which feel coarse and grainy to the touch.

Management
General
Treatment consists of application of medication as well as removal of nits (louse eggs). After application of medication, all nits should be combed out of the hair with a metal nit comb. Nit removal may be aided by prerinsing with a prerinse solution containing formic acid or dipping the comb in vinegar. Normal laundering

of clothes and bedclothes after treatment is sufficient to remove adult lice as well as nits.

Medication
The following medications may be used to treat pediculosis:

■ permethrin — apply after shampooing and rinsing hair (leave on for 10 minutes, and then rinse)

■ synergized pyrethrins 0.3% — apply to hair and, after 10 minutes, apply water to work up lather and then rinse; reapply in 7 to 10 days

■ lindane 1% — apply shampoo and rinse after 10 minutes, or apply lotion from neck down and remove after 8 to 12 hours

■ diphenhydramine — adults, 25 to 50 mg P.O. every 4 to 6 hours for itching; children age 6 and older, 12.5 mg P.O. every 4 to 6 hours.

Referral
■ Refer the patient to a dermatologist if conventional treatment is unsuccessful.

Follow-up
The patient needs to be seen if a secondary bacterial infection occurs.

Patient teaching
■ Teach the patient how to use the creams, ointments, powders, and shampoos that can eliminate lice. To prevent self-infestation, avoid prolonged contact with the patient's hair, clothing, and bed sheets.

Complications
■ Secondary bacterial infection

Special considerations
■ Ask the patient with pediculosis pubis for a history of recent sexual contacts so they can be examined and treated.

■ The patient should be tested for other sexually transmitted diseases, including human immunodeficiency virus and syphilis.

■ Inform schools if pediculosis is found in children.

HEALTHY LIVING To prevent the spread of pediculosis, examine all high-risk patients, especially elderly patients who depend on others for care or who are admitted from nursing homes, and people who live in crowded conditions.

•••••••••••

PHOTOSENSITIVITY REACTIONS

A photosensitivity reaction is a skin eruption that can be a toxic or allergic response to light alone or to light and chemicals. A phototoxic reaction is a dose-related primary response. A photoallergic reaction is an uncommon, acquired immune response that isn't dose-related — even slight exposure can cause a severe reaction.

Causes

Certain chemicals can cause a photosensitivity reaction, including dyes, coal tar, furocoumarin compounds found in plants, and drugs such as phenothiazines, sulfonylureas, sulfonamides, tetracycline, piroxicam, thiazide diuretics, antidiabetic agents, and diphenhydramine. Berlock dermatitis, a specific photosensitivity reaction, results from the use of oil of bergamot — a common component of perfumes, colognes, and pomades.

Clinical presentation

Phototoxic reaction occurs immediately and causes a burning sensation followed by erythema (sunburn-type reaction), edema, desquamation, and hyperpigmentation. Berlock dermatitis produces an acute reaction with erythematous vesicles that later become hyperpigmented.

Photoallergic reactions may take one of two forms. Developing 2 hours to 5 days after light exposure, polymorphous light eruption produces erythema, papules, vesicles, urticaria, and eczematous lesions on exposed areas; pruritus may persist for 1 to 2 weeks. Solar urticaria begins minutes after exposure and lasts about 1 hour; erythema and wheals follow itching and burning sensations.

Differential diagnoses

■ Contact dermatitis
■ Porphyria cutanea tarda
■ Variegate porphyria
■ Lupus erythematosus
■ Polymorphous light eruption

Diagnosis

Characteristic skin eruptions and patient history of recent exposure to light or certain chemicals suggest a photosensitivity reaction. A photopatch test for ultraviolet A (UVA) and ultraviolet B may aid diagnosis and may identify the causative light wavelength. Other studies must rule out connective tissue disease, such as lupus erythematosus and porphyrias.

Management
General

For many patients, treatment involves a sunscreen (skin protection factor of 30 to 50), protective clothing, and minimal exposure to sunlight. For others, progressive exposure to sunlight can thicken the skin and produce a tan that interferes with photoallergens and prevents further eruptions. If vesicular or weepy eruptions occur, cool wet dressings may be helpful. Photochemtherapy (psoralen plus UVA) therapy can be used as a treatment for solar urticaria.

Withdrawal of the causative agent, if possible, may also provide relief.

Medication

The following medications may be used to treat a photosensitivity reaction:
- triamcinolone 0.2% — apply to affected area b.i.d. to q.i.d.
- ibuprofen — 200 to 400 mg P.O. every 4 to 6 hours to relieve pain from the burn
- hydroquinone — apply to affected area q.d. to b.i.d. for hyperpigmentation.

Referral

- Refer the patient to a dermatologist for treatment.

Follow-up

The patient should be seen as determined by the dermatologist.

Patient teaching

- To prevent reactions, advise the patient to avoid prolonged exposure to light.
- Tell the patient to avoid being exposed to sunlight between 10 a.m. and 2 p.m.

Complications

- Skin cancer
- Hyperpigmentation
- Secondary bacterial infection

• • • • • • • • • • • •

PITYRIASIS ROSEA

Pityriasis rosea is an acute, self-limiting, inflammatory skin disease that produces a "herald" patch — which usually goes undetected — followed by a generalized eruption of papulosquamous lesions. Although this noncontagious disorder may develop at any age, it's most apt to occur in adolescents and young adults (primarily women). Incidence rises in the spring and fall.

Causes

The cause of pityriasis rosea is unknown, but the disease's brief course and the virtual absence of recurrence suggest a viral agent or an autoimmune disorder.

Clinical presentation

Pityriasis typically begins with an erythematous "herald" patch, which may appear anywhere on the body. Although this slightly raised, oval lesion is about ¾" to 2½" (2 to 6.5 cm) in diameter, approximately 25% of patients don't notice it. A few days to several weeks later, yellow-tan or erythematous patches with scaly edges (about ¼" to ⅜" [0.5 to 1 cm] in diameter) erupt on the trunk and extremities; rarely, they occur on the face, hands, and feet in adolescents. Eruption continues for 7 to 10 days, and the patches persist for 2 to 6 weeks. Occasionally, these patches are macular, vesicular, or urticarial. A characteristic of this disease is the arrangement of lesions along body cleavage lines, producing a pattern similar to that of a pine tree. Accompanying pruritus is usually mild but may be severe.

Differential diagnoses

- Syphilis
- Tinea corporis
- Seborrheic dermatitis
- Tinea vesicolor
- Viral exanthems
- Drug eruptions

Diagnosis

Characteristic skin lesions support the diagnosis.

Management

General

Treatment focuses on relief of pruritus with emollients, oatmeal baths, antihistamines, and occasionally exposure to ultraviolet light or sunlight.

Medication

The following medications may be used to treat pityriasis rosea:
- hydrocortisone cream — apply to affected area t.i.d. to q.i.d.
- diphenhydramine — 25 to 50 mg P.O. every 6 hours; children, 12.5 to 25 mg P.O. every 6 hours
- prednisone — up to 60 mg/day P.O. for severe inflammation.

Referral

- Refer the patient to a dermatologist if inflammation is severe and doesn't respond to treatment.

Follow-up

The patient should be seen monthly until lesions clear.

Patient teaching

- Reassure the patient that pityriasis rosea is noncontagious, spontaneous remission usually occurs in 4 to 8 weeks, and lesions generally don't recur.
- Urge the patient not to scratch. Advise him to avoid hot baths because they may intensify itching. Encourage the use of antipruritics.

Complications

- Secondary bacterial infection

• • • • • • • • • • • •

PSORIASIS

Psoriasis is a chronic, recurrent disease marked by epidermal proliferation. Its lesions, which appear as erythematous papules and plaques covered with silvery scales, vary widely in severity and distribution. Psoriasis affects approximately 8 of 10,000 people in the United States, and its incidence is higher in whites than in other races.

AGE ALERT Although this disorder is most common in young adults ages 15 to 35, it may strike at any age, including infancy.

Psoriasis is characterized by recurring partial remissions and exacerbations. Flare-ups are commonly related to specific systemic and environmental factors but may be unpredictable; they can usually be controlled with therapy.

Causes

The tendency to develop psoriasis is genetically determined. Researchers have discovered a significantly higher-than-normal incidence of certain human leukocyte antigens (HLAs) in families with psoriasis, suggesting a possible immune disorder. Onset of the disease is also influenced by environmental factors. Trauma can trigger the isomorphic effect or Koebner's phenomenon, in which lesions develop at sites of injury. Infections, especially those resulting from beta-hemolytic streptococci, may cause a flare of guttate (drop-shaped) lesions. Other contributing factors include pregnancy, endocrine changes, climate (cold weather tends to exacerbate psoriasis), and emotional stress.

Generally, a skin cell takes 14 days to move from the basal layer to the stratum corneum, where, after 14 days of normal wear and tear, it's sloughed off. The life cycle of a normal skin cell is 28 days compared with only 4 days for a psoriatic skin cell. This markedly shortened cycle doesn't allow time for the cell to mature. Consequently, the stratum corneum becomes thick and flaky, producing the cardinal manifestations of psoriasis.

Clinical presentation

The following signs and symptoms occur with psoriasis:

- itching
- pain from dry, cracked, encrusted lesions
- erythema
- well-defined plaques, which may cover large areas of the body. (See *Psoriatic plaques*.)

Psoriatic lesions most commonly appear on the scalp, chest, elbows, knees, shins, back, and buttocks. The plaques consist of characteristic silver scales that can either flake off easily or thicken, covering the lesion. Removal of psoriatic scales frequently produces fine bleeding points. Occasionally, small guttate lesions appear, either alone or with plaques; these lesions are typically thin and erythematous, with few scales.

Widespread shedding of scales is common in exfoliative or erythrodermic psoriasis and may also develop in chronic psoriasis.

Rarely, psoriasis becomes pustular, taking one of two forms. In localized pustular (Barber's) psoriasis, pustules appear on the palms and soles and remain sterile until opened. In generalized pustular (von Zumbusch's) psoriasis, which often occurs with fever, leukocytosis, and malaise, groups of pustules coalesce to form lakes of pus on red skin. These pustules also remain sterile until opened and commonly involve the tongue and oral mucosa.

In about 30% of patients, psoriasis spreads to the fingernails, producing small indentations and yellow or brown discoloration. In severe cases, the accumulation of thick, crumbly debris under the nail causes it to separate from the nail bed.

Some patients with psoriasis develop arthritic symptoms, usually in one or more joints of the fingers or toes or sometimes in the sacroiliac joints, which may progress to spondylitis. Such patients may complain of morning stiffness. Joint

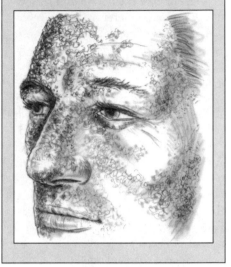

Psoriatic plaques

In this patient with psoriasis, plaques consisting of silver scales cover a large area of the face.

symptoms show no consistent linkage to the course of the cutaneous manifestations of psoriasis; they demonstrate remissions and exacerbations similar to those of rheumatoid arthritis.

Differential diagnoses
- Atopic dermatitis
- Seborrheic dermatitis
- Intertrigo
- Fungal infection
- Reiter's syndrome

Diagnosis
Diagnosis depends on patient history, appearance of the lesions and, if needed, the results of skin biopsy. Typically, serum uric acid level is elevated as a result of accelerated nucleic acid degradation, but indications of gout are absent. (HLA) −BW17, −B13, −B16, and −CW6, may be present in early-onset psoriasis.

Management
General
Treatment depends on the type of psoriasis, the extent of the disease, the patient's response to the disease, and the effect the disease has on the patient's lifestyle. No permanent cure exists, and all methods of treatment are merely palliative.

Removal of psoriatic scales necessitates application of occlusive ointment bases, such as petroleum jelly, salicylic acid preparations, or preparations containing urea. Baker P & S liquid (phenol, sodium chloride, and liquid paraffin) applied to the scalp at bedtime, or liquid carbonis detergens in an emollient base applied for 6 to 8 hours are also effective. These medications soften the scales, which can then be removed by scrubbing them carefully with a soft brush while bathing. No effective treatment exists for psoriasis of the nails.

Methods to retard rapid cell production include exposure to ultraviolet light (ultraviolet B [UVB] or natural sunlight) to the point of minimal erythema. Tar preparations or crude coal tar may be applied to affected areas about 15 minutes before exposure or may be left on overnight and wiped off the next morning. A thin layer of petroleum jelly may be applied before UVB exposure (the most common treatment for generalized psoriasis). Exposure time can increase gradually. Outpatient or day treatment with UVB avoids long hospitalizations and prolongs remission. Psoralen-plus-ultraviolet A (PUVA) therapy can also be implemented.

Medication
The following medications may be used to treat psoriasis:
- hydrocortisone 1% cream — apply to affected area t.i.d. to q.i.d.
- betamethasone cream — apply to affected area t.i.d. to q.i.d.
- calcipotriene 0.005% cream — apply to affected area b.i.d. for 6 to 8 weeks
- methotrexate — 10 to 25 mg/week P.O. for severe cases
- anthralin — apply and then wash off after 20 minutes; shouldn't be applied to unaffected areas or sensitive areas, such as the face and genitalia
- aspirin — 325 to 650 mg P.O. every 4 to 6 hours p.r.n.

Referral
- Refer the patient to a dermatologist if the condition involves a large body surface area.
- Refer the patient to the National Psoriasis Foundation for information support.

Follow-up
The patient should be seen in 2 to 3 weeks unless a bacterial infection occurs. Initially, the patient taking methotrexate should be evaluated weekly and then monthly for red blood cell, white blood cell, and platelet counts because cytotoxins may cause hepatic or bone marrow toxicity. Liver biopsy may be done to assess the effects of methotrexate.

Patient teaching
- Teach the patient correct application of prescribed ointments, creams, and lotions
- Caution the patient to avoid scrubbing his skin vigorously, to prevent Koebner's phenomenon.
- If a medication has been applied to the scales to soften them, suggest the patient use a soft brush to remove them.
- Caution the patient receiving PUVA therapy to stay out of the sun on the day of treatment and to protect his eyes with sunglasses that screen ultraviolet A for 24 hours after treatment. Tell him to wear goggles during exposure to this light.

Complications
- Pustular psoriasis
- Corticosteroid adverse effects
- Exfoliative erythrodermatitis

ROSACEA

Rosacea is a chronic skin eruption that produces flushing and dilation of the small blood vessels in the face, especially the nose and cheeks. Papules and pustules may also occur but without the characteristic comedones of acne vulgaris.

AGE ALERT Rosacea is most common in white women between ages 30 and 50.

When rosacea occurs in men, it's usually more severe and commonly associated with rhinophyma, which is characterized by dilated follicles and thickened, bulbous skin on the nose. Ocular involvement may result in blepharitis, conjunctivitis, uveitis, or keratitis. Rosacea usually spreads slowly and rarely subsides spontaneously.

Causes

Although the cause of rosacea is unknown, stress, infection, vitamin deficiency, menopause, and endocrine abnormalities can aggravate this condition. Anything that produces flushing—for example, hot beverages, such as tea or coffee; tobacco; alcohol; spicy foods; physical activity; sunlight; and extreme heat or cold—can also aggravate rosacea.

Clinical presentation

Signs and symptoms of rosacea include:
- periodic flushing across the central oval of the face
- telangiectasia
- papules
- pustules
- nodules.

Rhinophyma is commonly associated with severe rosacea but may occur alone. Rhinophyma usually appears first on the lower half of the nose and produces red, thickened skin and follicular enlargement. It's found almost exclusively in men over age 40.

Differential diagnoses
- Acne
- Folliculitis

Diagnosis

Typical vascular and acneiform lesions—without the comedones characteristically associated with acne vulgaris—and rhinophyma in severe cases confirm rosacea.

Management
General

Treatment may include electrolysis to destroy large, dilated blood vessels and removal of excess tissue in patients with rhinophyma.

Medication

The following medications may be given:
- tetracycline—initially 250 mg P.O. every 6 hours, then 125 to 500 mg/day or every other day
- doxycycline—initially 50 to 100 mg every 12 hours, then 100 mg/day P.O.
- isotretinoin—0.5 to 2 mg/kg/day P.O. in 2 divided doses for 15 to 20 weeks
- metronidazole 0.75% gel—apply to face 1 to 2 times daily.

Referral
- Refer the patient to a dermatologist if treatment is unsuccessful.

Follow-up

The patient should be seen in 5 weeks to assess treatment.

Patient teaching
- Instruct the patient to avoid hot beverages, alcohol, extended sun exposure, and other possible causes of flushing.

Complications
- Change in appearance
- Loss of self-esteem

• • • • • • • • • • •
SCABIES

Scabies is a skin infection that results from infestation with *Sarcoptes scabiei var. hominis* (itch mite), which provokes a sensitivity reaction. It occurs worldwide, primarily in environments marked by overcrowding and poor hygiene. It's commonly acquired by sleeping with or on the bedding of an infested individual. It can be endemic.

Causes

Mites can live their entire life cycles in the skin of humans, causing chronic infection. The female mite burrows into the skin to lay her eggs, from which larvae emerge to copulate and then reburrow under the skin. Initial contact with scabies organisms causes no symptoms. However, within about 30 days, some patients become allergic to mite product and develop severe pruritus. (See *Scabies: Cause and effect.*)

Scabies is transmitted through skin or sexual contact.

Clinical presentation

Scabies typically causes itching, which intensifies at night. Characteristic lesions are usually excoriated and may appear as erythematous nodules. These threadlike lesions are approximately ⅜″ (1 cm) long and generally occur between fingers, on flexor surfaces of the wrists, on elbows, in axillary folds, at the waistline, on nipples and buttocks in females, and on genitalia in males. In infants, the burrows (lesions) may appear on the head and neck.

Intense scratching can lead to severe excoriation and secondary bacterial infection. Itching may become generalized secondary to sensitization.

Differential diagnoses
- Pediculosis

- Other causes of pruritus

Diagnosis

Visual examination of the contents of the scabietic burrow may reveal the itch mite. If not, a drop of mineral oil placed over the burrow, followed by superficial scraping and examination of expressed material under a low-power microscope, may reveal mite ova or feces. However, excoriation or inflammation of the burrow often makes such identification difficult. If diagnostic tests offer no positive identification of the mite and if scabies is still suspected (for example, if family members and close contacts of the patient also report itching), skin clearing that occurs after a therapeutic trial of a pediculicide confirms the diagnosis.

Management
Medication

The following medications may be used to treat scabies:
- lindane cream — apply to the entire skin surface and remove after 8 to 12 hours
- crotamiton — apply to the entire skin surface, repeat in 24 hours, wash off 48 hours after 2nd application; may repeat in 7 to 10 days
- diphenhydramine — adults, 25 to 50 mg P.O. every 4 to 6 hours; children, 12.5 to 25 mg P.O. every 4 to 6 hours.

Referral
- Refer the patient to a dermatologist if the condition is resistant to conventional treatment.

Follow-up

The patient should be seen if bacterial infection occurs.

Patient teaching
- Contaminated clothing and linens as well as the clothes worn the 2 previous

Scabies: Cause and effect

Infestation with *Sarcoptes scabiei var. hominis* — the itch mite — causes scabies. This mite (shown enlarged below) has a hard shell and measures a microscopic 0.1 mm. The second illustration shows the erythematous nodules with excoriation that appear in patients with scabies. These lesions are usually highly pruritic.

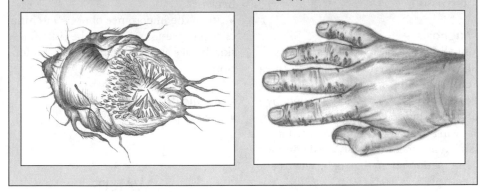

days must be washed in hot water the morning after treatment.

■ Tell the patient there is no need to dry-clean or fumigate his furniture or house.

■ Advise the patient to discontinue using the drug, thoroughly wash it off his skin, and report the reaction if skin irritation or hypersensitivity reaction develops.

Complications
■ Eczema
■ Pyoderma
■ Nodular scabies
■ Postscabetic pruritus

Special considerations
■ Family members and the patient's other close personal contacts should be checked for possible symptoms.

• • • • • • • • • • •

TINEA VERSICOLOR

Tinea versicolor (also known as pityriasis versicolor) is a chronic, superficial, fungal infection that may produce a multicol-

ored rash, commonly on the upper trunk. This condition, primarily a cosmetic defect, usually affects adolescents when sebaceous gland activity is at its highest, especially during warm weather. It's most prevalent in tropical countries. Recurrence is common.

Causes
The agent that causes tinea versicolor is *Malassezia furfur* (*Pityrosporum orbiculare*). Whether this condition is infectious or merely a proliferation of normal skin fungi is uncertain.

Clinical presentation
Tinea versicolor typically produces raised or macular, round or oval, slightly scaly lesions on the upper trunk. These lesions extend to the lower abdomen, neck, arms and, rarely, the face. They're usually tawny but may range from hypopigmented (white) patches in dark-skinned patients to hyperpigmented (brown) patches in fair-skinned patients. Some areas don't tan when exposed to sunlight, causing the cosmetic defect for which most

persons seek medical help. Inflammation, burning, and itching are possible but usually absent.

Differential diagnoses
- Vitiligo
- Seborrheic dermatitis
- Pityriasis

Diagnosis
Visualization of lesions during Wood's light examination strongly suggests tinea versicolor. Microscopic examination of skin scrapings prepared in potassium hydroxide solution confirms the disorder by showing hyphae, clusters of yeast, and large numbers of variously sized pores (a combination referred to as "spaghetti and meatballs").

Management
Medication
The following medications may be used in the treatment of tinea versicolor:
- selenium sulfide shampoo — apply and remove after 10 to 60 minutes once daily for 7 days
- sodium thiosulfate 25% solution — apply b.i.d. to affected areas for 2 to 4 weeks; or sulfur salicylic shampoo applied as a lotion h.s. and washed off each morning for 2 weeks
- ketoconazole cream — apply once daily for 2 weeks
- clotrimazole 1% cream — apply to lesions b.i.d. until resolved.

Referral
- Refer the patient to a dermatologist if diagnosis is uncertain.

Follow-up
The patient should be seen if the skin breaks and a secondary bacterial infection occurs.

Patient teaching
- Assure the patient that after his fungal infection is cured, discolored areas will gradually blend in after exposure to the sun or ultraviolet light.
- Teach the patient proper hand-washing technique, and encourage good personal hygiene.
- Stress the importance of not scratching or picking lesions to avoid the risk of skin breaks and secondary bacterial infections.

Complications
- Secondary bacterial infection

• • • • • • • • • • • •

WARTS

Warts, also known as verrucae, are common, benign, viral infections of the skin and adjacent mucous membranes. Although their incidence is highest in children and young adults, warts may occur at any age. The prognosis varies: Some warts disappear readily with treatment; others require more vigorous and prolonged treatment.

Causes
Warts are caused by infection with the human papillomavirus, a group of ether-resistant, deoxyribonucleic acid–containing papovaviruses. Mode of transmission is probably through direct contact, but autoinoculation is possible.

Clinical presentation
Clinical manifestations depend on the type of wart and its location:
- common (verruca vulgaris) — rough, elevated, rounded surface; appears most commonly on extremities, particularly hands and fingers; most prevalent in children and young adults

■ filiform—single, thin, threadlike projection; commonly occurs around the face and neck

■ periungual—rough, irregularly shaped, elevated surface; occurs around edges of fingernails and toenails; when severe, may extend under the nail and lift it off the nail bed, causing pain

■ flat (also known as juvenile)—multiple groupings of up to several hundred slightly raised lesions with smooth, flat, or slightly rounded tops; common on the face, neck, chest, knees, dorsa of hands, wrists, and flexor surfaces of the forearms; usually occur in children but can affect adults; distribution is often linear because these warts can spread from scratching or shaving

■ plantar—slightly elevated or flat; occurs singly or in large clusters (mosaic warts), primarily at pressure points of the feet

■ digitate—fingerlike, horny projection arising from a pea-shaped base; occurs on scalp or near hairline

■ condyloma acuminatum (moist wart)— usually small, pink to red, moist, and soft; may occur singly or in large cauliflower-like clusters on the penis, scrotum, vulva, and anus; may be transmitted through sexual contact, but is not always venereal in origin.

Differential diagnoses

■ Squamous cell carcinoma
■ Hypertrophic actinic keratoses
■ Condylomata lata
■ Molluscum contagiosum
■ Seborrheic keratosis
■ Varicella-zoster virus

Diagnosis

Visual examination usually confirms the diagnosis. Plantar warts can be differentiated from corns and calluses by certain distinguishing features. Plantar warts obliterate natural lines of the skin, may contain red or black capillary dots that

are easily discernible if the surface of the wart is shaved down with a scalpel, and are painful on application of pressure. Plantar warts and corns have soft, pulpy cores surrounded by thick callous rings; plantar warts and calluses are flush with the skin surface.

Recurrent anal warts require sigmoidoscopy to rule out internal involvement, which may necessitate surgery.

Management

General

Treatment of warts varies according to location, size, number, pain level (present and projected), history of therapy, patient age, and compliance with treatment. Most people eventually develop an immune response that causes warts to disappear spontaneously and require no treatment. Cryotherapy (liquid nitrogan) may be used-liquid nitrogen to kill the wart and the resulting dried blister needs to be peeled off several days later. If initial treatment isn't successful, it can be repeated at 2- to 4-week intervals. This method is useful for either periungual warts or for common warts on the face, extremities, penis, vagina, or anus.

Medication

The following medications may be used to treat warts:

■ 40% salicylic acid plasters—apply to site every 12 to 24 hours for 2 to 4 weeks
■ 25% podophyllin in compound with tincture of benzoin—for venereal warts: apply to site and remove after 4 hours; repeat every 2 to 4 days.

Surgical intervention

Electrodesiccation and curettage may be needed: High-frequency electric current destroys the wart and is followed by surgical removal of dead tissue at the base and application of an antibiotic ointment (such as polysporin), covered with a ban-

Removing warts by electrosurgery

1. Injection of 1% to 2% lidocaine under and around the wart, avoiding the wart itself

2. Electrodesiccation of the wart

3. Removal of the wart tissue with a curette and small, curved scissors

4. Light desiccation of the area to control bleeding and prevent recurrence

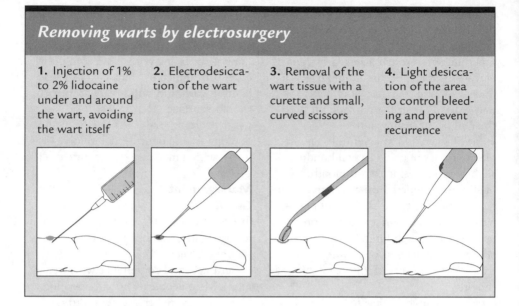

dage, for 48 hours. This method is effective for common, filiform and, occasionally, plantar warts. (See *Removing warts by electrosurgery.*)

Referral
▪ Refer the patient to a dermatologist, if necessary.

Follow-up
The patient should be seen in 2 weeks or sooner if secondary bacterial infection occurs.

Patient teaching
▪ During acid or podophyllum therapy, tell the patient to protect the surrounding area with petroleum jelly or sodium bicarbonate (baking soda).

Complications
▪ Recurrence
▪ Minor scarring with removal

Special considerations
▪ With genital warts, the patient's sexual partner may also require treatment.

•••••••••••••

SELECTED REFERENCES

Diseases, 3rd ed. Springhouse, Pa.: Springhouse Corp., 2001.

Fauci, A.S., et al., eds. *Harrison's Principles of Internal Medicine*, 15th ed. New York: McGraw-Hill Book Co., 2001.

Fitzpatrick, T.B., et al. *Color Atlas and Synopsis of Clinical Dermatology: Common and Serious Diseases*, 4th ed. New York: McGraw-Hill Book Co., 2001.

Fleischer, A.B., Jr. *20 Common Problems in Dermatology*. New York: McGraw-Hill Book Co., 2000.

Ignatavicius, D.D., et al. *Medical-Surgical Nursing Across the Health Care Continuum*, 3rd ed. Philadelphia: W.B. Saunders Co., 1999.

Rakel, R.E., ed. *Conn's Current Therapy 2001*. Philadelphia: W.B. Saunders Co., 2001.

White, G., and Cox, N. *Diseases of the Skin: A Color Atlas and Text*. St. Louis: Mosby–Year Book, Inc., 2000.

Trauma

Trauma is the third leading cause of death in the United States, outranked only by cardiovascular disease and cancer. In people under age 35, it's the leading cause of death.

• • • • • • • • • • • •
ASSESSMENT

Trauma care basics include triage; assessing and maintaining airway, breathing, and circulation (the ABCs); protecting the cervical spine; assessing the level of consciousness (LOC); and, as necessary, preparing the patient for transport and possibly surgery.

Three types of trauma exist: blunt trauma, which leaves the body surface intact; penetrating trauma, which disrupts the body surface; and perforating trauma, which leaves entrance and exit wounds as an object passes through the body.

Triage
Triage is the setting of medical priorities for emergency care by making sound, rapid assessments. In many cases, the need for triage arises at the scene of injury and con-

tinues in the emergency department. Following health care facility protocol, you'll decide which patient to treat first, which injury to treat first, how to best utilize other members of the medical team, and how to control patient and staff traffic.

In most cases, a victim is assigned to one of the following categories:
■ *emergent*—life-threatening or limb-threatening injury requiring treatment within a few minutes to prevent death or further injury; includes patients with respiratory distress, cardiopulmonary arrest, severe hemorrhage, or shock
■ *urgent*—serious but not immediately life-threatening injury that should receive treatment within 1 hour, for example, stable head, chest, or abdominal injuries and long bone fractures
■ *delayed*—minor injuries that can wait 4 to 6 hours for treatment, such as lacerations and abrasions
■ *indefinite*—treatment can wait indefinitely; patient can be referred to a clinic (in disaster or military situations, applies to patients with massive injuries who have minimal chance for recovery, even with immediate, vigorous care)
■ *deceased.*

Care of the trauma patient

Begin your care of an injured patient with a brief assessment of the ABCs: airway, breathing, and circulation.

Immobilize the patient's head and neck with an immobilization device, sandbags, backboard, and tape if this hasn't been done. Obtain cervical spine X-rays and rule out cervical spine injury before moving the patient again.

Monitor vital signs, assessing baseline readings, and note significant changes. The patient should be placed on a cardiac monitor and a pulse oximeter.

Assess LOC and pupillary and motor response to assess neurologic status. Assess decorticate or decerebrate responses. The patient doesn't have to have a head injury to exhibit an abnormal neurologic response. Any injury that impairs ventilation or perfusion can cause cerebral edema and can raise intracranial pressure. If the patient has neurologic symptoms and is hypotensive, look for an extracranial cause because intracranial bleeding usually isn't the cause of hypotension.

Assess arterial blood gas measurements, and calculate the effects of the supplemental oxygen to establish a baseline for oxygen and acid-base therapy. Multiple injuries always create a need for supplemental oxygen because of blood loss and overwhelming physiologic stress. Actually, a conscious multiple-injury patient should display compensatory hyperventilation. If he doesn't, expect neurologic involvement or chest injury.

Blood studies should be done for type and crossmatch, complete blood count, prothrombin time, partial thromboplastin time, platelet count, and routine blood studies, including amylase levels. Two I.V. lines with 14G or 16G catheters should be started for fluid resuscitation with normal saline or lactated Ringer's solution. Administer tetanus prophylaxis, if appropriate. (See *Managing tetanus prophylaxis*.)

Quickly and carefully look for multiple injuries by systematically examining the patient. If you detect no spinal injury, carefully logroll the patient to examine his back for other wounds.

In chest trauma, assess for open wounds, tension pneumothorax, hemothorax, cardiac tamponade, bruises and hematomas, flail chest, and fractured larynx. Cover open wounds and apply direct pressure to wounds as necessary. Insertion of chest tubes, needle thoracotomy, pericardiocentesis, cricothyrotomy, or tracheotomy may be necessary.

As indicated, an indwelling urinary catheter and a nasogastric tube should be inserted. Prophylactic antibiotics and appropriate diagnostic studies—such as X-rays, computed tomography scans, or excretory urography—should be initiated. Contact the appropriate medical or surgical specialist.

Because severe injuries commonly lead to shock, check skin temperature, color, and moisture.

In all cases of massive external bleeding or suspected internal bleeding, watch for hypovolemia and estimate blood loss. Remember, however, that a blood loss of 500 to 1,000 ml might not change systolic blood pressure, but it might elevate the pulse rate. Stay alert for signs of occult bleeding, which commonly occurs in the chest, abdomen, and thigh. Repeat abdominal examinations frequently to assess the patient for abdominal distention; this could be a sign of internal injuries and bleeding.

Increased diameter of the legs or abdomen usually means that blood has leaked into these tissues (as much as 4,000 ml into the abdomen, 3,000 ml into the chest, and 2,000 ml into a thigh). Such blood loss induces characteristic signs of hypovolemic shock.

Managing tetanus prophylaxis

HISTORY OF TETANUS IMMUNIZATION (NUMBER OF DOSES)	TETANUS-PRONE WOUNDS		NON-TETANUS-PRONE WOUNDS	
	Td*‡	TIG†‡	Td	TIG
Uncertain	Yes	Yes	Yes	No
0 to 1	Yes	Yes	Yes	No
2	Yes	No (Yes if 24 hours since wound was inflicted)	Yes	No
3 or more	No (Yes if more than 5 years since last dose)	No	No (Yes if more than 10 years since last dose)	No

*Td = Tetanus and diphtheria toxoids adsorbed (for adult use), 0.5 ml

†TIG = Tetanus immune globulin (human), 250 U

‡When Td and TIG are given concurrently, separate syringes and separate sites should be used. *Note:* For children younger than age 7, tetanus and diphtheria toxoids and pertussis vaccine, adsorbed (DPT), are preferred over tetanus toxoid alone. If pertussis vaccine is contraindicated, administer tetanus and diphtheria toxoids, adsorbed (DP).

If the patient has renal injuries or a fractured pelvis, look for the classic sign of retroperitoneal hematoma—numbness or pain in the leg on the affected side as a result of pressure on the lateral femoral cutaneous nerve in L1 to L3. Retroperitoneal bleeding may not cause abdominal tenderness. Although the initial resuscitation fluids are crystalloids, significant hypovolemia due to hemorrhage requires blood transfusion. A central venous pressure or pulmonary artery catheter should be considered to monitor circulating blood volume.

• • • • • • • • • • • •

ARM AND LEG FRACTURES

Arm and leg fractures usually result from trauma and commonly cause substantial muscle, nerve, and other soft-tissue damage. The prognosis varies with the extent of disablement or deformity, the amount of tissue and vascular damage, the adequacy of reduction and immobilization, and the patient's age, health, and nutritional status. Children's bones usually heal rapidly and with little deformity. Bones of adults in poor health and with impaired circulation may not heal properly. Severe open fractures, especially of the femoral shaft, may cause substantial blood loss and may be life-threatening. Types of fractures include open, simple,

Classifying fractures

One of the best-known systems for classifying fractures uses a combination of such terms as simple, nondisplaced, and oblique — to describe fractures. An explanation of these terms appears below.

GENERAL CLASSIFICATION OF FRACTURES

- *Simple (closed)* — Bone fragments don't penetrate the skin.
- *Compound (open)* — Bone fragments penetrate the skin.
- *Incomplete (partial)* — Bone continuity isn't completely interrupted.
- *Complete* — Bone continuity is completely interrupted.

CLASSIFICATION BY FRAGMENT POSITION

- *Comminuted* — The bone breaks into small pieces.
- *Impacted* — One bone fragment is forced into another.
- *Angulated* — Fragments lie at an angle to each other.
- *Displaced* — Fracture fragments separate and are deformed.
- *Nondisplaced* — The two sections of bone maintain essentially normal alignment.

- *Overriding* — Fragments overlap, shortening total bone length.
- *Segmental* — Fractures occur in two adjacent areas with an isolated central segment.
- *Avulsion* — Fragments are pulled from normal position by muscle contractions or ligament resistance.

CLASSIFICATION BY FRACTURE LINE

- *Linear* — The fracture line runs parallel to the bone's axis.
- *Longitudinal* — The fracture line extends in a longitudinal (but not parallel) direction along the bone's axis.
- *Oblique* — The fracture line crosses the bone at roughly a 45-degree angle to the bone's axis.
- *Spiral* — The fracture line crosses the bone at an oblique angle, creating a spiral pattern.
- *Transverse* — The fracture line forms a right angle with the bone's axis.

---

compound, impaction, avulsion, greenstick, compression, and intertrochanteric.

Causes

Most arm and leg fractures result from major traumatic injury, such as a fall on an outstretched arm, a skiing accident, or child abuse (suggested by multiple or repeated episodes of fractures). However, in a person with a pathologic bone-weakening condition, such as osteoporosis, bone tumors, metabolic disease, or long-term steroid use, a mere cough or sneeze can also produce a fracture. Prolonged standing, walking, or running can cause stress fractures of the foot and ankle — typically in soldiers, nurses, postal workers, and joggers. Brittle bones make an older person especially prone to fractures. Falling on an outstretched arm or hand or suffering a direct blow to the arm or shoulder is likely to fracture the radius or humerus.

Clinical presentation

Arm and leg fractures may produce:
- pain
- point tenderness

- pallor
- pulse loss
- paresthesia
- paralysis.

Other signs include:
- deformity
- swelling
- discoloration
- crepitus
- open wound
- loss of limb function.

Numbness and tingling, mottled cyanosis, cool skin at the end of the extremity, and loss of pulses distal to the injury indicate possible arterial compromise or nerve damage. Conduct a covert foot or arm neurologic examination, including motor and sensory function. Open fractures also produce an obvious skin wound.

Differential diagnoses
- Blunt trauma
- Soft tissue injury
- Dislocations
- Compartment syndrome
- Arthritis
- Gout
- Pseudogout
- Deep vein thrombosis
- Muscle spasm

Diagnosis

A history of traumatic injury and the results of the physical examination, including gentle palpation and a cautious attempt by the patient to move parts distal to the injury, suggest an arm or leg fracture.

Test range of motion and joint function. Make comparisons with the opposite body side if it's uninjured. Explore all open wounds.

Note: When performing the physical examination, also check for other injuries. Anteroposterior and lateral X-rays of the suspected fracture, as well as X-rays

---

Fat embolism

A complication of long bone fracture, fat embolism may also follow severe soft-tissue bruising and fatty liver injury. Posttraumatic embolization may occur as bone marrow releases fat into the veins. The fat can lodge in the lungs, obstructing the pulmonary vascular bed, or pass into the arteries, eventually disturbing the respiratory and circulatory systems.

Fat embolism occurs 12 to 48 hours after an injury, typically producing fever, tachycardia, tachypnea, blood-tinged sputum, cyanosis, anxiety, restlessness, altered level of consciousness, seizures, coma, and rash. Diagnostic test results reveal decreased hemoglobin, increased serum lipase levels, leukocytosis, thrombocytopenia, hypoxemia, and fat globules in urine and sputum. A chest X-ray may show mottled lung fields and right ventricular dilation. An electrocardiogram may reveal tachycardia and large S waves in lead I, large Q waves and an inverted T wave in lead III, and right axis deviation.

Although some treatment measures are controversial, they may include steroids to reduce inflammation, heparin to prevent thrombosis, and oxygen to correct hypoxemia. Expect to immobilize fractures early.

---

of the joints above and below it, confirm the diagnosis. (See *Classifying fractures.*)

Management

General

Emergency treatment consists of splinting the limb above and below the suspected fracture, applying a cold pack, and elevating the limb to reduce edema and pain.

Recognizing compartment syndrome

Compartment syndrome occurs when pressure within the muscle compartment, resulting from edema or bleeding, increases to the point of interfering with circulation. Crush injuries, burns, bites, and fractures requiring casts or dressings may cause this syndrome. Compartment syndrome most commonly occurs in the lower arm, hand, lower leg, and foot.

Symptoms include:
- increased pain
- decreased touch sensation
- increased weakness of the affected part
- increased swelling and pallor
- decreased pulses and capillary refill.

Treatment of compartment syndrome consists of:
- placing the limb at heart level
- removing constricting forces
- monitoring neurovascular status
- monitoring compartment pressures
- performing emergency fasciotomy.

In severe fractures that cause blood loss, apply direct pressure to control bleeding, and administer fluid replacement as soon as possible to prevent or treat hypovolemic shock.

After confirming a fracture diagnosis, treatment begins with reduction. Closed reduction is accomplished by manual manipulation. Administration of sedation and analgesia facilitates the muscle stretching necessary to realign the bone.

After open or closed reduction, the fractured arm or leg must be immobilized by a splint or a cast or with traction. X-rays are ordered to confirm that the reduction was successful and that proper bone alignment was achieved.

When a splint or cast fails to maintain the reduction, immobilization requires skin or skeletal traction using a series of weights and pulleys. In skin traction, elastic bandages and sheepskin coverings are used to attach traction devices to the patient's skin. In skeletal traction, a pin or wire inserted through the bone distal to the fracture and attached to a weight allows more prolonged traction.

Medication

The following medications may be used in the treatment of arm and leg fractures:
- tetanus (if immunization not current) — 0.5 ml I.M.
- ibuprofen — 200 to 800 mg P.O. every 6 hours
- codeine — 30 to 60 mg P.O. every 4 to 6 hours
- hydromorphone — adults, 2 to 4 mg P.O. every 4 to 6 hours
- heparin — 5,000 U S.C. every 12 hours for lower extremity fractures
- ampicillin — 1 to 2 g/day P.O. in divided doses.

Surgical intervention

When closed reduction is impossible, open reduction during surgery reduces and immobilizes the fracture by means of rods, plates, or screws. Afterward, a cast is usually applied. Surgery may also be needed to repair soft-tissue damage and thoroughly debride the wound.

Referral

- Refer the patient to an orthopedic surgeon.
- After cast removal, refer the patient to a physical therapist to restore limb mobility.

Follow-up

The patient should be seen as indicated by the orthopedic surgeon.

Patient teaching

- If the fracture requires long-term immobilization with traction, tell the patient to frequently change positions to increase comfort and prevent pressure ulcers. Encourage active range-of-motion exercises to prevent muscle atrophy. Encourage deep breathing and coughing to avoid hypostatic pneumonia.
- Urge adequate fluid intake to prevent urinary stasis and constipation.
- Tell the patient to immediately report signs and symptoms of impaired circulation. Warn him not to get the cast wet and not to insert foreign objects under the cast.
- Encourage the patient to start moving around as soon as he can. Teach the patient how to use crutches properly.

Complications

- Permanent deformity and dysfunction if bones fail to heal (nonunion) or heal improperly (malunion)
- Aseptic necrosis of bone segments from impaired circulation
- Hypovolemic shock
- Muscle contractures
- Renal calculi from decalcification
- Fat embolism (see *Fat embolism*, page 739)
- Compartment syndrome (see *Recognizing compartment syndrome*).

• • • • • • • • • • • •

BURNS

A major burn is a horrifying injury, requiring painful treatment and a long rehabilitation period. It's commonly fatal or permanently disfiguring and incapacitating (emotionally and physically). In the United States, about 2.2 million people suffer burns annually. Of these, about 100,000 are chemical burns and 300,000 are serious burns. Approximately 6,000 deaths occur, making burns the nation's third leading cause of accidental death.

Causes

Thermal burns, the most common type, commonly result from residential fires, automobile accidents, children playing with matches, improperly stored gasoline, space heater or electrical malfunctions, or arson. Other causes include improper handling of firecrackers, scalding accidents, and kitchen accidents (such as a child climbing on top of a stove or grabbing a hot iron). Some burns in children are traced to parental abuse.

Chemical burns result from the contact, ingestion, inhalation, or injection of acids, alkalis, or vesicants. Electrical burns usually occur after contact with faulty electrical wiring or high-voltage power lines; many children sustain them by chewing on electric cords. Friction (abrasion) burns happen when the skin is rubbed harshly against a coarse surface. Sunburn, of course, follows excessive exposure to sunlight.

Clinical presentation

Assessment is needed to determine the depth of skin and tissue damage. A partial-thickness burn damages the epidermis and part of the dermis, whereas a full-thickness burn affects the full dermis and, possibly, subcutaneous tissue. A more traditional method gauges burn depth by degrees. However, most burns are a combination of different degrees and thicknesses. (See *Gauging burn depth*, page 742.)

Burns are classified as follows:
- *First degree* — Damage is limited to the epidermis, causing erythema and pain.
- *Second degree* — The epidermis and part of the dermis are damaged, producing blisters and mild to moderate edema and pain.
- *Third degree* — The epidermis and the dermis are damaged. No blisters appear,

Gauging burn depth

One method of assessing a burn is by determining the burn's depth. A partial-thickness burn damages the epidermis and part of the dermis, whereas a full-thickness burn damages the epidermis, dermis, subcutaneous tissue, and muscle, as shown below.

Epidermis

Dermis

Subcutaneous tissue

Muscle

■ Damaged tissue ■ Dead tissue

Normal skin   Partial thickness   Full thickness

---

but white, brown, or black leathery tissue and thrombosed vessels are visible.

The size of a burn must be estimated; it's usually expressed as the percentage of body surface area (BSA) covered by the burn. The Rule of Nines chart usually provides this estimate, but the Lund-Browder classification is more accurate because it allows for BSA changes with age.

A correlation of the burn's depth and size permits an estimate of its severity, as follows:

■ *major* — third-degree burns on more than 10% of BSA; second-degree burns on more than 25% of adult BSA (more than 20% in children); burns of hands, face, feet, or genitalia; burns complicated by fractures or respiratory damage; electrical burns; all burns in poor-risk patients
■ *moderate* — third-degree burns on 2% to 10% of BSA; second-degree burns on

15% to 25% of adult BSA (10% to 20% in children)
■ *minor* — third-degree burns on less than 2% of BSA; second-degree burns on less than 15% of adult BSA (10% in children).

Other important factors in assessing burns include:
■ *Location* — Burns on the face, hands, feet, and genitalia are most serious because of possible loss of function.
■ *Configuration* — Circumferential burns can cause total occlusion of circulation in an extremity as a result of edema. Burns on the neck can produce airway obstruction, whereas burns on the chest can lead to restricted respiratory expansion.
■ *History of complicating medical problems* — Note disorders that impair peripheral circulation, especially diabetes, pe-

ripheral vascular disease, and chronic alcohol abuse.

- *Patient age* — Victims under age 4 or over age 60 have a higher incidence of complications and, consequently, a higher mortality.
- *Smoke inhalation* — This can result in pulmonary injury.
- *Other injuries* — Other injuries sustained at the time of the burn can affect the burn.

Differential diagnoses
- Ocular burns
- Caustic ingestion
- Exposure to hazardous materials
- Sunburn
- Chemical burn
- Thermal burn
- Electrical injury
- Smoke inhalation
- Abrasions
- Scalded skin syndrome

Management
General
Immediate, aggressive burn treatment increases the patient's chances of survival. Later, supportive measures and strict aseptic technique can minimize infection. Burns require comprehensive care and should be addressed at a facility specializing in burn care. (See *Managing burns with skin grafts*.)

Minor burns are treated with cool saline or compresses. Devitalized skin may need debridement. The wound may be covered with a nonstick dressing. Moderate and major burns require stabilization of airway, breathing, and circulation. Bleeding must be controlled and I.V. fluids started. (See *Fluid replacement after a burn*, page 744.) The burn should be covered with a dry, sterile sheet until the patient is transported to a burn facility.

When electrical or chemical burns occur, it's helpful to know the voltage or causative chemical involved. Thermal

Managing burns with skin grafts

When a patient has a limited, well-defined burn, he may need a temporary graft to minimize fluid and protein loss from the burn surface, to prevent infection, and to reduce pain. Types of temporary grafts include:
- allografts (homografts), which are usually cadaver skin
- xenografts (heterografts), which are typically pigskin
- biosynthetic grafts, which are a combination of collagen and synthetics.

To treat a full-thickness burn, a patient may need an autograft. This method uses the patient's own skin — usually a split-thickness graft — to replace the burned skin. For areas where appearance or joint movement is important, the autograft is transplanted intact. In flat areas where appearance is less critical, the graft may be meshed (fenestrated) to cover up to three times its original size.

When burns cover the entire body surface, the test-tube skin graft may provide lifesaving treatment. In this method, a small full-thickness biopsy yields epidermal cells that are cultured into sheets and then grafted onto the burns. According to its developers, this smooth, supple test-tube skin represents a major advance in the treatment of extensive burns.

burns may also be present if the patient's clothes ignited. Cardiopulmonary resuscitation is needed if ventricular fibrillation is present (usually with electrical contact). Chemical burns need irrigation with copious amounts of water or normal saline solution or a weak base (such as sodium bicarbonate) to neutralize hydrofluoric acid.

Fluid replacement after a burn

The commonly used Parkland formula is a guideline for fluid replacement for burn patients. Variations may be made depending on the patient's response to treatment.

Parkland formula:
4 ml/kg body weight × % body surface area burned

Over 24 hours, administer 4 ml lactated Ringer's solution per kilogram of body weight times the percentage of body surface area burned. Give one-half of the total amount of solution over the first 8 hours and the rest of the solution over the next 16 hours.

Medication

The following medications may be used in the treatment of burns:
- silvadene — apply to affected area b.i.d.
- erythromycin opthalmic ointment 0.5% — apply to affected eye t.i.d. or q.i.d. for ocular burns
- meperidine — adults, 50 to 100 mg P.O. or I.M. every 4 hours p.r.n.; children, 1.1 to 1.8 mg/kg P.O. or I.M. every 4 hours p.r.n.
- tramadol — 50 to 100 mg P.O. every 4 to 6 hours
- morphine — adults, 2.5 to 15 mg I.V., S.C., or I.M. every 4 hours p.r.n.; children, 0.1 to 0.2 mg/kg I.V. or S.C. every 4 hours
- tetanus — 0.5 ml I.M.
- acetaminophen — 325 to 650 mg P.O. every 4 hours p.r.n.
- ibuprofen — adults, 400 to 800 mg P.O. every 6 hours; children, 5 to 10 mg/kg every 4 to 6 hours.

Surgical intervention

Surgery may be needed for debridement of the wound.

Referral

- If the patient is immunocompromised, has second- or third-degree burns, or electrical or inhalation burns, refer him to a tertiary care center for treatment.
- Refer the patient to an ophthalmologist if he has ocular burns.
- Refer the patient to a plastic surgeon if necessary.
- Refer the patient to a psychologist for counseling, if necessary.

Follow-up

The type and extent of the burn determines follow-up care.

Patient teaching

- For minor burns, provide thorough teaching and complete aftercare instructions for the patient. Stress the importance of keeping the dressing dry and clean, elevating the burned extremity for the first 24 hours, taking analgesics as ordered, and returning for a wound check in 1 to 2 days.
- Teach the patient and family about the expected course of illness based on the extent of the burn.

HEALTHY LIVING Teach the patient the importance of having smoke detectors in every household and on every level of the dwelling. Tell him that an evacuation plan should be reviewed with family members to be used in case of fire.

Complications

- Wound infection
- Scarring
- Decreased mobility secondary to deformity
- Curling's ulcer
- Septic shock
- Psychological problems

CONCUSSION

Concussion is the most common head injury. A concussion results from a blow to the head that's hard enough to jostle the brain and make it strike the skull, causing temporary neural dysfunction, but not hard enough to cause a cerebral contusion. Most concussion patients recover completely within 24 to 48 hours. Repeated concussions, however, exact a cumulative toll on the brain.

Causes

A blow that causes a concussion is usually sudden and forceful, such as a fall to the ground, a punch to the head, or an automobile accident. Such blows also may result from child abuse. Whatever the cause, the resulting injury is mild compared to the damage done by cerebral contusions or lacerations.

Clinical presentation

A concussion may produce a short-term loss of consciousness and vomiting. The patient may also suffer from anterograde and retrograde amnesia, in which he can't recall what happened immediately after the injury, and also has difficulty recalling events that led up to the traumatic incident. The presence of anterograde amnesia and the duration of retrograde amnesia reliably correlate with the severity of the injury.

This type of injury commonly causes:
- irritability
- lethargy
- behavior out of character
- dizziness
- nausea
- severe headache.

Some children have no apparent ill effects, but many grow lethargic and somnolent in a few hours. All of these signs occur normally with a concussion. Post-concussion syndrome — characterized by headache, dizziness, vertigo, anxiety, and fatigue — may persist for several weeks after the injury.

Differential diagnoses
- Epidural hematoma
- Epidural or subdural infection
- Migraine headache
- Tension headache
- Hemorrhagic stroke

Diagnosis

Differentiating between a concussion and more serious head injuries requires a thorough history of the injury and a neurologic examination. Such an examination must evaluate the patient's level of consciousness, mental status, cranial nerve and motor function, deep tendon reflexes, and orientation to time, place, and person. If no abnormalities are found and if a severe head injury appears unlikely, the patient should be observed for signs of more severe cerebral trauma. Observation provides a baseline for gauging deterioration in the patient's condition. Whenever you suspect a severe head injury, obtain a computed tomography scan or magnetic resonance imaging to rule out fractures and more serious injuries.

Management
General

The patient with a concussion needs to rest quietly and be observed in case a more serious head injury develops. If the patient lost consciousness as a result of the injury, he should not participate in sports for 3 months following the injury.

Medication

Acetaminophen (325 to 650 mg P.O. every 4 hours) may be used to treat a concussion. For a child's dose, follow the directions on the package.

Referral
- Refer the patient to a hospital to determine the extent of the injury.

Follow-up
The patient should be seen if neurologic symptoms develop or if he continues to have head pain.

Patient teaching
- After discharge, instruct the patient to be alert for worsening of headache, vomiting, signs of an ear bleed, or cerebrospinal fluid leak. Be sure to give instructions for waking the patient every few hours at night for observation of mental state and administration of medication.

Complications
- Intercerebral hemorrhage
- Brain injury

•••••••••••••
HEAT SYNDROME

Heat syndrome may result from environmental or internal conditions that increase heat production or impair heat dissipation. The three categories of heat syndrome are heat cramps, heat exhaustion, and heatstroke. Heat cramps are severe muscle cramps that occur after exercising in extreme heat; they're caused by excessive fluid and electrolyte loss. Heat exhaustion is acute hyperthermia due to dehydration. This may progress to heatstroke. Heatstroke is extreme hyperthermia with thermoregulatory failure

Causes
Humans normally adjust to excessive temperatures by complex cardiovascular and neurologic changes that are coordinated by the hypothalamus. Heat loss offsets heat production to regulate the body temperature. It does this by evaporation

(sweating) or vasodilation, which cools the body's surface by radiation, conduction, and convection.

However, heat production increases with exercise, infection, and the use of certain drugs such as amphetamines, and heat loss decreases with high temperatures or humidity, lack of acclimatization, excess clothing, obesity, dehydration, cardiovascular disease, sweat gland dysfunction, and the use of such drugs as phenothiazines and anticholinergics. When heat loss mechanisms fail to offset heat production, the body retains heat and may develop heat syndrome.

Clinical presentation
For specific guidelines on recognizing and managing heat disorders, see *Managing heat syndrome*.

Differential diagnoses
- Adult respiratory distress syndrome
- Alcohol withdrawal syndrome
- Diabetic ketoacidosis
- Encephalitis
- Thyroid disorder
- Malaria
- Meningitis
- Myocardial infarction (MI)
- Neuroleptic malignant disorder
- Drug toxicity
- Septic shock

Diagnosis
Diagnosis is based on clinical presentation and related body temperature. For heat exhaustion, the core temperature is elevated but less than 103° F (39.4° C). In heatstroke, the core temperature is greater than 104° F (40° C).

Laboratory findings may include:
- complete blood count showing hemoconcentration
- electrolyte measurements showing elevated sodium and chloride levels.

Managing heat syndrome

TYPE AND PREDISPOSING FACTORS	CLINICAL PRESENTATION	MANAGEMENT
Heat cramps ■ Commonly affect young adults ■ Strenuous activity without training or acclimatization ■ Normal to high temperature or high humidity	■ Muscle twitching and spasms, weakness, severe muscle cramps ■ Nausea ■ Normal temperature or slightly elevated ■ Diaphoresis	■ Hospitalization is usually unnecessary. ■ Replace fluids and electrolytes. ■ Loosen the patient's clothing, and have him lie down in a cool place. Massage his muscles. If muscle cramps are severe, start an I.V. infusion with normal saline solution.
Heat exhaustion ■ Commonly affects young people ■ Physical activity without acclimatization ■ Decreased heat dissipation ■ High temperature and humidity	■ Nausea and vomiting ■ Decreased blood pressure ■ Thready, rapid pulse ■ Cool, pallid skin ■ Headache, mental confusion, syncope, giddiness ■ Oliguria, thirst ■ Elevated temperature ■ Muscle cramps	■ Hospitalization is usually unnecessary. ■ Immediately give salt tablets and a balanced electrolyte drink. ■ Loosen the patient's clothing, and put him in a shock position in a cool place. Massage his muscles. If cramps are severe, start an I.V. infusion. ■ If needed, give oxygen.
Heatstroke ■ Exertional type — commonly affects young, healthy people who are involved in strenuous activity ■ Classical type — commonly affects elderly, inactive people who have cardiovascular disease or who take drugs that influence temperature regulation ■ High temperature and humidity without any wind	■ Hypertension followed by hypotension ■ Atrial or ventricular tachycardia ■ Hot, dry, red skin, which later turns gray; no diaphoresis ■ Confusion, progressing to seizures and loss of consciousness ■ Temperature higher than 104° F (40° C) ■ Dilated pupils ■ Slow, deep respirations; then Cheyne-Stokes respirations	■ Hospitalization is needed. ■ Initiate ABCs of life support. ■ To lower body temperature, cool the patient rapidly with ice packs on arterial pressure points and hypothermia blankets. ■ To replace fluids and electrolytes, start an I.V. infusion. ■ Insert nasogastric tube to prevent aspiration. ■ Give diazepam to control seizures. ■ Monitor temperature, intake and output, and cardiac status. Give dobutamine to correct cardiogenic shock (vasoconstrictors are contraindicated).

Other abnormal findings need to be related to specific organ damage associated with the disorder.

Management

Specific management depends on the type of heat disorder. (See *Managing heat syndrome*, page 747.)

🔲 **CLINICAL CAUTION** Vigorous fluid replacement in elderly people or those with underlying cardiovascular disease may cause pulmonary edema.

Referral

■ Refer the patient to the hospital for treatment, if needed.
■ Refer the patient to social services depending on the cause of the heat disorder.

Follow-up

The patient should be seen 1 week after hospitalization.

Patient teaching

■ Tell the patient who has had heat cramps or heat exhaustion to exercise gradually and to increase his salt and water intake.
■ Tell the patient with heatstroke that residual hypersensitivity to high temperatures may persist for several months.
■ Remind the patient to drink 400 to 500 ml of cool fluids before exercise and 200 to 300 ml at regular intervals during exercise.

Complications

■ Major organ system failure
■ Cardiac arrhythmias
■ MI
■ Seizure
■ Coma
■ Pulmonary edema
■ Rhabdomyolysis
■ Disseminated intravascular coagulation

🔲 **HEALTHY LIVING** Heat disorders are easily preventable, so it's important to educate the public about the various factors that cause them. This information is especially vital for athletes, laborers, and soldiers in field training.

Special considerations

■ Advise the patient to avoid heat disorders by taking precautions in hot weather, such as wearing loose-fitting, lightweight clothing; resting frequently; avoiding hot places; and drinking adequate fluids.
■ Inform the patient who is obese, elderly, or taking drugs that impair heat regulation that he should avoid becoming overheated.
■ Educate the public, especially elderly people, on the use of fans, air conditioning, and adequate ventilation.

• • • • • • • • • • • •

INSECT BITES AND STINGS

Insect bites and stings are among the most common traumatic complaints. More serious bites and stings include those of ticks, brown recluse spiders, black widow spiders, scorpions, bees, wasps, and yellow jackets.

Clinical presentation

For specific signs and symptoms occurring from different bites and stings see *Comparing insect bites and stings*, pages 750 to 753.

Differential diagnoses

■ Angina
■ Cat-scratch fever
■ Cavernous sinus
■ Corneal laceration
■ Human bite
■ Rheumatoid arthritis
■ Snake bite

- Toxicity to unknown agent
- I.V. drug use
- Dermatosis

Diagnosis
Clinical presentation along with detailed history may help diagnosis.

Management
General
The initial management goal in treating a patient with an insect bite or sting is to support respiratory and cardiovascular function. Specific management depends on the source of the bite or sting. (See *Comparing insect bites and stings*, pages 750 to 753.)

Medication
The following medications may be used in treating a patient with an insect bite or sting:
- epinephrine — adults, 0.1 to 0.5 mg I.M., I.V., or S.C.; children, 0.01 ml/kg I.V. or S.C. for systemic reaction
- diphenhydramine — adults, 25 to 50 mg P.O., I.M., or I.V.; children, 5 mg/kg/day P.O., I.M., or I.V. in divided doses
- cimetidine — adults, 300 to 800 mg I.V. every 6 hours, or 400 mg P.O. b.i.d.; children, 5 mg/kg I.V. every 6 hours
- albuterol nebulizer treatment — adults, 2.5 mg in 3 ml normal saline solution every 15 to 30 minutes; children, 0.1mg/kg in 3 ml normal saline solution every 15 to 20 minutes for bronchospasm
- methylprednisolone — 2 to 60 mg/day P.O.; individualized dosage.

Referral
- Refer the patient to a hospital for treatment, if needed.

Follow-up
The patient may need to be seen, depending on the source of the bite or sting and the complications involved.

Patient teaching
- To reduce the risk of being bitten by a tick, tell the patient to keep away from wooded areas, to wear protective clothes, and to examine his body carefully for ticks after being outdoors.

HEALTHY LIVING Tell the patient to never pull a tick out of the skin. Instead, the patient should place petroleum jelly or mineral oil over the tick to cause suffocation. If the tick is pulled out, there is an increased chance of leaving the head imbedded in the skin. If suffocation isn't effective after 20 minutes, carefully pull the tick out with tweezers.

- To prevent brown recluse and black widow spider bites, advise the patient to spray infested areas, tuck pant legs into socks in such areas, wear gloves and heavy clothes when working around woodpiles or sheds, inspect outdoor work clothes for spiders before use, and discourage children from playing near infested areas.
- Tell the patient who is allergic to bee stings to wear a medical identification bracelet or carry a card and to carry an anaphylaxis kit. Explain how to use the kit and refer him to an allergist for hyposensitization.
- To prevent bee stings, warn the patient to avoid using fragrant cosmetics during insect season, to avoid wearing bright colors and going barefoot, and to avoid touching flowers and fruits that attract bees. Advise him to use insect repellent.

Complications
- Anaphylactic shock
- Death
- Arthritis
- Thrombocytopenia
- Hemolytic anemia
- Respiratory distress
- Neurologic disease
- Acrodermatitis chronica atrophicans

(Text continues on page 752.)

Comparing insect bites and stings

GENERAL INFORMATION	CLINICAL PRESENTATION

Hard tick

- Common in woods and fields throughout the Northeast and Midwest United States
- Attaches to host in any of its life stages (larva, nymph, or adult); fastens to host with its teeth, then secretes a cementlike material to reinforce attachment
- Flat, black speckled body about ¼" (6.3 mm) long; has eight legs
- Also transmits Rocky Mountain spotted fever and Lyme disease
- Most infestations from May to July
- 91% of cases occur in PA, NJ, NY, and MD

- Local reaction with no initial antibody response.
- Lyme disease has three distinct stages.
- Immunoglobulin (Ig) M antibody peaks 3 to 6 weeks after bite with a rise in IgG titers.
- Erythema migrans lesion with flulike symptoms occurs by the 9th day after bite. Pain, itching or paresthesia may be present.

Brown recluse (violin) spider

- Common to south-central United States; usually found in dark areas (outdoor privy, barn, or woodshed)
- Dark brown violin on its back; three pairs of eyes; female more dangerous than male
- Most bites occur between April and October.

- Venom is coagulotoxic. Reaction begins within 2 to 8 hours after bite.
- Localized vasoconstriction causes ischemic necrosis at bite site. Small, reddened puncture wound forms a bleb and becomes ischemic. In 3 to 4 days, center becomes dark and hard. Within 2 to 3 weeks, an ulcer forms.
- Minimal initial pain; increases over time.
- Other symptoms include fever, chills, malaise, weakness, nausea, vomiting, edema, seizures, joint pain, petechiae, cyanosis, and phlebitis.
- Rarely, thrombocytopenia and hemolytic anemia develop, leading to death within first 24 to 48 hours (usually in a child or patient with previous history of cardiac disease). Prompt and appropriate treatment results in recovery.

Black widow spider

- Common throughout the United States, particularly in warmer climates; usually found in dark areas (outdoor privy, barn, or woodshed)
- Female coal black with red or orange hourglass on ventral side; female larger than male (male doesn't bite)
- Mortality less than 1% (increased risk among elderly people, infants, and people with allergies)

- Venom is neurotoxic. Patient's age, size, and sensitivity determine the severity and progression of symptoms.
- Pinprick sensation, followed by dull, numbing pain (may go unnoticed).
- Edema and tiny, red bite marks.
- Rigidity of stomach muscles and severe abdominal pain (10 to 40 minutes after bite).
- Muscle spasms in extremities.
- Ascending paralysis, causing difficulty swallowing and labored, grunting respirations.
- Other symptoms include extreme restlessness, vertigo, sweating, chills, pallor, seizures (especially in children), hyperactive reflexes, hypertension, tachycardia, thready pulse, circulatory collapse, nausea, vomiting, headache, ptosis, eyelid edema, urticaria, pruritus, and fever.

MANAGEMENT	PATIENT TEACHING AND SPECIAL CONSIDERATIONS
■ Removal of tick ■ Antimicrobial therapy (doxycycline 100 mg P.O. b.i.d. for 21 days) for Lyme disease ■ Mechanical ventilation for respiratory failure	■ Follow precautions in removing ticks from skin. ■ To reduce risk of being bitten, teach patient to keep away from wooded areas; to wear light-colored, protective clothes; and to carefully examine body for ticks after being outdoors. ■ Tell patient to apply insect spray containing diethyltoluamide to skin and clothes when in high-risk areas.
■ Combination therapy with corticosteroids, antibiotics, antihistamines, tranquilizers, I.V. fluids, and tetanus prophylaxis ■ Dapsone 100 mg b.i.d. to suppress leukocyte response ■ Possibly surgical debridement and skin grafting for large ulcerative lesions ■ Possibly skin grafting for large chronic ulcer	■ Clean lesion with 1:20 Burow's aluminum acetate solution, and apply antibiotic ointment ■ Take complete patient history, including allergies and other preexisting medical problems. ■ Monitor vital signs, general appearance, and changes at bite site. ■ Reassure patient with disfiguring ulcer that skin grafting can improve appearance. ■ To prevent brown recluse bites, tell the patient to spray infested areas with creosote at least every 2 months, to wear gloves and heavy clothes when working around woodpiles or sheds, to inspect outdoor working clothes for spiders before use, and to discourage children from playing near infested areas.
■ Neutralization of venom using antivenin I.V., preceded by desensitization when skin or eye tests show sensitivity to horse serum ■ Calcium gluconate I.V. to control muscle spasms ■ Muscle relaxants such as diazepam for severe muscle spasms ■ Adrenaline or antihistamines ■ Oxygen by nasal cannula or mask ■ Tetanus immunization ■ Antibiotics to prevent infection	■ Take complete patient history, including allergies and other preexisting medical problems. ■ Have epinephrine and emergency resuscitation equipment on hand in case of anaphylactic reaction to antivenin. ■ Keep patient quiet and warm and affected part immobile. ■ Clean bite site with antiseptic; apply ice to relieve pain and swelling and to slow circulation. ■ Assess vital signs frequently during first 12 hours after bite. Symptoms usually subside in 3 to 4 hours. ■ To prevent black widow spider bites, tell patient to spray infested areas with creosote at least every 2 months, to wear gloves and heavy clothing when working around woodpiles or sheds, to inspect outdoor working clothes for spiders before putting them on, and to discourage children from playing near infested areas.

(continued)

Comparing insect bites and stings *(continued)*

GENERAL INFORMATION	CLINICAL PRESENTATION
Scorpion ■ Common throughout the United States (30 different species); 2 deadly species in southwestern states ■ Curled tail with stinger on end; eight legs; 3″ (7.6 cm) long ■ Most stings occur during warmer months. ■ Mortality less than 1% (increased risk among elderly people and children)	*Local reaction:* ■ Local swelling and tenderness, sharp burning sensation, skin discoloration, paresthesia, and lymphangitis with regional gland swelling. *Systemic reaction (neurotoxic):* ■ Immediate sharp pain; hyperesthesia; drowsiness; itching of nose, throat, and mouth; impaired speech (due to sluggish tongue); generalized muscle spasms (including jaw muscle spasms, laryngospasms, incontinence, and seizures); nausea; vomiting; and drooling. ■ Symptoms last 24 to 78 hours; bite site recovers last. ■ Anaphylaxis is rare. ■ Death may follow cardiovascular or respiratory failure. ■ Prognosis is poor if symptoms progress rapidly in first few hours.
Bee, wasp, yellow jacket ■ When honeybee (rounded abdomen) or bumblebee (over 1″ [2.5 cm] long; furry, rounded abdomen) stings, stinger remains in victim; bee flies away ■ Wasp or yellow jacket (slender body with elongated abdomen) retains stinger and can sting repeatedly ■ Venom composition varies among species ■ Bees account for 1 million stings each year	*Local reaction:* ■ Painful wound (protruding stinger from bees), edema, urticaria, and pruritus. *Systemic reaction (anaphylaxis):* ■ Symptoms of hypersensitivity usually appear within 20 minutes and may include weakness, chest tightness, dizziness, nausea, vomiting, abdominal cramps, and throat constriction. The shorter the interval between sting and systemic symptoms, the worse the prognosis. Without prompt treatment, symptoms may progress to cyanosis, coma, and death.

• • • • • • • • • • • •

MAMMAL BITES

Although seldom fatal, bites from animals or humans can cause injuries ranging from bruises and superficial scratches to severe crush injuries, deep puncture wounds, tissue loss, and severe damage to blood vessels. In the United States, 60% to 90% of animal bites come from dogs and about 10% come from cats; the third most common bites are from humans.

Surprisingly, human bites are feared most because of the great variety of infectious bacteria and viruses normally present in the oral cavity. Women have a higher incidence of being bitten by cats and men have a higher incidence of being bitten by dogs.

AGE ALERT Peak incidence of animal bites among children is between ages 5 and 14.

A dog bite may cause a crushing wound due to round teeth and strong jaws.

MANAGEMENT	PATIENT TEACHING AND SPECIAL CONSIDERATIONS
■ Antivenin (made from cat serum), if available (contact the Antivenin Lab, Arizona State University, Tempe) ■ Calcium gluconate I.V. for muscle spasm ■ Phenobarbital I.M. for seizures ■ Emetine S.C. to relieve pain (opiates such as morphine and codeine contraindicated because they enhance venom's effects)	■ Take complete patient history, including allergies and other preexisting medical conditions. ■ Immobilize patient and apply tourniquet proximal to sting. ■ Pack area extending beyond tourniquet in ice. After 5 minutes of ice pack, remove tourniquet. ■ Assess vital signs. Watch closely for signs of respiratory distress. (Keep emergency resuscitation equipment available.)
■ Antihistamines and corticosteroids (in urticaria) ■ Tetanus prophylaxis ■ In anaphylaxis, oxygen by nasal cannula or mask and epinephrine 1:1,000 S.C. or I.M. ■ In bronchospasm, albuterol and corticosteroids ■ In hypotension, epinephrine and isoproterenol	■ If stinger is in place, scrape it off. Don't pull it; this action releases more toxin. ■ Clean site and apply ice. ■ Watch patient carefully for signs of anaphylaxis. Keep emergency resuscitation equipment available. ■ Tell the patient who is allergic to bee stings to wear medical identification bracelet or carry card and to carry an anaphylaxis kit. Teach him how to use the kit, and refer him to allergist for hyposensitization. ■ To prevent bee stings, tell patient to avoid wearing fragrant cosmetics during insect season, to avoid wearing bright colors and going barefoot, to avoid flowers and fruit that attract bees, and to use insect repellent.

An adult dog exerts 200 to 400 pounds per square inch of pressure when it bites; therefore, damage to bone, vessels, muscle, tendons, and nerves may occur. Cat bites inoculate bacteria deep into tissue.

Bites on the hand have a higher infection incidence rate due to poor blood supply of the many structures. Nearly all infections are mixed because multiple organisms are found in animals' saliva. Clenched-fist injuries are the most serious because damaged joint capsules increase the risk of developing osteomyelitis and septic arthritis.

Unfortunately, many animals — usually wild ones — carry the rabies virus in their saliva and can transmit it by biting or licking an open wound. Rabies is rare in the United States, but it's always fatal unless treated. The risk of getting rabies from a dog is low but possible. Bats, skunks, and raccoons cause nearly all cases of rabies in the United States.

Human bites can infect other humans with diseases such as herpes simplex virus, cytomegalovirus, syphilis, tuberculosis and, possibly, acquired immunodeficiency syndrome.

Causes
Animal bites commonly occur when a sick or injured animal is trying to protect itself or when an animal is protecting its food, territory, or young. In most cases, human bites most often result from fights among school-age children and young adults.

Clinical presentation
A dog bite may cause bleeding, pain, tenderness, swelling, and decreased sensation at the injury site. A large dog usually inflicts a more severe wound than a smaller dog. A cat bite may cause small, deep puncture wounds.

A human bite may induce bleeding, which may be scant or profuse. If the bite results in a puncture wound or a tear, bleeding may occur immediately, with bruising and swelling appearing later. Assess the injured area for teeth marks.

Differential diagnoses
- Human bite
- Animal bite
- Cellulitis
- Fracture
- Trauma
- Osteomyelitis
- Tetanus
- Rabies

Diagnosis
Diagnosis is made depending on the history of the wound. X-rays of the injured area may be needed to determine the extent of damage. Wound or blood cultures may be taken to determine the specific antimicrobial therapy needed.

Management
General
If the bite wound isn't bleeding heavily (as with a puncture wound), wash it vigorously with soap and water for 5 to 10 minutes. Let it bleed a bit to help flush out pathogens. A syringe and catheter may be used to create a high-pressure water stream to clean the wound. If animal bite puncture wounds are simple and don't involve the hands, no other treatment is necessary. Human bites require wound cultures to rule out gram-negative organisms. Splint clenched-fist injuries and then elevate the hand; obtain an X-ray to rule out fractures.

CLINICAL CAUTION Don't scrub a bite wound; you could bruise the tissue. Also, don't tape the wound or seal it in any way — doing so increases the risk of infection. Apply an ice pack to the wound site for 20 minutes to decrease edema and pain.

Medication
The following medications may be used to treat patients with mammal bites:
- acetaminophen — adults, 325 to 650 mg P.O. every 4 hours; children, dosage per package directions
- ibuprofen — 200 to 400 mg P.O. every 4 hours
- tetanus toxoid — 0.5 ml I.M. for patients who have been immunized in the past but haven't had a booster within the past 10 years; 0.5 ml of tetanus toxoid and tetanus immune globulin for patients who haven't had an initial immunization series
- rabies prophylaxis if rabies is considered possible, given without delay; consult a health care provider before starting therapy (see *Guide to postexposure rabies prophylaxis*)
- erythromycin — adults, 250 to 500 mg P.O. every 6 hours; children, 30 to 50 mg/kg/day in 4 divided doses.

Guide to postexposure rabies prophylaxis

To make decisions about rabies treatment, consider the details of the exposure, the animal's species and vaccination status, and the prevalence of rabies in the region. The wound should be thoroughly cleaned with soap and water. All bites by an animal of questionable health or vaccination status require prompt evaluation. The table below provides general guidelines for the next actions to take. Note that the Food and Drug Administration (FDA) considers all three types of rabies vaccines equally safe and effective.

ANIMAL SPECIES	CONDITION OF ANIMAL AT TIME OF ATTACK	TREATMENT OF EXPOSED HUMAN
Wild Skunk Raccoon Bat Other carnivores	Considered rabid unless proven negative (the animal should be killed and the head tested immediately; observation not recommended)	Rabies immune globulin, human (RIG*) and human diploid cell vaccine (HDCV) or rabies vaccine, adsorbed (RVA**)
Domestic Cat Dog	Healthy and available: 10 days of isolation and observation	None
	Unknown (escaped)	Consult public health officials and a health care provider; if treatment is indicated, give RIG* and HDCV or RVA**
Other Livestock Gnawing animals (such as hamsters, rabbits, and beavers)	Rabies suspected or known	RIG* and HDCV or RVA** Consider individually

*RIG should be administered at the beginning of treatment. Administer 20 IU/kg I.M. This product isn't FDA-approved for intradermal use.

**HDCV or RVA are equally effective. Administer 1 ml of vaccine I.M. on days 0, 3, 14, and 28. If using HDCV, divide the dose in half, giving one-half I.M. and one-half infiltrated thoroughly around the wound. HDCV is the only rabies vaccine approved by the FDA for intradermal use.

Surgical intervention
Moderate to severe wounds should be debrided. If no signs or symptoms of infection appear after 2 days, the wound may be closed with sutures or tape strips.

Referral
■ Refer the patient to a plastic surgeon, if needed.

Follow-up
The patient should be seen within 2 to 3 days to evaluate the wound.

Patient teaching

- Tell the patient that symptoms of infection usually appear after 24 hours and to report them if they occur.

Complications

- Septic arthritis
- Osteomyelitis
- Soft tissue injury
- Sepsis
- Gas gangrene
- Death
- Hemorrhage

Special considerations

- Advise anyone who has witnessed an animal bite to tell the authorities where the incident occurred and the animal owner's name, if possible. If the animal was wild, tell them the animal's location at the time of the bite. Authorities try to capture the animal and then confine it for 10 days of observation. If it appears rabid, it's killed and its brain tissue is tested for rabies.

• • • • • • • • • • • •

RAPE TRAUMA SYNDROME

The term *rape* refers to illicit sexual intercourse without consent. It's a violent assault in which sex is used as a weapon. Rape results in varying degrees of physical and psychological trauma. Rape trauma syndrome occurs during the period following the rape or attempted rape; it refers to the victim's short-term and long-term reactions to the trauma.

In the United States, 1.3 adult women are raped every minute. The incidence of reported rape is highest in large cities and continues to rise. However, an estimated 80% to 90% of rapes are never reported. According to the U. S. Justice Department, 8% of all American women

will be victims of rape or attempted rape in their lifetime.

AGE ALERT Known victims of rape range in age from 2 months to 97 years. The age-group most affected is 10- to 19-year-olds. About one in seven reported rapes involves a prepubertal child; most of these cases involve manual, oral, or genital contact with the child's genitals by a member of the child's family.

More than 50% of rapes occur in the home; about one-third of these involve a male intruder who forces his way into the home. In about half of the cases, the victim has some casual acquaintance with the attacker. Most rapists are ages 15 to 24 and have planned the attack.

In most cases, the rapist is a man and the victim is a woman. However, rapes do occur between persons of the same sex, especially in prisons, schools, hospitals, and other institutions. Approximately 9% of reported rapes are from males. It's estimated that 1 million males in prison are raped each year.

The prognosis is good if the rape victim receives physical and emotional support and counseling to help her deal with her feelings. Victims who articulate their feelings are able to cope with fears, interact with others, and return to normal routines faster than those who don't.

Causes

Some of the cultural, sociologic, and psychological factors that contribute to rape are increasing exposure to sex, permissiveness, cynicism about relationships, feelings of anger, and powerlessness amid social pressures. Many rapists have feelings of violence or hatred toward women or sexual problems, such as impotence or premature ejaculation. They may feel socially isolated and be unable to form warm, loving relationships. Some rapists may be psychopaths who need violence for physical pleasure, no matter how it affects their victims; others rape to satisfy a need for power. Some were abused as children.

Clinical presentation

A rape victim may or may not appear injured. Immediate reactions to rape vary and include crying, laughing, hostility, confusion, withdrawal, or outward calm; anger and rage may surface later. A child may react differently from an adult. (See *If the rape victim is a child*.)

Being careful to avoid upsetting the victim as much as possible, obtain an accurate history of the rape, pertinent to physical assessment. (Remember, your notes may be used as evidence if the rapist goes to trial.) Physical injuries vary with each assault. Even if the victim wasn't beaten, the physical examination (including a pelvic examination) usually reveals signs of physical trauma, especially if the attack was prolonged. Depending on specific body areas attacked, a patient may have a sore throat, mouth irritation, difficulty swallowing, ecchymoses, or rectal pain and bleeding. If additional physical violence accompanied the rape, the victim may have hematomas, lacerations, bleeding, severe internal injuries, and hemorrhage; if the rape occurred outdoors, she may suffer from exposure. X-rays may reveal fractures. For a male victim, be especially alert for injury to the mouth, perineum, and anus. As ordered, obtain a pharyngeal specimen for a gonorrhea culture and rectal aspirate for acid phosphatase or sperm analysis.

Differential diagnoses

- Consenting sex among adults

Diagnosis

The patient's history is important in diagnosing rape. The presence of sperm is indicative of sexual activity. There may be evidence of trauma.

If the rape victim is a child

Carefully interview the child to assess how well she will be able to deal with the situation after going home. Interview the child alone, away from the parents. Tell the parents that this is being done for the child's comfort, not to keep secrets from them. Ask them what words the child is comfortable with when referring to parts of the anatomy.

HISTORY AND EXAMINATION

A young child places only as much importance on an experience as others do, unless there is physical pain. A good question to ask is, "Did someone touch you when you didn't want to be touched?" As with other rape victims, record information in the child's own words. A complete pelvic examination is necessary only if penetration has occurred; such an examination requires parental consent and an analgesic or a local anesthetic.

NEED FOR COUNSELING

The child and the parents need counseling to minimize possible emotional disturbances. Encourage the child to talk about the experience, and try to alleviate confusion. After a rape, a young child may regress; an older child may become fearful about being left alone. The child's behavior may change at school or at home.

Help the parents understand that it's normal for them to feel angry and guilty but warn them against displacing or projecting these feelings onto the child. Instruct them to assure the child that they're not angry with her; that the child is good and didn't cause the incident; that they're sorry it happened but glad the child is alright; and that the family will work the problems out together.

Management
General

Record the victim's statements in the first person, using quotation marks. Also document objective information provided by others. Never speculate as to what may have happened or record subjective impressions or thoughts. Include in your notes the time the victim arrived at the hospital, the date and time of the alleged rape, and the time that the victim was examined.

Many centers have certified forensic examiners and counselors to assist the general staff with rape victims. Follow the protocols and procedures of the institution.

Accuracy is essential. Most emergency departments have "rape kits," which include containers for specimens. (See *Legal considerations*.)

Most states require hospitals to report incidences of rape. However, the patient may not press charges and may not assist the police.

Treatment consists of supportive measures and protection against venereal disease, human immunodeficiency virus (HIV) testing, and, if the patient wishes, testing for pregnancy.

Medication

The following medications may be used in the treatment of rape victims:
- acetaminophen — 325 to 650 mg P.O. every 4 hours
- ibuprofen — 400 to 800 mg P.O. every 4 to 6 hours p.r.n.
- buspirone — 5 to 20 mg P.O. b.i.d. to t.i.d.
- alprazolam — 0.25 to 0.5 mg P.O. b.i.d. to t.i.d.
- diazepam — adults, 2 to 10 mg P.O. b.i.d. to q.i.d.; children, 1 to 2.5 mg P.O. t.i.d. to q.i.d.
- norgestrel or levonorgestrel, and ethinyl estradiol — 2 tablets P.O. immediately, plus 2 tablets 12 hours later to prevent pregnancy.

Referral

- Refer the patient to a hospital for examination and treatment.
- Refer the patient for psychological counseling, if needed, to cope with the aftereffects of the attack.
- Refer the patient and family to organizations such as Women Organized Against Rape or a local rape crisis center for support and information.

Follow-up

The follow-up depends on the victim and her request for follow-up testing for pregnancy or sexually transmitted diseases such as HIV.

Patient teaching
- Because cultures can't detect gonorrhea or syphilis for 5 to 6 days after the rape, stress the importance of returning for follow-up venereal disease testing.

Complications
- Injury
- Psychological problems
- Injury to self

• • • • • • • • • • • •

SPRAINS AND STRAINS

A sprain is a complete or incomplete tear in the supporting ligaments surrounding a joint that usually follows a sharp twist. A strain is an injury to a muscle or tendinous attachment. Both injuries usually heal without surgical repair.

Causes
Sprains and strains are the most common sport-related injuries. A sprain is the result of trauma, direct or indirect, that forces a joint out of position, causing damage to the supporting ligaments. A strain is the result of overuse of muscles and tendons. Intense training without adequate rest may precipitate a strain.

Clinical presentation
A sprain causes these signs and symptoms:
- local pain (especially during joint movement)
- swelling
- loss of mobility (which may not occur until several hours after the injury)
- black-and-blue discoloration from blood extravasating into surrounding tissues.

A sprained ankle is the most common joint injury. (See *Muscle-tendon ruptures.*)

Muscle-tendon ruptures

Perhaps the most serious muscle-tendon injury is a rupture of the muscle-tendon junction. This type of rupture may occur at any such junction, but it's most common at the Achilles tendon, extending from the posterior calf muscle to the foot. An Achilles tendon rupture produces a sudden, sharp pain and, until swelling begins, a palpable defect. Such a rupture typically occurs in men between ages 35 and 40, especially during physical activities such as jogging or tennis.

To distinguish an Achilles tendon rupture from other ankle injuries, perform this simple test: With the patient prone and his feet hanging off the foot of the table, squeeze the calf muscle. If this causes plantar flexion, the tendon is intact; if it causes ankle dorsiflexion, it's partially intact; if there's no flexion of any kind, the tendon is ruptured.

An Achilles tendon rupture usually requires surgical repair, followed first by a long leg cast for 4 weeks and then by a short cast for another 4 weeks.

A strain may be acute (an immediate result of vigorous muscle overuse or overstress) or chronic (a result of repeated overuse). An acute strain causes a sharp, transient pain (the patient may report having heard a snapping noise) and rapid swelling. When severe pain subsides, the muscle is tender; after several days, ecchymoses appear. A chronic strain causes stiffness, soreness, and generalized tenderness several hours after the injury.

Differential diagnoses
- Dislocation of joints
- Fracture

- Compartment syndrome
- Subluxation of joints
- Muscle spasm

Diagnosis

A history of a recent injury or chronic overuse, clinical findings, and an X-ray to rule out fractures establish the diagnosis.

Management

General

Treatment of sprains consists of controlling pain and swelling and immobilizing the injured joint to promote healing. Immediately after the injury, control swelling by elevating the joint above the level of the heart and by intermittently applying ice for 24 to 48 hours. To prevent a cold injury, place a towel between the ice pack and the skin. Support the joint using an elastic bandage. If the sprain is severe, immobilize the joint with a splint. If the patient has a sprained ankle, he may need crutch gait training. Patients with sprains seldom require hospitalization. An immobilized sprain usually heals in 2 to 3 weeks, after which the patient can gradually resume normal activities.

Medication

The following medications may be used to treat sprains and strains:
- ibuprofen — 200 to 400 mg P.O. every 4 to 6 hours
- codeine — adults, 15 to 60 mg P.O. every 4 to 6 hours; children, 3 mg/kg/day in divided doses every 4 hours.

Surgical intervention

Occasionally, torn ligaments don't heal properly and cause recurrent dislocation, requiring surgical repair. Some athletes may request immediate surgical repair to hasten healing; to prevent sprains, they may tape their wrists and ankles before

sports activities. Complete muscle rupture may require surgery.

Referral

- Refer the patient to an orthopedic surgeon if treatment is unsuccessful.
- Refer the patient for physical therapy, if needed.

Follow-up

The patient may need to be seen, depending on the type and extent of injury.

Patient teaching

- Tell the patient to elevate the joint for 48 to 72 hours after the injury (pillows can be used while sleeping) and to apply ice intermittently for 24 to 48 hours.
- If an elastic bandage has been applied, teach the patient to reapply it by wrapping from below to above the injury, forming a figure eight. For a sprained ankle, apply the bandage from the toes to midcalf. Tell the patient to remove the bandage before going to sleep and to loosen it if it causes the leg to become pale, numb, or painful.
- Instruct the patient to report if the pain worsens or persists; if so, an additional X-ray may reveal a previously undetected fracture.

Complications

- Arthritis
- Chronic joint instability

• • • • • • • • • • • • •

WOUNDS, OPEN TRAUMA

Open trauma wounds (abrasions, avulsions, crush wounds, lacerations, missile injuries, and punctures) are injuries that commonly result from home, work, or motor vehicle accidents and from acts of violence.

Clinical presentation

In all open wounds, the extent of injury needs to be assessed. Peripheral nerve damage is a common complication in lacerations and other open trauma wounds. Fractures and dislocations may also be present. Signs of peripheral nerve damage vary with location:

- *radial nerve* — weak forearm dorsiflexion, inability to extend the thumb in a hitchhiker's sign
- *median nerve* — numbness in the tip of the index finger; inability to place the forearm in a prone position; weak forearm, thumb, and index finger flexion
- *ulnar nerve* — numbness in the tip of the little finger, clawing of the hand
- *peroneal nerve* — footdrop, inability to extend the foot or big toe
- *sciatic and tibial nerves* — paralysis of the ankles and toes, footdrop, weakness in the leg, numbness in the sole.

Differential diagnoses

- Abdominal penetrating injury
- Acute respiratory distress syndrome
- Alcohol abuse
- Substance abuse
- Lactic acidosis
- Metabolic acidosis
- Mesenteric ischemia
- Necrotizing fascitis
- Abuse
- Hemorrhagic shock
- Sepsis

Diagnosis

History and clinical presentation of the wound diagnose open trauma wounds. With suspected nerve involvement, electromyography, nerve conduction, and electrical stimulation tests can provide more detailed information about possible peripheral nerve damage. A full trauma workup should be done as per facility protocol. X-ray, computed tomography scans, and ultrasound may provide information concerning the extent of the injury. Peritoneal lavage may be performed to diagnose an abdominal injury.

Management

General

Most open wounds require emergency treatment. (See *Managing open trauma wounds*, pages 762 to 764.)

Assessment of vital signs, level of consciousness, obvious skeletal damage, local neurologic deficits, and general patient condition determines the scope of treatment. The patient should be assessed at a certified trauma center by a multispecialty team. Information about the mechanism and time of injury and treatment already given may also guide treatment. If the injury involved a weapon, the police must be notified.

Medication

The following medications may be used in the treatment of patients with open trauma wounds:

- morphine — adults, 5 to 20 mg I.M., or S.C. every 4 hours or 2.5 to 15 mg I.V every 4 hours; children, 0.1 to 0.2 mg/kg I.M., or S.C. every 4 hours
- lorazepam — adults, 2 to 6 mg/day P.O. in divided doses
- cefazolin — adults, 1 to 12 g I.V. or I.M. in divided doses; children, 25 to 100 mg/kg/day in divided doses every 6 to 8 hours
- lidocaine local injection — adults, 1% solution injected into site; children, 0.5% to 1% solution injected into site
- tetanus — 0.5 ml I.M. if immunization isn't current.

Surgical intervention

Surgery may be required depending on the type of injury sustained.

(*Text continues on page 764.*)

Managing open trauma wounds

TYPE	CLINICAL ACTION
Abrasion ■ Open surface wounds (scrapes) of epidermis and possibly the dermis, resulting from friction; nerve endings exposed ■ Diagnosis based on mechanism of injury	■ Obtain a history to distinguish injury from second-degree burn. ■ Clean the wound gently with topical germicide and irrigate it. Too vigorous scrubbing of abrasions will increase tissue damage. ■ Remove imbedded foreign objects. Apply a local anesthetic or provide analgesia. ■ Apply a light, water-soluble antibiotic cream to prevent infection. ■ If the wound is severe, apply a loose protective dressing that allows air to circulate. ■ Administer tetanus prophylaxis if necessary.
Avulsion ■ Complete tissue loss that prevents approximation of wound edges, resulting from cutting, gouging, or complete tearing of skin; frequently affects nose tip, earlobe, fingertip, and penis ■ Diagnosis based on full-thickness skin loss, hemorrhage, pain, history of trauma; X-ray required to rule out bone damage	■ Check the patient history for bleeding tendencies and use of anticoagulants. ■ Record the time of injury to help determine if tissue is salvageable. Preserve tissue (if available) in cool saline solution for a possible split-thickness graft or flap. ■ Control hemorrhage with pressure, absorbable gelatin sponge, or topical thrombin. ■ Clean the wound gently, irrigate it with saline solution, and debride it if necessary. Cover it with a bulky dressing. ■ Tell the patient to leave the dressing in place until return visit, to keep the area dry, and to watch for signs of infection. ■ Administer analgesics and tetanus prophylaxis, if necessary.
Crush wound ■ Heavy falling object splits skin and causes necrosis along split margins and damages tissue underneath; may look like laceration ■ Diagnosis based on history of trauma, edema, hemorrhage, massive hematomas, damage to surrounding tissues (fractures, nerve injuries, or loss of tendon function), shock, and pain	■ Check the patient history for bleeding tendencies and use of anticoagulants. ■ Clean open areas gently with soap and water. ■ Control hemorrhage with pressure and cold pack. ■ Apply a dry, sterile bulky dressing; wrap the entire extremity in a compression dressing. ■ Immobilize the injured area and encourage the patient to rest. Assess vital signs, peripheral pulses, and circulation often. ■ Administer tetanus prophylaxis if necessary. ■ A severe injury may require I.V. infusion of lactated Ringer's or saline solution with a large-bore catheter as well as surgical exploration, debridement, and repair.

Managing open trauma wounds *(continued)*

TYPE	CLINICAL ACTION
Penetrating wound ■ Small-entry wounds that damage underlying structures, resulting from sharp, pointed objects ■ Diagnosis based on multiple considerations, including kinetic energy, hemorrhage (rare), deep hematomas (in chest or abdominal wounds), ragged wound edges (in bites), small-entry wound (in very sharp object), pain, and history of trauma; X-rays can detect retention of injuring object	■ Check the patient history for bleeding tendencies and use of anticoagulants. ■ Obtain a description of the injury, including mechanism of injury. ■ Assess the extent of the injury. ■ Don't remove impaling objects until the injury has been completely evaluated by the surgical specialist. ■ Thoroughly clean the injured area with soap and water. Irrigate minor wounds with saline solution during inspection and exploration. ■ Administer tetanus prophylaxis and, if necessary, a rabies vaccine. ■ Deep wounds that damage underlying tissues may require exploratory surgery; retention of the injuring object requires surgical removal and cosmetic repair.
Laceration ■ Open wound, possibly extending into deep epithelium, resulting from penetration with knife or other sharp object or from a severe blow with a blunt object ■ Diagnosis based on hemorrhage, torn or destroyed tissue, pain and history of trauma	*In lacerations less than 8 hours old and in all lacerations of face and areas of possible functional disability (such as the elbow):* ■ Apply pressure and elevate the injured extremity to control hemorrhage. ■ Clean the wound gently with saline solution or water; irrigate with normal saline solution. ■ As necessary, debride necrotic margins and close the wound, using strips of tape or sutures (primary closure). ■ A severe laceration with underlying structural damage may require surgery. *In grossly contaminated lacerations or lacerations more than 8 hours old (except lacerations of face and areas of possible functional disability):* ■ *Don't* close the wound immediately (delayed closure). ■ Instruct the patient to elevate the injured extremity for 24 hours after the injury to reduce swelling. ■ Tell the patient to keep the dressing clean and dry and to watch for signs of infection. *In all lacerations:* ■ Check the patient history for bleeding tendencies and anticoagulant use. ■ Determine the approximate time of injury and estimate the amount of blood lost. ■ Assess for neuromuscular, tendon, and circulatory damage. ■ Administer tetanus prophylaxis as needed. ■ Stress the need for follow-up and suture removal. ■ If the injury is the result of foul play, report it to the local authorities.

(continued)

Managing open trauma wounds (continued)

TYPE	CLINICAL ACTION
Missile injury ■ High-velocity tissue penetration such as a gunshot wound ■ Diagnosis based on entry and possibly exit wounds, signs of hemorrhage, shock, pain, and history of trauma; X-rays, complete blood count and differential, and electrolyte levels required to assess extent of injury and estimate blood loss	■ Check the patient history for bleeding tendencies and use of anticoagulants. ■ Control hemorrhage with pressure, if possible. If the injury is near vital organs, use large-bore catheters to start two I.V. lines, using lactated Ringer's or normal saline solution for volume replacement. Prepare for possible exploratory surgery. ■ Maintain a patent airway, and monitor for signs of hypovolemia, shock, and cardiac arrhythmias. Assess vital signs and neurovascular response often. ■ Cover a sucking chest wound during exhalation with an occlusive dressing taped on only three sides. ■ Clean the wound gently with saline solution or water; debride as necessary. ■ If damage is minor, apply a dry, sterile dressing. ■ Administer tetanus prophylaxis if necessary. ■ Obtain X-rays to detect retained fragments. ■ If possible, determine the caliber of the weapon. ■ Report the injury to the local authorities.

Referral
■ Refer the patient to a hospital for treatment.
■ Refer the patient for psychological counseling if needed.

Patient teaching
■ Teach the patient and family about the injury and potential outcomes.
■ Teach the patient about medications and their potential adverse effects.
■ Teach the patient about the specific care required for the injury.

Complications
■ Hemorrhage
■ Death

● ● ● ● ● ● ● ● ● ● ● ●

SELECTED REFERENCES

Dolan, B., and Holt, L. *Accident and Emergency Care: Theory into Practice.* Philadelphia: W.B. Saunders Co., 1999.

Harwood-Nuss, A.L. *The Clinical Practice of Emergency Medicine,* 3rd ed. Philadelphia: Lippincott Williams & Wilkins, 2000.

Oman, K.S., et al. *Emergency Nursing Secrets.* Philadelphia: Lippincott Williams & Wilkins, 2000.

Tintinalli, J., ed. *Emergency Medicine: A Comprehensive Study Guide,* 5th ed. New York: McGraw-Hill Book Co., 2000.

Immune disorders

The environment contains thousands of pathogenic microorganisms—viruses, bacteria, fungi, and parasites. Ordinarily, we protect ourselves from infectious organisms and other harmful invaders through an elaborate network of safeguards—the host defense system. Understanding how this system functions provides the framework for studying various immune disorders.

• • • • • • • • • • • •

HOST DEFENSE SYSTEM

The host defense system includes physical and chemical barriers to infection, the inflammatory response, and the immune response. Physical barriers, such as the skin and mucous membranes, prevent invasion by most organisms. Organisms that penetrate this first line of defense simultaneously trigger inflammatory and immune responses. Both responses involve cells derived from a hematopoietic stem cell in the bone marrow.

Chemical barriers include lysozymes (found in body secretions, such as tears, mucus, and saliva) and hydrochloric acid (found in the stomach). Lysozymes destroy bacteria by removing cell walls. Hydrochloric acid breaks down food and mucus that contain pathogens.

The inflammatory response involves polymorphonuclear leukocytes, basophils, mast cells, platelets and, to some extent, monocytes and macrophages.

The immune response primarily involves the interaction of lymphocytes (T and B), macrophages, and macrophage-like cells and their products. These cells may be circulating or may be localized in the tissues and organs of the immune system, including the thymus, lymph nodes, spleen, and tonsils. The thymus participates in the maturation of T lymphocytes (cell-mediated immunity); these cells are "educated" to differentiate "self" from "nonself." In contrast, B lymphocytes (humoral immunity) mature in the bone marrow. The key humoral effector mechanism is the production of immunoglobulin by B cells and the subsequent activation of the complement cascade. The lymph nodes, spleen, liver, and intestinal lymphoid tissue help remove and destroy circulating antigens in the blood and lymph.

The major histocompatibility complex

The major histocompatibility complex (MHC) is a cluster of genes on human chromosome 6 that plays a pivotal role in the immune response. Also known as human leukocyte antigen (HLA) genes, these genes are inherited in an autosomal codominant manner; that is, each individual receives one set of MHC genes (haplotype) from each parent, and both sets of genes are expressed on the individual's cells. These genes play a role in the recognition of self versus nonself and the interaction of immunologically active cells by coding for cell-surface proteins.

HLA antigens are divided into three classes:

- Class I antigens appear on nearly all of the body's cells and include HLA-A, HLA-B, and HLA-C antigens. During tissue graft rejection, they're the chief antigens recognized by the host. When killer (CD8+) T cells use a virally infected antigen, they recognize it in the context of a class I antigen.
- Class II antigens only appear on B cells, macrophages, and activated T cells. They include the HLA-D and HLA-DR antigens. Class II antigens promote efficient collaboration between immunocompetent cells. Helper (CD4+) T cells require that antigen be presented in the context of a class II antigen. Because these antigens also determine whether an individual responds to a particular antigen, they're also known as immune response genes.
- Class III antigens include certain complement proteins (C2, C4, and Factor B).

ANTIGENS

An antigen is any substance that can induce an immune response. T and B lymphocytes have specific receptors that respond to specific antigen molecular shapes (epitopes). In B cells, this receptor is an immunoglobulin (antibody) cell: immunoglobulin D (IgD) or IgM, sometimes referred to as a surface immunoglobulin. The T-cell antigen receptor recognizes antigens only in association with specific cell surface molecules known as the major histocompatibility complex (MHC). (See *The major histocompatibility complex*.) MHC molecules, which differ among individuals, identify substances as self or nonself. Slightly different antigen receptors can recognize a phenomenal number of distinct antigens, which are coded by distinct, variable region genes.

B LYMPHOCYTES

B lymphocytes and their products, immunoglobulins, contribute to humoral immunity. The binding of soluble antigen with B-cell antigen receptors initiates the humoral immune response. The activated B cells differentiate into plasma cells that secrete immunoglobulins or antibodies. This response is regulated by T lymphocytes and their products, lymphokines. These lymphokines, which include interleukin-2 (IL-2), IL-4, IL-5, and interferon-8 (IFN-8), are important in determining the class of immunoglobulins made by B cells.

The five known classes of immunoglobulins (Ig) — IgG, IgM, IgA, IgE, and IgD — are distinguished by the constant (C) regions of their heavy chains. However, each class has a kappa or a lambda light chain, which gives rise to many subtypes. The almost limitless combinations of light and heavy chains give immunoglobulins their specificity.

T LYMPHOCYTES

T lymphocytes and macrophages are the chief participants in cell-mediated immunity. Immature T lymphocytes are derived from the bone marrow. Upon migration to the thymus, they undergo a maturation process that depends on human leukocyte antigen (HLA) genes, which are products of the major histocompatibility complex. Thus, mature T cells can distinguish between self and nonself. T cells acquire certain surface molecules, or markers; these markers combined with the T-cell antigen receptor promote the particular activation of each type of T cell. T-cell activation requires presentation of antigens in the context of a specific HLA antigen. Helper T cells require class II HLA antigens; cytotoxic T cells require class I HLA antigens. T-cell activation also involves interleukin-1 (IL-1), which is produced by macrophages, and IL-2, which is produced by T cells.

Natural killer (NK) cells are a discrete population of large lymphocytes, some of which resemble T cells. NK cells recognize surface changes on body cells infected with a virus; then they bind to and in many cases kill the infected cells.

MACROPHAGES

Important cells of the reticuloendothelial system, macrophages influence both immune and inflammatory responses. Macrophage precursors circulate in the blood. When they collect in various tissues and organs, they differentiate into macrophages with varying characteristics. Unlike B and T lymphocytes, macrophages lack surface receptors for specific antigens; instead, they have receptors for the C region of the heavy chain (Fc region) of immunoglobulin, for fragments of the third component of complement (C3), and for nonimmunologic factors, such as carbohydrate molecules.

One of the most important functions of macrophages is the presentation of antigen to T lymphocytes. Macrophages ingest and process antigen, then deposit it on their own surfaces in association with HLA antigen. T lymphocytes become activated upon recognizing this complex. Macrophages also function in the inflammatory response by producing interleukin-1, which generates fever. In addition, macrophages synthesize complement proteins and other mediators that produce phagocytic, microbicidal, and tumoricidal effects.

CYTOKINES

Cytokines are low-molecular-weight proteins involved in the communication between cells. Their purpose is to induce or regulate a variety of immune or inflammatory responses. However, disorders may occur if cytokine production or regulation is impaired. Cytokines are categorized as colony-stimulating factors, interferons, interleukins, tumor necrosis factors, and the transforming growth factor.

COMPLEMENT SYSTEM

The chief humoral effector of the inflammatory response, the complement system consists of more than 20 serum proteins.

When activated, these proteins interact in a cascadelike process that has profound biological effects. Complement activation takes place through one of two pathways. In the classic pathway, binding of immunoglobulin M (IgM) or IgG and antigen forms antigen-antibody complexes that activate the first complement component, C1. This, in turn, activates C4, C2, and C3. In the alternate pathway, activating surfaces such as bacterial membranes directly amplify spontaneous cleavage of C3. Once C3 is activated in either pathway, activation of the terminal components—C5 to C9—follows.

The major biological effects of complement activation include phagocyte attraction (chemotaxis) and activation, histamine release, viral neutralization, promotion of phagocytosis by opsonization, and lysis of cells and bacteria. Other mediators of inflammation derived from the kinin and coagulation pathways interact with the complement system.

• • • • • • • • • • • •
POLYMORPHONUCLEAR LEUKOCYTES

In addition to macrophages and the complement system, other key participants in the inflammatory response are the polymorphonuclear leukocytes—neutrophils, eosinophils, and basophils.

Neutrophils, the most numerous of these cells, derive from bone marrow and increase dramatically in number in response to infection and inflammation. Highly mobile cells, neutrophils are attracted to areas of inflammation (chemotaxis); in fact, they're the primary constituent of pus.

Neutrophils have surface receptors for immunoglobulin and complement fragments, and they avidly ingest opsonized particles such as bacteria. Ingest-

ed organisms are then promptly killed by toxic oxygen metabolites and enzymes such as lysozyme. Unfortunately, neutrophils not only kill invading organisms but may also damage host tissues.

Also derived from bone marrow, eosinophils multiply in both allergic disorders and parasitic infestations. Although their phagocytic function isn't clearly understood, evidence suggests that they participate in host defense against parasites. Their products also may diminish the inflammatory response in allergic disorders.

Two other types of cells that function in allergic disorders are basophils and mast cells. (Mast cells, however, aren't blood cells.) Basophils circulate in peripheral blood, whereas mast cells accumulate in connective tissue, particularly in the lungs, intestines, and skin. Both types of cells have surface receptors for immunoglobulin E (IgE). When cross-linked by an IgE–antigen complex, they release mediators characteristic of the allergic response.

• • • • • • • • • • • •
TYPES OF IMMUNE RESPONSES

Because of their complexity, the processes involved in host defense and immune response may malfunction. When the body's defenses are exaggerated, misdirected, or either absent or depressed, the result may be a hypersensitivity disorder, autoimmunity, or immunodeficiency, respectively.

Hypersensitivity disorders
An exaggerated or inappropriate immune response may lead to various hypersensitivity disorders. Such disorders are classified as type I through type IV, although some overlap exists.

Type I hypersensitivity (allergic disorders)
In individuals with type I hypersensitivity, certain antigens (allergens) activate T cells. These cells, in turn, induce B-cell production of immunoglobulin E (IgE), which binds to the crystallizable fragment (Fc) receptors on the surface of mast cells. When these cells are reexposed to the same antigen, the antigen binds with the surface IgE, cross-links the Fc receptors, and causes mast cell degranulation with the release of various mediators. (Degranulation may also be triggered by complement-derived anaphylatoxins — C3a and C5a — or by certain drugs such as morphine.)

Examples of type I hypersensitivity disorders are anaphylaxis, hay fever (allergic rhinitis) and, in some cases, asthma.

Type II hypersensitivity (antibody-dependent cytotoxicity)
In type II hypersensitivity, an antibody is directed against cell surface antigens. (Alternatively, though, the antibody may be directed against small molecules adsorbed to cells or against cell surface receptors rather than against cell constituents themselves.) Type II hypersensitivity then causes tissue damage through several mechanisms. Binding of the antigen and the antibody activates complement, which ultimately disrupts cellular membranes.

Another mechanism is mediated by various phagocytic cells with receptors for immunoglobulin (Fc region) and complement fragments. These cells envelop and destroy (phagocytose) opsonized targets, such as red blood cells, leukocytes, and platelets. Antibody activity against these cells may be visualized by immunofluorescence. Cytotoxic T cells and natural killer cells also contribute to tissue damage in type II hypersensitivity.

Examples of type II hypersensitivity include transfusion reactions, hemolytic disease of the neonate, autoimmune hemolytic anemia, Goodpasture's syndrome, and myasthenia gravis.

Type III hypersensitivity (immune complex disease)
In type III hypersensitivity, excessive circulating antigen-antibody complexes (immune complexes) result in the deposition of these complexes in tissue — most commonly in the kidneys, joints, skin, and blood vessels. (Normally, immune complexes are effectively cleared by the reticuloendothelial system.) These deposited immune complexes activate the complement cascade, resulting in local inflammation. They also trigger platelet release of vasoactive amines that increase vascular permeability, augmenting deposition of immune complexes in vessel walls.

Type III hypersensitivity may be associated with infections, such as hepatitis B and bacterial endocarditis; certain cancers in which a serum sickness–like syndrome may occur; and autoimmune disorders such as lupus erythematosus. This hypersensitivity reaction may also follow drug or serum therapy.

Type IV hypersensitivity (delayed hypersensitivity)
In type IV hypersensitivity, an antigen is processed by macrophages and presented to T cells. The sensitized T cells then release lymphokines, which recruit and activate other lymphocytes, monocytes, macrophages, and polymorphonuclear leukocytes. The coagulation, kinin, and complement pathways also contribute to tissue damage in this type of reaction.

Examples of type IV hypersensitivity include tuberculin reactions, contact hypersensitivity, and sarcoidosis.

Autoimmune disorders

Autoimmunity is characterized by a misdirected immune response in which the body's defenses become self-destructive. The cause of this abnormal response remains puzzling. Recognition of self through the major histocompatibility complex is known to be of primary importance in an immune response. However, how an immune response against self is prevented and which cells are primarily responsible is still being studied.

Immunodeficiency

In immunodeficiency, the immune response is absent or depressed, resulting in increased susceptibility to infection. This disorder may be primary or secondary. Primary immunodeficiency reflects a defect involving T cells, B cells, or lymphoid tissues. Secondary immunodeficiency results from an underlying disease or factor that depresses or blocks the immune response. The most common forms of immunodeficiency are caused by viral infection (as in acquired immunodeficiency syndrome) or are iatrogenic in origin.

• • • • • • • • • • • •
ACQUIRED IMMUNODEFICIENCY SYNDROME

Currently one of the most widely publicized diseases, acquired immunodeficiency syndrome (AIDS) is characterized by progressive immunodeficiency. Although it's characterized by progressive destruction of cell-mediated (T-cell) immunity, it also affects humoral immunity and even autoimmunity because of the central role of CD4$^+$ T cells in immune reactions. The resultant immunodeficiency makes the patient susceptible to opportunistic infections, unusual cancers, and other abnormalities that define AIDS. (See *Common infections and neoplasms in AIDS.*) This syndrome was first described by the Cen-

ters for Disease Control and Prevention (CDC) in 1981. Since then, the CDC has declared a case surveillance definition for AIDS and has modified it several times, most recently in December 1999.

A retrovirus — type I human immunodeficiency virus (HIV) — is the primary etiologic agent for AIDS. Transmission of HIV occurs by contact with infected blood or body fluids and is associated with identifiable high-risk behaviors. As a result, HIV incidence is disproportionately high in homosexual and bisexual men, I.V. drug users, neonates of HIV-infected women, recipients of contaminated blood or blood products (dramatically decreased since the mid-1980s), and heterosexual partners of people in the former groups. Because of similar routes of transmission, AIDS shares epidemiologic patterns with hepatitis B and sexually transmitted diseases. The CDC estimates that 600,000 to 900,000 Americans are currently infected with HIV (with 200,000 being unaware of the infection); 23% are women.

AGE ALERT AIDS is the fifth leading cause of death among people ages 25 to 44 in the United States.

The natural history of AIDS begins with infection by the HIV retrovirus, which is detectable only by laboratory tests, and ends with the severely immunocompromised, terminal stage of the disease. Depending on individual variations and the presence of cofactors that influence progression, the time that elapses from acute HIV infection to the appearance of symptoms (mild to severe), to diagnosis of AIDS and, eventually, to death varies greatly. Recent advances in antiretroviral therapy and treatment and in prophylaxis of common opportunistic infections can delay the natural progression of HIV infection and prolong survival.

Causes

AIDS results from infection with HIV, which strikes cells bearing the $CD4^+$ antigen; the latter (normally a receptor for major histocompatibility complex molecules) serves as a receptor for the retrovirus and lets it enter the cell. HIV prefers to infect the $CD4^+$ lymphocyte but may also infect other $CD4^+$ antigen–bearing cells of the GI tract, uterine cervical cells, and neuroglial cells. After invading a cell, HIV either replicates, leading to cell death, or becomes latent. HIV infection leads to profound pathology either directly through the destruction of $CD4^+$ cells, other immune cells, and neuroglial cells or indirectly through the secondary effects of $CD4^+$ T-cell dysfunction and resultant immunosuppression.

The infection process takes three forms: immunodeficiency (opportunistic infections and unusual cancers), autoimmunity (lymphoid interstitial pneumonitis, arthritis, hypergammaglobulinemia, and production of autoimmune antibodies), and neurologic dysfunction (AIDS dementia complex, HIV encephalopathy, and peripheral neuropathies).

HIV is transmitted by direct inoculation during intimate sexual contact, especially associated with the mucosal trauma of receptive rectal intercourse; transfusion of contaminated blood or blood products (a risk diminished by routine testing of all blood products); sharing of contaminated needles; or transplacental or postpartum transmission from infected mother to fetus (by cervical or blood contact at delivery and in breast milk). Accumulating evidence suggests that HIV isn't transmitted by nonintimate family members or social contact. The average time between exposure to the virus and diagnosis of AIDS is 8 to 10 years, but shorter and longer incubation times have been recorded.

Common infections and neoplasms in AIDS

PROTOZOA
Pneumocystis carinii
Cryptosporidium
Toxoplasma gondii

FUNGI
Candida species
Cryptococcus neoformans
Histoplasma

MYCOBACTERIA
Mycobacterium avium-intracellulare
M. tuberculosis

VIRUSES
Cytomegalovirus
Herpesvirus

NEOPLASMS
Hodgkin's disease
Kaposi's sarcoma
Malignant lymphoma

Clinical presentation

HIV infection manifests itself in many ways. After a high-risk exposure and inoculation, the infected person usually experiences a mononucleosis-like syndrome, which may be attributed to flu or another virus. The patient may remain asymptomatic for years. In this latent stage, the only sign of HIV infection is laboratory evidence of seroconversion. When signs and symptoms appear, they can take many forms:

- persistent generalized adenopathy
- nonspecific signs and symptoms (weight loss, fatigue, night sweats, and fever)
- neurologic symptoms resulting from HIV encephalopathy
- opportunistic infection
- cancer.

The clinical course varies slightly in children with AIDS. Apparently, their incubation time is shorter, with a mean of 17 months. Signs and symptoms resemble those in adults except for findings related to sexually transmitted disease. Children show virtually all of the opportunistic infections observed in adults, with a higher incidence of bacterial infections:

- otitis media
- pneumonias other than *Pneumocystis carinii* pneumonia
- sepsis
- chronic salivary gland enlargement
- lymphoid interstitial pneumonia.

Differential diagnoses

- Dependent on the stage of the HIV infection
- Any prolonged illness without ready explanation

Diagnosis

The CDC defines AIDS as an illness characterized by one or more "indicator" diseases coexisting with laboratory evidence of HIV infection and other possible causes of immunosuppression. The CDC's current AIDS surveillance case definition requires laboratory confirmation of HIV infection in people who have a CD4+ T-lymphocyte count greater than 200 cells/µl or who have an associated clinical condition or disease. (See *Classification system for HIV infection and expanded AIDS surveillance case definition for adolescents and adults*.)

Antibody tests are the most commonly performed tests; they indicate HIV infection indirectly by revealing HIV antibodies. The recommended protocol requires initial screening of individuals and blood products with an enzyme-linked immunosorbent assay (ELISA) test. A positive ELISA test result should be repeated and then confirmed by an alternate method, usually the Western blot technique or an immunofluorescence assay. The radioimmunoprecipitation assay is considered more sensitive and specific than the Western blot technique. Because it requires radioactive materials, it's a poor choice for routine screening. In addition, antibody testing isn't reliable. People produce detectable levels of antibodies at different rates — a "window" varying from a few weeks to as long as 35 months in one documented case — so an HIV-infected person can test negative for HIV antibodies. Antibody tests are also unreliable in neonates because transferred maternal antibodies persist for 6 to 10 months. To overcome these problems, direct tests are used, including antigen tests (p24 antigen capture assay), HIV cultures, nucleic acid probes of peripheral blood lymphocytes, and the polymerase chain reaction. (See *Laboratory tests for diagnosing and tracking HIV and assessing immune status*, page 774.)

Additional tests to support the diagnosis and help evaluate the severity of immunosuppression include CD4+ and CD8+ T-lymphocyte subset counts; erythrocyte sedimentation rate; complete blood cell count; serum $beta_2$-microglobulin, p24 antigen, and neopterin levels; and anergy testing. Because many opportunistic infections in AIDS patients are reactivations of previous infections, patients are also tested for syphilis, hepatitis B, tuberculosis, toxoplasmosis and, in some areas, histoplasmosis.

Management

General

No cure has been found for AIDS, however, in 1998, the CDC recommended that all people who have symptomatic or HIV infection receive aggressive antiviral therapy. The nucleoside analogues (sometimes called reverse transcriptase inhibitors) have been the mainstay of AIDS therapy in recent years. These

Classification system for HIV infection and expanded AIDS surveillance case definition for adolescents and adults

DIAGNOSTIC CATEGORIES

CD4+ T-cell and clinical categories	Clinical category A: Asymptomatic, acute (primary) HIV or PGL	Clinical category B: Symptomatic, not (A) or (C) conditions	Clinical category C: AIDS-indicator conditions
(1) ≥ 500/µL	A1	B1	C1
(2) 200 to 499/µL	A2	B2	C2
(3) < 200/µL AIDS indicator T-cell count	A3	B3	C3

As of January 1, 1993, people with acquired immunodeficiency syndrome (AIDS) indicator conditions (clinical category C) and those in categories A3 or B3 were considered to have AIDS.

Clinical category A

Clinical category A includes one or more of the following in adults or adolescents with confirmed human immunodeficiency virus (HIV) infection and without conditions in clinical categories B and C:
- asymptomatic HIV infection
- persistent generalized lymphadenopathy (PGL)
- acute (primary) HIV infection with accompanying illness or history of acute HIV infection.

Clinical category B

Examples of conditions include but aren't limited to:
- bacillary angiomatosis
- candidiasis, oropharyngeal (thrush) or vulvovaginal (persistent, frequent, or poorly responsive to therapy)
- cervical dysplasia (moderate or severe) or cervical carcinoma in situ
- constitutional symptoms, such as a fever of 104° F (38.5° C) or diarrhea exceeding 1 month in duration
- hairy leukoplakia, oral

- herpes zoster (shingles), involving at least two distinct episodes or more than one dermatome
- idiopathic thrombocytopenia purpura
- listeriosis
- pelvic inflammatory disease, particularly if complicated by tubo-ovarian abscess
- peripheral neuropathy.

Clinical category C

Examples of conditions in adults and adolescents include:
- candidiasis of bronchi, trachea, lungs, or esophagus
- cervical cancer, invasive
- coccidioidomycosis, disseminated or extrapulmonary
- crytpococcosis, extrapulmonary
- cryptosporidiosis, chronic intestinal (exceeding 1 month's duration)
- cytomegalovirus disease (other than liver, spleen, or lymph nodes)
- cytomegalovirus retinitis (with loss of vision)
- encephalopathy, HIV-related

- herpes simplex with chronic ulcers (exceeding 1 month's duration) or bronchitis, pneumonitis, or esophagitis
- histoplasmosis, disseminated or extrapulmonary
- isosporiasis, chronic intestinal (exceeding 1 month's duration)
- Kaposi's sarcoma
- lymphoma, Burkitt's (or equivalent); immunoblastic (or equivalent); primary, of brain
- *Mycobacterium avium-intracellulare* or *M. kasasii*, disseminated or extrapulmonary
- *M. tuberculosis*, any site (pulmonary or extra pulmonary)
- *Mycobacterium*, other species or unidentified species, disseminated or extrapulmonary
- *Pneumocystis carinii* pneumonia
- pneumonia, recurrent
- progressive multifocal leukoencephalopathy
- *Salmonella* septicemia, recurrent
- toxoplasmosis of brain
- wasting syndrome due to HIV.

Adapted from Centers for Disease Control and Prevention, U.S. Department of Health and Human Services, 1993 revised classification system for HIV infection and expanded AIDS surveillance case definition for AIDS among adolescents and adults. MMWR CDC Recommendations and Reports 41 (RR-17), 1-19. From Smeltzer, S.C., and Bare, B.G. *Brunner & Suddarth's Textbook of Medical Surgical Nursing*, 9th ed. Philadelphia: Lippincott Williams & Wilkins, 2000.

Laboratory tests for diagnosing and tracking HIV and assessing immune status

TEST	FINDINGS IN HIV INFECTION
Human immunodeficiency virus (HIV) antibody tests	
▪ Enzyme-linked immunosorbent assay (ELISA)	▪ Positive results (must be confirmed by Western blot technique)
▪ Western blot technique	▪ Positive
▪ Indirect immunofluorescence assay (IFA)	▪ Positive results (must be confirmed by Western blot technique)
▪ Radioimmunoprecipitation assay (RIPA)	▪ Positive results (more sensitive and specific than Western blot technique)
HIV tracking	
▪ P24 antigen	▪ Positive for free viral protein
▪ Polymerase chain reaction (PCR)	▪ Detection of HIV RNA or DNA
▪ Branch DNA (bDNA)	▪ Detection of HIV RNA
▪ Nucleic acid sequence–based amplification (NASBA)	▪ Detection of HIV RNA
▪ Peripheral blood mononuclear cell culture for HIV-1	▪ Positive when two consecutive assays detect reverse transcriptase or p24 antigen capture assay in increasing magnitude
▪ Quantitative cell culture	▪ Increased viral load within cells
▪ Quantitative plasma culture	▪ Increased viral load by free infectious virus in the plasma
▪ β_2-microglobulin	▪ Increased protein with disease progression
▪ Serum neopterin	▪ Increased levels seen with disease progression
Immune status	
▪ Number of CD4+ cells	▪ Decreased
▪ Percentage of CD4+ cells	▪ Decreased
▪ CD4+:CD8+ ratio	▪ Decreased CD4+:CD8+ ratio
▪ White blood cell count	▪ Normal to decreased
▪ Immunoglobulin levels	▪ Increased
▪ CD4+ cell function tests	▪ Decreased ability of T4 cells to respond to antigen
▪ Skin test sensitivity reaction	▪ Decreased to absent

drugs, which include zidovudine (AZT), lamivudine, didanosine, stavudine, efavirenz, and zalcitabine, interfere with viral reverse transcriptase, which impairs HIV's ability to turn its ribonucleic acid into deoxyribonucleic acid for insertion into the host cell.

Medication

Antiretroviral therapy typically begins when the patient's CD4+ T-cell count drops to less than 500/µl or when the patient develops an opportunistic infection. Most clinicians recommend starting the patient on a combination of drugs in an attempt to gain the maximum benefit and to inhibit the production of resistant mutant strains of HIV. The drug combinations and dosages are then altered, depending on the patient's response.

Increasingly, changes in therapy are being based on the patient's viral load rather than on his CD4$^+$ T-cell count. Because the CD4$^+$ count is influenced by the total white blood cell count, changes in the CD4$^+$ count may have nothing to do with changes in the patient's HIV status. Many patients on antiretroviral therapy have their viral load checked every 3 months. Some antivirals that can be used include:

- zidovudine — 200 mg P.O. every 8 hours or 100 mg P.O. 5 times per day; if intolerant, decrease dose to 300 to 400 mg per day P.O. in divided doses
- didanosine — patients weighing more than 132 lb (60 kg), 200 mg P.O. every 12 hours; patients weighing less than 132 lb, 125 mg P.O. every 12 hours; children, 90 to 150 mg/m^2 P.O. every 12 hours
- zalcitabine — patients age 13 and older, 0.75 mg P.O. every 8 hours.

The increasing use of protease inhibitors (PIs), another class of antiretroviral agents, has greatly increased the life expectancy of AIDS patients. These drugs block the enzyme protease, which HIV needs to produce virions, the viral particles that spread the virus to other cells. PIs dramatically reduce viral load — sometimes to undetectable levels — but produce a corresponding increase in the CD4$^+$ T-cell count; in addition, because they act at a different site than nucleoside analogues, the PIs don't produce additional adverse effects when added to a patient's regimen. These drugs include:

- ritonavir — adults, 600 mg P.O. b.i.d.
- indinavir — 800 mg P.O. every 8 hours
- nelfinavir — adults, 750 mg P.O. t.i.d.; children, 20 to 30 mg/kg P.O. t.i.d.

Once antiviral therapy is initiated, treatment should be aggressive. Initially, highly active antiviral therapy, consisting of a triple drug therapy regimen — a PI and two nonnucleoside reverse transcriptase inhibitors — is recommended. In addition to these primary treatments, use anti-infectives to combat opportunistic infections (some are used prophylactically to help patients resist opportunistic infections) and antineoplastic drugs to fight associated neoplasms. Supportive treatments help maintain nutritional status and relieve pain and other distressing physical and psychological symptoms.

Referral
- Refer the patient to a specialist in HIV or AIDS treatment.
- For information and support, refer the patient and family to a local support group.

Follow-up
See the patient based on the stage of the infection or have him be seen by a specialist. Follow CD4$^+$ counts every 3 months.

Patient teaching
- Teach the patient about medications he's currently taking and adverse effects that may occur. Encourage him to follow the prescribed times in order to decrease adverse effects.
- Teach the patient and family members about modes of transmission and prevention.

Complications
- Opportunistic infections and malignancies
- Neuropsychiatric symptoms
- Thrombocytopenia
- AIDS meningoencephalitis

Special considerations
- Stress the importance of taking medication as prescribed. If the patient chooses to inconsistently take or restart his medication without consultation, he may become resistant to the medication.

HEALTHY LIVING Advise health care workers and the public to use precautions in all situations that risk exposure to blood, body fluids, and secretions. Diligently practice standard precautions to prevent the inadvertent transmission of AIDS and other infectious diseases that are transmitted by similar routes.

• • • • • • • • • • •

ALLERGIC RHINITIS

Allergic rhinitis is a reaction to airborne (inhaled) allergens. Depending on the allergen, the resulting rhinitis and conjunctivitis may occur seasonally (hay fever) or year-round (perennial allergic rhinitis). Allergic rhinitis is the most common atopic allergic reaction, affecting over 20 million Americans. It's most prevalent in young children and adolescents but can occur in all age-groups.

Causes

Hay fever reflects an immunoglobulin E (IgE–mediated) type I hypersensitivity response to an environmental antigen (allergen) in a genetically susceptible individual. In most cases, it's induced by windborne pollens: in the spring by tree pollens (oak, elm, maple, alder, birch, and cottonwood), in the summer by grass pollens (sheep sorrel and English plantain), and in the fall by weed pollens (ragweed). Occasionally, hay fever is induced by allergy to fungal spores.

In perennial allergic rhinitis, inhaled allergens provoke antigen responses that produce recurring symptoms year-round.

The major perennial allergens and irritants include dust mites, feather pillows, mold, cigarette smoke, upholstery, and animal dander. Seasonal pollen allergy may exacerbate signs and symptoms of perennial allergic rhinitis.

Clinical presentation

The following are signs and symptoms of seasonal allergic rhinitis:

- paroxysmal sneezing
- profuse watery rhinorrhea
- nasal obstruction or congestion
- pruritus of the nose and eyes
- pale, cyanotic, edematous nasal mucosa
- red and edematous eyelids and conjunctivae
- excessive lacrimation
- headache or sinus pain
- itching in the throat
- malaise.

In perennial allergic rhinitis, conjunctivitis and other extranasal effects are rare, but chronic nasal obstruction is common. In many cases, this obstruction extends to eustachian tube obstruction, particularly in children.

In both types of allergic rhinitis, dark circles may appear under the patient's eyes ("allergic shiners") because of venous congestion in the maxillary sinuses. The severity of signs and symptoms can vary from season to season and from year to year.

Differential diagnoses

- Chronic vasomotor rhinitis
- Infectious rhinitis
- Influenza
- Chronic sinusitis
- Deviated nasal septum
- Nasal polyps
- Rebound drug use (decongestant nasal sprays)
- Foreign body

Diagnosis

Microscopic examination of sputum and nasal secretions reveals large numbers of eosinophils. Blood chemistry shows normal or elevated IgE level. A definitive diagnosis is based on the patient's personal and family history of allergies as well as physical findings during a symptomatic phase. Skin testing paired with tested responses to environmental stimuli can pinpoint the responsible allergens given the patient's history.

Management
General
Treatment aims to control symptoms by eliminating the environmental antigen, if possible, and providing drug therapy and immunotherapy.

Medication
The following antihistamines may be used to treat allergic rhinitis:
- fexofenadine — 60 mg P.O. b.i.d.
- diphenhydramine — adults, 25 to 50 mg P.O. q.i.d.; children, 12.5 to 25 mg P.O. q.i.d.

Use the following steroids to treat allergic rhinitis:
- flunisolide — adults, 2 inhalations each nostril b.i.d.; children ages 6 to 12, 1 inhalation each nostril t.i.d.
- beclomethasone — adults, 2 inhalations each nostril b.i.d.; children ages 6 to 12, 1 inhalation each nostril t.i.d.
- triamcinolone — adults, 2 inhalations each nostril t.i.d.; children ages 6 to 12, 1 to 2 inhalations each nostril t.i.d.

Long-term management includes immunotherapy, or desensitization with injections of extracted allergens, administered before or during allergy season or perennially. Seasonal allergies require particularly close dosage regulation.

Referral
- Refer the patient to an allergist if conventional treatment is unsuccessful.

Follow-up
See the patient once every 2 weeks until symptoms improve.

Patient teaching
- Advise the patient to use intranasal steroids regularly for optimal effectiveness.
- To reduce environmental exposure to airborne allergens, suggest that the patient sleep with the windows closed, avoid the countryside during pollination seasons, use air conditioning to filter allergens and minimize moisture and dust, and eliminate dust-collecting items, such as wool blankets, deep-pile carpets, and heavy drapes, from the home.

Complications
- Sinusitis
- Otitis media
- Secondary infection
- Decreased pulmonary function
- Adverse effects of steroid medication
- Nasal polyps

Special considerations
- In severe and resistant cases, suggest that the patient consider drastic changes in lifestyle, such as relocation to a pollen-free area either seasonally or year-round.

• • • • • • • • • • • •

ANAPHYLAXIS

Anaphylaxis is a dramatic, acute atopic reaction marked by the sudden onset of rapidly progressive urticaria and respiratory distress. A severe reaction may precipitate vascular collapse, leading to systemic shock and sometimes death. Rapid assessment and intervention is essential.

Causes
The source of anaphylactic reactions is ingestion of or other systemic exposure to sensitizing drugs or other substances. Such substances may include serums (usually horse serum), vaccines, allergen

Penicillin guidelines

When administering penicillin or one of its derivatives, such as ampicillin or carbenicillin, follow these recommendations of the World Health Organization:

- Have an emergency kit available to treat allergic reactions.
- Take a detailed patient history, including penicillin allergy and other allergies. In an infant younger than 3 months old, check for penicillin allergy in the mother.
- Never give penicillin to a patient who has had an allergic reaction to it.
- Before giving penicillin to a patient with suspected penicillin allergy, refer the patient for skin and immunologic tests to confirm it.
- Always tell a patient that he's going to receive penicillin before he takes the first dose.
- Observe carefully for adverse effects for at least one-half hour after penicillin administration.
- Be aware that penicillin derivatives also elicit an allergic reaction.

extracts, enzymes (L-asparaginase), hormones, penicillin and other antibiotics, sulfonamides, local anesthetics, salicylates, polysaccharides, diagnostic chemicals (sulfobromophthalein, sodium dehydrocholate, and radiographic contrast media), foods (especially legumes, nuts, berries, seafood, and egg albumin) and sulfite-containing food additives, insect venom (honeybees, wasps, hornets, yellow jackets, fire ants, mosquitoes, and certain spiders) and, rarely, ruptured hydatid cyst.

A common cause of anaphylaxis is penicillin, which induces anaphylaxis in 1 to 4 of every 10,000 patients treated with it. Penicillin is most likely to induce anaphylaxis after parenteral administration or prolonged therapy and in atopic patients with an allergy to other drugs or foods. (See *Penicillin guidelines*.)

An anaphylactic reaction requires previous sensitization or exposure to the specific antigen, resulting in the production of specific immunoglobulin E (IgE) antibodies by plasma cells. This antibody production takes place in the lymph nodes and is enhanced by helper T cells. IgE antibodies then bind to membrane receptors on mast cells (found throughout connective tissue) and basophils.

On reexposure, the antigen binds to adjacent IgE antibodies or cross-linked IgE receptors, activating a series of cellular reactions that trigger degranulation — the release of powerful chemical mediators (such as histamine, eosinophil chemotactic factor of anaphylaxis, and platelet-activating factor) from mast cell stores. IgG or IgM enters into the reaction and activates the release of complement fractions.

At the same time, two other chemical mediators, bradykinin and leukotrienes, induce vascular collapse by stimulating contraction of certain groups of smooth muscles and by increasing vascular permeability. In turn, increased vascular permeability leads to decreased peripheral resistance and plasma leakage from the circulation to extravascular tissues, which lowers blood volume, causing hypotension, hypovolemic shock, and cardiac dysfunction.

Clinical presentation

An anaphylactic reaction produces sudden physical distress within seconds or minutes (although a delayed or persistent reaction may occur for up to 24 hours) after exposure to an allergen. The severity of the reaction is inversely related to the interval between exposure to the allergen and the onset of signs and symptoms.

The initial signs and symptoms of anaphylaxis include:

- feeling of impending doom or fright
- weakness
- sweating
- sneezing
- shortness of breath
- nasal pruritus
- urticaria
- angioedema.

Initial signs and symptoms are followed rapidly by symptoms in one or more target organs. Cardiovascular symptoms include:

- hypotension
- shock
- cardiac arrhythmias (if untreated, arrhythmias may precipitate circulatory collapse).

Respiratory symptoms can occur at any level in the respiratory tract and commonly include:

- nasal mucosal edema
- profuse watery rhinorrhea
- itching
- nasal congestion
- sudden sneezing attacks
- edema of the upper respiratory tract (resulting in hypopharyngeal and laryngeal obstruction — hoarseness, stridor, and dyspnea — early signs of acute respiratory failure, which can be fatal).

GI and genitourinary symptoms include:

- severe stomach cramps
- nausea
- diarrhea
- urinary urgency and incontinence.

Differential diagnoses

- Carcinoid syndrome
- Globus hystericus
- Pheochromocytoma
- Hereditary angioedema
- Serum sickness
- Other causes of shock (myocardial infarction, status asthmaticus, heart failure)

Diagnosis

Anaphylaxis can be diagnosed by the rapid onset of severe respiratory or cardiovascular signs and symptoms after ingestion or injection of a drug, vaccine, diagnostic agent, food, or food additive or after an insect sting.

Management

General

Maintain airway patency. Observe for early signs of laryngeal edema (hoarseness, stridor, and dyspnea), which will probably require endotracheal tube insertion or a tracheotomy and oxygen therapy.

In case of cardiac arrest, begin cardiopulmonary resuscitation, including closed-chest heart massage, assisted ventilation, and sodium bicarbonate; other therapy is indicated by clinical response. Watch for hypotension and shock, and maintain circulatory volume with volume expanders (plasma, plasma expanders, saline, and albumin) as needed. Stabilize blood pressure with the I.V. vasopressors norepinephrine and dopamine. Monitor blood pressure, central venous pressure, and urine output as a response index.

Medication

The following medications may be used to treat anaphylaxis:

- epinephrine 1:1,000 aqueous solution — 0.1 to 0.5 ml S.C. or I.M., repeated every 10 to 15 minutes p.r.n.
- diphenhydramine — 25 to 50 mg I.V., I.M., or P.O. every 6 hours for 24 hours
- cimetidine — 300 mg I.V. for one dose.

Referral

- The patient will need immediate referral to the hospital emergency department. Medical transport should be called, if appropriate.

Follow-up
The patient should be seen 72 hours after discharge from the hospital.

Patient teaching
- Tell the patient to wear a medical alert bracelet at all times.
- Teach the patient how to use an anaphylaxis kit, if appropriate.

Complications
- Cardiac arrest
- Respiratory failure (hypoxemia)
- Death

Special considerations
- If a patient must receive a drug to which he's allergic, prevent a severe reaction by making sure he receives careful desensitization with gradually increasing doses of the antigen or advance administration of steroids.

HEALTHY LIVING To prevent anaphylaxis, teach the patient to avoid exposure to known allergens. A person allergic to certain foods or drugs must learn to avoid the offending food or drug in all of its forms. For example, a patient allergic to insect stings should avoid open fields and wooded areas during the insect season. An anaphylaxis kit (epinephrine, antihistamine, and tourniquet) should also be carried whenever the patient with known severe allergic reactions goes outdoors. In addition, every patient prone to anaphylaxis should wear a medical identification bracelet identifying his allergies.

••••••••••••

ASTHMA

Asthma is a reversible lung disease characterized by obstruction or narrowing of the airways, which are typically inflamed and hyperresponsive to a variety of stimuli. It may resolve spontaneously or with treatment. Its symptoms range from mild wheezing and dyspnea to life-threatening respiratory failure. (See *Determining asthma's severity.*) Symptoms of bronchial airway obstruction may persist between acute episodes. Although asthma can strike at any age, half of all cases first occur in children under age 10; in this age-group, asthma affects twice as many boys as girls. It's estimated that 17 million Americans suffer from asthma.

Causes and pathophysiology
Extrinsic asthma results from sensitivity to specific external allergens. In cases in which the allergen isn't obvious, it's referred to as intrinsic asthma. Allergens that cause extrinsic asthma include pollen, animal dander, house dust or mold, kapok or feather pillows, food additives containing sulfites, and any other sensitizing substance. Extrinsic (atopic) asthma usually begins in childhood and is accompanied by other manifestations of atopy (type I, immunoglobulin E–mediated allergy), such as eczema and allergic rhinitis. In intrinsic (nonatopic) asthma, no extrinsic allergen can be identified. Most cases are preceded by a severe respiratory infection. Irritants, emotional stress, fatigue, exposure to noxious fumes, as well as changes in endocrine, temperature, and humidity, may aggravate intrinsic asthma attacks. In many asthmatics, intrinsic and extrinsic asthma coexist.

Several drugs and chemicals may provoke an asthma attack without using the IgE pathway. Apparently they trigger release of mast-cell mediators by way of prostaglandin inhibition. Examples of these substances include aspirin, various nonsteroidal anti-inflammatory drugs (such as indomethacin and mefenamic acid), and tartrazine, a yellow food dye. Exercise may also provoke an asthma attack. In exercise-induced asthma, bron-

Determining asthma's severity

ASSESSMENT	MILD ASTHMA	MODERATE ASTHMA	SEVERE ASTHMA	RESPIRATORY FAILURE
Signs and symptoms during acute phase	▪ Brief wheezing, coughing, dyspnea with activity ▪ Adequate air exchange ▪ Intermittent, brief wheezing; cough; or dyspnea once or twice per week ▪ Asymptomatic between attacks	▪ Respiratory distress at rest ▪ Hyperpnea ▪ Marked coughing and wheezing ▪ Air exchange normal or below normal ▪ Exacerbations that may last several days	▪ Marked respiration distress ▪ Marked wheezing or absent breath sounds ▪ Pulsus paradoxus > 10 mm Hg ▪ Chest wall contractions ▪ Continuous symptoms ▪ Frequent exacerbations	▪ Severe respiratory distress ▪ Impaired consciousness ▪ Severe wheezing; silent chest ▪ Use of accessory muscles of respiration ▪ Prominent pulsus paradoxus (30 to 50 mm Hg)
Diagnostic test results	▪ FEV_1 or peak flow 80% of normal values ▪ pH normal or increased ▪ PaO_2 normal or decreased ▪ $PaCO_2$ normal or decreased ▪ Normal chest X-ray	▪ FEV_1 or peak flow 60% to 80% of normal values; may vary 20% to 30% with symptoms ▪ pH generally elevated ▪ $PaCO_2$ increased ▪ $PaCO_2$ generally decreased ▪ Hyperinflation on chest X-ray	▪ FEV_1 or peak flow < 60% of normal values; may vary 20% to 30% with medications and up to 50% with exacerbations ▪ pH normal or reduced ▪ $PaCO_2$ normal or decreased ▪ $PaCO_2$ normal or increased ▪ Hyperinflation on chest X-ray	▪ FEV_1 or peak flow < 25% of normal values ▪ pH decreased ▪ PaO_2 < 60 mm Hg ▪ $PaCO_2$ > 40 mm Hg
Other assessment findings	▪ One attack per week (or none) ▪ Positive response to bronchodilator therapy within 24 hours ▪ No signs of asthma between episodes ▪ No sleep interruption or hyperventilation ▪ Minimal evidence of airway obstruction ▪ Minimal or no increase in lung volume	▪ Symptoms occurring more than twice per week ▪ Coughing and wheezing between episodes ▪ Diminished exercise tolerance ▪ Possible sleep interruption ▪ Increased lung volumes	▪ Frequent severe attacks ▪ Daily wheezing ▪ Poor exercise tolerance ▪ Frequent sleep interruption ▪ Bronchodilator therapy not completely reversing airway obstruction ▪ Markedly increased lung volumes	▪ Cyanosis ▪ Tachycardia

chospasm may follow heat and moisture loss in the upper airways.

The allergic response has two phases. When the patient inhales an allergenic substance, sensitized IgE antibodies trigger mast-cell degranulation in the lung interstitium, releasing histamine, cytokines, prostaglandins, thromboxanes, leukotrienes, and eosinophil chemotaxic factors. Histamine then attaches to receptor sites in the larger bronchi, causing irritation, inflammation, and edema. Inflammatory cells flow in during the late phase. The influx of eosinophils provides additional inflammatory mediators and contributes to local injury.

Clinical presentation

An asthma attack may begin dramatically, with simultaneous onset of many severe symptoms, or insidiously, with gradually increasing respiratory distress. It typically includes the following signs or symptoms or some combination of them:
- progressively worsening shortness of breath
- cough
- wheezing
- chest tightness.

During an acute attack, the cough sounds tight and dry. As the attack subsides, tenacious mucoid sputum is produced (except in young children, who don't expectorate). Characteristic wheezing may be accompanied by coarse rhonchi, but fine crackles aren't heard unless associated with a related complication. Between acute attacks, breath sounds may be normal.

The intensity of breath sounds in symptomatic asthma is typically reduced. A prolonged phase of forced expiration is typical of airflow obstruction. Evidence of lung hyperinflation (use of accessory muscles, for example) is particularly common in children. Acute attacks may be accompanied by tachycardia, tachypnea,

and diaphoresis. In severe attacks, the patient may be unable to speak more than a few words without pausing for breath. Cyanosis, confusion, and lethargy indicate the onset of respiratory failure.

Differential diagnoses
- Viral respiratory infection
- Chronic bronchitis
- Pneumonia
- Tuberculosis
- Cystic fibrosis
- Thyroid dysfunction
- Heart failure
- Foreign body aspiration

Diagnosis

Laboratory studies in patients with asthma commonly show abnormalities:
- Pulmonary function studies reveal signs of airway obstruction (decreased peak expiratory flow rates and forced expiratory volume in 1 second), low-normal or decreased vital capacity, and increased total lung and residual capacity. However, pulmonary function studies may be normal between attacks.
- Pulse oximetry may reveal decreased arterial oxygen saturation.
- Arterial blood gas analysis provides the best indication of an attack's severity. In acutely severe asthma, partial pressure of arterial oxygen is less than 60 mm Hg, partial pressure of arterial carbon dioxide ($PaCO_2$) is 40 mm Hg or more, and pH is usually decreased.
- Complete blood count with differential reveals increased eosinophil count.
- Chest X-rays may show hyperinflation with areas of focal atelectasis.

Management
General

Treatment of acute asthma aims to decrease bronchoconstriction, reduce bronchial airway edema, and increase pulmonary ventilation. After an acute episode, treatment focuses on avoiding or removing precipitating factors, such as environmental allergens or irritants.

If asthma is caused by a particular antigen, it may be treated by desensitizing the patient through a series of injections of limited amounts of the antigen. The aim is to curb the patient's immune response to the antigen.

Treatment of status asthmaticus consists of aggressive drug therapy: a beta$_2$-adrenergic agonist by nebulizer every 30 to 60 minutes, possibly supplemented with S.C. epinephrine, I.V. corticosteroids, I.V. aminophylline, oxygen administration, I.V. fluid therapy, and intubation and mechanical ventilation for hypercapnic respiratory failure (PaCO$_2$ of 40 mm Hg or more). (See *How status asthmaticus progresses*, page 784.)

Medication

The following beta$_2$-adrenergic agonists may be used to treat asthma:
- albuterol — nebulizer, adults and children over age 12, 2.5 mg t.i.d.; extended-release tablets, 4 to 8 mg every 12 hours; children under age 12, 4 mg every 12 hours; inhaler, adults and children over age 4, 1 to 2 inhalations every 4 to 6 hours
- pirbuterol — 1 to 2 inhalations every 4 to 6 hours
- salmeterol — 2 inhalations every 12 hours.

The following corticosteroids may also be used:
- beclomethasone — adults, 2 inhalations t.i.d. to q.i.d.; children ages 6 to 12, 1 to 2 inhalations t.i.d. or q.i.d

The following mast cell stabilizers may be used:
- cromolyn — 2 inhalations q.i.d.
- theophylline — 5 mg/kg P.O. followed by 3 mg/kg every 6 hours for two doses then 3 mg/kg every 8 hours.

For the most part, medical treatment of asthma attacks must be tailored to each patient. However, the following treatments are generally used:
- *Chronic mild asthma* — A beta$_2$-adrenergic agonist by metered-dose inhaler (alone or with cromolyn) may be used before exercise and exposure to an allergen or other stimuli to prevent symptoms; if symptoms occur, the beta$_2$-adrenergic agonist may be used every 3 to 4 hours.
- *Chronic moderate asthma* — For initial treatment, an inhaled beta-adrenergic bronchodilator, inhaled corticosteroid, and cromolyn may be used. If symptoms persist, inhaled corticosteroid dosage may be increased, and sustained-release theophylline or oral beta$_2$-adrenergic agonist (or both) may be added; short courses of oral corticosteroids may also be used.
- *Chronic severe asthma* — Initially, around-the-clock oral bronchodilator therapy with long-acting theophylline or beta$_2$-adrenergic agonist may be required, supplemented with inhaled beta$_2$-adrenergic agonist and inhaled corticosteroid with or without cromolyn; oral corticosteroid such as prednisone may be added in acute exacerbations.
- *Acute asthma attack* — Acute attacks that don't respond to self-treatment may require hospital care, beta$_2$-adrenergic agonists by inhalation or S.C. (in three doses over 60 to 90 minutes), and possibly oxygen for hypoxemia. If the patient responds poorly, systemic corticosteroids and, possibly, S.C. epinephrine may help. Beta$_2$-adrenergic agonist inhalation continues hourly. I.V. aminophylline may be added to the regimen and I.V. fluid therapy is started. Patients who don't respond to this treatment, whose airways remain obstructed, and who have increasing respiratory difficulty are at risk for status asthmaticus and may require mechanical ventilation.

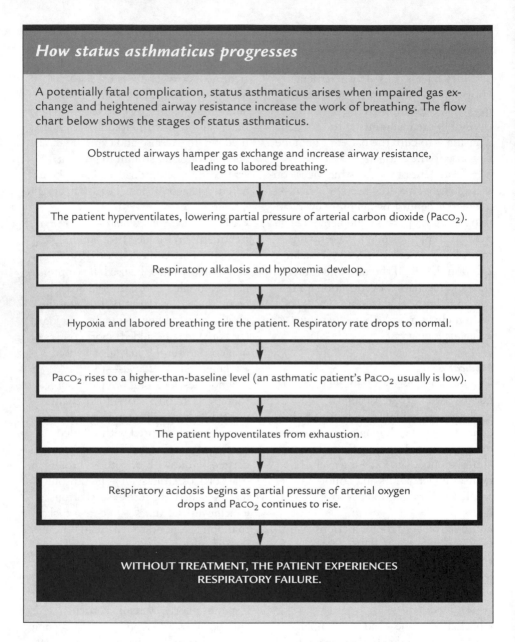

How status asthmaticus progresses

A potentially fatal complication, status asthmaticus arises when impaired gas exchange and heightened airway resistance increase the work of breathing. The flow chart below shows the stages of status asthmaticus.

Obstructed airways hamper gas exchange and increase airway resistance, leading to labored breathing.

↓

The patient hyperventilates, lowering partial pressure of arterial carbon dioxide ($PaCO_2$).

↓

Respiratory alkalosis and hypoxemia develop.

↓

Hypoxia and labored breathing tire the patient. Respiratory rate drops to normal.

↓

$PaCO_2$ rises to a higher-than-baseline level (an asthmatic patient's $PaCO_2$ usually is low).

↓

The patient hypoventilates from exhaustion.

↓

Respiratory acidosis begins as partial pressure of arterial oxygen drops and $PaCO_2$ continues to rise.

↓

WITHOUT TREATMENT, THE PATIENT EXPERIENCES RESPIRATORY FAILURE.

Referral

■ The patient may need to be referred to a pulmonologist for control of the disorder.
■ Refer the patient to the American Lung Association for information and support.

Patient teaching

■ If the patient is taking corticosteroids by inhaler, tell him to watch for signs of candidal infection in the mouth and pharynx. Tell him to use an extender device and to rinse his mouth afterward to help prevent it.

- Teach the patient proper use of an inhaler.
- Teach the patient and family about the disorder and potential emergent situations.
- Control exercise-induced asthma by instructing the patient to use a bronchodilator or cromolyn 30 minutes before exercise. Also, instruct him to use pursed-lip breathing while exercising.
- Teach the patient and his family to avoid known allergens and irritants.
- If the patient has moderate to severe asthma, explain how to use a peak flow meter to measure the degree of airway obstruction. Tell him to keep a record of peak flow readings and to bring it to medical appointments. Explain the importance of calling at once if the peak flow drops suddenly (may signal severe respiratory problems).
- Tell the patient to report a fever above 100° F (37.8° C), chest pain, shortness of breath without coughing or exercising, or uncontrollable coughing.
- Teach the patient diaphragmatic and pursed-lip breathing as well as effective coughing techniques.
- Urge the patient to drink at least 3 qt (3 L) of fluids daily to help loosen secretions and maintain hydration.

Complications
- Respiratory failure
- Atelectasis
- Adverse effects of medications
- Death
- Syndrome of inappropriate antidiuretic hormone

Special considerations
- Make sure that you emphasize to the patient the need for annual influenza immunization.

• • • • • • • • • • • •
CHRONIC FATIGUE AND IMMUNE DYSFUNCTION SYNDROME

Sometimes called chronic fatigue syndrome, chronic Epstein-Barr virus (EBV), or myalgic encephalomyelitis, chronic fatigue and immune dysfunction syndrome (CFIDS) is typically marked by debilitating fatigue, neurologic abnormalities, and persistent symptoms that suggest chronic mononucleosis. It's estimated that 422 of every 100,000 Americans are affected by this disorder.

AGE ALERT Chronic fatigue and immune dysfunction syndrome commonly occurs in adults under age 45, primarily in women.

Causes
The cause of CFIDS is unknown, but researchers suspect that it may be found in human herpesvirus 6, other herpesviruses, enteroviruses, or retroviruses. Rising levels of antibodies to EBV, once thought to implicate EBV infection as the cause of CFIDS, are now considered a result of this disease. CFIDS may be associated with a reaction to viral illness that's complicated by dysfunctional immune response and by other factors that may include gender, age, genetic disposition, prior illness, stress, and environment.

Clinical presentation
The characteristic symptom of CFIDS is prolonged, often overwhelming fatigue that's commonly associated with a varying complex of other symptoms. To aid identification of the disease, the Centers for Disease Control and Prevention (CDC) uses a "working case definition" to group symptoms and severity.

CDC criteria for diagnosing CFIDS

To meet the case definition of chronic fatigue and immune dysfunction syndrome (CFIDS) supplied by the Centers for Disease Control and Prevention (CDC), a patient must meet the following criteria:

▪ The patient has persistent or relapsing fatigue that's of new onset and is unexplained after clinical evaluation. This fatigue isn't resolved with bed rest and is severe enough to reduce or impair average daily activity and has persisted for at least 6 months.

▪ Four or more of the following signs and symptoms are also present and must not predate the fatigue:
– impairment of memory or concentration
– sore throat
– tender lymph nodes
– muscle pain
– multijoint pain without swelling or redness
– headaches of a new type, pattern, or severity
– unrefreshed sleep
– postexertional malaise lasting more than 24 hours.

Conditions that exclude a diagnosis of CFIDS

▪ Any active medical condition that may cause fatigue
▪ Diagnosed illness that may have relapsed or hasn't completely resolved
▪ Past or present diagnosis of major depressive disorder with psychotic or melancholic feature
▪ Alcohol or substance abuse within 2 years of onset of fatigue
▪ Severe obesity

Conditions that don't exclude a diagnosis of CFIDS

▪ Any condition that can't be confirmed by diagnostic tests
▪ Any condition receiving treatment that will alleviate all symptoms related to the condition
▪ Any condition that was treated with definitive treatment before the development of CFIDS symptoms
▪ Any isolated physical examination finding that's insufficient to suggest an exclusionary condition

Differential diagnoses
▪ Malignancy
▪ Autoimmune disease
▪ Localized infection
▪ Chronic or subacute bacterial infection
▪ Lyme disease
▪ Fungal disease
▪ Endocrine disorder
▪ Human immunodeficiency virus infection
▪ Psychiatric disease
▪ Chronic viral disease
▪ Chronic inflammatory disease
▪ Neuromuscular disease
▪ Drug dependency or abuse

Diagnosis
The cause and nature of CFIDS are still unknown, so no single test unequivocally confirms its presence. Therefore, the diagnosis is based on the patient's history and the CDC's criteria. (See CDC criteria for diagnosing CFIDS.) Because the CDC criteria are admittedly a working concept that may not include all forms of this disease and are based on symptoms that can

result from other diseases, diagnosis is difficult and uncertain.

Management
General
No treatment is known to cure CFIDS. For some patients, avoidance of environmental irritants and certain foods may help to relieve symptoms.

Medication
The following medications may be used to treat CFIDS:
- clonazepam — 0.25 to 1 mg b.i.d.; maximum 4 mg/day
- buspirone — 5 mg P.O. b.i.d. to t.i.d.
- fluoxetine — 20 to 80 mg/day P.O.
- ibuprofen — 200 to 400 mg P.O. every 4 to 6 hours
- poly I: poly C12U — twice weekly I.V. (experimental).

Referral
- Refer the patient to the CFIDS Association of America for information and support.
- Refer the patient for psychological counseling if appropriate.

Follow-up
The patient should initially be seen every 2 weeks, and then monthly depending on symptoms.

Patient teaching
- Encourage the patient to exercise as tolerated in order to avoid exacerbation of symptoms.
- Teach the patient coping strategies, such as relaxation techniques, in order to deal with disorder.

Complications
- Muscle wasting
- Severe depression
- Infection
- Socioeconomic problems

Special considerations
- CFIDS can be debilitating to the point that the patient may be bedridden. Treat each case individually, referring the patient to the appropriate resources and support.

••••••••••••

LATEX ALLERGY

Latex is a substance found in an increasing number of products both on the job and in the home. Also increasing is the number of latex allergies. Latex allergy is a hypersensitivity reaction to products that contain natural latex, which is derived from the sap of a rubber tree, not synthetic latex. These hypersensitivity reactions range from local dermatitis to a life-threatening anaphylactic reaction.

Causes
Approximately 1% of the population has a latex allergy; however, 17% to 25% of health care workers suffer from latex allergies. Anyone who is in frequent contact with latex-containing products is at risk for developing a latex allergy. (See *Products that contain latex,* page 788.) The more frequent the exposure, the higher the risk. The populations at highest risk are:
- medical and dental professionals
- workers in latex companies
- patients with spina bifida.

Other individuals at risk for latex allergy include:
- patients who have a history of asthma or other allergies, especially to bananas, avocados, tropical fruits, or chestnuts
- patients with a history of multiple intra-abdominal or genitourinary surgeries
- patients who require frequent intermittent urinary catheterization.

Products that contain latex

MEDICAL PRODUCTS
- Adhesive bandages
- Airways, nasogastric tubes
- Ambu bag
- Blood pressure cuff, tubing and bladder
- Catheters
- Catheter leg straps
- Dental dams
- Elastic bandages
- Electrode pads
- Fluid-circulating hypothermia blankets
- Hemodialysis equipment
- I.V. catheters
- Latex or rubber gloves
- Medication vials
- Pads for crutches
- Protective sheets
- Reservoir breathing bags
- Rubber airways and endotracheal tubes
- Tape
- Tourniquets

NONMEDICAL PRODUCTS
- Adhesive tape
- Balloons (excluding Mylar)
- Cervical diaphragms
- Condoms
- Disposable diapers
- Elastic stockings
- Glue
- Latex paint
- Nipples and pacifiers
- Rubber bands
- Tires

Clinical presentation

Early signs that a life-threatening hypersensitivity reaction may be occurring include hypotension, tachycardia, and oxygen desaturation.

Other clinical findings include:
- urticaria
- flushing
- bronchospasm
- difficulty breathing
- pruritus
- palpitations
- abdominal pain
- syncope.

Mild signs and symptoms may include:
- itchy skin
- swollen lips
- nausea
- diarrhea
- red, swollen, teary eyes.

Differential diagnoses
- Septic shock
- Myocardial infarction
- Dermatitis
- Asthma
- Anaphylaxis

Diagnosis

A patient who describes even the mildest symptoms during a history taking and physical assessment should be suspected of having a latex allergy. The patient may describe dermatitis or mild respiratory distress when using latex gloves, inflating a balloon, or coming in contact with other latex products.

A blood test for latex sensitivity can confirm the diagnosis. This test, which measures specific immunoglobulin E antibodies against latex, should be used only when latex allergy is suspected; it isn't recommended as a screening tool.

Management
General

The best treatment for latex allergy is prevention; the more a latex-sensitive person is exposed to latex, the worse his symptoms will become. To avoid exposure, advise the patient to substitute products made of silicone and vinyl for those made of latex. There's no known treatment for an allergic reaction to latex. Care is supportive in nature. The patient's airway, breathing, and circulation must be monitored. An artificial airway, oxygen therapy, cardiopulmonary resuscitation, and fluid management may be necessary.

Medication

When a latex allergy is suspected or known, the patient may receive medications before and after surgery or other invasive procedures.

The following medications may be used before surgery or other invasive procedures:
- prednisone — 5 to 60 mg/day P.O. (highly individualized)
- diphenhydramine — 25 to 50 mg P.O., I.M., or I.V. every 6 hours
- cimetidine — 300 mg I.V. before surgery.

The following medications may be used after surgery or other invasive procedures:
- hydrocortisone — 5 to 30 mg P.O. b.i.d. to q.i.d.
- diphenhydramine — 25 to 50 mg P.O., I.M., or I.V. every 6 hours
- famotidine — 20 mg P.O. or I.V. b.i.d.

During an acute reaction, administer epinephrine 0.1 to 0.5 mg S.C. or I.M., or use diphenhydramine, hydrocortisone, and famotidine, as mentioned above, which are commonly administered by I.V. infusion.

Referral

- The patient may need to be referred to a dermatologist or allergist for diagnosis.
- The patient may need psychological counseling to cope with lifestyle changes.
- Refer the patient to the American Latex Allergy Association for information and support.

Follow-up

Follow-up with the patient as needed to evaluate control of allergy.

Patient teaching

- Urge the patient to wear an identification tag mentioning his latex allergy.
- Teach the patient and family members how to use an epinephrine autoinjector.
- Teach the patient to be aware of all latex-containing products and to use vinyl or silicone products instead. Advise him that Mylar balloons don't contain latex.

Complications

- Anaphylaxis
- Respiratory distress
- Cardiovascular collapse
- Dermatitis

Special considerations

- Keep latex-free equipment available in your practice area at all times in order to conduct a complete examination on a patient with a latex allergy.

• • • • • • • • • • • •

LUPUS ERYTHEMATOSUS

A chronic inflammatory disorder of the connective tissues, lupus erythematosus appears in two forms. Discoid lupus erythematosus affects only the skin. (See *Discoid lupus erythematosus*, page 790.) Systemic lupus erythematosus (SLE) affects multiple organ systems, as well as the skin, and can be fatal. Like rheumatoid arthritis, SLE is characterized by recurring remissions and exacerbations that are especially common during the spring and summer. The annual incidence of SLE averages 27.5 cases per 1 million Whites and 75.4 cases per 1 million Blacks. SLE strikes 8 times more women than men, 15 times more during childbearing years. It occurs worldwide but is

Discoid lupus erythematosus

Discoid lupus erythematosus (DLE) is a form of lupus erythematosus marked by chronic skin eruptions that, if untreated, can lead to scarring and permanent disfigurement. About 1 of 20 patients with DLE later develops systemic lupus erythematosus (SLE). The exact cause of DLE is unknown, but some evidence suggests an autoimmune defect. An estimated 60% of patients with DLE are women in their late 20s or older. This disease is rare in children.

DLE lesions are raised, red, scaling plaques, with follicular plugging and central atrophy. The raised edges and sunken centers give them a coinlike appearance. Although these lesions can appear anywhere on the body, they usually erupt on the face, scalp, ears, neck, and arms or on any part of the body that's exposed to sunlight. Such lesions can resolve completely or may cause hypopigmentation or hyperpigmentation,

atrophy, and scarring. Facial plaques sometimes assume the butterfly pattern characteristic of SLE. Hair tends to become brittle or may fall out in patches.

As a rule, patient history and the appearance of the rash itself are diagnostic. Lupus erythematosus cell test is positive in fewer than 10% of patients. Skin biopsy of lesions reveals immunoglobulins or complement components. SLE must be ruled out.

Patients with DLE should avoid prolonged exposure to the sun, fluorescent lighting, or reflected sunlight. They should wear protective clothing, use sunscreening agents, avoid engaging in outdoor activities during periods of most intense sunlight (between 10 a.m. and 2 p.m.), and report any changes in the lesions. Drug treatment consists of topical, intralesional, or systemic medication, as in SLE.

most prevalent among Asians and Blacks. The prognosis improves with early detection and treatment but remains poor for patients who develop cardiovascular, renal, or neurologic complications or severe bacterial infections.

Causes

The exact cause of SLE remains a mystery, but evidence points to interrelated immunologic, environmental, hormonal, and genetic factors. Autoimmunity is thought to be the prime causative mechanism. In autoimmunity, the body produces antibodies against its own cells such as the antinuclear antibody. The formed antigen-antibody complexes can suppress the body's normal immunity and damage tissues. Patients with SLE produce anti-

bodies against many different tissue components, such as red blood cells (RBCs), neutrophils, platelets, lymphocytes, or almost any organ or tissue in the body.

Certain predisposing factors may make a person susceptible to SLE. Physical or mental stress, streptococcal or viral infections, exposure to sunlight or ultraviolet light, immunization, pregnancy, and abnormal estrogen metabolism may all affect the development of this disease.

SLE also may be triggered or aggravated by treatment with certain drugs—for example, procainamide, hydralazine, anticonvulsants and, less commonly, penicillins, sulfa drugs, and oral contraceptives.

Clinical presentation

The onset of SLE may be acute or insidious and produces no characteristic clinical pattern. However, its signs and symptoms commonly include:

- fever
- weight loss
- malaise
- fatigue
- rash
- polyarthralgia.

SLE may involve every body system:

- Joint involvement, in 90% of patients, is similar to that in rheumatoid arthritis.
- Skin lesions, in areas of the body exposed to light, occur that are most commonly an erythematous rash. Skin eruptions are commonly provoked or aggravated by ultraviolet rays.
- Facial areas, such as the nose and cheeks, are affected by the classic butterfly rash (occurring in fewer than 50% of patients; see *Butterfly rash*).
- Digits can be affected by the development of vasculitis, possibly leading to infarctive lesions, necrotic leg ulcers, or digital gangrene.
- Ears, nose, and digits may be affected by Raynaud's phenomenon (occurring in about 20% of patients).
- Mucous membranes may commonly appear with patchy alopecia and painless ulcers.

Constitutional signs and symptoms of SLE include:

- aching
- malaise
- fatigue
- low-grade or spiking fever
- chills
- anorexia
- weight loss.

Other signs and symptoms include:

- lymph node enlargement (diffuse or local and nontender)
- abdominal pain
- nausea

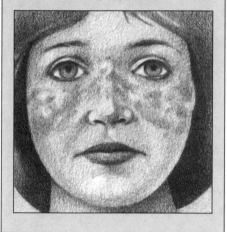

Butterfly rash

In the classic butterfly rash, lesions appear on the cheeks and the bridge of the nose, creating a characteristic butterfly pattern. The rash may vary in severity from malar erythema to discoid lesions (plaque).

- vomiting
- diarrhea
- constipation
- irregular menstrual periods or amenorrhea (during the active phase of SLE).

About 50% of SLE patients develop signs of cardiopulmonary abnormalities, such as:

- pleuritis
- pericarditis
- dyspnea
- myocarditis
- endocarditis
- tachycardia
- parenchymal infiltrates
- pneumonitis.

Renal effects may include:

- hematuria
- proteinuria
- urine sediment

Signs of systemic lupus erythematosus

Diagnosing systemic lupus erythematosus (SLE) is difficult because it often mimics other diseases; symptoms may be vague and vary greatly from patient to patient.

For these reasons, the American Rheumatism Association has issued a list of criteria for classifying SLE to be used for consistency in epidemiologic surveys. Four or more of the following signs and symptoms are usually present at some time during the course of the disease:

- malar or discoid rash
- photosensitivity
- oral or nasopharyngeal ulcerations
- nonerosive arthritis (of two or more peripheral joints)
- pleuritis or pericarditis
- profuse proteinuria (exceeding 0.5 g per day) or excessive cellular casts in urine
- seizures or psychoses
- hemolytic anemia, leukopenia, lymphopenia, or thrombocytopenia
- positive lupus erythematosus cell, anti-DNA, or anti-Sm test or chronic false-positive serologic test for syphilis
- abnormal titer of antinuclear antibody.

Differential diagnoses
- Influenza
- Pleuritis
- Pericarditis
- Pneumonia
- Renal failure
- Urinary tract infection
- Arthritis
- Seizure disorder
- Migraine headache
- Depression
- Actinic keratoses
- Polymorphous light eruption
- Drug eruptions
- Rosacea
- Sarcoid
- Tinea faciei
- Lupus vulgaris

Diagnosis
Diagnostic tests for patients with SLE include a complete blood count with differential (for signs of anemia and decreased white blood cell [WBC] count); platelet count (may be decreased); erythrocyte sedimentation rate (commonly elevated); and serum electrophoresis (may show hypergammaglobulinemia).

Specific tests for SLE include:
- antinuclear antibody, anti-DNA, and lupus erythematosus cell tests — positive in active SLE. Because the anti-DNA test is rarely positive in other conditions, it's the most specific test for SLE. However, if the patient is in remission, anti-DNA may be reduced or absent (correlates with disease activity, especially renal involvement, and helps monitor the response to therapy)
- urine studies — may show RBCs and WBCs, urine casts and sediment, and significant protein loss (more than 0.5 g in 24 hours)
- blood studies — decreased serum complement (C3 and C4) levels indicate active disease

- cellular casts (may progress to total kidney failure)
- urinary tract infection (may result from heightened susceptibility to infection).

Seizure disorders and mental dysfunction may indicate neurologic damage. Central nervous system involvement may produce emotional instability, psychosis, and organic mental syndrome. Headaches, irritability, and depression are common. (See *Signs of systemic lupus erythematosus.*)

■ chest X-ray—may show pleurisy or lupus pneumonitis

■ electrocardiogram—may show conduction defect with cardiac involvement or pericarditis

■ kidney biopsy—determines disease stage and extent of renal involvement.

Some patients show a positive lupus anticoagulant test and a positive anticardiolipin test. Such patients are prone to antiphospholipid syndrome (thrombosis and thrombocytopenia).

Management
General
The photosensitive patient should wear protective clothing (hat, sunglasses, long sleeves, and slacks) and use a screening agent with a sun protection factor of at least 15 when outdoors. Because SLE usually strikes women of childbearing age, questions about pregnancy commonly arise. Available evidence indicates that a woman with SLE can have a safe, successful pregnancy if she has no serious renal or neurologic impairment. If renal failure occurs, dialysis or kidney transplant may be necessary.

Medication
The following medications may be used in the treatment of lupus erythematosus:

■ aspirin—325 to 650 mg P.O. every 4 to 6 hours

■ triamcinolone 0.1%—apply to all active lesions b.i.d.

■ hydroxychloroquine—400 mg P.O. q.d. or b.i.d.

■ indomethacin—25 mg P.O. b.i.d. to t.i.d.

■ prednisone—60 mg/day P.O. then taper down (for acute exacerbations)

■ cyclosporine—1 to 4 mg/kg/day P.O.

Referral
■ Refer the patient to an immunologist for treatment.

■ The patient may need to be referred for physical therapy and occupational counseling as appropriate.

■ Refer the patient to the Lupus Foundation of America for information and support.

Follow-up
The patient should be seen by the specialist. If the patient is on hydroxychloroquine, ophthalmologic examinations should be performed every 6 months.

Patient teaching
■ Tell the patient to follow a balanced diet. Renal involvement may mandate a low-sodium, low-protein diet.

■ Urge the patient to get plenty of rest.

■ Tell the patient to apply heat packs to relieve joint pain and stiffness. Encourage regular exercise to maintain full range of motion (ROM) and prevent contractures. Teach ROM exercises as well as body alignment and postural techniques.

■ Explain the expected benefit of prescribed medications. Watch for adverse effects, especially when the patient is taking high doses of corticosteroids.

Complications
■ Diffuse proliferative glomerulonephritis
■ Renal failure
■ Urinary tract infection
■ Infection
■ Steroid adverse effects
■ Lupus arthritis

• • • • • • • • • • • •

RHEUMATOID ARTHRITIS

A chronic, systemic, inflammatory disease, rheumatoid arthritis (RA) primarily attacks peripheral joints and surrounding muscles, tendons, ligaments, and blood vessels. Spontaneous remissions and un-

Juvenile rheumatoid arthritis

Juvenile rheumatoid arthritis (JRA) is an inflammatory disorder of the connective tissues that's characterized by joint swelling and pain or tenderness affecting children younger than age 16. JRA may also affect organs such as the eyes, heart, lungs, liver, skin, and spleen.

Depending on the type, this disease can occur as early as age 6 weeks — although rarely before age 6 months — with peak onset between ages 1 and 3 and 8 and 12. JRA affects an estimated 70,000 to 100,000 children in the United States; overall incidence of JRA is twice as high in girls. Precipitating factors include viral or bacterial (particularly streptococcal) infection, trauma, and emotional stress, but their relationship to JRA remains unknown.

Three major types of JRA exist, including:

■ *systemic JRA* that may cause mild, transient arthritis or frank polyarthritis associated with fever or rash. Fever of 103° F (39.4° C) or higher occurs once or twice per day, causing an evanescent rheumatoid rash, and then rapidly returns to normal or subnormal.

■ *polyarticular JRA* that has an insidious onset and involves five or more joints commonly in the wrists, elbows, knees, ankles, and small joints of the hands and feet. Larger joints can also be af-fected, including the temporomandibular joints, cervical spine, hips, and shoulders, which become swollen, tender, and stiff.

■ *pauciarticular JRA* that involves few joints (usually no more than four), commonly affecting the knees and other large joints. Three subtypes of pauciarticular JRA include chronic iridocyclitis, sacroiliitis, and joint involvement without iritis.

Laboratory tests are useful for ruling out other inflammatory or even malignant diseases that can mimic JRA. Complete blood count shows decreased hemoglobin levels, neutrophilia, and thrombocytosis. Erythrocyte sedimentation rate and C-reactive protein, haptoglobin, immunoglobulin, and C3 complement levels may be elevated. X-rays in early stages reveal such changes as soft-tissue swelling, effusion, and periostitis in affected joints.

Successful management of JRA involves physical therapy, administration of anti-inflammatory drugs, nutrition and exercise, and regular eye examinations. Splints help reduce pain, prevent contractures, and maintain correct joint alignment. Surgery is usually limited to soft-tissue releases to improve joint mobility. Joint replacement is delayed until the child has matured physically and can handle vigorous rehabilitation.

predictable exacerbations mark the course of this potentially crippling disease. RA usually requires lifelong treatment and, sometimes, surgery. In most patients, the disease follows an intermittent course and allows normal activity, although 10% suffer total disability from severe articular deformity or associated extra-articular symptoms or both. The prognosis worsens with the development of nodules, vasculitis, and high titers of rheumatoid factor (RF). RA occurs worldwide, striking three times more females than males. This disease affects 2.1 million people in the United States alone.

AGE ALERT Although it can occur at any age, the peak onset period for RA in women is between ages 30 and 60. (See *Juvenile rheumatoid arthritis*.)

Causes and pathophysiology

The cause of the chronic inflammation characteristic of RA isn't known, but various theories point to infectious, genetic, and endocrine factors. Currently, it's believed that a genetically susceptible individual develops abnormal or altered immunoglobulin G (IgG) antibodies when exposed to an antigen. This altered IgG antibody isn't recognized as "self," and the individual forms an antibody known as RF against it. By aggregating into complexes, RF generates inflammation. Eventually, cartilage damage from inflammation triggers additional immune responses, including activation of complement. This in turn attracts polymorphonuclear leukocytes and stimulates release of inflammatory mediators, which enhance joint destruction.

Much more is known about the pathogenesis of RA than about its causes. If unarrested, the inflammatory process within the joints occurs in four stages. First, synovitis develops from congestion and edema of the synovial membrane and joint capsule. Formation of pannus — thickened layers of granulation tissue — marks the onset of the second stage. Pannus covers and invades cartilage and eventually destroys the joint capsule and bone. Progression to the third stage is characterized by fibrous ankylosis — fibrous invasion of the pannus and scar formation that occludes the joint space. Bone atrophy and malalignment cause visible deformities and disrupt the articulation of opposing bones, causing muscle atrophy and imbalance and, possibly, partial dislocations or subluxations. In the fourth stage, fibrous tissue calcifies, resulting in bony ankylosis and total immobility.

Clinical presentation

RA usually develops insidiously and initially produces nonspecific signs and symptoms, such as:

Joint deformities

In advanced rheumatoid arthritis, marked edema and congestion cause spindle-shaped interphalangeal joints and severe flexion deformities.

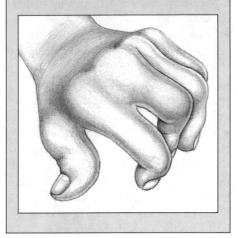

- fatigue
- malaise
- anorexia
- persistent low-grade fever
- weight loss
- lymphadenopathy
- vague articular symptoms.

Later, more specific localized articular symptoms develop, commonly in the fingers at the proximal interphalangeal, metacarpophalangeal, and metatarsophalangeal joints. These symptoms, which usually occur bilaterally and symmetrically and may extend to the wrists, knees, elbows, and ankles, have the following characteristics:

- The affected joints stiffen after inactivity, especially upon rising in the morning.
- The fingers may assume a spindle shape from marked edema and congestion in the joints. (See *Joint deformities*.)
- The joints become tender and painful, at first only when the patient moves them, but eventually even at rest. They

commonly feel hot to the touch. Ultimately, joint function is diminished.

Deformities are common if active disease continues:

- Proximal interphalangeal joints may develop flexion deformities or become hyperextended.
- Metacarpophalangeal joints may swell dorsally.
- Volar subluxation and stretching of tendons may pull the fingers to the ulnar side ("ulnar drift").
- The fingers may become fixed in a characteristic "swan's neck" appearance, or boutonnière deformity.
- The hands appear foreshortened and the wrists are boggy.
- Carpal tunnel syndrome from synovial pressure on the median nerve causes tingling paresthesia in the fingers.

The most common extra-articular finding is the gradual appearance of rheumatoid nodules—subcutaneous, round or oval, nontender masses—usually on pressure areas such as the elbows. Vasculitis can lead to skin lesions, leg ulcers, and multiple systemic complications. Peripheral neuropathy may produce numbness or tingling in the feet or weakness and loss of sensation in the fingers. Stiff, weak, or painful muscles are common.

Differential diagnoses

- Systemic lupus erythematosus
- Osteoarthritis
- Lyme disease
- Gout
- Pseudogout
- Polymyositis
- Scleroderma
- Chronic infection
- Reiter's syndrome
- Sarcoidosis

Diagnosis

Typical clinical features suggest RA, but a definitive diagnosis is based on laboratory and other test results:

- X-rays—in early stages, bone demineralization and soft-tissue swelling; later, loss of cartilage and narrowing of joint spaces; finally, cartilage and bone destruction and erosion, subluxations, and deformities
- RF test—positive in 75% to 80% of patients, as indicated by a titer of 1:160 or higher
- synovial fluid analysis—increased volume and turbidity but decreased viscosity and complement (C3 and C4) levels; white blood cell count commonly exceeds 10,000/µl
- serum protein electrophoresis—may show elevated serum globulins
- erythrocyte sedimentation rate—elevated in 85% to 90% of patients (may be useful to monitor the response to therapy because elevation commonly parallels disease activity)
- complete blood count—usually reveals moderate anemia and slight leukocytosis.

A C-reactive protein test can help monitor the response to therapy.

Management
General

Supportive measures include 8 to 10 hours of sleep every night, frequent rest periods between daily activities, and splinting to rest inflamed joints. A physical therapy program that includes range-of-motion exercises and carefully individualized therapeutic exercises forestalls loss of joint function; application of heat relaxes muscles and relieves pain. Moist heat usually works best for patients with chronic disease. Ice packs are effective during acute episodes.

Medication

For a list of appropriate medications for arthritis, see *Drug therapy for arthritis*.

Drug therapy for arthritis

DRUG AND DOSAGE	CLINICAL CONSIDERATIONS
aspirin *Dosage:* 325 to 1,000 mg P.O. every 4 to 6 hours	■ Don't use in patients with GI ulcers, bleeding, or hypersensitivity or in neonates. ■ Give with food, milk, an antacid, or a large glass of water to reduce adverse GI effects. ■ Monitor salicylate level. Remember that toxicity can develop rapidly in febrile, dehydrated children. ■ Teach the patient to reduce the dose, one tablet at a time, if tinnitus occurs. ■ Teach the patient to watch for signs of bleeding, such as bruising, melena, and petechiae. ■ Tell the patient to watch for adverse effects, such as GI disturbance and hypersensitivity reaction.
celecoxib *Dosage:* 100 to 200 mg P.O. b.i.d. **fenoprofen** *Dosage:* 300 to 600 mg P.O. t.i.d. to q.i.d. **ibuprofen** *Dosage:* 300 to 800 mg P.O. every 6 to 8 hours **naproxen** *Dosage:* 250 to 500 mg P.O. b.i.d. **piroxicam** *Dosage:* 20 mg/day P.O. **sulindac** *Dosage:* 150 to 200 mg P.O. every 12 hours **tolmetin** *Dosage:* 400 to 600 mg P.O. every 8 to 12 hours	■ Don't use in patients with renal disease, in asthmatics with nasal polyps, or in children. ■ Use cautiously in patients with GI and cardiac disease or in patients who are allergic to other nonsteroidal anti-inflammatory drugs (NSAIDs). ■ Give with milk or meals to reduce adverse GI effects. ■ Tell the patient that the drug effect may be delayed for 2 to 3 weeks. ■ Monitor kidney, liver, and auditory functions in long-term therapy. Stop the drug if abnormalities develop. ■ Use cautiously in elderly patients; they may experience severe GI bleeding without warning. ■ Tell the patient to watch for adverse effects such as central nervous system abnormalities.
hydroxychloroquine *Dosage:* initially 400 to 600 mg P.O. daily for 2 to 3 months, then 200 mg P.O. h.s.	■ Don't use in patients with retinal or visual field changes. ■ Use cautiously in patients with hepatic disease, alcoholism, glucose-6-phosphate dehydrogenase deficiency, or psoriasis. ■ Perform a complete blood count (CBC) and liver function tests before therapy and during chronic therapy. ■ Patients should have regular ophthalmologic examinations. ■ Tell the patient to take the drug with food or milk. ■ Warn the patient that dizziness may occur. ■ Tell the patient to watch for adverse reactions such as GI disturbances.

(continued)

Drug therapy for arthritis (continued)

DRUG AND DOSAGE	CLINICAL CONSIDERATIONS
gold sodium thiomalate *Dosage:* initially 10 mg I.M. followed by 25 mg in 1 week, then 25 mg weekly to total dose of 1 g, then 25 to 50 mg every 2 weeks for 2 to 20 weeks, then 25 to 50 mg every 3 to 4 weeks as maintenance therapy	■ Check urine for blood and albumin before each dose. If positive, hold the drug. Stress the need for regular follow-up, including blood and urine testing. ■ To avoid local nerve irritation, mix the drug well and give a deep I.M. injection in the buttock. ■ Advise the patient not to expect improvement for 3 to 6 months. ■ Tell the patient to report a rash, bruising, bleeding, hematuria, or oral ulcers. ■ Tell the patient to watch for and report adverse effects such as nitritoid reaction (flushing, fainting, and sweating).
methotrexate *Dosage:* 7.5 mg per week P.O. initially in single or divided doses, then decrease when response is obtained	■ Don't give to breast-feeding or pregnant women or to alcoholic patients. ■ Monitor uric acid levels, CBC, intake and output, and liver function tests. ■ Warn the patient to promptly report unusual bleeding (especially GI) or bruising. ■ Warn the patient to avoid alcohol, aspirin, and NSAIDs. ■ Advise the patient to follow the prescribed regimen. ■ Tell the patient to watch for adverse effects, such as difficulty breathing, hair loss, GI disturbance, rash, oral ulcers, and dizziness.
prednisone 5 to 60 mg per day P.O. (dosage is individualized)	■ Monitor glucose levels. ■ Always adjust to the lowest effective dose; gradually reduce drug dosage. ■ Most adverse reactions are dose or duration dependent. ■ For better results and less toxicity, order a once-daily dose in the morning. ■ Tell the patient to take with food to reduce GI irritation. ■ Tell the patient not to discontinue the drug abruptly or without consent of the health care practitioner.

Surgical intervention

Advanced RA may require synovectomy, joint reconstruction, or total joint arthroplasty.

Useful surgical procedures in RA include metatarsal head and distal ulnar resectional arthroplasty, insertion of a Silastic prosthesis between the metacarpophalangeal and proximal interphalangeal joints, and arthrodesis (joint fusion). Arthrodesis sacrifices joint mobility for stability and relief of pain. Synovectomy (removal of destructive, proliferating synovium, usually in the wrists, knees, and fingers) may halt or delay the course of this disease. Osteotomy (the cutting of bone or excision of a wedge of bone) can realign joint surfaces and redistribute stresses. Tendons may rupture spontaneously, requiring surgical repair. Tendon transfers may prevent deformities or relieve contractures.

Referral

■ The patient may need to be referred to a rheumatologist for treatment.

- The patient may need to be referred for physical and occupational therapy.
- Refer the patient and family to the Arthritis Foundation for information and support.

Follow-up

The patient should be seen by the health care provider according to the severity of symptoms.

Patient teaching

- Encourage a balanced diet, but make sure the patient understands that special diets won't cure RA. Stress the need for weight control because obesity adds further stress to joints.
- Urge the patient to perform activities of daily living.
- Teach the patient how to stand, walk, and sit correctly: upright and erect. Tell her to sit in chairs with high seats and armrests; she'll find it easier to get up from a chair if her knees are lower than her hips. If she doesn't own a chair with a high seat, recommend putting blocks of wood under the legs of a favorite chair. Suggest an elevated toilet seat.
- Instruct the patient to pace daily activities, resting for 5 to 10 minutes out of each hour and alternating sitting and standing tasks. Adequate sleep is important and so is correct sleeping posture. She should sleep on her back on a firm mattress and should avoid placing a pillow under her knees, which encourages flexion deformity.
- Teach the patient to avoid putting undue stress on joints, to use the largest joint available for a given task, to support weak or painful joints as much as possible, to avoid positions of flexion and promote positions of extension, to hold objects parallel to the knuckles as briefly as possible, to always use her hands toward the center of her body, and to slide — not lift — objects, whenever possible.

- Stress the importance of shoes with proper support.

Complications

- Temporomandibular joint disease
- Infection
- Osteoporosis
- Myositis
- Cardiopulmonary lesions
- Lymphadenopathy
- Peripheral neuritis
- Pericarditis
- Pulmonary nodules or fibrosis
- Pleuritis
- Scleritis
- Episcleritis
- Destruction of the odontoid process
- Cord compression

Special considerations

- Make sure the patient and family understand that RA is a chronic disease that requires major changes in lifestyle. Emphasize that there are no miracle cures, despite claims to the contrary.

• • • • • • • • • • • •

SCLERODERMA

Scleroderma is a diffuse connective tissue disease characterized by fibrotic, degenerative, and occasionally inflammatory changes in skin, blood vessels, synovial membranes, skeletal muscles, and internal organs (especially the esophagus, intestinal tract, thyroid, heart, lungs, and kidneys). Approximately 30% of patients with scleroderma die within 5 years of onset.

AGE ALERT Scleroderma, also known as progressive systemic sclerosis, affects more women than men, especially between ages 30 and 50.

Causes

The cause of scleroderma is unknown. This disease occurs in distinctive forms:

- CREST syndrome — a benign form characterized by calcinosis, Raynaud's phenomenon, esophageal dysfunction, sclerodactyly, and telangiectasia
- diffuse systemic sclerosis — characterized by generalized skin thickening and invasion of internal organ systems
- localized scleroderma — characterized by patchy skin changes with a droplike appearance known as morphea
- linear scleroderma — characterized by a band of thickened skin on the face or extremities that severely damages underlying tissues, causing atrophy and deformity (most common in childhood).

Other forms include chemically induced localized scleroderma, eosinophilia myalgia syndrome (recently associated with ingestion of L-tryptophan), toxic oil syndrome (associated with contaminated oil), and graft-versus-host disease.

Clinical presentation
Scleroderma typically begins with Raynaud's phenomenon — blanching, cyanosis, and erythema of the fingers and toes in response to stress or exposure to cold. Progressive phalangeal resorption may shorten the fingers.

Compromised circulation, which results from abnormal thickening of the arterial intima, may cause slowly healing ulcerations on the tips of the fingers or toes that may lead to gangrene. Raynaud's phenomenon may precede scleroderma by months or years.

Later symptoms include:
- pain, stiffness, and swelling of fingers and joints
- skin thickening produces taut, shiny skin over the entire hand and forearm
- facial skin becomes tight and inelastic, causing a masklike appearance and "pinching" of the mouth; as tightening progresses, contractures may develop.

GI dysfunction causes frequent reflux, heartburn, dysphagia, and bloating after meals. These symptoms may cause the patient to decrease food intake and lose weight. Other GI effects include:
- abdominal distention
- diarrhea
- constipation
- malodorous floating stools.

In advanced disease, cardiac and pulmonary fibrosis produces arrhythmias and dyspnea. Renal involvement is usually accompanied by malignant hypertension, the main cause of death.

Differential diagnoses
- Mixed connective tissue disease
- Sclerodermatomyositis
- Eosinophilia-myalgia syndrome
- Diffuse fascitis with eosinophilia
- Systemic lupus erythematosus
- Rheumatoid arthritis
- Polymyositis

Diagnosis
Typical cutaneous changes provide the first clue to diagnosis. Results of diagnostic tests include:
- blood studies — slightly elevated erythrocyte sedimentation rate, positive rheumatoid factor in 25% to 35% of patients, and positive antinuclear antibody test
- urinalysis — proteinuria, microscopic hematuria, and casts (with renal involvement)
- hand X-rays — terminal phalangeal tuft resorption, subcutaneous calcification, and joint space narrowing and erosion
- chest X-rays — bilateral basilar pulmonary fibrosis
- GI X-rays — distal esophageal hypomotility and stricture, duodenal loop dilation, small-bowel malabsorption pattern, and large diverticula
- pulmonary function studies — decreased diffusion and vital capacity
- electrocardiogram — possible nonspecific abnormalities related to myocardial fibrosis

■ skin biopsy — may show changes consistent with the progress of the disease, such as marked thickening of the dermis and occlusive vessel changes.

Management
General
Currently, no cure exists for scleroderma. Treatment aims to preserve normal body functions and minimize complications. Treatments vary according to symptoms.

Medication
The following medications may be used to treat scleroderma:
■ prednisone — 5 to 60 mg/day P.O. (highly individualized)
■ colchicine — 0.5 to 1.2 mg P.O., then 0.5 to 1.2 mg P.O. every hour until pain decreases or adverse effects occur
■ aspirin — 2.4 to 3.6 g/day P.O. in divided doses
■ recombinant human relaxin — experimental.

Referral
■ Refer the patient to a rheumatologist for treatment.
■ The patient may need to be referred for physical therapy.
■ Refer the patient to the Scleroderma Foundation for information and support.

Follow-up
The patient should be monitored frequently to evaluate the course of the disorder and the effectiveness of treatment.

Patient teaching
■ Teach the patient to avoid fatigue by pacing activities and organizing schedules to include necessary rest.
■ Tell the patient to follow a soft, bland diet with frequent small meals and plenty of fluids.
■ Tell patient that it's crucial not to smoke.

Complications
■ Renal failure
■ Respiratory failure
■ Flexion contractures
■ Disability
■ Arrhythmia
■ Obstructive bowel disease

Special considerations
■ Because of the debilitating nature of scleroderma, lifestyle changes may be necessary for the patient.
■ Blood platelet levels need to be monitored throughout drug therapy.

• • • • • • • • • • • •
SJÖGREN'S SYNDROME

The second most common autoimmune rheumatic disorder after rheumatoid arthritis (RA), Sjögren's syndrome (SS) is characterized by diminished lacrimal and salivary gland secretion (sicca complex). SS affects 2 to 4 million Americans and occurs mainly in women (90% of patients).

 AGE ALERT The average age of onset of SS is the late 40s.
SS may be a primary disorder or it may be associated with connective tissue disorders, such as RA, scleroderma, systemic lupus erythematosus (SLE), and polymyositis. In some patients, the disorder is limited to the exocrine glands (glandular SS); in others, it also involves other organs, such as the lungs and kidneys (extraglandular SS).

Causes
The cause of SS is unknown, but genetic and environmental factors probably contribute to its development. Viral or bacterial infection or perhaps exposure to pollen may trigger SS in a genetically susceptible individual. Tissue damage results from infiltration by lymphocytes or

from the deposition of immune complexes. Lymphocytic infiltration may be classified as benign, malignant, or pseudolymphoma (nonmalignant, but tumorlike aggregates of lymphoid cells).

Clinical presentation

About 50% of patients with SS have confirmed RA and a history of slowly developing sicca complex. However, some seek medical help for rapidly progressive and severe oral and ocular dryness, in many cases accompanied by periodic parotid gland enlargement.

Ocular dryness (xerophthalmia) leads to:
- foreign body sensation (gritty, sandy eye)
- redness
- burning
- photosensitivity
- eye fatigue
- itching
- mucoid discharge.

The patient may also complain of a film across his field of vision.

Oral dryness (xerostomia) leads to:
- difficulty swallowing and talking
- abnormal taste or smell sensation or both
- thirst
- ulcers of the tongue, buccal mucosa, and lips (especially at the corners of the mouth)
- severe dental caries.

Dryness of the respiratory tract leads to:
- epistaxis
- hoarseness
- chronic nonproductive cough
- recurrent otitis media
- increased incidence of respiratory infections.

Other effects may include:
- dyspareunia and pruritus (associated with vaginal dryness)
- generalized itching
- fatigue

- recurrent low-grade fever
- arthralgia or myalgia
- lymph node enlargement, which may be the first sign of malignant lymphoma or pseudolymphoma.

Specific extraglandular findings in SS include:
- interstitial pneumonitis
- interstitial nephritis (which results in renal tubular acidosis in 25% of patients)
- Raynaud's phenomenon (20%)
- vasculitis (which is usually limited to the skin and characterized by palpable purpura on the legs (20%)
- evidence of hypothyroidism related to autoimmune thyroid disease (about 50%)
- systemic necrotizing vasculitis (in a few patients).

Differential diagnoses
- SLE
- Multiple sclerosis
- RA
- Sarcoidosis
- Endocrine disorder
- Depression
- Adverse drug effects
- Cancer

Diagnosis

Diagnosis of SS rests on the detection of two of the following three conditions: xerophthalmia, xerostomia (with salivary gland biopsy showing lymphocytic infiltration), and an associated autoimmune or lymphoproliferative disorder.

Laboratory values include elevated erythrocyte sedimentation rate in most patients, mild anemia and leukopenia (30%), and hypergammaglobulinemia (50%). Autoantibodies are also common, including anti–SS-A (anti-Ro) and anti–SS-B (anti-La), which are antinuclear and antisalivary duct antibodies. Seventy-five percent to 90% of patients test positive for rheumatoid factor; 90% are positive for antinuclear antibodies.

Other tests help support this diagnosis. Schirmer's test and slit-lamp examination with rose bengal dye are used to measure eye involvement. Salivary gland involvement is evaluated by measuring the volume of parotid saliva and by secretory sialography and salivary scintigraphy. Lower-lip biopsy shows salivary gland infiltration by lymphocytes.

Management
General
Treatment is usually symptomatic and includes conservative measures to relieve ocular or oral dryness. Mouth dryness can be relieved by using a methylcellulose swab or spray and by drinking plenty of fluids, especially at mealtime. Meticulous oral hygiene is essential, including regular flossing, brushing, at-home fluoride treatment, and frequent dental checkups. Other treatment measures vary with associated extraglandular findings.

Medication
The following medications may be used to treat SS:
- pilocarpine hydrochloride — 5 mg P.O. t.i.d.
- ibuprofen — 200 to 600 mg P.O. every 6 to 8 hours.

Referral
- The patient may need to be referred to a rheumatologist for treatment.
- Refer the patient to the Sjögren's Syndrome Foundation for additional information and support.

Follow-up
The patient will need to be seen based on the extent of the symptoms.

Patient teaching
- Advise the patient to avoid drugs that decrease saliva production, such as atropine derivatives, antihistamines, anticholinergics, and antidepressants.
- If mouth lesions make eating painful, suggest high-protein, high-calorie liquid supplements to prevent malnutrition. Advise the patient to avoid sugar, which contributes to dental caries. Also, tell her to avoid tobacco, alcohol, and spicy, salty, or highly acidic foods, which cause mouth irritation.
- Tell the patient to instill artificial tears as often as every half hour to prevent eye damage (corneal ulcerations and corneal opacifications) from insufficient tear secretions. Suggest the use of sunglasses to protect the patient's eyes from dust, wind, and strong light. Moisture chamber spectacles may also be helpful. Because dry eyes are more susceptible to infection, advise the patient to keep her face clean and to avoid rubbing her eyes.
- Stress the need to humidify home and work environments. Suggest normal saline solution drops or aerosolized spray for nasal dryness. Advise the patient to avoid prolonged hot showers and baths and to use moisturizing lotions to help ease dry skin. Suggest K-Y lubricating jelly as a vaginal lubricant.

Complications
- Pulmonary infection
- Renal failure
- Lymphoma

URTICARIA AND ANGIOEDEMA

Urticaria, commonly known as hives, is an episodic, usually self-limited skin reaction characterized by local dermal wheals surrounded by an erythematous flare. Angioedema is a subcutaneous and dermal eruption that produces deeper, larger wheals (usually on the hands, feet, lips, genitals, and eyelids) and a more diffuse swelling of loose subcutaneous tissue. Urticaria and angioedema can occur simultaneously, but angioedema may last longer.

Causes

Urticaria and angioedema are common allergic reactions that may occur in 20% of the general population. One out of five people experience urticaria. The causes of these reactions include allergy to drugs, foods, insect stings and, occasionally, inhalant allergens (animal dander and cosmetics) that provoke an immunoglobulin E (IgE)–mediated response to protein allergens. However, certain drugs may cause urticaria without an IgE response. When urticaria and angioedema are part of an anaphylactic reaction, they almost always persist long after the systemic response has subsided. This occurs because circulation to the skin is the last to be restored after an allergic reaction, which results in slow histamine reabsorption at the reaction site.

Nonallergic urticaria and angioedema are probably also related to histamine release by some still-unknown mechanism. External physical stimuli, such as cold (usually in young adults), heat, water, or sunlight, may also provoke urticaria and angioedema. Dermographism urticaria, which develops after stroking or scratching the skin, occurs in as much as 20% of the population. Such urticaria develops with varying pressure, usually under tight clothing, and is aggravated by scratching.

Several different mechanisms and underlying disorders may provoke urticaria and angioedema. These include IgE-induced release of mediators from cutaneous mast cells; binding of IgG or IgM to antigen, resulting in complement activation; and such disorders as localized or secondary infections (such as respiratory infection), neoplastic diseases (such as Hodgkin's disease), connective tissue diseases (such as systemic lupus erythematosus), collagen vascular diseases, and psychogenic diseases.

Clinical presentation

The characteristic features of urticaria are distinct, raised, evanescent dermal wheals surrounded by an erythematous flare. These lesions may vary in size. In cholinergic urticaria, the wheals may be tiny and blanched, surrounded by erythematous flares.

Angioedema characteristically produces nonpitted swelling of deep subcutaneous tissue, usually on the eyelids, lips, genitalia, and mucous membranes. These swellings don't usually itch but may burn and tingle.

Differential diagnoses

- Insect bite
- Erythema multiforme
- Vasculitis and polyarteritis
- Systemic lupus erythematosus

Diagnosis

An accurate patient history can help determine the cause of urticaria. Such a history should include:

- medications, including over-the-counter preparations (vitamins, aspirin, and antacids)
- frequently ingested foods (strawberries, milk products, fish)
- environmental influences (pets, carpet, clothing, soap, inhalants, cosmetics, hair dye, and insect bites and stings).

Diagnosis also requires physical assessment to rule out similar conditions as well as a complete blood count, urinalysis, erythrocyte sedimentation rate, and a chest X-ray to rule out inflammatory infections. Skin testing, an elimination diet, and a food diary (recording time and amount of food eaten and circumstances) can pinpoint provoking allergens. The food diary may also suggest other allergies. For instance, a patient allergic to fish may also be allergic to iodine contrast materials.

Recurrent angioedema without urticaria, along with a familial history, points to hereditary angioedema. (See *Hereditary angioedema*.) Decreased serum levels of complement 4 (C4) and C1 esterase inhibitors confirm this diagnosis.

Management
General
Treatment aims to prevent or limit contact with triggering factors or, if this is impossible, to desensitize the patient to them and to relieve symptoms. Once the triggering stimulus has been removed, urticaria usually subsides in a few days — except for drug reactions, which may persist as long as the drug is in the bloodstream.

During desensitization, progressively larger doses of specific antigens (determined by skin testing) are injected intradermally.

Medication
The following medications may be used to treat urticaria or angioedema:
- epinephrine — 0.1 to 0.5 mg S.C. or I.M. (for severe reactions)
- hydroxyzine — 25 to 50 mg P.O. every 6 to 8 hours
- diphenhydramine — adults, 25 to 50 mg P.O. every 6 hours; children, 12.5 to 25 mg P.O. every 6 to 8 hours
- cimetidine — 300 mg I.V.
- methylprednisolone — 4 to 48 mg P.O. as a single dose or in divided doses.

Hereditary angioedema

A nonallergenic type of angioedema, hereditary angioedema results from an autosomal dominant trait — a hereditary deficiency of an alpha globulin, the normal inhibitor of C1 esterase (a component of the complement system). This deficiency allows uninhibited C1 esterase release, resulting in the vascular changes common to angioedema.

The clinical effects of hereditary angioedema usually appear in childhood with recurrent episodes of subcutaneous or submucosal edema at irregular intervals of weeks, months, or years, in many cases after trauma or stress. Hereditary angioedema is unifocal, without urticarial pruritus, but is associated with recurrent edema of the skin and mucosa (especially of the GI and respiratory tracts). GI tract involvement may cause nausea, vomiting, and severe abdominal pain. Laryngeal angioedema may cause fatal airway obstruction.

Treatment of acute hereditary angioedema may require androgens, such as danazol. Tracheotomy may be necessary to relieve airway obstruction resulting from laryngeal angioedema.

Referral
- The patient may need to be referred to an allergist for treatment.

Follow-up
Follow up with the patient according to his response to treatment.

Patient teaching
- Teach the patient to use an anaphylaxis pen, if appropriate.

■ Tell the patient to avoid known allergens.
■ Inform the patient about effective medication to use if he's accidentally exposed to allergens.

Complications
■ Severe systemic allergic reaction
■ Death

• • • • • • • • • • •
SELECTED REFERENCES

Braunwald, E., et al., eds. *Harrison's Principles of Internal Medicine*, 15th ed. New York: McGraw-Hill Book Co., 2001.

Busse, W.W., et al. "Pathophysiology of Severe Asthma," *Journal of Allergy and Clinical Immunology* 106(6):1033-42, December 2000.

Dolin, R., Masur, H., et. al. *AIDS Therapy.* New York: Churchill Livingstone, Inc., 1999.

Koopman, W.J. *Arthritis and Allied Conditions: A Textbook of Rheumatology*, 14th ed. Philadelphia: Lippincott Williams & Wilkins, 2001.

Lahita, R.G., et al. *Textbook of the Autoimmune Diseases.* Philadelphia: Lippincott Williams & Wilkins, 2000.

Smeltzer, S.C., and Bare, B.G. *Brunner & Suddarth's Textbook of Medical Surgical Nursing*, 9th ed. Philadelphia: Lippincott Williams &Wilkins, 2000.

Neoplasms

Primarily a disease of older adults, cancer is second only to cardiovascular disease as the leading cause of death in the United States (over 560,000 deaths annually). More than 67% of patients who die of cancer are over age 65. The most common cancers in the United States are prostate, breast, lung, and colorectal.

• • • • • • • • • • • •

OVERVIEW

Cancer results from a malignant transformation (carcinogenesis) of normal cells. A characteristic feature of cancer cells is their ability to proliferate uncontrollably, thus establishing themselves at other tissues to form secondary foci (metastasis). Additionally, cancer cells serve no useful purpose. (See *Comparing benign and malignant tumors*, page 808.) Cancer cells metastasize via the circulation through the blood or lymphatics, by unintentional transplantation from one site to another during surgery, and by local extension.

Classified by their histologic origin, tumors derived from epithelial tissues are called carcinomas; from epithelial and glandular tissues, adenocarcinomas; from connective, muscle, and bone tissues, sarcomas; from glial cells, gliomas; from pigmented cells, melanomas; and from plasma cells, myelomas. Cancer cells derived from erythrocytes are known as erythroleukemia; from lymphocytes, leukemia; and from lymphatic tissue, lymphoma.

What causes cancer?

Researchers have found that cancer develops from mutations within the genes of cells. Thus, cancer is a genetic disease. Cancer susceptibility genes are of two types. Some are oncogenes, which activate cell division and influence embryonic development, and some are tumor suppressor genes, which halt cell division.

These genes are typically found in normal human cells, but certain kinds of mutations may transform the normal cells. Inherited defects may cause a genetic mutation, whereas exposure to a carcinogen may cause an acquired mutation. Current evidence indicates that carcinogenesis results from a complex in-

Comparing benign and malignant tumors

CHARACTERISTIC	BENIGN	MALIGNANT
Growth	Slow expansion; push aside surrounding tissue but don't infiltrate	Usually infiltrate surrounding tissues rapidly, expanding in all directions
Limitation	Commonly encapsulated	Seldom encapsulated; in many cases poorly delineated
Recurrence	Rare after surgical removal	When removed only by surgery, commonly recur due to infiltration into surrounding tissues
Morphology	Cells closely resemble cells of tissue of origin	Cells may differ considerably from those of tissue of origin
Differentiation	Well differentiated	Variable
Mitotic activity	Variable	Extensive
Tissue destruction	Usually slight	Extensive due to infiltration and metastatic lesion
Spread	No metastasis	Spread via blood or lymph systems; establish secondary tumors
Effect on body	Cachexia rare; usually not fatal but may obstruct vital organs, exert pressure, produce excess hormones; can become malignant	Cachexia typical, with such symptoms as anemia, weight loss, and weakness; fatal if untreated

teraction of carcinogens and accumulated mutations in several genes.

In animal studies of the ability of viruses to transform cells, some human viruses exhibit carcinogenic potential. For example, the Epstein-Barr virus, the cause of infectious mononucleosis, has been linked to Burkitt's lymphoma and nasopharyngeal carcinoma.

High-frequency radiation, such as ultraviolet and ionizing radiation, damages the genetic material known as deoxyribonucleic acid (DNA), possibly inducing genetically transferable abnormalities.

Other factors, such as a person's tissue type and hormonal status, interact to potentiate radiation's carcinogenic effect. Examples of substances that may damage DNA and induce carcinogenesis include:

- asbestos — mesothelioma of the lung
- vinyl chloride — angiosarcoma of the liver
- aromatic hydrocarbons and benzopyrene (from polluted air) — lung cancer
- alkylating agents — leukemia
- tobacco — cancer of the lung, oral cavity and upper airways, esophagus, pancreas, kidneys, and bladder.

Diet has also been implicated, especially in the development of GI cancer as a result of a high animal fat diet. Additives comprised of nitrates and certain methods of food preparation—particularly charbroiling—are also recognized factors.

The role of hormones in carcinogenesis is still controversial, but it seems that excessive use of some hormones, especially estrogen, produces cancer in animals. Also, the synthetic estrogen diethylstilbestrol causes vaginal cancer in some daughters of women who were treated with it. It's unclear, however, whether changes in human hormonal balance retard or stimulate cancer development.

Some forms of cancer and precancerous lesions result from genetic predisposition either directly (as in Wilms' tumor and retinoblastoma) or indirectly (in association with inherited conditions such as Down syndrome or immunodeficiency diseases). Expressed as autosomal recessive, X-linked, or autosomal dominant disorders, their common characteristics include:

- early onset of malignant disease
- increased incidence of bilateral cancer in paired organs (breasts, adrenal glands, kidneys, and eighth cranial nerve [acoustic neuroma])
- increased incidence of multiple primary malignancies in nonpaired organs
- abnormal chromosome complement in tumor cells.

Immune response
Other factors that interact to increase susceptibility to carcinogenesis are immunologic competence, age, nutritional status, hormonal balance, and response to stress. Theoretically, the body develops cancer cells continuously, but the immune system recognizes them as foreign cells and destroys them. This defense mechanism, known as immunosurveillance, has two major components: cell-mediated immune response and humoral immune response. Their interaction promotes antibody production, cellular immunity, and immunologic memory. Presumably, the intact human immune system is responsible for spontaneous regression of tumors.

Theoretically, the cell-mediated immune response begins when T lymphocytes become sensitized by contact with a specific antigen. After repeated contacts, sensitized T cells release chemical factors called lymphokines, some of which begin to destroy the antigen. This reaction triggers the transformation of an additional population of T lymphocytes into "killers" of antigen-specific cells—in this case, cancer cells.

Similarly, the humoral immune response reacts to an antigen by triggering the release of antibodies from plasma cells and activating the serum-complement system, which destroys the antigen-bearing cell. However, an opposing immune factor, a "blocking antibody," enhances tumor growth by protecting malignant cells from immune destruction.

Theoretically, cancer arises when one of several factors disrupts the immune system:

- Aging cells, when copying their genetic material, may begin to err, giving rise to mutations. The aging immune system may not recognize these mutations as foreign and thus may allow them to proliferate and form a malignant tumor.
- Cytotoxic drugs decrease antibody production and destroy circulating lymphocytes.
- Extreme stress or certain viral infections can depress the immune system.
- Increased susceptibility to infection commonly results from radiation, cytotoxic drug therapy, and lymphoproliferative and myeloproliferative diseases, such

as lymphatic and myelocytic leukemia. These cause bone marrow depression, which can impair leukocyte function.

■ Acquired immunodeficiency syndrome weakens cell-mediated immunity.

■ Cancer itself is immunosuppressive; advanced cancer exhausts the immune response. (The absence of immune reactivity is known as anergy.)

Diagnostic methods

A thorough medical history and physical examination should precede sophisticated diagnostic procedures. Useful tests for the early detection and staging of tumors include X-ray, endoscopy, isotope scan, computed tomography scan, and magnetic resonance imaging, but the single most important diagnostic tool is a biopsy for direct histologic study of tumor tissue. Biopsy tissue samples can be taken by curettage, fluid aspiration (pleural effusion), fine-needle aspiration biopsy (breast), dermal punch (skin or mouth), endoscopy (rectal polyps), and surgical excision (visceral tumors and nodes).

An important tumor marker, carcinoembryonic antigen (CEA), although not diagnostic by itself, can signal malignancies of the large bowel, stomach, pancreas, lungs, and breasts. CEA titers range from normal (less than 5 ng) to suspicious (5 to 10 ng) to suspect (over 10 ng). CEA serves many valuable purposes:

■ as a baseline during chemotherapy to evaluate the extent of tumor spread

■ to regulate drug dosage

■ to prognosticate after surgery or radiation

■ to detect tumor recurrence.

Although no more specific than CEA, alpha-fetoprotein — a fetal antigen uncommon in adults — can suggest testicular, ovarian, gastric, and hepatocellular cancers. Beta human chorionic gonadotropin may point to testicular cancer

or choriocarcinoma. Other commonly used tumor markers include prostate-specific antigen (PSA) to detect and monitor prostatic cancer, and CA-125, useful for monitoring ovarian, colorectal, and gastric cancers.

Staging and grading

Choosing effective therapeutic options depends on correct staging of malignant disease, often with the internationally known TNM staging system (tumor size, nodal involvement, metastatic progress). This classification system provides an accurate tumor description that's adjustable as the disease progresses. TNM staging allows reliable comparison of treatments and survival rates among large population groups; it also identifies nodal involvement and metastasis to other areas.

Grading, another way to define a tumor, classifies the lesion according to corresponding normal cells, such as lymphoid or mucinous lesions; it compares tumor tissue to normal cells (differentiation); and it estimates the tumor's growth rate. For example, a low-grade tumor typically has cells more closely resembling normal cells, whereas a high-grade tumor has poorly differentiated cells.

Five major therapies

Cancer treatments include surgery, radiation, chemotherapy, biotherapy (also called immunotherapy), and hormonal therapy. Each therapy may be used alone or in combination, depending on the type, stage, localization, and responsiveness of the tumor and on limitations imposed by the patient's clinical status.

Surgery, once the mainstay of cancer treatment, is typically combined with other therapies. Surgery may be performed as a biopsy to obtain tissue for study; as continued surgery to remove the bulk of the tumor; or before chemotherapy or radiation to debulk the tumor in hope of a better outcome. Later, other therapies may be used to discourage proliferation of residual cells. Surgery can also relieve pain, correct obstruction, and alleviate pressure. Today's less radical surgical procedures (such as lumpectomy instead of radical mastectomy) are more acceptable to patients.

Radiation therapy aims to destroy the dividing cancer cells while damaging resting normal cells as little as possible. Therapeutic radiation is either particulate or electromagnetic. Both types ionize matter and have cellular DNA as their target.

Radiation treatment approaches include external beam radiation and intracavitary and interstitial implants. The latter therapy requires personal radiation protection for all staff members who come in contact with the patient.

Radiation may be used palliatively to relieve pain, obstruction, malignant effusions, cough, dyspnea, ulcerations, and hemorrhage; it can also promote the repair of pathologic fractures after surgical stabilization and delay tumor spread. (For localized adverse effects, see *Managing radiation's adverse effects*, page 812.)

Combining radiation and surgery can minimize radical surgery, prolong survival, and preserve anatomic function. For example, preoperative doses of radiation shrink a tumor, making it operable, while preventing further spread of the disease during surgery. After the wound heals, postoperative doses prevent residual cancer cells from multiplying or metastasizing.

Chemotherapy includes a wide array of drugs, which may induce regression of a tumor and its metastasis. It's particularly useful in controlling residual disease and, as an adjunct to surgery or radiation therapy, it can induce long remissions and sometimes effect cures, especially in patients with childhood leukemia, Hodg-

kin's disease, choriocarcinoma, or testicular cancer. As a palliative treatment, chemotherapy aims to improve the patient's quality of life by temporarily relieving pain and other symptoms.

Some major chemotherapeutic agents include:
- alkylating agents and nitrosoureas (inhibit cell growth and division by reacting with DNA)
- antimetabolites (prevent cell growth by competing with metabolites in the production of nucleic acid)
- Antitumor antibiotics (block cell growth by binding with DNA and interfering with DNA-dependent ribonucleic acid synthesis)
- plant alkaloids (prevent cellular reproduction by disrupting cell mitosis)
- steroid hormones (inhibit the growth of hormone-susceptible tumors by changing their chemical environment).

Adverse effects of chemotherapy vary. Although antineoplastic agents are toxic to cancer cells, they can also cause transient changes in normal tissues, especially among proliferating body cells. For example, antineoplastic agents typically suppress bone marrow, causing anemia, leukopenia, and thrombocytopenia; irritate GI epithelial cells, causing nausea and vomiting; and destroy the cells of the hair follicles and skin, causing alopecia and dermatitis.

Some I.V. chemotherapy drugs are irritants and still others are vesicants. Irritants cause pain at the injection site and along the vein but don't usually cause tissue necrosis. However, vesicants, if extravasated, may cause deep cutaneous necrosis requiring debridement and skin grafting.

Chemotherapeutic drugs can be given P.O., S.C., I.M., I.V., intracavitarily, intrathecally, intraperitoneally, topically, intralesionally, and by arterial infusion, depending on the drug and its pharmaco-

Managing radiation's adverse effects

AREA RADIATED	EFFECT	MANAGEMENT
Abdomen or pelvis	Cramps, diarrhea	Administer loperamide and diphenoxylate with atropine. Provide low-residue diet. Maintain fluid and electrolyte balance.
Head and neck	Alopecia	Gently comb and groom the scalp. Use a soft head covering.
	Mucositis	Provide non-alcohol-based mouthwash with viscous lidocaine; cool carbonated drinks; ice pops; soft, nonirritating diet; soft toothbrushes or swabs. Avoid spicy food and alcohol.
	Xerostomia (dry mouth)	Encourage good mouth hygiene; consider prescribing an oral saliva replacement.
	Dental caries	Apply fluoride to teeth prophylactically; provide gingival care.
Chest	Lung tissue irritation	Tell the patient to stop smoking and to avoid people with upper respiratory infections. Provide steroid therapy and a humidifier, if necessary.
	Pericarditis, myocarditis	Control arrhythmias with appropriate agents (procainamide, disopyramide phosphate); monitor for heart failure.
	Esophagitis	Give pain medication. Provide total parenteral nutrition. Maintain fluid balance.
Kidneys	Nephritis, lassitude, headache, edema, dyspnea, hypertensive nephropathy, azotemia, anemia	Maintain fluid and electrolyte balance. Watch for signs of renal failure. Consider prescribing erythropoietin.

logic action. Administration is usually intermittent to allow for bone marrow recovery between doses.

Biotherapy (also known as immunotherapy) relies on treatment agents known as biological response modifiers. Biological agents are usually combined with chemotherapeutic drugs or radiation therapy. Much of the work done in biotherapy is still experimental. However, the Food and Drug Administration has approved several new drugs, which are providing promising results. For example, rituximab — a monoclonal antibody — is effective for treatment of relapsed or refractory B-cell non-Hodgkin's lymphoma.

The main biotherapy agent classifications include interferons, interleukins, hematopoietic growth factors, and monoclonal antibodies. Interferons have antiviral, antiproliferative, and immunomodulary effects. Interleukins exert their effects on the T lymphocytes. Monoclonal antibodies, such as rituximab, provide the most tumor-specific therapy for cancer by selectively binding to tumor cell surfaces.

Although not used to treat cancer directly, hematopoietic growth factors are used to increase the patient's blood counts when chemotherapy or radiation causes a decrease.

Adverse effects of biotherapeutic agents mimic the body's normal immune response, with flulike symptoms being the most common.

Hormonal therapy is based on studies showing that certain hormones affect the growth of certain cancer types. For example, the luteinizing hormone–releasing hormone analogue leuprolide is used to treat prostate cancer. With long-term use, this hormone inhibits testosterone release and tumor growth. Tamoxifen, an antiestrogen hormonal agent, blocks estrogen receptors in breast tumor cells that require estrogen to thrive. Additionally, tamoxifen can be given prophylactically to women at high risk for breast cancer.

Some adverse effects of these hormonal agents include hot flashes, sweating, impotence, decreased libido, nausea and vomiting, and blood dyscrasias (with tamoxifen).

Maintaining nutrition and fluid balance

Tumors grow at the expense of normal tissue by competing for nutrients; consequently, the patient with cancer commonly suffers protein deficiency. Cancer treatments themselves produce fluid and electrolyte disturbances, such as vomiting and anorexia. Maintaining adequate nutrition, fluid intake, and electrolyte balance should be a major focus in cancer care.

Obtain a comprehensive dietary history to pinpoint nutritional problems and their causes such as diabetes; then help plan the diet accordingly. Advise the patient to:

- consume a liquid diet high in protein, carbohydrates, and calories if he can't tolerate solid foods (if he has stomatitis, recommend soft, bland, nonirritating foods)
- make mealtime as relaxing and pleasant as possible; encourage him to dine with others, if possible
- drink a glass of wine before dinner to stimulate the appetite and aid relaxation
- drink juice or other caloric beverages instead of water
- consume small, frequent meals if he can't tolerate normal ones
- avoid strong-smelling foods
- consume homemade food.

If the patient can't eat

The patient who has had recent head, neck, or GI surgery or who has pain when swallowing can receive nourishment through a nasogastric (NG) tube.

If an NG tube isn't appropriate, other alternatives are gastrostomy, jejunostomy and, occasionally, esophagostomy. These procedures make it possible for the patient to receive prescribed protein formulas and semiliquids, such as cream soups and eggnog; they also make it easier for the patient to feed himself.

Total parenteral nutrition

Commonly considered an important component of cancer care if the patient can't tolerate enteral nutrition, total parenteral nutrition (TPN) can improve a severely debilitated patient's protein balance. In doing so, TPN characteristically strengthens and conditions the patient, allowing him to better tolerate treatment.

TPN can produce a slight weight gain in the patient receiving radiation

Patient-controlled analgesia system

The patient-controlled analgesia (PCA) system is a popular option for pain treatment in cancer care. Clinical studies report that patients on PCA tend to titrate analgesic drugs effectively and maintain comfort without oversedation. They tend to use less of the drug than the amount normally given by I.M. injection.

PCA provides other significant advantages:
- Patients are alert and active during the day.
- Patients no longer need to suffer pain while awaiting their injections.
- Patients are free from pain caused by injections.

therapy, provide optimum nutrition for wound healing, and help the patient combat infection after radical surgery.

Pain control

Patients with cancer typically have a great fear of overwhelming pain. Therefore, controlling pain is a major consideration at every stage of managing cancer—from localized cancer to advanced metastasis. In patients with cancer, pain may result from inflammation of or pressure on pain-sensitive structures, tumor infiltration of nerves or blood vessels, or metastatic extension to bone. Such chronic and unrelenting pain can wear down the patient's tolerance to treatment, interfere with eating and sleeping, and color his life with anger, despair, and anxiety.

Narcotic analgesics, either alone or in combination with nonnarcotic analgesics, antianxiety agents, or tricyclic antidepressants are the mainstay of pain relief in patients with advanced cancer. In terminal stages of cancer, effective nar-

cotic dosages may be quite high because drug tolerance invariably develops. Provide such analgesics generously. Anticipate the need for pain relief, and provide it on a schedule that doesn't allow pain to break through. Don't wait to relieve pain until it becomes severe. (See *Patient-controlled analgesia system*.)

Nonpharmacologic pain-relief techniques can be used alone or, more commonly, in combination with drug therapy. Popular techniques include cutaneous stimulation, relaxation, biofeedback, distraction, and guided imagery.

Surgical excision of the tumor can relieve pressure on sensitive tissues and pain caused by inflamed necrotic tissue, treatment with antibiotics can combat inflammation, and radiation therapy can shrink metastatic tissue and control bone pain. When a tumor invades nerve tissue, effective pain control requires anesthetics, destructive nerve blocks, electronic nerve stimulation with a dorsal column or transcutaneous electrical nerve stimulator, rhizotomy, or chordotomy.

The hospice approach

A holistic approach to patient care modeled after St. Christopher's Hospice in London, hospice care provides comprehensive physical, psychological, social, and spiritual care for terminally ill patients. Although some hospices are located in inpatient settings, most hospice programs serve terminally ill patients amid the more familiar and relaxed surroundings of their own home.

The goal of the hospice care team is to help the patient achieve as full a life as possible, with minimal pain, discomfort, and restriction. Of the many medications provided for pain control, morphine is considered the drug of choice.

Hospice care also emphasizes a coordinated team effort to help the patient and family members overcome the severe anxiety, fear, and depression that occur with terminal illness. As a means to this end, hospice staffs encourage family members to help with the patient's care, thereby providing the patient with warmth and security and helping the family caregivers begin the grieving process before the patient dies.

Everyone involved in this method of care must be committed to high-quality patient care, unafraid of emotional involvement, and comfortable with personal feelings about death and dying. Good hospice care also requires open communication among team members, not just for evaluating patient care but also for helping the staff cope with their own feelings.

Psychological aspects

No illness evokes as profound an emotional response as the diagnosis of cancer. Patients express this response in several ways. A few face this difficult reality from the outset of diagnosis and treatment. Many use denial as a coping mechanism and simply refuse to accept the truth, but this stance is increasingly difficult for them to maintain. As evidence of the tumor becomes inescapable, the patient may plunge into deep depression. Family members may express denial in attempts to cope by encouraging unproven methods of cancer treatment, which can delay effective care. Some patients cope by intellectualizing about their disease, enabling them to obscure the reality of the cancer and regard it as unrelated to themselves. Generally, intellectualization is a more productive coping behavior than denial because the patient is receiving treatment. Be aware of the possible behavioral responses so you can identify them and then interact supportively with the patient and his family. For many malignancies, you can offer realistic hope for long-term survival or remission; even in

advanced disease, you can offer short-term achievable goals. To help a patient cope with cancer, make sure you understand your own feelings about it. Then listen sensitively to the patient so you can offer genuine understanding and support. When caring for a patient with terminal cancer, increase your effectiveness by seeking out someone to help you through your own grieving.

• • • • • • • • • • • •

BLADDER CANCER

Bladder tumors can develop on the surface of the bladder wall (benign or malignant papillomas) or grow within the bladder wall (generally more virulent) and quickly invade underlying muscles. Ninety percent of bladder tumors are transitional cell carcinomas arising from the transitional epithelium of mucous membranes. Less common are adenocarcinomas, epidermoid carcinomas, squamous cell carcinomas, sarcomas, tumors in bladder diverticula, and carcinoma in situ. Bladder cancer is more common in densely populated industrial areas. Cancer of the bladder is the most common cancer of the urinary tract.

AGE ALERT Bladder tumors are most prevalent in men over age 50.

Causes

Certain environmental carcinogens, such as 2-naphthylamine, benzidine, tobacco, and nitrates, predispose people to transitional cell tumors. Thus, workers in certain industries (rubber workers, weavers and leather finishers, aniline dye workers, hair-dressers, petroleum workers, and spray painters) are at high risk for such tumors. The period between exposure to the carcinogen and development of symptoms is about 18 years.

Squamous cell carcinoma of the bladder is most common in geographic areas where schistosomiasis is endemic. It's also associated with chronic bladder irritation and infection (for example, from renal calculi, indwelling urinary catheters, and cystitis caused by cyclophosphamide).

Clinical presentation

In early stages, approximately 25% of patients with bladder tumors have no symptoms. Commonly, the first sign is gross, painless, intermittent hematuria (in many cases with clots in the urine). Many patients with invasive lesions have suprapubic pain after voiding. Other signs and symptoms include:
- bladder irritability
- urinary frequency
- nocturia
- dribbling.

Differential diagnoses
- Urinary tract infection
- Pyelonephritis
- Incontinence

Diagnosis

Only cystoscopy and biopsy confirm bladder cancer. Cystoscopy should be performed when hematuria first appears. When it's performed under anesthesia, a bimanual examination is usually done to determine if the bladder is fixed to the pelvic wall. A thorough history and physical examination may help determine whether the tumor has invaded the prostate or the lymph nodes.

The following tests can provide essential information about the tumor:
- Urinalysis can detect blood in the urine and malignant cytology.
- Excretory urography can identify a large, early stage tumor or an infiltrating tumor, delineate functional problems in the upper urinary tract, assess hydrone-

phrosis, and detect rigid deformity of the bladder wall.
- Retrograde cystography evaluates bladder structure and integrity. Test results help to confirm the diagnosis.
- Pelvic arteriography can reveal tumor invasion into the bladder wall.
- Computed tomography scanning reveals the thickness of the involved bladder wall and detects enlarged retroperitoneal lymph nodes.
- Ultrasonography can detect metastasis beyond the bladder and can distinguish a bladder cyst from a tumor.

Management
General

Investigational treatments include photodynamic therapy and intravesicular administration of interferon alfa and tumor necrosis factor. Photodynamic therapy involves I.V. injection of a photosensitizing agent such as hematoporphyrin ether, which malignant cells readily absorb. Then a cystoscopic laser device introduces laser energy into the bladder, exposing the malignant cells to laser light, which kills them. Because this treatment also produces photosensitivity in normal cells, the patient must totally avoid sunlight for about 30 days.

Medication

Intravesicular chemotherapy is used for superficial tumors (especially those that occur in many sites) and to prevent tumor recurrence. This treatment involves washing the bladder directly with antineoplastic drugs, most commonly:
- thiotepa — 30 to 60 mg in 30 to 60 ml of normal saline solution instilled in the bladder for 2 hours weekly for 4 weeks
- doxorubicin — 60 to 75 mg/m^2 I.V. as a single dose at 21-day intervals *or* 20 mg/m^2/week *or* 25 to 30 mg/m^2/day for 2 to 3 consecutive days every 3 to 4 weeks

■ mitomycin — 10 to 20 mg/m² I.V. as a single dose and repeated every 6 to 8 weeks; dosage dependent on clinical and hematologic response and concurrent myelosuppressant therapy

■ bacille Calmette-Guérin — instilled into the bladder based on published protocols.

Surgical intervention

Superficial bladder tumors are removed by transurethral (cystoscopic) resection and fulguration (electrical destruction). This procedure is adequate when the tumor hasn't invaded the muscle.

If additional tumors develop, fulguration may have to be repeated every 3 months for years. However, if the tumors penetrate the muscle layer or recur frequently, cystoscopy with fulguration is no longer appropriate.

Tumors too large to be treated through a cystoscope require segmental bladder resection to remove a full-thickness section of the bladder. This procedure is feasible only if the tumor isn't near the bladder neck or ureteral orifices. Bladder instillation of thiotepa after transurethral resection may also help control such tumors.

For infiltrating bladder tumors, radical cystectomy is the treatment of choice. The week before cystectomy, treatment may include external beam therapy to the bladder. Surgery involves removal of the bladder with perivesical fat, lymph nodes, urethra, the prostate and seminal vesicles (in males), and the uterus and adnexa (in females). The surgeon forms a urinary diversion, usually an ileal conduit. The patient must then wear an external pouch continuously. Other diversions include ureterostomy, nephrostomy, vesicostomy, ileal bladder, ileal loop, and sigmoid conduit.

Treatment of patients with advanced bladder cancer includes cystectomy to remove the tumor, radiation therapy, and systemic chemotherapy with such drugs as cyclophosphamide, fluorouracil, doxorubicin, and cisplatin. This combination sometimes is successful in arresting bladder cancer. Cisplatin is the most effective single agent.

Referral

■ Refer the patient to a surgeon and oncologist for treatment.

■ The patient may need to be referred for follow-up home health care or to an enterostomal therapist.

■ Refer the patient to the American Cancer Society for information and support.

Follow-up

The patient should be seen as directed by the gynecologist.

Patient teaching

■ Advise the patient with a urinary stoma that he may participate in most activities except for heavy lifting and contact sports.

■ Teach the patient and family, if appropriate, about the urinary stoma and how to care for it.

Complications

■ Impotence
■ Infection
■ Metastasis
■ Anemia
■ Hydronephrosis
■ Urinary incontinence
■ Urethral stricture

Special considerations

■ Males are impotent following radical cystectomy and urethrectomy because these procedures damage the sympathetic and parasympathetic nerves that control erection and ejaculation. At a later date, the patient may desire a penile implant to make sexual intercourse (without ejaculation) possible.

CLINICAL CAUTION All high-risk people — for example, chemical workers and people with a history of benign bladder tumors or persistent cystitis — should have periodic cytologic examinations and learn about the danger of disease-causing agents.

• • • • • • • • • • • •

BRAIN TUMORS, MALIGNANT

Malignant brain tumors are common (slightly more so in men than women), occurring in about 4.5 persons per 100,000. These tumors may occur at any age. In adults, incidence is generally highest between ages 40 and 60. The most common tumor types in adults are gliomas and meningiomas, which usually occur supratentorially (above the covering of the cerebellum). Peak age in children is between ages 3 and 9. The most common types in children are astrocytomas, medulloblastomas, ependymomas, and brain stem gliomas. In children, brain tumors represent the second most common type of childhood cancer.

Causes
The cause of most brain tumors is unknown; however, exposure to ionizing radiation is a known environmental risk, and genetics and other environmental factors have been implicated. Additionally, most malignant tumors of the brain are of metastatic origin; 20% to 40% of patients with cancer develop brain metastasis.

Clinical presentation
Brain tumors cause central nervous system changes by invading and destroying tissues and by secondary effect, such as:

- compression of the brain, cranial nerves, and cerebral vessels
- cerebral edema
- increased intracranial pressure (ICP). (See *Comparing malignant brain tumors*.)

Generally, clinical features result from increased ICP; these features vary with the type of tumor, its location, and the degree of invasion. (See *What happens in increased ICP*, page 822.) Headaches that occur are usually deep aching pain, nonthrobbing, that worsens with coughing or straining. Onset of symptoms is usually insidious, and brain tumors are commonly misdiagnosed.

Differential diagnoses
- Subarachnoid hemorrhage
- Temperol arteritis
- Trauma
- Migraine
- Seizure disorder
- Psychiatric disease

Diagnosis
In many cases, a definitive diagnosis follows a tissue biopsy performed by stereotactic surgery. In this procedure, a head ring is affixed to the skull, and an excisional device is guided to the lesion by a computed tomography (CT) scan or magnetic resonance imaging (MRI).

Other diagnostic tools include patient history, neurologic assessment, skull X-rays, brain scan, CT scan, MRI, and cerebral angiography. Lumbar puncture shows increased pressure and protein levels, decreased glucose levels and, occasionally, tumor cells in cerebrospinal fluid (CSF).

Management
General
The mode of therapy depends on the tumor's histologic type, radiosensitivity, and location and may include surgery,

(*Text continues on page 821.*)

Comparing malignant brain tumors

TUMOR	CLINICAL FEATURES
Astrocytoma ■ Second most common malignant glioma (approximately 30% of all gliomas) ■ Occurs at any age; incidence higher in males ■ Usually occurs in white matter of cerebral hemispheres; may originate in any part of the central nervous system ■ Cerebellar astrocytomas usually confined to one hemisphere	*General:* ■ Headache; mental activity changes ■ Decreased motor strength and coordination ■ Seizures; scanning speech ■ Altered vital signs *Localizing:* ■ Third ventricle: changes in mental activity and level of consciousness, nausea, pupillary dilation and sluggish light reflex; later — paresis or ataxia ■ Brain stem and pons: early — ipsilateral trigeminal, abducens, and facial nerve palsies; later — cerebellar ataxia, tremors, other cranial nerve deficits ■ Third or fourth ventricle or aqueduct of Sylvius: secondary hydrocephalus ■ Thalamus or hypothalamus: variety of endocrine, metabolic, autonomic, and behavioral changes
Ependymoma ■ Rare glioma ■ Most common in children and young adults ■ Usually locates in fourth and lateral ventricles	*General:* ■ Similar to oligodendroglioma ■ Increased ICP and obstructive hydrocephalus, depending on tumor size
Glioblastoma multiforme (spongioblastoma multiforme) ■ Peak incidence at age 50 to 60 years; twice as common in males; most common glioma ■ Unencapsulated, highly malignant; grows rapidly and infiltrates the brain extensively; may become enormous before diagnosed ■ Usually occurs in cerebral hemispheres, especially frontal and temporal lobes (rarely in brain stem and cerebellum) ■ Occupies more than one lobe of affected hemisphere; may spread to opposite hemisphere by corpus callosum; may metastasize into cerebrospinal fluid (CSF), producing tumors in distant parts of the nervous system	*General:* ■ Increased intracranial pressure (ICP), nausea, vomiting, headache, papilledema ■ Mental and behavioral changes ■ Altered vital signs (increased systolic pressure; widened pulse pressure, respiratory changes) ■ Speech and sensory disturbances ■ In children, irritability, projectile vomiting *Localizing:* ■ Midline: headache (bifrontal or bioccipital); worse in the morning; intensified by coughing, straining, or sudden head movements ■ Temporal lobe: psychomotor seizures ■ Central region: focal seizures ■ Optic and oculomotor nerves: visual defects ■ Frontal lobe: abnormal reflexes, motor responses

(continued)

Comparing malignant brain tumors *(continued)*

TUMOR	CLINICAL FEATURES
Medulloblastoma ■ Rare glioma ■ Incidence highest in children ages 4 to 6 ■ Affects males more than females ■ Commonly metastasizes via CSF	*General:* ■ Increased ICP *Localizing:* ■ Brain stem and cerebrum: papilledema, nystagmus, hearing loss, flashing lights, dizziness, ataxia, paresthesia of face, cranial nerve palsies (V, VI, VII, IX, X, primarily sensory), hemiparesis, suboccipital tenderness; compression of supratentorial area produces other general and focal signs and symptoms
Meningioma ■ Most common nongliomatous brain tumor (15% of primary brain tumors) ■ Peak incidence among 50-year-olds; rare in children; more common in females (ratio 3:2) ■ Arises from the meninges ■ Common locations include parasagittal area, sphenoidal ridge, anterior part of the base of the skull, cerebellopontile angle, spinal canal ■ Benign, well-circumscribed, highly vascular tumors that compress underlying brain tissue by invading overlying skull	*General:* ■ Headache ■ Seizures (in two-thirds of patients) ■ Vomiting ■ Changes in mental activity ■ Similar to schwannomas *Localizing:* ■ Skull changes (bony bulge) over tumor ■ Sphenoidal ridge, indenting optic nerve: unilateral visual changes and papilledema ■ Prefrontal parasagittal: personality and behavioral changes ■ Motor cortex: contralateral motor changes ■ Anterior fossa compressing both optic nerves and frontal lobes: headaches and bilateral vision loss ■ Pressure on cranial nerves causes varying symptoms
Oligodendroglioma ■ Third most common glioma ■ Occurs in middle adult years; more common in women ■ Slow-growing	*General:* ■ Mental and behavioral changes ■ Decreased visual acuity and other visual disturbances ■ Increased ICP *Localizing:* ■ Temporal lobe: hallucinations, psychomotor seizures ■ Central region: seizures (confined to one muscle group or unilateral) ■ Midbrain or third ventricle: pyramidal tract symptoms (dizziness, ataxia, paresthesia of the face) ■ Brain stem and cerebrum: nystagmus, hearing loss, dizziness, ataxia, paresthesias of face, cranial nerve palsies, hemiparesis, suboccipital tenderness, loss of balance

Comparing malignant brain tumors *(continued)*

TUMOR	CLINICAL FEATURES
Schwannoma (acoustic neurinoma, neurilemoma, cerebellopontile angle tumor)	
■ Accounts for approximately 10% of all intracranial tumors ■ Higher incidence in women ■ Onset of symptoms between ages 30 and 60 ■ Affects the craniospinal nerve sheath, usually cranial nerve VIII; also, V and VII and, to a lesser extent, VI and X on the same side as the tumor ■ Benign, but commonly classified as malignant because of its growth patterns; slow-growing — may be present for years before symptoms occur	*General:* ■ Unilateral hearing loss with or without tinnitus ■ Stiff neck and suboccipital discomfort ■ Secondary hydrocephalus ■ Ataxia and uncoordinated movements of one or both arms due to pressure on brain stem and cerebellum *Localizing:* ■ V: early — facial hypoesthesia or paresthesia on side of hearing loss; unilateral loss of corneal reflex ■ VI: diplopia or double vision ■ VII: paresis progressing to paralysis (Bell's palsy) ■ X: weakness of palate, tongue, and nerve muscles on same side as tumor

radiation, chemotherapy, or decompression of increased ICP with diuretics, corticosteroids, or possibly ventriculoatrial or ventriculoperitoneal shunting of CSF.

Medication

Chemotherapy for malignant brain tumors includes the nitrosoureas that help break down the blood-brain barrier and allow other chemotherapeutic drugs to go through as well. Intrathecal and intra-arterial administration of drugs maximizes drug actions.

Palliative measures for gliomas, astrocytomas, oligodendrogliomas, and ependymomas include:

■ dexamethasone — 0.75 to 9 mg/day P.O. or 0.5 to 9 mg/day I.M.
■ mannitol — 1.5 to 2 g/kg I.V. of a 15% to 25% solution
■ phenytoin — 300 to 600 mg/day P.O. or I.V. in divided doses
■ famotidine — 20 mg P.O. or I.V. every 12 hours.

Surgical intervention

Treatment includes removing a resectable tumor; reducing a nonresectable tumor; relieving cerebral edema, increased ICP, and other symptoms; and preventing further neurologic damage.

A glioma usually requires resection by craniotomy, followed by radiation therapy and chemotherapy. The combination of nitrosoureas (carmustine [BCNU], lomustine [CCNU], or procarbazine) and postoperative radiation is more effective than radiation alone.

Surgical resection of low-grade cystic cerebellar astrocytomas brings long-term survival. Treatment of other astrocytomas includes repeated surgery, radiation therapy, and shunting of fluid from obstructed CSF pathways. Some astrocytomas are highly radiosensitive, but others are radioresistant.

Treatment of oligodendrogliomas and ependymomas includes resection and radiation therapy; for medulloblastomas, resection and possibly intrathecal infusion of methotrexate or another antineo-

What happens in increased ICP

Increased intracranial pressure (ICP) is the force exerted within the intact skull by intracranial volume: about 10% blood, 10% cerebrospinal fluid (CSF), and 80% brain tissue and water. The rigid skull allows little space for expansion of these substances. When ICP increases dramatically, brain damage can result.

The brain compensates for increases by regulating the volume of the three substances by limiting blood flow to the head, displacing CSF into the spinal canal, and increasing absorption or decreasing production of CSF. When compensatory mechanisms become overworked, small changes in volume lead to large changes in pressure.

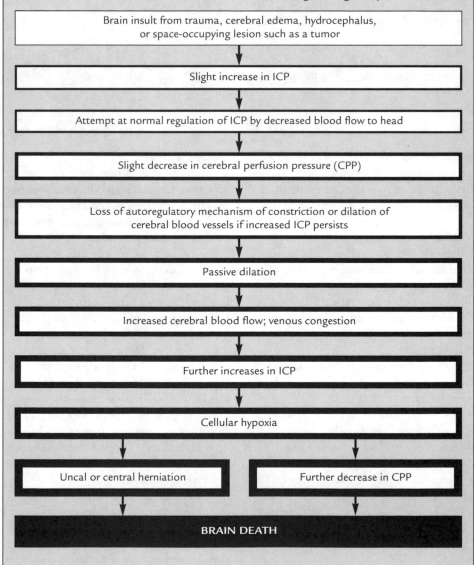

Brain insult from trauma, cerebral edema, hydrocephalus, or space-occupying lesion such as a tumor

↓

Slight increase in ICP

↓

Attempt at normal regulation of ICP by decreased blood flow to head

↓

Slight decrease in cerebral perfusion pressure (CPP)

↓

Loss of autoregulatory mechanism of constriction or dilation of cerebral blood vessels if increased ICP persists

↓

Passive dilation

↓

Increased cerebral blood flow; venous congestion

↓

Further increases in ICP

↓

Cellular hypoxia

↓   ↓

Uncal or central herniation   Further decrease in CPP

↓   ↓

BRAIN DEATH

plastic drug. Meningiomas require resection, including dura mater and bone (operative mortality may reach 10% because of large tumor size).

For schwannomas, microsurgical technique allows complete resection of the tumor and preservation of facial nerves. Although schwannomas are moderately radioresistant, postoperative radiation therapy is necessary.

Referral

- Refer the patient to a neurosurgeon and oncologist.
- Refer the patient for home care and physical, occupational, and speech therapy as appropriate.
- Refer the patient and family to the American Cancer Society for information and support.

Follow-up

The patient should be seen as directed by the specialist. After hospitalization, the patient should be seen within 2 weeks.

Patient teaching

- Teach the patient and his family signs of recurrence; urge compliance with the treatment regimen.
- Teach the family about any changes in function or personality that may occur as a result of brain tumor or surgery.

Complications

- Seizure
- Brain herniation
- Permanent neurologic loss
- Loss of ability to care for self

• • • • • • • • • • • • •

BREAST CANCER

Breast cancer is the most common cancer that affects women. Lifetime risk is 1 in 8. It occurs in men, but rarely.

AGE ALERT Breast cancer is the number two killer (after lung cancer) of women ages 35 to 54. It may develop any time after puberty, but the predominant age of occurrence is between 30 and 80, with peak occurrence between 45 and 65 years of age.

The 5-year survival rate for localized breast cancer has improved from the 1940s because of earlier diagnosis and the variety of treatments now available. According to the most recent data, mortality rates continue to decline in white women and, for the first time, are also declining in younger black women. Lymph node involvement is the most valuable prognostic predictor. With adjuvant therapy, a majority of women with negative nodes will survive 10 years.

Causes

The cause of breast cancer isn't known, but its high incidence in women implicates estrogen.

Certain predisposing factors are clear: Women at high risk include those who have a family history of breast cancer, particularly first-degree relatives (mother, sister, and maternal aunt).

Other women at high risk include those who:

- have long menstrual cycles or began menses early or menopause late
- have never been pregnant
- were first pregnant after age 30
- have had unilateral breast cancer
- have had ovarian cancer particularly at a young age
- were exposed to low-level ionizing radiation.

Inconclusive risk factors include exogenous estrogen, high-density fat, or high alcohol use.

Recently, scientists have discovered the BRCA1 and BRCA2 genes. These discoveries have made genetic predisposition testing an option for women at high risk for breast cancer.

Women at lower risk include those who:

- were pregnant before age 20
- have had multiple pregnancies
- are Native American or Asian
- are breast-feeding or using oral contraceptives (possibly).

Breast cancer occurs more commonly in the left breast than the right and more commonly in the outer upper quadrant. Growth rates vary. Theoretically, slow-growing breast cancer may take up to 8 years to become palpable at ⅜" (1 cm) in size. It spreads by way of the lymphatic system and the bloodstream, through the right side of the heart to the lungs, and eventually to the other breast, the chest wall, liver, bone, and brain.

Many refer to the estimated growth rate of breast cancer as "doubling time," or the time it takes the malignant cells to double in number. Survival time for breast cancer is based on tumor size and spread; the number of involved nodes is the single most important factor in predicting survival time.

Breast cancer is classified by histologic appearance and location of the lesion, as follows:

- adenocarcinoma — arising from the epithelium
- intraductal — developing within the ducts (includes Paget's disease)
- infiltrating — occurring in parenchyma of the breast
- inflammatory (rare) — reflecting rapid tumor growth, in which the overlying skin becomes edematous, inflamed, and indurated
- lobular carcinoma in situ — reflecting tumor growth involving lobes of glandular tissue

- medullary or circumscribed — large tumor with rapid growth rate.

These histologic classifications should be coupled with a staging or nodal status classification system for a clearer understanding of the extent of the cancer. The most commonly used system for staging cancer, before and after surgery, is the TNM (tumor size, nodal involvement, metastatic progress) staging system. (See *Staging breast cancer.*)

Clinical presentation

Warning signals of possible breast cancer include:

- lump (usually painless) or mass in the breast (a hard, stony mass is usually malignant)
- change in symmetry or size of the breast (usually enlargement)
- change in skin, thickening, scaly skin around the nipple, dimpling, edema (peau d'orange), or ulceration
- change in skin temperature (a warm, hot, or pink area; suspect cancer in a nonlactating woman past childbearing age until proven otherwise)
- unusual drainage or discharge (a spontaneous discharge of any kind in a non-breast-feeding, nonlactating woman warrants thorough investigation; so does any discharge produced by breast manipulation (greenish black, white, creamy, serous, or bloody); if a breast-fed infant rejects one breast, this may suggest possible breast cancer
- change in the nipple, such as itching, burning, erosion, or retraction
- pain (not usually a symptom of breast cancer unless the tumor is advanced, but it should be investigated)
- bone metastasis, pathologic bone fractures, and hypercalcemia
- edema of the arm
- axillary node enlargement.

Staging breast cancer

Cancer staging helps form a prognosis and a plan of treatment. For breast cancer, most clinicians use the TNM (tumor, node, metastasis) system developed by the American Joint Committee on Cancer.

PRIMARY TUMOR
TX — primary tumor can't be assessed
T0 — no evidence of primary tumor
Tis — carcinoma in situ: intraductal carcinoma, lobular carcinoma in situ, or Paget's disease of the nipple with no tumor
T1 — tumor 2 cm or less in greatest dimension
T1a — tumor 0.5 cm or less in greatest dimension
T1b — tumor more than 0.5 cm but not more than 1 cm in greatest dimension
T1c — tumor more than 1 cm but not more than 2 cm in greatest dimension
T2 — tumor more than 2 cm but not more than 5 cm in greatest dimension
T3 — tumor more than 5 cm in greatest dimension
T4 — tumor of any size that extends to the chest wall or skin
T4a — tumor extends to the chest wall
T4b — tumor accompanied by edema ulcerated breast skin or satellite skin nodules on the same breast
T4c — both T4a and T4b
T4d — inflammatory carcinoma

REGIONAL LYMPH NODES
NX — regional lymph nodes can't be assessed

N0 — no evidence of nodal involvement
N1 — movable ipsilateral axillary nodal involvement
N2 — ipsilateral axillary nodal involvement with nodes fixed to one another or to other structures
N3 — ipsilateral internal mammary nodal involvement

DISTANT METASTASIS
MX — distant metastasis can't be assessed
M0 — no evidence of distant metastasis
M1 — distant metastasis (including metastasis to ipsilateral supraclavicular nodes)

STAGING CATEGORIES
Breast cancer progresses from mild to severe as follows:
STAGE 0 — Tis, N0, M0
STAGE I — T1, N0, M0
STAGE IIA — T0, N1, M0; T1, N1, M0; T2, N0, M0
STAGE IIB — T2, N1, M0; T3, N0, M0
STAGE IIIA — T0, N2, M0; T1, N2, M0; T2, N2, M0; T3, N1 or N2, M0
STAGE IIIB — T4, any N, M0; any T, N3, M0
STAGE IV — any T, any N, M1

Differential diagnoses
- Abscess
- Fibroadenoma
- Ductal and lobular hyperplasia
- Sarcoma
- Lymphoma
- Metastatic disease to the breast

Diagnosis
The majority of breast masses are discovered by the patient. The most reliable method of detecting breast cancer is the monthly breast self-examination, followed by immediate evaluation of an abnormality. Other diagnostic measures in-

clude mammography, needle biopsy, and surgical biopsy. Mammography is indicated for any woman whose examination suggests an abnormality.

The value of mammography is questionable for women younger than age 35 (because of the density of the breasts), except those who are strongly suspected of having breast cancer. False-negative results can occur in as many as 30% of all tests. Consequently, with a suspicious mass, a negative mammogram should be disregarded, and a fine-needle aspiration or surgical biopsy should be done. Ultrasonography, which can distinguish a fluid-filled cyst from a tumor, can also be used instead of an invasive surgical biopsy.

Bone scan, computed tomography scan, measurement of alkaline phosphatase levels, liver function studies, and liver biopsy can detect distant metastasis. A hormonal receptor assay done on the tumor can determine if the tumor is estrogen- or progesterone-dependent. (This test guides decisions to use therapy that blocks the action of the estrogen hormone that supports tumor growth.)

HEALTHY LIVING Baseline mammography should be performed on women at age 40. It should then be done every 2 years until age 50 and then annually. Women with a family history of breast cancer and those who have had unilateral breast cancer should also have annual mammograms.

Management
General
Much controversy exists over breast cancer treatments. In choosing therapy, the stage of the disease, the woman's age and menopausal status, and the disfiguring effects of the surgery must be taken into consideration. Treatment of breast cancer may include a combination of treatments. Peripheral stem cell therapy may be used

for advanced breast cancer. Primary radiation therapy before or after tumor removal is effective for small tumors in early stages with no evidence of distant metastasis; it's also used to prevent or treat local recurrence. Presurgical radiation to the breast in inflammatory breast cancer helps make tumors more surgically manageable.

Medication
Chemotherapy, involving various cytotoxic drug combinations, is used as adjuvant or primary therapy, depending on several factors, including TNM staging and estrogen receptor status. The most commonly used antineoplastic drugs are:
- cyclophosphamide — initially, 40 to 50 mg/kg I.V. over 2 to 5 days or 1 to 5 mg/kg/day P.O.
- fluorouracil — 12 mg/kg/day I.V. for 4 days, then 1 day rest, then 6 mg/kg on days 6, 8, 10, and 12, then a single weekly maintenance dose of 10 to 15 mg/kg
- methotrexate — used in combination therapy
- doxorubicin — 60 to 75 mg/m^2/day I.V.; repeat every 21 days
- vinblastine — 3.7mg/m^2 I.V. weekly
- trastuzumab — 4 mg/ kg I.V. initially, then 2 mg/kg I.V. weekly
- prednisone — 5 to 60 mg/day P.O. (dose highly individualized).

Adjuvant treatment of choice for postmenopausal patients with positive estrogen receptor status is tamoxifen (10 to 20 mg P.O. b.i.d.); it has also been found to reduce the risk of breast cancer in high-risk women.

Surgical intervention
Surgery involves either mastectomy or lumpectomy. A lumpectomy may be done on an outpatient basis and may be the only surgery needed, especially if the tumor is small and there's no evidence of axillary node involvement. In many cas-

es, radiation therapy is combined with this surgery.

A two-stage procedure, in which the surgeon removes the lump and confirms that it's malignant and then discusses treatment options with the patient, is desirable because it allows the patient to participate in her plan of treatment. Sometimes, if the tumor is diagnosed as clinically malignant, such planning can be done before surgery. In lumpectomy and dissection of the axillary lymph nodes, the tumor and the axillary lymph nodes are removed, leaving the breast intact. A simple mastectomy removes the breast but not the lymph nodes or pectoral muscles. Modified radical mastectomy removes the breast and the axillary lymph nodes. Radical mastectomy, the performance of which has declined, removes the breast, pectoralis major and minor, and the axillary lymph nodes.

Postmastectomy, reconstructive surgery can create a breast mound if the patient desires and doesn't have evidence of advanced disease.

Referral
■ Refer the patient to a surgeon and an oncologist.
■ The patient may need to be referred to a plastic surgeon.
■ Refer the patient to the American Cancer Society Reach for Recovery for information and support.

Follow-up
The patient should be seen as directed by the specialist.

Patient teaching
■ Help the patient prevent lymphedema by instructing her to regularly exercise her hand and arm and to avoid activities that might cause infection or impairment in this hand or arm, which increases the

---

Postoperative arm and hand care

Hand exercises for the patient who's prone to lymphedema can begin on the day of surgery:
■ Have the patient open her hand and close it tightly six to eight times every 3 hours while she's awake.
■ Elevate the arm on the affected side on a pillow above the heart level.
■ Encourage the patient to wash her face and comb her hair — an effective exercise.
■ Measure and record the circumference of the patient's arm 2¼" (5.7 cm) from her elbow. Indicate the exact place you measured. By remeasuring a month after surgery and at intervals during and following radiation therapy, you'll be able to determine whether lymphedema is present. The patient may complain that her arm is heavy — an early symptom of lymphedema.
■ When the patient is home, she can elevate her arm and hand by supporting it on the back of a chair or couch.

---

chance of developing lymphedema. (See *Postoperative arm and hand care*.)
■ Remind the patient to not let anyone draw blood, start an I.V., give an injection, or take a blood pressure on the affected side because these activities will also increase the chances of developing lymphedema.

Complications
■ Metastasis
■ Infection
■ Psychological problems

HEALTHY LIVING Self-breast examination needs to be taught and encouraged for all women over age 20. It's the earliest way to detect breast cancer.

• • • • • • • • • • • •
CERVICAL CANCER

The third most common cancer of the female reproductive system, cervical cancer is classified as preinvasive or invasive.

Preinvasive carcinoma ranges from minimal cervical dysplasia, in which the lower third of the epithelium contains abnormal cells, to carcinoma in situ, in which the full thickness of epithelium contains abnormally proliferating cells (also known as cervical intraepithelial neoplasia [CIN]). Preinvasive cancer is curable 75% to 90% of the time with early detection and proper treatment. If untreated (and depending on the form in which it appears), it may progress to invasive cervical cancer.

In invasive carcinoma, cancer cells penetrate the basement membrane and can spread directly to contiguous pelvic structures or disseminate to distant sites by lymphatic routes. In almost all cases of cervical cancer (95%), the histologic type is squamous cell carcinoma, which varies from well-differentiated cells to highly anaplastic spindle cells. Only 5% are adenocarcinomas.

AGE ALERT Usually, invasive carcinoma occurs between ages 30 and 50; it rarely occurs in women younger than age 20.

Causes
Although the cause is unknown, several predisposing factors have been related to the development of cervical cancer: frequent intercourse at a young age (under age 16), multiple sexual partners, exposure to sexually transmitted diseases (particularly genital human papilloma virus [HPV]), and smoking.

Clinical presentation
Preinvasive cervical cancer produces no symptoms or other clinically apparent

changes. Early invasive cervical cancer causes:
- abnormal vaginal bleeding
- persistent vaginal discharge
- postcoital pain and bleeding.

In advanced stages, early invasive cervical cancer causes:
- pelvic pain
- vaginal leakage of urine and feces from a fistula
- anorexia
- weight loss
- anemia.

Differential diagnoses
- Severe cervitis
- Cervical polyps
- Carcinoma of endometrium

Diagnosis
A cytologic examination (Papanicolaou [Pap] test) can detect cervical cancer before clinical evidence appears. (Systems of Pap test classification may vary from hospital to hospital.) Abnormal cervical cytology routinely calls for colposcopy, which can detect the presence and extent of preclinical lesions requiring biopsy and histologic examination. Staining with Lugol's solution (strong iodine) or Schiller's solution (iodine, potassium iodide, and purified water) may identify areas for biopsy when the smear shows abnormal cells but there's no obvious lesion. Although the tests are nonspecific, they do distinguish between normal and abnormal tissues. Normal tissues absorb the iodine and turn brown; abnormal tissues are devoid of glycogen and won't change color. Additional studies, such as lymphangiography, cystography, and scans, can detect metastasis. (See *Staging cervical cancer.*)

Management
General
Appropriate treatment depends on accurate clinical staging. Preinvasive lesions

Staging cervical cancer

Cervical cancer treatment decisions depend on accurate staging. The International Federation of Gynecology and Obstetrics defines cervical cancer stages as follows.

STAGE 0
Carcinoma in situ, intraepithelial carcinoma

STAGE I
Cancer confined to the cervix (extension to the corpus should be disregarded)
STAGE IA — preclinical malignant lesions of the cervix (diagnosed only microscopically)
STAGE IA1 — minimal microscopically evident stromal invasion
STAGE IA2 — lesions detected microscopically, measuring 5 mm or less from the base of the epithelium, either surface or glandular, from which it originates; lesion width shouldn't exceed 7 mm
STAGE IB — lesions measuring more than 5 mm deep and 7 mm wide, whether seen clinically or not (preformed space involvement shouldn't alter the staging but should be recorded for future treatment decisions)

STAGE II
Extension beyond the cervix but not to the pelvic wall; the cancer involves the

vagina but hasn't spread to the lower third
STAGE IIA — no obvious parametrial involvement
STAGE IIB — obvious parametrial involvement

STAGE III
Extension to the pelvic wall; on rectal examination, no cancer-free space exists between the tumor and the pelvic wall; the tumor involves the lower third of the vagina; this includes all cases with hydronephrosis or nonfunctioning kidney
STAGE IIIA — no extension to the pelvic wall
STAGE IIIB — extension to the pelvic wall and hydronephrosis or nonfunctioning kidney, or both

STAGE IV
Extension beyond the true pelvis or involvement of the bladder or the rectal mucosa
STAGE IVA — spread to adjacent organs
STAGE IVB — spread to distant organs

may be treated with total excisional biopsy, cryosurgery, laser destruction, conization (and frequent Pap test follow-up).

Medication
Medications that may be used to treat cervical cancer include:
■ cisplatin — 100 mg/m^2 I.V. every 3 weeks
■ carboplatin — 360 mg/m^2 I.V. on day 1 every 4 weeks
■ methotrexate — 15 to 30 mg/day P.O. or I.M. for 5 days.

Surgical intervention
Therapy for invasive squamous cell carcinoma may include radical hysterectomy and radiation therapy (internal, external, or both).

Referral
■ Refer the patient to a gynecologist for treatment.
■ Refer the patient to the American Cancer Society for information and support.

Follow-up

The patient should be seen as directed by the gynecologist.

Patient teaching

■ After excisional biopsy, cryosurgery, and laser therapy, tell the patient to expect discharge or spotting for about 1 week afterward, and advise her not to douche, use tampons, or engage in sexual intercourse during this time. Tell her to watch for and report signs of infection. Stress the need for a follow-up Pap test and a pelvic examination within 3 to 4 months after these procedures and periodically thereafter.

■ If the patient is to have internal radiation therapy, teach her about the procedure and what to expect after the implant is inserted. Inform the family of safety precautions.

■ Tell the patient having radiation therapy to watch for and report uncomfortable adverse effects due to increased susceptibility to infection due to lower white blood cell count. Warn the patient to avoid persons with obvious infections during therapy.

■ Teach the patient to use a vaginal dilator to prevent vaginal stenosis and to facilitate vaginal examinations and sexual intercourse.

Complications

■ Ureteral fistula
■ Metastatic cancer
■ Hemorrhage
■ Pelvic infection
■ Loss of ovarian function
■ Uremia

• • • • • • • • • • • •
COLORECTAL CANCER

Colorectal cancer is the second most common visceral malignant neoplasm in the United States and Europe. Incidence is equally distributed between men and women. Colorectal malignant tumors are almost always adenocarcinomas. About half of these are sessile lesions of the rectosigmoid area; the rest are polypoid lesions.

Colorectal cancer tends to progress slowly and remains localized for a long time. Consequently, it's potentially curable in about 90% of patients if early diagnosis allows resection before nodal involvement. With improved diagnosis, the overall 5-year survival rate is about 60% for adjacent organ or nodal spread and greater than 90% for early localized disease. (See *Staging colorectal cancer*.)

Causes

The exact cause of colorectal cancer is unknown, but studies showing concentration in areas of higher economic development suggest a relationship to diet (excess saturated animal fat). Other factors that magnify the risk of developing colorectal cancer include:

■ other diseases of the digestive tract
■ age (over 40)
■ history of ulcerative colitis (average interval before onset of cancer is 11 to 17 years)
■ familial polyposis (cancer almost always develops by age 50).

Clinical presentation

Signs and symptoms of colorectal cancer result from local obstruction and, in later stages, from direct extension to adjacent organs (bladder, prostate, ureters, vagina, sacrum) and distant metastasis (usually liver). In the early stages, signs and symptoms are typically vague and depend on

Staging colorectal cancer

Named for pathologist Cuthbert Dukes, the Dukes' cancer classification system assigns tumors to four stages. These stages (with substages) reflect the extent of bowel-mucosa and bowel-wall infiltration, lymph node involvement, and metastasis.

STAGE A
Malignant cells are confined to the bowel mucosa, and the lymph nodes contain no cancer cells. Treated promptly, about 90% of these patients remain disease-free 5 years later.

STAGE B
Malignant cells extend through the bowel mucosa but remain within the bowel wall. The lymph nodes are normal. In substage B2, all bowel wall layers and immediately adjacent structures contain malignant cells, but the lymph nodes remain normal. About 63% of patients with substage B2 survive for 5 or more years.

STAGE C
Malignant cells extend into the bowel wall and the lymph nodes. In substage C2, malignant cells extend through the entire thickness of the bowel wall and into the lymph nodes. The 5-year survival rate for patients with stage C disease is about 25%.

STAGE D
Metastasized to distant organs by way of the lymph nodes and mesenteric vessels, malignant cells typically lodge in the lungs and liver. Only 7% of patients with stage D cancer survive 5 or more years.

---

the anatomic location and function of the bowel segment containing the tumor. Later signs or symptoms usually include:
- pallor
- cachexia
- ascites
- hepatomegaly
- lymphangiectasis.

Older patients may ignore bowel symptoms, believing that they result from constipation, poor diet, or hemorrhoids. Evaluate your older patient's responses to your questions carefully.

On the right side of the colon (which absorbs water and electrolytes), early tumor growth causes no signs of obstruction because the tumor tends to grow along the bowel rather than surround the lumen, and the fecal content in this area is normally liquid. It may, however, cause black, tarry stools; ane-

mia; and abdominal aching, pressure, or dull cramps. As the disease progresses, the patient develops:
- weakness
- fatigue
- exertional dyspnea
- vertigo
- diarrhea
- obstipation
- anorexia
- weight loss
- vomiting
- other signs or symptoms of intestinal obstruction.

In addition, a tumor on the right side may be palpable.

On the left side, a tumor causes signs of an obstruction even in early stages because, in this area, stools are of a formed consistency. It commonly causes rectal bleeding (in many cases ascribed to hem-

orrhoids), intermittent abdominal fullness or cramping, and rectal pressure. As the disease progresses, the patient develops:
- obstipation
- diarrhea or "ribbon" or pencil-shaped stools
- relief of pain with passage of a stool or flatus
- bleeding from the colon, with dark or bright red blood in the feces and mucus in or on the stools.

With a rectal tumor, the first symptom is a change in bowel habits, in many cases beginning with an urgent need to defecate on arising (morning diarrhea) or obstipation alternating with diarrhea. Other signs are blood or mucus in stool and a sense of incomplete evacuation. Late in the disease, pain begins as a feeling of rectal fullness that later becomes a dull, and sometimes constant, ache confined to the rectum or sacral region.

Differential diagnoses
- Constipation
- Irritable bowel syndrome
- Colitis
- Neoplasm from other primary site
- Infection

Diagnosis
Only a tumor biopsy can verify colorectal cancer, but other tests help detect it:
- Digital rectal examination can detect almost 15% of colorectal cancers.
- Hemoccult test (guaiac) can detect blood in stools.
- Proctoscopy or sigmoidoscopy can detect up to 66% of colorectal cancers.
- Colonoscopy permits visual inspection (and photographs) of the colon up to the ileocecal valve and gives access for polypectomies and biopsies of suspected lesions.
- Computed tomography scanning helps to detect areas affected by metastasis.

- Barium X-ray, using a dual contrast with air, can locate lesions that are undetectable manually or visually. Barium examination should follow endoscopy or excretory urography because the barium sulfate interferes with these tests.
- Carcinoembryonic antigen, although not specific or sensitive enough for early diagnosis, is helpful in monitoring patients before and after treatment to detect metastasis or recurrence.

Management
General
Radiation therapy induces tumor regression and may be used before or after surgery or combined with chemotherapy.

Medication
Chemotherapy is indicated for patients with metastasis, residual disease, or a recurrent inoperable tumor. Drugs used in such treatment commonly include:
- 5-fluorouracil — 12 mg/kg/day I.V. for 4 days; can repeat 6 mg/kg on days 6, 8, 10, 12; maintenance, 10 to 15 mg/kg/week as a single dose
- irinotecan — initially 125 mg/m^2 I.V. once weekly for 4 weeks then discontinue for 2 weeks then repeat cycle.

Surgical intervention
The most effective treatment of colorectal cancer is surgery to remove the malignant tumor and adjacent tissues and lymph nodes that may contain cancer cells. The type of surgery depends on the location of the tumor:
- Cecum and ascending colon — right hemicolectomy (for advanced disease) may include resection of the terminal segment of the ileum, cecum, ascending colon, and right half of the transverse colon with corresponding mesentery
- Proximal and middle transverse colon — right colectomy to include

transverse colon and mesentery corresponding to midcolic vessels, or segmental resection of transverse colon and associated midcolic vessels
■ Sigmoid colon — surgery is usually limited to the sigmoid colon and mesentery
■ Upper rectum — anterior or low anterior resection (newer method, using a stapler, allows for resections much lower than were previously possible)
■ Lower rectum — abdominoperineal resection and permanent sigmoid colostomy.

Referral
■ Refer the patient to a gastroenterologist and oncologist.
■ Refer the patient to the American Cancer Society for information and support.
■ The patient may need a referral to an enterostomal therapist.

Follow-up
The patient should be seen as directed by the specialist.

Patient teaching
■ If the patient is to have a colostomy, teach him and his family what to expect.
■ Tell the patient that he's at increased risk for recurrence and should have yearly screening and testing.

Complications
■ Obstruction
■ Perforation
■ Infection
■ Anastomotic stricture or leak
■ Pneumonia
■ Death

HEALTHY LIVING The American Cancer Society recommends fecal occult blood testing for everyone over age 50.

• • • • • • • • • • • •

ESOPHAGEAL CANCER

Esophageal cancer occurs worldwide, but incidence varies geographically. It's most common in Japan, China, the Middle East, and parts of South Africa.

AGE ALERT Esophageal cancer most commonly develops in men over age 60 and is almost always fatal.

Causes
The cause of esophageal cancer is unknown, but among predisposing factors are chronic irritation caused by heavy smoking and excessive use of alcohol, stasis-induced inflammation, nutritional deficiency, and diets high in nitrosamines. A genetic link has been proposed concerning an overexpression and mutation of the p53 tumor suppressor gene. Esophageal tumors are usually fungating and infiltrating. Most arise in squamous cell epithelium. However, the number of adenocarcinomas is greatly rising in the United States. Melanomas and sarcomas are few.

Regardless of type, esophageal cancer is usually fatal, with a 5-year survival rate of approximately 10% and regional metastasis occurring early via submucosal lymphatics. Metastasis produces such serious complications as tracheoesophageal fistulas, mediastinitis, and aortic perforation. Common sites of distant metastasis include the liver and lungs. (See *Staging esophageal cancer,* page 834.)

Clinical presentation
Dysphagia and weight loss are the most common presenting symptoms. Dysphagia is mild and intermittent at first, but it soon becomes constant. Pain, hoarseness, coughing, and esophageal obstruction follow. Cachexia usually develops.

Staging esophageal cancer

The TNM (tumor, node, metastasis) staging system accepted by the American Joint Committee on Cancer classifies esophageal cancer as follows.

PRIMARY TUMOR
TX — primary tumor can't be assessed
T0 — no evidence of primary tumor
Tis — carcinoma in situ
T1 — tumor invades lamina propria or submucosa
T2 — tumor invades muscularis propria
T3 — tumor invades adventitia
T4 — tumor invades adjacent structures

REGIONAL LYMPH NODES
NX — regional lymph nodes can't be assessed
N0 — no regional lymph node metastasis
N1 — regional lymph node metastasis

DISTANT METASTASIS
MX — distant metastasis can't be assessed
M0 — no known distant metastasis
M1 — distant metastasis

STAGING CATEGORIES
Esophageal cancer progresses from mild to severe as follows:
STAGE 0 — Tis, N0, M0
STAGE I — T1, N0, M0
STAGE IIA — T2, N0, M0; T3, N0, M0
STAGE IIB — T1, N1, M0; T2, N1, M0
STAGE III — T3, N1, M0; T4, any N, M0
STAGE IV — any T, any N, M1

Differential diagnoses
- Motility disorders of the esophagus
- Benign cause of dysphagia
- Mediastinal-pulmonary disease

Diagnosis
X-rays of the esophagus, with barium swallow and motility studies, reveal structural and filling defects and reduced peristalsis. Endoscopic examination of the esophagus, punch and brush biopsies, and exfoliative cytologic tests confirm esophageal tumors.

Management
General
Treatment of the patient with esophageal cancer includes diet adjustments and symptomatic treatment. The nutritional status of the patient needs to be addressed immediately.

Medication
Medications that may be used to treat esophageal carcinoma include:
- 5-fluorouracil — 12 mg/kg/day I.V. for 4 days; may repeat 6 mg/kg on days 6, 8, 10, and 12; maintenance, 10 to 15 mg/kg/week as a single dose
- metoclopramide — 1 to 4 mg/kg I.V. 30 minutes before chemotherapy, then repeat every 2 hours for 2 doses, then every 3 hours for 3 doses for nausea or 0.5 to 2 mg/kg P.O. every 3 to 4 hours.

Surgical intervention
Whenever possible, treatment includes resection to maintain a passageway for food. This may require such radical surgery as esophagogastrectomy with jejunal or colonic bypass grafts. Palliative surgery may include a feeding gastrostomy tube. Insertion of prosthetic tubes to bridge the tumor alleviates dysphagia.

Referral
▪ Refer the patient to a gastroenterologist and an oncologist for treatment.
▪ Refer the patient to the American Cancer Society for information and support.
▪ The patient may need a referral for home care.

Follow-up
The patient should be seen as directed by the specialist.

Patient teaching
▪ Promote adequate nutrition and assess the patient's nutritional and hydration status to determine the need for supplementary parenteral feedings.
▪ Instruct the family in gastrostomy tube care.

Complications
▪ Anastomotic leak or fistula
▪ Pneumonia
▪ Empyema
▪ Esophageal perforation
▪ Pneumonitis
▪ Pulmonary fibrosis
▪ Myelitis of the spinal cord
▪ Mediastinum perforation or tumor erosion from dislodged prosthetic tubes

• • • • • • • • • • • •

GASTRIC CARCINOMA

Gastric carcinoma is common throughout the world and affects all races; however, unexplained geographic and cultural differences in incidence occur — for example, a higher mortality in Japan, Iceland, Chile, and Austria. During the last 25 years, incidence in the United States has decreased by 50% and the resulting death rate is one-third what it was 30 years ago. Incidence is higher in males over age 40. Hispanics, Native Americans, and Blacks are twice as likely as Whites to develop gastric cancer. The prognosis depends on the stage of the disease at the time of diagnosis; however, the overall 5-year survival rate is approximately 19%.

Causes
The cause of gastric carcinoma is unknown. It's commonly associated with gastritis with gastric atrophy, which may result from gastric cancer and may not be a precursor state. Predisposing factors include environmental influences, such as smoking and high alcohol intake. Genetic factors have also been implicated because this disease occurs more commonly among people with type A blood than among those with type O; similarly it's more common in people with a family history of such carcinoma. Dietary factors also seem related, including types of food preparation, physical properties of some foods, and certain methods of food preservation (especially smoking, pickling, or salting). There's a strong correlation between infection with *Heliocobacter pylori* and distal gastric cancer.

According to gross appearance, gastric carcinoma can be classified as polypoid, ulcerating, ulcerating and infiltrating, or diffuse. The parts of the stomach affected by gastric carcinoma, in order of decreasing frequency, are the pylorus and antrum, the lesser curvature, the cardia, the body of the stomach, and the greater curvature. (See *Sites of gastric carcinoma*, page 836.)

Gastric carcinoma infiltrates rapidly to regional lymph nodes, omentum, liver, and lungs by the following routes: walls of the stomach, duodenum, and esophagus; lymphatic system; adjacent organs; bloodstream; and peritoneal cavity.

The decrease in gastric carcinoma in the United States has been attributed, without proof, to the balanced American diet and to refrigeration, which reduces nitrate-producing bacteria in food.

Sites of gastric carcinoma

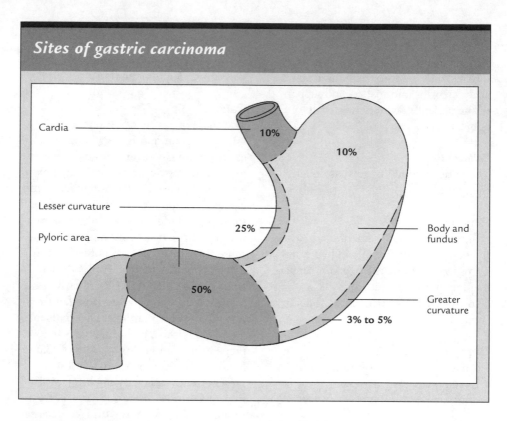

Cardia — 10%

10%

Lesser curvature — 25%

Pyloric area — 50%

Body and fundus

Greater curvature

3% to 5%

Clinical presentation

Early clues to gastric carcinoma are chronic dyspepsia and epigastric discomfort, followed in later stages by weight loss, anorexia, feeling of fullness after eating, anemia, and fatigue. If the carcinoma is in the cardia, the first sign or symptom may be dysphagia and, later, vomiting (commonly coffee-ground vomitus). Affected patients may also have blood in their stools.

The course of gastric carcinoma may be insidious or fulminating. Unfortunately, the patient typically treats himself with antacids or histamine-2 blockers until the symptoms of advanced stages appear.

Differential diagnoses

- Gastroesophageal reflux disease
- *H. pylori*
- Peptic ulcer disease
- Carcinoma of the colon
- Crohn's disease
- Gastric lymphoma

Diagnosis

Diagnosis depends primarily on reinvestigations of persistent or recurring GI changes and complaints. To rule out other conditions producing similar symptoms, diagnostic evaluation must include the testing of blood, stool, and stomach fluid samples.

Diagnosis of gastric carcinoma generally requires these studies:

- Barium X-rays of the GI tract with fluoroscopy show changes (tumor or filling defect in the outline of the stomach, loss of flexibility and distensibility, and abnormal gastric mucosa with or without ulceration).
- Gastroscopy with fiber-optic endoscopy helps rule out other diffuse gastric mucos-

Staging gastric carcinoma

The prognosis and treatment of gastric carcinoma depend on its type and stage. Using the TNM (tumor, node, metastasis) system, the American Joint Committee on Cancer describes the following stages of gastric carcinoma.

PRIMARY TUMOR

TX — primary tumor can't be assessed

T0 — no evidence of primary tumor

Tis — carcinoma in situ: intraepithelial tumor doesn't penetrate the lamina propria

T1 — tumor penetrates the lamina propria or submucosa

T2 — tumor penetrates the muscularis propria or subserosa

T3 — tumor penetrates the serosa (visceral peritoneum) without invading adjacent structures

T4 — tumor invades adjacent structures

REGIONAL LYMPH NODES

NX — regional lymph nodes can't be assessed

N0 — no evidence of regional lymph node metastasis

N1 — involvement of perigastric lymph nodes within 3 cm of the edge of the primary tumor

N2 — involvement of the perigastric lymph nodes more than 3 cm from the edge of the primary tumor or in lymph nodes along the left gastric, common hepatic, splenic, or celiac arteries

DISTANT METASTASIS

MX — distant metastasis can't be assessed

M0 — no evidence of distant metastasis

M1 — distant metastasis

STAGING CATEGORIES

Gastric carcinoma stages progress from mild to severe as follows:

STAGE 0 — Tis, N0, M0

STAGE IA — T1, N0, M0

STAGE IB — T1, N1, M0; T2, N0, M0

STAGE II — T1, N2, M0; T3, N0, M0

STAGE IIIA — T2, N2, M0; T3, N1, M0; T4, N0, M0

STAGE IIIB — T3, N2, M0; T4, N1, M0

STAGE IV — T4, N2, M0; any T, any N, M1

al abnormalities by allowing direct visualization and gastroscopic biopsy to evaluate gastric mucosal lesions.

■ Photography with fiber-optic endoscope provides a permanent record of gastric lesions that can later be used to determine disease progression and the effect of treatment.

Certain other studies may rule out specific organ metastasis: computed tomography scanning, chest X-rays, liver and bone scans, and liver biopsy. (See *Staging gastric carcinoma*.)

Management
General

Radiation has been particularly useful when combined with chemotherapy in patients who have unresectable or partially resectable disease. It should be given on an empty stomach and shouldn't be used preoperatively because it may damage viscera and impede healing.

Medication

Medications that may be used in the treatment of gastric cancer include:

■ 5-fluorouracil — 12 mg/kg/day I.V. for 4 days; may repeat 6 mg/kg on days 6, 8,

10, and 12; maintenance, 10 to 15 mg/kg/ week as a single dose
- metoclopramide — 1 to 4 mg/kg I.V. 30 minutes before chemotherapy, then repeat every 2 hours for 2 doses, then every 3 hours for 3 doses for nausea *or* 0.5 to 2 mg/kg P.O. every 3 to 4 hours
- carmustine (in combination with fluorouracil) — 75 to 100 mg/m² I.V. by slow infusion daily for 2 days; repeat every 6 weeks.

Surgical intervention

In many cases, surgery is the treatment of choice. Excision of the lesion with appropriate margins is possible in over one-third of patients. Even for patients whose disease isn't considered surgically curable, resection offers palliation and improves potential benefits from chemotherapy and radiation.

The nature and extent of the lesion determine what kind of surgery is most appropriate. Common surgical procedures include subtotal gastric resection (subtotal gastrectomy) and total gastric resection (total gastrectomy). When carcinoma involves the pylorus and antrum, gastric resection removes the lower stomach and duodenum (gastrojejunostomy or Billroth II). If metastasis has occurred, the omentum and spleen may also have to be removed.

If gastric cancer has spread to the liver, peritoneum, or lymph glands, palliative surgery may include gastrostomy, jejunostomy, or gastric or partial gastric resection. Such surgery may temporarily relieve vomiting, nausea, pain, and dysphagia, while allowing enteral nutrition to continue.

Referral

- Refer the patient to a surgeon and an oncologist for treatment.

- Refer the patient to the American Cancer Society for information and support.

Follow-up

The patient should be seen as directed by the specialist.

Patient teaching

- During radiation treatment, encourage the patient to eat high-calorie, well-balanced meals.
- After a total gastrectomy, teach patients an appropriate diet of small meals and vitamin supplements.

Complications

- Metastatic disease
- Anemia
- Pyloric stenosis

• • • • • • • • • • • • •

HODGKIN'S DISEASE

Hodgkin's disease is a neoplastic disease characterized by painless, progressive enlargement of lymph nodes, spleen, and other lymphoid tissue resulting from proliferation of lymphocytes, histiocytes, eosinophils, and Reed-Sternberg giant cells. The latter cells are its special histologic feature. Untreated Hodgkin's disease follows a variable but relentlessly progressive and ultimately fatal course. However, recent advances in therapy make Hodgkin's disease potentially curable, even in advanced stages; appropriate treatment yields a 5-year survival rate in approximately 80% of patients. The disease is most common in young adults, with a higher incidence in males than in females. It occurs in all races but is slightly more common in whites.

AGE ALERT The incidence of Hodgkin's disease peaks in two age-groups: ages 15 to 38 and after age

50 — except in Japan, where it occurs exclusively among people over age 50.

Causes
Although the cause of Hodgkin's disease is unknown, a viral etiology is suspected, with the Epstein-Barr virus as a leading candidate.

Clinical presentation
The first sign of Hodgkin's disease is usually a painless swelling of one of the cervical lymph nodes (but sometimes the axillary, mediastinal, or inguinal lymph nodes), occasionally in a patient who gives a history of recent upper respiratory infection. In older patients, the first signs and symptoms may be nonspecific:
- persistent fever
- night sweats
- fatigue
- weight loss
- malaise.

Rarely, if the mediastinum is initially involved, Hodgkin's may produce respiratory symptoms.

Another early and characteristic indication of Hodgkin's disease is pruritus, which, although mild at first, becomes acute as the disease progresses. Other signs and symptoms depend on the degree and location of systemic involvement.

Lymph nodes may enlarge rapidly, producing pain and obstruction, or enlarge slowly and painlessly for months or years. It isn't unusual to see the lymph nodes "wax and wane," but they usually don't return to normal. Sooner or later, most patients develop systemic manifestations, including enlargement of retroperitoneal nodes and nodular infiltrations of the spleen, the liver, and bones. Other signs and symptoms at this late stage include:

- edema of the face and neck
- progressive anemia
- possible jaundice
- nerve pain
- increased susceptibility to infection.

Differential diagnoses
- Other lymphomas
- Infected lymph node
- Other solid tumor metastasis
- Sarcoidosis
- Acquired immunodeficiency syndrome
- Drug reaction

Diagnosis
Diagnostic measures for confirming Hodgkin's disease include a thorough medical history and a complete physical examination, followed by a lymph node biopsy checking for Reed-Sternberg's abnormal histiocyte proliferation and nodular fibrosis and necrosis. (See *Reed-Sternberg cells,* page 840.)

Other appropriate diagnostic tests include bone marrow, liver, mediastinal, lymph node, and spleen biopsies and a routine chest X-ray, abdominal computed tomography scan, lung scan, bone scan, and lymphangiography to detect lymph node or organ involvement. Laparoscopy and lymph node biopsy are performed to complete staging.

Hematologic tests show mild to severe normocytic anemia; normochromic anemia (50% of patients); and elevated, normal, or reduced white blood cell count and differential showing any combination of neutrophilia, lymphocytopenia, monocytosis, and eosinophilia. Elevated serum alkaline phosphatase indicates liver or bone involvement.

The same diagnostic tests are also used for staging. A staging laparotomy is necessary for patients younger than age 55 or without obvious stage III or stage IV disease, lymphocyte predominance subtype

Reed-Sternberg cells

These enlarged, abnormal histiocytes (Reed-Sternberg cells) from an excised lymph node suggest Hodgkin's disease. Note the large, distinct nucleoli. Reed-Sternberg cells indicate Hodgkin's disease when they coexist with one of these four histologic patterns: lymphocyte predominance, mixed cellularity, lymphocyte depletion, or nodular sclerosis.

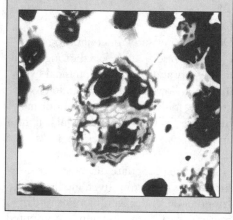

histology, or medical contraindications. Diagnosis must rule out other disorders that also enlarge the lymph nodes.

Management
General
Appropriate therapy (chemotherapy or radiation therapy, or both, varying with the stage of the disease) depends on careful physical examination with accurate histologic interpretation and proper clinical staging. (See *Staging Hodgkin's disease*.) Correct and timely treatment allows longer survival and even induces an apparent cure in many patients. Radiation therapy is used alone for stages I and II and in combination with chemotherapy for stage III. Chemotherapy is used for stage IV, sometimes inducing a complete

remission. New treatments include high-dose chemotherapeutic agents with autologous bone marrow transplantation or autologous peripheral blood stem cell transfusions. Biotherapy alone hasn't proven effective.

Medication
The well-known MOPP protocol (mechlorethamine, vincristine [Oncovin], procarbazine, and prednisone) was the first to provide significant cures to patients with generalized Hodgkin's disease. Another useful combination is ABVD (doxorubicin [Adriamycin], bleomycin, vinblastine, and dacarbazine). Dosages will vary according to patient.

Patient teaching
- Tell the patient to watch for and promptly report adverse effects of radiation and chemotherapy.
- Tell the patient to minimize adverse effects of radiation therapy by maintaining good nutrition, drinking plenty of fluids, pacing activities to counteract therapy-induced fatigue, and keeping the skin dry in irradiated areas.
- Control pain and bleeding of stomatitis by using a soft toothbrush, cotton swab, or anesthetic mouthwash such as viscous lidocaine (as prescribed); applying petroleum jelly to the lips; and avoiding astringent mouthwashes.

Complications
- Secondary malignancy
- Bone marrow suppression
- Anemia
- Sterility and gonadal dysfunction
- Immunosuppressed infections
- Thrombocytopenia purpura
- Coronary artery disease
- Pulmonary fibrosis

Staging Hodgkin's disease

Treatment of Hodgkin's disease depends on the stage it has reached — that is, the number, location, and degree of involved lymph nodes. The Ann Arbor classification system, adopted in 1971, divides Hodgkin's disease into the four stages below. Then doctors subdivide each stage into categories. Category A includes patients without defined signs and symptoms, and category B includes patients who experience such defined signs as recent unexplained weight loss, fever, and night sweats.

STAGE I

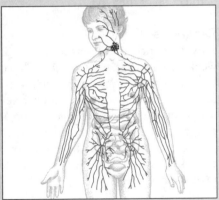

Hodgkin's disease appears in a single lymph node region (I) or a single extra-lymphatic organ (IE).

STAGE II

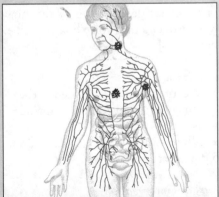

The disease appears in two or more nodes on the same side of the dia-phragm (II) and in an extralymphatic organ (IIE).

STAGE III

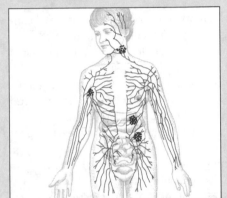

Hodgkin's disease spreads to both sides of the diaphragm (III) and perhaps to an extralymphatic organ (IIIE), the spleen (IIIS), or both (IIIES).

STAGE IV

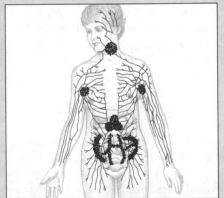

The disease disseminates, involving one or more extralymphatic organs or tis-sues, with or without associated lymph node involvement.

Special considerations

- If a female patient is of childbearing age, advise her to delay pregnancy until she experiences prolonged remission because radiation and chemotherapy can cause genetic mutations and spontaneous abortions.

• • • • • • • • • • • •

LARYNGEAL CANCER

The most common form of laryngeal cancer is squamous cell carcinoma (95%); rare forms include adenocarcinoma, sarcoma, and others. Such cancer may be intrinsic or extrinsic. An intrinsic tumor is on the true vocal cord and doesn't tend to spread because underlying connective tissues lack lymph nodes. An extrinsic tumor is on some other part of the larynx and tends to spread early. The ratio of male to female incidence is 3.8:1.

AGE ALERT Most victims of laryngeal cancer are between ages 50 and 65.

Causes

In laryngeal cancer, major predisposing factors include smoking and alcoholism; minor factors include chronic inhalation of noxious fumes and familial tendency. Cancer of the larynx rarely occurs in nonsmokers.

Laryngeal cancer is classified according to its location:
- supraglottis (false vocal cords)
- glottis (true vocal cords)
- subglottis (downward extension from vocal cords [rare]).

Clinical presentation

In intrinsic laryngeal cancer, the dominant and earliest symptom is hoarseness that persists longer than 3 weeks; in extrinsic cancer, it's a lump in the throat or pain or burning in the throat when drinking citrus juice or hot liquid. Later clinical effects of metastasis include:
- dysphagia
- dyspnea
- cough
- enlarged cervical lymph nodes
- pain radiating to the ear.

Differential diagnoses
- Acute or chronic laryngitis
- Benign vocal cord lesions
- Infection of the larynx

Diagnosis

Any hoarseness that lasts longer than 2 weeks requires visualization of the larynx by laryngoscopy. (See *Staging laryngeal cancer*.) Firm diagnosis also requires xeroradiography, biopsy, laryngeal tomography, computed tomography scan, or laryngography to define the borders of the lesion and chest X-ray to detect metastasis.

Management
General
The treatment goal is to eliminate the cancer and preserve speech. If speech preservation isn't possible, speech rehabilitation may include esophageal speech or prosthetic devices; surgical techniques to construct a new voice box are still experimental.

Medication
Medications that may be used in the treatment of laryngeal cancer include:
- cisplatin — 100 mg/m^2 I.V. every 3 weeks
- 5-fluorouracil — 12mg/kg/day I.V. for 5 days every 3 weeks.

Surgical intervention
Early lesions are treated with surgery or radiation, advanced lesions with surgery, radiation, and chemotherapy. In early stages, laser surgery can excise precancerous lesions; in advanced stages it can

Staging laryngeal cancer

The TNM (tumor, node, metastasis) classification system developed by the American Joint Committee on Cancer describes laryngeal cancer stages and guides treatment. The T stages cover supraglottic, glottic, and subglottic tumors.

PRIMARY TUMOR
TX — primary tumor unassessible
T0 — no evidence of primary tumor
Tis — carcinoma in situ

Supraglottic tumor stages
T1 — tumor confined to one subsite in supraglottis; vocal cords retain motion
T2 — tumor extends to other sites in supraglottis or to glottis; vocal cords retain motion
T3 — tumor confined to larynx, but vocal cords lose motion; or tumor extends to the postcricoid area, the pyriform sinus, or the preepiglottic space, and vocal cords lose motion; or both
T4 — tumor extends through thyroid cartilage or extends to tissues beyond the larynx (such as the oropharynx or soft tissues of the neck) or both

Glottic tumor stages
T1 — tumor confined to vocal cords, which retain normal motion; may involve anterior or posterior commissures
T2 — tumor extends to supraglottis or subglottis or both; vocal cords may lose motion
T3 — tumor confined to larynx, but vocal cords lose motion
T4 — tumor extends through thyroid cartilage or extends to tissues beyond the larynx (such as the oropharynx or soft tissues of the neck), or both

Subglottic tumor stages
T1 — tumor confined to subglottis
T2 — tumor extends to vocal cords; vocal cords may lose motion

T3 — tumor confined to larynx with vocal cord fixation
T4 — tumor extends through cricoid or thyroid cartilage or extends to tissues beyond the larynx, or both

REGIONAL LYMPH NODES
NX — regional lymph nodes can't be assessed
N0 — no evidence of regional lymph node metastasis
N1 — metastasis in a single ipsilateral lymph node, 3 cm or less in greatest dimension
N2 — metastasis in one or more ipsilateral lymph nodes, or in bilateral or contralateral nodes, larger than 3 cm but less than 6 cm in greatest dimension
N3 — metastasis in a node larger than 6 cm in greatest dimension

DISTANT METASTASIS
MX — distant metastasis unassessible
M0 — no evidence of distant metastasis
M1 — distant metastasis

STAGING CATEGORIES
Laryngeal cancer progresses from mild to severe as follows:
STAGE 0 — Tis, N0, M0
STAGE I — T1, N0, M0
STAGE II — T2, N0, M0
STAGE III — T3, N0, M0; T1, N1, M0; T2, N1, M0; T3, N1, M0
STAGE IV — T4, N0 or N1, M0; any T, N2 or N3, M0; any T, any N, M1

help relieve obstruction caused by tumor growth. Surgical procedures vary with tumor size and can include cordectomy, partial or total laryngectomy, supraglottic laryngectomy, or total laryngectomy with laryngoplasty.

- Refer the patient to a surgeon and oncologist for treatment.

Referral

- Refer the patient to the National Association of Laryngectomees for information and support.
- The patient may need to be referred to a speech therapist.

Follow-up

The patient should be seen as directed by the specialist.

Patient teaching

- Teach the patient about his illness and potential outcomes.
- Teach stoma care to the patient and family.

Complications

- Mucositis
- Hoarseness
- Tracheostomal stenosis
- Dysphagia
- Aspiration
- Radiation edema

• • • • • • • • • • • •

LEUKEMIA, ACUTE

Acute leukemia is a malignant proliferation of white blood cell precursors (blasts) in bone marrow or lymph tissue and their accumulation in peripheral blood, bone marrow, and body tissues. Its most common forms are acute lymphoblastic (lymphocytic) leukemia (ALL), abnormal growth of lymphocyte precursors (lymphoblasts); acute myeloblastic (myelogenous) leukemia (AML), rapid accumulation of myeloid precursors (myeloblasts); and acute monoblastic (monocytic) leukemia, or Schilling's type, marked by increase in monocyte precursors (monoblasts). Other variants include acute myelomonocytic leukemia and acute erythroleukemia.

Untreated, acute leukemia is invariably fatal, usually because of complications that result from leukemic cell infiltration of bone marrow or vital organs. With treatment, prognosis varies. In ALL, treatment induces remissions in 90% of children (average survival time: 5 years) and 65% of adults (average survival time: 1 to 2 years). Children between ages 2 and 8 have the best survival rate — about 50% — with intensive therapy. In AML, the average survival time is only 1 year after diagnosis, even with aggressive treatment. In acute monoblastic leukemia, treatment induces remissions lasting 2 to 10 months in 50% of children; adults survive only about 1 year after diagnosis, even with treatment.

Acute leukemia is more common in males than females, in whites (especially people of Jewish descent), in children (between ages 2 and 5; 80% of all leukemias in this age-group are ALL), and in persons who live in urban and industrialized areas. Acute leukemia ranks 20th in causes of cancer-related deaths among people of all age-groups. Among children, however, it's the most common form of cancer. It affects 6 out of 100,000 people.

Causes

Research on predisposing factors isn't conclusive but points to some combination of viruses (viral remnants have been found in leukemic cells), genetic and immunologic factors, and exposure to radiation and certain chemical. (See *Predisposing factors to acute leukemia*.)

The pathogenesis isn't clearly understood, but immature, nonfunctioning white blood cells (WBCs) appear to accumulate first in the tissue where they originate (lymphocytes in lymph tissue, granulocytes in bone marrow). These immature WBCs then spill into the bloodstream and from there infiltrate other tissues, eventually causing organ malfunction because of encroachment or hemorrhage.

Clinical presentation

Signs of acute leukemia are sudden onset of high fever accompanied by thrombocytopenia and abnormal bleeding, such as:
- nosebleeds
- gingival bleeding
- purpura, ecchymoses
- petechiae
- easy bruising after minor trauma
- prolonged menses.

Nonspecific signs and symptoms, such as low-grade fever, weakness, and lassitude, may persist for days or months before visible symptoms appear. Other insidious signs and symptoms include pallor, chills, and recurrent infections. In addition, ALL, AML, and acute monoblastic leukemia may cause:
- dyspnea
- anemia
- fatigue
- malaise
- tachycardia
- palpitations
- systolic ejection murmur
- abdominal or bone pain.

When leukemic cells cross the blood-brain barrier and thereby escape the effects of systemic chemotherapy, the patient may develop meningeal leukemia (confusion, lethargy, headache).

Differential diagnoses
- Other malignant disorder
- Aplastic anemia

Predisposing factors to acute leukemia

Although the exact causes of most leukemias remain unknown, increasing evidence suggests a combination of contributing factors.

ACUTE LYMPHOBLASTIC LEUKEMIA
- Familial tendency
- Monozygotic twins
- Congenital disorders, such as Down syndrome, Bloom syndrome, Fanconi's anemia, ataxia-telangiectasia, and congenital agammaglobulinemia
- Viruses

ACUTE MYELOBLASTIC LEUKEMIA
- Familial tendency
- Monozygotic twins
- Congenital disorders, such as Down syndrome, Bloom syndrome, Fanconi's anemia, ataxia-telangiectasia, and congenital agammaglobulinemia
- Ionizing radiation
- Exposure to the chemical benzene and cytotoxins such as alkylating agents
- Viruses

ACUTE MONOBLASTIC LEUKEMIA
- Unknown (irradiation, exposure to chemicals, heredity, and infections show little correlation to this disease)

- Mononucleosis
- Autoimmune thrombocytopenia purpura

Diagnosis

Typical clinical findings and bone marrow aspirate showing a proliferation of immature WBCs confirm acute leukemia.

An aspirate that's dry or free from leukemic cells in a patient with typical clinical findings requires bone marrow biopsy, usually of the posterior superior iliac spine. Blood counts show thrombocytopenia and neutropenia. Differential leukocyte count determines cell type. Lumbar puncture detects meningeal involvement.

Management
General
The plan of care for the patient with acute leukemia should emphasize comfort, minimize the adverse effects of chemotherapy, promote preservation of veins, manage complications, and provide teaching and psychological support. Many of these patients are children, so be especially sensitive to their emotional needs and those of their families. Bone marrow transplant may be possible. Transfusions of platelets to prevent bleeding and of red blood cells to prevent anemia may be needed.

Medication
Systemic chemotherapy aims to eradicate leukemic cells and induce remission (less than 5% of blast cells in the marrow and peripheral blood are normal). Chemotherapy is individualized and can be given in combination:
- Meningeal leukemia — intrathecal instillation of methotrexate or cytarabine with cranial radiation.
- ALL — vincristine, prednisone, high-dose cytarabine, L-asparaginase, AMSA, and daunorubicin. Because there's a 40% risk of meningeal leukemia in ALL, intrathecal methotrexate or cytarabine is given. Radiation therapy is given for testicular infiltration.
- AML — a combination of I.V. daunorubicin and cytarabine or, if these fail to induce remission, a combination of cyclophosphamide, vincristine, prednisone,

or methotrexate; high-dose cytarabine alone or with other drugs; amsacrine; etoposide; and 5-azacytidine and mitoxantrone.
- Acute monoblastic leukemia — cytarabine and thioguanine with daunorubicin or doxorubicin.

Treatment also may include antibiotic, antifungal, and antiviral drugs and granulocyte injections to control infection.

Referral
- Refer the patient to a hematologist or an oncologist for treatment.
- Refer the patient to the American Cancer Society for information and support.

Follow-up
The patient should be seen as directed by the specialist. If the patient is in remission, he should be seen monthly.

Patient teaching
- Teach the patient and his family how to recognize infection and abnormal bleeding and how to stop such bleeding.
- Promote good nutrition. Explain that chemotherapy may cause weight loss and anorexia, so encourage the patient to eat and drink high-calorie, high-protein foods and beverages. However, chemotherapy and adjunctive prednisone may cause weight gain, so dietary counseling and teaching are helpful.

Complications
- Infection
- Bleeding
- Sterility
- Pancreatitis

Special considerations
- Establish an appropriate rehabilitation program for the patient during remission.

LEUKEMIA, CHRONIC GRANULOCYTIC

Chronic granulocytic leukemia (CGL), also called chronic myelogenous (or myelocytic) leukemia, is characterized by the abnormal overgrowth of granulocytic precursors (myeloblasts, promyelocytes, metamyelocytes, and myelocytes) in bone marrow, peripheral blood, and body tissues. CGL is most common in young and middle-aged adults and is slightly more common in men than women; it's rare in children. In the United States, approximately 4,300 cases of CGL develop annually, accounting for roughly 20% of all leukemias.

CGL's clinical course proceeds in two distinct phases: the insidious chronic phase, with anemia and bleeding abnormalities and, eventually, the acute phase (blastic crisis), in which myeloblasts, the most primitive granulocytic precursors, proliferate rapidly. This disease is invariably fatal. Average survival time is 3 to 4 years after onset of the chronic phase and 3 to 6 months after onset of the acute phase.

Causes

Almost 90% of patients with CGL have the Philadelphia, or Ph1, chromosome, an abnormality discovered in 1960 in which the long arm of chromosome 22 is translocated, usually to chromosome 9. Radiation and carcinogenic chemicals may induce this chromosome abnormality. Myeloproliferative diseases also seem to increase the incidence of CGL, and some clinicians suspect that an unidentified virus causes this disease.

Clinical presentation

Typically, CGL induces the following clinical effects:

- anemia (fatigue, weakness, decreased exercise tolerance, pallor, dyspnea, tachycardia, and headache)
- thrombocytopenia, with resulting bleeding and clotting disorders (retinal hemorrhage, ecchymoses, hematuria, melena, bleeding gums, nosebleeds, and easy bruising)
- hepatosplenomegaly, with abdominal discomfort and pain in splenic infarction from leukemic cell infiltration.

Other signs and symptoms include:
- sternal and rib tenderness from leukemic infiltrations of the periosteum
- low-grade fever
- weight loss
- anorexia
- renal calculi or gouty arthritis from increased uric acid excretion
- prolonged infection and ankle edema (occasionally)
- priapism and vascular insufficiency (rarely).

Differential diagnoses

- Infection
- Anemia
- Viral induced cytopenia, lymphadenopathy, and organomegaly

Diagnosis

In patients with typical clinical changes, chromosomal analysis of peripheral blood or bone marrow showing the Philadelphia chromosome and low leukocyte alkaline phosphatase levels confirm CGL.

Other relevant laboratory results show:
- white blood cell (WBC) abnormalities—leukocytosis (leukocytes more than 50,000/μl, ranging as high as 250,000/μl), occasional leukopenia (leukocytes less than 5,000/μl), neutropenia (neutrophils less than 1,500/μl) despite high leukocyte count, and increased circulating myeloblasts

- hemoglobin—commonly below 10 g/dl
- hematocrit—low (less than 30%)
- platelets—thrombocytosis (more than 1million/µl) is common
- serum uric acid—possibly more than 8 mg/dl
- bone marrow aspirate or biopsy—hypercellular, characteristically shows bone marrow infiltration by significantly increased number of myeloid elements (biopsy is done only if aspirate is dry); in the acute phase, myeloblasts predominate
- computed tomography scan—may identify the organs affected by leukemia.

Management
General
During the acute phase of CGL, lymphoblastic or myeloblastic leukemia may develop. Treatment is similar to that for acute lymphoblastic leukemia. Remission, if achieved, is commonly short-lived. Bone marrow transplant may produce long asymptomatic periods in the early phase of illness but has been less successful in the accelerated phase. Despite vigorous treatment, CGL usually progresses after onset of the acute phase.

Medication
Aggressive chemotherapy has thus far failed to produce remission in CGL. Consequently, the goal of treatment in the chronic phase is to control leukocytosis and thrombocytosis. The most commonly used oral agents include:
- busulfan—4 to 8 mg/day P.O. until WBC count falls to 15,000/µl
- hydroxyurea—80 mg/kg P.O. every 3 days.

   Other medications that may be used include:
- aspirin—to prevent stroke if the patient's platelet count is over 1 million/µl

- allopurinol—to prevent secondary hyperuricemia or colchicine to relieve gout caused by elevated serum uric acid levels.

Surgical intervention
Local splenic radiation or splenectomy may be needed to increase platelet count and decrease adverse effects related to splenomegaly.

Referral
- Refer the patient to a hematologist or oncologist for treatment.
- Refer the patient to the American Cancer Society for information and treatment.

Follow-up
The patient should be seen as directed by the specialist.

Patient teaching
- To minimize bleeding, suggest a soft-bristle toothbrush, an electric razor, and other safety precautions.
- To minimize the abdominal discomfort of splenomegaly, provide small, frequent meals.
- Instruct the patient to use a stool softener or laxative to prevent constipation, as needed.
- Tell the patient to watch for and immediately report signs and symptoms of infection.
- Instruct the patient to watch for signs of thrombocytopenia, to immediately apply ice and pressure to an external bleeding site, and to avoid aspirin and aspirin-containing compounds because of the risk of increased bleeding.

Complications
- Infection
- Bleeding
- Thrombocytopenia

••••••••••••

LEUKEMIA, CHRONIC LYMPHOCYTIC

A generalized, progressive disease that's common in elderly patients, chronic lymphocytic leukemia (CLL) is marked by an uncontrollable spread of abnormal, small lymphocytes in lymphoid tissue, blood, and bone marrow. Nearly all patients with CLL are men over age 50. According to the American Cancer Society, this disease accounts for about one-fourth of all new leukemia cases annually.

Causes
Although the cause of CLL is unknown, researchers suspect hereditary factors (higher incidence has been recorded within families), still-undefined chromosome abnormalities, and certain immunologic defects (such as ataxia-telangiectasia or acquired agammaglobulinemia). The disease doesn't seem to be associated with radiation exposure. Prognosis is poor if anemia, thrombocytopenia, neutropenia, bulky lymphadenopathy, and severe lymphocytosis are present.

Clinical presentation
CLL is the most benign and the most slowly progressive form of leukemia. Clinical signs derive from the infiltration of leukemic cells in bone marrow, lymphoid tissue, and organ systems.

In early stages, patients usually complain of:
- fatigue
- malaise
- fever
- nodal enlargement
- susceptibility to infection.

In advanced stages, patients may experience:
- severe fatigue and weight loss
- liver or spleen enlargement

- bone tenderness
- edema from lymph node obstruction
- pulmonary infiltrates (may appear when lung parenchyma is involved)
- skin infiltrations, manifested by macular to nodular eruptions, which occur in about half the cases of chronic lymphocytic leukemia.

As the disease progresses, bone marrow involvement may lead to:
- anemia
- pallor
- weakness
- dyspnea
- tachycardia
- palpitations
- bleeding
- infection
- opportunistic fungal, viral, and bacterial infections (commonly occur in late stages).

Differential diagnoses
- Malignant lymphoma
- Hairy cell leukemia
- Other lymphoproliferative disorders

Diagnosis
Typically, CLL is an incidental finding during a routine blood test that reveals numerous abnormal lymphocytes. In early stages, white blood cell (WBC) count is mildly but persistently elevated. Granulocytopenia is the rule, but the WBC count climbs as the disease progresses. Blood studies also show hemoglobin levels less than 11 g, hypogammaglobulinemia, and depressed serum globulins. Other common developments include neutropenia (less than 1,500/µl), lymphocytosis (more than 10,000/µl), and thrombocytopenia (less than 150,000/µl). Bone marrow aspiration and biopsy show lymphocytic invasion.

Management

General

When chronic lymphocytic leukemia causes obstruction or organ impairment or enlargement, local radiation treatment can be used to reduce organ size.

Medication

Systemic chemotherapy includes alkylating agents, such as:

- chlorambucil — 0.1 to 0.2 mg/kg/day P.O. for 3 to 6 weeks, then adjusted for maintenance (usually 2 to 4 mg/day)
- cyclophosphamide — 40 to 50 mg/kg I.V. in divided doses over 2 to 5 days.

Other medications that may be used include:

- prednisone — 5 to 60 mg P.O.; highly individualized
- allopurinol — 200 to 300 mg/day P.O.

Referral

- Refer the patient to a hematologist or oncologist for treatment.
- Refer the patient to the American Cancer Society for information and support.

Follow-up

The patient should be seen as directed by the specialist.

Patient teaching

- Advise the patient to avoid aspirin and aspirin-containing products. Teach him how to recognize aspirin variants on medication labels.
- Tell the patient to avoid coming in contact with obviously ill people, especially children with common contagious childhood diseases.
- Urge the patient to eat high-protein foods and drink high-calorie beverages.
- Teach the patient the signs and symptoms of recurrence and tell him to report them immediately.

Complications

- Infection
- Secondary malignancy
- Cardiomyopathy
- Disseminated intravascular coagulation
- Pancytopenia

• • • • • • • • • • • •

LUNG CANCER

Even though it's largely preventable, lung cancer has long been the most common cause of cancer death in men; since 1987, it has also become the most common cause of cancer death in women. Lung cancer usually develops within the wall or epithelium of the bronchial tree. Its most common types are epidermoid (squamous cell) carcinoma, small cell (oat cell) carcinoma, adenocarcinoma, and large cell (anaplastic) carcinoma. Although the prognosis is usually poor, it varies with the extent of metastasis at the time of diagnosis and the cell type growth rate. Only about 14% of patients with lung cancer survive 5 years after diagnosis.

Causes

Most experts agree that lung cancer is attributable to inhalation of carcinogenic pollutants by a susceptible host. The most susceptible individual is a smoker over age 40, especially if he began to smoke before age 15, has smoked a pack or more per day for 20 years, or works with or near asbestos.

Pollutants in tobacco smoke cause progressive lung cell degeneration. Lung cancer is 10 times more common in smokers than nonsmokers; indeed, 80% of lung cancer patients are smokers. Cancer risk is determined by the number of cigarettes smoked daily, the depth of inhalation, how early in life smoking began, and the nicotine content of cigarettes. Two other factors also increase susceptibility: exposure to carcinogenic industrial and air pollutants (asbestos, uranium, arsenic, nickel, iron oxides, chromium, radioactive dust, and coal dust) and familial susceptibility.

Clinical presentation

Because early-stage lung cancer usually produces no symptoms, this disease may be at an advanced state at diagnosis. The following late-stage symptoms commonly lead to diagnosis:

■ Epidermoid and small cell carcinomas — smoker's cough, hoarseness, wheezing, dyspnea, hemoptysis, and chest pain
■ Adenocarcinoma and large cell carcinoma — fever, weakness, weight loss, anorexia, and shoulder pain.

In addition to their obvious interference with respiratory function, lung tumors may also alter the production of hormones that regulate body function or homeostasis. Clinical conditions that result from such changes are known as hormonal paraneoplastic syndromes:

■ Gynecomastia may result from large cell carcinoma.
■ Hypertrophic pulmonary osteoarthropathy (bone and joint pain from cartilage erosion due to abnormal production of growth hormone) may result from large cell carcinoma and adenocarcinoma.
■ Cushing's and carcinoid syndromes may result from small cell carcinoma.
■ Hypercalcemia may result from epidermoid tumors.

Metastatic signs and symptoms vary greatly, depending on the effect of tumors on intrathoracic and distant structures:

■ bronchial obstruction — hemoptysis, atelectasis, pneumonitis, dyspnea
■ recurrent nerve invasion — hoarseness, vocal cord paralysis
■ chest wall invasion — piercing chest pain, increasing dyspnea, severe shoulder pain, radiating down the arm

■ local lymphatic spread — cough, hemoptysis, stridor, pleural effusion
■ phrenic nerve involvement — dyspnea, shoulder pain, unilateral paralyzed diaphragm, with paradoxical motion
■ esophageal compression — dysphagia
■ vena caval obstruction — venous distention and edema of face, neck, chest, and back
■ pericardial involvement — pericardial effusion, tamponade, arrhythmias
■ cervical thoracic sympathetic nerve involvement — miosis, ptosis, exophthalmos, reduced sweating.

Distant metastasis may involve any part of the body, most commonly the central nervous system, liver, and bone.

Differential diagnoses

■ Metastatic cancer
■ Granuloma

Diagnosis

Typical clinical findings may strongly suggest lung cancer, but firm diagnosis requires further evidence through the use of the following tests:

■ Chest X-ray usually shows an advanced lesion, but it can detect a lesion up to 2 years before symptoms appear. It also indicates tumor size and location.
■ Sputum cytology, which is 75% reliable, requires a specimen coughed up from the lungs and tracheobronchial tree, *not* postnasal secretions or saliva.
■ Computed tomography (CT) scan of the chest may help to delineate the tumor's size and its relationship to surrounding structures.
■ Bronchoscopy can locate the tumor site. Bronchoscopic washings provide material for cytologic and histologic examination. The flexible fiber-optic bronchoscope increases the test's effectiveness.
■ Needle biopsy of the lungs uses biplane fluoroscopic visual control to detect pe-

ripherally located tumors. This allows firm diagnosis in 80% of patients.

■ Tissue biopsy of accessible metastatic sites includes supraclavicular and mediastinal node and pleural biopsy.

■ Thoracentesis allows chemical and cytologic examination of pleural fluid.

Additional studies include preoperative mediastinoscopy or mediastinotomy to rule out involvement of mediastinal lymph nodes (which would preclude curative pulmonary resection).

Other tests to detect metastasis include bone scan, bone marrow biopsy (recommended in small cell carcinoma), and CT scan of the brain or abdomen.

After histologic confirmation, staging determines the extent of the disease and helps in planning the treatment and predicting the prognosis. (See *Staging lung cancer.*)

Management
General
Recent treatment, which consists of combinations of surgery, radiation, and chemotherapy, may improve the prognosis and prolong survival. Nevertheless, because treatment usually begins at an advanced stage, it's largely palliative.

Preoperative radiation therapy may reduce tumor bulk to allow for surgical resection. Preradiation chemotherapy helps improve response rates. Radiation therapy is ordinarily recommended for stage I and stage II lesions, if surgery is contraindicated, and for stage III lesions when the disease is confined to the involved hemithorax and the ipsilateral supraclavicular lymph nodes.

Generally, radiation therapy is delayed until 1 month after surgery, to allow the wound to heal, and is then directed to the part of the chest most likely to develop metastasis. High-dose radiation therapy or radiation implants may also be used.

In laser therapy, still largely experimental, laser energy is directed through a bronchoscope to destroy local tumors.

Medication
Chemotherapy is individualized and may be given in combinations of fluorouracil, vincristine, mitomycin, cisplatin, and vindesine to produce a response rate of about 40% but have a minimal effect on overall survival. Promising combinations for treating small cell carcinomas include cyclophosphamide with doxorubicin and vincristine; cyclophosphamide with doxorubicin, vincristine, and etoposide; and etoposide with cisplatin, cyclophosphamide, and doxorubicin.

Surgical intervention
Surgery is the primary treatment for stage I, stage II, or selected stage III squamous cell carcinoma; adenocarcinoma; and large cell carcinoma, unless the tumor is nonresectable or other conditions rule out surgery.

Surgery may include partial removal of a lung (wedge resection, segmental resection, lobectomy, or radical lobectomy) or total removal (pneumonectomy or radical pneumonectomy).

Referral
■ Refer the patient to a surgeon and an oncologist for treatment.

■ Refer the patient to the American Cancer Society for information and support.

■ Refer smokers who want to quit to local branches of the American Cancer Society, Smoke Enders, I Quit Smoking Clinics, or I'm Not Smoking Clubs; suggest group therapy or individual counseling; or support the patient's use of smoking-cessation products.

Staging lung cancer

Using the TNM (tumor, node, metastasis) classification system, the American Joint Committee on Cancer stages lung cancer as follows.

PRIMARY TUMOR

TX — primary tumor can't be assessed or malignant tumor cells detected in sputum or bronchial washings but undetected by X-ray or bronchoscopy

T0 — no evidence of primary tumor

Tis — carcinoma in situ

T1 — tumor 3 cm or less in greatest dimension, surrounded by normal lung or visceral pleura; no bronchoscopic evidence of cancer closer to the center of the body than the lobar bronchus

T2 — tumor larger than 3 cm; one that involves the main bronchus and is 2 cm or more from the carina; one that invades the visceral pleura; or one that's accompanied by atelectasis or obstructive pneumonitis that extends to the hilar region but doesn't involve the entire lung

T3 — tumor of any size that extends into neighboring structures, such as the chest wall, diaphragm, or mediastinal pleura; tumor in the main bronchus that doesn't involve but is less than 2 cm from the carina; or tumor that's accompanied by atelectasis or obstructive pneumonitis of the entire lung

T4 — tumor of any size that invades the mediastinum, heart, great vessels, trachea, esophagus, vertebral body, or carina or tumor with malignant pleural effusion

REGIONAL LYMPH NODES

NX — regional lymph nodes can't be assessed

N0 — no detectable metastasis to lymph nodes

N1 — metastasis to the ipsilateral peribronchial or hilar lymph nodes or both

N2 — metastasis to the ipsilateral mediastinal or subcarinal lymph nodes or both

N3 — metastasis to the contralateral mediastinal or hilar lymph nodes, the ipsilateral or contralateral scalene lymph nodes, or the supraclavicular lymph nodes

DISTANT METASTASIS

MX — distant metastasis can't be assessed

M0 — no evidence of distant metastasis

M1 — distant metastasis

STAGING CATEGORIES

Lung cancer progresses from mild to severe as follows:

Occult carcinoma — TX, N0, M0

STAGE 0 — Tis, N0, M0

STAGE I — T1, N0, M0; T2, N0, M0

STAGE II — T1, N1, M0; T2, N1, M0

STAGE IIIA — T1, N2, M0; T2, N2, M0; T3, N0, M0; T3, N1, M0; T3, N2, M0

STAGE IIIB — any T, N3, M0; T4, any N, M0

STAGE IV — any T, any N, M1

Follow-up

The patient should be seen according to the oncologist's directions.

Patient teaching

■ Supplement and reinforce the information given to the patient by the health care team about the disease and the surgical procedure.

Complications

■ Metastatic disease
■ Death

Special considerations

■ Encourage patients with recurring or chronic respiratory infections and those with chronic lung disease who detect any change in the character of a cough to be evaluated promptly.

HEALTHY LIVING Educate high-risk patients in ways to reduce their chances of developing lung cancer.

• • • • • • • • • • • •

LYMPHOMA, MALIGNANT

Malignant lymphomas (also known as non-Hodgkin's lymphomas and lymphosarcomas) are a heterogeneous group of malignant diseases originating in lymph glands and other lymphoid tissue. Nodular lymphomas have a better prognosis than the diffuse form of the disease but, in both, the prognosis is worse than in Hodgkin's disease.

Malignant lymphomas are two to three times more common in males than in females and occur in all age-groups. Compared with Hodgkin's disease, they occur about one to three times more and cause twice as many deaths in children under age 15. Incidence rises with age (median age is 50). These lymphomas seem linked to certain races and ethnic groups, with increased incidence in whites and people of Jewish ancestry.

Causes

The cause of malignant lymphomas is unknown, although some theories suggest a viral source. Since the early 1970s, the incidence of these lymphomas has increased more than 80%, with about 53,000 new cases appearing annually in the United States. The reason for the increase is unknown, although it has been partly attributed to acquired immunodeficiency syndrome (AIDS).

Clinical presentation

Usually, the first indication of malignant lymphoma is swelling of the lymph glands, enlarged tonsils and adenoids, and painless, rubbery nodes in the cervical supraclavicular areas. In children, these nodes are usually in the cervical region, and the disease causes dyspnea and coughing. As the lymphoma progresses, the patient develops symptoms specific to the area involved and systemic complaints of fatigue, malaise, weight loss, fever, and night sweats.

Differential diagnoses

■ Hodgkin's disease
■ Other lymphomas
■ Infectious lymphadenopathy
■ Autoimmune disease
■ AIDS or human immunodeficiency virus infection

Diagnosis

Diagnosis requires histologic evaluation of biopsied lymph nodes; of tonsils, bone marrow, liver, bowel, or skin; or of tissue removed during exploratory laparotomy. (See *Classifying malignant lymphomas*.)

Other tests include bone and chest X-rays, lymphangiography, liver and spleen scan, computed tomography scan of the abdomen, and excretory urography. Laboratory tests include complete blood count (may show anemia), uric acid level (elevated or normal), serum calcium level (elevated if bone lesions are present), serum protein level (normal), and liver function studies.

Management

General

Radiation therapy is used mainly in the early, localized stage of the disease. Total nodal irradiation is generally effective for both nodular and diffuse histologies.

Classifying malignant lymphomas

Staging and classifying systems for malignant lymphomas include the National Cancer Institute's (NCI) system, the Rappaport histologic classification, and Lukes classification. (*Note:* The NCI also cites a "miscellaneous" category, which includes these lymphomas: composite, mycosis fungoides, histiocytic, extramedullary plasmacytoma, and unclassifiable.)

NCI	RAPPAPORT	LUKES
Low grade		
▪ Small lymphocytic	▪ Diffuse well-differentiated lymphocytic	▪ Small lymphocytic and plasmacytoid lymphocytic
▪ Follicular, predominantly small cleaved cell	▪ Nodular poorly differentiated lymphocytic	▪ Small cleaved follicular center cell, follicular only or follicular and diffuse
▪ Follicular mixed, small and large cell	▪ Nodular mixed lymphoma	▪ Small cleaved follicular center cell, follicular; large cleaved follicular center cell, follicular
Intermediate grade		
▪ Follicular, predominantly large cell	▪ Nodular histiocytic lymphoma	▪ Large cleaved or noncleaved follicular center cell, or both, follicular
▪ Diffuse, small cleaved cell	▪ Diffuse poorly differentiated lymphoma	▪ Small cleaved follicular center cell, diffuse
▪ Diffuse mixed, small and large cell	▪ Diffuse mixed lymphocytic-histiocytic	▪ Small cleaved, large cleaved, or large noncleaved follicular center cell, diffuse
▪ Diffuse large cell, cleaved or noncleaved	▪ Diffuse histiocytic lymphoma	▪ Large cleaved or noncleaved follicular center cell, diffuse
High grade		
▪ Diffuse large cell immunoblastic	▪ Diffuse histiocytic lymphoma	▪ Immunoblastic sarcoma, T-cell or B-cell type
▪ Large cell, lymphoblastic	▪ Lymphoblastic, convoluted or nonconvoluted	▪ Convoluted T cell
▪ Small noncleaved cell	▪ Undifferentiated, Burkitt's and non-Burkitt's diffuse undifferentiated lymphoma	▪ Small noncleaved follicular center cell

Medication

Chemotherapy is individualized and most effective with multiple combinations of antineoplastic agents. For example, cyclophosphamide, vincristine, doxorubicin, and prednisone can induce a complete remission in 70% to 80% of patients with nodular histology and in 20% to 55% of patients with diffuse histology. Other combinations—such as methotrexate, bleomycin, doxorubicin, cyclophosphamide, vincristine, and prednisone—induce prolonged remission and sometimes cure the diffuse form.

Referral
■ Refer the patient to an oncologist for treatment.
■ Refer the patient to the American Cancer Society for information and support.

Follow-up
The patient should be seen according to the oncologist's directions.

Patient teaching
■ Teach the family and patient about the illness and expected and potential outcomes.

Complications
■ Sterility
■ Immunosuppressed infections
■ Anemia
■ Bone marrow suppression
■ Idiopathic thrombocytopenia purpura

• • • • • • • • • • • •

MELANOMA, MALIGNANT

A malignant neoplasm that arises from melanocytes, malignant melanoma is relatively rare and accounts for only 1% to 2% of all malignancies. However, the incidence is greatly increasing with a noted 300% increase in the past 40 years. The four types of melanomas are superficial spreading melanoma, nodular malignant melanoma, lentigo maligna, and acral lentiginous melanoma. Melanoma is slightly more common in women than men and is rare in children. Peak incidence occurs between ages 50 and 70, although the incidence in younger age-groups is increasing.

Melanoma spreads through the lymphatic and vascular systems and metastasizes to the regional lymph nodes, skin, liver, lungs, and central nervous system (CNS). Its course is unpredictable, however, and recurrence and metastasis may not appear for more than 5 years after resection of the primary lesion. The prognosis varies with tumor thickness. Generally, superficial lesions are curable, whereas deeper lesions tend to metastasize. The Breslow level method measures tumor depth from the granular level of the epidermis to the deepest melanoma cell. Melanoma lesions less than 0.76 mm deep have an excellent prognosis, whereas deeper lesions (more than 0.76 mm) are at risk for metastasis. The prognosis is better for a tumor on an extremity (which is drained by one lymphatic network) than for one on the head, neck, or trunk (drained by several networks).

Causes
Several factors seem to influence the development of melanoma:
■ Excessive exposure to sunlight — Melanoma is most common in sunny, warm areas and usually develops on parts of the body that are exposed to the sun.
■ Skin type — Most persons who develop melanoma have blond or red hair, fair skin, and blue eyes; are prone to sunburn; and are of Celtic or Scandinavian ancestry. Melanoma is rare among blacks; when it does develop, it usually arises in lightly pigmented areas (the palms, plantar surface of the feet, or mucous membranes).
■ Hormonal factors — Pregnancy may increase risk and exacerbate growth.
■ Family history — Melanoma is slightly more common within families.
■ Past history of melanoma — A person who has had one melanoma is at greater risk for developing a second.

Clinical presentation
Common sites for melanoma are the head and neck in men, the legs in women, and the backs of persons exposed to excessive sunlight. Up to 70% arise

from a preexisting nevus. It rarely appears in the conjunctiva, choroid, pharynx, mouth, vagina, or anus.

Suspect melanoma when any skin lesion or nevus:

- enlarges
- changes color
- becomes inflamed or sore
- itches
- ulcerates
- bleeds
- undergoes textural changes
- shows signs of surrounding pigment regression (halo nevus or vitiligo; see *Recognizing potentially malignant nevi*, page 858).

Each type of melanoma has special characteristics:

- Superficial spreading melanoma, the most common, usually develops between ages 40 and 50. Such a lesion arises on an area of chronic irritation. In women, it's most common between the knees and ankles; in Blacks and Asians, on the toe webs and soles (lightly pigmented areas subject to trauma). Characteristically, this melanoma has a red, white, and blue color over a brown or black background and an irregular, notched margin. Its surface is irregular, with small elevated tumor nodules that may ulcerate and bleed. Horizontal growth may continue for many years; when vertical growth begins, prognosis worsens.
- Nodular melanoma usually develops between ages 40 and 50, grows vertically, invades the dermis, and metastasizes early. Such a lesion is usually a polypoidal nodule, with uniformly dark discoloration (it may be grayish), and looks like a blackberry. Occasionally, this melanoma is flesh-colored, with flecks of pigment around its base (possibly inflamed).
- Lentigo maligna melanoma is relatively rare. It arises from a lentigo maligna on an exposed skin surface and usually occurs between ages 60 and 70. This lesion looks like a large (3- to 6-cm) flat freckle of tan, brown, black, whitish, or slate color and has irregularly scattered black nodules on the surface. It develops slowly, usually over many years, and eventually may ulcerate. This melanoma commonly develops under the fingernails, on the face, and on the back of the hands.

Differential diagnoses

- Dysplastic nevi
- Vascular skin tumors
- Squamous cell carcinoma
- Basal cell carcinoma

Diagnosis

A *skin biopsy with histologic examination* can distinguish malignant melanoma from a benign nevus, seborrheic keratosis, and pigmented basal cell epithelioma; it can also determine tumor thickness. Physical examination, paying particular attention to lymph nodes, can point to metastatic involvement. (See *Staging malignant melanoma*, page 859.)

Baseline laboratory studies include complete blood count with differential, erythrocyte sedimentation rate, platelet count, liver function studies, and urinalysis. Depending on the depth of tumor invasion and metastatic spread, baseline diagnostic studies may also include chest X-ray and a computed tomography (CT) scan of the chest and abdomen. Signs of bone metastasis may call for a bone scan; CNS metastasis, and a CT scan of the brain.

Management
General

Deep primary lesions may merit adjuvant chemotherapy and biotherapy to eliminate or reduce the number of tumor cells. Clinical trials are currently under way to evaluate the effectiveness of isolated limb perfusion as chemotherapy for the man-

(*Text continues on page 860.*)

Recognizing potentially malignant nevi

Nevi (moles) are skin lesions that are commonly pigmented and may be hereditary. They begin to grow in childhood (occasionally they're congenital) and become more numerous in young adults. Up to 70% of patients with melanoma have a history of a preexisting nevus at the tumor site. Of these, approximately one-third are reported to be congenital; the remainder develop later in life.

Changes in nevi (color, size, shape, texture, ulceration, bleeding, or itching) suggest possible malignant transformation. The presence or absence of hair within a nevus has no significance.

TYPES OF NEVI

■ Junctional nevi are flat or slightly raised and light to dark brown, with melanocytes confined to the epidermis. Usually, they appear before age 40. These nevi may change into compound nevi if junctional nevus cells proliferate and penetrate into the dermis.
■ Compound nevi are usually tan to dark brown and slightly raised, although size and color vary. They contain melanocytes in the dermis and epidermis, and they rarely undergo malignant transformation. Excision is necessary only to rule out malignant transformation or for cosmetic reasons.
■ Dermal nevi are elevated lesions from 2 to 10 mm in diameter and vary in color from flesh to brown. They usually develop in older adults and generally arise on the upper part of the body. Excision is necessary only to rule out malignant transformation.
■ Blue nevi are flat or slightly elevated lesions from 0.5 to 1 cm in diameter. They appear on the head, neck, arms, and dorsa of the hands and are twice as common in women as in men. Their blue color results from pigment and collagen in the dermis, which reflect blue light but absorb other wavelengths. Excision is necessary to rule out pigmented basal cell epithelioma or melanoma or for cosmetic reasons.
■ Dysplastic nevi are generally greater than 5 mm in diameter, with irregularly notched or indistinct borders. Coloration is usually a variable mixture of tan and brown, sometimes with red, pink, and black pigmentation. No two lesions are exactly alike. They occur in great numbers (typically over 100 at a time), never singly, usually appearing on the back, scalp, chest, and buttocks. Dysplastic nevi are potentially malignant, especially in patients with a personal or familial history of melanoma. Skin biopsy confirms diagnosis; treatment is by surgical excision, followed by regular physical examinations (every 6 months) to detect new lesions or changes in existing lesions.
■ Lentigo maligna (melanotic freckles, Hutchinson freckles) is a precursor to malignant melanoma. (In fact, about one-third of them eventually give rise to malignant melanoma.) Usually, they occur in persons over age 40, especially on exposed skin areas such as the face. At first, these lesions are flat, tan spots, but they gradually enlarge and darken and develop black speckled areas against their tan or brown background. Each lesion may simultaneously enlarge in one area and regress in another. Histologic examination shows typical and atypical melanocytes along the epidermal basement membrane. Removal by simple excision (not electrodesiccation and curettage) is recommended.

Staging malignant melanoma

Several systems exist for staging malignant melanoma, including the TNM (tumor, node, metastasis) system, developed by the American Joint Committee on Cancer, and Clark's system, which classifies tumor progression according to skin layer penetration.

PRIMARY TUMOR
TX — primary tumor can't be assessed
T0 — no evidence of primary tumor
Tis — melanoma in situ (atypical melanotic hyperplasia, severe melanotic dysplasia), not an invasive lesion (Clark's level I)
T1 — tumor 0.75 mm thick or less that invades the papillary dermis (Clark's level II)
T2 — tumor between 0.75 and 1.5 mm thick, tumor invades the interface between the papillary and reticular dermis (Clark's level III), or both
T3 — tumor between 1.5 and 4 mm thick, tumor invades the reticular dermis (Clark's level IV), or both
T3a — tumor between 1.5 and 3 mm thick
T3b — tumor between 3 and 4 mm thick
T4 — tumor more than 4 mm thick, tumor invades subcutaneous tissue (Clark's level V), or tumor has one or more satellites within 2 cm of the primary tumor
T4a — tumor more than 4 mm thick, tumor invades subcutaneous tissue, or both
T4b — one or more satellites exist within 2 cm of the primary tumor

REGIONAL LYMPH NODES
NX — regional lymph nodes can't be assessed
N0 — no evidence of regional lymph node involvement
N1 — metastasis 3 cm or less in greatest dimension in any regional lymph node
N2 — metastasis greater than 3 cm in greatest dimension in any regional lymph node, in-transit metastasis, or both

DISTANT METASTASIS
MX — distant metastasis can't be assessed
M0 — no evidence of distant metastasis
M1 — distant metastasis
M1a — metastasis in skin, subcutaneous tissue, or lymph nodes beyond the regional nodes
M1b — visceral metastasis

STAGING CATEGORIES
Malignant melanoma progresses from mild to severe as follows:
STAGE I — T1, N0, M0; T2, N0, M0
STAGE II — T3, N0, M0
STAGE III — T4, N0, M0; any T, N1, M0; any T, N2, M0
STAGE IV — any T, any N, M1

CLARK'S LEVELS

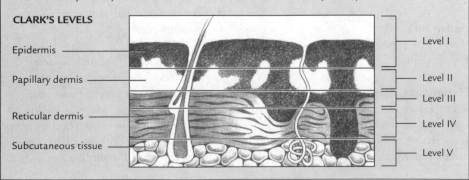

Epidermis
Papillary dermis
Reticular dermis
Subcutaneous tissue

Level I
Level II
Level III
Level IV
Level V

agement of malignant melanomas of extremities. Radiation therapy is usually reserved for metastatic disease. It doesn't prolong survival but may reduce tumor size and relieve pain.

Regardless of the treatment method, melanomas require close long-term follow-up to detect metastasis and recurrences. Statistics show that 13% of recurrences develop more than 5 years after primary surgery.

Medication

Medications that may be used to treat recurrent or metastatic carcinoma include:
- carmustine — 75 to 100 mg/m^2 I.V. infusion for 2 days; repeat every 6 weeks
- hydroxyurea — 80 mg/kg P.O. as a single dose every 3 days.

Surgical intervention

A patient with malignant melanoma requires surgical resection to remove the tumor. The extent of resection depends on the size and location of the primary lesion. Closure of a wide resection may require a skin graft. Surgical treatment may also include regional lymphadenectomy.

Referral

- Refer the patient to a dermatologist or surgeon for treatment.
- Make referrals for home care, social services, and spiritual and financial assistance as needed.

Follow-up

The patient should be seen as directed by the specialist.

Patient teaching

- Emphasize the need for close follow-up to detect recurrences early. Explain that recurrences and metastasis, if they occur, are commonly delayed, so follow-up must continue for years. Tell the patient how to recognize signs of recurrence.

HEALTHY LIVING To help prevent malignant melanoma, stress the detrimental effects of overexposure to solar radiation, especially to fair-skinned, blue-eyed patients. Recommend that they use a sunblock or sunscreen.

Complications

- Recurrence
- Metastasis
- Death

• • • • • • • • • • • •

PANCREATIC CANCER

A deadly GI cancer, pancreatic cancer progresses rapidly. Most pancreatic tumors are adenocarcinomas and arise in the head of the pancreas. Rarer tumors are those of the body and tail of the pancreas and islet cell tumors. The two main tissue types are cylinder cell and large, fatty, granular cell. The incidence of pancreatic cancer increases with age, peaking between ages 60 and 70. Geographically, the incidence is highest in Israel, the United States, Sweden, and Canada.

Causes

Evidence suggests that pancreatic cancer is linked to inhalation or absorption of the following carcinogens, which are then excreted by the pancreas:
- cigarettes
- food additives
- industrial chemicals, such as beta-naphthalene, benzidine, and urea.

Possible predisposing factors are chronic pancreatitis, diabetes mellitus, and chronic alcohol abuse (both pancreatitis and diabetes mellitus may be early manifestations of the disease as well).

Types of pancreatic cancer

TYPE AND PATHOLOGY	CLINICAL FEATURES
Head of pancreas ■ Commonly obstructs ampulla of Vater and common bile duct ■ Directly metastasizes to duodenum ■ Adhesions anchor tumor to spine, stomach, and intestines.	■ Jaundice (predominant sign) — slowly progressive, unremitting; may cause skin (especially of the face and genitals) to turn olive green or black ■ Pruritus — in many cases severe ■ Weight loss — rapid and severe (as great as 30 lb [13.6 kg]); may lead to emaciation, weakness, and muscle atrophy ■ Slowed digestion, gastric distention, nausea, diarrhea, and steatorrhea with clay-colored stools ■ Liver and gallbladder enlargement from lymph node metastasis to biliary tract and duct wall results in compression and obstruction; gallbladder may be palpable (Courvoisier's sign). ■ Dull, nondescript, continuous abdominal pain radiating to right upper quadrant; relieved by bending forward ■ GI hemorrhage and biliary infection common
Body and tail of pancreas ■ Large nodular masses become fixed to retropancreatic tissues and spine ■ Direct invasion of spleen, left kidney, suprarenal gland, diaphragm ■ Involvement of celiac plexus results in thrombosis of splenic vein and spleen infarction.	*Body* ■ Pain (predominant symptom) — usually epigastric, develops slowly and radiates to the back; relieved by bending forward or sitting up; intensified by lying supine; most intense 3 to 4 hours after eating; when celiac plexus is involved, pain is more intense and lasts longer ■ Venous thrombosis and thrombophlebitis — common; may precede other symptoms by months ■ Splenomegaly (from infarction), hepatomegaly (occasionally), and jaundice (rarely) *Tail* Symptoms result from metastasis: ■ Abdominal tumor (most common finding) produces a palpable abdominal mass; abdominal pain radiates to left hypochondrium and left side of the chest. ■ Anorexia leads to weight loss, emaciation, and weakness. ■ Splenomegaly and upper GI bleeding

Clinical presentation

The most common features of pancreatic carcinoma are:
■ weight loss
■ abdominal or low back pain
■ jaundice
■ diarrhea.

Other generalized effects include fever, skin lesions (usually on the legs), and fatigue. (See *Types of pancreatic cancer*.)

Islet cell tumors

Relatively uncommon, islet cell tumors (insulinomas) may be benign or malignant and produce signs and symptoms in three stages:
1. Slight hypoglycemia — fatigue, restlessness, malaise, and excessive weight gain
2. Compensatory secretion of epinephrine — pallor, clamminess, perspiration, palpitations, finger tremors, hunger, decreased temperature, and increased pulse and blood pressure
3. Severe hypoglycemia — ataxia, clouded sensorium, diplopia, episodes of violence, and hysteria.

Usually, insulinomas metastasize to the liver alone but may metastasize to bone, brain, and lungs. Death results from a combination of hypoglycemic reactions and widespread metastasis. Treatment consists of enucleation of tumor (if benign) and chemotherapy with streptozocin or resection to include pancreatic tissue (if malignant).

Differential diagnoses
- Pancreatitis
- Cholangiocarcinoma
- Choledocholithiasis
- Duodenal neoplasms
- Biliary tract stricture

Diagnosis
Definitive diagnosis requires a laparotomy with a biopsy.

Other tests used to detect pancreatic cancer include:
- ultrasound — can identify a mass but not its histology
- computed tomography scan — similar to ultrasound but shows greater detail
- angiography — shows vascular supply of tumor
- endoscopic retrograde cholangiopancreatography — allows visualization, instillation of contrast medium, and specimen biopsy
- magnetic resonance imaging — shows tumor size and location in great detail.

Laboratory tests supporting this diagnosis include serum bilirubin level (increased); serum amylase and serum lipase levels (sometimes elevated); prothrombin time (prolonged); aspartate aminotransferase and alanine aminotransferase levels (elevations indicate necrosis of liver cells); alkaline phosphatase level (marked elevation occurs with biliary obstruction); plasma insulin immunoassay (shows measurable serum insulin in the presence of islet cell tumors; see *Islet cell tumors*); hemoglobin level and hematocrit (may show mild anemia); fasting blood glucose level (may indicate hypoglycemia or hyperglycemia); and stools (occult blood may signal ulceration in GI tract or ampulla of Vater).

Management
General
Treatment of pancreatic cancer is rarely successful because this disease has usually widely metastasized at diagnosis. Therapy consists of surgery and, possibly, radiation and chemotherapy. Radiation therapy is usually ineffective except as an adjunct to chemotherapy or as a palliative measure. (See *Staging pancreatic cancer.*)

Medication
Standard chemotherapy for patients with locally unresectable cancer includes gemcitabine (1,000 mg/m² I.V. weekly for up to 7 weeks).

Other medications used in pancreatic cancer include:
- propantheline — 15 mg P.O. t.i.d. a.c. and 30 mg h.s.
- aluminum hydroxide — 500 to 1,500 mg P.O. 1 hour p.c. and h.s.

Staging pancreatic cancer

Using the TNM (tumor, node, metastasis) system, the American Joint Committee on Cancer has established the following stages for pancreatic cancer.

PRIMARY TUMOR
TX — primary tumor can't be assessed
T0 — no evidence of primary tumor
T1 — tumor limited to the pancreas
T1a — tumor 2 cm or less in greatest dimension
T1b — tumor more than 2 cm in greatest dimension
T2 — tumor penetrates the duodenum, bile duct, or peripancreatic tissues
T3 — tumor penetrates the stomach, spleen, colon, or adjacent large vessels

REGIONAL LYMPH NODES
NX — regional lymph nodes can't be assessed

N0 — no evidence of regional lymph node metastasis
N1 — regional lymph node metastasis

DISTANT METASTASIS
MX — distant metastasis can't be assessed
M0 — no known distant metastasis
M1 — distant metastasis

STAGING CATEGORIES
Pancreatic cancer progresses from mild to severe as follows:
STAGE I — T1, N0, M0; T2, N0, M0
STAGE II — T3, N0, M0
STAGE III — any T, N1, M0
STAGE IV — any T, any N, M1

- furosemide — 20 to 40 mg/day I.V. or P.O.
- insulin — dosage according to blood glucose levels.

Surgical intervention
Small advances have been made in the survival rate with surgery:
- Total pancreatectomy may increase survival time by resecting a localized tumor or by controlling postoperative gastric ulceration.
- Cholecystojejunostomy, choledochoduodenostomy, and choledochojejunostomy have partially replaced radical resection to bypass obstructing common bile duct extensions, thus decreasing the incidence of jaundice and pruritus.
- Whipple's operation, or pancreatoduodenectomy, has a high mortality rate but can produce wide lymphatic clearance, except with tumors located near the por-

tal vein, superior mesenteric vein and artery, and celiac axis. This rarely used procedure removes the head of the pancreas, the duodenum, and portions of the body and tail of the pancreas, stomach, jejunum, pancreatic duct, and distal portion of the bile duct.
- Gastrojejunostomy is performed if radical resection isn't indicated and duodenal obstruction is expected to develop later.

Referral
- Refer the patient to a surgeon and an oncologist.
- Refer the patient to the American Cancer Society for information and support.

Follow-up
The patient should be seen according to the surgeon and oncologist's directions.

Patient teaching

- Teach the family about the illness and expected and potential outcomes.
- Encourage the patient to follow a nutritious diet and eat small, frequent meals
- Teach the patient and family how to monitor blood glucose levels and administer insulin if appropriate.

Complications

- Metastatic disease
- Jaundice
- Diabetes
- Malnutrition
- Death

Special considerations

- If appropriate, discuss advance directives and hospice care with the patient and his family.

• • • • • • • • • • • •

PROSTATIC CANCER

Adenocarcinoma is the most common form of prostate cancer; sarcoma occurs only rarely. Most prostatic carcinomas originate in the posterior prostate gland; the rest originate near the urethra. Malignant prostatic tumors seldom result from the benign hyperplastic enlargement that commonly develops around the prostatic urethra in elderly men. Prostatic cancer seldom produces symptoms until it's advanced.

AGE ALERT Prostatic cancer is the most common cancer in men over age 50.

Causes

Four factors have been suspected in the development of prostatic cancer: family or racial predisposition, exposure to environmental elements, co-existing sexually transmitted diseases, and endogenous hormonal influence. Eating fat-containing animal products has also been implicated. Although androgens regulate prostate growth and function and may also speed tumor growth, no definite link between increased androgen levels and prostatic cancer has been found. When primary prostatic lesions metastasize, they typically invade the prostatic capsule and spread along the ejaculatory ducts in the space between the seminal vesicles or perivesicular fascia.

Incidence is highest in Blacks and lowest in Asians. In fact, Blacks have the highest prostate cancer incidence in the world and are considered at high risk for the disease. Incidence also increases with age more rapidly than other cancers.

Clinical presentation

Signs and symptoms of prostatic cancer appear only in the advanced stages and include:

- difficulty initiating a urine stream
- dribbling
- urine retention
- unexplained cystitis
- hematuria (rarely) (see *Staging prostatic cancer*).

Differential diagnoses

- Benign prostate growth
- Seminal vessicle enlargement
- Bladder cancer

Diagnosis

A digital rectal examination that reveals a small, hard nodule may help diagnose prostatic cancer.

A biopsy confirms the diagnosis. prostate-specific antigen (PSA) levels will be elevated in all, and serum acid phosphatase levels will be elevated in two-thirds of men with metastatic prostatic cancer.

Therapy aims to return the serum acid phosphatase level to normal; a subsequent rise points to recurrence. Mag-

Staging prostatic cancer

The American Joint Committee on Cancer recognizes the TNM (tumor, node, metastasis) cancer staging system for assessing prostatic cancer.

PRIMARY TUMOR
TX — primary tumor can't be assessed
T0 — no evidence of primary tumor
T1 — tumor an incidental histologic finding
T1a — three or fewer microscopic foci of cancer
T1b — more than three microscopic foci of cancer
T2 — tumor limited to the prostate gland
T2a — tumor less than 1.5 cm in greatest dimension, with normal tissue on at least three sides
T2b — tumor larger than 1.5 cm in greatest dimension or present in more than one lobe
T3 — unfixed tumor extends into the prostatic apex or into or beyond the prostatic capsule, bladder neck, or seminal vesicle
T4 — tumor fixed or invades adjacent structures not listed in T3

REGIONAL LYMPH NODES
NX — regional lymph nodes can't be assessed

N0 — no evidence of regional lymph node metastasis
N1 — metastasis in a single lymph node, 2 cm or less in greatest dimension
N2 — metastasis in a single lymph node, between 2 and 5 cm in greatest dimension, or metastasis to several lymph nodes, none more than 5 cm in greatest dimension
N3 — metastasis in a lymph node more than 5 cm in greatest dimension

DISTANT METASTASIS
MX — distant metastasis can't be assessed
M0 — no known distant metastasis
M1 — distant metastasis

STAGING CATEGORIES
Prostatic cancer progresses from mild to severe as follows:
STAGE 0 or STAGE I — T1a, N0, M0; T2a, N0, M0
STAGE II — T1b, N0, M0; T2b, N0, M0
STAGE III — T3, N0, M0
STAGE IV — T4, N0, M0; any T, N1, M0; any T, N2, M0; any T, N3, M0; any T, any N, M1

netic resonance imaging, computed tomography scan, and excretory urography may also aid diagnosis.

Elevated alkaline phosphatase levels and a positive bone scan point to bone metastasis.

Management
General
Management of prostatic cancer depends on clinical assessment, tolerance of therapy, expected life span, and the stage of

the disease. Treatment must be chosen carefully, because prostatic cancer usually affects older men, who commonly have coexisting disorders, such as hypertension, diabetes, or cardiac disease. Radiation therapy is used to cure some locally invasive lesions and to relieve pain from metastatic bone involvement.

Medication
Medications that may be used to treat prostate cancer include:

- estramustine — 10 to 16 mg/kg/day P.O. t.i.d. or q.i.d.
- flutamide — 250 mg P.O. every 8 hours
- mitoxantrone — 12 to 14 mg/m² I.V. every 21 days as an adjunct to corticosteroid therapy
- radionuclide strontium-89 — single injection.

If hormone therapy, surgery, and radiation therapy aren't feasible or successful, chemotherapy (using combinations of cyclophosphamide, doxorubicin, fluorouracil, cisplatin, etoposide, and vindesine) may be tried. However, current drug therapy offers limited benefit. Combining several treatment methods may be most effective.

Surgical intervention

Prostatectomy or orchiectomy may be done to reduce androgen production. Radical prostatectomy is usually effective for localized lesions.

Referral

- Refer the patient to a urologist and oncologist for treatment.
- Refer the patient to the American Cancer Society for information and support.

Follow-up

The patient should be seen as directed by the specialist.

Patient teaching

- Teach the patient and family about the illness and expected and potential outcomes.
- Tell the patient that urinary incontinence is common after surgery; teach exercises to improve bladder control.
- Teach the patient about adverse effects that may occur with hormone therapy.

HEALTHY LIVING The American Cancer Society advises a yearly digital examination for men over age 40, a yearly blood test to detect PSA in men over age 50, and ultrasound if abnormal results are found.

Complications

- Impotency
- Metastasis
- Pain
- Death

• • • • • • • • • • •

SQUAMOUS CELL CARCINOMA

Squamous cell carcinoma of the skin is an invasive tumor with metastatic potential that arises from the keratinizing epidermal cells. It usually occurs in fairskinned white males over age 60. Outdoor employment and residence in a sunny, warm climate (southwestern United States and Australia, for example) greatly increase the risk of developing squamous cell carcinoma.

Causes

Predisposing factors associated with squamous cell carcinoma include overexposure to the sun's ultraviolet rays, the presence of premalignant lesions (such as actinic keratosis or Bowen's disease), X-ray therapy, ingestion of herbicides containing arsenic, chronic skin irritation and inflammation, exposure to local carcinogens (such as tar and oil), and hereditary diseases (such as xeroderma pigmentosum and albinism). (See *Premalignant skin lesions*.) Rarely, squamous cell carcinoma may develop on the site of smallpox vaccination, psoriasis, or chronic discoid lupus erythematosus. All the major treatment methods have excellent cure rates; generally, the prognosis is better with a well-differentiated lesion than with a poorly differentiated one in an unusual location.

Premalignant skin lesions

DISEASE	CAUSE	PATIENT	LESION	TREATMENT
Actinic keratosis	Solar radiation	White men with fair skin (middle-aged to elderly)	Reddish brown lesions 1 mm to 1 cm in size (may enlarge if untreated) on face, ears, lower lip, bald scalp, dorsa of hands and forearms	Topical 5-fluorouracil, cryosurgery using liquid nitrogen, or curettage by electrodesiccation
Bowen's disease	Unknown	White men with fair skin (middle-aged to elderly)	Brown to reddish brown lesions, with scaly surface on exposed and unexposed areas	Surgical excision, topical 5-fluorouracil
Erythroplasia of Queyrat	Bowen's disease of the mucous membranes	Men (middle-aged to elderly)	Red lesions, with a glistening or granular appearance on mucous membranes, particularly the glans penis in uncircumcised males	Surgical excision
Leukoplakia	Smoking, alcohol, chronic cheek-biting, ill-fitting dentures, misaligned teeth	Men (middle-aged to elderly)	Lesions on oral, anal, and genital mucous membranes vary in appearance from smooth and white to rough and gray	Elimination of irritating factors, surgical excision, or curettage by electrodesiccation (if lesion is still premalignant)

Clinical presentation

Squamous cell carcinoma commonly develops on the skin of the face, the ears, the dorsa of the hands and forearms, and other sun-damaged areas. Lesions on sun-damaged skin tend to be less invasive and less likely to metastasize than lesions on unexposed skin. Notable exceptions to this tendency are squamous cell lesions on the lower lip and the ears. These are almost invariably markedly invasive metastatic lesions with a generally poor prognosis.

Transformation from a premalignant lesion to squamous cell carcinoma may begin with induration and inflammation of the preexisting lesion. When squamous cell carcinoma arises from normal skin, the nodule grows slowly on a firm, indurated base. If untreated, this nodule eventually ulcerates and invades underlying tissues. (See *Staging squamous cell carcinoma*, page 868.) Metastasis can occur

Staging squamous cell carcinoma

The American Joint Committee on Cancer uses the following TNM (tumor, node, metastasis) system for staging squamous cell carcinoma.

PRIMARY TUMOR
TX — primary tumor can't be assessed
T0 — no evidence of primary tumor
Tis — carcinoma in situ
T1 — tumor 2 cm or less in greatest dimension
T2 — tumor between 2 and 5 cm in greatest dimension
T3 — tumor more than 5 cm in greatest dimension
T4 — tumor invades deep extradermal structures (such as cartilage, skeletal muscle, or bone)

REGIONAL LYMPH NODES
NX — regional lymph nodes can't be assessed

N0 — no evidence of regional lymph node involvement
N1 — regional lymph node involvement

DISTANT METASTASIS
MX — distant metastasis can't be assessed
M0 — no known distant metastasis
M1 — distant metastasis

STAGING CATEGORIES
Squamous cell carcinoma progresses from mild to severe as follows:
STAGE 0 — Tis, N0, M0
STAGE I — T1, N0, M0
STAGE II — T2, N0, M0; T3, N0, M0
STAGE III — T4, N0, M0; any T, N1, M0
STAGE IV — any T, any N, M1

to the regional lymph nodes, producing characteristic systemic symptoms, such as:
- pain
- malaise
- fatigue
- weakness
- anorexia.

Differential diagnoses
- Basal cell carcinoma
- Actinic keratosis
- Malignant melanoma
- Keratoacanthoma

Diagnosis
An excisional biopsy provides definitive diagnosis of squamous cell carcinoma. Other appropriate laboratory tests depend on systemic symptoms.

Management
General
The size, shape, location, and invasiveness of a squamous cell tumor and the condition of the underlying tissue determine the treatment method used; a deeply invasive tumor may require a combination of techniques.

Medication
Chemotherapy is usually reserved for resistant or recurrent lesions.

Surgical intervention
Depending on the lesion, treatment may consist of wide surgical excision or electrodesiccation and curettage.

Referral
- Refer the patient to a dermatologist for treatment.

■ Refer the patient to the American Cancer Society for information and support.

Follow-up
The patient should be seen as directed by the dermatologist.

Patient teaching
■ Teach the patient and family about the illness and expected and potential outcomes.
■ Tell the patient that use of balsam of Peru, yogurt flakes, oil of cloves, or other odor-masking substances may help control odor caused by the lesion, although they may be ineffective for long-term use. Topical or systemic antibiotics also temporarily control odor and eventually alter the lesion's bacterial flora.

HEALTHY LIVING To prevent basal and squamous cell carcinoma, tell patients to:
■ avoid excessive sun exposure
■ wear protective clothing (hats, long sleeves)
■ periodically examine the skin for precancerous lesions; have any removed promptly
■ use strong sunscreening agents containing para-aminobenzoic acid, benzophenone, and zinc oxide; apply these agents 30 to 60 minutes before sun exposure
■ use lipscreens to protect the lips from sun damage.

Complications
■ Recurrence
■ Metastatic disease
■ Disfigurement
■ Depression

TESTICULAR CANCER

Malignant testicular tumors primarily affect young to middle-aged men and are the most common solid tumor in this group. (In children, testicular tumors are rare.) Most testicular tumors originate in gonadal cells. About 40% are seminomas — uniform, undifferentiated cells resembling primitive gonadal cells. The remainder are nonseminomas — tumor cells showing various degrees of differentiation. The prognosis varies with the cell type and disease stage. When treated with surgery and radiation, almost all patients with localized disease survive beyond 5 years. Incidence (which peaks between ages 20 and 40) is higher in men with cryptorchidism (even when surgically corrected) and in men whose mothers used diethylstilbestrol during pregnancy. Testicular cancer is rare in nonwhite males and accounts for less than 1% of male cancer deaths.

Causes
The cause of testicular cancer is unknown. It spreads through the lymphatic system to the iliac, para-aortic, and mediastinal lymph nodes and may metastasize to the lungs, liver, viscera, and bone.

Clinical presentation
The first sign is usually a firm, painless, and smooth testicular mass, varying in size and sometimes producing a sense of testicular heaviness. When such a tumor causes chorionic gonadotropin or estrogen production, gynecomastia and nipple tenderness may result. In advanced stages, signs and symptoms include:
■ ureteral obstruction
■ abdominal mass
■ cough
■ hemoptysis
■ shortness of breath

Staging testicular cancer

The TNM (tumor, node, metastasis) staging system adopted by the American Joint Committee on Cancer has established the following stages for testicular cancer.

PRIMARY TUMOR
TX — primary tumor can't be assessed (this stage is used in the absence of radical orchiectomy)
T0 — histologic scar or no evidence of primary tumor
Tis — intratubular tumor: preinvasive cancer
T1 — tumor limited to testicles, including the rete testis
T2 — tumor extends beyond tunica albuginea or into epididymis
T3 — tumor extends into spermatic cord
T4 — tumor invades scrotum

REGIONAL LYMPH NODES
NX — regional lymph nodes can't be assessed
N0 — no evidence of regional lymph node metastasis
N1 — metastasis in a single lymph node, 2 cm or less in greatest dimension

N2 — metastasis in a single lymph node, between 2 and 5 cm in greatest dimension, or metastasis to several lymph nodes, none more than 5 cm in greatest dimension
N3 — metastasis in a lymph node more than 5 cm in greatest dimension

DISTANT METASTASIS
MX — distant metastasis unassessible
M0 — no known distant metastasis
M1 — distant metastasis

STAGING CATEGORIES
Testicular cancer progresses as follows:
STAGE 0 — Tis, N0, M0
STAGE I — T1, N0, M0; T2, N0, M0
STAGE II — T3, N0, M0; T4, N0, M0
STAGE III — any T, N1, M0
STAGE IV — any T, N2, M0; any T, N3, M0; any T, any N, M1

- weight loss
- fatigue
- pallor
- lethargy.

Differential diagnoses
- Hernia
- Hydrocele
- Hematoma
- Spermatocele
- Syphilitic gumma
- Variocele
- Epididymitis

Diagnosis
Two effective means of detecting a testicular tumor are regular self-examinations and testicular palpation during a routine physical examination. Transillumination can distinguish between a tumor (which doesn't transilluminate) and a hydrocele or spermatocele (which does). Follow-up measures should include an examination for gynecomastia and abdominal masses.

Diagnostic tests include excretory urography to detect ureteral deviation resulting from para-aortic node involvement, urinary or serum luteinizing hormone levels, blood tests, lymphangiography, ultrasound, and abdominal computed tomography scanning. Serum alpha-fetoprotein and beta-human chorionic gonadotropin levels — indicators of testicular tumor activity — provide a baseline for measuring response to therapy and determining the prognosis.

Surgical excision and biopsy of the tumor and testis permits histologic verification of the tumor cell type—essential for effective treatment. Inguinal exploration determines the extent of nodal involvement. (See *Staging testicular cancer.*)

Management

General

The extent of surgery, radiation, and chemotherapy varies with tumor cell type and stage. Radiation of the retroperitoneal and homolateral iliac nodes follows removal of a seminoma. All positive nodes receive radiation after removal of a nonseminoma. Patients with retroperitoneal extension receive prophylactic radiation to the mediastinal and supraclavicular nodes.

Medication

Essential for tumors beyond stage 0, chemotherapy combinations include bleomycin, etoposide, and cisplatin; cisplatin, vindesine, and bleomycin; cisplatin, vinblastine, and bleomycin; and cisplatin, vincristine, methotrexate, bleomycin, and leucovorin. Chemotherapy and radiation followed by autologous bone marrow transplantation may help unresponsive patients.

Surgical intervention

Surgery includes orchiectomy and retroperitoneal node dissection. Most surgeons remove the testis, not the scrotum (to allow for a prosthetic implant). Hormone replacement therapy may be needed after bilateral orchiectomy.

Referral

- Refer the patient to an oncologist and surgeon for treatment.
- Refer the patient and his family to the American Cancer Society for information and support.

Follow-up

The patient should be seen according to the oncologist's and surgeon's directions.

Patient teaching

- Tell the patient to wear an athletic supporter until fully recovered from surgery.
- Teach the patient about chemotherapy, and how to deal with adverse effects that occur.

Complications

- Radiation nephritis
- Recurrent cancer
- Infertility

Special considerations

- Reassure the patient that sterility and impotence need not follow unilateral orchiectomy, that synthetic hormones can restore hormonal balance, and that most surgeons don't remove the scrotum. In many cases, a testicular prosthesis can correct anatomic disfigurement.

• • • • • • • • • • •

THYROID CANCER

Thyroid cancer occurs in all age-groups, especially in people who have had radiation treatment of the neck area. Papillary and follicular carcinomas are the most common types and are usually associated with a longer survival. Papillary carcinoma accounts for half of all thyroid cancers in adults; it's most common in young adult females and metastasizes slowly. It's the least virulent form of thyroid cancer. Follicular carcinoma is less common but more likely to recur and metastasize to the regional nodes and through blood vessels into the bones, liver, and lungs. Medullary carcinoma originates in the parafollicular cells derived from the last branchial pouch and contains amyloid and calcium deposits. It can produce calcitonin, histaminase, corticotropin (producing Cushing's syndrome), and prostaglandin E2 and F3 (producing diarrhea). This rare form of thyroid cancer is familial, is associated with pheochromocytoma, and is completely curable when detected before it causes symptoms. Untreated, it progresses rapidly. Seldom curable by resection, anaplastic tumors resist radiation and metastasize rapidly.

Causes
Predisposing factors include radiation exposure, prolonged thyroid-stimulating hormone stimulation (through radiation or heredity), familial predisposition, or chronic goiter.

Clinical presentation
The primary signs of thyroid cancer are a painless, hard nodule in an enlarged thyroid gland, or palpable lymph nodes with thyroid enlargement. Eventually, the pressure of such a nodule or enlargement causes hoarseness, dysphagia, dyspnea, and pain on palpation. If the tumor is large enough to destroy the gland, hypothyroidism follows, with its typical symptoms of low metabolism (mental apathy and sensitivity to cold). However, if the tumor stimulates excess thyroid hormone production, it induces symptoms of hyperthyroidism (sensitivity to heat, restlessness, and hyperactivity). Other clinical features include:
- diarrhea
- anorexia
- irritability
- vocal cord paralysis
- symptoms of distant metastasis.

Differential diagnoses
- Multinodular goiter
- Thyroid adenoma
- Thyroiditis
- Thyroid cyst
- Ectopic thyroid

Diagnosis
The first clue to thyroid cancer is usually an enlarged, palpable node in the thyroid gland, neck, lymph nodes of the neck, or vocal cords. A patient history of radiation therapy or a family history of thyroid cancer supports the diagnosis. However, tests must rule out nonmalignant thyroid enlargements, which are much more common. Thyroid scan differentiates between functional nodes (rarely malignant) and hypofunctional nodes (commonly malignant) by measuring how readily nodules trap isotopes compared with the rest of the thyroid gland. In thyroid cancer, the scintiscan shows a "cold," nonfunctioning nodule. Other tests include needle biopsy, computed tomography scan, ultrasonic scan, chest X-ray, serum alkaline phosphatase, and serum calcitonin assay to diagnose medullary cancer. Calcitonin assay is a reliable clue to silent medullary carcinoma. (See *Staging thyroid cancer.*)

Management
General
Thyroid cancer is most effectively treated with surgery. Chemotherapy may be used for symptomatic, widespread metastasis.

Medication
Medications that may be used to treat thyroid cancer include:
- propylthiouracil — initially, 100 mg P.O. t.i.d.; increase as needed to suppress synthesis of thyroid hormones
- radioactive iodine — 30 to 100 mCi P.O. with subsequent doses of 100 to 200 mCi
- doxorubicin — 60 to 75 mg/m² I.V. every 3 weeks.

Staging thyroid cancer

The classification and staging systems adopted by the American Joint Committee on Cancer describe thyroid cancer according to the tumor's (T) size and extent at its origin, its invasion of regional (cervical and upper mediastinal) lymph nodes (N), and the disease's metastasis (M) to other structures.

PRIMARY TUMOR
TX — primary tumor can't be assessed
T0 — no evidence of primary tumor
T1 — tumor 1 cm or less in greatest dimension and limited to the thyroid
T2 — tumor more than 1 cm but less than 4 cm in greatest dimension and limited to the thyroid
T3 — tumor more than 4 cm and limited to the thyroid
T4 — tumor (any size) extends beyond the thyroid

REGIONAL LYMPH NODES
NX — regional lymph nodes can't be assessed
N0 — no evidence of regional lymph node metastasis
N1 — regional lymph node metastasis
N1a — metastasis in ipsilateral cervical nodes
N1b — metastasis in bilateral, midline, or contralateral cervical or mediastinal lymph nodes

DISTANT METASTASIS
MX — distant metastasis can't be assessed
M0 — no evidence of distant metastasis
M1 — distant metastasis

STAGING CATEGORIES FOR PAPILLARY OR FOLLICULAR CANCER
Papillary or follicular cancer progresses from mild to severe as follows:
STAGE I — any T, any N, M0 (patient under age 45); T1, N0, M0 (patient age 45 or over)
STAGE II — any T, any N, M1 (patient under age 45); T2, N0, M0; T3, N0, M0 (patient age 45 or over)
STAGE III — T4, N0, M0; any T, N1, M0 (patient age 45 or over)
STAGE IV — any T, any N, M1 (patient age 45 or over)

STAGING CATEGORIES FOR MEDULLARY CANCER
Medullary cancer progresses from mild to severe as follows:
STAGE I — T1, N0, M0
STAGE II — T2, N0, M0; T3, N0, M0; T4, N0, M0
STAGE III — any T, N1, M0
STAGE IV — any T, any N, M1

STAGING CATEGORIES FOR UNDIFFERENTIATED CANCER
All cases are stage IV.
STAGE IV — any T, any N, any M

Surgical intervention
Surgical procedures used for thyroid cancer include:
■ total or subtotal thyroidectomy, with modified node dissection (bilateral or unilateral) on the side of the primary cancer (papillary or follicular cancer)

■ total thyroidectomy and radical neck excision (for medullary, giant, or spindle cell cancer)
■ radiation (^{131}I) with external radiation (for inoperable cancer and sometimes postoperatively in lieu of radical neck excision) or alone (for metastasis).

Referral
▪ Refer the patient to a surgeon and oncologist for treatment.
▪ Refer the patient to the American Cancer Society for information and support.

Follow-up
The patient should be seen as directed by the specialist.

Patient teaching
▪ Teach the patient and family about the illness and expected and potential outcomes.

Complications
▪ Recurrence
▪ Metastasis

• • • • • • • • • • • •

SELECTED REFERENCES

Abeloff, M.D., et al. *Clinical Oncology*, 2nd ed. New York: Churchill Livingstone, Inc., 2000.

DeVita, V.T., et al. *Cancer: Principles and Practice of Oncology*, 6th ed. Philadelphia: Lippincott Williams & Wilkins, 2001.

Dunne-Daly, C.F. "Principles of Radiotherapy and Radiobiology," *Seminars in Oncology Nursing* 15(4):250-259, November 1999.

Falk, K.M. "Cancer treatment" in *Principles of Practice for the Acute Care Nurse Practitioner*. Edited by Logan, P. Stanford, Conn.: Appleton & Lange, 1999.

Mauch, P.M., et al. *Hodgkin's Disease*. Philadelphia: Lippincott Williams & Wilkins, 1999.

Smith, R.A., et al. "American Cancer Society Guidelines for the Early Detection of Cancer," *CA-A Cancer Journal for Clinicians* 50(1):34-49, January/February 2000.

INDEX

• • • • • • • • •

i refers to an illustration; t refers to a table.

i refers to an illustration; t refers to a table.

i refers to an illustration; t refers to a table.

i refers to an illustration; t refers to a table.

i refers to an illustration; t refers to a table.

i refers to an illustration; t refers to a table.

i refers to an illustration; t refers to a table.

Metabolic, endocrine, and nutritional disorders
(*continued*)
protein-calorie malnutrition, 489-491
sodium imbalance, 500-503
Methicillin-resistant *Staphylococcus aureus* infection, 661-662
Migraine headache, 250
Mononucleosis, infectious, 662-664
Morbilli. *See* Rubeola.
Motion sickness, 594-595
Motor neuron disease, 228
Multiple neuritis. *See* Peripheral neuritis.
Multiple sclerosis
causes of, 257
clinical presentation of, 257
demyelination in, 258
diagnosis of, 257-258
management of, 259
patient teaching about, 259-260
special considerations for patient with, 260
Mumps, 664-666
Muscle strength, assessment of, 276-283i
Muscle-tendon ruptures, 759
Muscular dystrophy
causes of, 306
clinical presentation of, 306
diagnosis of, 306-307
introduction to, 305-306
management of, 307
patient teaching about, 307-308
special considerations for patient with, 308
Musculoskeletal disorders
assessment of, 273-275, 283-284
bursitis, 325-327
carpal tunnel syndrome, 284-286
clubfoot, 286-289
developmental dysplasia of the hip, 289-292
epicondylitis, 292-293
fibromyalgia syndrome, 293-297
gout, 297-301
herniated disk, 301-303
kyphosis, 303-305
muscular dystrophy, 305-308
Osgood-Schlatter, 308-309
osteoarthritis, 309-312
osteomyelitis, 312-314
osteoporosis, 314-316
Paget's disease, 316-318
scoliosis, 318-322
septic arthritis, 322-325
tendinitis, 325-327
Myasthenia gravis
causes of, 260
clinical presentation of, 260-261

Myasthenia gravis (*continued*)
diagnosis of, 262
impaired transmission in, 261
management of, 262-263
patient teaching about, 263
special considerations for patient with, 263
Myocardial infarction
causes and pathophysiology of, 114-115
clinical presentation of, 115
complications of, 117, 118-119t
diagnosis of, 115-116
management of, 116-117
patient teaching about, 117
Myocarditis, 119-121
Myxedema, signs of, 484i

N

Narcissistic personality disorder, 44
Nasal pack, inserting, 578i
Necrotizing fasciitis, 666-668
Neisseria gonorrhoeae, 530i
Neoplasms
in acquired immunodeficiency syndrome, 771
bladder cancer, 815-818
breast cancer, 823-827
cervical cancer, 828-830
colorectal cancer, 830-833
esophageal cancer, 833-835
gastric carcinoma, 835-838, 836i
Hodgkin's disease, 838-842, 841i
laryngeal cancer, 842-844
leukemia, 844-850
lung cancer, 850-854
malignant brain tumors, 818-823, 819-821t
malignant lymphoma, 854-856, 855i
malignant melanoma, 856-860, 859i
overview of, 807-815
pancreatic cancer, 860-864, 861t
prostatic cancer, 864-866
squamous cell carcinoma, 866-869
testicular cancer, 869-871
thyroid cancer, 871-874
Neuritis, peripheral, 263-264
Neurologic disorders
Alzheimer's disease, 225-227
amyotrophic lateral sclerosis, 227-229
assessment of, 213-225
Bell's palsy, 229-231
brain stem function evaluation for, 218i
cerebral palsy, 231-234
cerebrovascular accident, 234-238
down syndrome, 238-240
encephalitis, 240-242
epilepsy, 242-246

i refers to an illustration; t refers to a table.

i refers to an illustration; t refers to a table.

i refers to an illustration; t refers to a table.